WOMAN'S HEALTH AND MEDICAL GUIDE

Better Homes and Gardens®

WOMAN'S HEALTH AND MEDICAL GUIDE

Edited by
Patricia J. Cooper, Ph.D.

Illustrations by
Sandra McMahon
and
Lianne M. Krueger

Black and white
photography by
Fred Lyon

BETTER HOMES AND GARDENS® BOOKS
Editor: Gerald M. Knox
Art Director: Ernest Shelton

Associate Art Directors: Neoma Alt West, Randall Yontz
Copy and Production Editors: David Kirchner, Lamont Olson,
    David A. Walsh
Assistant Art Director: Harijs Priekulis
Senior Graphic Designer: Faith Berven
Graphic Designers: Alisann Dixon, Linda Ford,
    Lynda Haupert, Tom Wegner

Editor-in-Chief: James A. Autry
Editorial Director: Neil Kuehnl
Executive Art Director: William J. Yates

WOMAN'S HEALTH AND MEDICAL GUIDE
Copy and Production Editor: David Kirchner
Graphic Designer: Linda Ford

Director of Art Research: Patricia J. Cooper, Ph.D.
Editorial Assistant: Nancy Hubbell, M.A.
Editorial and Art Research Assistants:
    Marcia Stewart, M.A., Laurel Cook, Wendy Lewis

Exercise illustrations by Joe Isom
Color photographs by Mike Dieter

Special thanks to the following people for their valuable
assistance in producing this book: R. C. Strohman, Jim
Kunegenas, Katherine Marsh, Bill Allan, Lynda Haupert, Babs
Klein, Faith Berven, Angie Ford, Michael P. Scott, Rita Aero,
Danza Squire, Caroline Cooper, Willa Baker, Sheryl Ruzck,
Suzanne Fields, Sioban Harlow, Kim Fujishige, Mildred
Glacken, Marci Kremer, Jenny Strohman, Sue Williams,
Stephanie Harris; and the members of the Seminar on
Perspectives in Women's Health: Dr. Beverly Birns, Linda
Brod, Anne Lieberman, Donna Linson, Sara McIntire, Shirley
Middleton, Betty Wolff, Raydean Acevedo, Britt Trimble, Eva
Carrod, Norma Kobzina, Susan Downs, Charleen Kubota.

FOREWORD

Throughout human history, health has been prized above all else. Today we recognize that health can be enhanced and maintained with the kind of thoughtful, ongoing health care that is based on an understanding of how the whole person lives and functions through the life-span. From this perspective, women's health care differs significantly from that of men. Because women are biologically different, we need specific information about these differences, as well as a basic understanding of how a woman's body and mind function in health and disease.

This book was written for women—to assemble in one place most of what is known about our normal health and development and to provide the sort of knowledge that will give us confidence in making decisions and choices about our health care. The authors of the individual chapters—physicians, psychologists, and health care educators—have combined their expertise to produce a book about the whole woman in each stage of her life. This is a book for adolescents, for young women, for women contemplating childbearing, for women in the middle of their career years, and for old women—in short, for women of all ages and in all stages of life.

As a guide, this book will help you become a more active participant in your own health care. Each chapter contains practical and proven health care methods, as well as basic information about how your body and mind work. With this kind of knowledge comes a sense of self-confidence—in looking up symptoms when you feel ill, in forming questions about how your body is functioning, and in discussing your health care with physicians and psychologists. Background information in the book will help you interpret the answers you are given so that you can effectively cooperate with your physician and actively participate in choosing your treatment.

Taking charge of our health moves us further along the road toward full self-development. Personal growth and self-development have always presented us with the need to stretch our limits, and at no time in our history has this need been greater than it is now. In fact, this book arises precisely out of the growth opportunities now available to women.

To function as a whole woman in today's world requires an understanding of the basic biological and psychological facts of being female. With such an understanding, we can live in this world with wisdom and balance, continuing to care for ourselves and contributing to the lives of others as we respond to the new challenges of our expanded roles in life.

ACKNOWLEDGMENTS

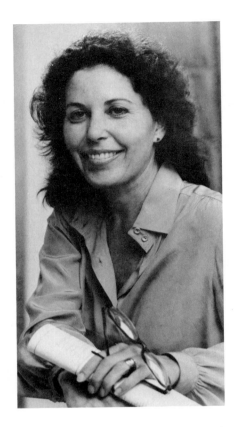

Patricia J. Cooper, Ph.D., the editor of the Better Homes and Gardens *Woman's Health and Medical Guide,* has had a distinguished career as a research biologist and educator in the biomedical sciences. She has served on the faculty at the University of Oregon Medical School and at the University of California at Berkeley, Departments of Zoology and of Health and Medical Sciences, where she currently teaches courses in embryology, human development, and women's health. Dr. Cooper is the author of numerous scientific papers and articles for women's magazines, and several books.

Peter L. Andrus, M.D., F.A.C.P. Assistant Professor of Community Medicine and Pediatrics, Baylor College of Medicine; Fellow, American College of Preventive Medicine; Fellow, American Academy of Pediatrics. Houston, Texas.

Sharon N. Andrus, R.N. Department of Psychology, University of Houston. Houston, Texas.

Patrick H. Beckham, M.D., F.A.C.P.S. Member, American Society of Plastic and Reconstructive Surgery; Member, American Association of Hand Surgery; President, Texas Society of Plastic Surgeons. Austin, Texas.

Beverly Birns, Ph.D. Coordinator, Women's Studies Program, Interdisciplinary Program in Social Sciences, State University of New York. Stony Brook, New York.

Vidal S. Clay, Ed.D. Lecturer in Human Development and Family Relations, University of Connecticut, Stamford, Connecticut; Lecturer, Graduate Center for Family Clinical Studies, University of Bridgeport. Westport, Connecticut.

Albert Decker, M.D., F.A.C.S., F.A.C.O.G. Executive Director, New York Fertility Research Foundation; Founding Member, New York Gynecological Society. New York, New York.

S. Jean Emans, M.D. Associate Chief, Adolescent Unit, Children's Hospital Medical Center. Boston, Massachusetts.

Jeanne Bunderson Ewing, Ph.D. Research Associate, University of California at Berkeley. Berkeley, California.

Cary E. Feibleman, M.D. Now in private practice associated with Memorial Hospital Medical Center of Long Beach, California; formerly Clinical Instructor, State University of New York at Buffalo. Long Beach, California.

Robert D. Friefeld, M.D. Member, American College of Physicians. Long Beach, California.

Doris Goodman, M.D. Staff Cardiologist and Director, Hypertension Program, Philadelphia V.A. Hospital; Fellow, American College of Cardiology; Fellow, American College of Physicians. Philadelphia, Pennsylvania.

Mary Gray, M.D., F.A.C.O.G. Member, Department of Obstetrics and Gynecology, Harvard Community Health Plan; Clinical Instructor, Harvard Medical School. Cambridge, Massachusetts.

Robert Hatcher, M.D., M.P.H. Associate Professor of Gynecology and Obstetrics, Emory University School of Medicine. Atlanta, Georgia.

Christine E. Haycock, M.D., F.A.C.S.M. Associate Professor of Surgery, New Jersey Colleges of Medicine and Dentistry, New Jersey Medical School; Chairwoman, Continuing Education Committee, American College of Sports Medicine. Newark, New Jersey.

F. Allan Hubbell, M.D. Adjunct Assistant Professor, Department of Internal Medicine, University of California College of Medicine. Irvine, California.

Nancy Cooper Hubbell. Psychologist in private practice; free-lance writer of health and psychology subjects. Long Beach, California.

Helen Singer Kaplan, M.D., Ph.D. Director, Human Sexuality Program, Cornell Medical Center. New York, New York.

Lucienne T. Lanson, M.D., F.A.C.O.G. Author of *From Woman to Woman: A Gynecologist Answers Questions About You and Your Body.* San Francisco, California.

Marjory Skowronski Lozen. Author of *Abortion and Alternatives.* Grass Valley, California.

Gay G. Luce, Ph.D. Founder and member of the Board of Directors of SAGE (Senior Actualization and Growth Explorations). Mill Valley, California.

Madeleine Reichert, D.M.H. Mt. Zion Hospital. San Francisco, California.

Anne Harris Rosenfeld. Free-lance writer specializing in health and mental health subjects; author of *New Views on Older Lives* and *Toward a Science of Psychiatry.* Washington, D.C.

Madeleine H. Shearer, R.P.T. Editor of *Birth and the Family Journal;* Member, American Society of Psychoprophylaxis in Obstetrics; Member, International Childbirth Education Association. Berkeley, California.

Gail Shierman, Ph.D. Assistant Professor of Physical Education, University of Oklahoma. Norman, Oklahoma.

Fredrick J. Stare, M.D. Professor of Nutrition, and founder and Chairman of the Department of Nutrition, Harvard School of Public Health; Member, American Institute of Nutrition. Boston, Massachusetts.

Justin J. Stein, M.D., F.A.C.R., F.A.C.S. Professor Emeritus, Radiological Sciences, University of California at Los Angeles; Professor, Radiological Sciences, University of California at Irvine; Past President, American Cancer Society. Long Beach, California.

Sarah Hall Sternglanz, Ph.D. Adjunct Assistant Professor, Department of Psychology, State University of New York. Stony Brook, New York.

Marcia Stewart, M.A. Health and Medical Sciences Program, University of California at Berkeley. Berkeley, California.

Louise B. Tyrer, M.D., F.A.C.O.G. Vice President for Medical Affairs of the Planned Parenthood Federation of America. New York, New York.

Myrna M. Weissman, Ph.D. Associate Professor of Psychiatry and Epidemiology, Yale University School of Medicine; Director, Depression Research Unit, Connecticut Mental Health Center. New Haven, Connecticut.

Elizabeth M. Whelan. Sc.D., M.P.H. Executive Director, American Council on Science and Health; Member, American Public Health Association; Member, Nutrition Today Association. New York, New York.

Juanita Williams, Ph.D. Professor of Psychology and Women's Studies, University of Southern Florida; Clinical Psychologist in private practice. Tampa, Florida.

Mildred Hope Witkin, Ph.D. Assistant Clinical Professor, Department of Psychiatry, Cornell University Medical College; Associate Director, Human Sexuality Program, the New York Hospital—Cornell Medical Center. In private practice in New York City and in Westport, Connecticut.

TABLE OF CONTENTS

LIST OF ILLUSTRATIONS

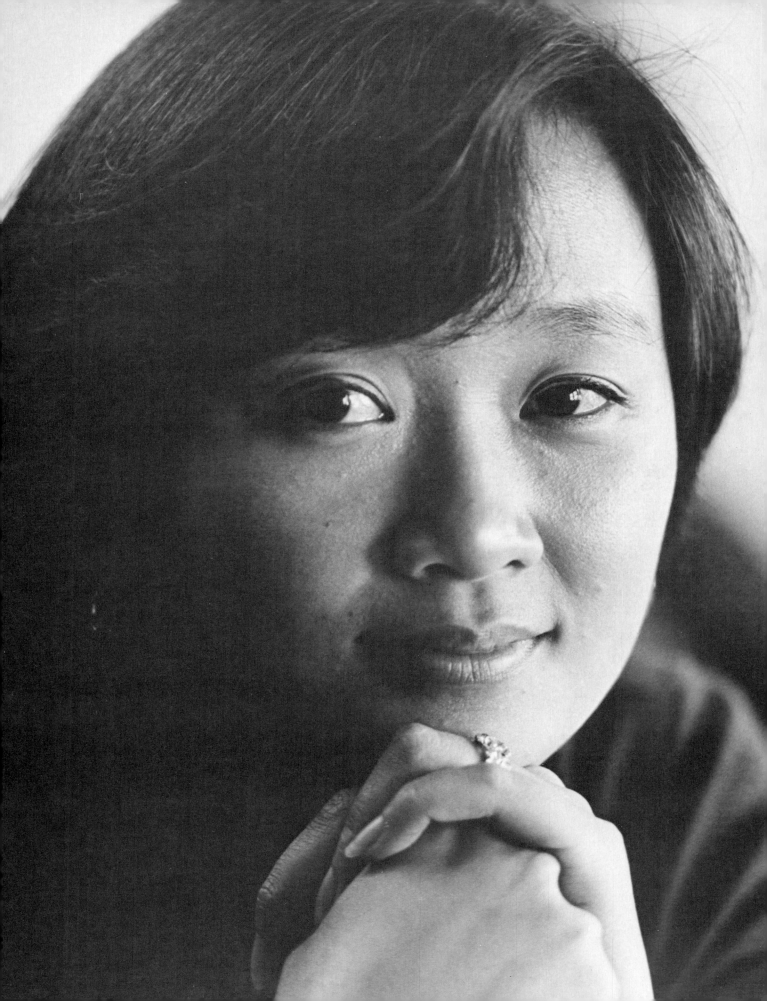

CHAPTER 1

WOMAN'S BODY

PATRICIA COOPER, Ph.D.

A woman's body, with its distinctively female features, is a product of many developmental interactions throughout our lives. While the physical characteristics that distinguish women from men can be readily seen and described, the subtler behavioral differences are not so easily defined. As women, we are products of our genes, certainly, but also of our own life experiences. Our femaleness is the result of, not only our physical bodies, but of our parents and how they raised us, the people we emulated as we grew up, our expectations of how women and men should behave, and our receptions in school and at work. As a unique individual, each woman has her own history that defines her expresssion of femininity and womanhood—the special marvel and wonder of her existence.

Woman's Body

From the moment of conception when the female sex is determined by the union of two X chromosomes, women are biologically distinct from men. This quintessential fact, so simple in its statement, determines the circumstances and experiences of our lives to a remarkable extent. Today we are just as fascinated with the subject of gender and the myriad differences between men and women as were our earliest human ancestors, who recorded their preoccupation with sexual distinctions in small statues, cave paintings, and ritual objects. Today we continue to represent human sexuality in art, and to investigate male-female differences in almost every field of human inquiry.

What is it that distinguishes a woman from a man? To what extent are sex differences due to learned behavior, and to what extent are they determined by our genes? What role do hormones play in determining sex differences, and what is the biological basis for femininity and masculinity? These questions, rephrased a hundred times throughout written history, continue to excite our interest and curiosity.

Today there is a new sense of interest and urgency in reviewing and reevaluating the old information about definitions of femininity. We're seeing expanding activity and innovative research in the field of woman's psychology, in the study of sex-role behavior, and in our understanding of how babies and children express sex differences. Patient advocate groups are improving medical care for women, and investigation continues into the role of socialization in sex differences. If traditional biological research has appeared to respond more slowly to the renewed interest in women, it is perhaps because in the last century the biological revolution already had outlined so clearly the distinctions between men and women from the cellular to the organismal level.

It is appropriate that this first chapter in a book on women's health begin with the questions and proceed to summarize our current knowledge in the hope of providing some answers. This chapter, then, will review the biological differences that make a woman different from a man—the obvious, basic facts of physical sex. Sex also will be discussed as part of an evolutionary continuum, for we should be reminded that, in terms of planetary history, life on our planet is only moments old, and human sexuality's span is the briefest of experiments. The biological facts about female sexuality provide basic knowledge for material covered in the remainder of the book, and serve as a necessary starting point for understanding how the body functions in health and disease.

At this point in history, women are creating a new image of the female—of a more self-reliant, aware, socially experimental creature. Women's interest in the basic facts about the conditions and functions of their bodies is leading to changes throughout all fields of

human endeavor. Women now need to better know about themselves precisely because they are in the midst of a great era of self-exploration and are beginning to take responsibility for their lives as they grow, develop, and thrust forward into new roles in society.

For the first time, women are beginning to take full responsibility for their reproductive function. Aided by new medical diagnostic tools, by changes in abortion laws, by contraceptive technology, by a new shared understanding between men and women about infant and child-care responsibilities, and by their own willingness to learn, women are making active, informed choices about whether to have children and how best to care for them.

Women have been leaders in preventive health and in self-care movements in the last decade. No longer willing to be passive participants in the doctor-patient relationship, they have formed study groups, written books, become patient advocates, and begun actively to explore the role they can play in their own health maintenance and disease treatment.

As they have moved into the work force, women have found themselves holding down two full-time jobs at once—caring for children and family, and developing a career or continuing their education. Women know they need all the body information, fitness, and health they can muster to meet their new challenges and roles in life with energy and enjoyment. Not satisfied with old roles, often with low profiles, with depression, and with unhappiness in personal, family, and work life, they are pressing forward to an experience of full mental and physical health. The ultimate responsibility for health rests with each of us, and basic knowledge of our bodies is part of what is required to reach our full growth potential.

Biological Sex

Sexual Evolution

The origins of the sexual differences between men and women can be best explained if we start with an understanding of the first living cells. As scientists have reconstructed events, life on this planet began with a fusion of organic molecules in a life-supporting atmosphere that produced the first living cell. Presumably, this earliest life form reproduced itself simply by splitting into two cells, for we see this type of reproduction in single-celled organisms today. Later in evolution, cells remained grouped together to form multicellular organisms and reproduced when part of the organism budded to one side and then broke away from the parent as a smaller but identical copy. Both types of reproduction just described are asexual— without male-female sexuality.

Sexual reproduction, which requires the union of male and female sex cells, came later in evolution when asexual organisms evolved specialized sex cells. At our present state of evolution, humans, as well as many other animals and plants, reproduce sexually. In sexual reproduction, the specialized sex cells have only *half* of the number of genes (and chromosomes) required to make a new organism. The other half must come from an equally specialized cell. When two such cells join and fuse, a new cell is created with the full number of chromosomes, hence the full complement of genetic material necessary to form a complete, new organism. Over the hundreds of millions of years that living organisms have evolved, sex cells also have evolved into two highly specialized cellular forms—the egg and the sperm.

Why did two separate sex cells evolve? Why does our particular life form consist of two sexual beings, each developing and carrying only one of these sex cells? Clearly, we can never satisfactorily answer these questions, but it seems obvious from our long study of ourselves and other living beings that the implications and advantages of sexual reproduction are far-reaching.

The formation of sex cells that contain only half of the genetic complement involves a random reshuffling of characteristics. The union of a single egg with a single sperm also is random. So genetic traits are thoroughly reshuffled for each individual, resulting in unique characteristics for each person born. Therefore, the progeny of sexually reproducing parents are *never* the same as the parents. This variation allows for members of a species to adapt to new environments. That is, as environments change, some of the offspring will "fit" the new changed environment because their individual characteristics are most suitable to that environment. Other offspring will not adapt to changes.

Humans have another trait related to sexuality and sexual reproduction that has greatly affected our evolution into beings with two distinct biological sexes. This is the trait of *internal fertilization* in which the union of egg and sperm takes place inside the female's body, as does the development of the baby. Internal fertilization, accomplished by intercourse between a man and a woman, greatly improves the chances for the union of egg and sperm in a nurturing, sustaining environment. To facilitate internal fertilization, distinct sexual anatomical differences have developed between males and females. Human and all mammalian females have developed a complex internal system to nurture and protect the developing embryo (see page 232). So human femaleness and maleness is the result of an evolutionary process developed over millions of years to ensure safe reproduction of the species.

Female Sexual Development

As already stated, your sex as a female begins with the union of egg and sperm, each carrying an X chromosome. Two X chromosomes determine the female sex (see page 485). But this is not the whole story, for genetic determination of female sex is only the beginning in a long series of events that lead to an adult's sexual identity. Biological sexuality depends not only on chromosomal sex, but on a continuous, harmonious unfolding of developmental patterns. Although not discussed in this chapter, sexual identity development also depends on psychological and social developmental processes. There is great variety in the social roles females play and also in the biological expression of femaleness. Female sexuality depends upon the expression of innumerable determinants along a developmental continuum.

Chromosomal or genetic sex. In the normal human egg, there are 23 chromosomes that carry all of the genetic information inherited from your mother. Twenty-two of these chromosomes are autosomes and one is a sex-determining chromosome, *the X chromosome.* The sperm also carries 23 chromosomes, 22 autosomes and one sex-determining chromosome that may be either *an X or a Y chromosome.* The Y chromosome, when united with an X chromosome, leads to male development. Two X chromosomes determine female development.

After the egg is fertilized, the new individual has 23 pairs of chromosomes, one of which is a pair of sex chromosomes. The latter are either an XX pair (female) or an XY pair (male). As the single cell begins to divide, each cell contains the full number of chromosomes. So every cell in a woman's body is female, containing two X chromosomes. The chromosomal sex of a person is then determined at fertilization, but the person's sexual identity may be far from completely developed. The next four months of fetal life will unfold a complex sequence of developmental steps leading to the differentiation of male and female sex organs (see page 487).

Internal and external sexual anatomy. All of the information for an individual's bodily development, including the instruction for sexual differentiation, are contained in the 23 pairs of chromosomes. But for the first two months of fetal life, the developing infant has no male or female sex organs. You can determine the sex of the infant only by examining the chromosomes in a cell (see page 489). During the third and fourth months of fetal life, however, sexual differentiation of female and male reproductive structures begins. See the diagram on page 486 for details of how female and male reproductive structures form from a mass of undifferentiated tissue. This development and growth of female sexual organs will continue throughout life, with

WOMAN'S BODY

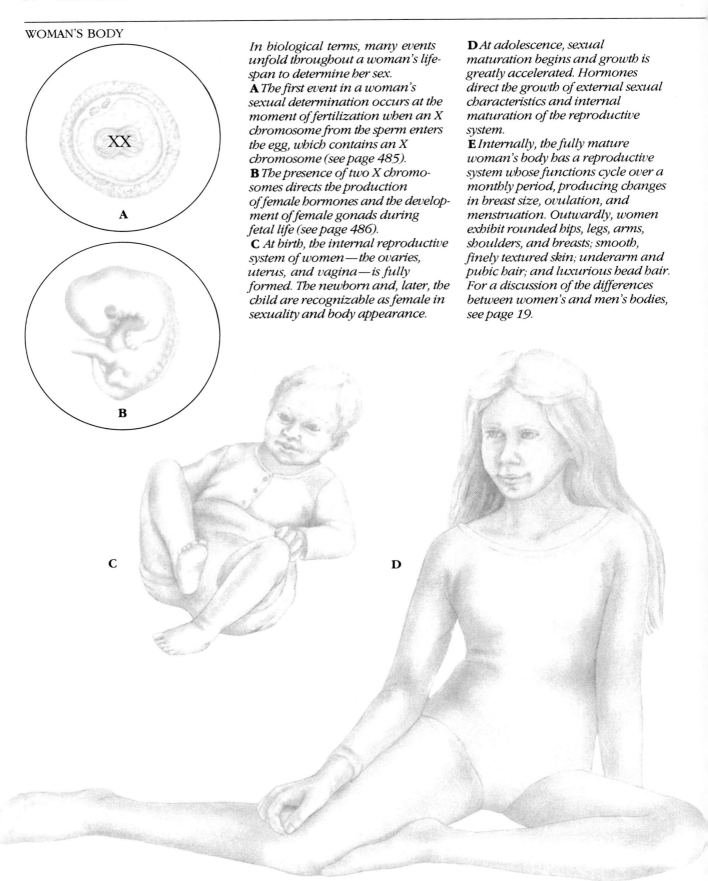

In biological terms, many events unfold throughout a woman's life-span to determine her sex.

A The first event in a woman's sexual determination occurs at the moment of fertilization when an X chromosome from the sperm enters the egg, which contains an X chromosome (see page 485).

B The presence of two X chromosomes directs the production of female hormones and the development of female gonads during fetal life (see page 486).

C At birth, the internal reproductive system of women—the ovaries, uterus, and vagina—is fully formed. The newborn and, later, the child are recognizable as female in sexuality and body appearance.

D At adolescence, sexual maturation begins and growth is greatly accelerated. Hormones direct the growth of external sexual characteristics and internal maturation of the reproductive system.

E Internally, the fully mature woman's body has a reproductive system whose functions cycle over a monthly period, producing changes in breast size, ovulation, and menstruation. Outwardly, women exhibit rounded hips, legs, arms, shoulders, and breasts; smooth, finely textured skin; underarm and pubic hair; and luxurious head hair. For a discussion of the differences between women's and men's bodies, see page 19.

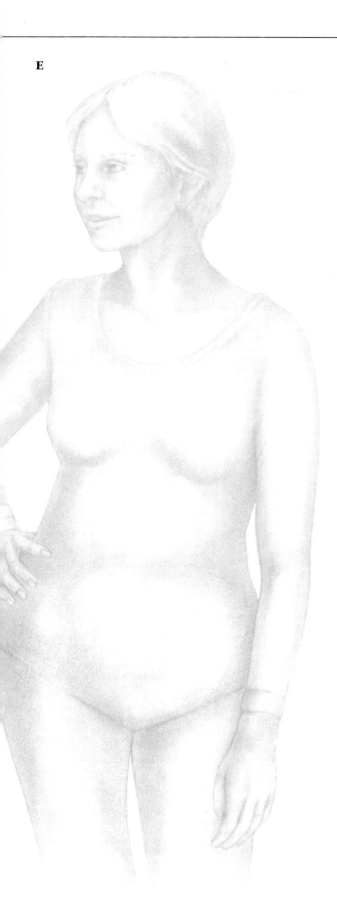

E

the reproductive system undergoing great changes at puberty, during pregnancy, and through menopause.

Endocrine or hormonal sexuality. As soon as the ovaries or testes begin to form in the two-month-old fetus, they begin to secrete chemical hormones that diffuse throughout the tissues of the infant's body. Males and females produce the same sex hormones; it is the *relative proportions* of the sex hormones that differ in males and females and that contribute to the continued development of a distinctively male or female body. Males produce higher proportions of androgens, particularly testosterone. Females produce higher proportions of estrogen and progesterone.

Sexual development at puberty. The secretion of hormones is greatly increased at adolescence, when the next major expression of female physical development takes place. In the relatively short span of several months to three years, a young girl's body changes by selective growth into the taller, heavier, more curved body of a sexually mature woman. Breasts develop; fat deposited beneath the skin rounds hips, legs, arms, and shoulders; and pubic hair and underarm hair appear. The reproductive system becomes functional as hormones direct the maturation and release of the first egg, signaling the onset of menstruation. The female body is now fully evident in terms of its sexuality.

From the perspective of biological development, then, woman's body can be defined as the product of an interaction of developmental systems over the life-span. Originally, femaleness is determined at conception by the meeting of two X chromosomes. Later in fetal life, the chromosomes direct the formation of female gonads—the ovaries. As ovarian cells differentiate, they produce female sex hormones, which further determine the development of internal and external female reproductive organs. At puberty, female hormones control changes that lead to the fully mature, reproductive woman's body.

Female-Male Differences

Women differ from men fundamentally in the development and function of their reproductive systems and in the appearance of their bodies. These differences are caused by the different sex chromosomes and the resulting proportional differences in hormone secretion, which, in turn, lead to developmental sexual distinctions. The physical structure of a woman's body does not necessarily dictate or determine behavorial differences. What constitutes feminine behavior and whether it is genetically or culturally determined is still a matter of debate and investigation (see page 92). However, the physical characteristics that distinguish women from men can be readily seen and measured.

The differences in male and female reproductive systems are discussed in detail on pages 484 to 487. Differences in secondary sexual characteristics are covered in the chapter on "Adolescence." But what are other key physical characteristics that distinguish women from men?

Women are, on the average, shorter and lighter than men. The average woman is almost five feet four inches tall and weighs 135 pounds, and the average man is just over five feet nine inches and weighs 162 pounds.

At adolescence, men's bones actually grow for a longer time than do women's, and the ratio of sex hormones dictates differences in muscle development at this time. Women seem to have a greater ratio of fat to muscle than do men. The differences in size and weight and the muscle-to-fat ratio in women and men have come under particular scrutiny recently as women's athletic participation undergoes revolutionary change.

What is a woman's physical potential, and how does it compare to a man's? Records to date indicate that men are 30 to 50 percent stronger than women in the upper body, yet women and men have the same strength potential in their legs. Research is active in the area of differences between women and men in body build, muscle characteristics, fat deposits, and cardiovascular endurance. As data collect and women continue toward equality in sports training, we can look forward to new information on these female-male differences.

The total average amount of fat in a woman's body differs from that in a man's. A woman's body is about 25 percent fat, compared to about 15 percent fat in a man. Men tend to carry fat in the stomach and chest areas, while women carry fat in the breasts and the hips. Also, women's shoulders are more rounded, narrow, and sloping due to a combination of differences in fat placement and muscle and skeletal mass.

Men have more muscle mass than women, although the type and quality of muscle fibers is the same in both sexes. Recently more women have begun to train their muscles with weights, a sport area previously almost exclusively dominated by men. Men develop very bulky muscles in weight training because of their high testosterone levels. Women who train their muscles using the same techniques gain strength and tone, but not greatly increased muscle size. This is because a woman's body contains only very small amounts of testosterone.

Women's body and facial hair is usually very faint and hardly noticeable, while their head hair is abundant and lasting. Men have pronounced body and facial hair, and their head hair may thin and disappear with age.

Women's necks are shorter and more rounded than men's, as are their legs, arms, hands, and feet. Men, with their deep voices, have a larynx one-third larger than women.

This brief review of the major physical distinctions between men and women does not begin to embrace the range of cultural and personal differences we see and experience daily. Yet if we were to stress the similarities between men's and women's bodies, we would come up with a much longer list than the account sheet of differences. In fact, when summarized in such a plain, factual manner, the differences between men and women seem rather small compared to our similar-ities—and to our common traits in the human species.

The Whole Woman

Biological sex is not the only expression of a woman's sexuality, nor is it the only component in the development of her sexual identity. How we are treated by members of our family, the way we see ourselves, and cultural expectations about how we should behave are all factors that influence our expression of sexuality. So also, a summary of female physical differences does not give a whole picture of woman's body.

Observe the woman on the next page sitting centered among the interlocking circles—symbols of parts of herself. This diagram represents an important concept: that a complete person is composed of many parts that function in unison to form a whole, living organism, a whole greater than the sum of its parts. The whole woman is all of these parts living together as one. The one is you. The one is Self.

The concept of wholism has profound implications for how we treat our bodies. The more we understand of our separate systems and how they influence our total health picture, the more tools we will have for choosing effective procedures to maintain our health and ensure our recovery from illness.

As research into optimal health and effective health care continues, it becomes ever clearer that all parts of the body are involved in maintaining health. The mind and body affect one another. The environment also acts upon the body, and we choose the environments in which we live. Emotional states, personal motivation, and even mental imagery contribute to how we respond to major illnesses and to surgery.

Thinking of yourself holistically ("wholistically") may prove useful in designing your own self-care system. For example, you may wish to quit smoking but find that your desire to quit is not enough. If substituting food and drink for a cigarette or entering a motivational program don't work for you, altering your life-style to remove the stress in your environment may do the trick. And when you've licked the habit, you'll not only have increased your self-esteem and well-being, but you'll have directly affected your respiratory, nervous, and circulatory systems—giving them a positive boost toward health and longer life. By considering all parts of your body and by looking at all the influences acting on you, you greatly increase your chances for effective health care.

In the remainder of the chapter, and in the remainder of the book, parts of the body and functions of the body are discussed separately. People often break down information into smaller and smaller units in order to study it in more detail. Keep in mind the picture of the whole body on the next page and reintegrate all of the details into your whole self.

THE WHOLE BODY

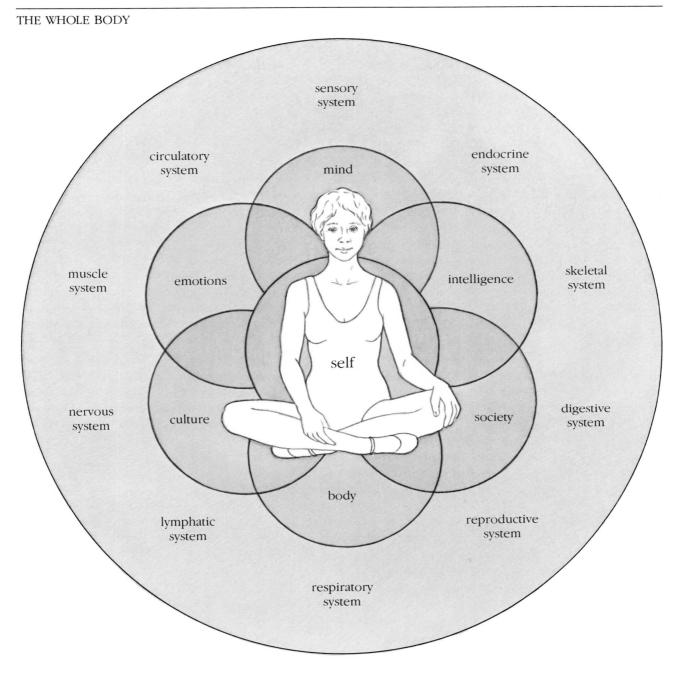

Health is a positive state of well-being—an enjoyable quality of life that you can experience. The first step toward full vitality and energetic enjoyment of your body is to accept your whole self in all of its parts: your mind, body, emotions, and the environment in which you find yourself. The second step is to come to an understanding about wholeness and health: in optimal health, all parts of your body act together in harmony to sustain your life and to increase your sense of well-being and balance. The third step is to become aware of how the parts of your Self interact at times when you feel comfortable and at ease, or times when you feel ill or tense. Notice how your feelings affect your appetite, how your mind can "forget" pain, and which environments make you feel energetic and confident.

Positive wellness is an achievement. To help yourself to optimal health, you must look at all parts of yourself—environment, personality, body, mind, and spirit—as an organic whole, determine which parts are out of balance, and begin actively to move yourself toward a balanced whole.

COMMUNICATION AND FEELING SYSTEMS

The nervous system of the human body is a network of immense complexity. Our understanding of how it works remains rudimentary, and among the most mysterious questions that we continue to ask are: "Where is the mind?" "Where does the Self reside?" and "What are feelings?" We know that the mind, consciousness, a sense of self, and feelings and communication are associated with the brain, nervous system, and sensory organs. But we must look to continued developments in science and technology as well as to further explorations into the nature of the mind, personality, and behavior to fully explain ourselves.

The nervous system is a means of communication within the body and with the outside world. Hormones (chemicals) also communicate messages, but not as rapidly as those sent by nerve transmission.

Data from our sensory organs—our ears, eyes, taste buds, and smell and touch receptors—rush signals to the brain where they are coordinated with dispatches from our muscles, lungs, and the cells throughout our body. We then act on this information through our behavior. Through this system, emotions are aroused and ideas conceived, memories are stored and images formed, pleasure is experienced, and words are processed.

As we think or feel and then speak to others, move our body in a telling way, or write a message, the nerve impulse that passes through this marvelous system moves out into the world from our center to affect people and objects in the world at large. So the nervous system can be thought of as a communication device that allows contact of our mind, senses, and feelings with ourselves and the outside world, while it in turn perceives, assesses, and acts on the many kinds of information coming into us.

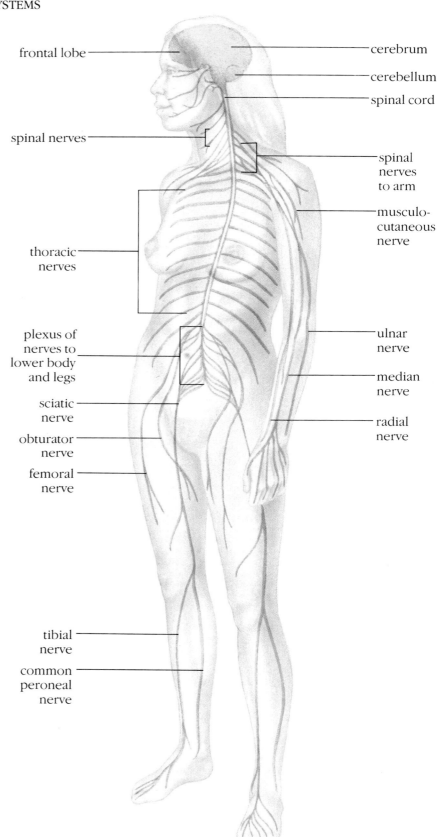

frontal lobe

cerebrum

cerebellum

spinal cord

spinal nerves

spinal nerves to arm

musculo-cutaneous nerve

thoracic nerves

plexus of nerves to lower body and legs

ulnar nerve

median nerve

radial nerve

sciatic nerve

obturator nerve

femoral nerve

tibial nerve

common peroneal nerve

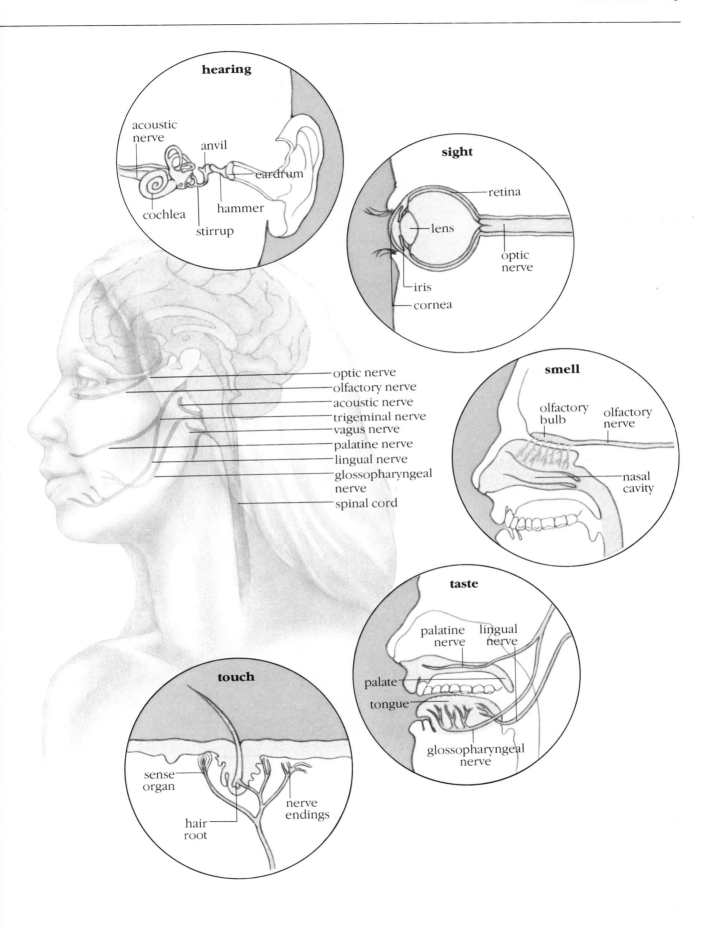

hearing

acoustic nerve

anvil

eardrum

hammer

cochlea

stirrup

sight

retina

lens

optic nerve

iris

cornea

optic nerve
olfactory nerve
acoustic nerve
trigeminal nerve
vagus nerve
palatine nerve
lingual nerve
glossopharyngeal nerve
spinal cord

smell

olfactory bulb

olfactory nerve

nasal cavity

taste

palatine nerve

lingual nerve

palate

tongue

glossopharyngeal nerve

touch

sense organ

hair root

nerve endings

MOVEMENT AND SUPPORT SYSTEMS

The support for the body resides in the bones. Bones are living tissue; even the minerals in bones are constantly being replaced. Tied to one another by ligaments, and fitted together at specialized junctions called joints, bones are glassy smooth at their ends, and are lubricated by fluid to greatly reduce the friction of bone against bone.

In the center of most bones is a red, spongy mass of tissue where fat is stored and blood is manufactured (in the sternum and ribs). A bone shaft is essentially a hollow cylinder. This construction accounts in great part for the amazing strength of bone, as well as its lightness. Another factor is the way in which minerals and protein fibers called collagen bind together to form an incredibly firm matrix.

The cranium protects the brain with eight thin pieces of platelike bone that meet at joints called sutures. At the base of the cranium, 26 beautifully constructed bones of the spine articulate the length of the body, with the last bone, or vertebra, anchored to the pelvis. Each vertebra is hollow, forming a bony ring; when all of the vertebrae are fitted together, they form a hollow column, the spinal column. Through the center of this hollow column passes the well-protected, delicate cord of nerves called the spinal cord.

The bones of the pelvis are firmly held together by cartilage. During the last months of pregnancy, the cartilage loosens, enlarging the pelvic opening and allowing some elasticity during delivery.

Bones originate in fetal life as cartilage. As childhood progresses, calcium and other minerals enter the cartilage cells, gradually changing them to bone. Some cartilaginous parts of bone remain and keep growing throughout life, such as the cartilage of the nose and that of the ears.

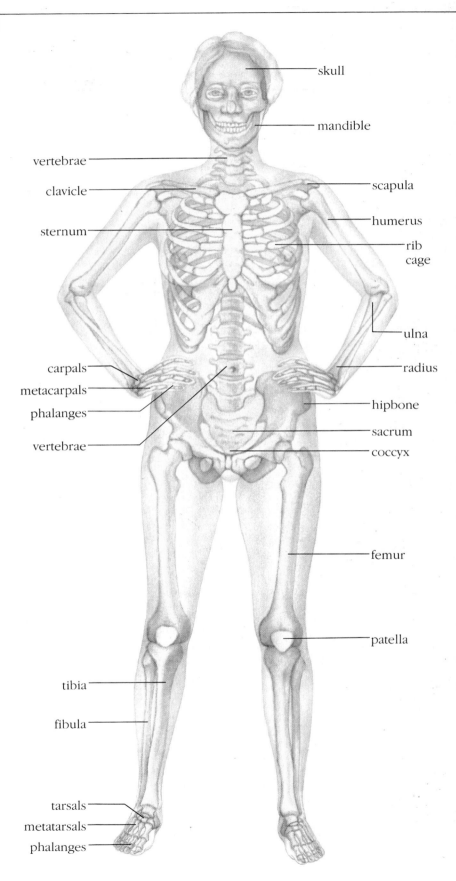

*Muscles, bones, and connective
tissue form the three basic elements
that support and move the body.
There are three types of muscles in
your body: skeletal muscles shown
here, which allow you to move at
will with speed, finesse, strength, and
skill; the visceral muscles, which
contract the stomach and intestines;
and the specialized cardiac muscles,
which pump blood throughout your
entire life-span.*

*Skeletal muscles act by contract-
ing, and usually are attached to two
or three bones by special connective
tissue called tendons. A single
muscle, such as a triceps muscle,
consists of thousands of muscle
fibers bound together with
connective tissue. Each fiber, in turn,
is composed of many fused muscle
cells. When you exercise, you add
protein to the muscle cells and the
diameter of the cells increases, but
no new muscle cells are made.*

*The contraction of a muscle is
triggered by a nerve impulse; the
strength of the contraction depends
on the number of muscle fibers that
are activated by the nerve impulse.
Many more fibers are activated
when you lift a heavy box than when
you lift a telephone receiver.*

*The smooth movements of the
body, which we call coordination,
depend on complex interaction
between the muscular, nervous, and
skeletal systems. Skeletal muscles
contract at the brain's command in
response to messages sent to them
from nerves. This contraction occurs
at the cellular level when the nerve
message is converted to chemical
energy, which, in turn, is converted
to the mechanical movement of
micro-fibers that slide past one
another in the nerve cell.*

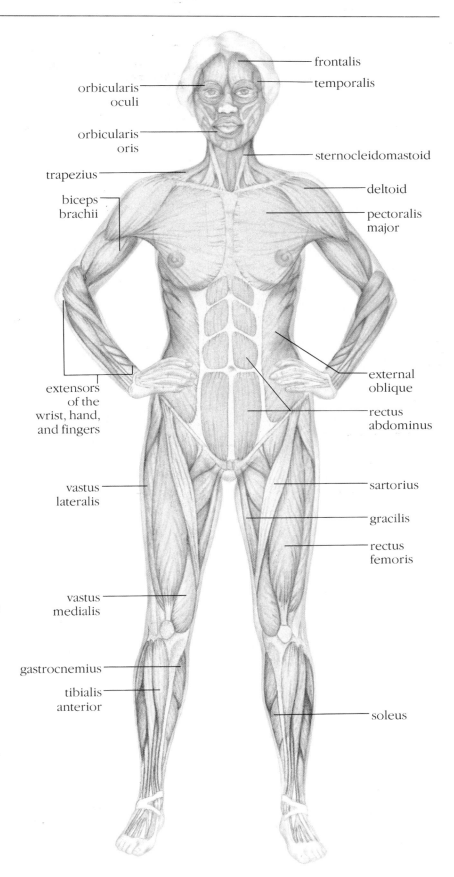

frontalis

temporalis

orbicularis
oculi

orbicularis
oris

sternocleidomastoid

trapezius

deltoid

biceps
brachii

pectoralis
major

extensors
of the
wrist, hand,
and fingers

external
oblique

rectus
abdominus

vastus
lateralis

sartorius

gracilis

rectus
femoris

vastus
medialis

gastrocnemius

tibialis
anterior

soleus

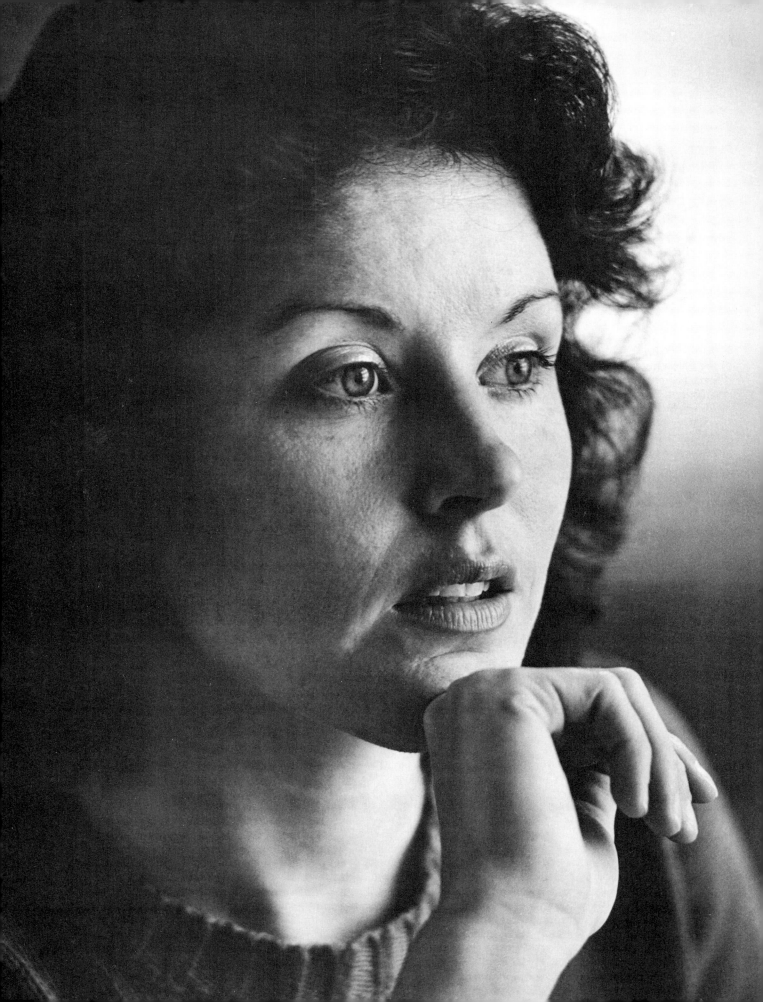

CHAPTER 2

WOMAN'S PSYCHOLOGY

JUANITA H. WILLIAMS, Ph.D

Throughout history, myths and beliefs about woman's nature have attempted to explain her behavior. But myths and beliefs are not science. Woman's psychology is the science that seeks an understanding of women by describing their behavior—not by describing myths and stereotypes.

There is an amazing diversity among women. Each of us is unique. From the moment of our conception, we differ in our genetic heritage, the circumstances of our births, and the patterns of our lives. We live in families, as single parents, with friends, or alone. We are healthy and handicapped, brave and afraid, rich and poor. We work at home and in thousands of different jobs outside the home.

But with all of our differences, we share with each other the distinctively female events of our bodies and our minds. These common events and experiences make up a shared female culture that helps us to understand each other, even as we acknowledge and respect our differences.

Woman's Psychology

Psychology is a science whose goal is the understanding and prediction of human behavior. Only within the last decade has the psychology of women begun to attract the attention of scientists and researchers. Before the women's movement, which has had far-reaching effects on the behavioral sciences as well as on many other areas of our lives, knowledge about women and our behavior was sparse indeed, and much of the information we thought we knew was unreliable and of questionable validity.

Beliefs, Myths, Stereotypes

The subject of woman and her behavior has always excited and mystified philosophers, theologians, and other commentators on the human condition, most of whom have been male. Beliefs about woman and her "nature" have been important in providing a semblance of understanding of women and their place in society. But beliefs are not science; they are simply personal or shared ideas about the world or some aspect of it.

What are some of these beliefs about woman and her behavior?

● Woman is a mysterious and unpredictable creature who can never be understood because she is a different order of being. To the ancient Egyptians, she was "a dark river whose twisting men know not." Sigmund Freud, the founder of psychoanalysis, echoed this theme in the last of his papers on women when he spoke of femininity as a riddle to men.

● Woman is a seductress, a cunning weaver of intrigues, whose main purpose in life is to ensnare man and to bring about his downfall. Her power is in the attractiveness of her body, which she uses to lure and captivate man. You'll recall that it was because of various enchantresses, from the nymph Calypso to the Sirens, that it took Odysseus ten years to return home from the Trojan War. It was this view of woman that brought about the witch mania of the fifteenth to seventeenth centuries, and resulted in the deaths of millions of women who were thought to have unholy powers because of their alliance with the devil. Stories of Delilah, Salome, Eve, and devil women and whores of all ages resonate through history in our literature and our cultural productions.

● Woman is a necessary evil in man's world. She has two values: her reproductive capacity and her sexual assets. Necessary for the continuity of human life on earth, and to gratify man's lust, she was otherwise an intrusive nuisance in his world. The poet John Milton in *Paradise Lost* has Adam ask, after the transgression, why did God
...Create at last
This noveltie on Earth, this fair defect
Of Nature, and not fill the world at once
With men as Angels without Feminie,
Or find some other way to generate
Mankind....
And the German philosopher Nietzsche wrote: "Man should be trained for war and woman for the recreation of the warrior; all else is folly.... The true man wants two things: danger and play. For that reason he wants woman, as the most dangerous plaything."

● Woman is an exalted being, more spiritual and morally pure than man. The embodiment of virtue, she is charged with maintaining the moral fiber of the society and with inculcating its values in the young. This image of woman on a pedestal, the "angel in the house," has represented the socially approved style of being female. The code of chivalry required that courtly deference, protection, and attention be paid to the lady. In exchange for these graces, she would stay in her place and carry out the mandates of this pedestal life-style, caring for the home and its inhabitants and maintaining domestic serenity.

Other stereotypes of woman include the Virgin, the Old Maid, the Shrew, and the Earth Mother. These are just a few of the ways whereby women have been categorized and "understood."

In general, however, myths and stereotypes about woman describe her in one of two ways: idealization or disparagement. She is either worshipped and adored as an exalted, sentimentalized vision (man's "better half"), or she is belittled as a case of arrested development, somewhere between man and child, or as an agent of those darker forces that man fears he will never be able to control. All of these ways of explaining woman have existed from earliest times, and continue to appear in the popular culture, in music, television, and literature—even as science begins to remove the veils and help us to present ourselves to the world as the fully human persons we are.

From infancy through maturity to old age, women in America live lives of exceptional diversity. Each of us is unique. There is no "typical" American woman. From conception onward, we differ in our genetic heritage, the circumstances of our birth, the families we become part of, the experiences we have as children, and the patterns of our maturing lives. Our homes are in suburbs and ghettos, on ranches and in mountain valleys. We live in intact families, as sole parents, with a friend or lover, or alone. We have no children, only one, or many. We are healthy and handicapped, brave and afraid, and living at all levels of affluence and poverty. We are workers at home and in thousands of different kinds of jobs outside the home.

But with all of our differences, we have our commonalities, too. We share with each other the distinctively female events of our bodies: menstruation, pregnancy, childbirth, lactation, and menopause. These are exclusively in the female realm, with no counterparts in the male's experience of his body. In addition, the social influences—family forms, schools, media, religion, government, and work settings, complex as they are—have in common certain patterns of values and expectations that help shape the kinds of experiences we have and the ways we live our lives. These common events and experiences suggest a shared female culture that helps us to understand each other, even as we acknowledge and respect our differences.

Thus, while no two lives are alike, we can discern patterns that fit the lives of many of us today. These have changed radically in the past few decades, and are changing still. Life for American women today is a series of stages and transitions, of developments and plateaus, of changes and challenges.

A Life Cycle of Change

The term life cycle refers to an individual's life history or "career," from birth to death. It consists of the various roles, statuses, and relationships that the person experiences as she moves through the developmental periods of her life in the process of aging. The typical life cycle of the American woman has changed dramatically in the last few decades. Compared to their mothers and grandmothers, young women today will live longer, marry later, have fewer children, and be better educated. They also are more likely to enter the labor force, and to work for a greater part of their lives.

Traditionally the life cycle of the American woman was almost synonymous with the family cycle. It was assumed from her birth that she would marry in her late teens and have a family, and her socialization, education, and training prepared her for these lifelong roles of wife and mother. The traditional woman was rarely employed outside the home, and although her work in the home was often highly productive, she received no wages and was thus entirely dependent economically upon her husband. Women who never married or who were widowed had access only to menial and low-paying jobs. In a time when a woman's identity was largely derived from that of her husband, their status was unenviable at best.

Not only were there social sanctions against employing women outside the home, but opportunities were sharply restricted. Until recently, most jobs were segregated on the basis of sex, and women were not permitted to work in male-dominated jobs that were higher paying. Instead they were limited to traditionally female jobs such as nursing, teaching, and clerical work, and to low-paying factory jobs. Further, higher education was not available to women at all until the mid-nineteenth century. Inasmuch as girls were going to grow up to be wives and mothers anyway, it was thought that they did not need much formal education beyond what was needed to prepare them for those roles. Indeed, it was widely believed that intellectual exertion was damaging to a young woman's health, that it would disrupt her menstrual cycle, and perhaps even make her infertile.

The life expectancy for women is now 76 years, an increase of 20 years since 1920. The median age for first marriage for women has increased a full year since 1950, while among 20- to 24-year-olds, the number of women remaining single is up by one-third. Women are postponing having children after marriage, and according to Department of Labor statistics, more than half expect to have no more than two. Voluntary childlessness is another rapidly increasing phenomenon: the number of wives under 30 who expect to remain childless has increased by one-fourth in the past five years.

While the educational levels of both men and women have risen greatly in the past three decades, the increase has been greater for women. In the first half of the 1970s, the number of women in college increased by 30 percent, compared to an increase of only 12 percent for men. And women now seem to be less likely to give up their educational endeavors during the years of marriage and childbearing. Between 1970 and 1974, the college enrollment of women aged 25 to 34 more than doubled. The number of women in law and medical schools has risen from about 5 percent in 1960 to about 20 percent today. Since education is generally held to be the key to economic independence and upward mobility in our society, these figures suggest that women's goals have shifted dramatically in the direction of acquiring skills that will make it possible for them to take care of themselves, and to live richer, more interesting lives.

Employment outside the home has become an increasingly important part of women's lives in recent years. More than half of all adult women are now in the labor force, and the increase has been greatest among married women with children. Reasons for this include increased opportunities for education and training, later marriage, fewer children, a higher divorce rate, and women's desire for economic independence and the personal satisfactions of a career.

Women's evolution from traditional to contemporary life cycles has occurred only within the past two or three decades, and its trends have changed our lives and our society. One effect has been a blurring of distinctions among women across marital categories; married women as well as their unmarried sisters now have jobs and careers. To some extent, too, the life-styles of women and men are more alike than before, especially in dual-career families in which economic responsibility as well as housework and child care are shared.

We are now ready to look at the contemporary life cycle of American women and at the psychological significance of its major stages and events from infancy to old age. Though each of us has had her own unique experience of growing up female, we also have much in common as we share the special consequences of the passage to womanhood.

Psychology of the Life Cycle

Infancy

When a healthy baby is born, the first question likely to be asked is "Is it a boy or a girl?" Its sex is its most important characteristic, and a major determinant of how the baby will grow up and the kind of life experiences it will have. Even in infancy, many psychological features are different for girls and boys. An observer might have difficulty identifying the sex of newborns in a hospital nursery since diaper-clad babies do not look or behave differently by sex. But the adults in their lives know what their sex is, and before the babies go home from the hospital, their parents are thinking about them and behaving toward them differently, just because of their sex.

Studies have shown a widespread parental preference for boys over girls. In the United States, most people want their firstborn to be a boy, and also choose boys as only children. People who want three children are more likely to want two boys and one girl rather

than two girls and one boy. Men tend to prefer boys more than women do. Also, Catholics and Jews prefer boys, while Protestants are more likely to continue childbearing in order to have at least one child of each sex. An interesting finding in a Hawaiian study revealed that boys were valued because they would carry on the family name, while girls were valued for "girlish" traits, such as obedience, neatness, and cuteness. The value of boys appeared to lie in the adults they would become; of girls, in their childhood contributions as household helpers and companions to the mother.

Though boys are favored, newborn girls have certain advantages over them. Girls have fewer congenital defects and physical problems of all kinds than boys do. And the death rate from miscarriages and stillbirths is much lower for girls; almost 33 percent more boys than girls die in their first year of life.

As just noted, parents respond differently to boys and girls from the first minutes and hours of life. In one study, 30 pairs of first-time parents were interviewed in the 24 hours after their child's birth. Half had boys, half girls. The boy and girl babies did not differ in length, weight, or physical condition. The parents were asked to rate their new babies on the extent to which they matched 18 descriptive adjectives, such as firm-soft, cuddly-not cuddly, strong-weak, and so on.

Girls were much more likely than boys to be described as little, beautiful, pretty, and cute, and as resembling their mothers. They also were described as softer, finer-featured, and more inattentive. Boys were seen as bigger, stronger, hardier, and more alert. And the study found that fathers were much more extreme than mothers in rating their infants in the direction of sex stereotypes. The implications of this study are that parents "see" boy and girl babies differently from birth, and develop different expectations and patterns of behavior toward them.

These differences in the perceptions of newborns are the basis for other differences in the ways girls and boys experience infancy. Differences in clothing and toys are commonly observed. More important are the different ways that mothers interact with boy and girl babies. (Fathers have little to do with infants. In one study, fathers interacted with their babies for an average of only 27 seconds a day!) Mothers talk more to girl babies, who are more attentive to verbal stimulation than boy babies are. But mothers hold boy babies more, perhaps because they are more restless and demanding of attention. Later in the first year, mothers hold boys less, and are more likely to encourage their independent and exploratory behavior. Girls stay closer to their mothers when they reach the toddler stage, and mothers are more accepting of their displays of dependency behavior.

What about psychological sex differences in infancy? Are boys and girls different from each other during the first years of life? The available research provides no clear-cut answers. A few studies have found that boy babies are more wakeful and fretful in the first months of life, and that girl babies are more sensitive to touch. These findings are not reliable, though, and lead us to conclude that demonstrable, clear-cut sex differences in behavior in infants have not been found. The most important thing to remember in this and later discussions of sex differences is that differences within a sex are always greater than differences between the sexes. Males and females overlap greatly on all measures of psychological characteristics.

Little girls, then, may not be the favored sex in the eyes of potential parents, but they are favored by nature to be healthier, and have fewer problems than boys have. Ironically, they begin life being treated as though they are weaker, smaller, more fragile, and less attentive than boys. More than anything else, this differential treatment may account for the different choices that females and males make later, and for some of the differences in the ways they spend their lives.

Girlhood

From birth onward, children receive thousands of noncontradictory messages that relate to their sex category. By the time they reach their third birthday, most children have developed a gender identity—an internalized knowledge of their sex category. They also can identify others by sex, and they know which clothes, toys, and other items are appropriate for boys and girls by cultural definition. The little girl's gender identity is normally congruent with her sexual body, with her genetic and hormonal status, her genitalia, and her internal reproductive structures. It is less dependent upon these, however, than it is upon her assigned sex category and the messages she gets from her environment about what sex she is.

Socialization processes are responsible in large part for the development of specialized interests, personality, skills, and behaviors that differentiate girls from boys. Children are taught how to be girls and boys in our society. "Boys don't cry" and "Girls play with dolls" are just two examples of the ways we socialize children into appropriate sex-role behaviors. In general, little girls have much more leeway with respect to sex-role behavior than little boys do. Society tolerates girls who are tomboys more readily than it does boys who are sissies. A young girl may dress in pants and boots, play active sports, and ride her horse bareback at breakneck speed, but a young boy may not with impunity play with dolls and dress in his sister's bikini.

Sex-related preferences for toys and activities appear around age three. In nursery schools, the little girls are in the doll corner playing house, while the boys are outside, roughhousing, tumbling about, and playing with cars and trucks.

In middle childhood, however, a phenomenon appears that continues to differentiate the sexes into adulthood: a preference by girls for the masculine role and a less-clear identification with the feminine role. Boys do not usually show cross-sex preferences, and are more likely to identify unambiguously with the masculine role. Studies have shown that when children could show a preference for being male or female, only one boy in ten chose female, while one girl in three chose male. Also, a study of toy preferences among four- to seven-year-olds found that boys preferred boys' toys much more than girls preferred girls' toys. As adults, most women can recall a period in their younger lives when they envied males, or wished they had been born male. Men rarely report wishes to have been born female.

What could bring about this disenchantment with the female condition? Quite possibly, girls see at an early age that the male role has higher status and greater rewards. When asked, girls commonly refer to the greater freedom that boys have, and see them as leading more interesting lives and being less hovered over and protected by parents. That females have historically had lesser status and have been perceived as inferior to males could contribute to the generalized feelings of inferiority reported by many girls and young women, particularly those who have been socialized into a traditional pattern of femininity. We shall return to this topic later.

As we saw earlier, psychological sex differences have not been demonstrated in young infants. Some such differences do emerge in early and middle childhood, but these are not so many or so great as many people believe. Current research on sex differences in children shows three areas of intellectual skills where sex differences are fairly well established: verbal ability, mathematical ability, and spatial ability. The first of these favors girls; the other two, boys. Verbal ability includes vocabulary, speech fluency, language comprehension, and reading. Mathematical ability includes arithmetic computations and mathematical reasoning. Spatial ability usually means being able to see the relationships between shapes and objects in space. Tests for this ability use mazes, form matching, and block-design copying.

These differences as measured by tests are fairly clear-cut by middle childhood. It is important to note again that we are talking about differences in the average performances of groups; the differences within a sex are always greater than the differences between males and females as groups. Some girls score higher in math and spatial ability than most boys do, and some boys have higher verbal ability than most girls do. The great variability of individuals is reflected in a story told about the English literary figure Samuel Johnson who, when asked who is brighter, men or women, replied, "Which man? Which woman?"

As for personality, the evidence is quite strong that boys are more aggressive than girls are. It is widely believed that boys are more physical in their aggressiveness, while girls resort to less-physical means, such as cattiness and verbal abuse. But several studies have found boys to be higher in both physical and verbal aggression. This sex difference, which has been observed across many cultures, as well as animal species, appears in humans at around age two. At one time, it was believed that the potential for aggression was the same in both sexes, but that it was inhibited in girls for social reasons yet allowed to become manifest in boys. However, recent research suggests that boys are, if anything, more likely to be punished for aggressive acts than girls are, and that parents strive to suppress aggressive behavior in both sexes.

The fact that this difference appears early in life and is observed in other cultures and animal species suggests that it derives in part from a biological basis. At the same time, we know that human behavior is highly malleable, and that societies by their child-rearing practices can raise their children, both boys and girls, to be aggressive or peaceable in their interactions with others.

Probably the most important thing that girls learn in the years of middle childhood is what it means to be female in our society. Most if not all societies assign different roles to males and females, though the content of these roles may differ from one group to another. We already have noted the traditional role for women in our society. Typically, young girls learned early what their destiny was to be, and their training was consistent with this goal. In recent years, however, there has been some blurring of sex roles, with more girls planning nontraditional careers, for example. But tradition dies hard; a walk through a department store or toy department still clearly demonstrates the differentiation of our products and activities along sex lines.

This would cause no consternation if it could be shown that identification with the so-called feminine role were healthy for girls. But this is not the case. Many studies have shown that girls who identify with feminine mothers (self-abnegating, unassertive, dependent on the husband, etc.) are less well-adjusted than are girls who identify with masculine mothers or fathers. This is probably because the latter have better-developed self-concepts and coping skills, with perhaps a more active problem-solving orientation toward life. In any case, the sex of the parent that the girl models is not important. Girls can learn the social skills and competencies they need to take care of themselves from a variety of people, regardless of their sex.

Girls learn about the role of the proper female from many sources. We have seen the effects of family perceptions and expectations. Later, a girl is exposed to the influences of school, television, books, and her peers. A 1972 study of prizewinning children's books showed that the women in them were dull, neat, and passive, and were identified mostly by their relationship to a male. Working women did not exist, nor did divorced mothers. Another study of school readers for grades one to six found that the ratio of boy-centered to girl-centered stories was 5 to 2; of male biographies to female biographies, 6 to 1; and of male folk or fantasy stories to female folk or fantasy stories, 4 to 1.

In addition, teachers tend to give more attention, both positive and negative, to boys. Boys are more likely to be reprimanded for disobedience and rowdy behavior, girls for lack of knowledge. This greater attention that boys receive could enhance feelings of importance, as well as reinforce a degree of resistance to authority and a desire for autonomy. For girls, the criticism for lack of knowledge could contribute to low self-esteem and lack of confidence.

In any case, though girls generally get better grades all through school than boys do, the bright ones are less likely to achieve to their potential. A study of gifted children that followed them to adulthood found that the girls were more gifted artistically, and that the seven most talented writers were girls. But as adults, all of the artists and writers among them were men. Almost half of the men had high-level occupations, compared with only 11 percent of the females, most of whom were teachers.

In recent years, some efforts have been made to reduce or eliminate sex-role stereotyping from children's books and television shows. Mothers now may be dressed in something other than an apron, and they may be employed in jobs other than housework. Fathers may help with child care, and may even do kitchen duty. While these efforts are laudable, the institutions of society change slowly, and relatively few girls seem to be getting the message that they can aspire to the same goals that attract their brothers. Our goal is a society wherein all the conditions for the acquisition of competence and self-confidence are provided equally for girls and boys. When this happens, we shall then see what the contributions of nature to woman's "place" really are.

Adolescence

At around age eleven, girls begin a growth spurt that signals the onset of puberty. For the next two years, girls are on the average taller and heavier than boys, whose entry into puberty comes later. Puberty is a developmental period whose most important event for girls is the menarche, the onset of the menses. Other physical events of this period include the development of the secondary sex characteristics: breast growth, increase in subcutaneous fat, appearance of body hair, maturation of the genitalia, and the characteristic shaping of the body.

Adolescence is generally considered to begin with puberty and to include the growth years when the body is maturing physically, to about age 18. As a developmental period, it has a reputation for being particularly difficult, fraught with conflicts with authority, with the dimensions of dependence-independence, with identity crises, with emerging sexuality, with fears and hopes for the future, and with anxieties about interpersonal skills and relations with others.

There is some evidence that this turbulent model of adolescence is an invention of Western society, with its practice of prolonging the dependency of the young and delaying their entry into the status of productive adults. In societies where girls are not educated and marry young, they move from childhood into motherhood seeming not to experience, at least psychologically, the qualities associated with this time of life in our culture.

Adolescence is a critical period in the life cycle of women in our society. It is when sexual and reproductive functions become salient, and relationships with males become infused with ambivalence, conflict, and desire. A girl's personal identity and destiny are not yet clarified, and the relationship with her parents is still marked by old dependencies and struggles to break away. In addition, the hormonal and other physical changes of her body contribute to her concern with herself, with her appearance and social impact, and to rapid changes in moods, tastes, and personal style.

Menarche is probably the most observable symbol of a girl's entry into the status of woman. In many societies, it is an occasion for special treatment. Seclusion, special efforts to prevent the girl from contaminating food, purification rituals, and celebrations are among the cultural devices that accompany the event. In our society, pleasurable experiences of menarche are not very common. Many girls are not prepared for it, and do not know the relationship between menstruation, sex, and reproduction.

The events of puberty are vivid reminders to the girl of her development toward womanhood, of her sexual potential, and of her capacity for motherhood. At the same time, she has not yet developed an independent identity, a sense of who she is and what she will do with her life. Some have suggested that girls do not push toward identity development as early as boys do,

deferring a definition of themselves until they find a mate to whom they can adapt. No doubt this has traditionally been the case. The girl grows up under the protection and guidance of her father, who then gives her away to a man who takes on her care, gives her his name, his opinions, ideas, and identity. Others have suggested that she *ought* to defer her identity formation for those very reasons. Today, while themes of liberation, careers, open marriages, and keeping one's own name are very much in the air, observation supports the continued finding that the formation of intimate relationships, especially with the opposite sex, are still very important preoccupations for adolescent girls.

Novelist Jessamyn West provided a touching example of this in a short story about a young girl who is alone in the house. She occupied herself at first with copying poems into her notebook and writing some of her own:
"I was lithe and had dreams
Now I am fat and have children."
Soon she abandoned her writing and went into her mother's room where she took off her clothes and wrapped herself in a lace shawl of her mother's. As she admired herself in the mirror, she fantasized about him who was yet to come:
"She loaned him her eyes that he might see her, and to her flesh she gave this gift of his seeing. She raised her arms and slowly turned and her flesh was warm with his seeing. Somberly and quietly she turned and swayed and gravely touched now thigh, now breast, now cheek, and looked and looked with the eyes she had given him."

One sees in this excerpt the mood changes, the experimenting with various selves, and the intense narcissism that are part of the adolescent girl's experience.

To the extent that girls do delay a commitment to themselves, and that the formation and nourishing of relationships are of major importance to them, they may set their life goals at a level below their abilities, and thus achieve less than they are capable of achieving. Some researchers have spoken of this conflict between a young woman's affiliative needs and her achievement needs. If a young woman sees that a commitment to a difficult goal, such as preparation for a profession, will interfere with her chances of making a successful marriage, she may abandon or put off her ambitions in the service of her stronger need at that time. As with other observations we have made in this chapter, social changes have eroded the old forms, and one sees new life-styles emerging. Young women seem to be detaching themselves from the traditional expectations that were bound up with the feminine role. Recent studies strongly emphasize that generalizations about girls should be avoided. There is no composite American girl. Yet there are prevalent values that seem to be shared by young girls from different backgrounds.

These, perhaps more than anything else, inform us of the nature of the adolescent experience for girls today in America:

- **Autonomy.** Adolescent girls want a voice in their own destiny, insisting on their right to be an individual equal with all others.
- **Family life.** They value family life and having children in a harmonious setting where man and woman live in a relationship based upon mutual trust and respect. They proclaim no manifesto for women's liberation, but insist on cooperation, sharing, and the value of choice in having children.
- **Material goods.** They want comfortable housing, the opportunity to travel, good clothes, and cars. The less affluent value these more than the affluent, the latter either rejecting material values or taking them for granted.
- **Education.** They see education as an important part of their lives, especially as a way of fulfilling individual capacities and life goals.
- **Honesty.** They see honesty and trust as the cornerstone of human relations. They despise phoniness, and are willing to return trust by being trusting.
- **Justice.** They are strong supporters of equal treatment of all people regardless of race, sex, or national or ethnic origins. At times, these concerns lead to conflict with their elders, but also to bonds with older people who share their commitment to the ideal of social justice.
- **Cooperation.** They stress the importance of people cooperating instead of competing.
- **Intimacy.** They want relationships to be honest, open, and gentle. They favor physical displays of warmth and affection among families, friends, and lovers. Although they do not consider premarital sex a sin, they think it ought to be part of a genuine and responsible relationship.
- **Meaning in life.** They struggle, as adolescents always have done, with the effort to make sense out of their existence and to find meaning in the confusion they experience as life. They are aware of the conflicting expectations placed on them. Some cope well, others poorly. But they are looking for something to believe in, at a time when old structures and sanctions seem not to be viable any more, and older heads than theirs also are joined in the search.

Adolescence. As adults we tend to forget its special anguish and its special beauty. It passes, finally, but our experience of that time of our lives shapes important perceptions of ourselves and our personal world.

Maturity

About 80 percent of American women between the ages of 25 and 34 now have at least a high school education. Graduation from high school is somewhat of a rite of passage in our society. It occurs for most people near their eighteenth birthday, the legal age for admission to adult status. From high school, women go on to college or some other kind of training, they get jobs and go to work, or they marry and start a family. In various combinations, these three scenarios account for the way most adult women spend their time.

Although American women live lives of great diversity, making generalizations difficult, they do experience transitions and stages during their adult lives that define their more important roles at certain times. From the multidimensional life of the young adult, they move to a new identity in marriage; from the role of young wife to that of new mother; from the role of nurturer and caretaker of the young to an expansion into community and work roles. As women get older, perhaps experiencing divorce or widowhood, the roles of mother and wife may become less important or disappear altogether. The woman of today can expect to live for 46 years after her last child begins school, which opens vast possibilities for exploration of herself and her potential, and for involvement in the larger world outside the home.

We shall now turn our attention to some of the psychological aspects of pregnancy and motherhood, the role of housewife and its adaptations, and some variants of the old roles that reflect women's changing values about themselves and their lives.

Pregnancy and childbirth are major developmental events that most women experience at least once. The motivation for having children is still strong in our culture. Becoming a mother means taking pride in this new status. Motherhood can provide feelings of expansion of the self to important primary group ties through which one's needs for affection and belonging can be met. The challenges of rearing children, the satisfactions that can come with creative effort, and the development of competence as a mother come into play.

A woman's psychological adjustment to pregnancy depends on several factors that vary in importance for each individual. Physical changes include elevation in hormone levels, especially estrogen, and changes in body size and shape. Some studies have found that pregnant women have an increased biologic vulnerability to mood swings because of these biochemical alterations. Changes in the figure are dramatic in the second and third trimesters, affecting the woman's perceptions of her body. An emotionally secure woman who is bearing a wanted child may well be proud of the visible evidence that she is pregnant, while a woman whose self-evaluation is tied to conventional ideas of feminine attractiveness might be anxious about the effects of pregnancy on her figure.

Pregnancy makes demands on a woman's body and her psychological well-being. Women who are emotionally stable, with positive attitudes toward themselves and their lives, will handle the increased stresses of pregnancy without difficulty. But women who have experienced severe life stresses, who are anxious and fearful about pregnancy, or who have a history of psychological illness are more likely to have troublesome pregnancies.

Situational factors affect women's reactions to pregnancy, too. Whether or not the child is planned and wanted, the woman's relationship with her husband, the presence of other children, the effect of pregnancy on the woman's work and her life-style, economic factors—all of these come into play and interact with physical changes and her typical adaptation to stress to further influence her psychological response at this time.

Finally, a woman's reaction to pregnancy is partly dependent on intrapsychic factors that may be largely unconscious. Pregnancy can activate old dependency needs left over from childhood. Sometimes a woman experiences ambivalence about sharing the love she receives from others with a new life. Attitudes toward her mother can be reactivated, too, as she now assumes for the first time an equal status, with its requirement for abandoning the self-centered concerns of childhood and its possibility of establishing a mature relationship with her own mother.

In discussing these sources of woman's psychological reactions to pregnancy—physical changes, previous psychological adjustment, situational variables, and intrapsychic events—we should note that they are not unique to pregnancy. These same influences affect a woman's responses and adaptations to many of the events and stages of her life, such as childbirth, mothering, self-development, menopause, and aging. It is the interactions among them, and their relative strength for an individual woman, that determine how she will adapt to the exigencies of her life.

Most women continue to view the role of mother as the most important of their adult lives, especially when children are young. Women's feelings about motherhood range from ecstasy to despair as they center a significant part of their adult years around their children's development and well-being.

The reasons for the salience of the mother role are not found in a "maternal instinct," but rather in social conventions and conditions. Young mothers continue to be the primary caretakers of children, who are mostly their responsibility even if they spend part of the day elsewhere while mother works. Too, children are seen as a very important part of today's family, and children's physical and mental health often are seen as causally related to the quality of the mothering they receive. While this may be unjust, it seems still to be the norm that mothers get most of the blame as well as the praise for how children turn out.

What does motherhood mean to women?

A recent study found that women could identify several consequences that came directly from their status as mothers. One was the need, at least partially, to give up their own interests and desires in the service of caring for their child. This meant a change in their identity and sense of self, at least for a while. The women saw another consequence as growth, maturing into a more competent adult, and becoming less childish and selfish. They also saw that their personal world was more constricted with the advent of children. They had less freedom and less discretionary time, but hoped for more freedom and time for themselves later. Finally, they commented upon the additional work required to take care of children, which required a shift in how they spent their time. The children came first, and housework, recreation, and time with husband, neighbors, and relatives (as well as time spent on oneself) all had to fall into place after the needs of the children were met.

In the long run, children are a source of great satisfaction for most women. Mothering, in addition to its headaches and aggravations, has strong achievement connotations that often are overlooked in contemporary analyses of women's roles. However, women are making major changes in this role in the direction of spending far less of themselves and their time in it. Instead, they are deciding that it will be just one of the ways they spend their time.

The psychology of the mature woman includes her experience of marriage, her relationships with men in and out of marriage, her sexuality, her work and its role in her life, and the quality of the adaptations she makes as she moves through her life cycle. The sexuality and mental health of women are discussed in other parts of this book. We shall now look briefly at some facets of marriage and divorce, some adaptations and alternatives to traditional forms, and at the meaning and importance of work to women today.

No typical pattern of marriage can describe the experience of the majority of American women. Only 16 percent of us live in the traditional nuclear family in which the man is the breadwinner, the woman is occupied with her domestic roles of wife and mother, and at least one child rounds out the picture. Marital styles may range from rigid role segregation wherein the husband is the dominant decision maker and the wife is dependent and submissive, to a co-equal sharing of roles with emphasis on individual growth and fulfillment for both parties.

The pattern of traditional marriage contains certain expectations, values, and ideals that are now being questioned by many. These include sexual exclusivity, the importance of children, the relegation of tasks by sex, the dominance of the husband, and the belief that all one's needs will be met by the other partner. Such a marriage is clearly restrictive of personal freedom and even growth, though its constraints may not be onerous to many.

A contemporary life-style is exemplified by the so-called open marriage. This is a relationship based on equality and freedom for both partners. It includes role flexibility, privacy, open and honest communication, and conditions for the development of individual potential and autonomy. The possibility of such a marriage is dependent upon educational, sexual, and economic freedom for women. Such a model may be more attractive to younger people who are less hampered by past experience. In any case, it is one alternative to more traditional styles, which up to now have had little competition.

Since one marriage in three now ends in divorce, many women are finding themselves unmarried again in their mature years. Divorce is always difficult. In addition to the concerns of finances and children, there are the emotional consequences: feelings of failure and rejection, loneliness, and anxiety about meeting people and forming new relationships. Divorce no longer carries the stigma it once did, but it still makes great demands on the coping skills of the woman who experiences it. Older single women have learned to take care of themselves and to cope with life alone, and some studies show that they are happier than their married counterparts. The divorced woman has typically not had this training. While some are overwhelmed by the demands of their new life, others find it a growth-enhancing experience wherein they develop new skills and competencies and increase their self-esteem.

The emergence of women into roles of economic productivity outside the home has resulted in adaptations of life-styles that are somewhere in between the traditional assignment and the brave new world of open marriage. What happens around the house when married women go to work? The research in this area leads to two conclusions: first, such women do less housework than they did when they were not working, and their husbands do more; and second, domestic chores and child care continue to be primarily the woman's responsibility.

A study of a group of highly educated professional women found four types of marriages: traditional, neotraditional, egalitarian, and matriarchal. In the traditional household, the professional woman's career had the status of a hobby; her husband paid the bills, while her major duties were still centered around the home and children. In the neotraditional family, the woman contributed income to the family and took part in making important decisions. Her husband "helped out" with the chores, though they were still in her domain. Only one family was found to be truly egalitarian, with a sharing of roles both in and outside the home. Matriarchal families were those in which the wives made more money than their husbands. In these, too, the women had the major responsibility for the household and the well-being of its occupants.

What motivates women to work outside the home? We have seen that half of all adult women are employed, and that 60 percent of these women are married. Research has shown that the reasons women work are threefold: money, the nature of the housewife-mother role, and personality factors. Most women work out of economic necessity. The single, divorced, or widowed woman works to support herself. The married woman works to supplement her husband's income, to provide some luxuries, or to send the children to college. Too, a paycheck can enhance feelings of personal worth and self-esteem. It is tangible evidence that someone is willing to pay for one's labor, often heretofore taken for granted as a contribution made in the name of love.

Many women do not find basic housework very interesting or creative. They may prefer to pay others to do it, while they themselves are doing another kind of work outside the home. Also, the exclusive company of small children with their unending demands can be tedious and nerve-wracking, even to dedicated mothers. Some women say that they are better mothers if they are away from their children for part of the day. Another factor is that children do grow up, go to school, and leave home, giving women who want it the chance to fill the void with paid employment.

Some women work because of their own personal needs and motivations. A need for achievement, personal fulfillment, creativity, status, and social contact—all of these can promote women into the working world. Some women have unusually high energy levels, with such an active orientation toward life that the narrow prescriptions of their domestic roles cannot contain them. And in latter days another factor has evolved—social pressure on women to be employed outside the home. This view comes in part from the feminist movement, which deplores the economic dependence of women on men, and encourages women to seek equal power and autonomy with men—things difficult to achieve without one's own income. In any case, it is rare today to meet a college-educated woman who openly avows that her goal in life is to be a wife and mother.

Most young women today intend to combine work with marriage. Birth control, delayed marriage, optional motherhood, and new technologies that free women from household drudgery have all combined to make this expectation a real possibility for large numbers of women. As in other areas of our lives, the ability to decide and to choose for ourselves what we will do with our lives is what is important. The content of those choices should be dictated by no one other than the woman who will live with them.

We have been talking about some of the nodal events and stages in the lives of adult women. Our discussion of necessity has been brief and somewhat cursory. The interested reader will find in-depth examinations of these and other issues in the suggested reading lists beginning on page 667.

Aging

The aging process in women has biological, psychological, and social consequences, each of which is important in mediating a woman's adaptations during the second half of her life.

As we age, we experience certain physical changes, as every woman knows. Skin and blood vessels lose their elasticity, muscular strength decreases, fat deposits increase, and the ovaries secrete less estrogen with the cessation of ovulation, an event associated with the loss of fertility. Women enter the period of the climacterium, whose major biological event is the menopause, the cessation after some forty years of the menstrual cycle.

Many women fear the aging process, with its physical changes. There have been good reasons for this in our society, which adulates youth, not age. The model for feminine beauty has typically been the "girl"—slim, feminine, and above all young. Women have been regarded as less physically attractive and desirable as they move past youth. Aging mothers and grandmothers are not seen as sex objects. Women have been mostly valued for their sexual and reproductive abilities, both of which are expressed in the context of youth. And unfortunately, in our society, women have not been encouraged to develop those qualities that are

enhanced by age, such as intellectual competence, wisdom, and creative skills of all kinds. Also, at the same time a woman is losing her youthful face and body, she may be losing other important functions as well: children leave home, and husbands go away or die. What she perceives as her purpose in life may be lost.

Studies of normal, healthy women during the climacterium are sparse. Recent studies support the finding that healthy women move through the climacterium without significant distress. One study of 100 women in the climacterium found only 4 percent who mentioned the menopause as a worry. More important concerns were widowhood, cancer, children leaving home, or just getting older. But almost all saw positive values in their stage of life. These included elimination of the fear of pregnancy, freedom from the nuisance of menstruation, more freedom and time with their husbands, and improved health and feelings of well-being.

Some women, however, experience psychological reactions associated with aging, and the most common of these is depression. See the chapter on "Depression" for a discussion of this problem.

Thus, older women are very likely to end their lives living alone. While this may sound dismal, with strong negative connotations, it shares with all the stages of life the possibility of being interesting, productive, and creative. The earlier stages of life lead inevitably to this one, and for that reason they should not be just antecedent to it but preparatory for it. "The last of life for which the first was made ..." is not an idle fantasy in societies that accord respect and honor to older people, that provide for them productive roles, and that believe that knowledge of one's usefulness invests life with meaning.

The psychology of women through the life cycle is better understood today than ever in human history. Even so, because of our enormous diversity even in our own society, to say nothing of other cultures whose ways are different, we can make few generalizations and we leave the subject with few verities. In some ways, then, the work of understanding falls back on the individual woman. She knows herself and her life better than anyone else does. Before understanding, though, comes awareness, a raising of the consciousness to look at our history, at the ways we have been explained in the past, at the common events of our lives, and at the impact upon us of social and cultural beliefs, attitudes, and conditions.

This is the best time ever to be a woman. We are living longer and healthier lives, we are getting better educations and work opportunities, we have more and freer choices of life-styles, and we are more liberated than ever before from old dependencies and from the exigencies of our bodies. All of these portend intriguing possibilities for those of us who are growing up female.

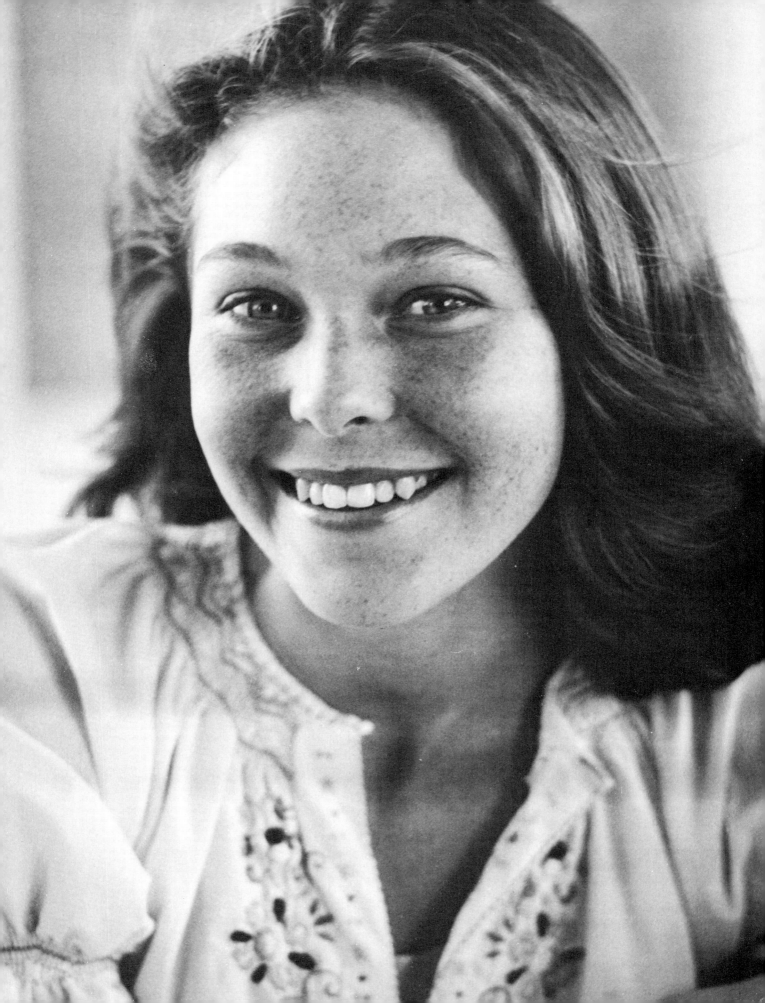

CHAPTER 3

NUTRITION

FREDRICK J. STARE, M.D.
ELIZABETH M. WHELAN, Sc.D., M.P.H.

Health is not simply the absence of sickness. It is a state of energy and vitality that allows us to sleep well, perform physical and mental tasks efficiently, and keep disease at bay. And proper nutrition is as vital to our health as is oxygen to our very life.

Eating is something we do every day—something that can either build and maintain our health or seriously undermine it. Eating *well* involves a knowledge of the caloric requirements necessary to maintain an ideal weight while also providing energy to carry us through a full day's activity. Eating *well* requires a knowledge of how to choose nutritional foods and how to prepare them to retain their nutrients.

As women, we have special nutritional needs and caloric requirements at various stages in our lives. Particularly in the childbearing years, it is essential to know how nutritional needs vary with pregnancy, the menstrual cycle, and lactation. And at all times, it is important to appreciate the value of eating well, with discernment and restraint.

Nutrition

The food you eat is a very personal matter. Normally, most people resist following a diet outlined completely and specifically by someone else. The complaints about food that are so common in college dormitories and other institutionalized settings illustrate the emotional value people place upon selecting their own foods. Menus planned for groups of people may be nutritionally adequate in every way, yet they may fail to allow for the fact that one or more of the included foods may not be eaten for cultural or personal reasons— and planned but uneaten food serves no nutritional purpose. Clearly, then, it is necessary to provide guidelines for each individual to use in planning their daily food intake. Although the merits of good nutrition are gaining ever-increasing recognition, it is the application of this knowledge to daily living that must be achieved.

Nutrition is vital to good health for people of all ages. Poor nutritional habits play a role in the causation of a number of common disorders such as coronary heart disease, obesity, tooth decay, osteoporosis, diabetes, vision problems, kidney disease, digestive disorders, allergies, sexual problems, increased fatigue, and social-psychological problems. Recently, evidence has suggested that dietary factors may be causally related to cancer of the breast and colon.

Except for some differences in calorie requirements, men and women have generally the same nutritional needs. But as we'll point out here, women, particularly during the childbearing years, are under additional stress nutritionally because of blood loss during the menstrual cycle, and the added nutritional requirements of pregnancy and lactation.

To appreciate the importance of nutrition, we must have some understanding of basic nutritional requirements, of which protein, fat, carbohydrate, vitamins, minerals, and water are the major components. Only the first three provide calories—that is, energy—but they can be utilized only in conjunction with the others. Except for water, these major components are comprised of some 50 specific nutrients, and no single food contains all of them in appropriate quantities. Thus, to be well nourished, one must eat a variety of foods selected from what most nutritionists refer to as the Basic Four Food Groups.

The Basic Four Food Groups

Nearly three decades ago, the United States Department of Agriculture devised the Basic Seven Food Groups to explain the variety needed in the diet to achieve good nutrition—a plan that was actually a simplification of the earlier Basic Eleven Food Groups. Despite this improvement, it soon became apparent that using a system with seven categories still presented more of a challenge than most people were willing to accept. Therefore, Harvard's Department of Nutrition suggested a daily food guide comprised of four basic food groups. At about the same time, the U.S.D.A. also settled on the same "Basic Four," and this plan was subsequently adopted by most nutrition education groups in the United States.

The Basic Four is a simple device for planning adequate nutrition on a daily basis; it outlines the variety of foods that will provide a "balanced diet," including the 50 or so essential nutrients. Although not structured to enumerate all foods needed daily, it does provide a very practical framework for meal planning. Sugar or refined fats and oils are not included because these substances, although they are important in nutrition, provide mainly calories and usually are not lacking in American diets.

The meat group includes meats, poultry, fish, eggs, and legumes such as dried beans, peas, and nuts—all good sources of protein. In addition, these foods supply vitamins of the B complex, such as thiamine, riboflavin, niacin, B_6, and B_{12}, and the mineral iron.

Milk and milk products supply more calcium per serving than any other food. Indeed, it is difficult to meet the recommendations for calcium without the use of milk or cheese. In addition, these foods provide valuable sources of protein, many of the B vitamins (especially riboflavin), vitamin A (if the milk is whole milk), and vitamin D (if it has been added to the milk as it should be). If you choose skim milk, dry skim milk powder, or low-fat milk (which we recommend you do), be sure to select those labeled as having vitamins A and D added, since the original vitamins are removed along with the fat in these types of milk. Adults and weight-conscious girls seem particularly disposed to omitting milk from their daily eating pattern. The new low-fat milks, with fewer calories and less cholesterol, or fat-free skim milk are good solutions.

Breads and cereals are often misunderstood and inaccurately described as fattening, overprocessed, almost worthless, and full of air and additives. Far from the truth! Breads and cereals are valuable sources of carbohydrate, protein, thiamine, riboflavin, niacin, and iron. In fact, it is difficult to obtain a sufficient quantity of thiamine and iron (particularly for a woman) if this group is excluded from the diet.

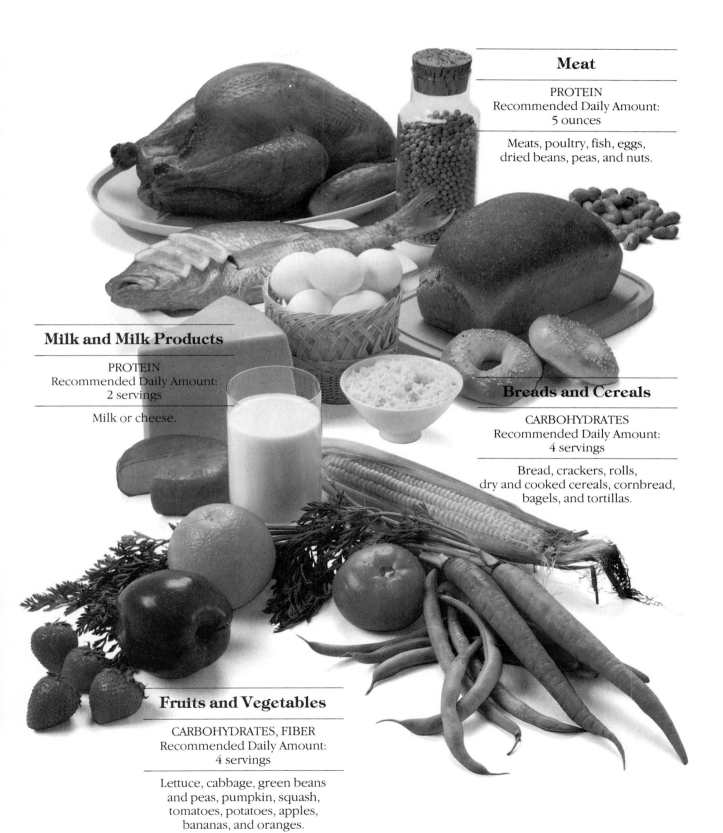

Meat

PROTEIN
Recommended Daily Amount:
5 ounces

Meats, poultry, fish, eggs,
dried beans, peas, and nuts.

Milk and Milk Products

PROTEIN
Recommended Daily Amount:
2 servings

Milk or cheese.

Breads and Cereals

CARBOHYDRATES
Recommended Daily Amount:
4 servings

Bread, crackers, rolls,
dry and cooked cereals, cornbread,
bagels, and tortillas.

Fruits and Vegetables

CARBOHYDRATES, FIBER
Recommended Daily Amount:
4 servings

Lettuce, cabbage, green beans
and peas, pumpkin, squash,
tomatoes, potatoes, apples,
bananas, and oranges.

Bread and cereals are important for a nutritionally balanced diet. For weight loss and overall health, it may be better to include a slice of bread in your daily diet, at 65 or 70 calories per slice, rather than an extra serving of meat at 75 to 90 calories per ounce.

While nutritional specialists recommend whole grain breads for their important vitamin and mineral content and the roughage provided, white breads outsell whole grain breads. Since important vitamins and minerals—thiamine, riboflavin, niacin, and iron—are partially removed when flour is milled, enrichment laws have been enacted in about half the states (in the others, enrichment is done voluntarily). These laws require the replacement of important vitamins and minerals to equivalent levels of whole wheat flour or bread when flour is milled for white bread.

Fruits and vegetables meet your needs for 100 percent of vitamin C, at least 60 percent of vitamin A, and much of your requirement for fiber.

Dietary surveys indicate that C is the vitamin most often found lacking in diets of all age groups. Vitamin A is often in short supply in diets of the elderly. How easily these shortages could be corrected! One serving of a vitamin-C-rich food daily and one serving of a vitamin-A-rich food at least every other day are sufficient for almost everyone. Two or three additional servings of vegetables or fruit complete the daily suggested quantities of fruit and vegetables. In addition to vitamins A and C, fruits and vegetables provide important amounts of minerals, folic acid, fiber (bulk), and carbohydrate. They also add texture, color, and variety—important psychological values of any diet.

Other Foods

Few of us eat without including a myriad of fats, sugars, spreads, dressings, and "complements" to our foods. Think of all those desserts, beverages (alcoholic and otherwise), and snacks! Indeed, these additions may increase the caloric value of daily foods by 25 percent or more. To put things in perspective, when the need arises to cut calorie intake, the "other foods" should be the ones sacrificed, not those from the four basic food groups. The illustration on page 49 shows how quickly calories add up from extra foods, such as sour cream on a baked potato.

Getting the Most Out of Food You Buy

Knowing which foods to select is only part of the nutrition process. You also must know how to preserve and prepare foods so that you end up *eating* the nutrients, instead of throwing them away.

Eat produce while it is fresh, since fruits and vegetables lose some of their nutrients as they lose freshness. Remember, too, that different parts of a plant have different nutrient contents. For example, leafy parts of collard greens, turnip greens, and kale have much more vitamin A than the stems. The outer leaves of lettuce are coarser than the tender inner leaves, but they contain more calcium, iron, and vitamin A, and so should be eaten along with the inner leaves.

Prepare your vegetables correctly. Cook them only until tender, in just enough water to prevent scorching, and use a pan with a tight-fitting lid. That way, you'll minimize your loss of the B vitamins, vitamin C, and some minerals. If you like potatoes, remember that in boiling peeled potatoes, or in whipping them afterwards if they're boiled in their skins, you lose much of their vitamin C. Keep the vitamin content high by boiling or baking potatoes with their jackets on.

Never store fruit juices or partly-used fruit uncovered or unwrapped—particularly those of the citrus variety. Exposure to air destroys their vitamin C content.

Don't keep foods in the freezer or on your shelves too long. Mark them with dates as you put them away. Keep canned foods cool (but not at freezing temperatures) and frozen foods cold, preferably at 0 degrees Fahrenheit or lower.

Current Nutritional Concerns

Today a growing number of women and men are concerned about the relationship of nutrition and good health. A number of current books claim to offer shortcuts to good health through diets composed of large amounts of one kind of food and none of certain others. The fact is, there are no shortcuts to good health. The best advice is to eat a well-balanced diet from the four basic food groups.

Here we'd like to focus on five specific concerns: salt and sugar, vitamins and minerals, fats in the diet, chemicals in food, and obesity and weight loss, and attempt to separate fact from fiction.

Salt and Sugar

We know that simple table salt (sodium chloride), which is present in all living things, may bring on problems if it is consumed in substantial quantities. Animal studies have demonstrated that excess salt intake interferes with growth and raises blood pressure. In humans, we know that congestive heart failure can be aggravated by high salt levels. Toxemia of pregnancy, certain types of kidney diseases, and hypertension can frequently be relieved by a drastic reduction in daily salt consumption.

Furthermore, natural everyday sodium chloride is habit forming, and many doctors recommend that less salt be given to infants and children to avoid this habit. Salt overdosing in children (which has happened when salt was mistaken for sugar) results in vomiting, fever, respiratory distress, and convulsions.

Unlike salt, there seems to be no health hazard associated with a moderate use of sugar; approximately 1 to 2 tablespoons per day with meals or in cooking constitute an important source of energy. Sugar is a pure digestible carbohydrate—and an important nutrient in our diet when used in moderation.

But what about the potential health hazards posed by sugar? While sugar is not a cause of diabetes, high levels of sugar consumption may aggravate the disease. And for many people, sugar may accelerate dental decay—more so when excessively consumed in "snacks" than when used in moderation at mealtime.

Vitamins and Minerals

If you believed everything you read today about vitamin supplements, you would be convinced that they, alone, and preferably in quantity, are magic tablets.

The truth about vitamins is twofold: we *do* need them, but unless you have a medically diagnosed vitamin deficiency, you will get all the vitamins and other nutrients you need from a well-balanced diet. Indeed, you can cause yourself real harm by self-medication with massive amounts of vitamins—particularly the fat-soluble vitamins (such as A and D), which are not excreted from the body.

Both minerals and vitamins are important for a proper balance of chemicals in your body. Minerals necessary for good health include calcium, sodium, phosphorus, magnesium, and zinc. See page 44 for recommended daily amounts of minerals for women.

Vitamins and How They Affect Your Health

A Promotes vision and healthy skin.
SOURCES: Liver, eggs, milk, butter, cheese, yogurt, carrots and other yellow vegetables, green leafy vegetables.

B Promotes healthy skin, especially around the mouth, nose, and eyes. Promotes a well-functioning nervous system.
SOURCES: Milk, whole grain cereals and breads (wheat germ, bran), meat, poultry, fish, vegetables (beans, peas).

C Promotes the healing of wounds, and strong teeth and bones.
SOURCES: Citrus fruits and juices, tomatoes, bean sprouts, green leafy vegetables, strawberries, cantaloupe.

D Promotes strong bones and teeth.
SOURCES: Milk, eggs, meat, cheese, butter, sunlight shining on bare skin, fish-liver oils, canned tuna, sardines.

E Assists vitamins A and C, certain fats, and the red blood cells in performing their specified roles in the body.
SOURCES: Whole grains, whole cereals, vegetable oils, eggs, liver, fruits, vegetables, seeds, nuts, wheat germ, and navy beans.

K Is needed in the blood-clotting mechanism.
SOURCES: Green plants such as spinach, cabbage, and kale; also produced by the bacteria normally inhabiting the intestines.

Vitamins and Minerals for Women*

	Age	Weight	Height	Energy	Fat-Soluble Vitamins			Ascorbic Acid	Folacin
					Vitamin A Activity	Vitamin D	Vitamin E Activity		
	Years	lbs.	in.	kcal	IU	IU	IU	mg	mg
Women	11-14	97	62	2,400	4,000	400	10	45	400
	15-18	119	65	2,100	4,000	400	11	45	400
	19-22	128	65	2,100	4,000	400	12	45	400
	23-50	128	65	2,000	4,000		12	45	400
	51+	128	65	1,800	4,000		12	45	400
Pregnant				+300	5,000	400	15	60	800
Lactating				+500	6,000	400	15	60	600

*Based on U.S. Recommended Daily Allowances

Vitamin A is essential for growth, vision, and healthy skin. A physician can detect vitamin A deficiency by noting problems in the functioning of the central nervous system, a condition that results when soft bones grow faster than spinal bones and, in the process, pinch important nerves. Without vitamin A, secretions that normally bathe the eyes dry up, irritating the corneas and impairing vision. Night blindness is a well-known manifestation of the deficiency. You should, however, have no difficulty in getting necessary amounts of vitamin A if you follow a well-balanced diet. Liver, so commonly associated with its high iron content, is also an excellent source of this vitamin. Vitamin A is additionally found in whole dairy products (but not in skimmed products unless they have been fortified). And, of course, carrots have almost become famous as a source of this vitamin. Likewise, all other deep yellow and dark green vegetables supply the yellow pigment known as carotene from which your body makes its own vitamin A. Don't be fooled because the dark green vegetables don't seem to be the right color—they contain the green pigment chlorophyll, which masks the presence of the carotene. But beware of high-dose supplements—they could mean trouble.

Vitamin B complex. The various B vitamins play a number of important roles. They help maintain healthy skin (especially around the mouth, nose, and eyes) and a well-functioning nervous system, working with carbohydrates for energy in the body. Vitamin B is a complex of 15 different substances that are classed together because they occur together in the same kinds of food. The most important B vitamins are thiamine, riboflavin, pyridoxine (B_6), pantothenic acid, niacin, folic acid, and cobalamin.

Generally, if your diet includes milk, whole grain foods, meat (occasionally liver), poultry, fish, and vegetables, you have no need to be concerned about getting enough of any B vitamin. Vitamin B_{12} deficiency is a definite problem for vegetarians who exclude products such as eggs and milk from their diets in addition to direct meat sources. This vitamin is found only in products of animal origin and too little of it will result in pernicious anemia.

Vitamin C (ascorbic acid) has historically been linked with its deficiency disease, scurvy, the scourge of sailors who took voyages of many weeks without fresh fruit. Its exact functions in the body are not fully understood, but we do know it is necessary for the healing of wounds. Citrus fruits and juices are high in vitamin C, and deficiencies in this country today are very rare. What about colds and vitamin C? Unfortunately, this vitamin has little to do with either the prevention or cure of the common cold. Studies show that at most, it might slightly reduce the duration of the cold, but most physicians today do not recommend vitamin C overdosing. Not only do they feel it is a waste of money, but the side effects are at this point unknown.

Water-Soluble Vitamins					Minerals					
Niacin	Ribo-flavin	Thiamine	Vitamin B_6	Vitamin B_{12}	Calcium	Phos-phorus	Iodine	Iron	Mag-nesium	Zinc
mg	mg	mg	mg	mg	mg	mg	mg	mg	mg	mg
16	1.3	1.2	1.6	3.0	1,200	1,200	115	18	300	15
14	1.4	1.1	2.0	3.0	1,200	1,200	115	18	300	15
14	1.4	1.1	2.0	3.0	800	800	100	18	300	15
13	1.2	1.0	2.0	3.0	800	800	100	18	300	15
12	1.1	1.0	2.0	3.0	800	800	80	10	300	15
+2	+0.3	+0.3	2.5	4.0	1,200	1,200	125	18+	450	20
+4	+0.5	+0.3	2.5	4.0	1,200	1,200	150	18	450	25

Vitamin D is required for the formation of strong bones and teeth; it is necessary to form the protein that is associated with the metabolism of calcium. You undoubtedly have heard of rickets, a disease caused by insufficient vitamin D in growing children. It is characterized by poor bone calcification and results in enlarged joints, bowed legs, and knock-knees. Vitamin D is unique in that it is not only consumed in the diet, but your body also can produce it from the action of the sun's ultraviolet rays on certain compounds in your skin. Usually we get sufficient amounts of this vitamin from a combination of sources. In our modern diets, the richest source is milk that has been vitamin D fortified. It also occurs in limited amounts in other animal foods such as eggs, meat, cheese, and butter. The same warning that was offered for vitamin A must also be made for vitamin D: this is another fat-soluble vitamin that can build up in the body and cause problems. You won't get too much vitamin D—or too little—if you eat a variety of foods and/or get out in the sun.

Vitamin E is a fat-soluble chemical in the alcohol family. Its chief function is to assist vitamins A and C, certain fats, and the red blood cells in performing their specified roles in the body. Health food "pill pushers" have erroneously touted this one as a "super vitamin" that can make you sexually young, improve sperm quality, prevent miscarriage and ulcers, ease arthritis pain, treat cancer and cirrhosis of the liver, both cure and prevent heart disease, and generally promote physical endurance. Exciting as these claims may sound, they are, unfortunately, contrary to nutritional fact. Vitamin E overdosing poses the same hazards as excesses of other fat-soluble vitamins. It is virtually impossible for an adult to develop a deficiency, since sources of this vitamin surround us. Indeed, early researchers in the 1930s who attempted to study the effects on laboratory animals who were deprived of it, discovered that their most difficult task was planning a diet that would cause vitamin E deficiency!

Vitamin K is still another fat-soluble vitamin. Although present in many foods, our main source is produced by the bacteria normally inhabiting the intestines. In other words, our bodies already have sufficient amounts of this vitamin without dependence on any outside sources.

Vitamins B_{15} and B_{17} are figments of the imaginations of food faddists and health charlatans. There are no such vitamins to be found!

"Chemicals" in Food

With the additive scare that has gripped Americans in recent years, you might believe that any strange-sounding chemical on a food label is dangerous. But before you reject processed foods—for instance, the new artificial egg substitutes for persons limiting their dietary cholesterol—because the label says: "Contains vegetable lecithin, mono- and diglycerides, xanthan gums, trisodium and triethyl citrate," and an array of other polysyllabic items, you should know that natural eggs (even organic ones laid by happy hens) contain, among other things, ovalbumin; conalbumin; mucin; lecithin; fatty, butyric, and acetic acids; zexanthine; and phosphates. Indeed, all foods and all living things contain chemicals.

You will continue to read and hear stories about how additives are dangerous. But those who uniformly condemn additives overlook the fact that the fortification of foods with vitamins C and D and iodine has all but eliminated the scourges of scurvy, rickets, and goiter. The mineral nutrient fluoride added to water (fluoridation) decreases tooth decay by half or more. The reality is that we know more about additives (which make up less than 1 percent of our diet) than we do about the basic chemistry of food itself.

Fats

In studying the subject of dietary fats, researchers have distinguished three different types, and have shown a relationship between blood levels of a substance called cholesterol and the intake levels of these individual fats.

Cholesterol is an organic waxy compound that is found only in foods of animal origin, and is also manufactured by several body tissues, particularly the liver. Egg yolks are the single most important food source of cholesterol because they contain generous quantities of it, and because they are a common and frequent item of the diet.

But other substances, namely those *saturated* fats found in meat, whole milk, cream, and butter products, and a few vegetable oils (coconut and palm) also have the ability to raise blood cholesterol levels. This is not because these fats are rich in cholesterol, but because they serve as the starting material for synthesizing cholesterol in the body. *Polyunsaturated* fats are of vegetable origin—for instance, soya, corn, sunflower, and cottonseed oils—and tend to lower blood cholesterol when they replace some of the saturated fats. *Monounsaturated* fats (such as olive oil) also tend to lower blood cholesterol when they replace saturated fats, but less so than the polyunsaturated fats.

Three decades of research in animals and humans strongly suggest that high dietary intake of cholesterol and saturated fats is one of the risk factors in coronary heart disease because it accelerates the development of atherosclerosis, a condition in which the arteries become narrow and obstructed. This paves the way for increased likelihood of heart attack or cerebral hemorrhage (stroke). Evidence now accumulating indicates that too much fat and cholesterol in the diet also play an important role in developing certain types of cancer—of the ovary, colon, breast, and uterus—possibly by overstimulating the endocrine glands.

In everyday terms, this means emphasizing main dishes low in saturated fat, such as fish, poultry, and veal instead of a steady diet of beef. You needn't eliminate beef from your diet, but you should choose leaner cuts, drain fat from drippings before you make a gravy, and drain fat from broiled meat before you add a sauce. Use polyunsaturated margarines instead of butter. Eat fewer egg yolks—preferably not more than two or three "visible" eggs a week (that is, not counting those used in baking and elsewhere). The American Heart Association recommends that you keep your cholesterol intake under 300 mg per day. Given that an egg yolk contains about 270 mg of cholesterol, you can see one obvious example of where your cholesterol-watching should be. Visit your doctor or local health clinic to have your cholesterol level measured. And for help in interpreting the results, contact the local chapter of the American Heart Association.

Obesity and Weight Control

Why do so many of us have to wage an ongoing battle against excess poundage? The answer is simple: we eat more than we need. We consume tasty but very caloric foods and generally lead sedentary lives.

If you are a woman of medium frame, five-feet five-inches in height (in shoes with two-inch heels), and age 25 or over, your desirable weight range in ordinary clothing is 116 to 130 pounds. If you are 10 to 20 percent over this "desirable weight," you are overweight. An excess of more than 20 percent means you are obese. But generally, if you are carrying excess fat, you know it without performing calculations.

Obesity is a serious problem. Throughout much of our world's history, plumpness has been symbolic of social status and affluence, but today it is both physically and medically unattractive. It is in itself a serious problem, but moreover, it causes an increase in the frequency and seriousness of most other diseases. Studies have shown that risk of heart disease is four times greater in persons with high blood pressure than in those with normal blood pressure, and extra pounds increase the risk of developing elevated blood pressure by two to three times. Obesity also means greater likelihood of elevated blood cholesterol, stroke, diabetes, and problems during pregnancy.

There are still other "survival factors": many employers avoid hiring the overweight. It's partly a matter of appearance, but many persons also relate fatness with laziness and assume that obesity may be a sign of physical or psychological conditions that could interfere with work. Additionally, recent studies suggest that college admission chances may be diminished among obese high school seniors. Of course, overweight can be a social problem throughout life.

Shedding Excess Weight

If you are among the overweight and decide it's time to do something about it, we suggest you first see your physician for advice—particularly if you are in the "obese" category. But if you have only a few pounds to shed, you can safely do it alone if you follow the sensible guidelines offered below. Be aware that dieting has become big business in the United States—and much of it is something less than legitimate. There are diet clinics and diet books advocating every imaginable sort of lose-weight-quick scheme, and they range all the way from just plain silly to downright dangerous. Many of the fad diets are nothing other than planned malnutrition, so it should be no surprise that once the diet is terminated (and most cannot be adhered to for very long), the lost weight is promptly replaced. Be realistic. It took weeks or months—or longer—to put on those extra pounds; there are no "miracle methods" for stripping them off again, especially if you intend to keep them off.

The key to successful, safe weight control is simple: body fat can be lost only when calorie expenditure exceeds calorie intake. If you eat more calories than your body requires, the extras are changed into fat. If you eat less than your body requires, the energy comes from stored fat. If you eat just what you need, you are in balance; you do not gain and you do not lose. In other words, to reduce you must eat less and exercise more.

The National Academy of Sciences recommends that women in the 19-to-22 age group who weigh about 122 to 128 pounds consume about 2,100 calories (see page 51); a man in the same age group with a weight of about 150 pounds should consume about 3,000 calories. But you must keep in mind that calorie needs decline sharply with age—and your desirable weight does not change after age 25.

We have already discussed the Basic Four Food Groups in some detail. If you find yourself a bit (or more) overweight, your body still requires a balanced diet selected from the Basic Four. Keep the portions smaller, cut out (or at least cut down) on the high-calorie foods, and skip the nonessential extras such as dressings, gravies, and rich desserts. And don't forget that alcoholic beverages can use up a good part of your daily calorie allowance in short order!

Get a bathroom scale—and use it. It is the best type of calorie counter there is. Exercise twice as much as usual, and you are well on your way to safe, permanent weight loss. The benefits—both social and medical—are well worth your efforts.

Ideal Weights for Women

| | WEIGHT IN POUNDS | | |
Height	Small Frame	Medium Frame	Large Frame
4'8"	92-98	95-107	104-119
4'9"	94-101	98-110	106-122
4'10"	96-104	101-113	109-125
4'11"	99-107	104-116	112-128
5'0"	102-110	107-119	115-131
5'1"	105-113	110-122	118-134
5'2"	108-116	113-126	121-138
5'3"	111-119	116-130	125-142
5'4"	114-123	120-135	129-146
5'5"	118-127	124-139	133-150
5'6"	122-131	128-143	137-154
5'7"	126-135	132-147	141-158
5'8"	130-140	136-151	145-163
5'9"	134-144	140-155	149-168
5'10"	138-150	144-159	153-173

If you are a woman between 18 and 25 years of age, subtract one pound from the chart weight for each year under 25.

A chart such as this one is intended only as a rough guide for checking your weight against the healthy average in the United States. Your own mirror and your sense of well-being are still the best guides to your correct weight.

200-CALORIE PORTIONS OF DIFFERENT FOODS

You will probably be surprised to know how little it takes of some foods, such as butter and bread, to add up to 200 calories, and how much it takes of others, such as vegetables, to equal the same number of calories. A calorie guide for different kinds of food is an important purchase for dieters.

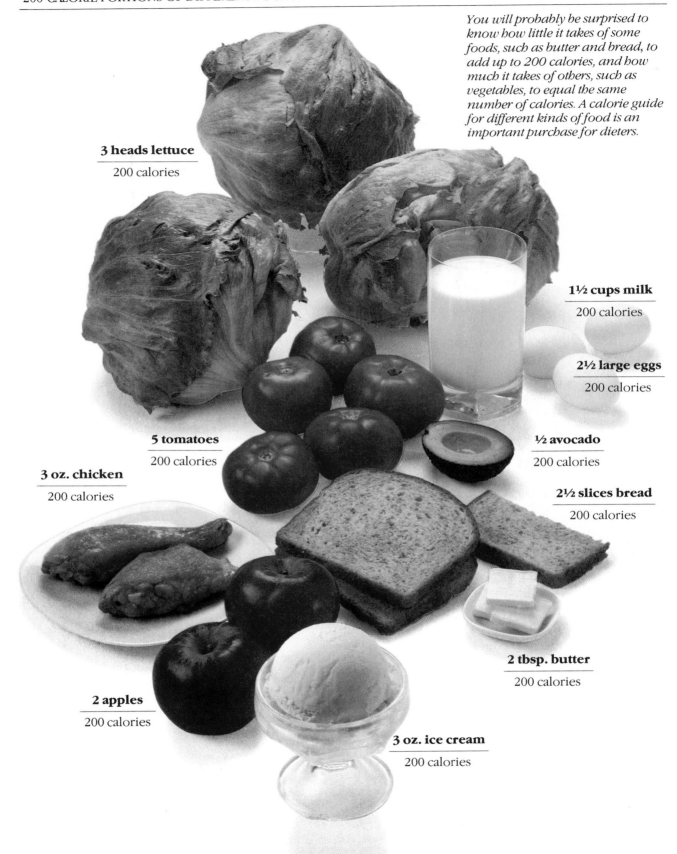

3 heads lettuce
200 calories

1½ cups milk
200 calories

2½ large eggs
200 calories

5 tomatoes
200 calories

½ avocado
200 calories

3 oz. chicken
200 calories

2½ slices bread
200 calories

2 tbsp. butter
200 calories

2 apples
200 calories

3 oz. ice cream
200 calories

HOW CALORIES ADD UP QUICKLY

You may not always realize how quickly calories add up at mealtime. The examples below show how simple it is to add hundreds of calories to one basic meal.

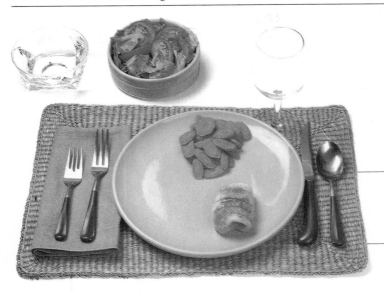

½ tomato	**20**
lettuce	**10**
carrots	**20**
3 ounces fish	**300**

TOTAL CALORIES **350**

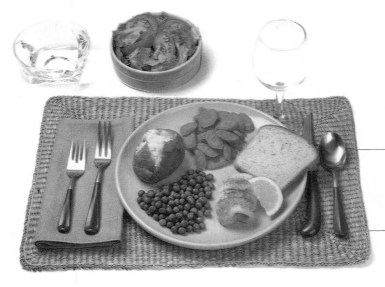

½ tomato	20
lettuce	10
carrots	20
3 ounces fish	300
baked potato	**150**
½ cup peas	**60**
1 slice bread	**80**
lemon wedge	**10**

TOTAL CALORIES **650**

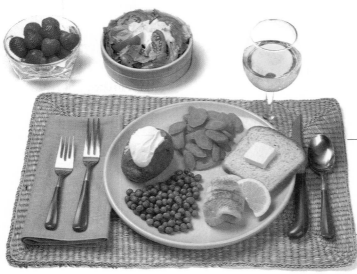

½ tomato	20
lettuce	10
carrots	20
3 ounces fish	300
baked potato	150
½ cup peas	60
1 slice bread	80
lemon wedge	10
6 ounces wine	**150**
1 cup strawberries	**60**
salad dressing	**100**
sour cream	**100**
1 tablespoon butter	**100**

TOTAL CALORIES **1,160**

Women tend to put on weight during different periods of their lives, especially when pregnant, while taking the pill, when cooking for a family, or at any time of little exercise (see page 54). It is important that you be aware of these sensitive periods of life, as well as any other time you begin to gain weight.

If you decide you want to diet and have more than five pounds to lose, see your doctor to determine what type of diet and exercise program is appropriate for your health and medical history. The diet you select depends also on your age, life-style, and emotional and psychological needs.

Dieting is often difficult. You may find that joining a diet group such as Weight Watchers or TOPS (see page 379) provides the support you need to start and stay with a new eating and exercise regime.

Calories Burned During Physical Activity

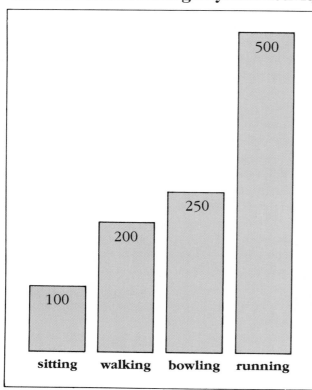

Physical exercise plays an important part in weight control and weight loss. The more physically active you are, the greater the number of calories burned, as shown here for an average woman five-feet five-inches tall and weighing 130 pounds. The numbers refer to the number of calories burned per hour.

For more detailed information on calories and exercise, see page 76 of the "Fitness" chapter.

Words of Wisdom for Dieters

Here is the collected, distilled wisdom of behavioral scientists and generations of dieters for staying with your decision to lose weight. Pick and choose to meet your individual needs.

- Exercise instead of eating. Jog. Dance. Go for a walk.
- Remove "extra" food from your environment. Keep only enough diet food for a day on hand.
- When you feel like eating, grab a carrot or a piece of celery.
- Relax. Learn exercises that remove tension and stress, and perform them when you feel like eating (see page 110).
- Eat slowly. Be conscious of the texture, smell, and taste of what you eat.
- Keep a detailed daily diary of what you eat, when you eat, and how you feel about it.
- Count calories.
- Don't skip breakfast.
- Weigh yourself every morning.
- Buy clothing a size smaller and keep it in a visible spot.

Anorexia Nervosa

On the other end of the spectrum is anorexia nervosa, a psychological disturbance in which the victim appears to have developed an abnormal fear of eating. It is most commonly seen in teen-age women, particularly those who have had a history of overweight problems. They begin a reducing diet—often of the "fad" variety—and continue to starve themselves long after their desirable weights have been reached. Even after becoming patently underweight, they still see themselves as "fat" and view any amount of body flesh with revulsion. Medical help and counseling are essential for treatment of this condition, which results in irregular menstruation, skin discoloration, and constipation, among other negative health effects. There are many cases on record of teen-age women who have literally starved themselves to death.

A number of theories have been advanced about what triggers anorexia nervosa. One is that a teen-age girl may rebel against perceived over-restrictions placed on her by family, school, friends, and society in general by exercising peculiar forms of control over the one thing that is exclusively her own: her body. Another theory involves a fear of approaching adulthood or, more specifically, womanhood. In losing extraordinary amounts of weight, all the feminizing curves are lost, and the teen-ager begins to look like a little girl again. Keep in mind that these are theories only. As with any psychological disorder, only a professional can determine the cause or causes and prescribe a suitable course of treatment.

Relative Calorie Needs Over the Life-Span

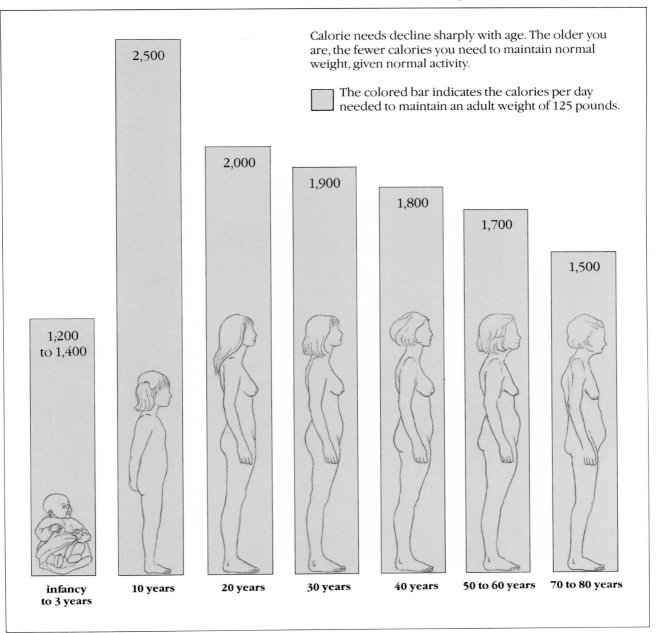

Calorie needs decline sharply with age. The older you are, the fewer calories you need to maintain normal weight, given normal activity.

The colored bar indicates the calories per day needed to maintain an adult weight of 125 pounds.

2,500

2,000

1,900

1,800

1,700

1,500

1,200 to 1,400

infancy to 3 years

10 years

20 years

30 years

40 years

50 to 60 years

70 to 80 years

Special Concerns of Women

Iron Deficiency

Iron, one of the body's most important nutrients, is also one of the most frequently deficient in our diets—especially for women—because it is so poorly absorbed. Only about 10 percent of our average iron intake is actually used. Iron is absorbed better from some foods than others. For example, it is absorbed better from meat than from green vegetables. So while you may be consuming what you think are perfectly adequate amounts of iron, you still may be deficient.

Iron is needed chiefly in the production of hemoglobin, that part of the red blood cells that picks up oxygen in the lungs and distributes it to the cells, where it is required for utilization of glucose, fats, and proteins. It is also an essential part of some enzyme systems and myoglobin, the red pigment of muscles. Because of periodic blood losses during menstruation, as well as the demands of pregnancy and lactation, a woman's daily iron requirement is almost twice that of a man—the Recommended Dietary Allowance (RDA) for men being 10 mg; for women, 18 mg, a difficult amount to consume in the average diet. This may account for women having been dubbed "the weaker sex" so many years ago: they probably were!

Iron-deficiency anemia is one of the most prevalent nutritional disorders in the United States today, with females decidedly more prone than males. When deficiency occurs, the red cells are reduced in number, and are paler and usually smaller. Hemoglobin consequently is also lowered. Sufficient oxygen cannot reach the cells, and the result is lethargy, weakness, and lightheadedness. The victim usually tires very easily and suffers from shortness of breath.

The causes are many. Do not decide on your own that simply because you are a woman experiencing some of the above symptoms, you can self-prescribe an iron supplement and your problem will be solved. The *symptoms* may respond dramatically to increased iron levels, while the *cause* may go untreated, only to grow worse. The various causes present different blood pictures, so a trip to your doctor is necessary for proper diagnosis and treatment.

The problem of widespread iron deficiency was first recognized in the 1930s and during World War II, when breads and other cereal products were legally required to be enriched with a certain amount of iron. At that time, these products constituted approximately 40 percent of the average American's diet, and for a while the trouble was alleviated. But today, such products only account for about 20 percent of the average diet (bread being undeservedly viewed by many as "fattening"), and iron deficiency is again a problem.

It has been suggested that new legislation be passed that would increase iron enrichment in breads and cereals by three times the current amounts. However opposition to increased iron enrichment has developed along two lines: additional iron would shorten the "shelf life" of these products by causing the fat in them to become rancid more quickly, and it would aggravate disease for the small number of persons who suffer from hemochromatosis, a condition in which high iron levels cause destruction of liver cells. As in many areas, risk-versus-benefit must be considered here. Fat rancidity can be avoided by more judicious planning, so that iron-enriched foods are sold and used within a shorter time period. And those who suffer from hemochromatosis simply can avoid products that contain high amounts of iron.

In the meantime, maintain your necessary iron levels by consuming sufficient amounts of meat, especially liver; beans and peas; dark green leafy vegetables; prunes; raisins; and whole grain or enriched cereals, breads, and pasta. Your doctor will advise if you also require an iron supplement.

"The Pill"

General side effects of birth control pills have received a great deal of attention (see page 168). What hasn't been discussed very often in the popular media, though, is the effect they have on nutritional status and body metabolism in general. Given that over fifty metabolic changes occur when you take oral contraceptives, the topic merits some serious attention.

Because hormone levels among pill users are elevated (due to daily ingestion of synthetic hormones), it is tempting to say the metabolic and nutritional changes that occur during pill use are like being "a little bit pregnant." In some senses this is true: there is fluid retention, breast enlargement, and weight gain in both circumstances (during pregnancy, the net weight gain is about ten pounds; during pill use, usually about six pounds). But the analogy doesn't hold up much further than that. There are some nutritional pluses and minuses associated with pill use, and not all of them parallel the metabolic events and needs of the pregnant woman.

If you take birth control pills, your body will need less of certain minerals—and at least one vitamin. Your iron needs, for instance, will be decreased. This is of particular interest in that iron deficiency, as we have mentioned, is the most widespread nutritional problem in women. Unlike the circumstances of oral contraceptive use, iron deficiency is aggravated by pregnancy, but when you are taking the pill, there is no growing fetus to nurture. In addition, there is considerably less blood loss during each menstrual period compared to the bleeding in non-pill cycles.

Further, unlike pregnancy, pill use does not appear to drain calcium supplies. Indeed, the pill seems to increase the intestinal absorption of calcium and decrease its removal from bones. The presence of estrogen in oral contraceptives also is associated with marked increases in the serum level of copper, a trace mineral necessary for the formation of hemoglobin.

A plus that could possibly be a minus is vitamin A. Levels of this nutrient are increased with pill use (and during pregnancy) due to the effects of higher levels of estrogen. But excessive levels of vitamin A can be toxic and particularly damaging to the liver, the organ in which it is stored. Thus, if you are on oral contraceptive therapy, you should not be taking high-dose supplements of this vitamin.

On the minus side, vitamin B_6 plays an important role in protein metabolism, especially in the conversion of the amino acid tryptophan to the vitamin niacin. There is evidence that pill users (and pregnant women) often experience some deficiency in this vitamin, although it is usually only a slight one. True deficiencies, which occur infrequently in this country, are characterized by hyperirritability, convulsions, and anemia.

There have been a number of suggestions in medical literature that slightly-lower-than-normal levels of vitamin B_6 (and possibly of some other nutrients as well) account, at least in part, for the symptoms of depression, tiredness, lethargy, sadness, or loss of libido that are reported in some 10 to 50 percent of oral contraceptive users. The explanation here is that there is some impairment of the metabolism of tryptophan in the brain that results in these behavioral changes. But there have been few studies made of this subject, and since depression can be induced by so many factors, it is difficult to attribute it exclusively to a dietary cause. Thus, the relationship here of depression and vitamin B_6 deficiencies remains a speculative one.

You can get vitamin B_6 from a variety of sources: meats are particularly high, but other good sources include whole grains, bananas, lima beans, cabbage, potatoes, spinach, liver and kidneys, and milk and milk products.

Folacin, another B vitamin, plays a vital role in the formation of nucleic acids, necessary for all cell growth and production, and in the degradation of amino acids. A number of studies have indicated that women on the pill have lower-than-average serum levels of folacin (although not all of them do).

Again, although pill users could probably benefit from eating more foods that contain folacin, there is little reason to believe that a serious deficiency will develop if you are eating anything that approaches a balanced diet. Folacin deficiencies generally occur only in conjunction with other health problems—sickle-cell anemia, alcoholism, leukemia, and pellagra. When they do occur, the symptoms include lesions of the alimentary canal and diarrhea, the latter condition leading to further depletion of the body's supply of folacin (and many other nutrients).

About 20 percent of the oral contraceptive users tested have enlarged cervical and vaginal cells, an early sign of slight folacin deficiency. But probably the greatest risk relates to pregnancy: during early pregnancy, significant amounts of this nutrient are critical. If a woman who has been on the pill for a number of years becomes pregnant immediately after discontinuing it, she might not be fully nutritionally prepared for a healthy pregnancy.

Where do you find a good supply of folacin? Spinach and other green leafy vegetables are good sources, as are mushrooms, liver, kidneys, and various fruits and vegetables. There are smaller amounts in meats and cereals. An important factor to remember in planning a diet rich in folacin is that the amount present in the food served may be highly variable, depending on the preparation procedures you use. If carelessly prepared, foods can lose up to 90 percent of their folacin content. Avoid storing fresh produce for more than a few days, and cook these foods for the shortest possible time.

Vitamin B_{12} is needed to ensure the health of all body cells, but is particularly important to the nervous system, the bone marrow, and the digestive tract. About half of all pill users have lower-than-average serum levels of B_{12}, although the actual tissue levels of this vitamin appear not to be affected. Again, true deficiencies are rare, but when they do occur, pernicious anemia develops (so named because until fairly recently, it was invariably fatal). The red blood cells become significantly larger, and other symptoms become evident, such as fatigue, glossitis (smoothness of the tongue), sore and cracked lips, and decreased hydrochloric acid in the stomach.

Foods of animal origin contain varying but generally significant amounts of vitamin B_{12}. As we mentioned earlier, unless you are a strict vegetarian, you should have no problem getting enough of this nutrient.

What should you eat while you're on the pill? The nutritional and general metabolic implications of oral contraceptive use are just now being understood. In addition to a pill user's decreased needs for iron, calcium, copper, and vitamin A, and her increased needs for vitamins B_6, B_{12}, and folacin, there may in the future be other nutrients that are shown to need adjustment in oral contraceptive therapy. For example, there is now limited evidence that estrogen increases the rate of ascorbic acid breakdown, thus increasing the dietary need for vitamin C. And it has been known for a number of years that estrogen stimulates the blood levels of triglycerides (fatty acids), though it does not have any consistent effect on cholesterol levels. The significance, if any, of this increase in triglycerides is not yet known.

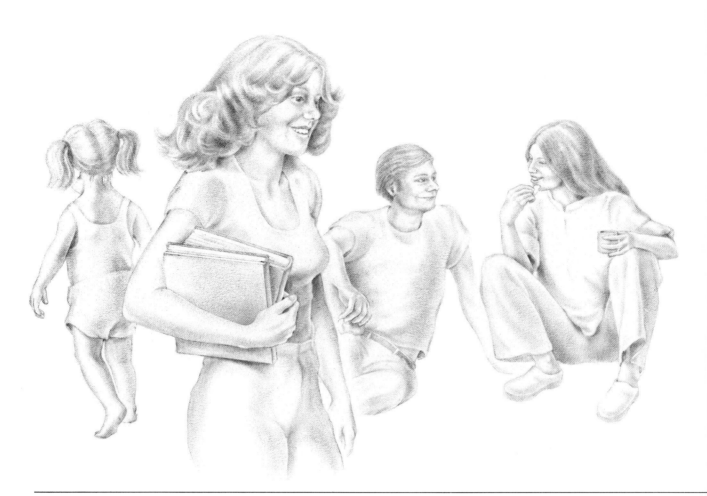

Weight-Gain Periods in the Life-Span

There are particular periods in the life-span when women are especially susceptible to weight gain. It is important to watch your weight during these times.

During childhood. Our eating habits are determined as early as infancy. Parents often reward children with food. Overweight children tend to gain excess weight throughout life, often for psychological gratification.

During adolescence. At puberty, growth spurts, sex hormone activity, and deposition of fat in the hips and breasts may lead to wide variation in eating habits and nutritional needs. These major physical changes, when added to psychological stress, may lead to overeating by teen-agers.

During young-adulthood. Eating out, entertaining, dinner parties, and a social life centered around food may combine with a decrease in the physical activity of the teen years, and often result in the beginning of adult weight problems.

During pregnancy. For many women, lifetime weight problems begin with pregnancy. A balanced diet is critical for you and your child's health, but watch carefully for excessive weight gain (see pages 56, 240, and 283).

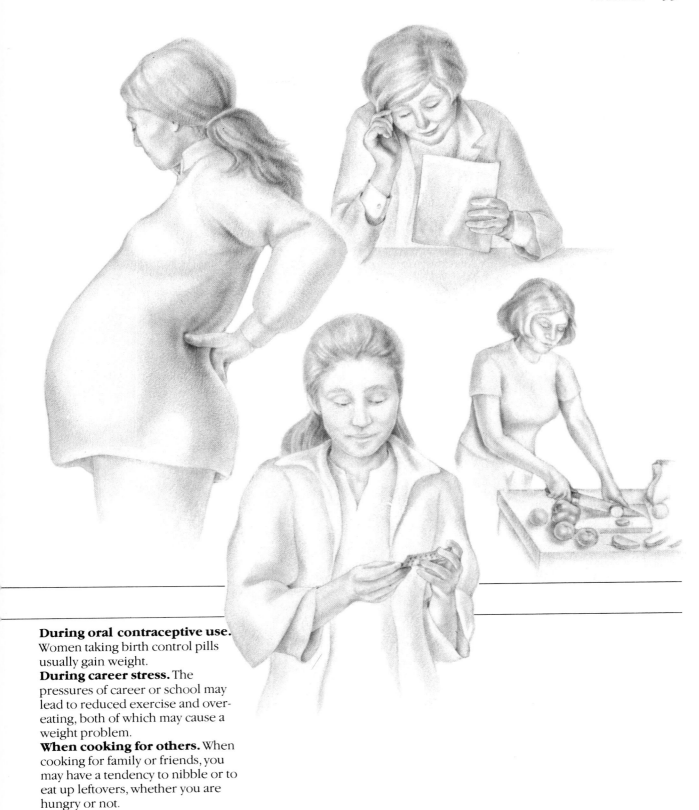

During oral contraceptive use.
Women taking birth control pills
usually gain weight.

During career stress. The
pressures of career or school may
lead to reduced exercise and overeating, both of which may cause a
weight problem.

When cooking for others. When
cooking for family or friends, you
may have a tendency to nibble or to
eat up leftovers, whether you are
hungry or not.

In the meantime, the most practical advice for a woman on the pill is to eat, in moderation, a variety of foods, making sure that she gets a bit more of those foods rich in vitamins B₆, B₁₂, and folacin. More and more physicians are now acknowledging that dietary assessment and nutritional counseling are essential components of family planning, and that they must necessarily keep attuned to the possibility that some specific minor deficiencies might develop.

Do you need vitamin or mineral supplements to compensate for some of the nutritional effects of oral contraceptives? The *Journal of the American Dietetic Association* recently supplied an interim answer to this question: "Until further information is available, no definitive recommendation regarding use of nutritional supplements can be made." Until one is made, you're better off not buying supplements unless they're recommended by your physician. Instead, spend your money in the grocery store on enjoyable foods that are also nutritious.

Nutrition During Pregnancy

Although it may come as a surprise to you, in your first two months of pregnancy, you don't need anything but a normal well-balanced diet. It is in the third month that your nutritional needs begin to change. But contrary to what you may have heard (and perhaps hoped for), you do not need significantly greater quantities of food while you are pregnant.

The National Academy of Sciences recommends that a typical woman five-feet five-inches tall and normally weighing about 128 pounds requires approximately 2,100 calories a day when she is not pregnant or when she is just one to two months pregnant; 2,400 calories when she is three or more months pregnant; and 2,600 to 2,800 calories when she is breast-feeding. You can get your 2,400 calories in well-balanced form by having each day two to four glasses of skim or low-fat milk; two servings of meat, chicken, or fish; one egg; four servings of fruits and vegetables (including citrus fruit and dark green leafy or yellow vegetables); and four servings from the bread and cereal category (see page 41).

Again, you don't have to eat *more* food to meet the needs of pregnancy—you just need to follow the "variety and balance" rule. Unfortunately, it is difficult to follow this rule and stay within the calorie limit if you attempt to include the "non-necessary food items" such as rich desserts, mayonnaise, salad dressings, or (although they are not technically foods) cocktails.

If you are pregnant, your doctor has probably told you that during your entire pregnancy you should put on no more than a total of 23 to 26 pounds, and that the weight should be gained primarily during the fifth to ninth months. (You may come to despise the scale in his office.) For the past fifty years, obstetricians have been encouraging patients to limit their weight gain—sometimes severely. Early in the century, the advice had some very immediate, practical applications; large babies often presented obstetrical complications, and since there is a relationship between the baby's birth weight and the amount of weight the mother gains, caloric restriction was essential. More recently, however, advice about weight control was based on the theory that excessive weight gain led to acute toxemia of pregnancy. Today this theory is no longer accepted; the strict warnings you routinely receive as you step off the scale are mostly related to your own general health and the knowledge that for many American women, lifetime weight problems begin with pregnancy.

Your attempts to keep your diet balanced and stay within reasonable calorie boundaries may be threatened to some extent by that almost-exclusive-to-pregnancy phenomenon known as the "food craving." The reason for such cravings is not understood, but they have been observed for years. Perhaps there is some biological cause, but more likely it is a psychological phenomenon of wanting to indulge yourself, or perhaps using food to allay any fears and anxieties that confront you at the moment. While you might say "absolutely ridiculous" to the notion of strawberry shortcake at 4 a.m. when you're not pregnant, you may now think, "Well, I guess it's okay, considering my condition."

Unless food cravings truly get out of control, either by straining your budget (a continued desire for lobster can definitely have this effect) or by precluding a well-balanced, moderate diet, these cravings shouldn't cause concern. After all, they're almost a matter of tradition.

Right now is a good time to muster all the motivation you possibly can to avoid the "well-I'm-pregnant-so-I-should-indulge-myself" pitfall. Pregnancy is a time when you want to pamper yourself and have other people show you special considerations. But those considerations should not include extra-rich desserts and two helpings of everything preceding them. "Eating for two" does *not* mean eating for two adults.

Vitamin Supplements During Pregnancy

Although your obstetrician will probably offer you vitamin supplements, you should be aware that this is more likely to be an "insurance policy" rather than a necessity. The National Research Council recently looked into the desirability of vitamin supplements in pregnancy and concluded that they were generally of "questionable value," the exceptions being iron and possibly the B vitamin, folic acid (folacin), both of which are difficult to get in sufficient amounts from a normal well-balanced diet. For more information on nutrition during pregnancy, see the "Pregnancy" chapter, beginning on page 220.

You'll want to take your own doctor's advice on the subject of supplements and feel comfortable with the knowledge that, while they may not help a great deal if you are eating properly, they can't hurt you or the baby. Beware of self-prescribing your own "megavitamins." As at any other time, those *can* be hazardous—and under these circumstances, to two (or possibly more) persons instead of one.

Nausea During Pregnancy

Some 60 percent of women experience nausea of some kind during the first two or three months of pregnancy. Often referred to as "morning sickness," it could just as accurately be called "any-time-of-the-day sickness." Not only is the discomfort itself somewhat worrisome, but likewise there is frequent concern that the growing fetus will suffer.

Generally speaking, there is no cause for alarm if you were in reasonably good health before pregnancy. During these early months, your nutritional needs have not yet increased; by the time they do, nausea problems will, in all likelihood, have disappeared.

The physiological reason for the nausea and vomiting of early pregnancy is clear: digestive processes are slowed down during the first months, and because of a decrease in production of stomach acid, the food just sits there, producing a sensation of fullness.

Psychoanalysts have offered elaborate explanations for such nausea, many of which are sheer nonsense. Simply put, this is a normal and temporary physical reaction that can usually be dealt with quite easily. Eat small amounts of food frequently instead of forcing three large meals on yourself, and alternate solid and liquid foods at the same meal. Avoid rich, greasy menus that are hard to digest even in a non pregnant state. Instead, try nibbling on crackers or lightly buttered toast. If nausea is not controlled in this manner, tell your physician and he may prescribe some perfectly harmless anti-nausea medication.

Alcohol Consumption During Pregnancy

While alcohol does not strictly belong in the category of nutrition (unless it contributes too many calories to the diet), it can have a profound effect on the future health of your child.

Children born to women who drink excessively during pregnancy exhibit a pattern of physical and mental birth defects collectively referred to as the "fetal-alcohol syndrome" (FAS). Growth deficiency is one of the most prominent symptoms, with affected babies being abnormally small at birth, especially in head size. Unlike many small newborns, these youngsters never catch up to normal growth. FAS babies usually have narrow eyes and low nasal bridges with short upturned noses. Almost half have heart defects, which in some cases require surgery.

What should you decide about alcohol use during pregnancy? You might want to consider abstaining completely from all forms of alcohol, especially in the first three months of your pregnancy when the most fundamental structural fetal development takes place. (You might have this issue solved for you if general nausea has been a problem.) But if you choose not to abstain, drink moderately, certainly no more than two, or occasionally three, ounces of 80-proof liquor a day. Drink *even less* during the first three months.

Women have consumed small amounts of alcohol during pregnancy for years without apparent harm to the growing fetus. But large amounts of alcohol and pregnancy definitely do not mix.

Nutrition After Pregnancy

For many women, the extra pounds that linger on after the baby is born are in themselves enough to initiate an acute attack of postpartum depression. Somehow you can delude yourself during the pregnancy itself, rationalizing every extra calorie by thinking "it's for the baby" and assuming that all the fat will naturally melt away immediately after the birth. But reality tends to set in the day you dress to leave the hospital: you may have asked your husband to bring over some chic outfit you've been eager to get into for months and find, to your dismay, that while your abdomen is considerably flatter than it was the week before, you are much larger than when you embarked upon the road to motherhood.

Dietary Needs of Pregnant Women

First two months

Eat a normal, well-balanced diet.

Third month to delivery

Calorie needs. You may consume an extra 300 calories per day.
Nutritional needs. Special vitamin needs include iron and folacin.

Dietary Needs of Lactating Women

Calorie needs. You may consume an extra 350 to 450 calories per day.
Nutritional needs. Eat a high-protein diet containing phosphorus, calcium, iron, vitamin A, thiamine, and ascorbic acid.

At that point, it's a bit late to be considering the well-established guidelines for nutrition and weight control during pregnancy. While your doctor probably told you during pregnancy that you should put on no more than 23 to 26 pounds, what he or she probably didn't tell you is that most women do put on considerably more than that. The median weight gain is actually 29 pounds, and by definition, that figure indicates that 50 percent of all pregnant women put on even more.

The depressing news is that the extra pounds simply do not come off immediately after you deliver. Generally, you can count on losing about 11 pounds as soon as the baby is born (7 ½ for the baby, 1 ½ for the placenta and membranes, and 2 for the amniotic fluid), and in the next 12 days, another 7 or so pounds (accounted for by accumulated water in your body tissues, the increased weight of the uterus and breasts, and increased blood volume). But from then on, you're on your own. The only way you are going to return to your normal weight—or perhaps do better than that, taking this opportunity to shed even more extra pounds—is by going on an after-pregnancy diet.

Breast-Feeding

What type of diet is appropriate for a woman who's just had a baby? Obviously, if you are planning to breast-feed, no low-calorie diet is recommended. The mother's diet during lactation must be sufficient to satisfy her needs as well as those of the growing infant. Generally speaking, the caloric needs of lactation can be met if 50 calories for every pound the baby weighs or gains are added to the 2,400 calories allowed during the latter part of pregnancy. (If you normally weigh 128 pounds and are nursing a 7-pound baby, your calorie calculation would then be 2,400 plus 350, or 2,750.) When you begin supplementing the infant's diet, you have to reduce the number of calories you eat.

Actually, the intake of protein is more important than the calorie intake. Your physician will recommend a high-protein diet that also offers significant amounts of calcium, phosphorus, iron, vitamin A, thiamine, and ascorbic acid. You usually can meet these requirements by slightly increasing the amounts of milk, cheese, eggs, whole wheat breads and cereals, and citrus juices you would (or should) normally be eating (see page 44).

If you stick to this regimen while breast-feeding, *you will lose weight,* since lactation requires a substantial number of calories. Of course, if you continue to succumb to some of the high-calorie food cravings of pregnancy, you will continue to gain weight.

Bottle-Feeding

If you are bottle-feeding your baby—or have recently terminated breast-feeding—you only need a well-balanced, low-calorie diet based on the Basic Four Food Groups discussed earlier in this chapter. As a general rule, your after-pregnancy diet should consist of five ounces from the meat group, two servings from the milk category, four from fruits and vegetables, and two to four from the bread and cereal group.

But in addition to following good nutritional guidelines and watching calories during the after-birth period, you'll want to enjoy your meals. The early days of parenthood are a very special time, and there *is* room in an effective after-pregnancy diet for some leeway—for example, a glass of wine with dinner and a cocktail on weekends—or, if you don't drink alcohol, treat yourself to an extra-special dessert or hors d'oeuvre.

Tips for After-Pregnancy Dieting

No matter how eager you are to return to your regular dress size, don't be taken in by one of the many fad diets now being promoted. Beware particularly of the "low-carbohydrate" versions. Right after you've had your baby, you'll need all the energy you can muster. If you severely restrict carbohydrates, not only will you be embarking on an ineffective long-term solution to your weight problem, but you'll also be inviting trouble. You need carbohydrates to provide the "brain food" to keep you going, and if you are following the baby's schedule, that means you'll need your energy both day and night.

• If you are choosing carefully from the Basic Four Food Groups, you don't need any special vitamin supplements in the postpartum period. But if you do have some prenatal vitamins left over, many physicians recommend that you keep taking them until they're used up, just in case your attempts at calorie restriction lead to a slightly unbalanced nutrient intake.

• As soon as you decide to fight your fat, stock up on calorie-saving foods: skim milk, cottage cheese, plain yogurt, and fresh fruits and vegetables (fill in here with frozen and canned varieties if your favorites are out of season). Also try some of the imitation products—margarines, mayonnaise, gelatin desserts—that offer great calorie savings compared with their "real" counterparts.

• Increase your normal intake of fruits and vegetables and other high-fiber foods to ensure that you are not bothered by constipation, a problem frequently encountered in the first postpartum months.

• Beware of the "middle-of-the-night snacking syndrome." Just because your baby needs to be fed at 2 a.m. doesn't mean that you have to eat, too. If you fear that opening the refrigerator to get the formula will prove simply irresistible to you, have it well stocked with "free foods" such as carrots, cucumbers, tomatoes, watercress, lettuce, and celery.

• Make an effort to cut back on your portions—put half as much as you usually would on your plate.

• Don't be overly enthusiastic about supplementing your after-pregnancy diet with vigorous exercise. Check with your doctor before you begin any exercise program. Chances are, he or she will want you to take it easy for at least six weeks. For information on exercise during and after pregnancy, see the chapters on "Pregnancy," "Labor and Delivery," and "Fitness."

• Take a critical look at your husband's weight. It is not uncommon for the dietary splurges of your pregnancy to affect him as well. If he is overweight, he too may benefit from the after-pregnancy diet.

• Most important, accept the fact that you are no longer pregnant. You have no reason for deluding yourself anymore. You may have been eating for two for nine months, but for the next few months, if you want to return to your regular weight, you are going to have to eat for less than one.

The Golden Years

Life-style changes in the later years often create many nutritional problems for the elderly, ranging from severe underweight to obesity, and from digestive malfunctions to varying degrees of malnourishment.

After age 25, the average American's calorie needs decrease by about 5 percent every ten years. Notice that we say *average*. While this decrease is due in part to a slowing of the metabolic processes, calorie requirements also depend on how much exercise you get. It should be apparent, however, that if you are near retirement age, you simply don't need to eat as much as you used to (see page 51).

But too often, as you find yourself with more and more time on your hands, you may fill too many of the empty hours by trying out all those scrumptious recipes you've been saving up. Or, conversely, perhaps you feel there's no longer any reason to bother preparing properly balanced meals—and then, with appetite never quite satisfied, you tend to "nibble" a good part of the day. Partially, the obvious solution in both cases is to find something besides food to focus your attention on.

Perhaps your problem is exactly the opposite, particularly if you live alone. Sitting down to eat at an otherwise empty table may simply take away your appetite entirely. Here again, only a little effort is required: try exchanging dinner or lunch visits with one or two neighborhood friends on a regular basis. Get out the good silver, put candles on the table, and float a flower at each place setting. (After all, who deserves elegance more than you?) Study some gourmet cookbooks or magazine illustrations for fancy serving ideas and new menu combinations. Even if one of you is on a special diet, this should present no unsolvable problem. If it is difficult to compromise on the entire menu, an extra dish or two can always be prepared—even if it means two entrées.

For both the underweight and the overweight, appetite can be helped back into more normal bounds by including more activity in your life. A daily walk or two is healthful for anyone; light gardening can be most rewarding; outdoor games such as shuffleboard and croquet offer fresh air and mild exercise without being exhausting. Religious and political organizations, volunteer workers in a hospital or school, arts and crafts groups—all would welcome your knowledge and talents and provide the kind of stimulation we all need to promote good health.

Of course, there are other health problems commonly found in the elderly. Ill-fitting dentures or poor teeth often prevent proper eating habits (another reason for fluoridated water), causing too little food to be eaten, too lopsided a diet, or inadequate chewing ability—a frequent cause of digestive upsets. This is a problem that must be corrected—for your general good health as well as to help you again enjoy a greater variety of foods.

Care should be taken to see that sufficient amounts of iron and vitamins A and C are consumed regularly. (See the specific sections earlier in this chapter for foods rich in these nutrients.) Calcium levels, too, tend to fall too low in the elderly, contributing to osteoporosis (brittleness of the bones), a condition far more common in older women than in men. More dairy products are indicated here. Also take special care to minimize your intake of saturated fat.

Remember to drink plenty of water and other fluids. Together with whole grain breads and cereals, and fibrous fruits and vegetables, it will help perk up a too-sluggish digestive system and prevent constipation.

A word needs to be said, also, about the health food stores and mail order catalogs promising to sell you the Fountain of Youth. However unfortunately, there just isn't one! If you think you need food supplements of any kind, consult your doctor. He may recommend a simple vitamin/mineral supplement, but other than that, your money is better spent on nutritious, wholesome, enjoyable food judiciously selected from the Basic Four Food Groups.

Nutrition in the golden years is the same as for all other age groups—you just need a little less of it.

In summary, good health is best promoted by choosing a wide variety of foods from the Basic Four Food Groups to supply the some-50 known nutrients required physiologically by the body. Taste, smell, color, texture, temperature, and certain other factors provide psychologic values.

The key to improving nutritional levels in general lies in improving nutrition education programs. Eating patterns represent an accumulation of habits learned throughout one's lifetime. If nutrition is carefully taught to children from the earliest years, good dietary patterns can be encouraged while food habits are still developing. Hopefully, then, good nutrition will become "second nature"—and many of our current problems of overweight and diet-related diseases will never get a foot in the door.

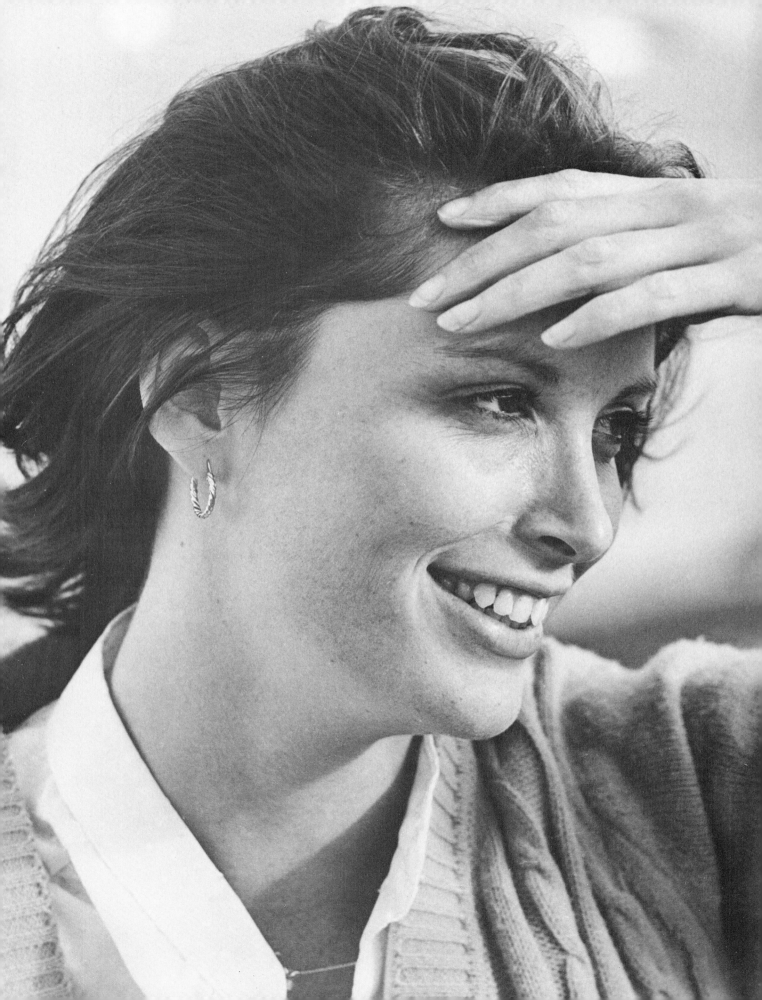

CHAPTER 4

FITNESS

CHRISTINE E. HAYCOCK, M.D., F.A.C.S.M.
GAIL SHIERMAN, Ph.D.

No two people think of fitness in exactly the same way. To some, it means jogging five miles a day through town. To others, fitness may be a quiet session of yoga practiced at home. And to still others, it may mean lifting weights at the local gym. The point is, there are almost as many ways to achieve fitness as there are benefits of being fit. With a minimum of effort, you can design a lifelong fitness program tailored to your abilities, interests, life-style, and even your personality that will begin to pay off the very first day.

Fitness

No doubt you've been hearing and reading a great deal about fitness in the past few years. As a nation, we're becoming more fitness-conscious. People are jogging, playing tennis, and working out in record numbers in an attempt to reap the rewards of good health, weight control, improved appearance, higher energy, and just a feeling of well-being.

Most people approach exercise with intermittent bursts of enthusiasm and activity. The weekend athlete may get quite a workout for two days, only to sit behind her desk for the next five days, mistakenly thinking she's working toward total fitness. But total fitness requires more than a weekend bike ride or round of tennis. In order to attain it, it's important to know what constitutes a fit body, how to assess and monitor fitness, and most of all, how to design a lifelong and regular *exercise program that suits your life-style.*

Body Fitness

Think of body fitness as a state of well-being that lets you function at your optimum level. A woman who is fit will be able to carry on everyday work and leisure activities without undue fatigue or stress. In addition, she'll have energy in reserve to better deal with emergency situations when they arise.

There are degrees of fitness that vary from person to person and from time to time, but they share one important, undeniable characteristic: they improve the quality of your life.

Parameters of Fitness

The three main components of fitness are muscular strength and endurance, flexibility, and cardiovascular endurance. Some physical fitness advocates also include motor-ability components such as power, speed, and agility, but these are secondary considerations for most adults.

Strength is the ability to contract a muscle or muscle group against resistance, as measured in one all-out effort. Strength is specific to the muscle or muscle group that's being used. For example, just because you can do 50 sit-ups doesn't mean that you're strong throughout your body. Measuring strength is difficult and requires specialized equipment. There's no quick and easy way to measure the strength of individual muscles at home. However, you can get some indication of your strength by lifting weights of known poundage, or having a weight-training center test you on various pieces of apparatus. The object of such a strength test is to see how much weight you can lift in one all-out effort. This will involve some trial and error on your part, and so it's wise to seek expert advice from trained personnel before using the equipment.

Another aspect of muscular strength is endurance—the ability to repeat a particular exercise. For example, if you can do more than one sit-up, you're exhibiting the endurance of your abdominal muscles. You can develop muscular endurance by repeating an exercise more often each time you do it. Throughout this chapter, we'll use the term "strength" to mean muscular strength *and* endurance.

Flexibility (stretching ability) is the second component of fitness and is defined as the maximum range through which you can move each joint without straining it or its surrounding muscles. Just as strength is specific to a given muscle, flexibility is specific to a given joint. Being able to do a back bend doesn't mean that the other joints of your body are as flexible. One common flexibility test is bending over to touch your toes; it demonstrates the flexibility of your back and the backs of your legs.

Later in this chapter, we'll list exercises that increase flexibility, and that will give you a better idea of how well your own joints move (see page 64).

Cardiovascular endurance (circulatory-respiratory endurance or aerobic capacity) is the third component of fitness. This is the ability of the heart and vessels to deliver oxygenated blood to the heart and to the muscles of the body. The more efficient the heart and lungs become, the easier it is to participate in prolonged, continuous physical activity. A very effective way to measure cardiovascular endurance is to see how far you can run in a specified time (see page 74).

Weight and body fat. The three components of fitness (strength, flexibility, and cardiovascular endurance), along with a proper diet, also are the means by which you can control your weight. While it's important for a woman to achieve and maintain her optimum weight in order to function well and efficiently, it's sometimes hard to know what that optimum weight is. Universally applicable charts of height and ideal weight are difficult to construct because individuals vary so greatly. However, a range of ideal weights for particular heights and body types is given on page 47.

Body composition depends upon your percentage of body fat, the weight of this fat, and your lean body weight. Of course, excess fat adversely affects your health. An acceptable amount of body fat in women is approximately 25 percent; ideally, a woman should have 16 to 20 percent of body fat.

Measuring body fat usually requires trained personnel who either use instruments to measure the skin-fold thickness at known fat deposit sites (the triceps, shoulder blade, abdomen, or hips) or who utilize an underwater weighing technique. A simple test you can do yourself is to pinch the skin of the back of your upper arm at its midpoint. If the skin thickness measures over one inch, you're probably overweight.

THE THREE MAIN COMPONENTS OF FITNESS

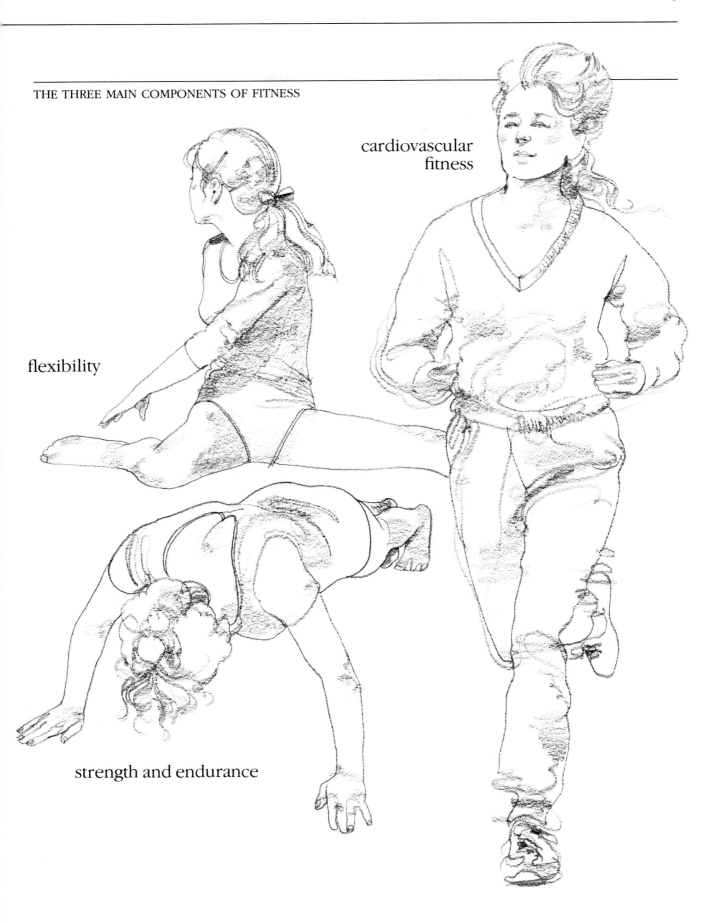

cardiovascular
fitness

flexibility

strength and endurance

How Fit Are You?

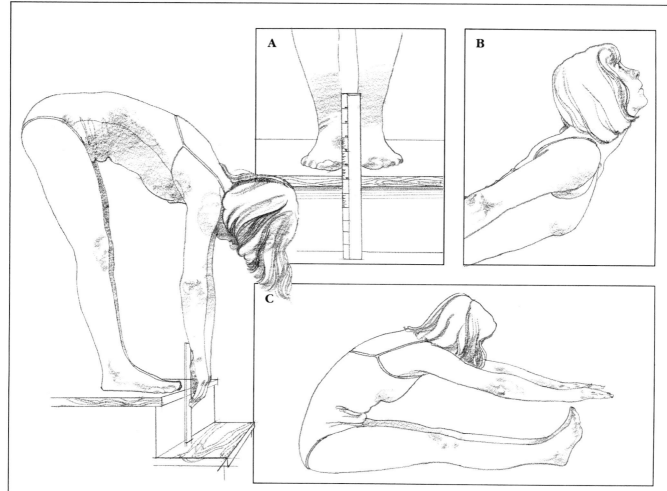

Knowing how fit you are before you begin your exercise program will let you measure your improvement as you progress. The following tests are easy to perform and give you good base-line measurements of your own muscular strength and endurance, flexibility, and cardiovascular fitness. Other ways to measure these three main components of fitness are shown on pages 72, 68, and 77.

Flexibility

Full trunk flexibility. (A) Stand on a stool to which you have attached a ruler, as shown. With heels together, toes near the edge, and knees locked, slowly relax and bend all the way over. Have a friend read your score where your fingertips touch the ruler. Any score greater than six is excellent, four to six is good, and any lower score or no score at all means you need stretching exercises.

Lower back. (B) Lie on your stomach with your feet anchored under a sofa and carefully arch up as high as possible, looking up.

Have a friend measure the distance from your chin to the floor with a piece of string. If your chin is 20 inches off the floor, excellent; 10 to 15 inches, good; under five inches, keep working.

Backs of legs. (C) Sit as shown, turn your toes straight up to the ceiling, and see how far past your toes you can reach. If you reached eight inches past your toes, you have excellent flexibility; four inches, good flexibility. If you couldn't reach your toes, flexibility exercises are a must.

Cardiovascular Fitness

The step test. On a low bench, stool, or step that is 16 inches high, step up and down using first one foot and then the other. Continue at a rate of about two to three seconds for each up-and-down sequence. Give it your best effort and stop when exhausted.

Now take your pulse at the carotid artery for 10 seconds and multiply the figure by six to get your pulse rate per minute.

Excellent . . . . **under 140**
Good . . . . **140 to 170**
Fair . . . . **170 and up**

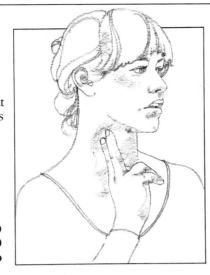

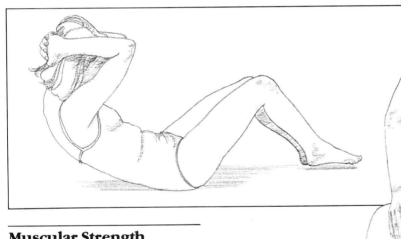

Muscular Strength

Abdominal muscles. (A) Complete 25 sit-ups with your knees bent and your hands behind your head. Anchor your feet under a sofa or have someone hold your feet. If you can complete all 25 without stopping, your abdominal muscles are in good shape.

Upper arms and shoulders. (B) Stand between two sturdy straight-back chairs (preferably with two assistants seated in them to keep them steady) and suspend yourself between them by placing your hands on the top rails. Bend your elbows out as shown and lift your feet off the floor. If you can hold this position for 30 seconds, your upper arms and shoulders are in average shape.

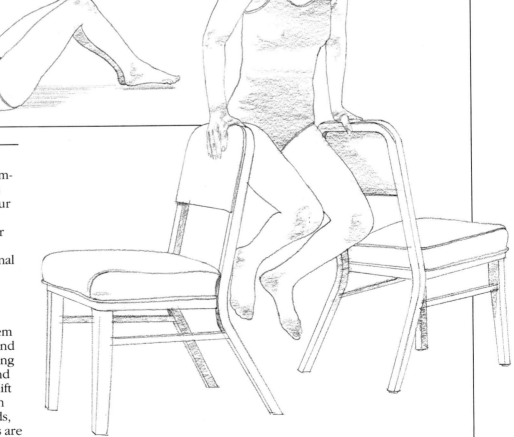

Benefits of Fitness

Being fit has many benefits. For one, a fit body lets you adapt more readily to stress, and in a related way, can help you relax. You'll find that involvement in any type of physical activity heightens your awareness of your body. With this awareness comes the ability to sense tension in particular muscles or areas of your body. If you can pinpoint tense muscles, you can learn, with some practice, to consciously relax them (see page 110). You'll also discover that you fall asleep faster and sleep better when you've included some form of physical activity in your daily routine.

Fitness, then, can improve the overall quality of your life. As your body works more efficiently, you'll find you have more energy to devote to work or recreation. And because fitness also improves the appearance of the body, it can do wonders for your self-image, too. As you become more fit, you'll undoubtedly add your own benefits to this list.

Achieving Fitness

There are almost as many ways to build and maintain body fitness as there are people who seek it. A good general program will include exercises to promote all aspects of fitness: muscular strength, flexibility, cardiovascular endurance, and relaxation.

It's up to you to decide how to maintain your own level of fitness. You can easily find a successful program to reflect your unique personal preferences. But regardless of the type of exercise program you choose, you must maintain it to achieve the desired outcome—a totally fit body.

Monitoring Fitness

To be sure you're getting the most from your exercise program, you'll want to monitor your level of fitness in such a way that your progress is easy to follow. The amount of time necessary to gain maximum benefit from an exercise session is an important consideration. Generally, exercising vigorously for 30 minutes each day is sufficient to build and maintain body fitness.

But what is "vigorous"? The average woman's maximum heart rate is about 190 beats per minute; during a 30-minute exercise session, your heart rate should be at least 70 percent of that maximum. Consequently, if you can maintain your heart rate at about 135 beats per minute for 30 minutes, you'll get the most benefit from your exercise program. Check your pulse periodically during exercising to be sure your heart rate is staying high enough (see page 77).

When you keep your heart beating at the proper rate, physiological changes will occur within your body as it learns to respond to physical stress in a more efficient way. You can participate in more vigorous activity, or you can remain active longer before fatigue sets in. This is called the "training effect," and is the goal the physically active person should work toward. It has been shown that 30 minutes of vigorous activity done three times a week can produce the same training effect as exercising five or six times a week.

Designing an Exercise Program

Remember that a general exercise program consists of exercises for building strength and flexibility for all parts of the body while also increasing cardiovascular endurance. Various kinds of exercise can be combined into an optimum fitness program that also suits your life-style.

Isometric and isotonic exercises may fit well in your fitness program. Isometrics, although popular years ago, have not received as much attention lately. In an isometric exercise, the muscle contracts but no movement takes place. A good example is pushing the palms of the hands together. The muscles of the arms and chest tighten, yet no movement occurs. Isometric exercises should be held for 10 seconds each time for maximum strength gain, which is their only benefit.

Isotonics is the term applied to exercises that involve movement; when the muscle contracts, movement occurs. Although any kind of movement is considered isotonic, including all of the general exercises listed in this chapter, the term is generally applied to exercises using gym equipment such as the Universal Gym, the Nautilus equipment, and free weights (barbells and dumbbells). This equipment provides the needed resistance in isotonic exercises, which are claimed to be better for building strength.

Weight training for women is becoming increasingly popular, and several myths concerning its effects already have been dispelled. But to repeat, women will *not* develop the bulging muscles men do. The hormone testosterone, which is believed to cause muscle enlargement, is abundant in men. Women, however, have only a very small amount of this hormone, so muscle enlargement is almost impossible.

Sports and physical activity may be a large part of your fitness program. Individual sports vary in their contributions to total fitness. Remember to keep in mind the three major components of fitness—strength, flexibility, and cardiovascular endurance.

Bicycling and jogging or running promote good cardiovascular endurance, but not flexibility. Walking and running strengthen the lower part of the body, but do nothing for the strength and flexibility of the upper part. Bicycling is somewhat better for strengthening both upper and lower parts of the body, especially on bicycles with dropped-style handlebars.

Swimming is by far the best all-around activity for achieving fitness since it promotes cardiovascular endurance, requires strength from all parts of the body, and puts the joints through their full range of motion when several different strokes are used.

Individual and team sports vary greatly in their benefits. When a skill level is involved, it's often difficult to accurately measure the benefits derived from a particular sport (see page 71). If you prefer sports to general exercise, be sure to pick one that suits you. If that sport doesn't fulfill all of the requirements for maintaining fitness, supplement it with a few specific exercises listed in the General Exercise Program (see page 82).

Aerobic dance is popular today and is an excellent source of fitness. Essentially this type of exercise involves dance patterns, moves, and routines set to currently popular music. Aerobic dance increases the heart rate so that a "training effect" occurs, and it maintains flexibility. An aerobic dance workout strengthens the lower part of the body a bit more than the upper part.

Yoga is another popular form of exercise, excellent for obtaining and maintaining flexibility as well as for training the mind in concentration. Yoga does not promote cardiovascular endurance, however. You may want to use yoga for flexibility and relaxation and choose another activity for cardiovascular endurance and strength.

Maintaining Your Fitness Program

The key to maintaining your fitness program is to design it to be satisfying, enjoyable, convenient, and compatible with your life-style. Make exercise a positive habit in your life. In the early stages of your program, use these suggestions to help you make exercise a habit you can stick with.

Exercise with a partner. Associate with people who will support your efforts by encouraging you.

Set aside a specific exercise time every day, and keep to your schedule. People who have been exercising for years claim that the first six months are the most difficult; after that it becomes a habit.

Find a good place to exercise. Where you exercise depends on your individual fitness program and may have some bearing on how well you're able to maintain it. If you choose tennis as your activity, obviously, you're limited to tennis courts. Aerobic dance requires ample space to move plus a provision for music. And weight training requires the specialized apparatus and equipment usually found at fitness centers or school gyms.

For general exercises, too, where you exercise depends on the type of exercise you choose. If you prefer doing exercises on a mat, most gyms, community centers, or YWCA/YMCAs will have adequate facilities.

The best place to exercise may be your own home. Yoga, for example, is especially suited to quiet home surroundings. You need only a warm room and a mat or carpeting. If you exercise at home, try to set aside a time when you won't be disturbed.

Local universities and community centers generally conduct exercise classes—either free or at a nominal cost. As for health clubs and health spas, we advise you to check them out thoroughly before joining. Make sure you'll patronize the club frequently—at least twice a week—to make it worth the price of membership. Talk to other members before joining, and schedule a visit at the time of day you're most likely to use the facilities in order to see how crowded the club is likely to be.

Rules for Exercising

Following these simple general rules will add to the safety and enjoyment of any exercise, sport, or physical activity you begin.

1) You should be certain that exercise will present no hazard to your health. Your physician should help you estimate your present level of fitness—possibly with stress testing—and give you an idea of where to begin.

2) After you find the type of physical activity you enjoy, engage in it with as much vigor and enthusiasm as possible. However, don't continue any activity if you experience excessive stress or pain. Each woman must find her own optimum level of activity. While your program shouldn't be too easy for you, it also must not be so hard that you're uncomfortable.

3) Make your exercise program progressive. Begin at an easy pace and gradually increase the effort required as you become better conditioned. Also, begin with easy exercises and work up to harder ones.

If you want to attain top training shape once you've attained a high degree of overall fitness, begin to apply the overload principle to your activity. This involves doing the exercise or activity until you become tired, and then doing it a little longer, as well as trying to increase the intensity of the effort. For example, if you can run a mile in 12 minutes, next time try running the same distance in 11 minutes and 50 seconds.

4) Wear clothing that will allow freedom of movement, and a good support bra; there should be no binding anywhere. Material that contains some cotton will absorb perspiration.

5) Use the proper sports equipment. Don't skimp on good shoes, for example. Find a reputable sporting goods store and buy the equipment that fits your individual needs.

6) Whenever you exercise in a different location than usual, acclimate or adjust to the new environment. Take into consideration the heat, humidity, and altitude, and begin less strenuously than usual.

7) Breathe when you exercise. *Don't hold your breath at any time.*

Stretching Exercises

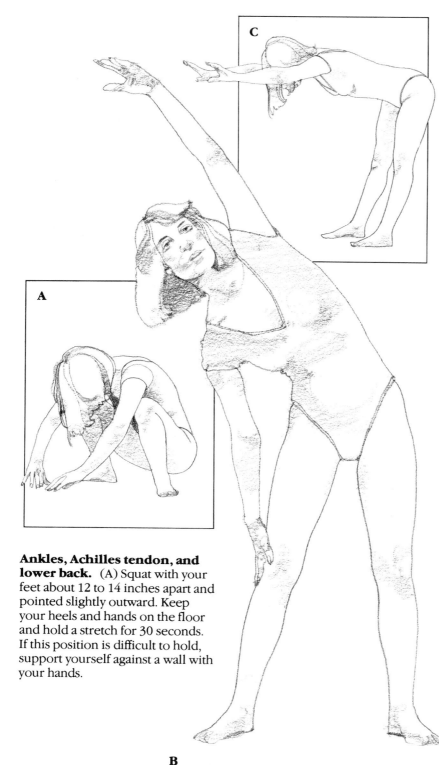

Flexibility, one of the three major components of fitness, is achieved and maintained through a routine of stretching movements. The simplest forms of stretching are the natural movements you make after you've been still for a while — yawning, twisting your torso, or stretching your arms over your head. These stretching movements relieve cramped muscles and are relaxing as well. Other movements, such as touching your toes or reaching for the sky, stretch joints, ligaments, and tendons, and help to maintain normal flexibility and ease of movement.

The following stretching exercises go still further toward promoting flexibility fitness. You can do them by themselves each day for 15 minutes, or as warm-ups for more strenuous exercise, such as jogging, cycling, or swimming.

Do each exercise slowly, concentrating on the muscles being stretched. Breathe regularly and naturally. Learn to recognize the precise amount of tension that indicates stretching of muscles; you should feel the sensation of stretching diminish the longer you hold the stretch. Then you know the muscle is relaxing in the stretch; it feels good. You may want to close your eyes to better concentrate on this subtle sensation. Listen to the message of your own muscles, and don't compare your flexibility to anyone else's.

Shoulders, waist, and arms. (B) Stand with your feet about 12 inches apart. Raise your arms overhead and clasp your hands loosely. Bend slowly to one side from the waist and hold for 10 to 15 seconds. Repeat on the other side. Be sure to keep your legs straight and your body forward. An alternate way to do this stretch is to keep one arm flat against your side and stretch the other arm over your head as far as possible. Repeat five times on each side.

Ankles, Achilles tendon, and lower back. (A) Squat with your feet about 12 to 14 inches apart and pointed slightly outward. Keep your heels and hands on the floor and hold a stretch for 30 seconds. If this position is difficult to hold, support yourself against a wall with your hands.

Arms, shoulders, and back.

(C) Bend at the waist so your upper body is parallel to the floor. Stretch your arms forward, about shoulder-width apart, and reach for an imaginary support that is in front of you, at approximately shoulder height and a foot or so away. Keep your arms and legs straight, and your head and chest down. Hold for 15 seconds.

Straighten and repeat, again reaching for the imaginary support a foot above you. Repeat two to three times, holding for 15 seconds.

Conclude by "shaking out" your arms and hands.

Calf.

(D) Stand, facing a wall about three to four feet away. Bend your right leg and keep your left leg straight behind you for support and balance. Do not lift your heels off the floor. Lean against the wall in this position, hands clasped, and rest your head on your arms. Move your hips slowly forward. You will feel a stretch in the back (calf) of your left leg. Hold for 30 seconds. Alternate legs and repeat.

Hamstrings and upper back.

(E) Sit on the floor with your feet spread apart and reach first for one foot, and then the other. Keep your knees straight. Repeat five times with each leg.

Remain sitting, and stretch one leg out straight, foot upright. Bring the sole of your other foot to rest along the inside of your straight leg. Keep your back straight and lean slightly forward from the waist, with your head bent slightly forward. You'll feel the pull in the hamstring of your straight leg. Hold for 30 seconds and repeat with the other leg.

Groin muscles.

(F) Lie on your back in a relaxed position. Bend your knees and put the soles of your feet together. Hold the stretch for 30 seconds.

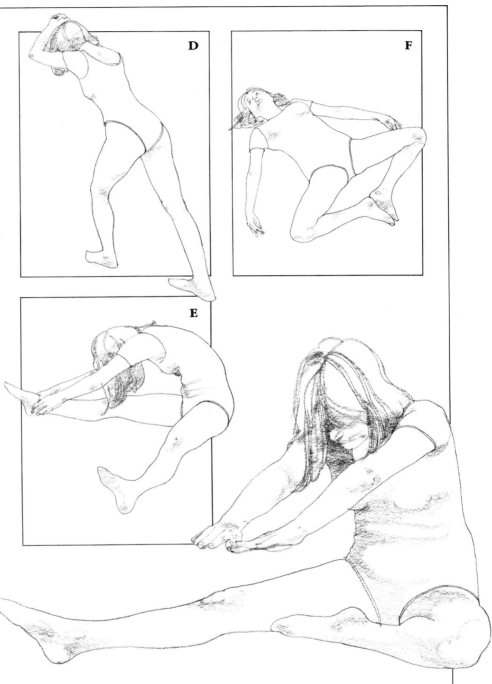

Stretching Exercises continued

Spine. (A) Sit and hug your knees with your arms. Make your body into a ball and rock slowly back and forth. Repeat, gently, five times.

Straighten your legs and bring them up over your head. Bend your knees and place your hands on the back of your hips for balance. Hold your knees to the ground, behind your head, for 20 to 30 seconds. As you become more flexible, do this with straight legs instead of bent knees.

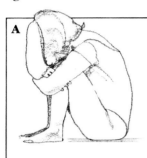

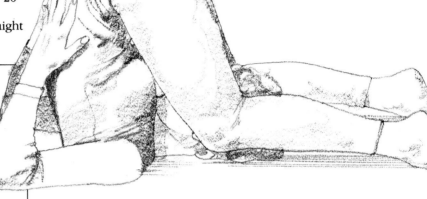

Thigh. (B) Lie on your side in a straight line and rest your head upon your arm. Grasp your foot and pull your upper leg gently toward your hip. Hold for five seconds. Repeat on your other side.

Legs. (C) Lie on your back in a relaxed position, with both legs straight. Try to keep your head on the floor as you pull your left leg toward your chest. Hold for 20 seconds and repeat the movement with your right leg.

Total body stretch. (D) Lie on your back, with your arms and legs straight. Point your fingers and toes, and stretch as much as possible. Hold for five seconds and relax. Repeat three to five times.

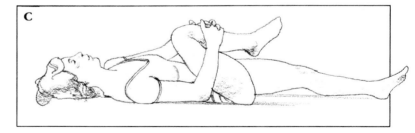

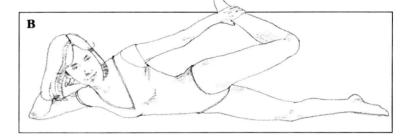

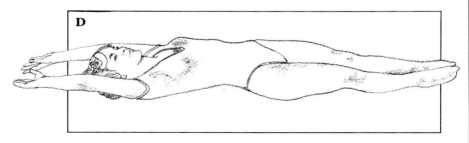

Ten Sports: How They Promote Fitness

FITNESS ELEMENTS	alpine skiing*	nordic skiing*	swimming	tennis	walking
Cardiorespiratory endurance	16	19	21	16	13
Muscular endurance	18	19	20	16	14
Muscular strength	15	15	14	14	11
Flexibility	14	14	15	14	7
Balance	21	16	12	16	8
Weight control	15	17	15	16	13
Muscle definition	14	12	14	13	11
Digestion	9	12	13	12	11
Sleep	12	15	16	11	14

FITNESS ELEMENTS	basketball	bicycling	bowling	handball/ squash	jogging
Cardiorespiratory endurance	19	19	5	19	21
Muscular endurance	17	18	5	18	20
Muscular strength	15	16	5	15	17
Flexibility	13	9	7	16	9
Balance	16	18	6	17	17
Weight control	19	20	5	19	21
Muscle definition	13	15	5	11	14
Digestion	10	12	7	13	13
Sleep	12	15	6	12	16

Individual and team sports vary greatly in their benefits. A team of medical experts assessed several different sports on the basis of nine elements necessary for fitness, such as cardiorespiratory endurance. An activity rating of 21 indicates maximum benefit from this activity.

*Alpine skiing refers to downhill and slalom skiing. Nordic skiing refers to cross-country skiing and jumping.

Weight Training for Women

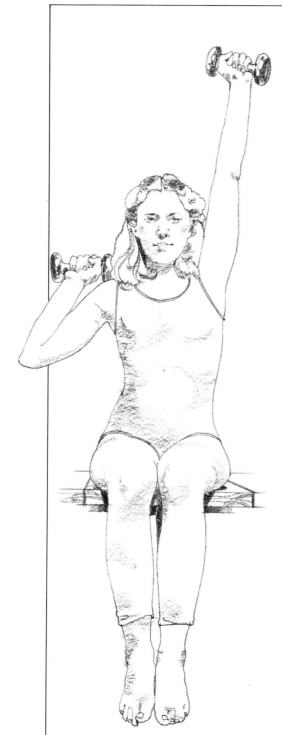

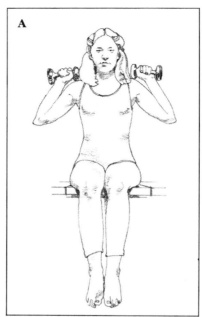

A

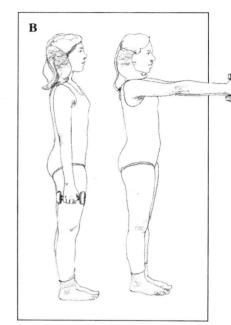

B

An ideal conditioning program for women includes weight training combined with an aerobic exercise, such as running or bicycling. Weight training will develop your muscular strength and endurance to a maximum and still let you retain grace and flexibility. Aerobic exercises help you maintain cardiovascular fitness and a high energy level.

Weight training routines use equipment in graduated weights—such as dumbbells and pulley devices—to selectively stress and strengthen muscle groups: the neck and shoulders, chest, back, stomach, arms, and legs. Some examples of dumbbell and pulley routines to firm up different parts of your body are shown here. Trained personnel at a local weight training center, gym, or YWCA/YMCA will help you develop an individual routine. You

should work all of your muscles by developing a total body program—for example, moving from station to station on a Universal Gym.

Remember, it's important to start weight training within your own capacity in order to avoid muscle injury—overload in steps (see page 67). Also, be sure to warm up before lifting weights; loosen up with jumping jacks, perform several lifting exercises without weights, and use the stretching exercises on page 68. Perform weight lifting exercises slowly and deliberately, concentrating on the muscles being developed. Repeat each exercise until the muscle is too tired to support another lift. When you reach this fatigue point, you will feel a hot or burning sensation in the muscle. Do not continue exercises if you feel pain.

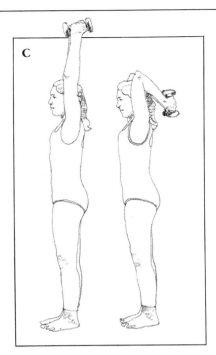

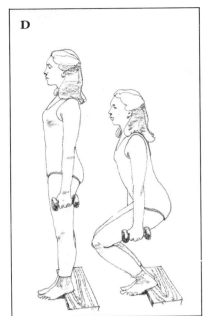

Dumbbell squat. (D) To develop your entire leg, particularly the thighs and buttocks, stand with your feet shoulder width apart on a thick book or 2x4 board. Holding weights as shown, keep your back straight and squat until your thighs are level with your knees. Stand slowly.

Lunge. (E) To firm your thighs and buttocks, stand with your feet slightly apart, a five-pound weight in each hand, and step forward with your right foot, bending both knees. Return to the starting position and alternate feet. Keep your head and back straight.

Sitting lift. (A) To strengthen and firm the shoulders and the backs of the upper arms, sit on a bench and grip five-pound dumbbells with your palms facing forward. Fully extend the weights overhead, first one hand and then the other. Keep your back straight.

Arms forward. (B) To firm the shoulders and upper arms, stand with your back straight, pelvis tucked in, and feet comfortably apart. Lift five-pound dumbbells straight forward as shown.

Triceps press. (C) To firm the backs of the upper arms, stand erect or sit on a bench. Grip five-pound dumbbells as shown and raise them over your head. Lower the dumbbells slowly behind your head, with elbows pointed upward; return your arms upward until your elbows are straight.

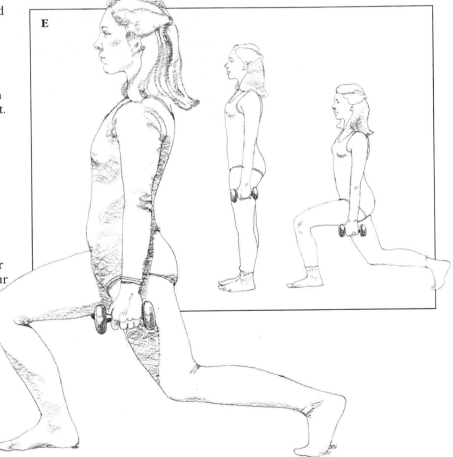

The Woman Runner

Deciding to run. Making the decision to start running is probably the most difficult part of this sport. Your motivation may come from enthusiastic friends who run and who extol the personal rewards of running: "You'll feel better," "It's a great way to lose weight," or "Running is relaxing." Health and medical experts provide further motivation by pointing out the physical benefits of running—strengthened cardiovascular endurance and improved stamina and overall health. In fact, running contributes more to your physical fitness and burns up more calories than any other sport (see page 71).

Once you've made the decision, you're on your way to becoming a runner!

Check with your doctor. While runners come in all ages and shapes, running is not recommended for all women. If you are over 40 or have health problems, such as diabetes, high blood pressure, or obesity, you should check with your doctor before running. An exercise stress (treadmill) test of the heart may be recommended.

What to wear. After you have medical clearance, the next step is to buy a good pair of running shoes for the necessary cushioning and support of your feet. For your comfort and to help prevent injury, good running shoes are a must. Go to a sporting goods or runners' store, explain to the salesclerk that you are a beginner, and specify what kind of surface you'll be running on. Try on a lot of different styles and ask questions. You don't need fancy clothes for running—the most important thing is that you wear something comfortable, such as a cotton or nylon tricot T-shirt and loose shorts. A good support bra is very important. On cold days, wear layers of clothing, including a sweat shirt and tights. If you run at dawn or dusk, increase your visibility by wearing bright clothing.

Warm up. Before you go out to run, warm up by doing 10 minutes of stretching exercises. Concentrate on your legs and stretch your hamstrings and calf muscles. Toe-touching and sit-ups are also good. This warm-up will give your heart a chance to adjust to the higher work load of running.

Where and when to run. Where and when you run is an individual choice. You may choose to run alone or with a friend, to run around a high school track, on park trails, city streets, or just around your neighborhood; to run at dawn or dusk or sometime in between—it's up to you.

Do be sensible about running, though. Try to run early in the morning and in the evening in hot weather. And avoid running in isolated spots.

How to run. There's really no special way to run. Simply alternate feet and land flat-footed on your heels first (don't run on your toes). Relax your arms and body, and don't slouch—good upright posture is important. Jog or run at a speed that feels comfortable to you and allows normal breathing and talking. Just do what feels natural.

How long to run. If you're a beginning runner, start slowly in building up your endurance and conditioning level. On your first few times out, try running for 10 to 15 minutes or about one mile. Don't strain. You may choose to alternately walk and run this distance the first few times.

Run regularly. While you may want to vary where and when you run, running regularly is important. To reap the full physical and psychological benefits from running, and to maintain and improve your condition and progress, run regularly, three or four times a week. (On non-running days, be sure to get some other form of exercise, such as swimming or dancing.)

Apply the overload principle (see page 67) and adapt to running. You can measure your progress by taking your pulse and figuring out your maximum heart rate (see page 77). You may want to keep a runner's diary to record your progress and running experiences.

Cool down. Just as important as a warm-up before running is a cool down afterwards. Stop running before you reach home. Walk a bit to allow your breathing and heart rate to return to normal. Or, go through some post-run stretching and relaxing exercises.

Joys of running. Now don't you feel great? Actually, you may feel some aches and pains the first few weeks of running, especially if you smoke or are out of shape. Listen to your body and slow down a bit. A hot bath after running will help ease sore muscles. Remember that the first six to eight weeks of running will be the hardest—after that, it only gets easier! Running is not meant to be torture, but exhilarating and energizing.

Running is a lifetime sport. For a minimum investment in time and money, running will provide great personal satisfaction and improve your physical capabilities, conditioning, and sense of well-being.

For more information. There are many good books available on running. See the list of references for this chapter. Also, check local adult education programs and your YWCA/YMCA for information about running classes.

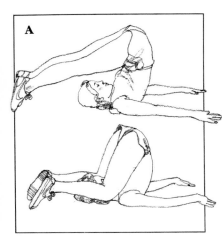

A

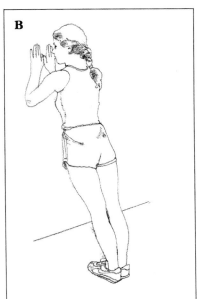

B

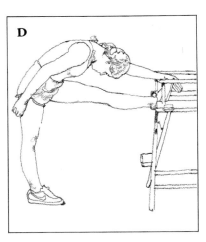

D

Before running, every runner should do 10 minutes of warm-up exercises, stretching the back of the legs and the lower back muscles. These same exercises after running, plus others for the front of the legs and the abdominal muscles, assure balanced muscle development and joint flexibility. Do these exercises slowly, holding the stretches for 30 seconds and taking 10 to 30 seconds to move into new positions.

A Lying on a thick pad, bring your legs over your head and try to touch your toes to the floor. Try to keep your legs straight. Then bend your legs to bring your knees alongside your ears and relax in this position.

B To do wall push-ups, lean in until you feel the stretch in the back of your legs.

C With your legs bent, slowly sit up to an upright position. Lie down slowly and repeat.

D With your knees locked, place one leg on a low stool, a chair, or a support of whatever height you find comfortable. Bend over toward your knee until you feel a strong stretch.

C

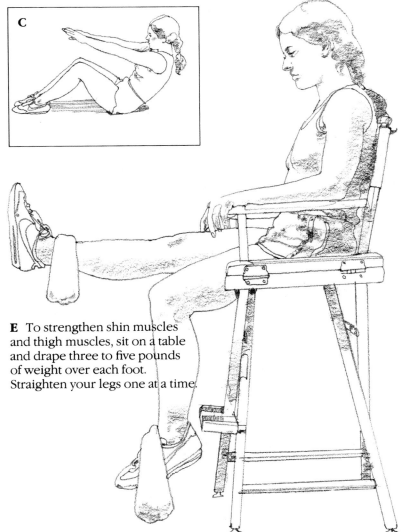

E To strengthen shin muscles and thigh muscles, sit on a table and drape three to five pounds of weight over each foot. Straighten your legs one at a time.

Exercise and Calorie Expenditure

	calories used per hour by weight groups			
	120 POUNDS	140 POUNDS	160 POUNDS	180 POUNDS
Sedentary activity • sleeping • eating • reading • watching television • playing a musical instrument	40-90	50-100	60-100	70-120
Light activity • cooking • ironing • typing • dressing • shopping with a light load	100-140	120-160	140-180	160-200
Moderate activity • walking moderately fast • gardening • cleaning floors • doing carpentry work • playing table tennis	150-190	200-240	220-260	260-300
Vigorous activity • swimming • playing golf • dancing • bicycling • playing volleyball	200-340	260-400	300-440	340-480
Strenuous activity • running • playing tennis • downhill skiing • hill climbing	over 350	over 450	over 550	over 650

All physical exercise uses energy and burns up calories. The actual number of calories needed for activity each day depends on your basal metabolism and body weight, and how long and hard you engage in physical activity.

This chart shows exercise and calorie expenditures for different body weights.

Using Your Pulse as an Indicator of Cardiovascular Fitness Improvement

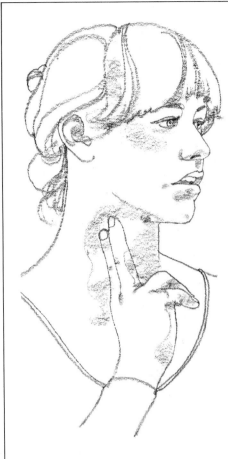

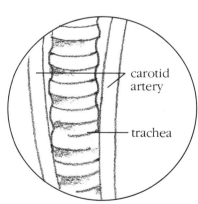

carotid artery

trachea

Cardiovascular fitness is one of the three major components of overall fitness. You may already have taken the test that indicates your level of cardiovascular fitness (see page 65). Following the instructions given here, you'll be able to use your pulse rate as a precise guide for measuring your cardiovascular fitness improvement.

How to count your pulse. Learn to count your pulse at the carotid artery, where you can clearly feel your pulse rate (which is the same as your heart rate). With your fingers, find your Adam's apple and the firm tube of the trachea above and below it. Move your fingers to one side of the trachea and press to feel your pulse in the carotid artery. Take your pulse for 10 seconds and multiply by six to obtain your pulse rate for one minute.

When to count your pulse. To monitor your cardiovascular fitness, begin a movement that is easy and that increases your heart rate. After 10 minutes, immediately count your pulse. Don't delay even for a second, as the pulse rate falls off rapidly after exercise. Multiply by six to obtain your count for one minute, and using the chart that follows, check to see if you are in the target zone. The target zone represents the heart rate you must maintain for 30 minutes each day to obtain maximum cardiovascular fitness.

If you are not in the target zone after 10 minutes of movement, exercise more vigorously. You may even need to jog or dance to move into your target zone. Adjust your exercise pattern and monitor your pulse count until you know you are within your target zone for a full 30 minutes each day.

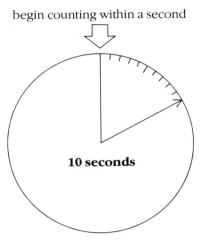

begin counting within a second

10 seconds

$$\text{total count at 10 seconds} \times 6 = \text{pulse rate per minute}$$

Using your pulse as a training guide. As your cardiovascular condition improves, you'll notice that you are moving faster and with greater ease to stay in your target zone. You're experiencing the first signs of being in condition. Take your resting pulse rate while sitting relaxed and calm. As your condition improves, your resting pulse count will drop, another indicator of improved cardiovascular fitness.

Heart rate for women for CV conditioning		
AGE	TARGET ZONE	MAXIMUM RATE
25	130-157	185
30	126-153	180
35	123-149	175
40	119-145	170
45	116-140	165
50	112-136	160
55	109-132	155
60	105-128	150
65	102-123	145

Exercise During and After Pregnancy

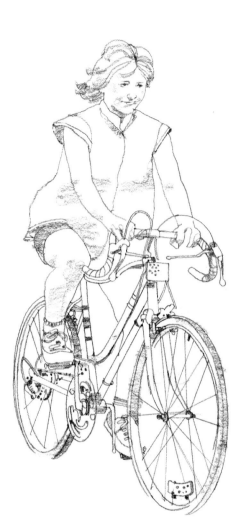

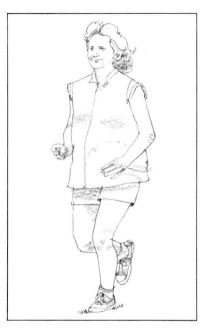

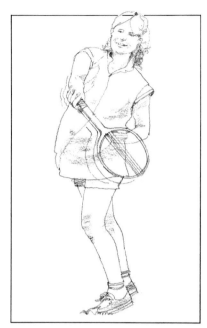

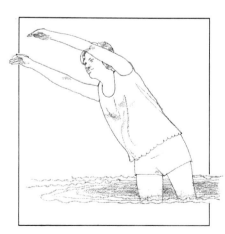

During pregnancy, exercise is vital for good maternal health, and a healthy birth and recovery. Obstetricians and sports physiologists generally agree that exercises and sports are safe and healthful for pregnant women as long as they feel comfortable doing them.

Physical exercise helps women adjust to the hormonal and physical changes of pregnancy (in muscles, joints, and tissues) as well as the emotional and psychological changes. Swimming is probably the sport best suited to pregnancy because the water helps support the woman's additional weight and takes some of the burden off of pelvic ligaments.

Exercise provides extra support for the growing baby by strengthening abdominal muscles as well as muscles supporting the backbone and the pelvic floor—areas that are put under great stress in pregnancy. Specific exercises for strengthening these muscles are shown in the "Labor and Delivery" chapter.

Danger to the fetus from normal sports activity is minimal because the uterus is one of the best protected organs in a woman's body. Still, your sports participation during pregnancy should be determined on an individual basis and always with your physician's approval. Be sure to stop a particular exercise or sport if you experience spotting, pains, or anything out of the ordinary.

Running. You can and should run while pregnant.

Swimming is probably the sport best suited to pregnancy.

Bicycling. Pregnant women can enjoy bicycling through the ninth month of pregnancy.

Tennis. Women tennis buffs and professional players continue sets throughout pregnancy, adjusting their pace, rhythm, and balance to compensate for changes in weight distribution.

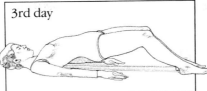

1st day

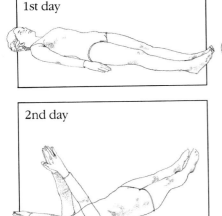

2nd day

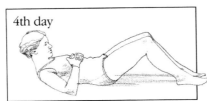

3rd day

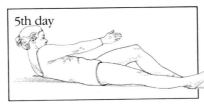

4th day

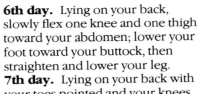

5th day

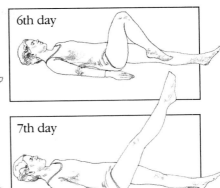

6th day

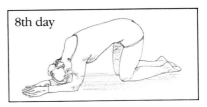

7th day

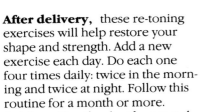

8th day

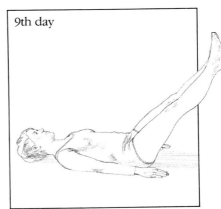

9th day

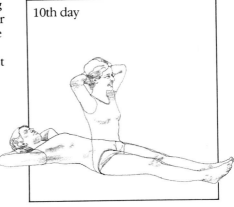

10th day

After delivery, these re-toning exercises will help restore your shape and strength. Add a new exercise each day. Do each one four times daily: twice in the morning and twice at night. Follow this routine for a month or more.

1st day. Breathe deeply, expanding your abdomen. Hiss as you slowly exhale, then forcibly draw in your abdominal muscles.

2nd day. Lying on your back with your legs slightly parted, place your arms at right angles to your body and slowly raise them, keeping your elbows stiff. When your hands touch, lower your arms gradually.

3rd day. Lying with your arms at your sides, draw your knees up slightly, and arch your back.

4th day. Lying with your knees and hips flexed, tilt your pelvis inward and tightly contract your buttocks as you lift your head.

5th day. Lying with your legs straight, raise your head and left knee slightly, then reach for (but do not touch) your left knee with your right hand. Repeat, using your right knee and your left hand.

6th day. Lying on your back, slowly flex one knee and one thigh toward your abdomen; lower your foot toward your buttock, then straighten and lower your leg.

7th day. Lying on your back with your toes pointed and your knees straight, raise one leg and then the other as high as possible, using your abdominal muscles (but not your hands) to slowly lower your legs.

8th day. Leaning on your elbows and knees, keep your forearms and lower legs together. Hump your back upward, strongly contracting your buttocks and drawing in your abdomen. Then relax and breathe deeply.

9th day. Same as the 7th day, but lift both legs at once.

10th day. Lying on your back with your arms clasped behind your head, sit up and lie back slowly. At first, you may have to hook your feet under furniture.

Yoga

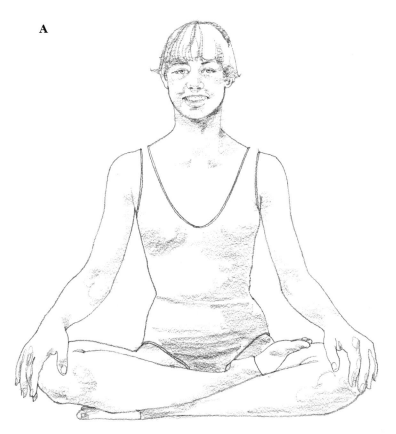

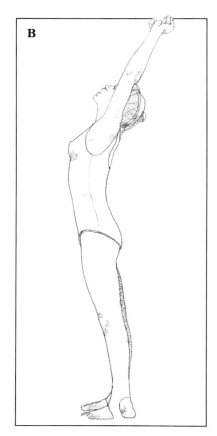

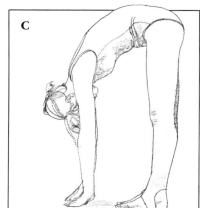

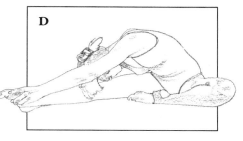

Yoga means "union." The practice of yoga combines specific methods designed hundreds of years ago in India to develop and unify every aspect of the individual—physical, emotional, spiritual, and intellectual. Over the ages, yoga has proved so successful that many of our modern exercise programs in the West are based on yogic techniques.

Yoga exercises are particularly useful for beginning exercisers. Simple yoga exercises are excellent for flexibility; many pinpoint areas of muscular tension, allowing you to concentrate on alternate stretching and deep relaxation of stress points in your body.

The following exercises involve deep breathing, stretching, and deep relaxation.

Sitting posture. (A) Sit comfortably on the floor, with your legs crossed, hands on your knees, and your spine straight. This is a discipline exercise for sitting still.
Backward bend. (B) Inhale. Stretch up and then back over your head; tighten your buttocks and arch your back. Hold only for a few seconds.
Spinal stretch. (C) Stand erect; slowly drop your chin, head, shoulders, and arms forward. Be relaxed and limp. Let your trunk hang forward. Feel the stretching and lengthening in your spine, and the blood flow to your face and head. Slowly uncurl back to the starting position.
Flexibility. (D) Assume position D and slowly reach out as far as you can over one straight leg. Do not bounce; stop and hold at a comfortable stretch. Repeat over your other leg.

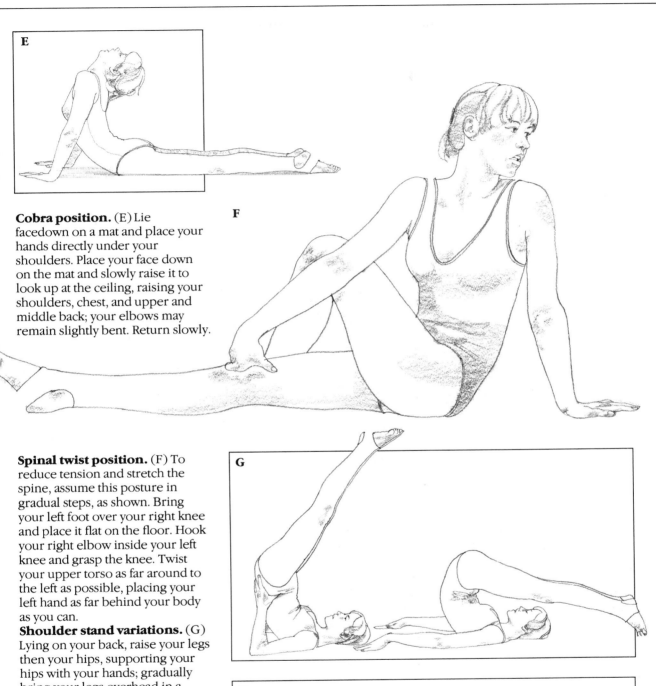

Cobra position. (E) Lie facedown on a mat and place your hands directly under your shoulders. Place your face down on the mat and slowly raise it to look up at the ceiling, raising your shoulders, chest, and upper and middle back; your elbows may remain slightly bent. Return slowly.

Spinal twist position. (F) To reduce tension and stretch the spine, assume this posture in gradual steps, as shown. Bring your left foot over your right knee and place it flat on the floor. Hook your right elbow inside your left knee and grasp the knee. Twist your upper torso as far around to the left as possible, placing your left hand as far behind your body as you can.

Shoulder stand variations. (G) Lying on your back, raise your legs then your hips, supporting your hips with your hands; gradually bring your legs overhead in a straight or bent position, as shown. Hold, then return slowly, lowering your legs to the floor.

Modified locust. (H) Lie face-down on a mat. As shown, raise your chin, then both legs, keeping your knees straight. Hold for a few seconds, then slowly return.

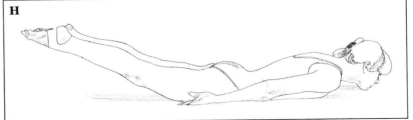

A General Exercise Program

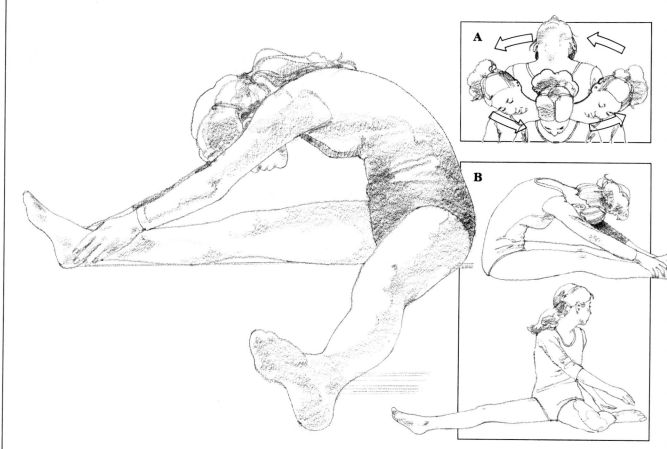

The following exercises include movements to promote muscular strength and endurance as well as flexibility. But for total body fitness, remember to combine them with an activity that produces a training effect to increase and maintain cardiovascular fitness.

Execute each exercise as specified by the directions, and move quickly from one exercise to the next. All flexibility movements should be executed through the full range of motion of the joints involved. Make sure that the pelvis is in proper alignment by keeping the seat tucked in.

Head circles: for relaxation. (A) Sitting comfortably and straight, drop your head forward. Circle to the side, back, and front. Repeat in each direction several times, concentrating on relaxing your neck and shoulder muscles.

Hamstring stretches: for stretching the backs of the legs. (B) Sit on the floor with your legs together, straight out in front of you. Grasp your lower legs with your hands and slowly but firmly pull your trunk down to your legs. Try to touch your head to your knees. Do not point your toes. Pull as far as you can, and then hold that position for a count of 10. Relax and do this several times, attempting to bend further each time.

Variations: a. Sit with your legs straight and apart, executing the same technique as above over each leg separately. b. Sit with one leg straight out in front and the other leg bent to the side (in a hurdle position). Grasp the forward leg, and pull as described above. Add a twist to the bent-leg side between pulls. Repeat several times, alternating legs.

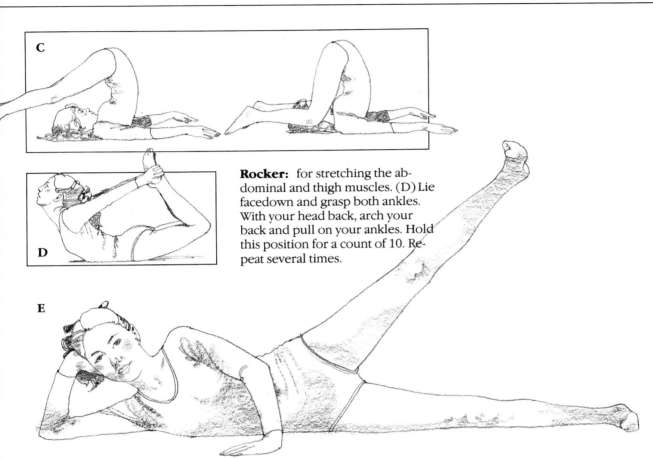

Rocker: for stretching the abdominal and thigh muscles. (D) Lie facedown and grasp both ankles. With your head back, arch your back and pull on your ankles. Hold this position for a count of 10. Repeat several times.

Plough or half-back somersault: for stretching the backs of the legs and the back. (C) Begin in a sitting position with your legs together and straight out in front of you. Lean forward to build momentum, and roll backward, keeping your legs straight. Try to touch the floor with your toes, still keeping your legs straight. Hold this position for a count of 10, and return to the starting position. Variations: a. Hold the backward position for a count of 10. Then bend your knees and try to place them on the floor beside your ears. b. Keeping your legs straight, roll over backwards, touch your toes to the floor, and return upright immediately. Repeat several times. This method of doing the exercise not only stretches your hamstrings but strengthens your abdominal muscles as well.

Side leg lifts: for strengthening the outside of the thigh and stretching the inside of the thigh. (E) Lie on one side with your top arm out in front of you for balance. Lift your top leg at a moderate speed as far as it will go. Repeat several times on each side. Do not rotate your leg outward; keep your foot pointing straight ahead, not toward the ceiling.

Trunk twists: for stretching the thigh muscles. (F) Stand with your feet shoulder-width apart and your hands on your hips. Twist twice to one side and then to the other side. Twist further on the second twist. Repeat several times with each side.

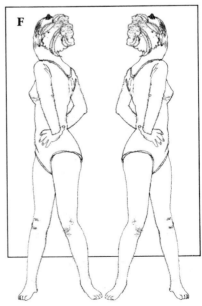

A General Exercise Program continued

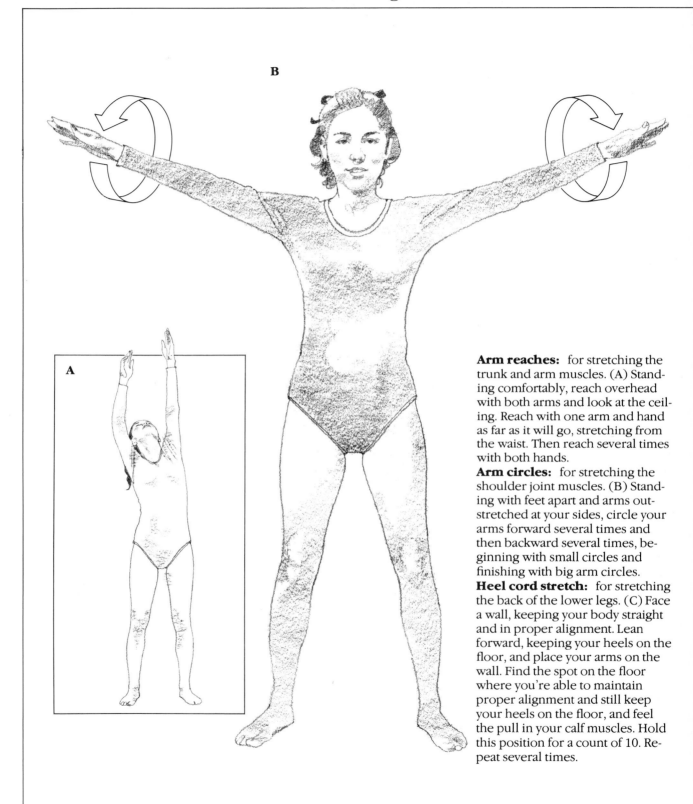

Arm reaches: for stretching the trunk and arm muscles. (A) Standing comfortably, reach overhead with both arms and look at the ceiling. Reach with one arm and hand as far as it will go, stretching from the waist. Then reach several times with both hands.

Arm circles: for stretching the shoulder joint muscles. (B) Standing with feet apart and arms outstretched at your sides, circle your arms forward several times and then backward several times, beginning with small circles and finishing with big arm circles.

Heel cord stretch: for stretching the back of the lower legs. (C) Face a wall, keeping your body straight and in proper alignment. Lean forward, keeping your heels on the floor, and place your arms on the wall. Find the spot on the floor where you're able to maintain proper alignment and still keep your heels on the floor, and feel the pull in your calf muscles. Hold this position for a count of 10. Repeat several times.

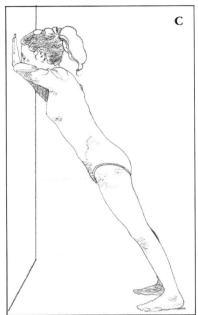

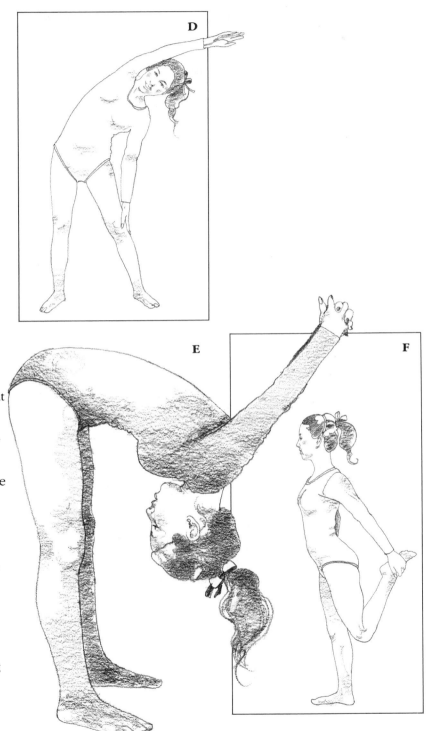

Side bends: for stretching the sides of the trunk. (D) Stand with your feet apart and bend to one side, sliding that arm down your leg while your other arm is straight overhead next to your ear. Slide your arm down as far as it will go; hold for a count of 10 and rest. Repeat several times, alternating sides.

Back arm pull: for stretching the arms, chest muscles, and legs. (E) Standing comfortably, grasp both hands behind your back. Keeping your arms straight, bend over and try to roll your arms back and upward as far as you can. Repeat several times, holding for a count of 10 each time.

Thigh stretches: for stretching the thigh. (F) Standing, bend one leg backward and grasp your ankle. Pull your foot toward your buttocks as far as you can, holding the stretched position for a count of 10. Repeat the movement several times for each leg.

A General Exercise Program continued

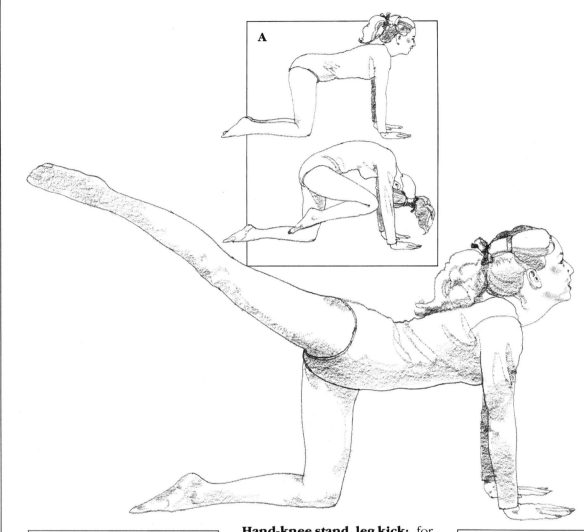

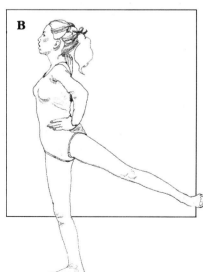

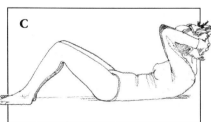

Hand-knee stand, leg kick: for strengthening the legs, buttocks, and back. (A) Get down on the floor on your hands and knees. Bring one knee off the floor toward your chest. Bend your head down, trying to touch your nose to your knee. Then kick the leg backward, rotating the leg out while raising your head. Repeat 10 times with each leg.

Leg swings: for strengthening and stretching the thigh muscles and buttocks. (B) Holding onto a doorknob or bar, swing your outside leg forward and backward, rotating the leg outward as you swing backward. Repeat several times on each side.

Sit-ups: for abdominal strength. (C) Lie down with your knees *bent* and your hands behind your head. Sit up. Repeat. If this is too hard, fold your arms across your chest and try to sit up.

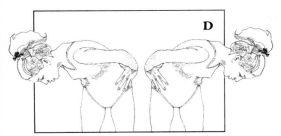

Trunk circles: for stretching the trunk muscles. (D) Standing with your feet shoulder-width apart and your hands on your hips, move your trunk in a circle forward, to one side, back, to the other side, and back to the front. Repeat several times in each direction.

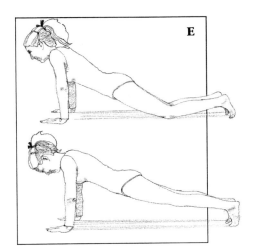

Push-ups: for strengthening the arms and shoulder girdle. (E) Modified: Lie facedown with your hands on the floor under your shoulders. Keeping the body in a straight line (hips in) and your knees on the floor, push your body up until your arms are straight. Repeat. Regular: If the modified push-up is too easy, try this one. Lie facedown and place your hands under your shoulders. Keeping your body straight, push up until your arms are straight. Repeat if possible. Work up to 12 push-ups.

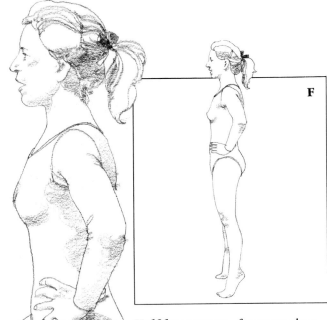

Half-leg squats: for strengthening the legs. (F) There are four counts to this exercise. Standing with your feet shoulder-width apart and your hands on your hips, rise on your toes (count 1), bend your knees to a half-squat position (count 2), rise up on your toes again (count 3), and return to the starting position (count 4). Repeat several times, keeping your back straight and seat tucked in.

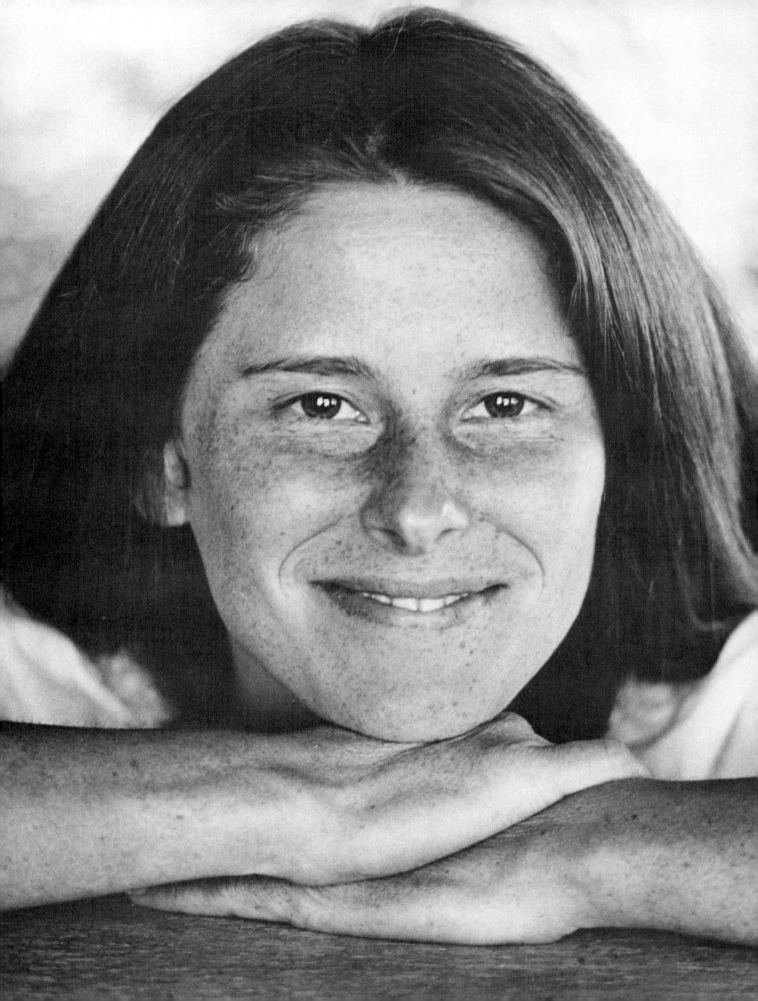

CHAPTER 5

MENTAL HEALTH

BEVERLY BIRNS, Ph.D.
SARAH HALL STERNGLANZ, Ph.D.

Who has ever heard a completely satisfactory definition of mental health? Certainly, it is harder to define than physical health. Still, most women would agree that a mentally healthy person is able to both give and receive love, is capable of being close to other people, has a realistic view of the present and future, is competent and can meet the demands of everyday life, has the self-confidence necessary to feel worthwhile, and is engaged in some kind of satisfying work.

But this definition cannot apply to all people in all situations. As women, we may find that the roles society expects of us conflict with our own perception of what it means to be mentally healthy. Questioning the validity of those expectations and accepting responsibility for resolving those conflicts can be the first step toward improving our mental health.

Mental Health

"Mrs. Smith, you are in perfect health." These are the words that we most often hear after the physical has been done, the history taken, and all the tests completed. If no illness is found, then health is assumed. Traditionally, the concept of health has been closely connected with the concept of disease. We do not typically visit a physician, or for that matter even think about our health, unless there is something wrong. We experience a symptom—a fever, a headache, dizziness, a lump, or some sign that something is not right—and we seek the help of a doctor. Doctors, in the course of their training, are taught to identify and treat the many diseases that can occur. However, doctors receive little training with regard to health maintenance, and so it's not surprising to hear them define health as "the absence of disease."

However, as hospital costs soar and many diseases seem too hard to cure, there is currently a trend to think more about health as a positive state, to be studied, understood, and sought after. In addition, many of us are beginning to take more responsibility for our own health. We are learning more about nutrition and exercise, and about the way that our bodies function.

To be healthy is not simply not to be sick. When we are healthy, we feel well, eat well, sleep well, and also try to maintain our feeling of well-being. We understand that we are most likely to stay well if we get enough exercise, eat properly, and avoid cigarettes and other harmful substances. How, then, does this concept of health apply to mental health?

Defining Mental Health

The concept of mental health is even more complicated than that of physical health. We usually can tell when someone is mentally ill, and could therefore define mental health as some people define physical health, as the absence of mental disease. However, who among us has ever heard a doctor state, "Mrs. Smith, you are in a state of perfect mental health"? Clearly, we know even less about mental health than we do about physical health. We have no thermometers or physical ways of measuring mental health. In some countries, the word does not even exist. Perhaps it was Freud who gave the briefest definition. He defined mental health in

terms of the ability to love and to work. Others add such concepts as self-esteem and maturity. At best, it is a difficult concept to define and there is little agreement in the field about what mental health is. Mental health, even more than physical health, has many in-betweens. For instance, we all have good days and bad days. Sometimes we feel happy and sometimes blue. Some signs of mental health might be enjoying your job, being in love or very happy with your friends or relatives, enjoying your children, or finding many sources of pleasure in life. In order to better understand the remainder of the chapter, we will nevertheless try to define what we mean when we speak of mental health.

Different theories of personality talk about different sides of the mentally healthy personality. In general, however, there is some agreement as to what a mentally healthy person is like.

A person may be considered mentally healthy if they have a realistic view about the present and future; if they are competent and can meet the demands of everyday life; if they have the self-confidence necessary to feel that they are worthwhile; and if they are capable of being close to other people, and are able to both give and receive love. Another trait frequently included is the ability to enjoy life.

Although this definition lists several points that are useful in defining mental health, it also presents many problems. One problem is trying to apply a single definition to all people in all situations. Clearly, this would be a false view of human nature. Although being a loving person may be important in the vocational work of a nurse or teacher, it is not essential for the work of a computer analyst or a railroad engineer. And although enjoying life is certainly important, it would seem to be odd in a person who is living with a terminally ill child or who is facing long-term unemployment.

Another problem is that many people think of mental health as the same thing as being well-adjusted. Again, although it may feel more comfortable to do what is expected of us, there are times when being well-adjusted may not mean you are mentally healthy at all. This is particularly true for women. For most of our lives, we have been told that being a well-adjusted woman means being happily married and a good mother. At times, being happily married and a good mother may be a sign of good mental health. However, if we remain in a poor marriage, let's say "for the sake of the children," this may indeed lead to *poor* mental health. Thus, there can't be one definition of mental health that applies to all people and all situations. Our individual qualities, our life goals, and our life circumstances all influence our mental health at any one time.

Developmental Stages

The parts of the mentally healthy personality that we have discussed so far do not appear fully formed in the adult. The chapter on "Adolescence" thoroughly describes how women grow and develop from girlhood. Therefore, this chapter will just touch on some of those important stages.

As young infants, we are born helpless and totally dependent on the care of others, both for our survival and our feelings of well-being. It may be that in these early months we begin to develop some basic ideas about the people in our world. If, as infants, we are fed when we are hungry and our other basic needs for warmth and comfort are met, then it's likely that we will develop a sense of being comfortable in the world. The skills that we need for living take many years to learn. In the early years, as we are learning to talk and walk and take care of ourselves, encouragement of these skills leads us to feel that we are competent people. During the school years, we continue to learn skills for working with the world of objects, but we also learn how to get along with other people who are our own age, and begin to think about the importance of friendship and getting along with others. Later on, as adolescents, we begin to ask many questions, such as "What kind of a person am I? What kind of a life do I want? Do I plan to work? to marry? to have children?" It is at this stage that the lives of boys and girls and their ideas about the future become very different. As most boys become concerned with their future careers, their question becomes "How will I earn a living?" But for many young women, even those planning to work, there is a much greater concern with "Who will I marry?"

It is during adolescence that both males and females become involved in close friendships and frequently fall in love. And it is as young adults that we become able to give and receive love on an equal basis. Only when we develop this ability to share feelings and genuinely love and care for others are we able to become good parents—caretakers of children who require great love and giving of self to ensure their proper development. From this, it would seem that both males and females should develop similar skills—competence, independence, concern for others, and an ability to manage one's own life.

It is now very important to see how people in general, and particularly those who devote their lives to helping other people, view the mental health of males and females.

Myths of Mental Health

Attitudes of Professionals

From our description so far, it seems that men or women could rate high on an index of mental health. Being able to take care of oneself and lead a productive life, having close loving relationships with other people, and being caring and helpful to others, as well as having a strong sense of one's own identity, could describe any "mentally healthy" person. It's important to know, however, that a recent study of mental health professionals showed that they did not agree with this idea. It showed, rather, that mental health professionals, like most of the rest of us, hold very stereotypic and traditional views of what mentally healthy men and women should be like.

The first part of the study consisted of asking several hundred people to describe men and women using a long list of adjectives. Some of the words were sensitive, emotional, aggressive, talkative, shy, etc. From the very long original list, 41 items were found that most people believed would tell men from women. The first finding was that most people agreed that men and women were different in many ways. Men were considered to be aggressive, independent, dominant, direct, and not emotional. The women were called sneaky, talkative, submissive, very emotional, not self-confident, gentle, tactful, quiet, and aware of the feelings of others. In general, the characteristics of men were more desirable.

The next part of the study explored the attitudes of mental health professionals, the people who are responsible for treating people with psychological problems. One group of therapists was asked to describe a mature, healthy, socially competent adult using the same list of words. Another group was asked to describe a healthy woman, and a third group, a healthy man. The groups that defined men and adults used the same words. Healthy adults and men and were both described as independent, competent, objective, and not overly emotional. However, the group asked to define a healthy mature woman described someone who is *not* independent, *not* self-confident, who is very emotional, cries easily, is gentle, quiet, and submissive. Thus, according to these mental health professionals, doctors, and social workers, a woman can be either mentally healthy or feminine, but not both. To be feminine, they say, is to be low in self-confidence, submissive, and very emotional.

The Role of Socialization

During infancy and early childhood, children of both sexes are treated differently in many ways. In regard to independence and the learning of many basic skills, the sexes are not treated alike. For example, most mothers are sensitive to the cries of hunger or pain of boys and girls, but they respond more frequently when a baby boy cries. Children of both sexes are toilet-trained and encouraged to walk and talk and to learn reading and writing. However, girls are encouraged to develop verbal skills while boys get attention for practicing math and physical skills. In addition, boys get attention for destructive and aggressive behavior that can lead to elementary school problems, while "naughty" girls do not.

As children grow up, they are taught to become adults by assuming different roles. For boys, being able to cope is strongly encouraged as they approach adolescence. Boys are more often encouraged to do well in school than girls are, and their intellectual efforts are more often praised. For girls, who at first do well in school, academic success is less often encouraged as they move into adolescence. Instead, it is relating to other people and caretaking that are encouraged. The doll play of early childhood gives way to baby-sitting by high school. Very often, girls who have earned excellent grades in school begin to do less well than boys, either to win the boys' favor or simply because no one seems that enthusiastic about their academic achievement.

During adolescence, when most boys are trying to decide on their future employment, careers, or professions, girls become more concerned with who and when they will marry. If they are planning to work, this is usually seen as a temporary situation. Even when girls have clear career interests and hopes, these still are seen in relation to marriage and family plans. Thus, even in this period of struggle for equal rights for women, both parents and teachers still encourage different behaviors in males and females, and even doctors and therapists tend to describe mentally healthy adult men and women differently. Are the mental health professionals correct? Should women be more emotional and men more objective? Is competence and assertiveness a positive sign of mental health for men and not for women?

Three Mental Health Skills

Our view of mental health is that the characteristics of someone who is mentally healthy should be the same for men *and* women. These qualities are important in any occupation or role, and at all times in the life cycle. They determine not only what you do with your life but the quality of your life as well. There are three of these characteristics: 1) the person in relation to the physical world, 2) the person in relation to other people, and 3) the person in relation to the self. Now let's look at these skills that are so important to mental health.

The Physical World

The woman who learns to master her physical environment, how to deal with the complexities of modern life, and how to make things work is the woman who is most likely to be able to cope with problems, whether they are concerned with the management of the home, the difficulties of raising a family, or managing the world of work. Being skillful in dealing with the objects in your environment has a direct relation to your mental health and the quality of your life. Let's see how these skills develop and then how they influence your mental health.

Beginning in infancy, one of the first and most important tasks of growing up is learning to control our physical environment. Infants learn to hold their own bottle and later to use a knife and fork. Even later, we learn to tie shoes, work zippers, turn on the light, and dial a phone. Still later, we learn how to use a stove, a laundry machine, and if we live in the suburbs or the country, we learn to drive a car.

While as women we learn to operate a great variety of machines, we rarely learn how the stove works, how to repair a broken light switch, and even more rarely, how to fix our cars or change a flat tire. Besides the time and money that we would save if we could change a flat tire, think of how much better we would feel about ourselves if we did not have to wait endlessly for that kind of help.

Women are now beginning to say that they want to learn how to build and repair things. It is only within the last ten years that a young New York City high school student insisted in a court of law that she had as much right to study shop as her brothers. The girl won her lawsuit, but in many schools and homes, it still is assumed that girls do not need to understand as much about the world of things as boys do. A large study of children's textbooks, as well as other studies of parents' and teachers' behaviors, indicates that the general view of men and women in this society is that the men are the builders, architects, engineers, doctors, lawyers, politicians, factory workers, and bankers. Men are the explorers and the decision-makers. Men make war, but also determine the conditions of peace. Women are taught that they do not require the same skills that men do to function in society.

At most times in history, women *did* need to know the same skills as most men. Men and women farmed the food that they ate, grew the cotton and wove the cloth, and both even shared in some of the child care, although women have always done most of this activity. It is only since the industrial revolution, when men (and some women) went out to work in the factories and most women remained at home, that women became less involved in the production of things. As it became possible to buy "manufactured" clothing and mass-produced food, women's skills became more narrow. Women then became principally involved in cooking, cleaning, and child care.

However, in recent decades we increasingly have become a technological society. Many women are in the work force and many require mechanical skills. One example would be the saleswoman in the local department store. Selling used to involve knowing where the merchandise was, receiving money, and returning change. However, today a simple purchase made with a credit card involves a fairly complex computerized cash register.

The situation for women who are primarily homemakers is also machine-oriented. Many women no longer breast-feed babies and must therefore know how to make formulas, as well as the principles of sterilization. Even laborsaving devices such as washing machines now often involve dials and switches and knowledge about which detergents and water temperatures are most suitable for which types of fabrics. Although it is certainly true that housework is less physically draining than it was 100 years ago, it requires a very different set of skills, and many of these involve knowledge of science, math, and technology.

Let us return to our concern with the relationship between being competent in dealing with objects and the issue of mental health. Even though some mental health professionals still may believe that the mentally healthy woman is someone who is passive, submissive, docile, caring, and not at all independent, current research indicates that this is not the case. In fact, the women who rate themselves very high on "feminine" characteristics turn out to be the ones who are most likely to bring their children to mental health clinics for help. Furthermore, very "feminine" women are less likely to play with a baby or a little kitten when given the opportunity to do so than are women who rate themselves high on some of the feminine traits but also on some of the masculine traits.

Our point is that for a woman to be mentally healthy, she must feel that she is a capable human being, and in today's society that involves a considerable knowledge about how the objects in our environment work, and how we can best manage them.

Women and Interpersonal Relations

Being able to have good relationships with others is an important part of mental health. However, because of the way we are brought up, as women we sometimes tend to overdo this—that is, to always put our own needs second to those of other people. Let us see how this behavior can both be a great strength and at times interfere with our mental health.

One of our shared human characteristics is our interdependence with other human beings—the human smile, human language, and the verbal sharing of our past, present, and future. Just as our adjustment to life depends on being comfortable in the world of things, so does it depend on our having peaceful, friendly, and at times, loving relationships with other people. We may understand the technology of the computer and all the machines that exist, but if we don't solve the problems of war and domestic violence, then mental health will no longer be an issue, since our very survival will be threatened.

The nature of our relations with others varies enormously. There are the casual encounters that occur many times in the course of the day—the greeting of the postman or the casual talk of people waiting for a bus or standing in line at the check-out counter. Then there are the other somewhat less-casual contacts of people who work in the same office or building or live in the same neighborhood, but who do not necessarily seek each other out as close friends. Next there are the more complicated relationships of people who work together very closely, such as a medical team in an emergency room, or the teachers in a school whose work depends on a certain degree of positive interaction. The family is clearly the most closely knit group of people, who depend on each other in many ways. It is in the family that people often experience the most loving and warm relations, but also the most complicated and frequently angry feelings. Some or all of these ways of relating to people may involve many and changing feeling states. They range from feeling happy around other people to sometimes feeling frustrated when people want us to do things or act in ways that are unacceptable to us.

Our relations with others are determined partly by chance factors and partly by intellectual factors, such as appreciation of the same music or an interest in religion or politics. But most of all in the relations that we choose, there is always a factor that involves feelings. A recent example comes from the mouth of a four-year-old little girl who announced one day when she returned from nursery school that she knew which boy she was going to marry when she grew up. Her mom asked her how she could tell, and she responded,

"When he tells stories, I always laugh, and when I tell stories, he always laughs." Even as adults we seek out people who make us laugh and avoid those who are sour and bitter. Clearly, other people contribute to our feelings of happiness or sadness, contentment or dissatisfaction. Our mental health is much improved if we are surrounded by people with whom we get along and who contribute to our happiness and joy in life. Our relations with others are a function of who the others are, but also of our ability to tolerate differences and to be able to understand the differing needs of other people.

Since the world of people is considered woman's place, as women, we sometimes overlearn the lessons of how to respond to the needs of others. Just as men are supposed to construct the world of work, women are expected to understand and take care of everyone's emotional needs. Women are supposed to be the caretakers—of the children, of their husbands, of the family, the school, the hospital, and the community. It is women who tend to the home, where the best and the worst of human emotions are expressed.

How does it happen that it is women who are expected to be the "keepers of the domestic tranquility"? And what does this mean for the mental health of women? Early in life, parents spend more time encouraging girl babies to smile than they do boys. As little children, it is girls who are given the dolls to dress, feed, care for, and love. We also are given the toy irons, dishes, pots and pans, and the nurse's kits that will help teach us the skills we will need as adults to take care of others. Our teachers make us the monitors when they leave the room because they know that we will try to keep the classroom orderly, and in our teens we become the baby-sitters because we are considered to be responsible and caring. As we learn to darn the torn cloth and wash the cut knees, we also learn to mend the hurt feelings.

Being able to settle disputes is a very important and valuable social skill, whether it concerns sisters and brothers who are fighting over who gets the first piece of pie, or neighbors disputing how late and how loud the stereo is played. Likewise, being helpful and cheerful when others are hurt, sad, or upset is fine in a friend. Being able to comfort and help those who are in need is a trait that we should encourage in both women and men. This ability, more frequently associated with women, is cause for pride in the "female sex." Why, then, should we consider this a mental health problem if it is such a desirable trait?

We said at the beginning that very often women learn the lesson of pleasing and caring for others too well. This means that very often we smile when we are really feeling hurt (or even angry) because we have learned that people like us best when we are smiling, and we want to be liked. For instance, a wife who smiles even when her husband is being unkind, may ultimately no longer know what she really feels, and may also ultimately live with very angry feelings that she may take out on someone else, express in devious ways, or turn in on herself. At other times when the demands placed on us are too great, we nonetheless go on trying to please everyone "to keep peace in the family." As psychiatrist Jean Baker Miller writes, women who come for therapy frequently think that they are not good-enough wives, or good-enough mothers. Of course there are some women who might not be "good" wives or mothers, but more often women have the expectation that they should be all things to all people, a goal that nobody can reach. It also is interesting that this concern with not being good enough to others is rarely expressed by men, even though it must surely be true of some of them.

Complete commitment to the needs of other people, particularly if it means neglecting oneself, has been shown to have a bad effect on mental health. As an example, the mother of a young infant who is very sick might feel that his care is entirely her responsibility. However, anyone who has ever stayed up three sleepless nights in a row knows that it is not possible to do justice to the baby, other family members, or oneself with little or no sleep. It would be far better to ask the baby's father or a baby-sitter, if necessary, to relieve you for a few hours so you can catch up on your sleep. A study on this subject divided women into two groups—those whose lives were spent taking care of other people and those who, although wives and mothers, maintained other outside interests. Those women who gave all of themselves to the needs of others were the ones who were the most unhappy when there was a shift in their lives, whether it was the children leaving home or a divorce.

From these studies and from our own everyday experience, we can see that as women we are expected to be skillful in dealing with other people and meeting the needs of other people. Although skills in these areas are of great importance to both men and women, they frequently become the only interest of some women. Not being able to express our own feelings and needs, then, can be bad for our mental health.

Self-Esteem

We may manage the objects in our physical world fairly well, and we may get on very well with our family and many close friends, but if our self-esteem is low, our mental health is bound to suffer. Each day we spend many hours doing activities concerned with things—

whether they are typewriters, dishwashers, computers, or electrical appliances. We spend many hours each day engaged in activities with other people, from the first good morning to the last good night. However, no matter how we occupy our waking hours, there is one aspect of our lives that is always with us and that is our *self*.

What then is this "self" or self-esteem, as it is commonly called? It is the way we think and feel about ourselves. Early in childhood and even as adults, the way others see and think about us has a profound influence on what we think and feel about ourselves. For instance, if when we were children, our parents made a big fuss about us because we were very pretty, or because we were very nice to others, or because we won all the awards in school, our self-esteem was high. Unfortunately, as children, females get much less attention paid to them for their actions than do male children, so it is not surprising that as adults, many of us have trouble with this important part of our lives. It is also important to note that self-esteem isn't something that is established for all time in childhood. As adults, if we do any one thing exceptionally well—or for that matter, several things—and if these achievements are noted by others, our self-esteem may rise.

At all times in our lives, the way we feel about ourselves will determine decisions that we make. If we feel that we are being a very good mother to our first child, this will make it more likely for us to have a second. If we decide to return to school after many years' absence and get an A in our first course, we may feel ready to take additional courses. If, however, we are unhappy in our marriage, we are bound to see some of the fault as being our own, and our feelings about ourselves as "wives" may influence our decisions about whether or not to remarry. Thus, we tend to engage in those activities and seek out those people who tend to make us feel good about ourselves, to hold ourselves in "high esteem."

If we learn as young children to believe that we are beautiful and that all we need to do is smile and the world will love us, then we may grow up to think physical beauty is very important, and we may look for happiness through being a cheerleader, the "most beautiful girl" in the class, etc. Although this may work for some women, it can lead to many difficulties. If you continue to think beauty is your most important asset, you will worry and become depressed as it begins to fade. If you later decide that your face is not the "real you," you still may worry, since you may never know if you are valued for your actions or just for your pretty face.

By the same token, some of us are encouraged to do well in school and to be proud of the fact that we are considered "smart." This view of ourselves also leads to certain kinds of behavior and life choices. It may mean that we will grow to need to be very good in school and that we can only be happy as an adult if we can do work that requires being intellectual. If we are encouraged and have the necessary money, we may become highly educated and get the opportunity to use our education. Then we may feel good about ourselves because we do rewarding work. Whatever values we learn as youngsters are bound to have a strong effect on the kind of life and the quality of life we lead. One thing is clear: whatever attitudes we have learned about ourselves are bound to have an influence on all parts of our lives, the friends we choose, the grades we get in school, the men that we marry (or our not marrying at all), and on whether we view life as an exciting experience or a chore to be endured.

Self-esteem is a very important part of mental health. If all of our self-esteem is bound to one activity, trait, or person, changes that may occur can be disastrous. For instance, if our self-esteem as a youngster is based on being very beautiful, then as we age and our looks are no longer those of a movie star, we may be in severe trouble. Likewise, if our self-esteem is based only on what our husbands say, our self-esteem may suffer if this source of support should shift. Thus, it is the woman who has many sources of life satisfaction, who enjoys many things, and who feels good about herself in many different situations that is ahead. Because she knows that she is really a valuable and valued person for many of the things she does and for her many enjoyable relationships with people, she is most likely to have a high level of self-esteem and also of mental health.

Now let's look at some of the life situations that many women experience as adults and see how these concepts apply to the mental health of women in different stages of the life cycle.

Women's Life Situations

We said earlier that different situations will cause different problems for your mental health. One of the most important things that affects your mental health is the role you are living at the time. In the course of our lives, we play many different roles. A role in real life, as in a play, tells us how to behave and how to act to other people. You began by playing the roles of child and daughter. Later you probably took on the roles of wife and mother. In each case, society told you to do certain things *just because* you were in that role. Children should obey their parents. Wives should help and encourage their husbands. Mothers should take care of their children.

Sometimes it's easy to follow these rules, sometimes not. Some roles and their rules are easy for one person but hard for another. If you are in a role whose rules are easy for you to follow, you are probably happy and your mental health is good. If you move into a role that is hard for you, your mental health may suffer. It is important for you to know your own strengths and weaknesses so that you will be able to spot problems before they overwhelm you. In some cases, you may even want to avoid roles that would be hard for you.

Sometimes, of course, you will disagree with what society says you should do. For example, if two roles are in conflict about what you should do, you may have to refuse to follow one. If your husband abused your children, it would be hard to both encourage and help him and still take care of the children. At other times, you may think the role is wrong in what it tells you to do. When you cannot keep up with the demands and needs of a role, when you disagree with a role, when two roles tell you to do different things, or when you are not getting any or enough pleasure from a role, your mental health will suffer. A woman who might be very healthy and happy in one role might be miserable in another. For these reasons, it's important to look at frequent roles or life situations and to see what problems each of them is likely to create.

The four roles we will discuss here are those of the single working woman, the wife, the mother, and the formerly married (widowed or divorced) woman. These are roles that almost all women will play. For each of them, we will discuss common problems and how to recognize them. We will discuss why these situations cause trouble for your mental health and how you might try to solve problems as they come up. We also will talk about why you might sometimes have trouble realizing that you are in trouble and why you might sometimes be embarrassed or afraid to look for help. In one chapter we cannot cover every problem you might have or every role you might be in, but after you read this material, you should be better able to look at your own life situation and see where the problems lie.

The Single Working Woman

People have a lot of different ideas about the single working woman. At one point, people think of her as a swinging single; at the next, as an old maid. Employers think she is flighty and likely to leave her job when she marries or "for no good reason." There is a general feeling that she is "in a holding pattern" waiting for a man to arrive and decide the pattern of her life. People think that the single man is happy about being single; the single woman, unhappy.

In fact, psychologists and sociologists now know that the mental health of single women is better than that of single men. Perhaps it is not surprising that women are choosing to stay single longer and are marrying later. It is also not true that single women are a bad risk for employers. They do not change jobs any more often than men with the same type of jobs.

Problems of the single working woman. Being a single working woman does not always mean that you will be mentally healthy, of course. Earlier, we said that the healthy personality is one that can work well with both the world of objects and the world of people, and that also has a strong sense of self-esteem. The woman with a healthy personality must exercise all three "muscles" and must also hear from the rest of the world that she is doing well. Being a working woman is likely to give us a chance to work with the world of objects. Being a single woman might seem to mean that you would have less chance to relate to people closely than, say, a mother. As we shall see, because of the jobs women hold, this is not necessarily true. Finally, we may find that the single woman's self-esteem seems low; again, this relates, at least in part, to the kind of work women commonly do.

We have said that working successfully in the world of objects and/or interpersonal skills is one source of self-esteem. Why then is the self-esteem of the single woman low? Most of the jobs that women hold demand a relatively low level of skills and thus can be mastered by most women. On the other hand, these jobs are not held in high status by the culture at large, so that many women's job-related sense of self-esteem is low. "Only a secretary" is a typical description from a person with such a problem. The obvious solution—to change fields or to rise to the top of one's field (to be the owner of a restaurant rather than a waitress in it)—has been blocked by our culture until recently. Jobs were open in only a few fields for most women. Obviously, many of the women who took these jobs would rather have been doing something else.

Possible solutions. What can we do about this? First, let's look at the woman who is happy in the job she has and whose self-esteem is high. Most women work in the helping professions. They are teachers, nurses, secretaries, or beauticians. This kind of work may make you happy either because you were raised to feel it is important and useful or because you enjoy working with and helping other people. The beautician who listens to her clients' problems or the secretary who serves as an "office wife" are examples of people who enjoy this kind of role.

Problems arise for women from two sources: 1) the job may not live up to expectations (two years as one of 20 in a typing pool offers little scope for personal interaction with your boss; being a floater in a hospital may have the same effect on a nurse), or 2) the same kind of emotional demands that you get at work also may be made at home. A single woman caring for an aging parent may find that the demands of the parent for caretaking leave little left for the job, or vice versa. Similarly, when a woman marries, or especially when she has children, she may find the multiple demands too much. At this point, she may prefer a job that can be done in an efficient manner with little emotional involvement—and at this point, she may become dissatisfied with the barriers that keep her in her earlier emotionally demanding and satisfying work.

There also exists a second category of woman who is happy in her work—one who has a nontraditional job and enjoys it. Women who have been in this type of work from the beginning of their careers, so far as we know, have usually had an unusual family background. Often they are the oldest girl or the only child, with no brothers. Their fathers and mothers treated them somewhat like sons and encouraged them to learn masculine skills, such as risk-taking. These women marry late and do not usually have children of their own.

If you are happy in your work and social relations, no problems exist. But what if you are one of the many women in a low-valued (and usually low-paying!) job who is receiving few satisfactions or too many demands? Your choices depend on your problem.

Problem 1. You essentially like your job, but the social interaction you expected is not there.

In this case, you have three choices. You may hunt for a new job, you may look for your social rewards outside of work, or you may try to revise your job to suit your needs. If you have not job-hunted recently, your library should have numerous guides to help you begin. If you decide to do your helping and caretaking outside of work, there also are many options, either through volunteer work or often within your own extended family. Some appropriate volunteer projects are joining Big Sisters, foster grandparenting, doing orphanage work, tutoring disadvantaged children, and visiting hospitals or nursing homes. A program that allows you to develop one-to-one relations is probably best. If you are sure you could cope with it, another possibility is single-parent adoption. The children available usually are school age and/or handicapped. In many places, financial assistance is available to help parents overcome the handicaps.

If you decide to try to revise your job to suit your needs, first take a long look at your company. Is it possible? Have other people done it either where you work or at similar places? Remember, your goal is your personal mental health and well-being, and they will not be improved if you fail at this attempt due to unrealistic expectations. For example, it may be impossible to develop personal relationships with patients if you work in the emergency room of a major hospital.

If you decide that your goal is reasonable, see your supervisor, but first develop some *specific* suggestions that you think will help (e.g., instead of having one aide do all of the temperatures and one do all of the bedpans, why not have each aide assigned to do everything for a small number of patients). If possible, involve some of your co-workers so that your supervisor will see that at least some will be willing to make the changes you suggest. If your supervisor fears a loss of efficiency, suggest a trial period of a month or so. If you work in a traditional female profession, the development of good relations with the patients/clients/students is probably one of your supervisor's goals, too, so he or she should be interested in your ideas.

Finally remember that before you take *any* action, it can't hurt to talk it over with a friend you respect, preferably not someone who is personally involved in the change this will make in your life (e.g., not a co-worker or close relative). This person may be able to point out things you have overlooked and save you much later pain. Maintaining and improving your mental health is one of the things friends are for, so take advantage of it!

Problem 2. You have or have developed social and/or caretaking responsibilities elsewhere, and now you want a job that is less emotionally demanding, more intellectually challenging, more highly valued, and/or better paying.

Your basic problem is that you would like to transfer from traditionally female work to traditionally male work. In the past, this has been close to impossible because there have been no such routes for advancement or transfer. This is changing somewhat, but there is still a long way to go. School principals and hospital administrators are usually still men who have advanced through traditionally male paths. Your simplest path in these times of affirmative action is probably to transfer yourself into one of the male pathways and then move up. Additional education might make this change possible. For example, move from copywriting to sales; company presidents usually are recruited from the financial side of a company. Similarly, there are more future career choices open to the telephone line repair person than to the operator (and usually at higher pay). Trying to become the first hospital administrator ever to come straight from the nursing staff will be frustrating; it might be better for your mental health to take courses in hospital administration.

Specific advice depends on your company. Possible sources besides friends are your union, your company's affirmative action officer, or, if things look bleak, a local chapter of the National Organization for Women, American Civil Liberties Union, or a similar group. It may take some extra work to remove yourself from a traditionally female job if you no longer like it (or never liked it), but it should be possible. If your work is not satisfying you, your unhappiness and irritation are symptoms of the threat to your mental health—and you should try to act on these warnings.

The Married Woman

Almost every woman in this country marries at least once. Even those who divorce usually remarry (often to the same man). Most young girls are brought up to think that marriage is the most important thing that can happen to a woman (except possibly for motherhood), and for many women, that is true. Choosing the right husband may be the most important mental health decision you ever make. Being married to a good person may not guarantee happiness, but being married to a person who is bad for you certainly will make you miserable.

What is the married woman like? In storybooks, the married woman is a housewife, busy all day making a home ready for her husband to come home to. She hopes to have children soon if she is young, or grandchildren soon if her own children are grown. If her husband is retired, she is also his full-time companion as they enjoy their golden years together. She is part chef, part gardener, part interior designer, and part mistress, and her husband is the most important person or thing in her life. In turn, her husband is supposed to admire her for what she does and to feel that she makes all his hard work worthwhile.

In real life, very few childless wives lead a life like this. For example, among young married women, most work. Few husbands today earn enough so that the couple can afford to pass up her earnings—either to save for a down payment for a house or just to meet daily costs. Even among those couples who do not need the wife to work, most women who worked before marriage continue to do so because they want to. A second difference is that today young couples tend to put off having children longer. A final difference is that many women today do not find helping and encouraging their husband the most important things in their lives. They look for a more equal relationship, one in which help and encouragement go in both directions.

Problems of the married woman. One problem comes from a feeling that even if you are working full-time, your house and husband should be cared for in the same way as if you were home all day. Women's groups call this "trying to be Superwoman." There are some good and some bad ways to handle this problem, and we will discuss them and their relationship to your mental health.

A second problem comes up when the husband either does not admire his wife either as a person or a wife, or does like her but never tells her about it. He still may need her and may want to stay married to her because he needs a companion, a housewife, or even a person to put down, beat up, or feel superior to. He may never praise her or say good things to her. When you have a husband who rarely or never gives you any emotional support or help, it can be extremely destructive to your mental health. If you have made your husband very important in your life and if he thinks badly of you (or acts as if he does), then you will think badly of yourself—your self-esteem will be seriously hurt. Again, we will discuss good and bad ways to get out of this situation.

A third general problem comes up when the husband and wife have different ideas about what is supposed to happen in a marriage. One may be trying to live a "storybook" marriage, while the other is trying for something different. Psychologists would say that husband and wife have different expectations—they expect different things from their marriage. If you and your husband cannot agree on where you are going, you can't possibly agree on how to get there. A marriage stuck at this point will make you both miserable and damage your mental health, and calls for much discussion about your ideals and goals, or counseling from a minister, doctor, or professional.

Problem 1. The "Superwoman" problem. This is a very common problem among working wives, and almost everyone falls into this trap sooner or later. If they do not talk about it before marriage, both husband and wife usually agree that the wife is responsible for all inside housework except repairs. Studies of working wives show that they do almost as much housework as do women who stay home, while their husbands do very little more than the husbands of wives who stay home. If she is working a 40-hour week, the woman must then do her housework during her "free" time at night and on weekends. She gets little rest and relaxation, nor does she get "special credit" in their marriage because both partners assume she should do the housework, and because housework in general is considered unimportant.

This situation is not good for your mental health. Everyone needs a certain amount of rest, and everyone needs to have extra work noticed and praised, or resentment about doing it will grow. A worse danger yet lies in the fact that most women can manage this double load if their standards for housework are not extremely high. This means that when a child arrives, she may attempt to continue in the same way, just adding child care to the list of tasks. Almost no woman can do this successfully, but it is easy to be sucked into trying if you are used to doing all the housework in addition to a paid job.

What can you do about this? Essentially, you must discuss the situation and negotiate with either your husband or yourself to change it. Where does the problem lie? Do you have rigid standards that you are driving yourself to meet? The average working wife does X hours of housework per week. What do you do? Do you wax the kitchen floor once a week? Do you think the two of you really scuff it up that much? Don't you think two hours on Saturday would be better spent on a picnic or a movie rather than on your stripping off the "waxy yellow buildup"? Does your husband care? If not, why do you?

Often we have learned certain rules that were made for different situations. If your mother had eight children, it may have made sense to wax once a week or to wash the windows frequently—but when was the last time you put a jelly fingerprint on the kitchen window? Make a list of all your housework and go through it, ideally with your husband, and eliminate or plan to do less often as many items as possible. Go by what is important to the both of you and no one else.

At this point, consider the option of sharing the housework. How do you feel about it? Must you personally clean your own toilet bowls to be happy? Suppose you had a bad back or a weak heart. Would you then feel guilty about having someone else do your heavy cleaning? Isn't your mental health as important as your physical health? Are you one of the rare women who really enjoys every housework task? Isn't there something you'd rather do that would make you happier and improve your mental health?

Suppose you have decided that there are some chores that must be done but that you would not do if you had your "druthers." How do you get rid of these tasks? Find someone else to do them. Pay someone if you can—if there are only a few specific tasks, hire a local teen-ager once a week or so.Even a regular cleaner may not be as expensive as you think. Trade off with a friend. Let her or him wax your floors while you scour his or her bathtubs.

Convince your husband that it is his house, too, and that he should do an equal amount to support and maintain it. If he feels that he does an equal amount outside the home (and if you believe him), offer to trade tasks to get rid of particularly horrible ones. There must be something he hates. Perhaps he'd rather clean toilets than gutters. There are few outside tasks that an average woman can't do easily. Is vacuuming a two-story house with a 50-pound upright cleaner really less strenuous than shoveling snow off the sidewalk? If there is something you both hate, take turns (this also may persuade your husband that some tasks are worth paying to have done).

In some families, it works best to have both people take turns on every chore. In others, you may each specialize—but if you each have special chores, be sure to take account of how often each must be done. Leaf raking may be a big job but it usually only has to be done once or twice a year, and it is clearly less work than cooking every night. A positive aspect of talking about all this with your husband is that it makes you talk about yourselves and your ideas to each other. It also is good practice if you are likely to have children or grandchildren to care for.

What do you do if your husband refuses to do "women's work"? This depends on how you feel about it and about him. It is possible that you may be able to change his mind if the two of you can talk to someone he respects—a minister, doctor, marriage counselor, or friend. An important point to remember is that the way you and your husband act toward each other early in your marriage is probably the way you will act later. Old habits are hard to change. Such a man also may be unwilling to help with child care later. Only you can decide how important his help (or lack of it) is to you.

Problem 2. Your husband does not admire you as a wife or a person.

Almost every husband acts like this some of the time. Men are not usually brought up to praise and encourage other people. If your husband has this problem in a mild way—perhaps just a difficulty in saying words of praise and thanks—marriage counseling is likely to help. The difficulty will be to get him to the counseling. If he is unwilling to see a professional counselor, he might still be willing to see your minister or doctor. If they cannot help you themselves, they might at least persuade him to accept counseling.

In some cases, however, the problem is more serious. The husband may not only not praise and thank his wife, he may instead constantly tell her how terrible she is at everything. If she has no close family or friends, she may begin to believe him. No one can live healthily with such a constant threat to their self-esteem. If this happens to you, in self-defense you will either decide that your husband is unimportant or you will look for others to tell you that you're a good person. If you do neither, you may become dangerously depressed. The first two solutions are likely to end your marriage, but the last could end you. A man who feels this way also may beat his wife.

You may feel that you are not a good person and that he is right, but try to remember that if you have lived with him long, you are in no condition to judge. Such men usually feel this way about all or most women. It probably has little to do with you personally. If you do not receive strong support from outside your marriage, you will, of course, be brainwashed by the one important person in your life, your husband. You should seek help from a professional at once to try to gather strength to change this situation. If you can get your husband to join you in seeing a marriage counselor, you should; if, as is likely, you can't, you should see someone yourself.

In many areas, special programs and halfway houses exist for battered wives, and these often are open to the psychologically battered as well as the physically battered. The halfway houses provide a safe stopping place if you are thinking of leaving your husband, where you (and you children) can stay if you have nowhere else to go. If your husband will not change, separation and/or divorce may be the only mentally healthy answer for you.

Marriage after the children have left. A lot has been written about the "empty nest" syndrome, the idea being that women feel useless once their children are gone. While some women do feel this way, most are not too bothered by it. In fact, psychologists have found that most people feel less stress and generally are more pleased with their lives once the children *have* left home.

A problem that may arise some time after the children have left is difficulty due to the husband's retirement. When the children leave, most women take stock and decide how to organize their lives and what to work for. Having a husband suddenly always around, often feeling somewhat depressed and useless, can be surprisingly irritating. Since you know about when you will "retire" from mothering and when your husband will retire from his job, try to plan what you will do then. There are now many books and advice services for retired mothers and retired employees. Good sources to check are your library, local colleges, and the local department of social services.

Motherhood

Motherhood, too, comes in many flavors, each with its own problems and satisfactions. One may be the traditional mother, home with the preschoolers (or home with the adolescent, which is quite different); the working mother, balancing the demands of work and family; or the single mother, who is usually also the working mother without the help and demands of a spouse, and so on.

We will discuss the problems of each of these groups and you will notice a certain similarity in our advice to all three. If you need help, one of your best sources is one or more other mothers in the same situation. Because our society tells us that women naturally love and know how to mother, many women are afraid to talk to their friends about their feelings about mothering. In this case, society plainly has told us wrong—after all, even rats, cats, and gorillas do a better job on their second children than on their first. Humans have the advantage of being able to think and talk to each other. We owe it to ourselves and to our children to know when we need help and to seek it.

The problems that mothers encounter are usually of three kinds: 1) the demands and needs of the children are too great for the mother to handle, 2) she is worried that she is not good at this important job, or 3) even if she is mothering well, her self-esteem suffers because of the low value society places on this role. All mothers of young children also have in common that they almost never have enough sleep. Being tired not only makes any problem look bigger, it also makes problems. Something that you could handle easily if you were fresh, you handle badly if you are tired.

Home with the children. Although we have been trained to think of this situation as the ideal way of life, in fact most mothers work. Even 40 percent of the mothers of preschoolers work. Indeed, if you come late to motherhood so that you can have a house in a "nice" neighborhood, you may find yourself the only mother on the block who's home. In her excellent book on child-rearing, *Right from the Start,* Selma Greenberg talks a lot about the importance of raising children around other people who are raising children.

Why is this considered to be so important? If a mother and child(ren) are alone together for long stretches, the limits on the mother's ability to give to her children will sooner or later be passed, however loving she may be. At this point, if you are a wise woman, you do what you should have done earlier—visit a friend with a child—or at least you put the child in his or her room until you are calm. If you are unwise and don't separate yourself from your child for a few minutes, one may have the beginnings of child abuse. Because of our society's emphasis on motherhood, even feeling briefly that you want to be left alone is likely to make you feel guilty and a failure as a mother.

What is surprising is that our culture is alone in suggesting that mother and child spend all their time together. In other cultures and, in fact, in essentially all of the monkey and ape species, children are never raised alone. Other adults and other children are always around to take up much of the child's time. This is the normal and maybe the "right" way to raise children, not the way the magazines and TV ads suggest. Children need other people, especially other children to play with. Even little babies can make friends and entertain each other. You have only to watch twins play together to see that. If you have no friends with similarly aged children, it will still be of benefit to your mental health and your child's to have a sitter for an hour every day or two, just to provide a break for you and variety for your child.

Mothering is your job now, but it is not a job that is best done with *constant* attention. Strengthening your friendships with others also makes it easier to deal firmly with your child. If you depend too much on your child for love and affection (and this is easy to do), the first rejections that happen as the child develops an independent personality ("If you won't let me have candy, I hate you, Mommy.") are hard to view in a commonsense way. Finally, having a companion will encourage you to explore new and different places with your child and increase your ability to interact in the world of objects. There are few things worse for your sense of self-esteem than the feeling that you are not fit to go to a museum or to be waited on at a restaurant because you have a small child with you.

If you have no suitable friends to share with, try to find some. Visit a local playground at the same time each day. Check to see if there is a Mother Center or similar support group in your area. Use your mother or sisters if you can talk easily to them. Try to find at least one person with whom you can share the bad as well as the good sides of your mothering experience. It will keep you from becoming exhausted, it will give you a much more realistic idea of how well you are doing at child-rearing, and it may even do something to help you to understand society's mixed view of mothering as woman's highest calling vs. being "only a mother."

Where, you may wonder, is the father in all of this? Ought he not to be doing this, too? It would be nice, but for most families today, it is not possible. The father in our culture is likely to be far from you and the children from nine to five, just when you need him the most. Further, unless he spends as much time with the children as you do, he won't understand your passion for even a short break (the average American father spends only 30 minutes a day with his children) or any of your mixed feelings about the children (he may have his own, but they will be different). Finally, he will lack the objectivity, the outside point of view, that your friend may have; after all, they are his children, too.

The working mother has a different set of problems. Whether or not the demands on her ability to deal with people are too great depends on the type of job she holds. If her job is relatively impersonal or can be made so, then as long as she is rested and healthy, she usually is able to deal with her children's demands for love and affection. If her job takes too much out of her, she has the choices that were described earlier for the single woman.

The working mother's problem is much more likely to be a feeling that she is not doing a good job at work and/or with her children. If her job is the type that usually demands after-hours work, she will not easily be able to do it. On the other hand, she may feel very worried and/or guilty about the care her children are receiving. For those mothers who are working because they want to, it should be some consolation to know that studies have shown that children whose mothers are doing what they (the mothers) want to do are happiest. This is not much help to those who work only because they must; but it is perhaps a warning to try not to pass any resentment on to the children.

It is good to remember that there are many kinds of child care other than yours. Aside from relatives, these include 1) having someone (such as an older person, another woman with children, or a college student) come to your house, 2) taking your child to a day-care center, or 3) taking your child to someone else's house (family day care). Much work still needs to be done, but so far psychologists have found that day-care center children are not hurt (and are often improved) either intellectually or socially by their experience. Day-care center children also are just as attached to their mothers as home-raised children. Almost no work has been done on home day care or baby-sitters, but as these are more homelike settings, any effects should be less. It may be a good idea to use at least two sitters rather than only one—then if the sitter quits, as often happens, the child will not be nearly as upset as if the sitter had been the only other caretaker.

The single mother has the most difficult problem of all. She is often a working mother as well, but has no partner with whom she can share housework, child care, etc. She is usually poor (because women are not paid well and because the father often is behind in his support payments) and so cannot hire help. The best solution, at least for the mother of preschoolers, is usually to live near or with relatives or other women in the same situation. Because of the large emotional and financial strain she lives under, good friends and close relatives are especially important. If you are a single mother, you also may find it very helpful to meet with groups of people in the same situation. Your church, YWCA, or a local college may sponsor such groups. If they don't, you might suggest that one be started. Parents Without Partners has chapters all over the country, and sponsors social meetings as well as speakers who can address your problems.

The lesbian mother. About 5 percent of American women are lesbians and prefer to have their basic sexual attachments with other women. Many of these women also are mothers because they did not find out they were lesbian or become lesbian until after they married and had children. Psychologists have concluded that lesbian women usually are no different than other women in any way relating to mental health, but that they do have one special set of problems. These problems are caused by the fact that, in most communities, lesbianism is not accepted. Lesbians also have a special problem relating to motherhood—the fear that someone who objects to their sex life will take their children away from them. This is not because lesbians are bad mothers; from what we know, we can say that, as mothers, lesbians are just as good (and just as bad) as other women.

The reason usually given for taking away the children of lesbian mothers is the fear that their children also will become homosexual. We do not yet know what causes homosexuality, but recent work by Dr. Richard Green makes it clear that having a lesbian mother does *not* make a child homosexual. If you are a lesbian mother and your mental health is being disturbed by the fear that your ex-husband or his parents or anyone else might try to get custody of your child, you should see a lawyer. If you don't want to see a local lawyer, contact a lesbian rights group in the nearest big city for the name of a sympathetic lawyer. If he or she is not familiar with Dr. Green's work, inform him or her, as it is expected to be very useful in potential court cases.

If you cannot find a local branch of the Daughters of Bilitis or similar groups, contact the local branch of NOW for suggestions. If you are openly lesbian, lesbian organizations also will have useful ideas for dealing with the pressures put on your children by other children or unfriendly neighbors. Children aside, it is probably a good idea for you to make contact with a lesbian organization for your own mental health. It is not easy to be lesbian (just as it is not easy to be a black or an immigrant) because ignorant, fear-filled people may make your life difficult. It's good to know of a group of like-minded women to whom you may turn for help and support.

The Formerly Married Woman

Most women in the United States marry, and most also will either be widowed or divorced. The average American married woman spends the last 13 years of her life as a widow. If she is an older woman (over 65), she probably will not remarry since there are so many more unmarried women of this age than men. Every married woman, then, should plan on being single again.

Problems of the formerly married woman. People tend to have very different ideas of the divorcée and the widow. We think of the widow as older and devastated by grief, while we think the divorced woman is younger, sexually freer, and "manhunting"—in short, the gay divorcée. While there may be a little truth to this idea, often it is completely wrong. Many women are now divorced after 20 to 40 years of marriage. Since women tend to marry older men, many widows are not elderly. If the divorce comes as a surprise to the woman (often the case), the shock may be as great as that of a sudden death. Similarly, because of the level of medical care today, "sudden" death has become less common. Often there is time for good-byes to be said and peace to be made, and for the woman to move slowly into widowhood. In other words, your feelings may be very similar whether you are divorced or widowed—feelings of loss if you loved your spouse, or feelings of relief and guilt if you did not.

Other people will treat you very differently, however. Every culture has a ritual for dealing with death. Relatives gather and offer support. Neighbors take over the cooking. Old friends come and reminisce about the good times in the past, either to the widow or in a public eulogy. Some sort of service is held, followed by a gathering or wake. For some time afterward, people make a special effort to include the widow in neighborhood activities.

The divorcée, however, is left to herself except for her closest friends. If anything, people are likely to blame her for not keeping her marriage together, or other women worry that she now will be after their husbands. If, in addition, she has young children, the divorcée usually will have more financial problems than the widow. Most men do not keep up on either their alimony or child support payments. Depending on where she lives, the divorcée may have difficulty finding government help if her ex-husband is supposed to support her. A widow usually receives insurance payments, and if not, the government is likely to believe that the widow has no other source of income.

In other words, both the widow and the divorcée have lost the person who was a major source of interpersonal satisfaction. In addition, the unwilling divorcée has received a major blow to her self-esteem; even the willing divorcée must feel some response to society's disapproval and some doubts about her ability to choose a good husband. People recognize the widow's problem and try to cushion her by surrounding her with love and support. People do little or nothing for the divorcée.

Possible solutions. What can be done about this? Unfortunately, until it happens to them or to a close friend, most people do not think about either problem. By the time the problem comes up, it's hard to be rational enough to do anything about it. Since every woman who marries is likely to have one or the other happen to her, it's a good idea to talk to a friend in each situation and to read some of the popular books on these topics. You will find out practical things, such as the fact that in many states if you have all of your money in joint accounts, you will not be able to make withdrawals because the death of one of you "freezes" a joint account. You will receive practical advice such as, for widows, not to make any major decisions or to move for at least a year. You also will learn to deal with your emotions, such as the rage that the widow may feel over being abandoned. Often, simply knowing that others also have these problems is comforting.

You also will learn to take advantage of whatever help is offered. People often will go out of their way to help shortly after the event. At the time, you may not feel like participating, but if you don't accept such an offer, it's unlikely to be repeated later when you would appreciate it more. There are also informal groups of newly single women that meet at women's centers, YWCAs, adult educational centers, and so on. As we have said earlier, the best place to find help with your problem is often through other women. Knowing how badly others feel also will let you judge whether or not you or your children need professional help.

Problems and Solutions

In this section we will discuss some specific events in the lives of women that may cause mental health problems, and also the many possible sources of help that can be found when we feel that we are "in trouble."

Women always have helped other women who were in need. Prior to this century, women delivered the babies and attended to postpartum needs. They also helped each other at other physically or emotionally stressful periods. When families were large, young girls learned about child-rearing and childbirth within the family, before they were involved in marriages and had families of their own. Women always could turn to their mothers, sisters, cousins, and friends at times of stress.

Problems

Many aspects of contemporary life have changed the nature of the stresses on the lives of young women. One major change that influences our mental health is the mobility of the American family. Many American families move every few years, creating many problems of adjustment. Since these moves usually are related to the man's job, it is the woman who has to deal with the new living place, the children's adjustment to new schools and friends, and her own feelings about being

uprooted. Thus, when a woman is most in need of help from close friends and relatives, she might be very far from these familiar helpmates. This sudden change of place and people frequently is a serious threat to a woman's mental health.

Another fairly frequent source of stress for women is television and popular literature and the way they often greatly romanticize many of the roles we play. Two important examples relate to marriage and family life. Most women believe that marriage is the most important event in their lives. Furthermore, we all are raised with a very romantic view of marriage. Since we live at a time when marriages are not prearranged, we marry out of free choice—ideally, when we are in love. This is true for both men and women. However, since work often is a very important part of men's lives, the marital relationship is usually of greatest importance to women.

Therefore, if it seems that marriage does not follow the storybook form of "they lived happily ever after," it usually is the woman who feels more unhappiness and guilt. If, when she marries, she assumes the major responsibility for making the marriage a good one, then even minor flaws or problems will be perceived as due to a fault in her ability to be a good wife. As the current divorce statistics remind us, marriage is not simple, and happiness is not guaranteed. The joining together of man and wife can begin the most rewarding of human relationships, but this is not necessarily so. It often is the difference between the false expectations of what marriage is about and the reality that becomes a source of a woman's unhappiness and a threat to her mental health.

Childbirth is another event in a woman's life that is frequently looked forward to with great joy (although this is not always the case, such as when babies are unplanned). We may have been told since childhood that motherhood will be the absolute fulfillment of our lives. Childbirth is itself a joyous experience for some women. However, for many others, even those who look forward to the birth of a child, it may be painful and upsetting. Very often women are medicated and sometimes even tied down so that the experience becomes one of loneliness and helplessness.

Because so few women are realistically prepared for this event, there often is a feeling of strangeness and self-criticism when the initial feeling of pride and pleasure becomes what is frequently experienced as the "blues." Many physicians believe that this common occurrence is due to the sudden change in hormones that occurs with the birth process. Since many women don't know how frequent and normal these feelings are, they may be a cause for further feelings of the "blues" and self-criticisms.

One of the major problems for women's mental health at this time, as at other critical points, is that since we don't expect there to be any problems, when they do occur, they lead us to feelings of self-criticism, guilt, and self-blame. It is when we feel that we are the victims of circumstances that our mental health suffers the most. As soon as we feel that we are more in control of the events in our lives, our feelings and our mental health improve. This is why the new childbirth methods emphasize the woman's participation in childbirth, and her husband's as well.

As mentioned earlier, being a mother presents both the possibility of many happy experiences as well as the possibility of mental health problems for us. We are not all equally prepared for, or by nature equally suited to, the tasks of motherhood. Even more important, not all babies are born the same. Some are born to be "very easy" infants and children, whereas others are very difficult to please from the beginning. Again, if we do not feel that we are being "good mothers" in the ways the books describe, we are filled with feelings of guilt, self-rejection, and self-criticism, all of which have a bad influence on our mental health.

These are but a few examples of events that may present problems for women who are normally happy and healthy. The recognition that we have a problem is often the first step toward a solution. Knowing that other people share this problem is also helpful. Although we all like to think that we can solve our own problems as they occur, there are times in the lives of each of us when the problems seem to pile up and the solutions are just about impossible for us to see. When these situations occur, often it is time to seek help.

Self-Help Groups

The best help for people with problems is very often provided by others who have had to cope with the same problem, and have done so successfully. Based on this very simple but very good idea, many self-help groups have been formed in the United States in recent years. The idea behind all of these groups is that many serious problems do not require the help of paid experts, who may have studied the problem, but who do not know it firsthand. Instead, many believe that help can best be offered by those who have successfully overcome the problem themselves.

Self-help groups are, by definition, groups of people who share a problem that they want to overcome, and who expect to give and receive help among others like themselves. The oldest self-help group is Alcoholics Anonymous, founded many years ago and still one of the most successful methods for the treatment of alcoholism. Currently there are not only groups for the alcoholics themselves, but also for the wives and even the children of alcoholics.

Parents Without Partners is another such group through which people who are facing similar difficulties related to being a single parent can come together and share ideas and provide support with one another. Part of the success of these groups comes from breaking down the feelings of isolation and guilt that people develop when they are faced with diffculties that undermine mental health.

Perhaps the biggest change that came about for women concerning self-help groups came with the growth of the women's movement. Prior to Betty Friedan's book, *The Feminine Mystique,* women who were not totally satisfied with their role of wife and mother were considered to be "maladjusted." Hundreds of books, almost all of them written by men, had stated that the ultimate goals of all "normal" women are a home, a husband, and lots of children to take care of. Although there were always some women who rejected some or all of this prescription, they were considered to be unusual, unfeminine, deviant, or sometimes "sick." The popularity of *The Feminine Mystique,* the development of the women's movement, and the steadily increasing number of women in the work force indicated that not all was working as it was described in the 50s. Many women must work, others choose to work, and increasingly women are beginning to realize that even if they spend part of their lives as homemakers, there are many years left after the last child is in school, and that the quality of their lives will depend on choices that they can make.

The Women's Movement

In many important ways, the women's movement has had a major effect on the mental health of women. One of the major themes of the women's movement is taking a new look at women's roles and the right of each woman to consider each decision that involves her life in a serious way. Perhaps the biggest change has been to encourage women to think about themselves as *active* participants in their lives rather than to passively accept events as they occur as if they had no control over them.

What, then, is the nature of the women's groups that are changing our lives? At some time in your life, you probably have been a part of an informal women's group, commonly called the "coffee klatch," a group of friends and neighbors who share recipes, ideas, and complaints and problems related to husbands and children. The new "consciousness-raising groups," as they have come to be called, differ from the traditional groups in many respects. In CR groups, women get together on a regular basis to discuss their past, present, and future lives. They discuss the aspects of their lives that they feel are working well and those aspects that they would like to change. Sometimes these discussions center around earlier events in their lives that are still affecting them; sometimes the discussions are about marriage, children, or work. They discuss the roles that have been prescribed for them and changes that they would like to see in their own lives. In these groups, women come to realize that many aspects of their lives that they felt were personal problems are also problems for other women. The words began to change from what is wrong with *me* to what is wrong with the system.

By sharing ideas and feelings, many women are beginning to try to make changes in their own lives to make them more pleasurable and also more productive. Individual problems are viewed as common problems, and new solutions are being sought. Again, the major message of the women's movement is for women to change from being passive bystanders to *active* participants in their lives. For many, this has led to big changes; changes in their marriage, in their child-rearing, and also in their personal goals and actions. For some, it has meant returning to school; for others, work; and for still others, real attempts to change marriages that were not working well, or child-rearing practices that were faulty. For many women, it has meant considering choices for the first time in their lives, and this has proved a source of strength to them. Most women who have participated in CR groups have found them to be of great help to their mental health. However, this is not always the case.

Beyond Self-Help Groups

For many of us, there comes a time in our lives when self-help groups, best friends, and even a loving family are not able to help us with our problems. It may be the death of someone we love very much, a child with a serious disease or condition, a threatened or broken marriage, or possibly some psychological problem that makes us feel overwhelmed by our feelings of despair. Depression and psychosomatic problems are frequent in women (see page 410). In times gone by, the family doctor or minister was frequently helpful in these situations, and even today it is to physicians and the clergy that most people turn when serious problems arise.

Sometimes help is available from these sources. But all too often, doctors prescribe pills (which may offer relief but do not solve the problem), most frequently to women who present serious sleeping or eating problems or who feel very anxious or always tired and "down." There are times when the best favor that we can do for ourselves is to seek the help of people who have been trained to deal with problems. The important thing is to know when a problem is serious and then to find out where to get help. Even those people who ultimately commit suicide frequently could have been helped with their problems had they found the right kind of help.

Counseling services are provided by many social service agencies; your doctor or minister might be able to recommend one to you. If your problems involve your children, the school may suggest an agency that might be able to help you. Many agencies recognize the fact that many American marriages face very serious problems and provide services to those in need. Seeking help from professionals does not mean that you are "crazy." Remember what we said at the beginning of the chapter: mental health is not something that we each have a certain amount of—it is an ideal. Facing up to mental health problems when they become serious is the first step in seeking help. Help in the form of someone who can listen to what you say, who will not judge you critically, and who will help you figure out solutions to problems can be very useful. For all people, but particularly for women, finding the "right" helping person is very important.

As we discussed earlier, some professionals still hold very old-fashioned views about what healthy women are like. If you are asking someone to help you make important decisions or to help you figure out problems that disturb you, it's important that you and that person share certain values. For instance, if your marriage has become absolutely intolerable to you and you really feel that it must be ended, then to choose as a counselor someone who believes that it is never justifiable to divorce may not be a good choice. Likewise, if you feel that you want to make changes in your life that will lead to your being a more independent, autonomous, competent, and assertive person, then a therapist who believes that a mentally healthy woman is one who necessarily devotes all of her time and energy to her husband and children and is always smiling and pleasant might not be the one to help you.

Of major importance to people seeking help from mental health professionals is the fact that, as with your physical health, you have a right and an obligation to yourself to know the qualifications and beliefs of the person that you are consulting. The most important person to be considered is *you.* The more responsibility you are willing to take for the choices that you make, including the choice of who is the best person to help you, the more active and independent you will be.

Mental health for women may mean taking charge of our lives. We may choose to remain sensitive and caring, but also independent, competent, and self-confident. Hopefully, as we approach our standards of mental health, we still will have a world with many kinds of people in it and with varying traits, but these traits will no longer be considered "male" traits or "female" traits, but simply traits that we value in anyone.

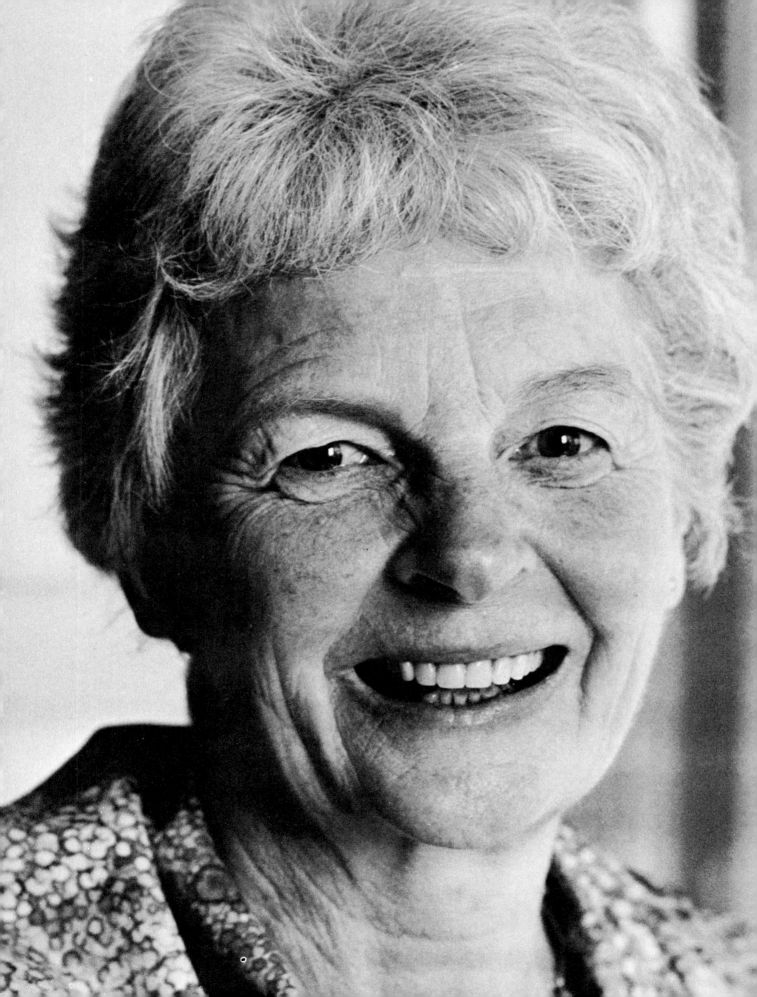

CHAPTER 6

SELF-AWARENESS

GAY G. LUCE, Ph.D.

Have you ever had a day filled with ease and pleasant tasks—a day of rewarding, quiet conversations that left you with a real sense of accomplishment? On such a day, you were relaxed. You felt good about yourself. You were self-aware.

Many of us have chosen to live complicated lives filled with job pressures, competition, and people to care for. Often we become so busy that we lose the ability to become quiet and self-aware. We forget how to relax and be with ourselves, while still accomplishing all that we need to do.

With a little practice, we can learn how to relax, exchanging habits that cause tension and dullness for ones that leave us even-tempered and alert. Once we notice that our days are full of stress, that our bodies feel tense, and that our minds seem clouded with emotions and worries, we have taken the first step toward learning how to relax.

Self-Awareness

All of us can remember special days when everything seemed to flow with extraordinary ease. The world around us seemed particularly crisp and sparkling, even though it may not have been sunny. On such days we accomplished our mundane tasks with grace, and even seemed to know what other people were feeling and thinking without having to be told. We could sense what was going on behind us without looking, and we incorporated interruptions from phones, children, and peers as part of our "dance."

On such a day, everything seems to happen in a comfortable rhythm: if we drive, there are no surprises or jarring moments. The pace at work is pleasant. We are aware of a kind of radiant energy within and a balance that is sometimes called "centering."

We also can remember the converse, days when everything seemed to be happening too fast and caught us always unprepared, when we had to make an effort to focus our attention, and found ourselves irritated and tangled by interruptions. We may have felt sluggish and awkward, had small accidents, cut fingers, or dropped things. From the start, nothing seemed to go right. Worrisome and irritating events piled up until we became increasingly tense, exhausted, and out of phase with the world.

We Americans tend to choose complicated lives. When we first go to school as children, we find ourselves in competition for success. In our jobs and even in our families, there are similar pressures. After awhile, deep satisfaction and harmony seem to be less dominant in living than pressure and limitation. We tend to look at our lives and notice that they are full of what we call stress.

Stress is the way we react to challenge and overload. It is within us, and not a property of our environment. To a great degree, stress is molded by our habits of thinking and behavior. We may not be able to change all the difficult aspects of our lives, but we can change our reactions to them, and thus diminish the stress. To do this, we must become aware of ourselves. Many of our tension habits are not conscious. For example, reading this chapter could be very stressful and fatiguing if you do it in a state of tension. Tension uses energy. You can test the amount of energy it takes to be tense by doing a simple experiment right now.

Making Tension Conscious

Clench your fists hard and hold them clenched. Now clench your jaw. Silently mouth the sounds of the words as you read. Read the next paragraph of this chapter this way and see what happens. Many people find reading a fatiguing activity. Here are some things they can do to ease their stress.

Relaxation

Antidotes to stress and exhaustion come from relaxation. However, not everyone knows how to relax. Many people—doctors included—think of relaxation as a state of near collapse. We have the image of a beer drinker in a reclining chair in front of the television, or the tennis player or marathon runner after a meet. Many of us think of relaxation as near sleep, but that is sedation, collapse, somnolence—not relaxation. To feel relaxation, pick up a cat, soft yet alert, or hold a baby and feel the fluid and supple body. Watch an adult who works steadily and tirelessly day after day, never irritated and never ill. The marks of relaxation are resilience, even-temperedness, acceptance, non-judgment, and alertness without nervousness. A relaxed person is not rigid, not always controlling, not hypercritical, and is able to be firm without being hostile.

If you have been holding your fists and jaw tightly clenched, and have been mouthing the words to yourself—stop.

With your eyes closed, feel your jaw, your hands, and your arms. Do you notice some warmth, tingling, or a sense of relief? How much of the previous paragraph on relaxation do you recall? Was it an effort to concentrate? Was the experience familiar? In other words, do you sometimes clench without realizing that you are tense? Many people have a different breathing pattern when they are tense. Did you notice your breathing rhythm? Did you hold your breath? In addition to physical sensations, there are often emotions associated with tension. Did you feel any tinge of emotion, such as anger? If you can't answer these questions, it's important for you to repeat this test and watch yourself closely. Then observe yourself throughout your ordinary day to see whether you notice these patterns of tension.

Four Kinds of Relaxation

Relaxation is not simple physical passivity, but is a state of equilibrium. Full, deep relaxation throughout a lifetime implies that a person is relaxed in four levels: physical, emotional, mental, and spiritual. They are interconnected, although the concept may seem unfamiliar. A few brief examples may help.

If you suppress your emotions, you hold them with your muscles, and even if you are not aware of it, you cannot relax those muscles. If your mind is busy judging, anticipating, making plans, or comparing, again your feelings and muscles will be engaged. Moreover, your mind is not relaxed and you cannot give full attention to what you are doing. Of course, the bottom line on deep relaxation is spiritual. If you cannot trust the universe, the nature that created you, you will have to be tense and actively trying to control forces and events that are, indeed, beyond control. Some people buy insurance so that they will be repaid if it rains on their vacation. We have to trust that there are many things we do not understand, and that we try to control only to our own detriment and tension. Being born implies physical death. If we try to avoid confronting it or make death a tragedy, we create tension for ourselves. Similarly, there is much in life we cannot rationally understand, yet in a state of spiritual relaxation, we may find we have knowledge that does not come from reasoning. This may seem a strange definition of relaxation. However, a state of acceptance of the inevitable has important consequences in the quality of one's experience. If you need surgery, you will heal faster in a state of relaxed acceptance, rather than in one of worry or resistance. You also will experience less pain.

People who express deep satisfaction and beauty in their lives are not necessarily people whose lives have been easy, but they usually are people with a certain trust in themselves, others, and the universe as a whole.

Physical Relaxation

When you are physically relaxing, you pass through a gateway to deeper relaxation states. In commonplace situations, everyone experiences the pleasure and release of stopping after prolonged exertion. It might be playing tennis, carrying a child, or sitting too long in one position. The rhythm of life involves change, from a state of contraction to a state of expansion or relaxation. We instinctively seek the contrast.

In physical relaxation, we soften our hold on muscles, and this in turn quiets our minds. Muscle tension is like static. It sends messages to our brains that interfere with other messages, as you may have noticed when you tried to read with your jaw and fists clenched.

Commonly, people go around holding muscles tight without knowing it. They know they are tired at night, but they don't realize that their entire physiology is affected by that unconscious tension. Not only do they burn up extra calories by contracting their muscles, but their body chemistry changes as well. Contracted tense muscles put out a different chemistry than relaxed muscles. A body in tension has a different hormonal balance, too. Nonetheless, most of us are so accustomed to our tensions, to the way we ordinarily feel, that we don't know we aren't relaxed. We aren't aware of the feelings that lie beneath the shield, nor do we even question our habitual attitudes toward our lives.

Since physical relaxation is an important first step in reaching the deepest levels of relaxation, we include the following exercises for you to practice. Choose one and repeat it daily for two weeks before attempting to decide how well it works.

Attitudes Toward Exercise

Initially it is not so important which exercise you choose to practice. You are acquiring balance. You might try thinking of living your life as walking on a tightrope. To do it with pleasure and ease, you need to be balanced, relaxed, and totally focused.

In practicing the relaxation exercises that will improve our sense of balance, it's helpful to remember that our minds and our attention are every bit as important as our muscles. Just as a single mental distraction can wreak havoc on the high wire, continued distractions will interfere with relaxation. Choose an exercise and give it your full attention.

Practicing these exercises will not always make you feel better. In fact, each time you do them, you will feel different. Don't expect a particular result. The real result will be cumulative and will affect your entire life.

Practicing relaxation sometimes may make you aware of tensions you overlooked before. Many people only begin to notice their tension after they've gained some mastery of a relaxation technique and thus have a way of recognizing it. Usually it leads to greater emotional relaxation and then to a deeper sense of comfort and a renewed energy.

You must be the judge. Only you can feel the inside of your body. Only you can know whether or not an exercise is doing you good. If you decide that it is harmful for you, stop at once. There are many relaxation techniques, and you should practice only the ones that suit you. If you don't find one in this chapter, an abundant literature from all over the world is available to choose from.

Physical Relaxation Exercises

Preparation

You should wear loose clothing, and remove any jewelry, your glasses, watch, and shoes. This is important. Your body is exquisitely sensitive. The prick from a hairpin, binding from a tight waistband, or the pressure of a watchband will send messages to your brain that will interfere with your best ability to detect what is happening.

Make certain that you will be uninterrupted for at least 40 minutes. Turn off the phone, and keep pets and children away, too. This is your time.

Posture

Lie flat on your back. Let your legs spread just enough so that they are not touching. Place small pillows under your head and your knees. The idea is to have your spine as straight as possible. Your arms should be at your sides, not touching your body.

Begin By Closing Your Eyes

Pay attention to every part of your body, relaxing as much as you can. If you're not quite comfortable, move around until you are. See if you can feel a wave of relaxation spreading up the entire length of your body from your heels and legs, over your hips, your stomach, your chest and back, your arms and shoulders, and finally to your neck and face.

Relaxation

Relaxation is the lack of worry, effort, and trying. Don't worry too much about doing the exercise right. Actually, if you try to do it "right," you'll automatically tense. Relaxation is a paradox: you need to allow yourself to relax, but without going to sleep. Allow yourself to empty your mind of all lists and conversations, things to do, and fantasies. Let them drift away. This is your time to begin learning the skill of deep relaxation.

Left forearm. 1. Lie with your arm relaxed beside you, palm down. Bend your left hand backward from the wrist, keeping the rest of your arm at rest. What do you feel in your upper forearm? Hold your left hand up for one to two minutes, then let it drop. Pay close attention to the sensations in your forearm. The change of sensation when you drop your hand is relaxation.

2. Repeat this three times with your left hand. After the third time, feel your entire body. See if you can experience heaviness and warmth throughout your body. Now see whether you detect any difference between your left and right arms. Compare the way they feel in detail.

3. Repeat this exercise with your right hand.

Both forearms and muscle groups. Flexor and extensor muscles, sometimes called opposing muscle groups, are involved in almost every movement we make. After working the muscles in one direction, you now can do the opposing motion. Prepare as you did the first time, and when you are lying comfortably with your arms at rest, palms down, begin as you did the first time.

1. Lift your left hand backward at the wrist, hold it for one to two minutes, and pay attention to all of the sensations in your arm. Relax your hand and pay attention to your upper forearm. Do this three times only on the left side.

2. Now turn your left arm over, palm up. Bend your left hand forward from the wrist, paying attention to all of the sensations in your forearm. Hold your hand that way for two to three minutes, then relax. Concentrate your attention on the sensations you feel in your arm.

3. Now lie quietly and compare your left arm with your right arm. Do they feel different? What is the difference? Give yourself plenty of time to compare your two arms.

4. Now turn your attention to your right arm, and repeat steps one through three. Lie quietly and compare both arms.

It's up to you to do this exercise thoroughly. Clinicians may ask a person to do this very slowly, adding only one muscle group at a time. Some people may need a week or two on the first exercise without going on to the second. The important thing to learn is to discriminate among subtle sensations and to detect and allow the feeling of letting go.

The feet. 1. Lying comfortably and prepared, place your full attention on your feet. Clench your toes and curl the arch of your left foot away from your face. Hold this position for one to two minutes, paying close attention to the feelings in your leg.

2. Relax your left foot, and feel the sensations in your leg. Compare your left foot with your right foot and see if both legs feel the same.

3. Now clench your right foot, and hold for one to two minutes.

4. Relax your right foot, and compare your feet and your legs.

5. Lying comfortably, again bring your full attention to your left foot. Bend the toes toward your face, moving your foot forward from the ankle, and hold for one to two minutes. Observe the sensations in your leg as you hold the position and after you relax. Compare your feet and legs.

6. Repeat steps one through five with your right foot. Again, compare both feet and legs, going over them mentally and noting the subtlest details.

If you wish to learn more relaxation exercises, you will find excellent instructions in *You Must Relax* by Dr. Edmund Jacobson, originator of these exercises.

Whole-Body Relaxation: I

The following exercise can be done at any time. It is especially effective as a means of falling asleep if done in bed at night.

1. Do your usual preparation and get into a comfortable posture, lying on your back. In this exercise, you will activate both sides of your body at once.

2. Clench your toes, then bend them back toward your face. Hold them, and then release.

3. Bend your toes back, and then your instep. Hold and release.

4. Clench your toes and your instep, and bend your foot back at the ankle. Hold and release. You can begin to see the principle. This is a cumulative exercise. You will tense accumulated muscle groups as you move up the body. At each repetition, add another muscle group: calf muscles, thighs, buttocks and lower back. stomach muscles, and chest muscles. Next make fists. Finally, add arm, neck, and jaw muscles successively.

5. In the last step of this cumulative exercise, tighten your feet, legs, lower back, buttocks, stomach, arms, shoulders, neck, and jaw, frown hard, and tightly press your eyes closed. Hold yourself very tight, feeling the intensity of it, and then let go.

Follow the sensations that travel through your body—the heaviness, warmth, tingling, and expanded feelings. Follow whatever sensations occur with your full attention.

WHOLE-BODY RELAXATION

Practicing relaxation sometimes may make you aware of tensions you overlooked before. Many people only begin to notice their tension after they've gained some mastery of a relaxation technique and thus have a way of recognizing tension. Usually this leads to greater emotional relaxation and then to a deeper sense of comfort and a renewed energy. To find out how this works, follow the steps above and on the next page.

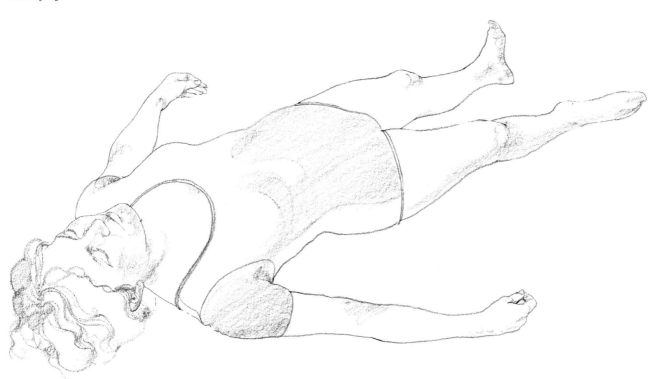

Whole-Body Relaxation: II

When you have learned to tense and release your entire body and are familiar with the sensations of relaxation that follow release, you will be ready to add this exercise.

1. With your eyes closed and lying still, feel the heaviness in your feet, legs, buttocks, and back. Feel the weight and the relaxation of your abdomen and chest. Feel the weight of your back, shoulders, and arms. Feel their warmth. Feel your neck and shoulders, and the weight of your head. Allow your face to feel like a jar of cold honey that is melting in the sun. As you move your attention over your face, feel the sunlight on it, and feel it melting. Feel your eyes, floating and relaxed. Let your jaw relax so that your mouth hangs open. If you are deeply relaxed, you may even drool like a baby. Take a deep breath into your abdomen and allow a wave to come up your body, a wave of warmth and deep, pleasant relaxation.

2. Closely follow the sensation of your breath. Feel it coming into your nose, dividing and passing down your throat into your lungs. Feel the filling of your abdomen, the pause when your lungs are full, and then the long, slow exhalation, with its pause as your lungs are emptied. Discover the character of your breath. What part of the breath cycle do you enjoy the most? Do you feel more relaxed after you inhale, or after you exhale?

Breathing and Feeling

Breathing is a key to the quality of our lives. Not only is it vital to our physical survival, but it also is a signal to the state of our feelings. We can hear the emotions in the breathing of another person—the caught breath of a child in excited anticipation; the silence among people holding their breaths in a tense moment; the sighs of relief or of sadness; the rapid, shallow breaths of anxiety or crying; or the slow, even breathing of a sleeping person or animal.

Where do you breathe? Place your hand on your collarbone and close your eyes. Take 15 breaths so shallow that you only move the hand on your collarbone, not your chest or abdomen. Write down how that makes you feel.

Now place your hand on the middle of your chest and take ten breaths. See how that feels. Do not let your diaphragm move.

Place your hand on your stomach and take ten breaths, moving your hand but not your lower belly. How does that feel?

Place your hand about three finger widths below your navel and breathe so that your belly moves your hand. See how this feels. Deep belly breathing is something to practice in bed at night or in the morning. Once you can take 15 deep breaths into your lower abdomen without holding your hand on your belly to check its movement, you will have an automatic circuit breaker for tense moments in your life. Practice at home.

During the day, whenever you hit a bad moment, take six deep breaths, keeping your mind on the sensation of breathing. Many people have been surprised at the potency of this simple exercise. When you are stopped in traffic or have to wait in line, breathe and pay attention to your breathing. If someone starts an argument and you feel your temper rising, this is another opportunity to pay attention to your breathing.

Many of us take shallow breaths as a way of controlling our feelings. This is the root of much of our tension. Not only do we deprive ourselves of the oxygen of full deep breathing, but we also tense and compress ourselves to hold back the feeling.

Our culture and the upbringing of most Americans urge us to hold back certain feelings. We should be nice, not angry. We should not be crybabies. We should not be too overtly loving lest our affection be mistaken for a sexual overture. We should not express fear, or helplessness, or rage, or deep pleasure. We should reserve our tears for tragedy, and expend our anger only in political causes or competitive sports.

As children, we may rebel at first, being too overwhelmed by our feelings to be "nice," but eventually most of us learn to control our feelings. We control our feelings with our muscles. To control tears, for instance, we may compress the chest and throat, virtually stop breathing, and hold the chin steady with a stiff upper lip.

Rage, too, we control by contracting and tightening the muscles of the neck, the hands, the chest, and the jaw. We may control fear by compressing our stomachs. After a while, this becomes such a habitual way of breathing that we are unaware that we are "doing anything." We think that our lack of feeling is just "the way we are." No wonder we're surprised to learn as adults that this "normal way of being" actually is a state of continued tension or stress.

Many women have extremely tight jaws, having clenched their teeth to hold back negative feelings day after day while serving their families. This tension of prolonged politeness may, according to some doctors, develop into a painful condition in later life known as temporal mandibular joint disease. Lifelong tensions, of which we are unaware, can be sources of chronic ailments in old age.

It is clear that our muscles remain tense as long as we hold back our feelings, even though we may not consciously feel that inner musclar tension. What can we do about it? We cannot become volatile infants, spraying our frustrations and negativity on the people around us. But we can find an acceptable way to express a negative emotion. We also can be aware of the negative emotion within us and simply accept the fact that it is there.

Many people fear that expressing a negative emotion might make them a negative person. This is an ironic fear, for a negative emotion is not your identity. When you are sad, is that sadness your identity? If we do not get involved in our emotions, whether negative or sad, thinking them to be our identity, they will pass in the manner of clouds in the sky. In ancient Chinese medicine, it is said that a healthy person should spend about a fifth of each day in a state of anger, fear, grief, joy and compassion, or some variant. Within some limits, the freedom to express our human feelings assures us of a flow of energy and can prevent us from becoming stuck in any particular feeling.

Spend one day watching your feelings and notice how quickly they change.

Expressing Feelings

Expressing feelings is a crucial step in deep relaxation. Crying, for instance, is a reflex that allows our nervous system to discharge tension. If you hold back your tears, you may feel the tension as a mild headache or sore throat. Similarly, if you compress aggression, you may feel some pain in the chest. In Europe, Japan, and other countries where a relaxation procedure called Autogenic Training is used in treating psychosomatic illnesses, people might be advised deliberately to cry for a few minutes each day or to shout their aggressions into a tape recorder. Dr. Wolfgang Luthe, researcher and translator of the volumes on Autogenic Training, often teaches patients how to cry for a few minutes as a means of releasing their inner tension.

WHERE DO YOU BREATHE?

Breathing is a key to the quality of our lives. Not only is it vital to our physical survival, but it also is a signal to *the state of our feelings. See the instructions at left for a simple test that demonstrates proper breathing.*

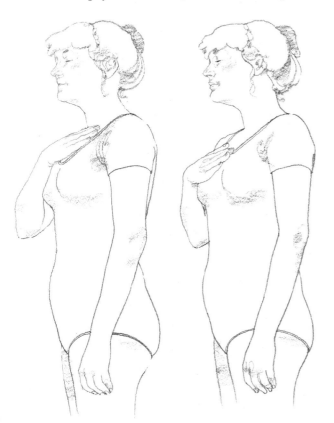

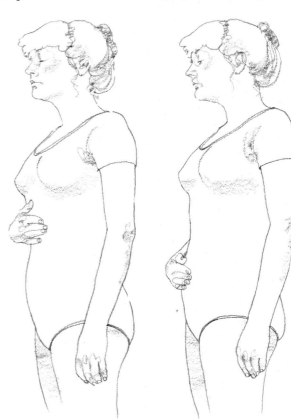

Fear of expressing feeling is a silent bondage. It is often rationalized as a fear of becoming destructive. There are many ways to handle negative emotions without hurting other people or destroying relationships. You can express virtually any feeling imaginable as long as you do not blame anyone else or make others responsible for your feelings. The feeling is yours. If you learn to communicate clearly, you can relieve other people of even the slightest embarrassment by stating how you feel. "When I see my parents fight, I get upset, and I feel angry and fearful and helpless, and I feel like crying."

Most people will bless you for expressing your feelings clearly and taking responsibility for them. It gives them permission to be human too, and to feel their feelings instead of stifling them.

The Feelings in Your Breath

One exercise that has helped many people to discover their withheld feelings is very simple.

1. Make sure you will not be interrupted and that you feel safe and private.

2. Sit with your eyes closed and take a few deep breaths. Now, as you exhale, sigh loudly, giving *voice* to the exhalation. Listen to your *voice*. Repeat the sigh, loudly making whatever sound you feel like. Do it again, listening to the sound you make. Make 20 sounds, without trying to control them. Just let them come out. Listen to them.

If you are sad, your sounds may help you to release your sadness and tears. If you are happy, you may find yourself laughing. Laughter and tears are both ways of releasing tension.

Discharging Tension

Talking is another way of discharging tension. Did you ever notice how a nervous person at a party might talk nonstop? Have you ever felt something so intensely that you just had to tell a friend? Have you ever noticed yourself becoming uncomfortable in a situation where you had to remain still to be polite, but developed an urge to move, becoming restless? Have you ever "run off" a strong feeling, or exercised away some emotion? Physical activity, an old avenue of release from stress, is another way of discharging tension. Some of the old prescriptions for releasing emotional and sexual tension are still more valid than tranquilizers. You can run around the block, run up and down stairs, skip rope, or play tennis. One woman who commutes an hour to work rolls up the windows of her car and sings and shouts and screams until she has vocalized any unspent feelings.

As you relax, by definition, you will allow yourself the freedom of expressing feelings. And as that happens, your feelings will no longer seem so important. By learning to watch your feelings, without becoming attached to them, you increasingly will begin to know and to trust yourself.

Watching Your Feelings

There are literally hundreds of thousands of exercises for watching one's feelings that have been devised by people from different cultures around the world. The following exercise is simple.

If you have heart disease or neck or back symptoms that prevent you from standing in this kind of position, do not do this exercise at all. If for some other reason you cannot do this exercise standing, you can do it sitting.

1. Stand with your feet a little wider apart than your shoulders, and firmly planted. Take a deep breath and exhale loudly, flinging your arms upward, with your hands open. Stand in that position for about ten minutes, although the length of time you stand is not important. When you first want to lower your hands because your arms feel tired, stay up a little longer.

Notice your sensations and your feelings, and the thoughts that come into your mind. If you feel some fatigue, or if the muscles in your arms begin to ache, notice the thoughts and feelings you experience when you consider yourself pained.

At first you may think you cannot stand there any longer, but if you continue for just a bit, you may feel as if you could hold the position forever.

2. When you decide to lower your hands, place them over the center of your chest and sit down with your eyes closed for 10 to 15 minutes. Pay close attention to all of your subtle feelings.

If you do this exercise daily for a week, you'll begin to notice that there are feelings behind all physical sensations, and you'll discover ever-changing subtleties. You also will notice ways that the exercise can change your sense of vitality and your own feeling state.

Quieting the Mind

If you've been doing some of the exercises in this chapter, you may be aware that there are periods after relaxation when there isn't much on your mind. As you relax more deeply, you can begin to experience the freshness and vitality of your existence because your mind will be clearer. No longer will it be like a dirty windowpane between you and your experiences. Instead it will be quieter and not so full of static from irrelevant streams of thought.

Contemplation is a simple method for quieting and cleaning the mind. In order to be able to repeat the practice of contemplation at any time, you may want to select a small object for contemplation, one you can take with you at all times. The palm of your dominant hand, a ring you always wear, or your left thumbnail are objects always at hand. A leaf, a piece of tree bark, or an unshelled nut are other easily carried, readily accessible objects for contemplation.

Practice three times every day, ten minutes at a time.

1. Do your preparation for relaxing. Find a comfortable sitting position from which you will not have to move. Concentrate on your breathing until you feel yourself relaxed.

2. Caress the object with your eyes. If you begin to think about it, allow yourself to return to a practice of merely caressing it with your vision. Thoughts and feelings may come; let them pass by. If you float off on a daydream, bring yourself back to looking at your chosen object.

You may think this is exceedingly boring. That's fine: continue. Most of us are not used to being quiet and alert. Our inner judgments will all rise up in protest. For ten minutes at a time, let those judgments pass through but do not act on them. Set a small alarm so that you can sit for ten minutes. Don't get up early.

Your body may start to give your messages—aching, itching, or wanting to move. Sit still. Observe the protests of your body, and continue caressing your object with your eyes.

You may begin to see "changes" in the object you're contemplating, or have experiences of color, imagery, and form. Let these pass, too.

You may get sleepy. Keep caressing the object, and if you are still sleepy after the ten minutes, take a nap then.

When you have done this for several weeks, you will have a portable method for regaining the stillness of mind you knew as a child or experienced on those vibrant, memorable summer days when the entire world seemed touched with grace.

As you use meditation and contemplation to gain deeper knowledge of yourself and the meaning of your life, and as the habits of relaxation begin to give you inner spaciousness, you will begin to have a different attitude about your own thoughts. You will see that many of our distresses are imaginary, vague fears that make us wary of coming disaster, nervous in cars or elevators, or jumpy in the dark. The real traumas we experience are few and far between, and usually do not last long. They are a minuscule part of our experience compared to the imaginary fears constructed by our minds with the help of our culture. Still, these imaginary fears make us tense and insecure, and we wander through our lives holding endless mental conversations about how we might make our lives better or avoid depression or disaster.

Perspective Exercise

You can relax into the universe as a whole. Think of your position in the universe now, sitting in a room or outside. Close your eyes and rise up a thousand feet in your imagination. Now rise up a mile into the air, look down, and pinpoint your location. In your imagination, go higher so that you can see your location on the earth as a whole. Such imagery can bring you a new sense of perspective.

A simple breathing exercise can deepen into most profound relaxation with the help of perspective imagery.

You need fifteen uninterrupted minutes for this exercise, which can be done lying or comfortably sitting.

1. Begin to pay attention to your breathing, inhalation, and exhalation. Draw your breath down into your abdomen until deep abdominal breathing becomes easy and automatic.

2. Feel the air coming into your lungs and bringing energy into your body. The oxygen in the air is literally the fire of your life, burned in every cell. It is generated by a process that combines sunlight and the chlorophyll of plants on earth. Whenever you inhale, you are inhaling the product of the sun's light. As you inhale, imagine that sunlight coming from across space into your body.

3. As you exhale, imagine breathing out toward the sun. Now you can begin to extend the image. First you are taking in energy from the solar system, and then you can begin to take in energy from beyond, from farther into the galaxy. As you exhale, you can begin to imagine that you are exhaling to the edges of the universe. Breathe deeply, from the cosmic energy beyond the solar system, and exhale back into the depths of the universe.

4. After about ten minutes, return your mind to your location. Feel the air around you. Listen to the sounds. You may feel like a great antenna, inhaling the starlight, or a flower or a tree. Whatever your unique quality of feeling may be, it is a key you can use for entering the deepest level of relaxation.

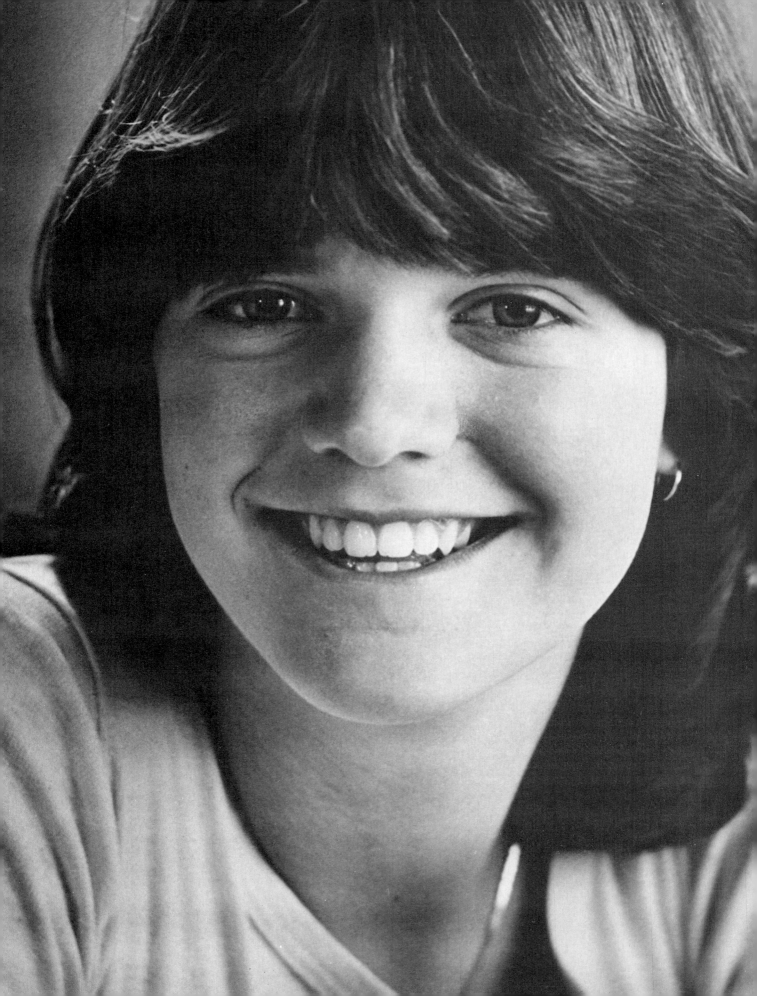

CHAPTER 7

ADOLESCENCE

PATRICIA COOPER, Ph.D.

Between the ages ten and sixteen, a girl leaves childhood and advances rapidly toward full womanhood. Looking back as an adult, she may marvel at the changes that occurred in her body and how she took them all for granted. She will come to realize that, just as her body quickly changed, so did her interests and her roles in life.

If you are now experiencing this marvelous transition, you are already developing new strengths and skills as well as assessing your talents and appearance. You may feel a new love for yourself and for life. Of course, you also may feel overwhelmed at times. But given enough time for growth, the uncertainties of adolescence always give way to the competence and confidence of adulthood.

Adolescence

Between the ages of 11 and 15, young women go through one of the most dramatic growth periods of life. Called puberty or adolescence, it is the time in the life-span when sexual maturation occurs, menstruation begins, and body growth is greatly accelerated. Puberty is second only to birth as the most dramatic physical transition in our lives, and the visible body alterations of puberty are equaled only by the changes that occur during pregnancy.

This chapter provides information about the normal physical changes of adolescence, and offers explanations for some of the more puzzling events that occur in our bodies as we become sexually mature.

If you are a girl going through adolescence, the material that follows may help to reassure you that the big changes occurring in your body are a cause for celebration. Puberty happens to everyone. Although it is a perfectly normal sequence in the greater pattern of life, when you are right in the middle of it, you may feel like the only person in the world who is going through these changes. Part of the excitement is seeing and feeling yourself change — sometimes in ways that cause intense self-consciousness. Step back, gain a little distance, and remember that this is just a passing stage that everyone goes through.

Information always increases self-confidence, and the facts presented in this chapter will answer questions adolescents often ask about puberty—questions you may not think to ask your parents or doctor.

If you have passed adolescence, this chapter may remind you of information you would like to pass on to your daughter or another young girl. It's important to tell young people all the details of the sexual changes they can expect in adolescence before the changes occur. A girl should know about menstruation before she has her first period, and about contraception and intercourse before first ovulating. And, boys and girls should be aware of changes they will begin to feel in their relationships with one another. A thorough understanding of the physical changes underlying these new and powerful emotions will go a long way toward stabilizing a young person in this challenging life transition.

Synopsis of Events

A great deal of research has been devoted to discovering how sexual maturity comes about, and yet we know only a small part of the story. For example, we do not know why puberty begins, or what initiates the elegant, rhythmic interaction of hormones and tissue growth that leads to the first menstrual period, the menarche. Over the years, theorists have suggested that height, genetic programs, climate, and emotions are initiating factors. Some interesting new research suggests that reaching a critical body weight triggers the onset of menstruation. There is a time in adolescence when fat tissue in a girl has increased by 125 percent since childhood. The theory is that this fat deposition, which in turn leads to a weight gain, is the initiating factor in menarche. The critical weight is about 94 to 103 pounds, which is the average weight at menarche.

Whatever the original trigger for puberty, we do know that sometime around age nine, the hypothalamus signals the pituitary gland to begin a stepped-up secretion of luteinizing hormone and follicle-stimulating hormone. These hormones cause the ovaries, relatively quiescent in their growth since birth, to begin maturing. In the process, the ovaries produce the sex hormones estrogen and progesterone, which are released in the bloodstream for distribution throughout the body. The diagrams on pages 126, 128, and 129 are helpful in visualizing these events.

As the powerful chemicals reach their target cells, the whole body begins to go through one of the most beautiful of its transformations. The limbs become longer, and the torso rounder in some parts and more lean in others. The breasts swell, and the hair becomes more luxurious as it changes texture and color. Look around at young people in puberty and notice how their faces change almost weekly. People who were taller than everyone else in their group one year may be average height the next. Voices go through all sorts of dynamics as they deepen. Skin may break out in the most annoying manner, and new hair begins to grow in the armpits and groin. You can appreciate that just adjusting one's self-image and maintaining some balance through this period takes considerable time and thought.

Around age twelve, a growth spurt occurs in girls that continues until they reach full height. This growth spurt may add 12 to 18 inches of height in the space of a single year, a growth rate equaled only during prenatal development and between the ages of two and three years in childhood.

Stepped-up hormone secretion stimulates the growth of muscle and fatty tissue, changing the shape and contours of the body. The proportions of the body change, too, and the large head of infancy and childhood suddenly tops a much longer and fuller body.

Apocrine glands under the arms begin to function, and sweat may have a distinctive new odor. Hormones cause the secretion of extra oils from the sebaceous glands, leading to pimples (see page 564).

Around the middle of the adolescent span, menarche occurs in women. Menarche is the first time the wall of the uterus sheds its cellular lining, leading to the first bleeding of the menstrual cycle. As the reproductive cycle begins in women, other parts of the body fall into the monthly rhythm. Skin changes, emotional states, variations in energy levels and in feelings of well-being, and changes in breast size reflect this monthly rise and fall of female hormones. Small wonder that the adolescent years are among the most puzzling, exciting, and outright confusing years of our lives.

Transition from Childhood

During the period from birth to adolescence, each organ system continues to grow and differentiate. Under the influence of *growth hormone* secreted by the pituitary, the brain expands in size, and bone, cartilage, and connective tissue build a sturdy and flexible framework for the child's body. Muscles multiply as the soft round shape of the baby changes to a wiry, longer, more-defined shape of the child (see page 121).

Thyrotrophic hormone secreted by the thyroid gland assists growth hormone in regulating growth during this period of life. Both hormones also have broader regulatory functions in the body. Growth continues throughout the adolescent period until the full adult height of the individual is reached at about age 17 or 18 for girls.

Sex hormones secreted at the onset of adolescence result in the maturation of the genitals, the development of the internal reproductive organs, and the appearance of secondary sexual characteristics. All of these changes are discussed in more detail later.

Puberty has been occurring at younger and younger ages throughout the Western world during this century. In the year 1900, the average age for the onset of menstruation in girls was 14.2 years. In European countries, earlier menarche is even more striking. In Norway in 1840, the average girl began to menstruate at age 17, as compared to age 13 today. The best guess as to why this is happening is that better nutrition and health care in infancy and childhood have caused the age of onset to change.

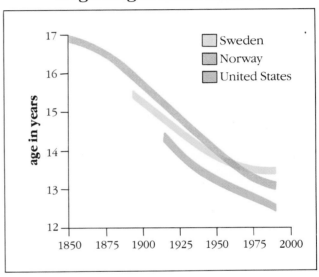

Beginning of Menstruation

Since 1850, menarche has occurred at earlier and earlier ages. In Norway in 1850, the average age at menarche was 17 years; in the United States today, it is between 12 and 13 years. Menarche, the first menstrual period, takes place some three years after pubertal changes begin in girls, at around age 10.

There is an indication that menarche is now stabilizing at around age 11 to 12, and that the average age of menarche is becoming similar in all countries. It is quite unlikely that the age of onset of menarche will continue to lower, as human genetic factors probably ensure a sufficiently long period of development prior to reproductive maturity. Through our evolution, we seem to have arrived at a fixed genetic time of around 10 years of childhood to attain the development necessary for our survival as adult, reproductive humans. For it is during this period that humans pass on the cultural information, the intellectual skills, and the emotional molding that have been responsible for the sustenance and advancement of our species.

The Average Age of Puberty Changes

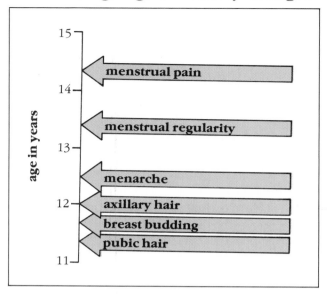

This chart depicts the average age at which the major events of puberty occur. See the chart on menarche below for the range of ages at which this one event of puberty may take place.

Range of the Age of Menarche

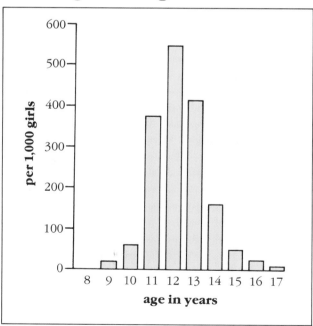

This chart illustrates how a single event in puberty, the first menstrual period, may vary in the age of onset from girl to girl. The age at which each individual goes through a growth spurt, acquires secondary sexual characteristics, and gains weight also is variable during the period of adolescence.

Maturation Through Puberty

Before discussing the major changes of menstruation and reproductive maturity in detail, let's consider the year-to-year changes that occur through the adolescent span of 10 to 18 years of age. The pituitary hormone secretion that initiates puberty actually begins around age eight or nine. All of these ages are approximate. The time change from child to adolescent to adult is quite variable among cultures and from woman to woman.

Secondary Sexual Characteristics

One of the major indices of a girl's passage through puberty is the physical development of characteristics that clearly identify her as a woman. These secondary sexual characteristics—breasts, pubic hair, full hips, and curvy limbs—distinguish our sex. Men also develop secondary sexual characteristics at puberty (see page 123). Internally, reproductive organs develop, leading to the production of mature eggs in women and of sperm in men.

The lower chart at left gives some idea of how menarche varies in onset from individual to individual. In addition, full height may be reached as early as age 11 and as late as age 18, and breasts may start to bud for some girls at age 10 and for others not until age 14. All of these variations are perfectly normal.

The drawings at right summarize the progression of puberty, emphasizing the secondary sexual characteristics. The age breakdown is only a guideline to when the changes may be expected.

Physical Changes in Adolescence

8 to 10 years. Puberty is not visible on the outside unless the girl is an early starter. There is no breast development or pubic hair, and no axillary hair (hair under the arms). The body shape is still that of late childhood. Average height is between 50 and 55 inches, and average weight is between 55 and 70 pounds.

11 to 12 years. Most young women will know that puberty has started by now. Breasts begin to swell out from the chest, and nipples begin to stand out. The areolae may enlarge in diameter. There is a little growth of pubic hair along the labia (lips of the vagina). Hips become a little fuller and broader. Other people begin to notice these secondary sexual characteristics at around this age. The voice lowers slightly, although not as much as in a boy at puberty. Menstrual periods may begin. The average weight in this period is 70 to 80 pounds, and the average height is about 60 inches.

PHYSICAL CHANGES IN ADOLESCENCE

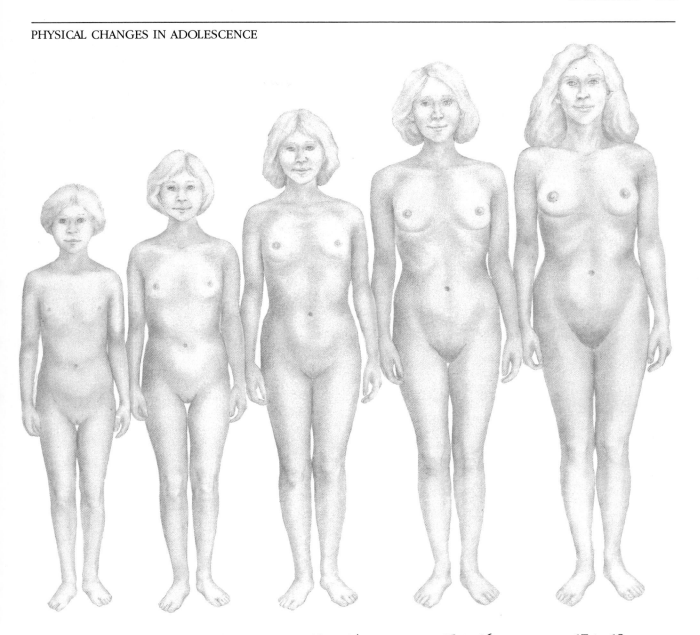

8 to 10 years	**11 to 12 years**	**13 to 14 years**	**15 to 16 years**	**17 to 18 years**
PREPUBERTY	EARLY PUBERTY	MID-PUBERTY	LATE PUBERTY	ADULTHOOD
• Body shape is that of late childhood.	• Breasts begin to bud. • The pelvis begins to grow. • Pubic hair appears. • Menstruation may begin.	• Breasts continue to grow. • Body shape is more curved. • The pelvis grows. • Pubic and axillary hair thicken. • Menstruation is under way.	• Reproductive system maturation is almost complete. • The body is fuller. • Breasts are more completely formed.	• The reproductive system is complete. • Full adult height and weight are reached. • Menstrual periods are regular.

13 to 14 years. By this age, it is very clear to the young woman and to others that puberty is in full flower. This is the age when most women begin to have regular periods. Breasts are fuller; darker and coarser (often curly) pubic hair begins to spread up from the vaginal area across the V-shaped area called the "mound of Venus." The body flourishes, growing rounder and taller (average weight is 110 pounds and average height is 63 inches). With regular periods, mature ova burst from the ovary at day 14 of the cycle, making pregnancy possible.

15 to 16 years. By now the reproductive system has matured at every level, and the young girl looks like a young woman. Breasts continue to swell and change: the nipples become quite prominent, and the areolae often form a small mound. Little raised bumps called papillae are evident on the areolae. See the opposite page for illustrations of these changes. Pubic hair continues to thicken and spread upward and outward toward the thighs.

17 to 18 years. All the curves and proportions of the adult body are now complete. Height has leveled off at full adult stature, and weight generally stabilizes at around 115 to 130 pounds. Breasts, pubic hair, and axillary hair also are fully developed.

The Growth Spurt for Boys and Girls

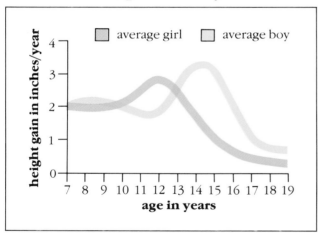

Adolescent girls grow tall before adolescent boys. An average girl will gain the most height between ages 12 and 13, and an average boy between ages 14 and 15.

Growth Spurt

In addition to the other physical changes that take place during puberty, a spurt in height and an increase in weight accompany the increase in sex hormones. The first rush of growth is around the time that breasts begin to swell, and by the mid-teens, a woman's body usually has reached full adult height, weight, and proportions. Your final height depends primarily on three factors: 1) the genetic factor—that is, the height you inherited from your mother, father, and grandparents, 2) the age at which you began the growth spurt, and 3) the time at which closure of your bones began and was completed.

As the illustrations on page 124 indicate, you gradually reach your adult height and weight from the years of early childhood to age 18, but the major growth spurt for girls is at around age 12, and for boys at around age 14, as shown above. A girl who has an early puberty will tend to be shorter than average, although from the ages of 10 to 12, she may be the tallest girl in her group.

Leg growth accounts for the first increase in height. At the same time, arms, hands, and feet are lengthening. This is the time when a young person may be called a "gangling adolescent," or when you are likely to hear, "She's all hands and feet." The spine then begins to lengthen. Growth in the bones of legs and arms slows and ceases as the growth plates in the bones close; however, the spine continues to grow until late puberty. An early maturer will finish her growth before a girl who started maturing later.

Where does the energy for such spectacular growth come from? From food, of course. Nutritional needs for adolescents will vary widely, just as for adults, and depend on each individual's activity level and body size. See the chapter on "Nutrition," beginning on page 40, for the recommended daily calorie intake and nutritional requirements of teen-agers.

Menstruation

Most women vividly remember their first period and the feelings and events surrounding it. If it did not come as a shock, it still probably came as a surprise, for the first period usually appears without warning: one day you find blood between your legs. This can be startling and even frightening if a girl is not expecting this first menstruation. If she *is* expecting menarche, and is dreading it because friends or relatives have treated menstruation as something dangerous, uncomfortable, or even taboo, the experience can be one of unease and confusion.

Actually, menarche is a time to accept and celebrate womanhood. But before a girl deals with her first menstrual cycle, it's important for her to have the straightforward biological facts as well as some practical tips for handling this important event.

BODY CHANGES AT PUBERTY IN YOUNG MEN AND WOMEN

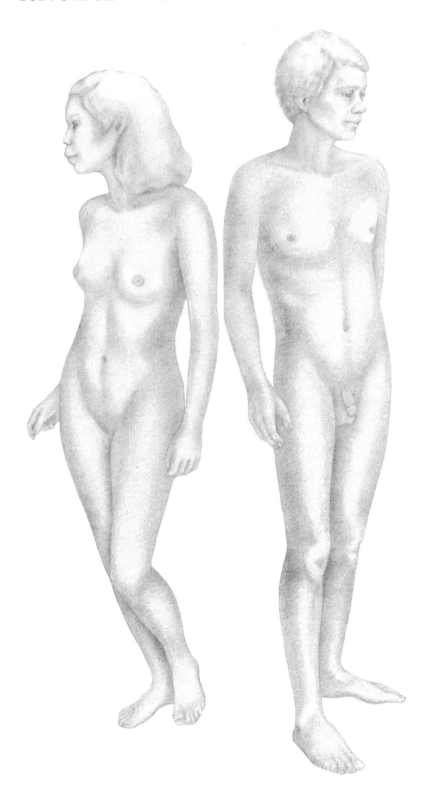

Boys and girls go through puberty at about the same ages, eight to 18 years, and sex hormone secretion is responsible for the changes in both young men and young women. Obviously, the physical changes that a girl goes through are not the same ones that a boy experiences. Female development is primarily due to the large quantities of estrogen hormone young women produce, and male development, to young men's production of testosterone.

In young men at puberty, centers in the brain stimulate the pituitary to produce hormones that greatly increase the amount of male hormones secreted. The testes mature and produce mature sperm, and externally, the penis and scrotum begin to enlarge. Pubic hair appears, as well as facial hair and hair on the chest and under the arms. In general, body hair increases and head hair begins to decrease. The voice deepens as the larynx enlarges. Muscles begin to develop in the arms, legs, and chest, and the shoulders broaden. Fat deposits shift into patterns that are characteristically male.

In young women at puberty, body hair also increases but remains fine and light; head hair becomes more luxurious. Hair appears under the arms and in the pubic area. Breasts develop and body contours become more rounded and filled-out as fat deposits increase in specifically feminine patterns. Female hormone secretion leads to the maturation of the ovaries, eggs, uterus, and vagina.

Menarche

The first period — the first bleeding — occurs at around age 12 or 13 and is called *menarche*. The blood between the legs comes from inside the body in the uterus, flows out the cervix, down the vaginal canal, and finally outside the body. Tissues filled with tiny blood vessels break away from the wall of the uterus every 28 days, and blood mixed with cell debris flows to the outside of the body. So the process of having a period occurs about every 28 days from the time you are around 12 to the time you are around 50. Having your first period means you are capable of getting pregnant. To put it another way, once you start having periods,

you know that an egg you have been carrying inside your body since birth is mature and ready to be fertilized.

At the time of your first period, you may experience cramps or aches in your womb that feel almost like stomach aches. And for weeks before your first period, you may feel sleepy, unusually hungry, or irritable. These symptoms clear up as soon as you begin bleeding. Some young women have slight cramps or a feeling of low energy before each period. Others experience almost no changes in body and emotions before a period. Each woman learns her own individual feelings and body rhythms connected with the menstrual cycle by observing her cycle over a few years.

Growth from Age Six to Eighteen

Physical growth in adolescence results in weight gain, height increase, and a change in body proportions. This chart shows how the body is transformed from relatively straight and thin to more curvy, with longer legs and arms. During adolescence, a girl's average height increases from about 45 inches to 65 inches, and her average weight goes from about 47 pounds to 120 pounds.

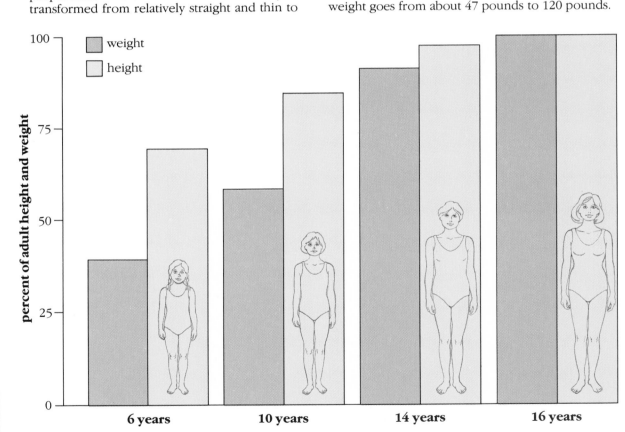

The next period may not return in exactly 28 days, for individuals vary in the length of their menstrual cycle. In the first two years of menstruation, periods often may be spaced irregularly. After two or three years, however, most adolescents begin to cycle with their own regularity. The chapter on "Adolescent Reproductive Problems" discusses abnormal states that might be signaled by changes in the cycle during puberty.

The Cycle

The menstrual cycle, also called the female reproductive cycle, is a smoothly integrated sequence of events that involves all the systems of a woman's body. The normal menstrual cycle that you experience every month is an excellent example of holistic health (see page 20). For the system to work effectively, each part must function correctly in a whole, healthy person. Specifically, the ovary and uterus are directed by the brain through chemicals released into the bloodstream and through the nervous system; glands turn their secretions on and off in a timed sequence. Your breasts swell, and your feelings, emotions, and behavior change with the cycle. Each part is regulated by the rhythm of the whole cycle.

The menstrual cycle is so integral to a woman's body that it is discussed throughout this book in connection with woman's psychology (see page 28), pregnancy (see page 220), birth control (see page 164), abortion (see page 206), infertility (see page 514), and reproductive problems (see page 496). In this chapter, we will discuss parts of the cycle, their separate functions, and then how the parts fit together in the whole, integrated cycle.

Before we plunge into this rather technical discussion, an obvious question should be raised: What is a menstrual cycle for? Simply put, the purpose of the cycle is to produce a baby. This does not mean that your purpose is to produce a baby, for that is a matter of choice. But in our human history, the reproductive cycle has evolved in the human male and female solely to ensure the continuation of the species.

A knowledge of the menstrual cycle allows every woman to assume responsibility for having children or for not having children. For with this knowledge comes the ability to choose appropriate methods of birth control. If you are just entering adolescence, it is important to understand the cycle so that you fully grasp that having the first period means that the first mature egg has been ovulated. Now you must take the responsibility for making mature decisions about your sexual behavior. And these choices and decisions are as much a part of the natural development of adolescence as the beginning of the menstrual cycle.

Starting to Menstruate

The first menstrual period, or menarche, is an important event in a young woman's life, and a real cause for celebration. But as you can appreciate, it can come as quite a shock to find yourself bleeding if you are not prepared for it.

Straightforward information should be shared with adolescent girls before their menarche occurs about:

- where menstrual blood comes from
- how long bleeding will last
- why menstruation happens
- how the menstrual cycle is related to pregnancy.

Preparation for menstruation should include information on the different types of tampons and napkins used to absorb blood. Adolescent girls often wish to practice with various types of tampons and napkins. A girl approaching menarche might keep a supply of these in her room, and take them with her on trips in anticipation of menstruation. Contact a school nurse or a sympathetic teacher if you are at school without supplies when menstruation begins.

The best person to communicate the facts about menstruation to an adolescent girl is usually her mother; in fact, this sharing can promote a special closeness between mother and daughter. Some women may find it difficult to talk about menstruation and sexuality, feeling embarrassed or uncomfortable with the subject. If so, adolescent girls will find the diagrams and text in this and other books informative and helpful in learning about the important and exciting changes that occur in their bodies at menarche.

GROWTH OF THE OVARY AND EGG

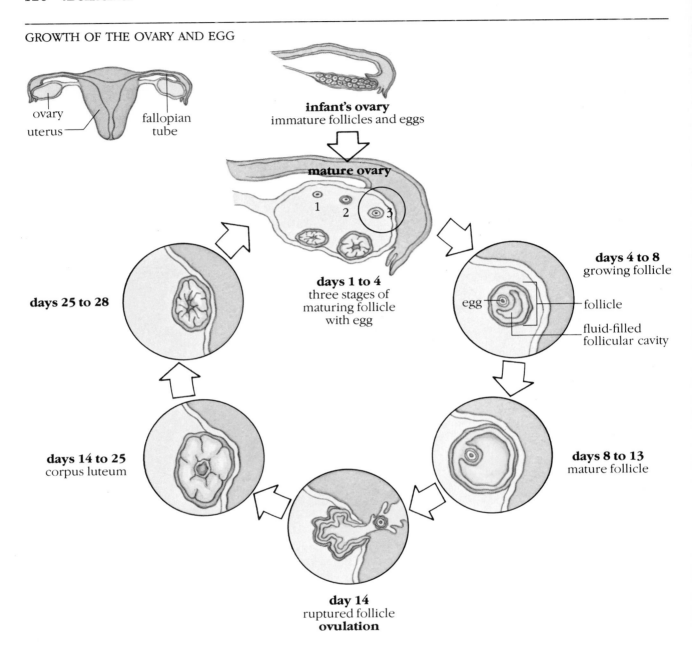

ovary
uterus — fallopian tube

infant's ovary
immature follicles and eggs

mature ovary

1 2 3

days 1 to 4
three stages of maturing follicle with egg

days 25 to 28

days 4 to 8
growing follicle

egg — follicle

— fluid-filled follicular cavity

days 14 to 25
corpus luteum

days 8 to 13
mature follicle

day 14
ruptured follicle
ovulation

By the end of two months of development, the female fetus has a tiny, almond-shaped ovary filled with future eggs or ova. At birth, the infant's ovaries contain a total of about 500,000 immature eggs—all the eggs a woman will have in her lifetime. From this point on through childhood, the eggs change very little. But at the onset of puberty, when eggs begin to mature, the immature eggs can take one of two paths. Many die and degenerate in the ovary (at the end of puberty, only about 35,000 of the original 500,000 remain), and the rest may become mature eggs, ovulated during the menstrual cycle. Of the large number initially present, only about 500 eggs are ever ovulated and have a chance for fertilization.

At puberty, with the maturation of the sexual organs, an egg begins to mature inside a compartment called a follicle. The cells of the follicle are specialized for protection, nutrition, and maturation of the egg growing within the fluid-filled follicular space.

At day one of the menstrual cycle, the follicle-stimulating hormone from the pituitary causes a follicle, with an egg inside, to start growing. As it enlarges, it moves toward the ovary surface, and finally on day 14, the follicle breaks open through the ovary wall, releasing the egg directly into the mouth of the oviduct. The egg then moves down the fallopian tube (see page 226) where it may be fertilized. If so, the follicle, which transforms into a corpus luteum, will grow larger into the corpus luteum of pregnancy (not shown here). If the egg is not fertilized, the corpus luteum will shrink and degenerate at the end of the menstrual cycle.

The brain has an active role in the reproductive cycle. This may seem odd at first, because the menstrual cycle just seems to happen naturally, without thought. And indeed it does. When we are healthy and feeling well, a lower part of the brain called the hypothalamus acts automatically to initiate the cycle. But as we will see later, under certain conditions, conscious parts of the brain can affect the hypothalamus and, in turn, the reproductive cycle.

The hypothalamus of the brain acts like a gland in the cycle, sending chemical messages to the pituitary gland, which lies snugly against it (see page 604). The messages begin puberty; they are delivered via the bloodstream, and they direct the pituitary to release luteinizing hormone (LH) and follicle-stimulating hormone (FSH). The ovary and uterus are stimulated by these hormones, as we will see in the next sections. The hypothalamus, in turn, is sensitive to estrogen secreted by the ovary. Each part of the cycle influences some other part in this feedback system (see page 128).

Now that we understand the chemical connection of the pituitary to the brain, it's easy to grasp how hormones and their flow may be affected by conscious thoughts. Many women have known through common sense and intuition that their emotional state, or the stress of work, affects their monthly cycle.

Under usual conditions, the cycle repeats itself automatically, but now extensive scientific research supports the observations that emotions, stress, anxiety, and environmental factors such as light, heat, and noise affect whether a cycle is "late" or "irregular." Conscious centers in the brain also affect other parts of the reproductive cycle. See page 155 for a discussion of how emotional, interpersonal, and environmental states can affect milk letdown in nursing mothers.

The anterior pituitary produces the hormones FSH (follicle-stimulating hormone) and LH (luteinizing hormone) only on signal from the brain and its hypothalamus. Only when these hormones begin to be secreted can puberty occur; so the brain controls not only the menstrual cycle, but menarche as well. The chain of events of the cycle so far is that the brain stimulates the hypothalamus, which secretes specific chemicals into the anterior pituitary gland, which, in turn, initiates the production of the hormones FSH and LH (see pages 128 and 607). But there are two other extremely important hormonal components, the ovarian hormones.

The ovary responds to the pituitary hormones by beginning to develop a mature egg enclosed in a follicle capsule (see pages 126 and 129). The mature egg is released into the oviduct after two weeks, and the follicle changes into a mass of hormone-secreting tissue. The hormones produced are estrogen and progesterone, and the tissue is called the corpus luteum. These hormones change the lining of the uterus to make it receptive to the implantation of the fertilized egg. When pregnancy does not occur, the corpus luteum ceases to produce estrogen and progesterone, and the lining of the uterus is sloughed off 14 days after ovulation — a menstrual period.

The ovarian hormones have another very important function in the cycle other than turning on the uterus. The two ovarian hormones control the output of pituitary hormones by signaling both the pituitary and the hypothalamus as to the amount of hormones needed from those two sources. That is, the ovarian hormones form a feedback loop or feedback control to other parts of the cycle. This is what causes the menstrual cycle to repeat itself month after month.

The uterus is the last component of the cycle that we will discuss in order to understand how all the pieces fit into a functioning whole. Let's arbitrarily pick a point in the cycle to begin a discussion of changes in the uterus— the point at the end of a menstrual cycle when the endometrium or uterine lining has been stripped to a very thin layer of cells. Under the influence of estrogen from the ovaries, the cells begin to rebuild a thick endometrium once again. By day 13 of the cycle, this spongy layer is quite thick and ready to receive and implant a fertilized egg.

If implantation occurs, the endometrium becomes even thicker and undergoes the changes necessary for a successful nine months of pregnancy. If implantation does not occur, the blood vessels that supply the endometrium begin to constrict (because of hormonal feedback) and the blood flow is not sufficient to keep the cells alive. The endometrium begins to deteriorate, slough off into the uterine cavity, and finally to flow out the cervix as a mixture of blood, mucus, and tissue— the menstrual period.

The cervix, the lower part of the uterus, also changes cyclically in the way it secretes mucus into the vagina. See page 518 for an illustration of changes in the cervix during the menstrual cycle.

The whole cycle functioning as a unit is more than the sum of the parts we have just described. To form a fully functional menstrual system, all of the parts must be put together into the whole, healthy body of one woman where they interact to support a fully reproductive human being.

The chart on page 129 shows the whole system diagrammatically for greater intellectual understanding, but only you, observing and participating in this great cycle in your own life, can fully appreciate its complexity and significance.

THE MENSTRUAL CYCLE

The diagram of the menstrual system at right shows how the various parts interrelate to produce a whole cycle. The brain, glands, ovaries, and uterus all interact in cyclic rhythm, directed by the hormones they produce. All organs in the body respond to some extent to the monthly cycle, for the hormones produced are carried throughout the body in the circulatory system.

By convention, the first day of the menstrual cycle is defined as the first day of bleeding. The use of 28 days also is a convention, as the length of the cycle varies from woman to woman. The hypothalamus of the brain stimulates the anterior pituitary to produce hormones that cause maturation of the egg in the ovary. The ovary also secretes hormones that cause the uterine lining to grow, leading eventually to a period or perhaps to pregnancy if intercourse happens at or near ovulation. Ovarian hormones also have a feedback effect on the brain, as shown in the diagram of the cycle within a woman's body.

The colored arrows on this page represent the site of production and the target organs of hormones produced in the menstrual cycle. On the adjacent page, the same colors are used to show the levels of hormones as they vary throughout the cycle. Refer to page 125 for an explanation of the hormone action.

pituitary hormones

 LH

 FSH

ovarian hormones

 progesterone

 estrogen

hypothalamus
pituitary

ovary

uterus

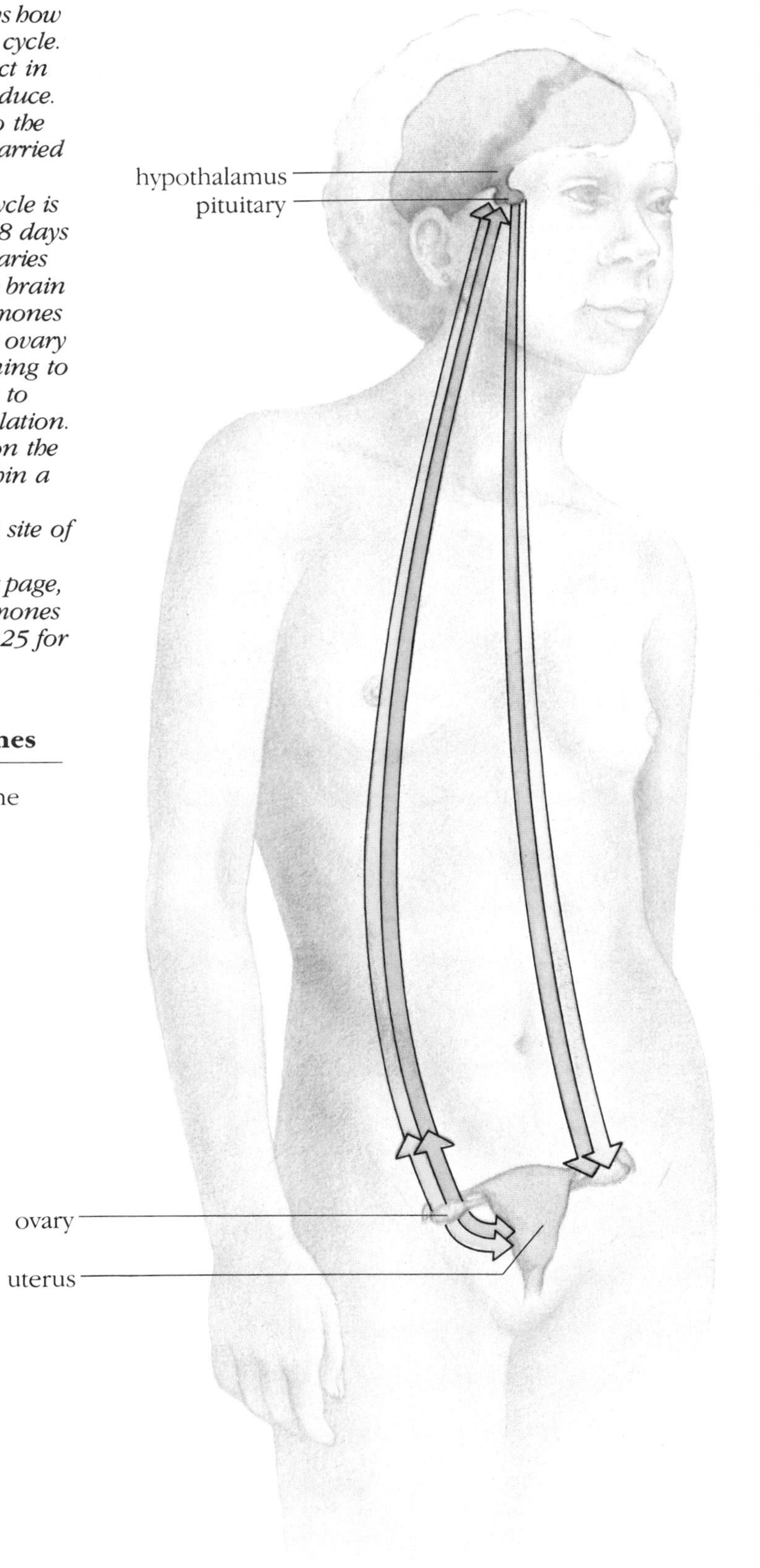

days 1 to 4

- The uterine lining breaks down (menstruation).
- An egg within its follicle starts to grow, stimulated by the secretion of FSH.

days 21 to 28

- If the egg is not fertilized and does not implant, the corpus luteum shrinks, and estrogen and progesterone levels fall.
- Menstruation occurs.

days 5 to 12

- Estrogen stimulates the uterine lining to begin to repair and grow after menstruation.
- The follicle continues to grow and produce estrogen.

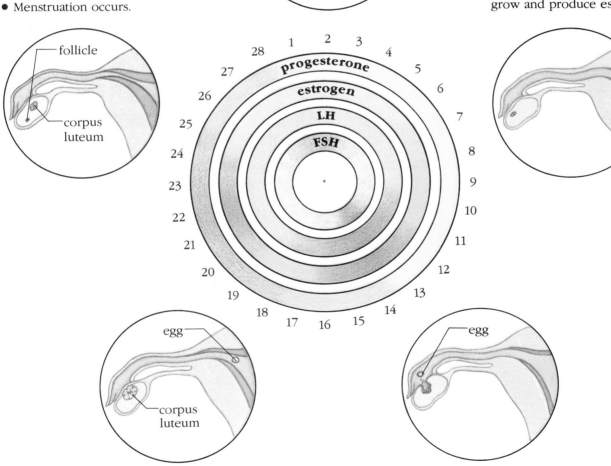

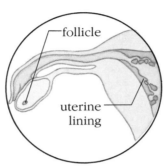

days 15 to 20

- The egg, if fertilized, implants in the uterine wall.
- The corpus luteum produces the hormones progesterone and estrogen.

days 13 to 14

- Luteinizing hormone causes the follicle to burst, releasing an egg into the fallopian tube. The follicle becomes a corpus luteum.

Adolescent Emotional Development

PATRICIA COOPER, Ph.D. AND NANCY C. HUBBELL

During the years between ages ten and 18, a young woman is expected to "grow up." Not only does she go through change physically, she also moves from the relative dependence of childhood to the independence of a person who can take care of herself. She becomes a woman.

Society expects a young person to behave like an adult during middle and late adolescence. Does this external pressure on adolescents, coupled with the young person's internal changes, mean that adolescence has to be a time of upheaval and crisis? Is there always storm and stress associated with this phase in the life-span?

It appears from research that most adolescents do not undergo severe stress in their teens. In fact, although a natural uprootedness seems to characterize this time of transition, most adolescents are equal to the task of assuming adult roles, becoming independent, and forging a sense of personal identity.

Experts agree that adolescence is a time when an individual passes through several key growth phases. Sometimes these are referred to as the tasks of adolescence. It is further generally agreed that if the adolescent meets these growth challenges successfully, she will be well on her way toward full self-reliance, maturity, and growth toward young adulthood. In the usual sequence of normal development from ages ten to 18, the adolescent will:

- achieve a personal identity and independence
- develop further intellectually
- undergo further social and moral development
- become sexually aware
- determine and play a sexual role
- make educational and vocational choices.

Personal identity formation is a new task for the adolescent. For the first time, she begins systematically to think about who she has been, to reflect on who she is, and to plan who she will become. No wonder that she may suddenly appear self-absorbed or acutely self-conscious. She is behaving normally for this stage. The stereotype of the young girl talking for hours on the phone with friends and analyzing and discussing her behavior in detail makes good sense in the light of identity formation. In the laboratory of peer group opinion and behavior, she is testing how she appears in public. She is listening to how her friends see her. The task of personal identity formation has the teen-ager taking the experience of childhood, the teachings of parents, and the idea of who she wants to become and integrating these into her daily behavior. In the process, she may act out many different roles, seeming to change her personality, opinions, goals, and moods with alarming rapidity.

Independence is expected to happen for the child in a rapid five- to eight-year span. At the end of adolescence, most families and cultural groups expect a young person to be physically and sexually mature, self-reliant, and confident about his or her further education and vocation.

Recent studies indicate that, for the most part, girls achieve their independence more easily than boys do. Various reasons have been advanced to explain this difference, among them that women are trained to be less self-assertive and so have an easier time passing into traditional cultural roles of maturity. Physically, boys have strong aggressive impulses that emerge at puberty, and these drives often bring them into greater conflict with the rules and laws of adult culture.

Regardless of these differences in boys and girls, both sexes benefit from having fair, nurturing parents who themselves present a good model for independence and self-reliance.

Intellectual development. Changes in how we think occur in stages throughout childhood and adolescence. The adolescent begins to think in ways that were impossible before. She reaches what is called the stage of "formal operational thought" and becomes capable of reasoning logically and abstractly about issues. She can construct a hypothetical situation and seek solutions to problems in a systematic way. She can imagine systems of values, and how they might affect societies and relationships. She begins to view the world at large.

These changes in ways of thought affect how the adolescent looks at society and also her morality. She now begins to make moral judgements about herself and others.

Moral values. In adolescent research, two stages of moral reasoning are recognized: conventional and autonomous morality. In childhood, the child acts morally out of fear of being punished. In early adolescence, the child becomes able to take into account the opinions of others and the rules of society.

The adolescent is said to be in the new stage called conventional morality. Now a young adolescent is able to think about morality in a larger framework, to reason about it. A young woman at this stage will generally talk about good and bad behavior, and will try to follow, first, the rules laid down by her parents, and second, those of her peers. She wants to be a good girl, to do what is right, and to follow the rules.

Later in adolescence, she will begin to consider the rules of society. She will analyze how they conflict with her parents' rules or those of her peers. She generally will have respect for law and order. All of these stages are those of conventional moral development.

Later, some adolescents enter a more advanced stage of moral development. A young woman may examine the laws of society and the rules of her parents in the light of her own developing ideas of right and wrong. That is, she may develop a system of personal ethics based on universal moral principles, and supported by her ability to observe, reason, abstract, and make moral judgments. This stage of autonomous morality may not follow the conventional moral stage until young adulthood, or at all.

Sexual expression. Is there a new morality among teen-agers? In studies of teen-age girls, a desire for greater openness about sexual matters has been voiced again and again. Young people generally discuss sex more openly than did their age group ten years ago. And both boys and girls say that their greatest anxiety does not come from their emerging sexuality but from "not knowing the facts." Adolescents want sufficient, accurate information about all aspects of sexual functioning.

Studies conducted over the last ten years show an increasing tendency for young people to feel that sexual matters are a private concern and should not be regulated by anyone but the parties directly involved. The majority of adolescents feel that abortion is a matter for the individual to decide, and that premarital sex for young people is all right if they are in love with each other.

As it seems unlikely that these trends in sexual development at adolescence will reverse, it is most important for adolescents to become informed and responsible about their sexual relationships.

Sexual roles. A major part of developing a personal identity is how we define our sexual identity. What it means to be female, to be a woman, is undergoing scrutiny as never before in history (see page 28). In our culture today, the female is given a lot of room to define her roles, and she is indeed thinking of new ways to define and express them. One study showed that many girls have strong, traditional sex role expressions (usually based on their mother as a model) and plan to marry and have a family as their goal. But an equally large number placed self-reliance and independence on a par with marriage and family as their goals. A third group of girls in this study did not wish to identify with the standard feminine role at all.

Vocational choice represents one of the last steps in the development of independence. And it is often delayed into the early twenties as young people interpose college education before a career and economic independence.

Again, in this area we find that studies of adolescents show a difference in male and female behaviors around educational and vocational choices. Adolescent girls' career choices are less stable and realistic than those of boys in the early years of adolescence (ages ten to 14). Early on, boys tend to make educational plans that reinforce their vocational plans. That is, they decide on a career and fit their education to it. Girls may choose a career direction later. More often, they attend college and choose a vocation that does not always coincide with their college training.

Certainly, girls' role models are changing as more women successfully combine careers with raising a family, or as they pursue fulfilling lives that do not include having children. As careers for women become more desirable in terms of personal satisfaction, women will begin to seek career guidance earlier in adolescence, and will more consciously direct their vocational and educational development.

The adolescent experience. Media images and folklore to the contrary, it appears that most young people do not undergo severe stress through adolescence. Their values tend to be rather closely aligned to those of society in general and to those of their parents in particular. The image of flaming youth in wholesale rebellion against parental values and authority simply is not borne out by research.

From the outside, adolescence may appear tumultuous as we watch the physical changes, the experiments with roles, the emergence of new behavior, the expression of novel feelings and moods, and the reflective withdrawal into self-study. But for the adolescent, these changes are normal and feel part and parcel of her life and growth.

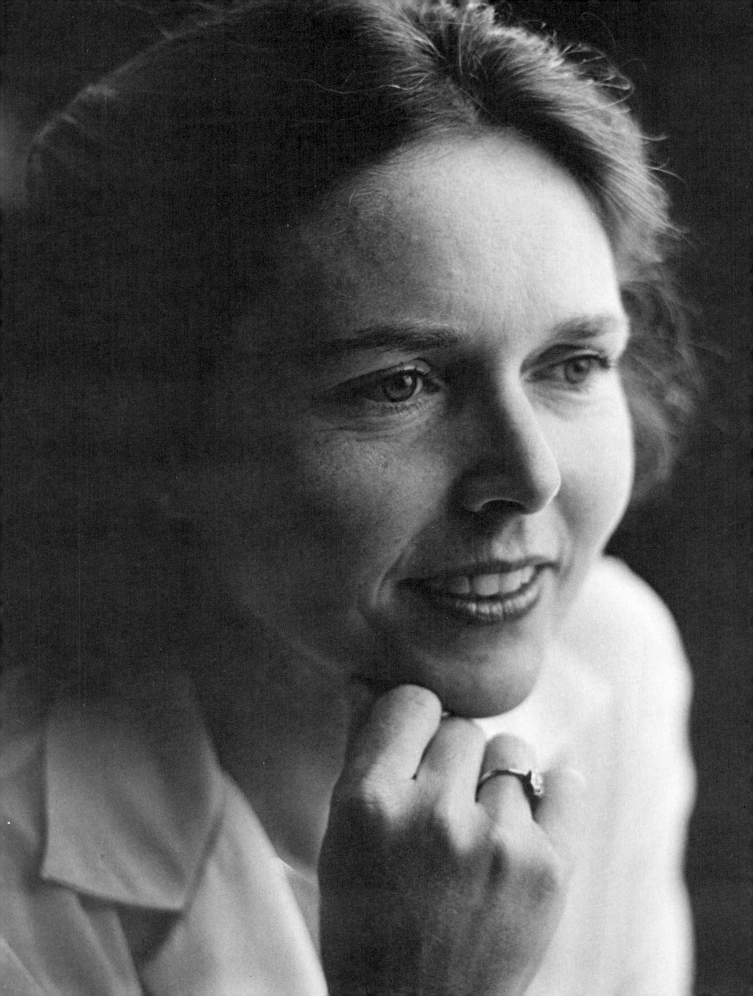

CHAPTER 8

SEXUALITY

HELEN SINGER KAPLAN, M.D., Ph.D.

MILDRED HOPE WITKIN, Ph.D.

Sexuality is an innate part of what makes us human, and sexual expression can be as diverse and individual as the varieties of human nature. But one idea that we all seem to agree on is that although two people can share a sexual experience for a variety of reasons, if it fails to give pleasure to both of them, then something is amiss.

Some people experience conflicts or problems in their sexual development that get in the way of the constructive reasons for having sex—namely, having children, experiencing pleasure, and expressing love. By better understanding your own sexuality, you can gain a greater awareness and appreciation of your partner's sexuality as well.

Sexuality

It's hard to imagine that there was a time less than fifty years ago when the word "sex" was barely mentioned, except as a synonym for gender. In the Age of Victoria, only adult males were "permitted" to have sexual feelings; women were supposed to be untainted by such "low, base appetites," and children were supposed to be completely "innocent," innocent meaning ignorant of sex. Beginning with Freud, of course, sexual attitudes changed, and we now acknowledge that it is normal and natural *for women, men, and children to experience sexual feelings.*

Sexuality involves pleasurable sensations in the body, especially—but not exclusively—in the genital regions. These normal, pleasurable feelings *are present from birth. In fact, about half of all male infants are born with their penises erect, and about half of all female infants are born with lubricated vaginas.*

It's also normal and natural for some form of sexuality to remain throughout our lives. Infants in the crib stimulate themselves by rubbing their genitals against the mattress or by using their hands directly. Young children play "doctor" and other games of sexual exploration. And adolescents, capable of full sexual intercourse, experience an explosion of sexuality. Barring physical or emotional problems, our capacity and desire for sexual expression remain with us until death.

Men and women are born sexual creatures and remain so all their lives. Sexuality is innate, part of what makes us normal human beings. But being sexual doesn't imply desiring sex all the time, just as a woman's ability to have multiple orgasms doesn't mean that she always must have an orgasm or that only one orgasm per lovemaking session is insufficient.

"Normal" human sexual practices differ widely from generation to generation, place to place, and culture to culture. Our sexual expression and preferences are shaped to a great extent by experience and learning. In contrast, animal sexuality is governed much more by physical factors, such as hormones. Thus, animals mate only when they are in "heat" (that is, fertile), and do so in a highly stereotyped manner.

But even with all the differences among humans, some aspects of sex appear to be constant across most cultures and time periods. One is the idea that sex should be pleasurable. Two people can make love for a variety of reasons, but if it doesn't give pleasure to them—both of them—something is wrong.

Procreation, pleasure, and the expression of love are the constructive reasons for having sex. However, *sometimes sex is used for other purposes, such as reducing tension, or dominating or manipulating a partner—nonloving uses that can lead to problems. Sex should not be a proving ground for a man's virility or a woman's devotion; it should not be a privilege to claim or a right to exercise; it should not be a means to obtain a reward or impose a punishment; it should not be something to do because everybody else does it. Sex should be an expression of mutual love and caring, a giving and receiving of pleasure—pleasure in the body and pleasure in the relationship.*

The fact that sex is preeminently an expression of a female-male relationship also is fairly constant across cultures. In terms of how most people in the world behave today and have behaved in the past, "normal" sex involves one man and one woman. The evolutionary reasons why this is so are obvious. More important is the fact that most people simply obtain the greatest physical and emotional gratification from sex as a couple with a partner of the opposite sex.

However, some people experience problems and conflicts in their sexual developments. They may be blocked in their heterosexual expression, and seek other ways of feeling sexual pleasure. Such sexual variations include homosexuality, sadism, masochism, exhibitionism, voyeurism, and even more unusual sexual practices.

Society traditionally has taken a moralistic and punitive attitude toward sexual variations, even though the scientific view holds that they are the product of psychological conflict and not a matter of sin or wrongdoing. "Normal" people also experience sexual conflicts, but usually express them in the form of harmless sexual fantasies.

This book is intended for women. But the female-male relationship is such a central aspect of a woman's sexuality that we have devoted considerable space to a discussion of sexuality in men. The best sexual partners—which is to say, those who obtain the most gratification for themselves and provide the greatest satisfaction to their partners—are those who are aware of the other's sexuality.

Making Love

What is normal sex? That's a question people frequently ask sex therapists when what they really mean is what is the "normal" frequency of intercourse, what are the "normal" positions and practices, what is the "normal" amount of time spent in foreplay and coitus, or what is the "normal" behavior of a couple after intercourse. The answer is that there *are* no simple norms. Whatever gives pleasure to both partners and is not destructive to either may be considered normal. If a couple persists in sexual behavior that pleases one partner and not the other, then the relationship is probably headed for trouble.

Sexual response consists of three phases: desire, excitement, and orgasm. Desire is principally a function of the brain; excitement and orgasm reflect physiological changes in the genital organs. During excitement the genitals swell; during orgasm genital muscles contract.

Sex normally begins with desire, which can arise spontaneously in both women and men. It's just as natural for a woman to make a sexual overture as for a man. Some fortunate couples are perfectly synchronized in their desire for each other. When one feels amorous, the other responds. But a certain sexual imbalance is well within normal limits. It's normal for one partner to experience desire before the other; to proceed through foreplay to intercourse with one partner wanting sex more than the other; or for either partner occasionally to have intercourse without a specific desire for sex but wanting mostly to give pleasure to the other.

On the other hand, it's not normal to have sex when one or both partners find the act repugnant, although many women (and men) do so just to please their partners or to keep the peace. Sexuality should not be a submission to another's desires, but a sensitive cooperation to obtain mutual pleasure. Similarly, although it is certainly normal for one partner not to respond with desire to the other's overtures every time, it is not normal for this to persist over lengthy periods. There is no obligation to have sex whenever the other proposes it, but if one partner proposes constantly and the other constantly refuses, something is wrong. Similarly, lack of desire in both partners over a long period of time is another sign of trouble.

Sometime during the course of normal lovemaking coitus will occur—the penis will enter the vagina. Coitus can take place at any time from the beginning of excitement to *after* the woman has had an orgasm. And it can occur—normally—under a variety of conditions: at morning, noon, or night; in the bedroom, living room, kitchen, garden, or garage; with manual or oral stimulation before coitus involving the genitals, anus, or any other area, and engaged in by either partner. If both partners agree to and take pleasure from the activity, all of these behavior patterns are "normal."

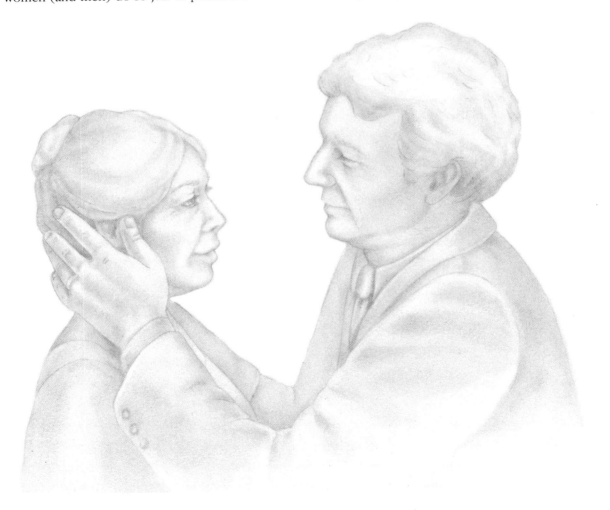

Further, any coital position that satisfies both partners is normal. Of the probably hundreds of variations, four are more or less basic, and the reader might wish to experiment with all of them.

The female-superior position (woman on top) allows greatest stimulation for the woman and rather less for the man, and may be very useful when the woman is "slow" and the man is "fast." It gives some women a feeling of being in control of the sexual activity, providing a sense of security that allows them greater freedom of response. Many women also welcome the chance this position gives them to exercise their sexual creativity, usually to the pleasure of both partners. In addition, the female-superior position leaves the man's hands free, allowing him to fondle the woman's breasts or engage in similar activities.

The male-superior position (man on top) provides greatest stimulation for the man, and somewhat less for the woman. This is the traditional position of intercourse for American men, and many men feel that it is the only really "masculine" position—a view that has no basis in biology and few parallels in other cultures. The male-superior position does offer the man more freedom for his own sexual creativity, and many women prefer it because they feel comfortable experiencing the man in a position of strength and control.

There should be no confusion about the word "superior" in these descriptions; it is simply Latin for "top." The bottom position is, of course, in no way "inferior" or secondary, and the bottom partner is not expected to be passive, submissive, yielding, surrendering, or anything other than an active participant. Further, neither the top nor bottom position is more "masculine" or "feminine" than the other. Position is solely a matter of preference and mutual accord.

The lateral (side-to-side) position offers intermediate stimulation to both sexes, but may be the least stimulating of all to the woman. Since it also is the least strenuous position, it's often used when one or both partners are physically tired, when one or both are obese, or when the woman is pregnant. The hands of both partners are free, but since the greatest freedom of thrusting occurs when the upper bodies are separated, the partners may be out of easy reach.

The rear-entry position offers very good stimulation for the penis, and good stimulation for the clitoris. It is preferred by many men who find themselves excited both by the prospect of rear entry and the sight of the woman's anal area. (It should be understood that we are talking about vaginal intercourse and not anal intercourse.) As has already been mentioned, sexual imagery or fantasy, which either partner may experience during any and all phases of lovemaking, is a normal phenomenon that can enhance the pleasure of sex.

When the intensity of sexual excitement reaches a peak, orgasm occurs—muscular contractions at the base of the penis in the man, and muscular contractions surrounding the vagina in the woman. It is neither necessary nor particularly normal for a man and woman to reach a peak of sexual excitement at the same time, and thus to have simultaneous orgasms (it's not abnormal either, of course). It is certainly well within the range of normality for women to have orgasms before or after their partners, and for these orgasms to occur before or after coitus. By manual or oral stimulation, the man can help the woman to orgasm before he enters and has his own. Or he can have his orgasm during coitus and then orally or manually help the woman to orgasm. These practices are by no means unusual alternatives.

Lifelong Sexual Development

Humans are born sexual creatures and remain so until death. However, sexuality changes during one's lifetime, and the course of sexuality is different in men and women.

Sex and aging in women. During early childhood, girls (and boys as well) experience diffuse sexual pleasures. They masturbate (although more boys masturbate than girls), have fantasies, and enjoy sex play. It's not until adolescence that gender differences in the development of sexuality begin to appear. Girls generally are slower to awaken to sexuality, and their orgastic urge apparently is less intense. While 90 percent of normal boys masturbate, about 30 to 40 percent of girls either do not masturbate at all or do not begin to masturbate until they have an intense sexual experience.

The first coital experiences of girls and boys also tend to differ. A boy may be shy or clumsy, and ejaculate more rapidly than he would like, but he usually has an orgasm the first time he attempts intercourse. This is not so for girls. In a girl's experiences before coitus, petting and genital stimulation might have been highly arousing, yet never have led to orgasm. Even a girl's first coital experiences frequently are disappointing and do not lead to orgasm—or even to pleasurable vaginal sensations. In fact, intercourse may be physically uncomfortable and cause the girl alarm at her failure to enjoy the experience.

In our culture, women tend to reach the peak of their responsiveness in their late thirties and early forties. Kinsey reports more women having extramarital affairs at this time, and Masters and Johnson observed intense and rapid responsiveness, especially after the birth of several children. Vaginal lubrication occurs almost instantly, and multiple orgasms are common. Many (but not all) women in this age group seem to have more interest in sex and to experience easier orgasms than when they were younger.

As with age-related sexual changes in men, we don't know whether the greater sexual responsiveness of the 30- to 40-year-old woman is determined primarily by biological or psychological factors. Certainly, it may result from a gradual loss of inhibitions, and greater security about being acceptable and pleasing to the man. For women, learning and experience seem to be of greater importance in becoming a sexual being than for men, whose sexuality seems more closely organized around their biologic urges.

Sexually, the woman's response to menopause is quite variable, and depends on her emotional state and the relationship with her partner. The abrupt end of menstruation produces a drastic decrease in the levels of two hormones, estrogen and progesterone. In some women, this is accompanied by irritability, depression, and large swings in mood. (A few women experience similar periods of tension during their monthly "mini-menopause"—the eight-day period around menstruation that also is characterized by a drop in estrogen and progesterone levels.)

On the other hand, increased irritability is by no means the same as decreased desire. In fact, from a physiological standpoint, desire should *increase* at menopause. The reason is that another hormone, androgen, which is responsible for sexual desire in women *and* men, decreases very slightly at menopause, while estrogen, which tends to cancel out androgen, decreases sharply. Some women do, in fact, seek increased sexual activity at these times, but this, of course, depends to a great extent on the attitude (and availability) of a partner.

Past menopause, women experience great variations in sexual responsiveness. Women now depend for sex on a dwindling supply of men, whose own sexual needs may have declined markedly. A woman who maintains regular sexual activity tends to maintain her sexual responsiveness; otherwise, sexuality declines significantly. Apart from the effects of opportunity, a gradual physical decline in sex seems to occur in women as well as men, but more slowly. Vaginal lubrication tends to be less prompt, and orgastic contractions become less vigorous and frequent, declining from five to seven contractions at age 30 to two or three at age 70. The general physiological heightening that accompanies sexual excitement becomes less pronounced, and erotic sensations seem to become less intense.

In sharp contrast to men, however, elderly women remain quite capable of enjoying multiple orgasms; in fact, studies indicate that 25 percent of women 70 years old masturbate. Nevertheless, many women cease to have intercourse during their 50s and 60s. Almost certainly, this abstinence arises from social and psychological factors. When elderly women lose their partners, they tend not to seek replacements unless they are unusually secure.

Sex and aging in men. Unlike women, whose sexual urges appear to rise gradually from puberty and peak at 35 to 45, men experience a sudden, dramatic increase of libido at puberty. In fact, in terms of sexual reactivity and potency, males reach their peak at 17 to 18 years of age, and decline thereafter.

At 17 to 18 years, the length of the refractory period (the time between an orgasm and the next erection) can be less than a minute. Erection is practically instantaneous upon almost any kind of stimulation, mental or physical: young men often are embarrassed at being stimulated to erection just by the vibrations of riding a bus. The frequency of orgasm also is high: four to eight orgasms a day are not uncommon. Detumescence, or emptying of blood from the penis, is slow, so the youth may retain much of his erection for half an hour or so after ejaculating.

From this peak, there is a gradual decline. The refractory period grows longer, more time or stimulation is needed to have an erection, the penis empties of blood more rapidly, and the number of orgasms needed to satisfy the man decreases. Sexual desire—at least, the desire to have sex as often as possible—also begins to diminish slowly.

Youth is a peak age for sexual fantasies and sexual thoughts in general; with age, the fantasies grow fewer. Physiologically, sexual pleasure in youth is sharply focused in the genital area; but as the man grows older, sexual pleasure becomes more generally sensuous and diffuse. Further, orgasm per se gradually assumes less importance. The force of the ejaculatory spurt diminishes, to a seepage in some cases, and some elderly men experience what Masters and Johnson call a "paradoxical refractory" period: if they lose an erection during foreplay, they require 12 to 24 hours before they can have another. It's just as though they had ejaculated.

Because the effects of sexual aging are so much more pronounced in men than in women, the quality of an elderly couple's lovemaking depends to a great extent on how they cope with the man's altered capabilities. When these limitations are properly viewed, the elderly couple can enjoy a fully rewarding sex life indefinitely.

The Biology of Sex

Because sex is a physical event, or at least the physical expression of desire, we need to know something about the biology of human sexuality in order to understand it properly. And the biology of sex involves the brain as well as the genitals.

Sexual Anatomy

Woman's anatomy. The genital organs of the woman are, primarily, the vagina, the vulva, and the clitoris; their anatomical relationship to the "reproductive" organs—the uterus—and to the bladder and excretory organs is shown on page 444. Note that the clitoris is surrounded by a fold of skin, the clitoral hood, which in turn is connected to the labia minora encircling the vagina. During coitus, the penis tends to move the labia minora, which causes the clitoral hood to move and thus stimulates the clitoris.

Man's anatomy. The genital organ of the man is, primarily, the penis. Its relation to the testicles, in which sperm are produced, and to the reproductive and excretory organs, is shown on page 203. The penis is composed of the glans, the shaft, and the base. At its tip is the glans, the most sensitive and erotically responsive part of the penis. At its base, the corpus spongiosum ends in a bulbous enlargement that contains powerful muscles; essentially, ejaculation consists of the rhythmic contractions of these bulbar muscles. Two other cylinders, the corpora cavernosa, are specifically adapted for erection. They consist of tiny caverns and a network of specialized blood vessels. Erection occurs when these caverns fill with blood.

The brain. Sexual desire seems to originate in certain centers of the brain. Unless these "sex centers" of the brain are active, a person does not experience desire or feel "sexy." And, of course, the brain mediates all of the emotions experienced in all aspects of sexuality, as well as most of the behavior patterns. In addition, involuntary reflexes, which in many cases need not involve the brain per se, sometimes can be controlled by cortical centers.

Sexual Physiology

Desire. Sexual desire is an appetite, which is physically similar to hunger, the appetite for food. One feels sexual desire only when certain parts of the brain are "turned on" or activated. In the case of sexual appetite or desire, the sex centers are "turned on" by a variety of factors: love, a certain time period, an attractive partner, etc. They also can be "turned off" by a variety of factors, both physical and emotional: anger, fear, depression, certain drugs, illnesses, and hormone deficiencies.

In humans, desire implies not only an urge for sex but also an urge to obtain reciprocity, an attempt to stimulate desire in the partner. This is exactly in accord with other mammals, where certain hormones produce estrus in the female and cause her to feel desire, and also secrete a substance that stimulates desire in the male. In animals, desire is triggered mainly by smell and special courtship behavior. Human sexual desire is not that simple, and involves complex emotional factors.

The expression of desire between two people is sex, or what we have been calling making love. For many people, love for one's partner makes sex more enjoyable, but it need not be present during actual lovemaking. However, it's normal for people having intercourse to feel affection for each other, though otherwise they might be indifferent. Even people who are active antagonists can have satisfying sex if they can set aside their antagonisms at least long enough for the required collaboration. Nor is it necessary for partners, even loving partners, to concentrate on each other during sex; images of different people or fantasies of having sex with others are quite common. What *is* necessary for pleasure in the sex act is the ability to give the erotic drive preference over other concerns, and to give the partner enough scope to do likewise.

Excitement. Physiologically, the principal goal of excitement is to prepare the partners for coitus, when the penis enters the vagina; it is to this end that the penis grows stiff and the vagina becomes lubricated. Since coitus involves strenuous activity, the bodies of both partners prepare themselves for unusual exertion; breathing becomes heavier, the heart beats faster, sending more blood to the organs; blood pressure increases; and many other changes occur.

Physiologically and psychologically, excitement lasts until orgasm, although sometimes it is divided into a preliminary phase and a plateau phase. Barring organic impairment, the physiological events are the same for most people. But in terms of attitudes, emotions, and behavior, the excitement phase can differ enormously among different people, and among the same people at different times.

Physical as well as emotional factors can interfere with the excitement phase. In women, a low estrogen level, such as occurs after menopause, may hinder lubrication of the vagina. In men, who need a high-blood-pressure system in the penis to achieve erection, certain drugs and illnesses can cause impotence. In both women and men, many psychological factors—in fact, any cause of fear or stress at the time of lovemaking—can interfere with the delicate reflexes that prepare the sex organs for intercourse.

Excitement in women. In women, the principal expression of excitement is genital swelling and lubrication of the vagina. This happens when the vaginal area becomes engorged with blood as a result of psychological and/or physical stimulation.

In its resting stage, the vagina is collapsed, quiescent, pale, and only slightly moist. But in response to stimulation (primarily of the clitoris), it expands and balloons into an internal "erection" that not only can accommodate an erect penis but also can stimulate it. The vagina enlarges just enough to hug the penis, regardless of penile size. While the vagina swells, capillaries in the circumvaginal plexus become filled or engorged with blood (a process known as vasocongestion) and the plexus expands, causing a secretion on the walls of the vagina. This is the "lubrication" that facilitates the entry of the penis.

As the woman's excitement grows, the walls of the uterus also become engorged with blood, and the uterus enlarges. It, too, begins to rise from its dormant position and lift out of the pelvic cavity, presumably in order to increase the likelihood of fertilization.

In addition to these largely internal and unperceived changes, engorgement and swelling of the lower external genital tract contribute to the woman's erotic pleasure and set the stage for her orgasm. Corresponding to vascular engorgement of the penis that causes erection in the male, the tissues that surround the vaginal opening become swollen and engorged, forming an "orgasmic platform." As excitement intensifies, the external tissues surrounding the vaginal entrance—the labia, the bulbs of the vestibule, the lower third of the vagina, and the perineum—become engorged with blood, brightly colored, and swollen and thickened.

Although the genitals of both women and men derive from the same embryonic tissue, there are sharp differences in the spread of the vasocongestive response. In men, vasocongestion is confined primarily to the penis; in women, it is more diffuse and less localized. Unlike men, women have no specific structures that fill with blood; rather, they experience a general swelling and engorgement of the internal and external genitals and the pelvic area. The thickening of the orgasmic platform results from the swelling of the blood vessels that surround the vaginal barrel and the bulbs of the vestibule. And vaginal lubrication is produced by local vasocongestion of the vaginal walls.

Excitement in men. In men, the principal expression of excitement is erection of the penis, produced by physical and/or psychological stimulation. In addition, the scrotum thickens and flattens out, and the testes begin to rise from their generally drooping position. During the peak of excitement but before orgasm and ejaculation, the penis excretes a drop of clear liquid (Cowper's fluid, which is not semen).

As discussed earlier, the penis consists of three "cylinders," the top two of which, the corpora cavernosa, are specifically adapted for erection. They contain tiny caverns and specialized blood vessels. When the penis is not erect, the caverns are collapsed and blood flows quietly through them. With erotic excitement, the veins in the penis open wide, and blood pours through them and into the caverns. The blood is prevented from running back by special valves that close by reflex action. The result is erection. When the valves do not close, or when they open too early, impotence occurs. Under normal circumstances, the valves close during excitement. Blood is pumped into the penis but cannot return. Under the pressure of the blood, particularly in the caverns of the corpora

cavernosa, the small, flaccid penis extends to the limits of its sheath, and also becomes hard and firm. The glans also enlarges but does not harden, which prevents it from hurting the woman when it enters the vagina.

Once erection has been attained, it can last for long periods of time. Indeed, it is this ability to maintain an erection without ejaculating that enables men to engage in erotic "courtship" activities, or foreplay, that are needed to prepare the more slowly aroused woman for intercourse. For most of his life, the man is physically capable of losing and regaining his erection several times during foreplay. With increasing age, however, it may take longer to regain an erection once it is lost.

Orgasm

It seems safe to say that no area of human sexuality has aroused more controversy, bred more myths, or inspired more ignorance masquerading as dogma than the area of orgasm—especially the female orgasm. Books have been written about women's orgasms, and often have managed only to add confusion to uncertainty. Fortunately, enough is known about orgasms in women (as well as in men) to provide a clear picture of what they are and what causes them. In both men and women, orgasm is produced by the contraction of genital muscles; and although male and female orgasms seem very different from each other, they actually share many similarities.

Orgasm in men. The male orgasm is designed to deposit semen deep into the vagina near the cervix of the uterus, where the possibility of fertilization is greatest. The orgasm itself has two phases, emission and ejaculation. Emission is entirely internal, and consists of the contraction of reproductive organs. The contraction is under the control of the autonomous (involuntary) nervous system, and cannot be brought under conscious control. The function of emission is to collect the various components of the ejaculate—the sperm and the prostatic fluid—from their storage depot in the seminal vesicles and deliver them to the bulbar urethra, in time to be expelled by the powerful ejaculatory mechanism.

Emission occurs a split second before ejaculation; and although men are not aware of the physiological events, they experience emission as a sensation of "ejaculatory inevitability," in the words of Masters and Johnson. From that point on, they cannot control ejaculation.

Ejaculation follows emission almost immediately: the bulbar muscles at the base of the penis begin to contract, involuntarily, at intervals of 0.8 second. These contractions squeeze the base of the penis and the urethra, forcing the semen, with its cargo of sperm, to spurt out. However, although ejaculation is an involuntary reflex, unlike emission it *can* be brought under voluntary control. In fact, most men who suffer from premature ejaculation can learn to control the ejaculatory reflex with the help of treatment.

Following orgasm, the blood drains from the penis, leaving it limp and flaccid. The man then enters a "refractory" period, during which he is physically unable to have another erection. The length of the refractory period varies with age and other factors, and can be as little as a minute (or even less) for a youth at the peak of sexual prowess, or as much as 24 hours (or more) for an elderly man.

Orgasm in women. In contrast to men, orgasm is relatively hidden in women, allowing them to hide their orgasms, or rather, their lack of orgasms. Clearly, both sexually and otherwise, the woman who fakes orgasms for her partner's sake may be doing herself an injustice. At the very least, it prevents her partner from knowing that he may not be providing adequate stimulation.

Physiologically, orgasm in women consists of reflexive, involuntary, rhythmic contractions of the muscles and thickened tissue surrounding the vaginal inlet—the pelvic muscles. Unlike the two phases of the male orgasm, emission and ejaculation, the woman's orgasm has only one phase that is analogous to ejaculation.

In the woman, the perineal, bulbar, and pubococcygeal muscles, the muscles of the perineal floor, and, to a lesser extent, the lower vaginal muscles (see page 225) contract rhythmically every 0.8 second against the thickened tissues surrounding the vagina. These contractions apparently are sensed by deep pressure proprioceptive receptors (organs that detect muscle and tendon movement), as well as by peripheral sensory receptors, to create the orgasmic experience.

The uterus also contracts during orgasm; however, women generally are not acutely aware of these contractions, except occasionally as a vague, diffuse, pleasurable feeling. Sometimes when the estrogen level is low (after menopause, for example), the uterine contractions may be painful—like menstrual cramps—to some women.

How many women have orgasms? Estimates vary widely. Kinsey believed that 90 percent of women ultimately were able to have orgasms during coitus; later researchers have found that only 35 percent of women had orgasms during coitus. Other clinical experience suggests that 8 to 10 percent of women have never had orgasms at all, and that of the remaining 90 percent, about half do not have orgasms during coitus by thrusting alone. In other words, it seems that less than half the women of America regularly have orgasms during intercourse through the unaided action of the penis; the others either do not have any orgasms, or need clitoral stimulation to bring orgasms about.

Do orgasms occur in the clitoris or the vagina? Although women lack an emission phase, orgasm in women is otherwise almost precisely analogous to orgasm in men. All orgasms occur at a peak of sexual excitement, and in most men this peak arises through stimulation of the glans and shaft of the penis. (Some men can have orgasms solely through fantasies, as can some women.) However, although it is the sensation in the glans and shaft that triggers the male

orgasm, the motor part of the orgasm actually occurs in the bulbar muscle. That is to say, stimulation of one part of the penis leads to orgasm in another part.

The mechanism is exactly the same in women. Erotic sensations and sexual excitement are felt in the clitoris (which is analogous to the glans of the penis), and this clitoral stimulation triggers orgasm. The motor part of the orgasm itself, however, occurs in muscles, as it does in men—the muscles in and surrounding the vagina. In fact, the rate of muscular contractions in women is exactly the same as in men, one about every 0.8 second.

So, for both women and men, orgasm is a reflex, and like every other reflex has both a sensory and a motor part: a part for sensation, the "itch," and a part for expression, the "scratch." In women, the sensation involves the clitoris; the expression, the muscular contractions of the vagina. "Vaginal orgasms" really are the same as "clitoral orgasms," and women who experience "vaginal" orgasms—without direct clitoral stimulation—are not necessarily more mature or less neurotic than those who need direct clitoral stimulation. Nor are there personality correlations associated with the need for clitoral stimulation. The woman who enjoys or needs direct clitoral stimulation is neither more nor less erotic, intelligent, mature, free of sexual hang-ups, neurotic, or angry at men than the woman who climaxes on coitus alone. In fact, the woman who can enjoy the greatest variety of sexual stimulation is probably sexually the most free.

Although orgasm generally is considered to be the climax of the sexual experience, the muscular contractions that typify orgasm really don't signify the end of lovemaking. Strictly speaking, lovemaking does not end until the bodies of the woman and man return to their normal or resting state.

For most women, sexual desire after orgasm ebbs gradually, in concert with a more gradual return of the body to its resting state. As a consequence, although many women feel satisfied after an orgasm, many others would welcome further stimulation and more orgasms. The desire for multiple orgasms does not mean that the initial orgasm was inadequate, nor that a multiple-orgastic woman is sexually superior to one who is content with a single climax.

Sexual Problems

Sexual problems are not a disgrace or a cause for shame or guilt, and by no means are they always associated with major emotional problems. Many couples live together for all of their lives with one or both of the partners in some way "dysfunctional." And there are some sexual conditions that are not considered dysfunctions at all, although popular mythology may hold them to be. Primary among these are partners not having simultaneous orgasms and, for the woman, not having orgasms during intercourse. As already mentioned, these conditions are well within the range of normality. It also is normal for a woman not to have an orgasm every time she has intercourse or to desire multiple orgasms as often as possible, just as it is normal for men occasionally to experience impotence.

Dysfunctions can occur in any of the three stages of sexual activity: desire, excitement, or orgasm.

Lack of Desire

Lack of desire can be global or situational in nature. That is, the individual may never or only very rarely desire sexual pleasure (global lack of desire), or may find herself or himself "turned off" only under certain circumstances or with certain partners (situational lack of desire). In addition to some illnesses and drugs, depression may inhibit sexual desire. Anger or hostility also is a common cause of lack of sexual interest. Finally, anxiety and fear—fear of rejection, fear of intimacy, unconscious guilt originating in childhood, and fear of sex with the opposite gender—are other factors that may be present when sex has gone out of a relationship.

Dysfunctions of Excitement

In women and men, dysfunctions of excitement are characterized physiologically by a failure or deficiency of the vasocongestive response. In women, the dysfunction of excitement is lack of arousal, or frigidity; in men it is impotence.

Lack of arousal. The inhibited woman derives little if any pleasure from sexual stimulation; she essentially is devoid of sexual feelings. On a physiological level, she may show no signs of genital vasocongestion in response to sexual stimulation, or she may respond only partially, with light vaginal lubrication, and then only because the thrusting penis produces a "mechanical" reaction. On the other hand, some inhibited women do enjoy the nonerotic physical aspects of sexual contact, the touching and closeness that accompany coitus.

Further, although there is no necessary connection between inhibition of the excitement phase and orgastic dysfunction, such women usually are anorgastic as well. Still, some women appear to have orgasms even while lacking both the psychological signs of excitement and the physiological signs, including lubrication.

Finally, women who suffer from inhibition of the excitement phase can be divided into two classes: those with a primary problem, who have never experienced erotic pleasure with any partner in any situation; and those whose problem is secondary, who have experienced sexual pleasure at least to some extent. Typically, women with secondary problems were capable of being aroused by petting before they were married, but lost the ability to respond later when coitus became the supreme goal of sex.

Some women with secondary excitement-phase problems are unresponsive only in specific situations. They may be enraged or even nauseated by the prospect of intercourse with some partners, but feel instantly aroused, and become lubricated, when other men they find more attractive merely touch their hand.

Impotence. Impotence in men is analogous to lack of arousal in women. It, too, is characterized by an absence of the vasocongestive response: the impotent man does not have an erection, or loses his erection before penetration. Also, just as frigidity occurs in primary and secondary forms, so does impotence. Men who suffer from primary impotence have never been potent with a woman, although some may have good erections by masturbating and even have spontaneous erections in other situations. Men with secondary impotence previously have been potent.

Although about 85 percent of cases of impotence are psychological in origin, many are not. The normal need for additional stimulation of the penis as men age is sometimes interpreted as impotence, but of course it is not. However, certain diseases, such as diabetes mellitus, thyroid disorders, and multiple sclerosis, can cause symptoms of impotence in some men. Certain drugs, such as those used in the treatment of high blood pressure, also can cause men to become impotent. In addition, some men (though not many) are born with or develop medical problems that prevent the penis from erecting. Such an impotent man often can still ejaculate. Where organic problems play a role, the impotence may be only partial, and the man may be able to have usable erections.

Dysfunctions of Orgasm

In women, the basic orgasmic dysfunction is the inability to have orgasms. In men, there are two orgastic dysfunctions, premature ejaculation and retarded ejaculation.

Lack of orgasm in women. Orgastic difficulties probably are the most prevalent sexual complaint of women, and also the one that causes the most confusion. The inability to have an orgasm may arise primarily from physiological reasons (insufficient clitoral stimulation) or from psychological reasons. Both causes may be working at the same time: the woman is not stimulated enough *and* she is too anxious or angry to relax.

The amount of stimulation required to bring about orgasms varies enormously. The same woman may climax easily during coitus with a beloved partner, yet require lengthy, direct clitoral stimulation when making love with someone she does not care for.

Physiological differences among women may provide part of the answer, but it's likely that psychological and cultural factors play a tremendous—and probably decisive—role in facilitating or inhibiting the woman's orgasm.

Vaginismus. Vaginismus is a conditioned spasm of the muscle surrounding the vaginal entrance that prevents penetration. The vaginal opening literally closes so tightly that intercourse is impossible. Hence, vaginismus is a common cause of unconsummated marriages, often lasting many years, even though it is one of the dysfunctions most successfully treated.

In addition to the physical symptom, women with varying degrees of vaginismus usually are phobic regarding coitus and penetration, and intercourse usually is painful. On the other hand, they are not necessarily frigid or anorgastic, and many are sexually responsive. They may be orgastic upon clitoral stimulation, enjoy sexual play, and seek sexual contact—as long as it does not lead to intercourse.

Premature ejaculation. In men, the most common sexual dysfunction is premature ejaculation, failure to establish voluntary control over the ejaculatory reflex during intense sexual excitement. Estimates of the number of men who are premature ejaculators range as high as 90 percent. No real connection has been found between prematurity and any kind of neurosis: premature ejaculators can be perfectly normal otherwise, while highly neurotic men can have superb ejaculatory control.

Retarded ejaculation. The man with retarded ejaculation has no problem with erections but finds it difficult or impossible to have orgasms, especially during coitus. Although in rare cases, retarded ejaculation may have an organic component, in the overwhelming majority of instances, it is caused by psychological problems alone. This is attested to by the great variety of situations in which retarded ejaculation is seen to occur.

Some men have retarded ejaculation only with certain women, and have normal ejaculations otherwise. A more common situation is when the man cannot reach orgasm *during intercourse,* even though he makes every effort to do so, and even though he may be able to ejaculate on manual or oral stimulation by the same partner. Other men become inhibited at the mere touch of their partner, and have to withdraw from coitus and masturbate themselves to orgasm, with the woman looking on. Some men cannot even tolerate the presence of a woman, and must go off alone before they can masturbate to ejaculation. And finally, there are some men, very few, who have never had an orgasm under any circumstances.

Physical Causes

Although the majority of sexual problems are psychological in origin—lying within the individual, the relationship, or both—many are attributable to physical or "medical" factors. Under this heading are included drugs, illnesses, and stress and depression.

Psychoactive Drugs

Considerable information and misinformation exists on the effects of different drugs on libido and performance, but in most cases the results are ambiguous. If any general conclusion can be drawn, it is that the moderate use of certain drugs possibly may enhance desire, but the heavy, frequent, or addictive use of any drug is practically certain to depress libido and hinder sexual performance.

Alcohol. Alcohol is the drug most frequently taken by Americans. Its basic effect is that of a depressant; it decreases the activity of brain centers responsible for anxiety. Although there is no evidence that alcohol actually stimulates sexuality, in small amounts it may help the user to lose some inhibitions and so to become more aware of sexual feelings and more able to act on them. In large amounts, however, alcohol depresses behavior in general, including sexual behavior. Typically, libido and performance both suffer.

Barbiturates and similar drugs. Barbiturates, sedatives, tranquilizers, and other "downers" have effects similar to those of alcohol: small doses may release inhibitions, but large doses tend to depress sexual behavior.

Marijuana and other hallucinogens. The effects of marijuana, LSD, and similar drugs on sexuality are unclear. Some users claim that they increase desire and/or pleasure—the latter because of heightened awareness of bodily sensations. Other users report no such responses, and still others say that hallucinogens lower their libido and reduce their interest in sex. The only sure conclusion is that the sexual response to hallucinogens is wholly individual and unpredictable.

Cocaine and amphetamines. Users of cocaine and amphetamines report, with some consistency, that sex is more exciting and desire more insistent when these drugs are taken in moderate dosages. However, the addicted person tends to crave the drug more than sex, and his or her libido usually is lowered. This pattern seems to continue as dosage increases.

Narcotics. Narcotics of all kinds are known to depress sexual desire, and may cause the symptoms of impotence in men.

Illness

Some illnesses, or the medications involved in their treatment, also have a negative effect on sexual desire or functioning. Almost always, it is the man who is most affected, since the erection of the penis is physiologically more complicated than vasocongestion of the vaginal area.

Diabetes. Diabetes mellitus causes the symptoms of impotence in many of its male victims. In fact, the onset of diabetes often is first signaled by problems with erections, which should prompt a physical examination and initiate the steps necessary for maintaining general health. Some men report total erectile failure; others report a range of difficulties, from only slight loss of stiffness to almost complete flaccidity. However, even though erectile problems may exist, the man usually retains his ability to have orgasms and to ejaculate. With counseling and a good relationship, the diabetic couple can have highly gratifying sexual experiences.

High blood pressure (hypertension). The drugs used in treating hypertension are lifesaving, but unfortunately often cause erectile problems in men. In addition, vascular problems in the penis may interfere with the erection mechanism in patients with high blood pressure. Other relatively unusual conditions and medications that also may cause or contribute to loss of potency or loss of libido include endocrine, liver, and neurologic problems. If either loss of potency or loss of libido seems to occur in an otherwise healthy relationship, the affected partner should have a physical examination by a physician who is expert in evaluating sexual problems.

Depression

Depression, stress, and fatigue can profoundly damage sexuality, and masked depression and tension states frequently are underlying causes of sexual dysfunctions. When a patient is severely depressed, sex is the furthest thing from his or her mind. Even moderately depressed patients lose interest in pursuing sexual activity and are very difficult to arouse. So are men and women who have been under chronic and relentless fatigue and stress, such as involved in active combat or the emotional crises attending a difficult divorce or a job loss.

The mechanism by which such emotional states impair sexuality is not clearly understood. However, it is known that depression retards all functions that preserve both self and species. Thus, the depressed person loses his appetite, suffers from constipation and sleep disturbance, experiences a slowing of thinking and movement, and is impaired in other vital functions. Not surprisingly, then, depression also has a devastating effect on sexual functioning. The pain of depression extinguishes libido, makes the depressed person resistant to arousal, and actually may impair vasocongestive sexual response. Erection in the male is especially vulnerable. There is some evidence that hormonal as well as psychological factors may play a role in the diminished sexuality of depressed patients.

Psychological Causes

The psychological origins of sexual dysfunctions can be either superficial or deep, and derive from the individual's personal problems or from difficulties in the relationship.

Superficial Problems

The four most common superficial problems that may cause sexual problems are fear of failure, demand for performance, excessive need to please the partner, and a condition termed "spectatoring." All, in effect, are different manifestations of one underlying cause— anxiety.

Fear of failure. Anticipation of being unable to perform the sexual act is perhaps the greatest immediate cause of impotence and, to some extent, of orgastic dysfunction as well. Once a man has experienced an episode of erective failure, the worry that it will happen again may cloud subsequent sexual experiences. Not surprisingly, the worry often is accompanied by fear, and by the tendency to concentrate attention on the state of his erection, which ensures the fulfillment of the prophecy. In effect, a vicious cycle is set up, which can perpetuate itself indefinitely. Generally speaking, fear of failure afflicts men more than women.

Demand for performance. Closely related to the sexual difficulties resulting from fear of failure are those that frequently follow a command or request to perform sexually. Not uncommonly, the sexual history of an impotent man reveals that the initial episode of erective failure occurred when the man attempted coitus at a partner's demand. But erections just don't work that way. A guilt-provoking or hard-to-refuse request for sex may create such conflict, fear, or anger in a person that sexual responsiveness in that situation is totally precluded. As with fear of failure, the demand for performance is particularly damaging to men. A woman can fake excitement (without lubrication) as well as orgasm, and so at least can simulate sexual performance, but a man cannot fake an erection.

Demands for sexual performance may result in transient episodes of impotence that may escalate via the fear of failure mechanism into serious impotence of the male, or into a habitual response pattern in the woman. Similarly, the demand for coital orgasm in a woman who has difficulty producing this response pattern may have a very destructive effect on her sexual adequacy. Unfortunately, it is not always the partner who makes demands on an individual; often enough, the demands for super-performance are self-imposed.

Excessive need to please the partner. The wish to give enjoyment and pleasure to the partner is not only desirable and healthy, but is a prerequisite for good lovemaking. However, the *compulsion* to please, to perform, or to serve—and not to disappoint—can be a severe source of disruptive emotion.

The other side of the need to please is the fear of rejection, and women are particularly vulnerable to rejection anxiety. Often a result of low self-esteem as well as desire to please, rejection anxiety has destroyed the sexual adequacy of many women.

Spectatoring. To enjoy good sex, one must be able to suspend all distracting thoughts and lose oneself in the erotic experience. People who are anxious about sexuality frequently remain outside themselves, keep tight control over their emotions, and continually observe their own sexual reactions—a practice that Masters and Johnson have termed "spectatoring." The tendency to preside as a judge of one's own lovemaking is highly destructive to sexuality. Spectatoring is very often evoked by other problems: the man with fear of failure or performance anxiety will monitor himself to make sure that he is "up to par"; the woman with rejection anxiety will constantly scan the total event to make sure that nothing "bad" is happening. The result is to prolong—not correct—the dysfunctional condition.

Deep Problems

Of course, more severe neurotic problems and profound sexual conflict also can result in sexual dysfunctions. These are rooted in early childhood and cause the afflicted individual to sabotage his or her own sexual happiness and fulfillment. Most sexual problems are multi-causal, the result of combinations of various circumstances and problems.

Interpersonal Problems

These are the problems that can turn two apparently "normal" and well-matched partners into fighting, bickering, enraged antagonists. Of the wide range of interpersonal problems, several are common.

Lack of trust. A trusting, loving relationship is essential to good sexual functioning. For a woman, a feeling of trust seems necessary for her to abandon herself to sexual pleasures. In fact, recent evidence indicates that trust may be one of the most important factors in determining orgasic capacity in women. Lack of trust may have originated in a woman's early upbringing, in which case it is an intrapsychic problem. Or, a woman may find herself in a relationship that just isn't conducive to trust. The frustration of one partner by the other in the sexual sphere is especially conducive to lack of sexual trust.

Power struggle. Violent power struggles transpire between some couples. Often each partner is entirely unaware of the struggle, yet each is dominated by the need to control the other, and conversely to avoid being dominated. Incredible anger and rage may be mobilized by power struggles. When such a struggle is a dominant theme in a couple's relationship, other important life goals become secondary. Thus, one or both partners may sacrifice his or her sex life to gain control over the other, or to avoid being dominated.

"Contractual" disappointments. The "marriage contract" concept is often useful in understanding and resolving hostilities and anxieties that get in the way of good sexual functioning. When we get married, we psychologically sign a marriage contract—"to love, honor, and obey, till death do us part." Some of the terms are consciously agreed upon (such as household work and budget maintenance) but most of the terms are beyond the awareness of both parties. For example, a couple's behavior may be governed by such covert agreements as: "I will buy you beautiful things and take care of you; in return, you will put me first in all things. (If you make me jealous, I will deprive you.)" When such contracts work, the marriage is a happy one. Trouble occurs when these contracts are mutually contradictory or impossible to fulfill. Then, if one partner gives according to the contract but fails to receive in return, he or she may become enraged and depressed without clearly understanding why. And sexual problems may result.

Failure of communication. Poor communication often contributes to and perpetuates sexual difficulties. To be an effective lover, one must know what excites the other, what turns him or her off, and how the other is responding as they are making love. Sexually dysfunctional couples often fail to effectively communicate with each other about these matters. They operate in the dark or, even worse, are guided by false assumptions about their partner's sexual responses.

Such communicative difficulties may stem from a variety of causes. Commonly they arise from culturally induced attitudes of shame and guilt. At other times, the failure to communicate is rooted deeply in the relationship. Such couples have general communication difficulties, and lack of openness in the sexual area is just one part of the larger problem. But whatever the cause, ignorance of the partner's sexual personality that results from poor communication is a prominent factor in sexual problems.

Intrapsychic problems, or the individual's psychic problems, may be superficial or profound, or at some intermediate level. For our purposes, we can think of superficial problems as those that are readily resolvable by sex therapy with little or no need for "depth psychology" approaches. Deeper problems are those that may require some or substantial amounts of therapy that elucidates hidden emotional factors.

Most modern specialists in sex therapy do not attempt complete resolution of profound intrapsychic problems when they occur in sexually dysfunctional patients. Rather, the therapist attempts to offer just enough insight, or awareness, or ability to bypass the intrapsychic inhibition, to allow the therapy to proceed. In the majority of cases, this is indeed possible, and the patient is discharged from sex therapy with the sexual dysfunction resolved, even though the more profound problem may remain. In other cases, the basic problem must be resolved first.

Treating Sexual Problems

Resolving a particular sexual problem depends first on pinpointing its cause. Is it primarily physical or psychological in origin? Physical causes sometimes can be solved by medical and drug therapies, or by surgery; clearly, such treatment can be offered only by qualified physicians. And, depressed and anxious patients whose problems are psychologically rooted frequently must be given medication for their depression before they can respond to sexual therapy.

Psychosex and Therapy

Until the publication in 1970 of *Human Sexual Inadequacy* by Masters and Johnson, the occurrence of sexual problems was generally considered a side effect of a more profound intrapsychic problem. Thus, treatment of the sexual dysfunction per se generally was not undertaken; instead, it was assumed that the sexual difficulty would be resolved along with the underlying difficulty. This usually meant "deep" analysis. The two disadvantages of this approach were that relief of the sexual dysfunction often did not automatically follow resolution of the deep problem, and that usually very long periods of time were required for treatment.

Modern treatment of sexual problems employs the principles of brief therapy. It attempts to alleviate the sexual symptoms directly without trying to reconstruct the couple's relationship or even the entire personality of either partner. Brief therapy consists of a combination of sexual exercises and psychotherapy. The exercises are designed to modify the couple's specific problem, such as anorgasmia or lack of desire, and are carried out in the privacy of the couple's home. Any emotional problems, conflicts, or misunderstandings that these exercises evoke are then discussed in office sessions with the therapist.

A great many couples are helped by these brief psychosexual treatment methods. But some, whose sexual problems are the product of the deeper kinds of intrapsychic or relationship difficulties already mentioned, require more extensive help.

Aging

We have previously described the course of sexual development in women and men, including the changes brought about by age. To repeat: aging appears to affect the sexuality of men more than of women. Among the changes it brings are a greater length of time required to regain an erection once it has been lost (sometimes up to 24 hours longer) and the need for greater direct stimulation of the penis to produce an erection initially. Do these changes imply a diminution of sexual satisfaction? The answer, broadly speaking, is that a couple can adjust to the loss of the man's physiological capability without any lessening of the *quality* of the sexual relationship. Indeed, sexuality can become more sensuous and pleasurable when the ejaculatory pressure becomes less urgent.

The principal barriers to the full enjoyment of sex among the elderly are psychological, and originate in the diminished self-concept experienced by men and women in a youth-oriented society that has unfortunate attitudes concerning the elderly.

This is especially true of men. A man in his middle fifties can no longer avoid facing the idea of death or of his own limitations. Socially and in business, he may feel his power and authority slipping, and see his place taken by younger men. His energy level may decline, leaving him less capable of physical exertion. At the same time, he may think others treat him as a diminished being, more and more irrelevant to the important business of life. Of course, he is acutely aware that society views sex in the elderly as ludicrous. If the aging man doesn't have exceptional inner resources and above all a supportive, encouraging relationship, depression and anxiety may result, leading to the "superficial" intrapsychic problems noted earlier: fear of failure, performance anxiety, and spectatoring. These, in turn, may lead to impotence and/or loss of desire.

The woman, in turn, becomes anxious about her husband's sexual decline and may falsely attribute it to the loss of her youthful appearance. She reasons that she must be unattractive, and is therefore rejected as a sexual partner.

With adequate communication, these attitudes might never occur. But unfortunately, such a man and woman typically do not communicate. They enter a conspiracy of silence, and the combination of anxiety and lack of communication can destroy their sexuality. It is difficult for a woman to be generous, seductive, and responsive if she thinks the man is slow because he is indifferent to her.

For these couples, knowledge, communication, and concern create a marvelous therapy. The man can help the woman have multiple orgasms, manually or orally, even though he has only one (or none) himself. And the woman can explore new forms of stimulation and sexual activities with the aging man. Couples can learn ways of using the differences and changes to enhance their closeness and increase the pleasure they can give each other. Lovemaking techniques can accommodate each partner's changing needs, and the relationship can be enriched by a sensitive and mutually generous adaptation of each partner to the other.

Thus, with new trends in sexual therapy, and with a modern view of sexuality and a knowledge of the reality of sexual functioning, a man and woman can and should look forward to sexual fulfillment throughout their life together.

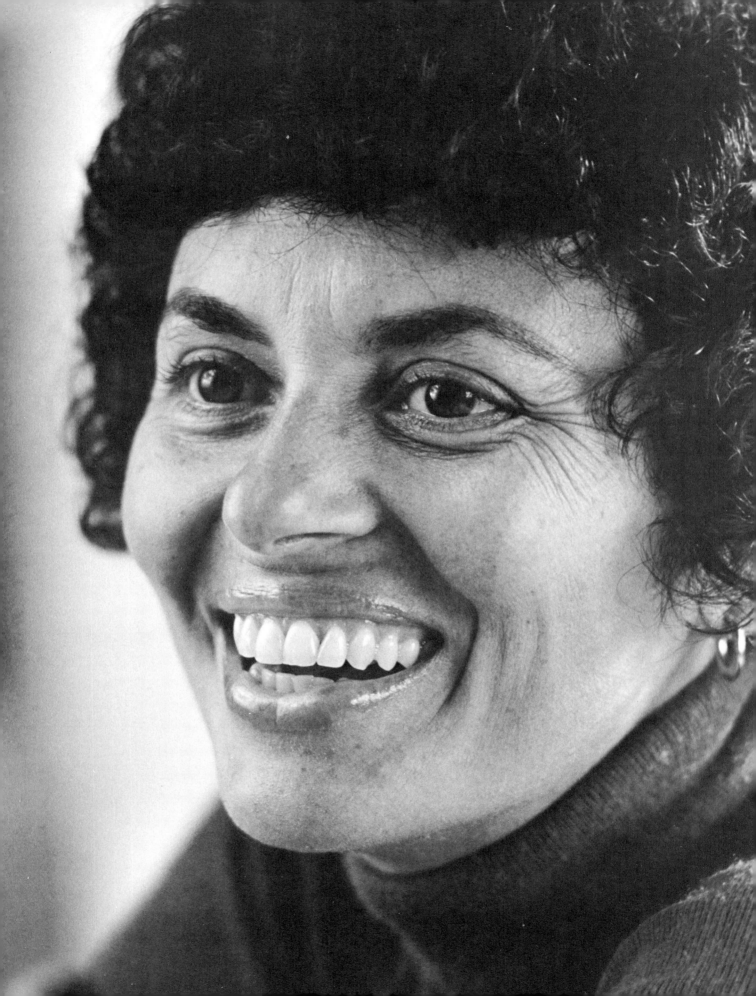

CHAPTER 9

BREASTS

NANCY COOPER HUBBELL

Breasts are uniquely feminine parts of our bodies, and as such are associated with beauty, sexuality, motherhood, and health throughout our lives.

As babies, girls, and women, we can see our breasts change—from their early swelling during puberty to their decrease in size in old age. Our breasts react to hormonal changes associated with the menstrual cycle, and to other changes in our lives. During pregnancy and nursing, our breasts are the source of food for our babies.

An understanding of the structure, function, and health of the breasts can give us an even greater appreciation of this important aspect of our femininity.

Breasts

Of all the external signs of the female form, breasts are the most visibly distinguishing feature of our sex. When we speak of normal breasts, we generally understand "normal" to mean breasts that are healthy and free of disease, without regard to whether they are large or small, sagging or budding, pendulous or rounded. Yet, every woman, from the time her breasts begin to develop, is quite sensitive to the look and feel of her own breasts, as well as to the perceptions and judgments of others.

Ideally, the state of having normal, healthy breasts would include both the absence of disease and a clear, self-accepting image of our breasts. But because a woman's attitude toward her breasts in health and disease is so heavily influenced by society, it's not possible to discuss normalcy without considering the complex interrelationship of physical, psychological, and social factors that shape our sense of what is normal. Consider, for example, the image of breasts and sex in our culture.

We may know from our own experience that breasts can be sexually stimulated, or that we feel our femininity is related to breast size and shape, but we're constantly confronted with an exaggeration or distortion of these feelings whenever we move outside of our own experience. In popular American culture, the breasts are a symbol of sex; the media stereotype is one of large, firm, exposed breasts that are essentially sexual playthings. The danger of such a stereotype is that it may lead us to think that breasts can be healthy and normal only if they correspond to this image.

Another common image is that of the nursing breast. This powerful image of a baby at its mother's breast, where the breast symbolizes mothering and nurturing, has been recorded throughout human history, and evokes for many women the pleasurable feelings associated with nursing an infant.

In the mid-twentieth century, a frightening image of the breast has arisen—that of the malignant breast. Breast cancer is taken up in detail in the chapter on "Breast Disease." All of these images are interrelated and confront us frequently—whether on television, in newspapers and magazines, in social interactions, or in our private reflections. It's small wonder that we are all concerned about our breasts.

Each specific concern that a woman has regarding her breasts reflects the complex nature of these interrelated images. Take, for example, the simple question of whether or not to breast-feed. A woman who is considering breast-feeding her newborn baby will perhaps think first of whether or not nursing her child will change the appearance of her breasts, and her

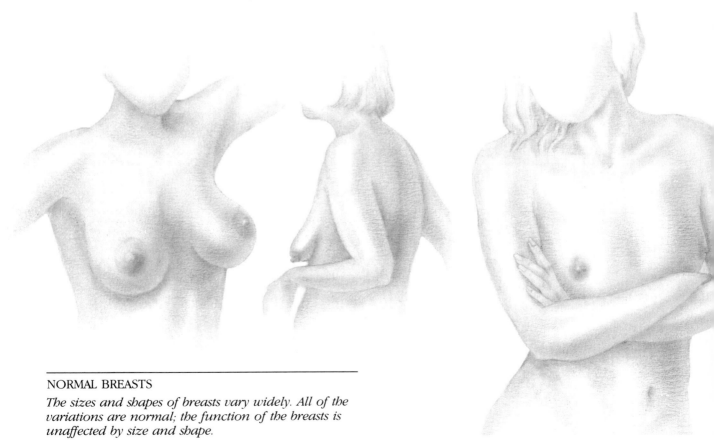

NORMAL BREASTS

The sizes and shapes of breasts vary widely. All of the variations are normal; the function of the breasts is unaffected by size and shape.

decision is immediately colored by the cultural norms of beauty she has absorbed throughout her life. She may consider how breast-feeding will affect her sexual relationship with her partner, again focusing on others' reactions more than on her own feelings and needs. Or she may wonder if breast-feeding is associated with breast disorders or diseases.

On another level, a woman's concern for her infant may prompt her to weigh the benefits of nursing in terms of the child's health and nutrition, psychological well-being, and the quality of the mother-child relationship in these early developmental months. Finally, she may reflect on what her parents and family want her to do, what her doctor recommends, or what her husband desires.

This discussion of the normal, healthy breast will help you relate your concerns about your breasts to your own feelings and needs. This is the first step toward developing a new sense of responsibility for your health and a positive attitude toward the beauty and function of your individual type of breasts. In turn, this awareness may help you to better enjoy your own sexual responsiveness, to feel confident in making decisions about breast-feeding, and generally, to positively claim and appreciate this significant aspect of womanhood.

Structure and Appearance

To best understand the structure of the breast, it's helpful to describe it in terms of its primary function for human survival—the production and delivery of milk to an infant. Likewise, an understanding of breast structure and development can help you resolve any questions or concerns you might have about the appearance of your breasts.

Structure of the Breast

The nipple delivers the milk to the baby. Typically, the nipple protrudes from the dark area surrounding it (the areola), but it may lie flat or it may be inverted (sunk into the areola). Regardless of the appearance of the nipple, it contains 15 to 25 small openings through which milk is conducted to its surface. The nipple is amply supplied with nerve endings and blood vessels. When the nipple is stimulated (for example, by the baby's sucking motions), blood flows to the vessels in the nipple causing it to become erect and protrude from the areola.

The areola is also a functional part of the breast. The little bumps in the areola are oil glands that enlarge

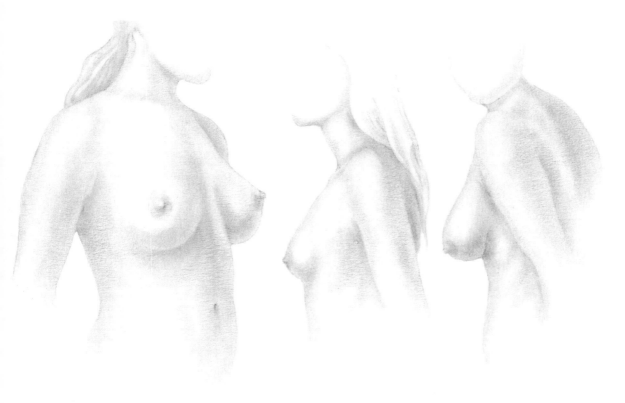

during pregnancy and secrete a substance that lubricates and protects the nipple during nursing.

Both the nipple and the areola are darker than the skin of the breast. This darker color apparently serves as a visual cue to the nursing baby; in order to bring milk from the reservoirs located directly behind the areola, the baby's mouth must encompass both the nipple and the areola. These reservoirs serve as storage pools for the milk that has made its way from the milk-producing glands located within the breast. When the baby sucks, the milk in the pools behind the areola is forced into the baby's mouth through the nipple. Each of the 15 to 25 openings on the nipple connects through a series of branching channels or ducts to its own milk-producing lobe. The milk is actually produced in these lobes in tiny structures called *alveoli.* The lobes do not become fully developed until pregnancy, when they enlarge to begin milk production.

The lobes are surrounded by *fat,* which provides protection for the delicate glandular tissue, gives mass to the breast, and provides its smooth contour. The amount of fat in the breast varies from woman to woman and accounts for differences in breast size.

The breasts are supported by *muscles* and *ligaments* that attach to the ribs, collarbone, and upper arm.

Development of the Breast

Breast development actually begins before birth. When you were born, the milk ducts in your breasts were already formed. Throughout childhood, they remained inactive, awaiting the stimulation necessary for their further development. This stimulation is provided by chemical substances called hormones, which are secreted into the bloodstream by the endocrine glands at the time of puberty; the pituitary gland and ovaries are endocrine glands that are instrumental in the development of breasts (see page 501).

The signal for development to begin comes from the pituitary gland, which stimulates the ovaries to increase production of the sex hormone, estrogen. The first sign of this increased production is the development of breasts, and it is at this point that we may first become concerned about their appearance. Development may be noticeable as early as age eight or nine or as late as age fifteen or sixteen, but it typically occurs between ages eleven and thirteen. In any case, some breast development will have taken place before the onset of the first menstrual period.

The first thing you will notice is that the nipple and areola will begin to stand out. Then the breasts themselves will begin to stand out from the chest. Growth of the ducts and lobes occurs from the nipple inward, with fat accumulating around the lobes to provide protection as they grow. The amount of fat accumulation determines how large your breasts will become.

As soon as breast development is under way, breast self-examination should be learned and practiced (see page 158). An early start will enable you to feel comfortable about touching and examining your breasts —a practice that should be continued throughout your life. Although it's very unlikely that you'll encounter any abnormalities during adolescence, examining your breasts from an early age will enable you to become so thoroughly familiar with how they look and feel to the touch that you'll instantly know when you see or feel something "abnormal."

Concerns About Appearance

Sizes and shapes of breasts vary widely (see page 148). All of these shapes and sizes are normal, and the function of the breasts is unaffected by such variation. Yet most of us are concerned at some time in our lives with the size and shape of our breasts. Some women feel embarrassed that their breasts are larger than they feel is normal or "acceptable," while others are concerned that their breasts are too small. And nearly every woman has compared her breasts from their earliest development to some "ideal" of current fashion, wondering whether her breasts conform to this ideal.

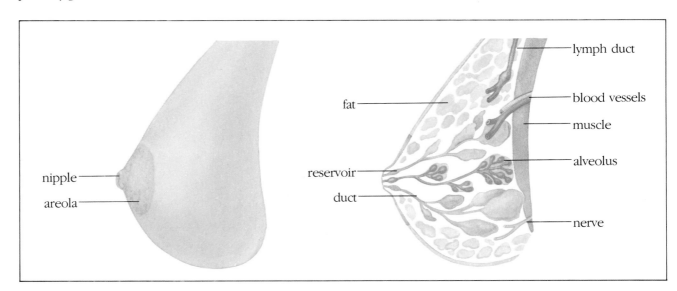

THE SUPPORTIVE STRUCTURES OF THE BREASTS

The breasts are supported by muscles and ligaments attached to the collarbone, the humerus or upper arm bone, the sternum, and the ribs.

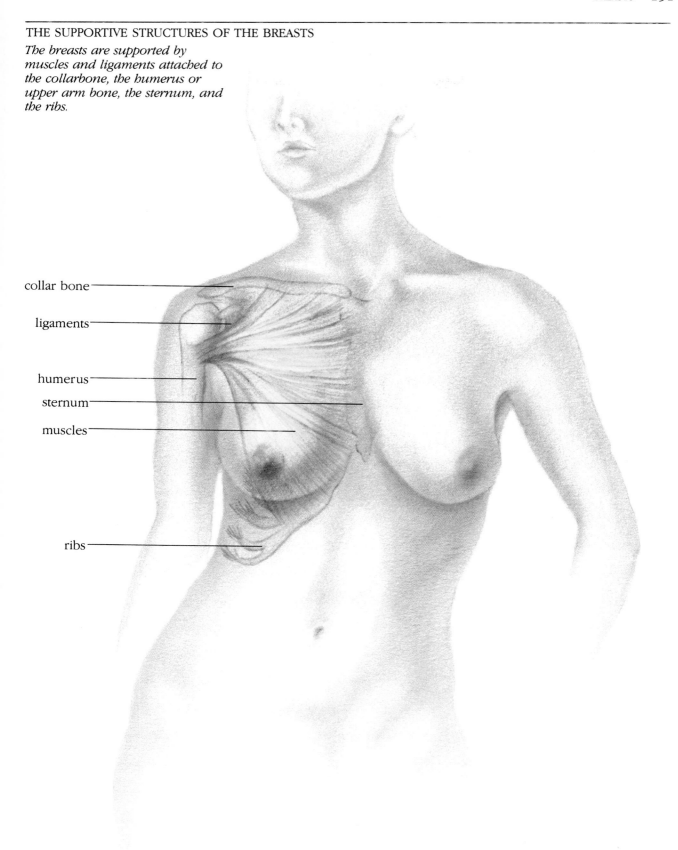

collar bone

ligaments

humerus

sternum

muscles

ribs

BREAST CHANGES THROUGH THE LIFE-SPAN

Breasts vary in shape and size through the life-span. Changes also occur in the nipples, areolae, and *lactation glands. The amount of fat in breasts varies, and accounts for differences in size.*

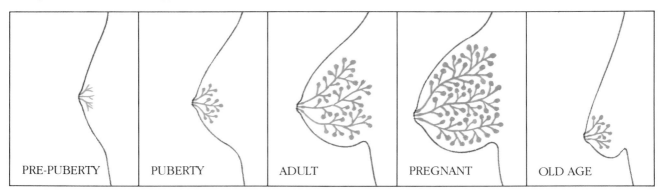

| PRE-PUBERTY | PUBERTY | ADULT | PREGNANT | OLD AGE |

In reality, your breasts needn't conform to any other standards than your own physical and mental sense of pleasure, health, and well-being. If your breasts are healthy and are functioning normally, then they should become part of your positive self-image—they're beautiful, as all healthy bodies are beautiful.

Although the amount of glandular tissue in your breasts has some effect on their size, fatty tissue accounts for most of this variation. The amount of fat in the breasts is determined in part by heredity, and in part by overall body size. A woman who is overweight may develop excess fatty deposits in her breasts, just as she will store excess fat in other areas of her body.

Since the amount of glandular tissue in the breasts continually varies with the level of the sex hormone estrogen in the normal monthly menstrual cycle, an increase or decrease in breast size often follows an increase or decrease of this hormonal level. In addition, the increased hormonal level that comes with pregnancy also results in an increase in the amount of glandular tissue in the breasts and, consequently, increased breast size (see above).

Breast sag concerns some women. As you will recall, the breasts are supported by muscles and ligaments. Whether or not they sag is partially dependent on the elasticity of this support structure, which in turn is affected by heredity, insofar as heredity influences the size, shape, and anatomy of the breasts and supportive tissue. As might be expected, small breasts or broad-based breasts are less likely to sag than large breasts or narrow-based breasts.

Wearing a bra can provide additional, external support to prevent breast sag. The question of whether or not to wear a bra is mostly a matter of comfort. A well-fitting bra may provide comfortable support, particularly for women who have large breasts and for women who are pregnant or breast-feeding. Exercises designed to tone the supporting muscles of the breasts also can help prevent breast sag (see pages 72). But because the strain on supportive tissue is greater during exercise, many women find it more comfortable to wear a bra while engaged in sports or physical activity.

Pregnancy and breast-feeding do not necessarily lead to sagging breasts, but since breasts do become heavier and larger during pregnancy, the extra support of a good bra may prevent undue strain on muscles and ligaments (see page 151).

Sexuality

Breasts are erogenous zones, and as such they enable us to experience many pleasurable feelings. Certain observable physiological changes take place in the area of the breasts during lovemaking, although women vary greatly in their subjective responses to breast stimulation. These responses run the gamut from women who reach orgasm through breast stimulation alone, to women who derive little or no satisfaction from such activity.

Masters and Johnson, in their book *Human Sexual Response,* describe the physiological changes that breasts undergo within the context of the four stages of lovemaking: the excitement phase, the plateau phase, orgasm, and resolution. These changes occur in conjunction with changes in other parts of the body, and result from increased muscular tension and the rush of blood to certain tissues during sexual excitement.

During the excitement phase, the nipples become erect and may transmit messages of excitation to other parts of the body. As blood rushes to the breasts in response to stimulation, the veins become more prominent and the breasts may increase in size.

The plateau phase extends the excitement phase. Blood continues to rush to the breasts, which may enlarge by as much as 25 percent. The areolae also may increase in size.

me and breasts of many women.

Just prior to orgasm, a pink flush appears on the chest and breasts of many women.

During the resolution phase following orgasm when muscular tension relaxes, the heart rate and blood pressure decrease and the flush goes away. The areolae and breasts gradually return to their normal pre-arousal state, but the nipples may remain erect for several hours.

The extent of our discussion of breasts as they relate to sexuality will depend upon how we define sexuality. If we define sexuality simply as a sensual, pleasurable experience that encompasses both physical and emotional gratification, we find that we are sexual beings in a number of different contexts. In other words, the changes described above can occur through self-stimulation as well as through lovemaking with a partner.

During breast-feeding, for example, some women experience some or all of these sexual responses—up to and including orgasm. Many more women might also experience this degree of arousal, had they not learned from attitudes of others that it represents an "inappropriate" response. Again, women's reactions vary greatly; most women who breast-feed experience feelings of physical and emotional gratification, but not sexual arousal. In any case, whenever breast-feeding is pleasurable for mother and baby, the mother-child bond is strengthened.

There is no "right" or "wrong" response in your experience of breast pleasure. Just be assured that whatever your body is feeling is private to you and is acceptable simply by being.

The Lactating Breast

Many useful books have been written to guide women who wish to breast-feed their infants. Breast-feeding is not the specific focus of this section; rather, we shall discuss the process of lactation (milk production) as a normal function of the breast.

Lactation—The Production of Milk

We have discussed the structures within the breast that secrete and deliver the milk, but what controls its production? The process of milk production is related to childbirth in a variety of ways. You will recall that the milk-producing lobes of the breast do not become fully operational until pregnancy, when they enlarge to begin milk production. These suitably developed lobes begin the actual production of milk when stimulated by a complex of lactogenic hormones (hormones that induce milk secretion).

Estrogen was responsible for stimulating the growth of glandular tissues of the breast during pregnancy, but estrogen also inhibits the production of milk. So once the growth of tissue is completed (around the fifth or sixth month of pregnancy), the ovaries decrease their production of the sex hormones estrogen and progesterone.

Milk Production in the Breasts

Pregnancy	
1 to 6 months	• Growth of glandular tissue in the breast
6 to 9 months	• Colostrum and milk-producing units (alveoli) increase in size and number
8 to 9 months	• Colostrum is produced in alveoli and may drip from the breast

Birth	
	• Colostrum is released through the nipple when baby sucks
	• Milk production in alveoli

Nursing	
2 to 3 days	• Milk letdown
	• Breast engorgement
3 days to 24 months, or until nursing ends	• Milk continues to be produced in alveoli
	• Milk is released through the nipple when baby nurses

The Milk Letdown Reflex

Positive environment

The milk letdown reflex is triggered by the baby sucking at the breast, or perhaps even by the sight, sound, or smell of a baby.

Negative environment

The milk letdown reflex may be "blocked" if the nursing mother experiences distraction, anxiety, fatigue, or embarrassment.

The hypothalamus signals the pituitary gland to release the hormone oxytocin into the bloodstream.

The hypothalamus receives "negative" nerve impulses, and blocks lactation hormones.

Systems function

Oxytocin reaches the breasts, where it causes the cells lining the alveoli to contract.

When the alveoli cells contract, milk is forced into the ducts, and then into the reservoirs behind the areola.

The baby's sucking causes milk to flow from these reservoirs into its mouth.

Systems fail

Baby receives milk

Baby does not receive milk

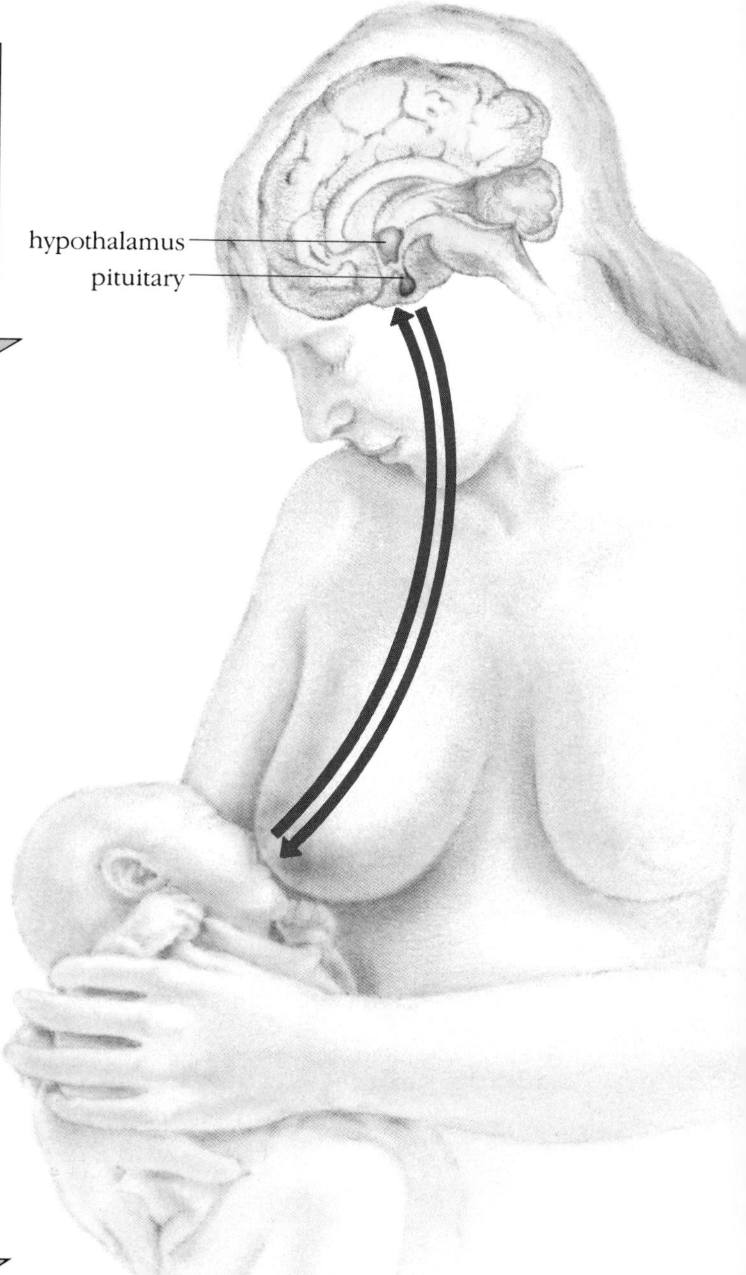

hypothalamus
pituitary

When the baby begins to nurse, messages go to the brain. In the brain, the hypothalamus sends messages to the pituitary gland, which, in turn, signals the breast to let down the milk.

At this time, the placenta (the organ through which the mother supplies oxygen and nourishment to the fetus) takes over hormone production, including production of a new hormone, human placental lactogen, which stimulates the development of alveoli.

You will remember that alveoli are the small sacs in the breast in which milk is produced. Once they are fully formed, the alveoli produce colostrum, which is the forerunner of the milk to come. (Late in pregnancy, this clear or yellowish liquid may drip from your breasts.) Colostrum differs from the milk secreted later in that it contains more protein, but both colostrum and milk contain antibodies that protect the newborn from disease. Your breasts will continue to produce colostrum until the milk yield begins, approximately three days after childbirth.

After delivery, the levels of estrogen and progesterone in your bloodstream decrease sharply—a signal for the hypothalamus (a major control center at the base of the brain) to allow the pituitary gland to release another hormone, prolactin. Prolactin stimulates the alveoli to produce milk.

Prolactin will continue to be released, and the alveoli will continue to produce milk as long as the breasts are suckled. In this way, the supply of milk is very conveniently controlled by the demand for it.

The Milk-Ejection Reflex

The release of milk from the breasts is controlled by the milk-ejection reflex (also called the letdown reflex). The nipple and areola contain receptors that respond to the mechanical pressure of the baby's sucking by sending nerve impulses to the hypothalamus. In turn, the hypothalamus signals the pituitary gland to release into the bloodstream another hormone, oxytocin.

Oxytocin flows through the bloodstream to the breasts, where it causes contractions of the cells lining the alveoli. These contractions force milk from the production site in the alveoli into the ducts. Contractions of the ducts continue to force the milk to the reservoirs behind the areola, and the baby's continued sucking brings the milk from the reservoirs into its mouth. Milk flow begins anytime from several seconds to several minutes after sucking begins.

Physiologically, the hypothalamus is informed by specific nerve impulses to begin the chain of events that results in the ejection of milk from the breasts. But the hypothalamus also is highly sensitive to emotional and psychological messages. Because of this sensitivity, the hypothalamus may trigger the milk-ejection reflex in the absence of nerve impulses set off by the baby's sucking. For example, once your body has experienced this reflex, you may eject milk at the mere sight, sound, or smell of a baby. Conversely, if you're under stress, the hypothalamus may fail to trigger the reflex despite your baby's sucking. Embarrassment, distraction, or fatigue are often sufficient to inhibit the milk-ejection reflex.

Other Effects of Lactogenic Hormones

Prolactin is maintained at high levels in the body as long as breast-feeding continues. But since prolactin tends to inhibit the function of the ovaries, most breast-feeding mothers do not ovulate or menstruate for several months after giving birth. Pregnancy, of course, is impossible without ovulation. However, lactation is *highly unreliable* as a method of birth control because it is impossible to predict when a particular woman will begin ovulating. Accordingly, as soon as a woman resumes intercourse following childbirth, she should consider some method of birth control. (Be aware that oral contraceptives inhibit the production of milk and thus may not be the best method to use at this time.)

Oxytocin, the hormone that induces uterine contractions, is involved at the time of labor and just after birth when the placenta is expelled. It continues to be produced during lactation, however, and helps the uterus to return more quickly to its normal size.

Care of the Lactating Breast

Breast support. Lactating breasts are subject to particular stresses that can be prevented or relieved by special care. As mentioned previously, wearing a supportive bra can provide a great deal of comfort as breasts get heavier toward the end of pregnancy.

You may purchase a nursing bra after the eighth month of pregnancy, since your breasts probably won't enlarge further. But be sure that the cup of the bra supports most of the weight, not the straps; if the straps leave indentation marks on your shoulders, the fit is not correct. Likewise the cups should not exert binding pressure on the breasts or nipples, and the band should fit snugly but, again, without binding. If the band "rides up" in the back, the fit is not proper.

Some nursing bras are fitted with plastic liners that prevent milk from leaking through your clothes, causing discomfort and embarrassment. On the other hand, plastic tends to trap moisture next to your skin and nipples, and can cause chapping. You might try a plastic-lined cup and, if chapping develops, simply remove the plastic liners.

Engorgement is a painful swelling of the breasts that may occur three to five days after the birth of your baby. The breasts may feel congested, hard, and tender to the touch. These symptoms are caused by the pressure of increased fluid in the breast tissue, as well as by increased blood circulation and the volume of milk being produced in the breast.

Some women choose to feed their babies "on demand" to relieve this sensation of engorgement. But the woman who is not nursing also will feel this discomfort until her milk "dries up." If the breast is not suckled, the alveoli will not be stimulated to produce milk and the engorgement gradually will subside. Until this happens, some doctors prescribe estrogen, by mouth or by injection, to inhibit milk production.

THE LACTATING BREAST

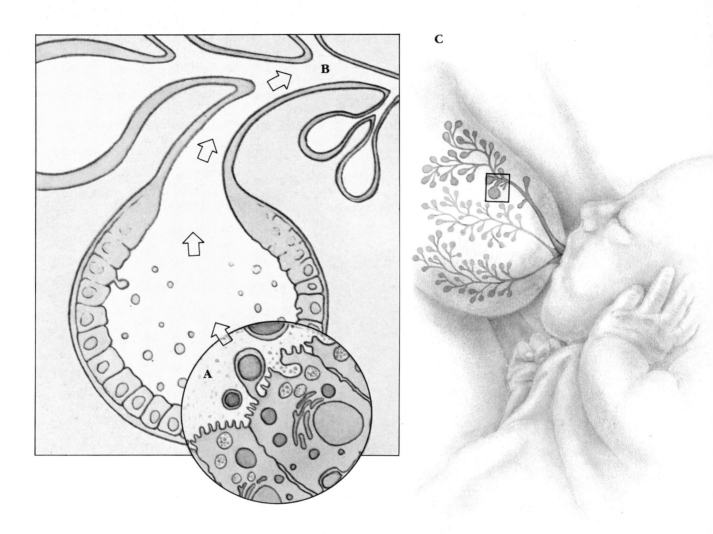

A *Cells lining the alvelolus produce milk, which is forced into the duct when the alveolus contracts.*

B *Contractions of the ducts then move the milk on its way to the reservoirs behind the areola.*

C *The baby's sucking brings milk from the reservoirs in the breast into its mouth.*

The following simple remedies may prove helpful for nursing and non-nursing mothers during this period of engorgement :
• Wear a bra that provides good support and doesn't bind the breasts.
• Ask your doctor about taking a mild pain reliever, such as aspirin. But remember that if you're nursing, any substance you ingest will reach your infant through your milk.
• Alternate applications of hot and cold compresses to ease the discomfort. To apply heat, wrap a hot water bottle in a towel, use a heating pad, or take a hot shower. (Do not use any heat compress for more than 20 to 30 minutes at a time, and never use it so hot that it can burn your skin.) Use ice packs for cold applications.
• Release (express) the milk manually from your breasts. With clean hands, place your thumb at the top of the areola and your fingers at the bottom; press gently backward, toward the chest wall. Continue this movement at different spots around the areola.

There may be times when you're unable to nurse your baby and thus relieve the pressure of engorgement. The baby may not be well, hospital regulations may space feeding times far apart, or you may be away for a single feeding when your baby also is able to feed from a bottle. At these times, you can express milk manually and still be ready when it is next time to feed your baby. In some cases, particularly before your milk supply has become regulated, the baby will not empty the breasts at each feeding. For this reason, it's important to alternate breasts at frequent intervals so that the baby doesn't leave you with one breast relaxed and the other engorged. You also can express milk manually after a feeding to be sure that your breasts are fully emptied and that you'll be comfortable until the next feeding.

Clogged ducts may cause small, tender, red lumps to appear on the breasts of a nursing woman. You can unblock the ducts and obtain relief by minimizing pressure on the affected area and by keeping the milk flowing. Again, alternate breasts frequently to assure that the baby is not exerting constant pressure on an affected duct. You also should be certain that your bra is not too tight, for it, too, can exert pressure on the ducts. Finally, you can nurse the baby for a longer period and feed it more frequently (assuming the baby will cooperate), and if necessary, empty the breasts manually after each feeding.

Sore nipples may cause you some discomfort early in nursing. To minimize it, late in your pregnancy take preventive measures to toughen the nipples and decrease their sensitivity. Wash the nipples briskly with a washcloth, roll them between your thumb and forefinger for a few minutes each day, rub them with a towel, or occasionally don't wear a bra.

Once you begin nursing, don't use anything harsh or drying on the nipples, including soap. Apply mild creams only if needed. Secretions from the areolae will keep the nipples clean and lubricated. To prevent chapping, keep the nipples dry and change bra linings frequently. And if your nipples are especially sensitive, don't use plastic bra liners.

Infection can be very painful and seriously disrupt or even halt your efforts to breast-feed. Unlike the discomfort of engorgement, the breast feels extremely heavy and "feverish." And rather than being relieved by the baby's sucking, the discomfort may be aggravated to the point where you won't want to nurse the baby at all.

Clearly, the best cure is prevention. Be sure that your nursing bras are clean and dry. Should you develop an infection, however, have it checked by your physician. If you are conscientious in your desire to breast-feed your child, the infant can probably be weaned to a bottle for a short time until you can again begin nursing. In fact, it's wise to introduce your baby to a bottle at some early point, just in case something happens to prevent your nursing for one or more feedings.

Health Care of the Breasts

From our discussion of the changes that occur as the breasts develop and perform their function of milk production, you've seen that the breasts are not static. They're constantly undergoing changes associated with different phases of the menstrual cycle and with different stages of life. As functioning, changing parts of your body, your breasts need continuing care and attention in order to remain healthy.

You Are Responsible

Finding a lump in a breast is the most common health concern women have about their breasts.

If you develop a lump in one of your breasts at some time in your life, it's very likely that you'll discover it yourself. In fact, 95 percent of breast lumps are self-discovered. This discovery most often occurs accidentally while a woman is bathing or dressing, rather than systematically while she is examining her breasts. Since so few lumps are initially discovered by doctors, it is clear that, whether you like it or not, you are responsible for the health care of your own breasts. But the fact remains: most women do not practice regular monthly breast self-examination.

Barriers to Overcome

Some of the psychological barriers to regular breast self-examination can be dealt with easily; others not so easily. For example, lack of information about the importance and the technique of breast self-examination is a barrier. Women who lack this information aren't likely to practice regular self-examination. This chapter and the "Breast Disease" chapter will provide information about the importance of breast self-examination, as well as the techniques of self-examination. You will learn what to look for, what to feel for, when to begin examining your breasts, and what changes you may expect throughout your lifetime. But if at all possible, you'll find it helpful to receive instruction in breast self-examination from a physician, a nurse, or another person who is trained to show you exactly how to examine your own breasts.

Our attitudes and feelings are barriers that may be more difficult to remove.

Many women will have to change a lifelong habit of placing the sole responsibility for their health upon their doctors. It's important to know that a doctor cannot monitor your breasts as closely as you can. He may examine your breasts only once or twice a year, and in doing so, he must take into account the wide variation among women's breasts. You, on the other hand, can become an expert on your own breasts. You can learn to detect any slight change in your breasts and can call it to the attention of your doctor. Your description of the difference you have found can be most helpful in establishing a diagnosis of a particular lump or suspected abnormality.

In addition, if your doctor doesn't examine your breasts as part of your regular checkup, don't feel hesitant about asking him to do so. It's his professional obligation to examine your breasts and to instruct you in the technique of self-examination.

Most of us fear finding lumps in our breasts because we equate lumps with cancer. Illogical though it may be, fear that we might find a lump may keep us from regularly examining our breasts. Knowledge can help overcome this fear. Actually the vast majority of lumps (around 90 percent) are *not* cancerous (see pages 545 and 546)

Don't be afraid. Learn the technique of breast self-examination and practice it regularly. It's not difficult, and you'll gain confidence as you learn the simple method and begin practicing it. The most effective way to protect yourself against breast cancer is to closely monitor your own breasts, bringing any abnormality to the attention of your doctor.

Some women may feel uncomfortable about touching their breasts or are embarrassed about seeking instruction in breast self-examination. For these women, there are women's health collectives and self-help groups that provide instruction in self-examination for women of all ages in an encouraging and supportive atmosphere. And again, it may be helpful to remember that doctors stress breast self-examination as the single most important thing a woman can do to protect herself against breast cancer.

When to Begin

You should begin examining your breasts as soon as their development becomes apparent. Self-examination should then be practiced for the rest of your life. So whatever your age, begin now.

We know that changes occur in the breasts during different phases of the menstrual cycle. In order to become familiar with your own breast changes, it's a good idea to begin by examining your breasts every few days throughout your cycle.

During each monthly cycle, your body produces the female hormones, estrogen and progesterone. These hormones are instrumental in preparing your body for a possible pregnancy. This preparation for pregnancy affects the breasts by causing some growth of the blood vessels and the gland ducts. As a result of this growth, before your period begins each month, you may notice a general thickening and enlargement of your breasts, and they may feel painful or tender to the touch.

Once your period begins, your breasts will begin to return to their previous state. About a week following your period, your breasts will be at their "quietest" stage. This is the time you should examine them each month. At this quiet stage, your breasts will not be as tender or as full, and it will be easier for you to detect any changes in texture, shape, or contour. With practice, you'll be able to recognize what is normal for your breasts during this particular phase of your cycle, and any changes will become readily apparent.

Techniques of Self-Examination

Breast self-examination consists of examination both by sight and by touch. There is a wide range of individual variation in the way breasts look and feel, so remember that your task is to become familiar with your own breasts and to know what is normal for you. In this way, you'll be able to detect any differences that were not present before.

Examination by sight requires a mirror and a good light. Stand in front of the mirror with your arms resting at your sides and look at your breasts.

However your breasts look is normal for you. One breast may be larger than the other or one or both nipples may be inverted. These characteristics all fall within the range of normal variations. Remember, you are concerned with detecting any *changes* that occur in the appearance of your breasts. For example, if you have never had an inverted nipple and one nipple begins to retract, this is a change that should be brought to the attention of your doctor.

Look for changes in breast contour, size, or shape. For example, is there a bulge in one breast but not in the other? Is the skin puckered or dimpled?

Inspect the nipples for any changes. Are the nipples scaling? Is there a discharge? Are the nipples symmetrical, or is one pointing to one side?

In order to explore the entire breast, repeat the examination with arms extended over your head. Then place your hands firmly on your hips, and flex your chest muscles. Repeat the examination once more in this position.

It is important to remember that any changes you note in the appearance of your breasts do not necessarily mean that something is wrong. However, they should be brought to the attention of your doctor just in case a problem exists.

Examination by touch (palpation) is the second part. Self-examination is most effective when done in a position that best enables you to feel any lumps, knots,

or thickenings in your breasts. When you lie down, you will notice that your breasts spread out and flatten on your chest. Likewise, when you place one hand beneath your head, the breast on that side distributes itself more evenly on the chest wall. If your breasts are large, you may find that placing a folded towel or a small pillow beneath the shoulder of the side you're examining also will help.

Assume the position described above to continue examining your breasts. Using the flat part of your fingers, examine the right breast with the left hand and the left breast with the right hand. Gently press the breast tissue against the chest wall, paying particular attention to the texture of the breast tissue.

In order to ensure a thorough examination, it may be helpful to picture your breast as the face of a clock. Begin at the outermost edge of your breast at the 12 o'clock position. Now, move around this outer edge to the 1 o'clock position, gently pressing and noticing the structure of the breast. Continue examining in this manner. Around the lower edge of the breast, you may notice a firmness that was not apparent at the top of the breast. This is the normal glandular structure in this area, and not a cause for concern.

BREAST SELF-EXAMINATION BY SIGHT

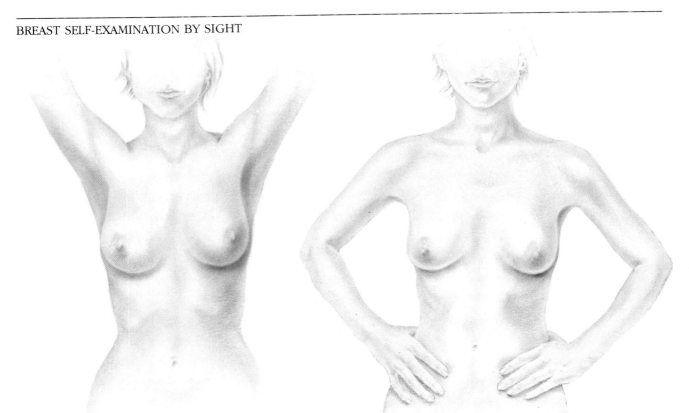

Stand in front of a mirror in good light. Extend your arms over your head to entirely expose both breasts. Look for any changes in the appearance, contour, size, and shape of your breasts and nipples.

Now, with hands placed on the hips and your chest muscles flexed, repeat the sight examination.

BREAST SELF-EXAMINATION BY TOUCH

Lying on your back with one hand beneath your head, use the flat part of your other hand to press your breast against the chest wall. Feel for any knot, lump, or thickening. Continue pressing in a circular pattern around the breast to thoroughly examine all breast tissue. Now examine your other breast.

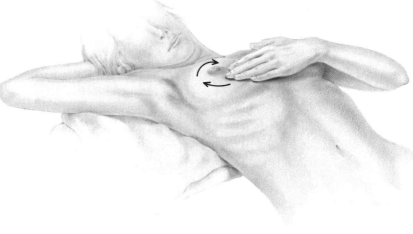

Gently squeeze the nipple to check for any discharge. Repeat the nipple examination on the other breast.

This part of the examination can be done most effectively in the bath or shower, using soapy fingers.

Place one hand behind your head, and move the flat part of your fingers over each part of your breast, using a circular motion. Move from the outermost part to the nipple, checking for any lump, knot, or thickening. Repeat this touch examination on the other breast.

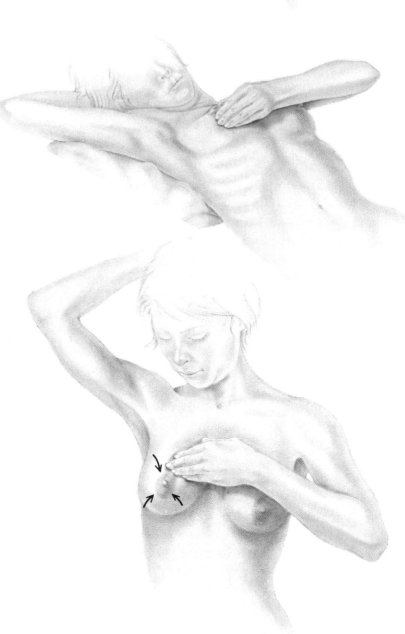

When you again reach the 12 o'clock position, move about an inch toward the center of your breast and begin another circle. Continue examining your breast in concentric circles until you reach the nipple.

Gently squeeze the nipple to check for any discharge. Only a very small percentage of breast cancers are associated with a discharge, but you still should report any findings to your doctor.

Repeat the entire examination on the opposite breast. The final part of the exam can be done in the bath or shower. Your fingers will glide more easily over wet, soapy skin.

Put your right hand behind your head, and with your left hand, place the flat part of your fingers on your right breast. Using a circular motion, move your fingers gently over each part of your breast from the outermost part to the nipple. Again, feel for any lump, knot, or thickening. Repeat the examination on your left breast.

There is no single description of how normal breast tissue feels, so at first you may wonder whether or not what you're feeling is normal. Give yourself time to become thoroughly familiar with your own breasts. Then, if you feel unsure or uneasy about anything you detect, ask questions of your doctor. But by all means, continue to examine your breasts. You'll gradually become familiar with your own normal breast tissue so that any abnormality that may occur will be apparent.

Remember that the abnormalities you might detect are probably not cancer, but only by bringing them to the attention of your doctor can you rule out that possibility.

Variations Throughout Your Life-Span

As we've noted, our breasts undergo changes that are associated with different stages of our reproductive lives. Some of these changes are predictable and are illustrated on page 152; others are discussed below.

Variations during pregnancy are perhaps the most dramatic of these changes. Fullness and tenderness similar to premenstrual symptoms appear around the fifth week of pregnancy. Around the same time, the nipples and areolae enlarge and darken. The little bumps in the areolae (called the glands of Montgomery) also enlarge. These changes may, in fact, provide a clue to pregnancy.

If you examine your breasts regularly, these changes will not escape your notice, although the fullness and tenderness may make self-examination more difficult. In addition, as your pregnancy progresses, you may notice that your breasts become more nodular. That is, you may begin to notice a lumpy texture to your breasts. This change in texture is to be expected and is the result of the enlargement of the milk-producing glands. The glandular tissue will continue to enlarge throughout your pregnancy, and by delivery, it will have replaced most of the fatty tissue in the breast.

As the blood supply to the breasts increases in preparation for milk production, the veins in the breasts become more prominent.

During the latter part of your pregnancy, you may notice a discharge from your nipples during self-examination. This discharge is called colostrum and is perfectly normal (see page 286).

Variations during lactation are similar to those of pregnancy (see page 155 for information on breast care during lactation). Your breasts still will be enlarged. During the time your breasts are producing milk, they will be quite heavy, and the glandular tissue will be prominent.

As you begin to wean your baby (or even if you don't breast-feed), your milk will gradually "dry up." The hormonal balance in your body will change, and your breasts will return to their pre-pregnancy state. If you have been breast-feeding, it may take several months for your breasts to return to their former size. Glandular tissue will become smaller, and the fatty tissue will once again become predominant in your breasts. You also may notice that your breasts are less firm than they were before you became pregnant—a normal development.

Variations during and following menopause also are important to note. Once your body no longer prepares for a possible pregnancy each month, glandular tissue in the breasts begins to shrink. Around the age of menopause (45 to 55 years), women's breasts lose tone and become less firm because of this shrinkage and the breakdown of fibrous supportive tissue. A decrease in breast fullness actually makes self-examination easier. This is fortunate because the risk of breast cancer increases with age (see page 546), and it's especially important to perform regular self-examination after menopause.

Regular Medical Checkups

Regular medical checkups are an essential part of maintaining breast health. Once-a-year visits to your doctor should become a part of your routine health care, and at this visit, you should request a complete physical checkup. If necessary, remind your doctor that a breast examination is part of any complete physical checkup.

Keep a record of any changes that you notice during your monthly self-examination, and report any abnormalities immediately to your doctor. Know your rights and responsibilities as a patient and exercise them (see page 394). If you find a lump and have it diagnosed right away, you'll have time to get a second opinion if you want one. You'll also have time to learn about the treatment options for your particular condition and to decide which one is right for you. You are the only one who can make these decisions, so give yourself ample time by minimizing the delay between discovery and diagnosis.

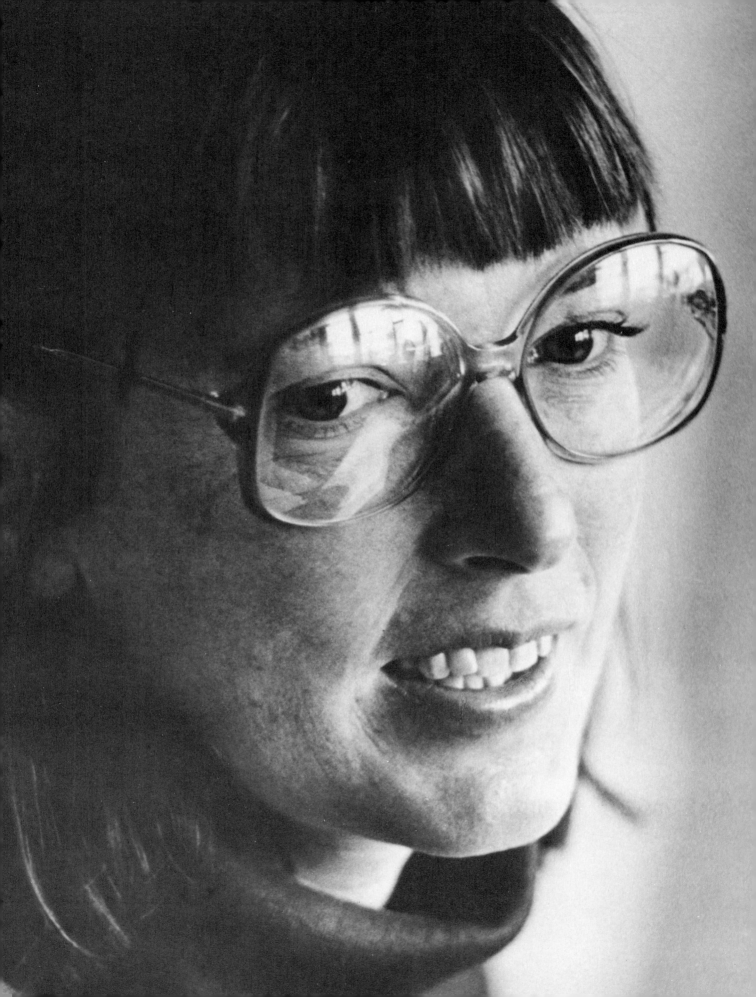

CHAPTER 10

BIRTH CONTROL

ROBERT HATCHER, M.D., M.P.H.

Throughout history, women and men have attempted to control reproduction. But only with recent developments in contraceptive technology has the personal control of reproduction become possible. This control has had a far-reaching impact on women's freedom of choice and on our relationships with men.

Individuals vary widely in their feelings about contraception and the methods they use. It is important to understand your reasons for using contraception and to explore many avenues of advice and counsel in deciding on the most suitable method of birth control for you.

Birth Control

Family planning is extremely important to the physical health of women, of men, and of children. It comes as no great surprise that to be successful in planning your family, you need to be adequately informed about the various birth control methods available. Providing that information is a primary goal of the family planning services in your community, and the purpose of this chapter.

In general, no one method of birth control is "good" or "bad"; each method currently available has its strong advocates. For some, a given method simply may be ineffective or inconvenient; for others, it may even be dangerous.

In addition, different stages of your reproductive life may dictate different methods of birth control. A particular method may be the best one for you at one time in your life, but not the best at another time. Changes in the patterns of your sexual activity may make one method more acceptable than another, or changes in your health may necessitate a change of birth control method. Some couples even use two methods of birth control simultaneously to increase contraception effectiveness, and you may wish to consider that approach.

Finally, if you are currently using a method of birth control with which you are satisfied, you may be interested in learning more about what are considered to be its advantages and disadvantages.

In order to decide upon the best method for you at any given time in your life, or to fully evaluate the method you now use, you need to know:

• the effectiveness of the method

• the convenience of use of the method as it relates to your sex life

• the side effects of the method—both detrimental and beneficial.

In addition, the method of birth control you choose must be used correctly in order to maximize its effectiveness. While this chapter does not provide instructions on how to use each method of birth control—some being extremely complicated or quite specific—we will give a few of the most important tips that apply to each method.

Where to Go for Help

There are many sources of help for couples seeking guidance with birth control planning. It's wise to know where to go in your community for birth control information, and it is particularly important to find a birth control center as soon as you move to a new community. If you note one of the danger signals of using IUDs or pills, you will know where to find help.

Planned Parenthood affiliates are present in many large communities throughout the country (see page 374). They provide free advice and inexpensive birth control procedures. Often, Planned Parenthood Clinics offer free birth control pills, pregnancy tests, Pap smears, and VD screening and treatment. In addition, health departments and hospitals have family planning programs, and many give out birth control information, as well as make arrangements for a person to use the contraceptive methods discussed in this chapter.

Many women go to their obstetrician/gynecologist to obtain a pelvic examination and to discuss contraceptive options. General practitioners, internists, and pediatricians also are able to deliver birth control services and perform pelvic examinations.

Clinics that perform abortions often are very willing to give pregnancy tests to determine whether a woman is pregnant and to provide contraceptive services if she is not. Some abortion clinics also provide sterilization procedures and sexual counseling, as well as family planning services.

In almost any community in the country, a local Catholic church has information on natural family planning. Churches often sponsor natural family planning groups that meet regularly.

Women's health clinics also may provide contraceptive services (see page 370). Inquire about self-help groups for women interested in natural or rhythm methods. In many areas, women's groups provide birth control information and mutual support.

For women or men who prefer to base decisions on their own private reading, see the suggested sources listed in the section beginning on page 667.

The Relative Effectiveness of Various Birth Control Methods

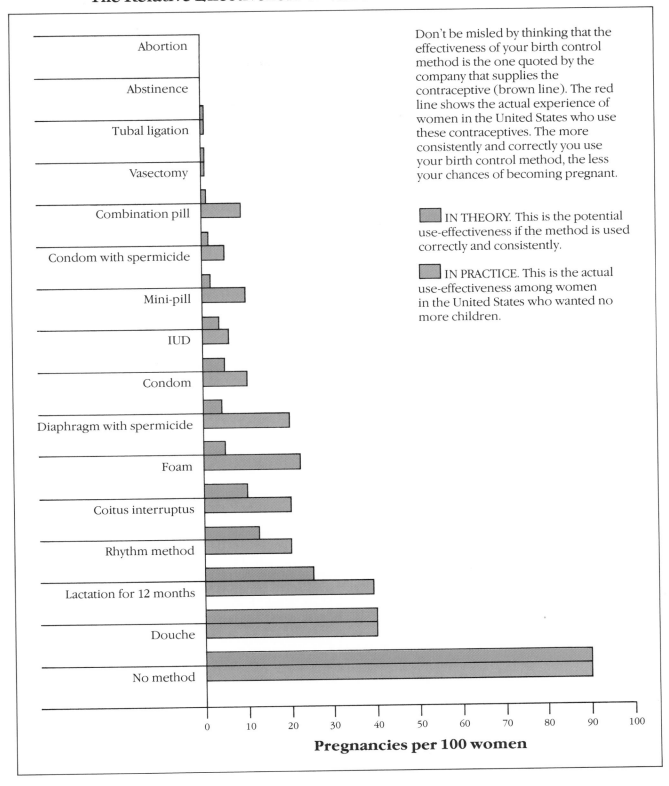

Don't be misled by thinking that the effectiveness of your birth control method is the one quoted by the company that supplies the contraceptive (brown line). The red line shows the actual experience of women in the United States who use these contraceptives. The more consistently and correctly you use your birth control method, the less your chances of becoming pregnant.

IN THEORY. This is the potential use-effectiveness if the method is used correctly and consistently.

IN PRACTICE. This is the actual use-effectiveness among women in the United States who wanted no more children.

Pregnancies per 100 women

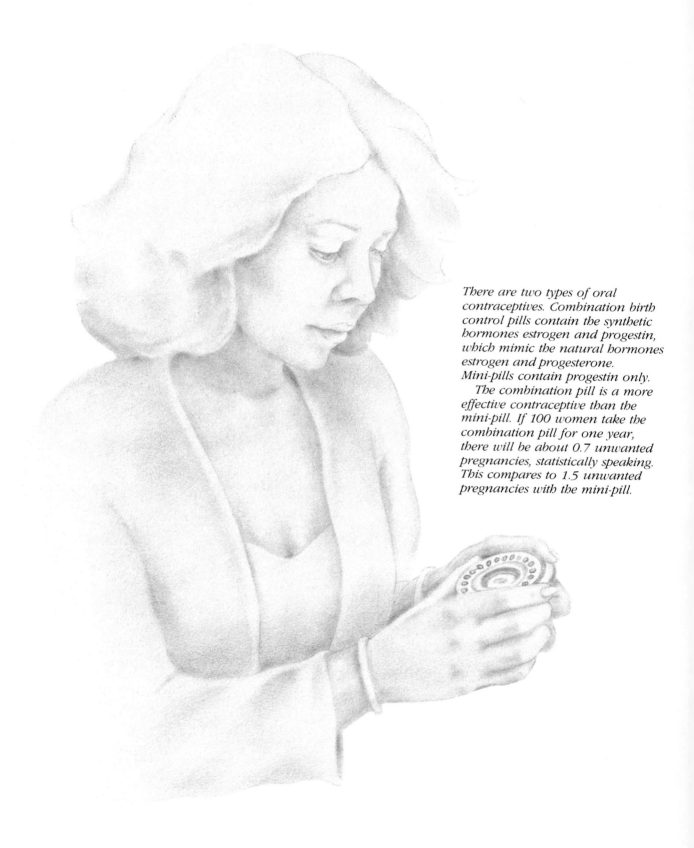

There are two types of oral contraceptives. Combination birth control pills contain the synthetic hormones estrogen and progestin, which mimic the natural hormones estrogen and progesterone. Mini-pills contain progestin only.

The combination pill is a more effective contraceptive than the mini-pill. If 100 women take the combination pill for one year, there will be about 0.7 unwanted pregnancies, statistically speaking. This compares to 1.5 unwanted pregnancies with the mini-pill.

Oral Contraceptives

Combination Pills

As early as 1937, it was determined that the hormone classified as *progesterone* could cause a woman to stop ovulating. Because of the rapid shift of priorities brought about by the Second World War, however, research that would apply this information to the development of oral contraceptives was terminated. It was not until the 1950s that field trials of oral contraceptives began, and not until 1960 that the birth control pill first gained Food and Drug Administration approval in the United States.

Birth control pills contain synthetic estrogen and progesterone, which are natural hormones produced by your body. The man-made compounds are so similar in chemical composition to the natural hormones made by your body, that when the synthetic hormones are ingested orally in the birth control pill, they mimic the effect of the natural hormones. The synthetic hormone that mimics estrogen is called by the same name, *estrogen,* while the synthetic hormone that mimics progesterone is called by a slightly different name, *progestin.* Birth control pills, then, contain two synthetic hormones, estrogen and progestin.

The pills marketed in 1960 contained a great deal more estrogen and progestin than do those manufactured today. Since 1960, there has been a steady decline in the dosage of hormones in oral contraceptives. The lower-dose oral contraceptives that combine estrogen and progestin are almost as effective as the pills marketed in 1960, and have fewer side effects.

There are now approximately 10 to 12 million women in the United States who are using birth control pills. Of this number, one to two million are actually very poor candidates for this method of contraception—a serious problem that women and their physicians must confront. Women considering the pill should read this chapter carefully, as well as other discussions of hormone pills included in the chapters on "Menopause" and "Circulatory Disorders."

Oral contraceptives usually stop ovulation by their action on the hypothalamus and the pituitary gland (see page 169), but they also have effects on cervical mucus and on the lining of the uterus. It is the combination of these three effects that makes it remarkably unlikely that a woman who uses the pill properly will become pregnant.

Effectiveness. Birth control pills are 99.66 percent effective in preventing conception if used correctly. It goes without saying that their effectiveness decreases significantly if they are taken incorrectly.

TYPES OF BIRTH CONTROL PILLS

COMBINATION PILLS *contain both estrogen and progestin, although the ratio of these hormones varies with the brand used. The pills are taken for 21 days of each 28-day cycle, leaving seven days when they are not taken. Some brands provide placebo pills that do not contain any hormones for use on these seven days. These placebos, shown here in pink, are color-coded to differentiate them from hormone-containing pills. If you are taking a combination pill, you will bleed on the days that you take the placebo pills, shown here in pink. This is referred to as withdrawal bleeding because the pink pills contain no hormones, and the withdrawal of the hormones causes some uterine bleeding. It is not true menstruation because oral contraceptives do not allow the uterus to build up a thick lining, as would occur in normal cycles. MINI-PILLS, which contain only progestin, usually are sold in packages of 28. One pill is taken on each day of a 28-day cycle. If you are taking progestin-only or mini-pills, you will have a high rate of irregular menstrual bleeding.*

COMBINATION PILLS

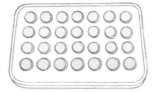

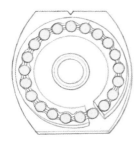

sun	mon	tue	wed	thu	fri	sat
					1	2
3	4	5	6	7	8	9
10	11	12	13	14	15	16
17	18	19	20	21	22	23
24	25	26	27	28	29	30

MINI-PILLS

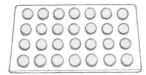

Convenience of use. The pill is taken on a daily regimen unrelated to the timing of sexual intercourse. Some couples feel that such a contraceptive, which is not used immediately prior to intercourse, allows greater spontaneity.

This method does require the assistance of a physician in prescribing the pills, however. In addition, some degree of advance planning is required during the first month of pill use. During this first cycle, oral contraceptives are slightly less effective, and many physicians advise using a second method of birth control simultaneously. After the first cycle, a woman must remember to take the pill each day as directed.

Beneficial side effects. Oral contraceptive use remarkably diminishes the menstrual cramps many women experience cyclically.

The amount of blood lost during the menstrual cycle falls to approximately 20 cc in contrast to 30 to 35 cc among nonusers. Thus, a good deal less iron is lost each month, and there is less incidence of iron-deficiency anemia.

The pill-taking regimen regulates the menstrual period—one of the most important non-contraceptive benefits in the view of most women on the pill. Acne also tends to improve in oral contraceptive users. And because ovulation does not occur, the pain that some women experience at the time of ovulation is absent. A woman using oral contraceptives is approximately 75 percent less likely to develop a functional ovarian cyst (see page 455).

Detrimental side effects. Some of these effects are transient, disappearing after a few cycles of use. Others appear to remain consistent over time. Perhaps the worst problems are those that tend to worsen over time.

Initial, often transient effects among pill users are nausea, cyclical weight gain, and heightened fullness and tenderness of the breasts. Breakthrough bleeding also tends to occur early in the use of oral contraceptives.

Sometimes women notice immediately that contact lenses fail to fit because of estrogen-related fluid retention that causes a change in the shape of the cornea.

Women who are breast-feeding may find that the pill causes a decrease in the amount of breast milk produced (see page 289). Most physicians recommend that nursing mothers use alternative methods of birth control.

Problems that remain consistent over time usually appear early in the course of pill use.

Some women who have previously experienced orgasm may find that they do not have orgasms while taking the pill. Other women may notice that their interest in having sex is diminished while taking the pill. If either of these problems occurs, the pill user must be aware that they could be caused by oral contraceptives. The problem may be alleviated by switching to another pill, or pill use may need to be discontinued altogether.

Among women who notice that their complexion changes for the worse, acne tends to appear fairly early in pill use and remains constant over time.

Headaches also may occur and remain about the same in incidence, intensity, and duration throughout a woman's use of birth control pills.

Problems that tend to worsen over time are of the greatest concern to women and their physicians.

The headaches that some women experience during the week when they are *not* taking oral contraceptives tend to worsen over time. Severe migrainelike headaches can be a serious contraindication, and should be reported to your physician.

Monilia vaginitis may occur more frequently in pill users, and may worsen over time. Monilia is an infection caused by a yeastlike organism, and is accompanied by severe itching of the genital area and by a white, cheesy vaginal discharge.

The menstrual period may become more and more scanty, or may stop entirely.

The risk that a woman who takes pills will develop a number of even more serious problems increases over time. That is, the longer a woman uses the pill, the more risk she assumes that she will develop such serious complications as cardiovascular problems, gallbladder disease, and hepatic adenoma (benign tumor of the liver).

Women who take oral contraceptives increase their risk of developing cardiovascular problems, including heart attacks, strokes, blood-clotting problems in the legs and abdomen, hypertension, migraine headaches, and vascular problems in the arteries and veins supplying the eyes.

The death rate is higher among pill users, primarily because of these cardiovascular complications. Statistically, figures reported for women in their early reproductive years are approximately five deaths out of every 100,000 women using the pill. For women who are older, the risk of death increases remarkably; it is also far greater for women who have used pills continuously for five years or more, and for women who are heavy smokers. The overall increase in mortality rates for women who have used the pill is approximately one death per 5,000 per year. For women who have used pills continuously for five or more years, the rate is approximately one death in 2,000 per year—far in excess of the risk of death from pregnancy.

It would be most desirable if one could tell a woman using pills that, once she has been using them for six months and has not experienced any major or minor problems, she can rest assured that the pills are perfectly safe and effective for her. But this is not the case. A woman who uses birth control pills must be wary of complications occurring at any time during the course of oral contraceptive use.

HOW BIRTH CONTROL PILLS PREVENT PREGNANCY

Birth control pills that contain the synthetic hormones estrogen and progestin prevent pregnancy in the following ways:
THE BRAIN *The pill is ingested, and the hormones dissolve and enter the bloodstream. The hormones reach the hypothalamus in the brain and the anterior pituitary gland near the brain. They then give a signal to the hypothalamus, which in turn sends a signal to the anterior pituitary*

gland, inhibiting the production of hormones that normally would stimulate the ovary to produce a mature egg and release it into the oviduct.
THE OVARY *Due to a lack of hormones from the anterior pituitary gland, the ovary does not release the egg. That is, ovulation does not occur. Obviously, if a mature egg is not ovulated into the oviduct, fertilization and pregnancy cannot occur.*

THE UTERUS *Even if by some rare accident ovulation occurs while a woman is taking birth control pills, the hormones in the pills act directly on the lining of the uterus to keep it in a state that makes implantation of a fertilized egg impossible.*
THE CERVIX *The progestin in the pill produces a thick cervical mucus that is hostile to sperm, further reducing the chances for pregnancy to occur.*

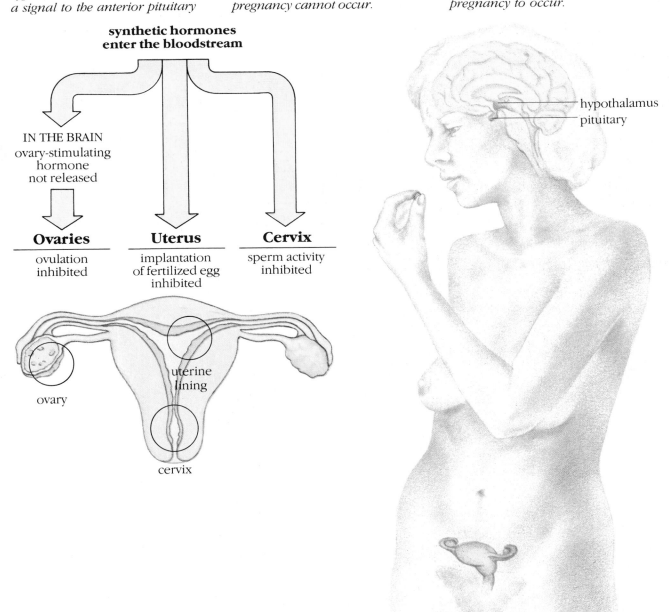

synthetic hormones enter the bloodstream

IN THE BRAIN
ovary-stimulating hormone not released

Ovaries
ovulation inhibited

Uterus
implantation of fertilized egg inhibited

Cervix
sperm activity inhibited

ovary

uterine lining

cervix

hypothalamus
pituitary

DANGER SIGNALS OF PILL COMPLICATIONS

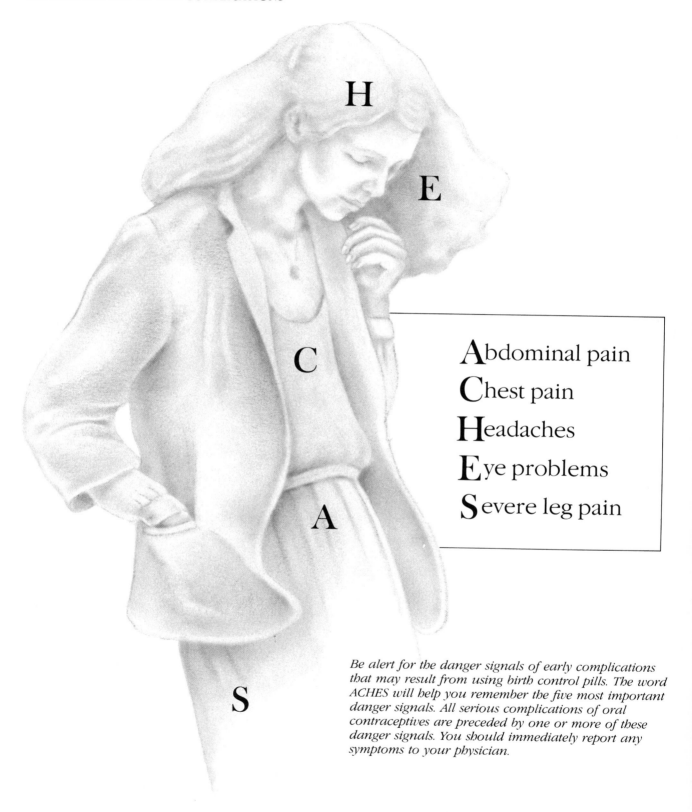

Abdominal pain
Chest pain
Headaches
Eye problems
Severe leg pain

Be alert for the danger signals of early complications that may result from using birth control pills. The word ACHES will help you remember the five most important danger signals. All serious complications of oral contraceptives are preceded by one or more of these danger signals. You should immediately report any symptoms to your physician.

The early danger signals of oral contraceptive use are extremely difficult to interpret. The word ACHES will help you to remember the five most important danger signals—early signs of potentially catastrophic problems from oral contraceptives—that must be reported to your physician: abdominal pain, chest pain, headaches, eye problems (such as blurred vision, loss of vision, or spots in front of the eyes), and severe leg pain.

Virtually all serious complications are *preceded* by one or more of these early danger signals. If you are extremely conscientious in looking for these danger signals, and if you report them to a physician who recognizes that they may be caused by oral contraceptives, most of the serious complications attributed to the pill can be avoided.

Oral contraceptives are but one of the causes of each of these danger signals, however, and a physician may not immediately associate the two unless the patient brings it to his or her attention.

Contraindications to pill use have increased to the extent that one wonders whether, in ten years' time, any woman will be considered a good candidate for pill use. Whether or not you have started taking the pill, one way to determine whether or not its use is contraindicated for you is to ask yourself these questions:

- Have you ever been told that you should not take oral contraceptives because of a blood-clotting problem, a stroke, or a heart attack?
- Do you have active liver disease at the present time from a condition such as hepatitis or mononucleosis?
- Are you being treated for a malignancy of the breast or reproductive system?
- Do you have severe headaches of any kind? Have your headaches been described by a doctor as migraine?
- Is your blood pressure abnormally high, or do you have hypertension?
- Have you ever been told that you are a prediabetic or a diabetic? Does diabetes run in your family?
- Have you ever had gallbladder disease?
- Do you have sickle-cell disease?
- Are you currently using a long leg cast or any other type of cast that immobilizes you significantly?
- Are you considering having surgery in the next month?
- Are you age 35 or older?
- Are you currently nursing a baby?
- If you already are taking the pill, have you become more depressed while using oral contraceptives?

You should speak to your physician about the questions that you have answered "yes," and ask about the questions you cannot answer.

Problems after stopping oral contraceptives also may arise for some women. For example, some women may develop post-pill absence of menstruation—a particular problem for the woman who wants to become pregnant soon after discontinuing pills. Some physicians strongly recommend that oral contraceptive users wait until they have had several regular periods after discontinuing pills before trying to become pregnant. Other women may lose a small amount of hair or develop acne following pill discontinuation.

Finally, and perhaps most seriously, it now appears that some women, particularly those who have used oral contraceptives for five years or longer, remain at a slightly increased risk of developing cardiovascular complications, such as heart attacks and strokes, even after they have stopped taking pills.

Unfortunately, the pill user is exposed to a media blitz regarding oral contraceptives, and sometimes the information she receives is rather confusing. On the whole, the media have been effective in warning women about problems resulting from pill use, and have helped many individuals. However, all too often, a specific news story is very one-sided in its approach. One week, a local newspaper article may be extremely positive about oral contraceptives, listing the benefits of this method, its effectiveness, and its popularity with American women. The next week, a new article may appear that is extremely negative, referring to problems with liver tumors, strokes, and heart attacks.

The problem is that a woman may read only one of these two articles. It would certainly be helpful if all media coverage of oral contraceptives presented a balanced picture. However, it is much more newsworthy to present extremes, and the pill user may find such an approach confusing.

In addition, the warnings on the oral contraceptive package insert that is provided with all birth control pills may frighten some women. It is important that you read this information very carefully. When questions arise, feel free to return to the clinic or physician's office where the pills were prescribed and seek answers.

Important tips for pill users.

- Pay close attention to the five danger signals of oral contraceptive complications (see opposite), and return to your clinician should you develop Abdominal pain, Chest pain, Headaches, Eye problems (such as loss of vision, blurred vision, or spots in front of the eyes), or Severe leg pain. Remember the word ACHES to remind you of these important pill danger signals.
- Learn how to use a second method of birth control, since there is a very strong likelihood that you will not use oral contraceptives for the entirety of your reproductive years. Many women who discontinue pills before they have completed even a single year of oral contraceptive use become pregnant simply because they are not comfortable with other means of birth control. Familiarity with a second method of birth control also gives you a backup method should you miss any pills out of the daily regimen. Finally, during your first cycle of pill use, a backup method always should be used in addition to oral contraceptives.
- *When you are seen by a doctor for other problems, be sure to mention that you are using birth control pills.*

Progestin-Only or "Mini-Pills"

When oral contraceptives were first marketed in the United States, the pills contained estrogen and progestin. From 1960 until 1973, pills marketed in the United States had progressively decreasing amounts of both the estrogen and the progestational agent, but continued to combine the two.

In 1973, three "mini-pills"—Micronor, Nor-QD, and Ovrette—became available. In contrast to the combined pill, these mini-pills contain progestin only.

The mini-pills operate in several ways. They may, as in the case of the original oral contraceptives, stop ovulation, but this effect occurs in only one-third of the women who take mini-pills. And like the first pills, mini-pills also may produce a thick cervical mucus that is "hostile" to sperm, making it more difficult for sperm to get through the cervical canal, up into the uterus, and into the fallopian tubes. Mini-pills also affect a complex process called *capacitation.* Sperm that are deposited in the vaginal tract must become activated in order to cause fertilization. This process of activation is called capacitation, and is blocked by the presence of progestational agents, such as those in the mini-pill. Finally, mini-pills disrupt the maturation of the lining of the uterus (the endometrium) in such a way that implantation of a fertilized egg cannot occur. In other words, the mini-pill has multiple effects that combine to prevent conception.

The main advantage of taking mini-pills rather than the combined oral contraceptives revolves around the mini-pill's absence of estrogen. Because of this absence, users of mini-pills are less likely to develop cardiovascular complications such as heart attacks, strokes, thromboembolic events, or blood clots than are users of combined oral contraceptives. In addition, other side effects associated with estrogen-containing pills—headaches, cyclic weight gain, nausea, chloasma or the mask of pregnancy (darkening of the skin of the face), high blood pressure, and breast swelling and tenderness—are less likely to occur.

Effectiveness. Mini-pills are 98.5 to 99 percent effective if used correctly and consistently. Pregnancy *may* occur even if mini-pills are taken correctly, however. The 1 to 1.5 percent pregnancy rate is a good bit higher than the .34 percent pregnancy rate for the combined pill, but both rates are extremely low. It should be noted that these statistics apply only to groups of women who use pills or mini-pills *correctly and consistently.* Mini-pill users who miss a single pill or two are far more likely to conceive. If a pill is missed, a backup method of birth control must be used.

Convenience of use. Like combined pills, the daily regimen of mini-pill use is unrelated to the time of sexual intercourse. Mini-pills are taken every single day, without a "week off," and thus eliminate the potential confusion of counting days. For the first two to three months of using mini-pills, a backup method of birth control also should be used. In addition, some physicians recommend that you continue using a backup method at mid-cycle—days 10 through 18 after the first day of your last menstrual period.

As with the combined pills, a physician's assistance is required both in prescribing mini-pills and in monitoring your health while you are taking them.

Beneficial side effects. As with the combined pills, the use of mini-pills may decrease menstrual cramps, although less predictably so than with combined pills.

Detrimental side effects. Although the mini-pill has few serious side effects, women who have had a stroke, a heart attack, or a thromboembolic complication still should consider themselves poor candidates for its use until we know for certain that mini-pills will not produce the complications associated with estrogen-containing pills. For the present, physicians generally are guided by the principle that the absolute contraindications for combined pills are also absolute contraindications for mini-pills.

Irregular menstrual periods are quite common with mini-pill use, in contrast to the regulated menses produced by the combined birth control pills.

Intermittent "spotting" may occur in mini-pill users.

Important tips for mini-pill users.

● Don't miss a single mini-pill. Mini-pills must be taken every single day, *even during your period.*

● A backup method of birth control should be used consistently during the first two to three months of taking mini-pills. Thereafter, you may want to use a backup method of birth control at mid-cycle—days 10 through 18 after the first day of your last menstrual period.

● If you do not have a period within 45 days of your last one, immediately go to a physician to determine whether or not you are pregnant.

Alternatives to the Pill

All too many women, especially young women, think of birth control pills as the only means of birth control available to them. It is important to recognize that many other contraceptive options are available today.

In addition to the woman who has not looked at all of the options available are those women who, despite the occurrence of complications or the presence of contraindications, push the physician to continue prescribing pills. Physicians also need to assume part of the responsibility in these cases. In some instances, a physician also may have considered oral contraceptives to be the only approach to contraception.

A number of options do exist, and it is important that women be informed in order to make decisions about the method they will use at any given time in their lives.

Intrauterine Devices (IUDs)

The first IUDs were marketed in the United States in the early 1960s. At the present time, there are three to four million women in this country who are using IUDs.

As the name suggests, IUDs are devices that are inserted into the uterus to prevent conception. Currently, there are two basic types of IUDs: those that are medicated (with copper or progesterone) and those that are non-medicated. Non-medicated IUDs have an advantage in that they need not be removed after a given period of time, as is necessary with medicated IUDs.

Strange as it may seem, we still do not understand completely how intrauterine devices work. Most researchers believe that they establish an inflammatory reaction within the uterus and thus prevent implantation of the fertilized egg. This inflammatory reaction, resulting from the presence of a foreign body, is not the same as that associated with a bacterial infection.

Effectiveness. Used correctly, IUDs are 97 to 99 percent effective. There are very few mistakes that a user of an IUD can make and, therefore, the effectiveness rate, even when careless errors are included, is well above 90 percent.

Convenience of use. The IUD is inserted by a clinician and, once it is known that the device can be tolerated, requires little attention. Initially, the IUD user is asked to check, at least once a month after her menstrual period, that the strings of the IUD are present at the mouth of the cervix. She should return for a checkup several weeks after IUD insertion and thereafter, once each year.

IUD insertion is a one-time event and thus, like the pill, is not related to the actual timing of sexual intercourse.

Beneficial side effects. One IUD, the Progestasert-T, may decrease menstrual cramps.

Detrimental side effects. Infections of the uterus or fallopian tubes are the most serious problems associated with IUDs. Such infections can cause such severe pelvic infections as to require a hysterectomy.

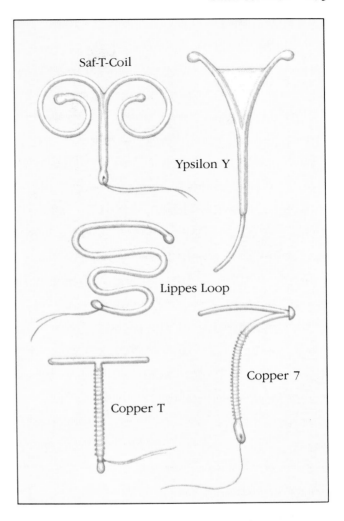

FIVE TYPES OF INTRAUTERINE DEVICES

A number of different types of intrauterine devices effectively prevent conception. The Copper T, Copper 7, Lippes Loop, Saf-T-Coil, and Ypsilon Y are shown here in their approximate size. The exact size and type of IUD that's right for you depends on several factors, including your pregnancy history and the depth of your uterus. Your physician chooses the one to be used, based on his or her familiarity with each type, and on your individual physical requirements.

INSERTING AN IUD

A flexible rod called a uterine sound is inserted in the uterus to determine its length and position.

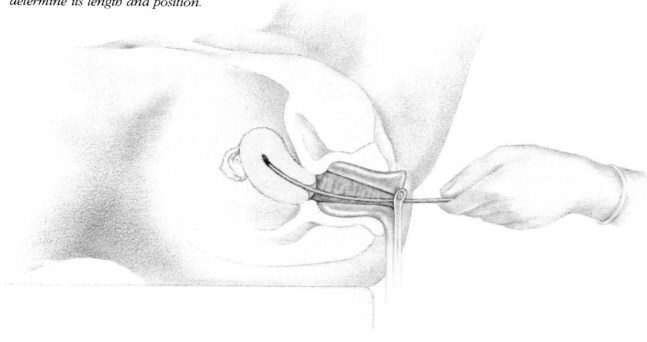

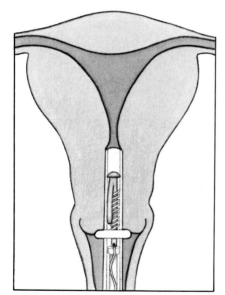

The IUD is elongated in an inserter, which enters the uterus through the cervix.

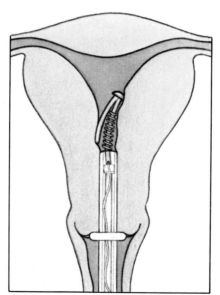

When the inserter is withdrawn, the IUD resumes its original shape. (This is a Copper 7 IUD.)

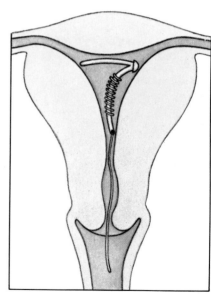

When the IUD is in place within the uterus, the tail or string hangs through the cervical os into the vagina.

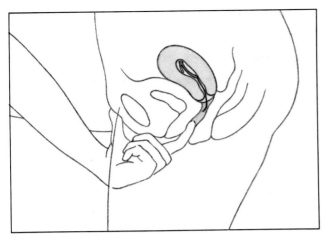

CHECKING PLACEMENT OF AN IUD
The string of a properly placed IUD can be felt within the vagina using the fingers. It is important to check the string each month after your menstrual period to ensure that the IUD remains in place.

The IUD is not the recommended method of contraception for teen-agers, or for women who hope to become pregnant in the future. This is because of the potential complications of infection that may result in tubal scarring, causing infertility.

Menstrual cramps are more frequently experienced by IUD users. Menstrual periods last longer, and there is increased blood loss and the possibility of iron-deficiency anemia.

Although far less common than with oral contraceptives, deaths have occurred from IUD use.

The danger signals for the IUD user are: Abdominal pain, Bleeding, Chills or fever, and a bad vaginal Discharge. Both the IUD user and her physician may overlook or underestimate a vaginal discharge as the sign of a potentially serious problem with an IUD, but this symptom merits close examination.

Important tips for IUD users.
● To remember the important danger signals of IUD complications, think of ABCD:
Abdominal pain, **B**leeding, **C**hills or fever, **D**ischarge.
● Use a simultaneous backup method of birth control for the first four to twelve weeks of IUD use. Thereafter, also consider using a backup method during mid-cycle when ovulation is most likely to occur.
● If your period is late and you think you might be pregnant, immediately go to your physician to have the pregnancy confirmed and the IUD removed. If the IUD is left in place during pregnancy, infectious problems can be particularly severe.

How Safe Is an IUD?

1   INFECTION Almost all forms of pelvic inflammatory disease, particularly gonorrhea, are more severe in women with IUDs. When untreated infection spreads from the uterus to the tubes, ovaries, and pelvis, it can cause sterility and even death.
2   PERFORATION If the IUD is not inserted properly, it can be pushed through the wall of the uterus.
3   BLEEDING AND PAIN Sometimes the heavy bleeding and cramping experienced during the first few months after insertion do not subside.
4   EXPULSION The IUD may come out accidentally, especially during menstruation.

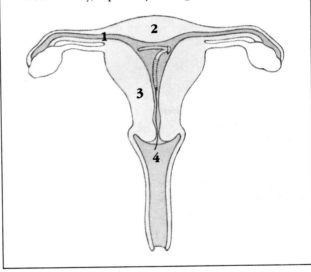

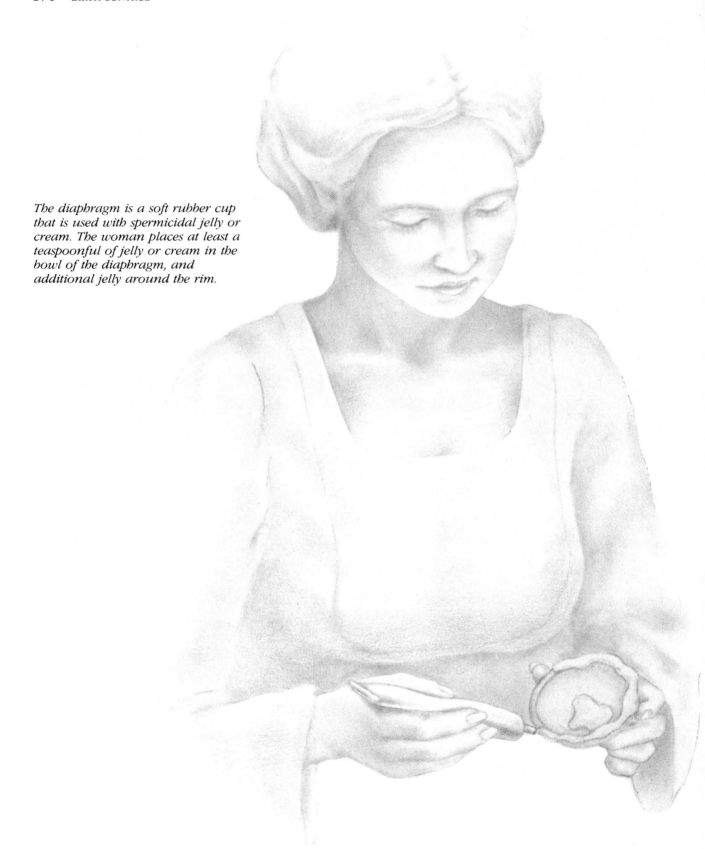

The diaphragm is a soft rubber cup that is used with spermicidal jelly or cream. The woman places at least a teaspoonful of jelly or cream in the bowl of the diaphragm, and additional jelly around the rim.

The Diaphragm

The diaphragm is another barrier method of birth control. When filled with spermicidal jelly and placed over the mouth of the cervix, it combines mechanical and chemical protection against conception.

Used in some form since 1882, the diaphragm seems to be gaining popularity in this country.

Effectiveness. The diaphragm has a very high effectiveness rate when used consistently and correctly—around 97 percent. Many types of user errors can occur with the use of diaphragms, however, and when these are taken into account, the effectiveness rate drops to only 80 to 85 percent. To be fully effective, the diaphragm must be properly fitted by a clinician, properly placed in the vagina before intercourse, and replenished with a spermicidal agent before each act of intercourse. In addition, the diaphragm must be left in place for six to eight hours after intercourse.

Convenience of use. The diaphragm can be inserted several hours (two to six hours) prior to sexual intercourse. Many women insert the diaphragm immediately before having sex, and because of the chemical activity of the jelly, this practice may make this method slightly more effective. If the diaphragm is inserted several hours prior to intercourse, additional spermicidal jelly can be inserted with an applicator just prior to intercourse.

A physician, clinician, or nurse practitioner must fit a woman for a diaphragm, and the size should be rechecked if the woman gains or loses 15 pounds, has an abortion, or gives birth.

Like any rubber product, the diaphragm requires careful maintenance (washing, thorough drying, and dusting with cornstarch—*not* talcum—after removal). Because rubber products deteriorate over time, it is also important to hold the diaphragm up to a strong light periodically in order to look for holes either in the middle of the diaphragm or at the junction of the "bowl" and the firm rim.

Inserting and removing the diaphragm requires some practice initially. Until you have practiced insertion and removal several times, you should use a backup method of birth control simultaneously. Of course, you must keep the diaphragm, the spermicidal jelly, and the jelly applicator handy to ensure consistent use.

Beneficial side effects. Using a diaphragm acquaints a woman with her sexual anatomy, a useful understanding for her to have.

As a barrier across the cervix, the diaphragm holds back the menstrual flow, and has been used by women who wish to feel more comfortable having sexual intercourse during periods.

Again, since the diaphragm covers the cervix, it may decrease the likelihood of a woman developing cervical inflammation and certain vaginal infections.

Detrimental side effects. In some women, the pressure of the diaphragm on the urethra invites urinary tract infections. Women who use the diaphragm should look for changes in their pattern of urination as an early sign of such infections.

Allergic reactions to the diaphragm itself rarely occur. Any allergy that results is usually to the spermicidal agent, and may be alleviated by using a different spermicide. If the allergy is to the rubber, then use of the diaphragm must be discontinued.

DIAPHRAGM EQUIPMENT AND CARE

Your diaphragm will come with a small case to protect it, and an inserter or introducer if it is a coil or flat spring diaphragm. The arch spring diaphragm, which is the most commonly used, does not require an inserter. You can buy a tube of contraceptive jelly or cream that comes with an applicator at any drugstore.

If you take a few extra minutes to care for your diaphragm, it will last longer, and there will be less chance of accidental pregnancy caused by holes or tears. When you first get the diaphragm, examine it for holes, tears, or puckered areas, especially around the rim. Return it if you suspect any irregularities. Each time you wash your diaphragm, repeat this inspection. Check to see if it will hold water without leaking, and hold it up to a light to see pinholes and tears.

After each use, wash the diaphragm and applicator with warm water and a pure soap. Detergent soaps, cold cream soaps, and soaps containing petroleum should not be used because they weaken the rubber. Thoroughly towel-dry the diaphragm.

Before returning the diaphragm to its case, you may want to dust it with cornstarch to be sure it is completely dry. Do not use scented talcs or baby powder, because they, too, will weaken the rubber. Keep the diaphragm in its case, away from direct heat sources.

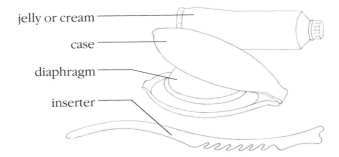

jelly or cream

case

diaphragm

inserter

INSERTING THE DIAPHRAGM

With one hand, pinch the rim of the diaphragm together with your thumb and middle finger, while holding the index finger on the rim. Stand with one foot propped at chair-seat height and insert the diaphragm as far into the vagina as it will go, pushing against the rim with the index finger.

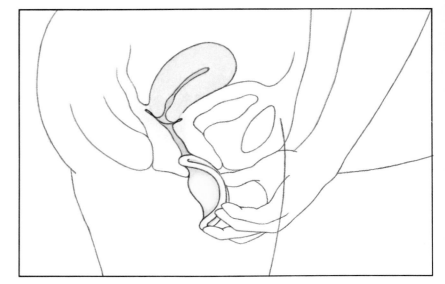

Tuck the front rim of the diaphragm above the ridge of the pubic bone, and press the back rim up behind the cervix.

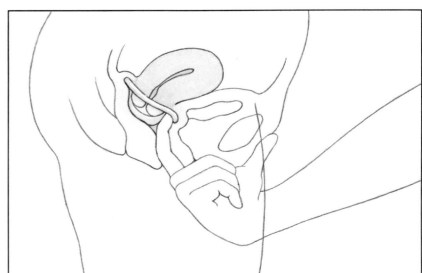

Check that the diaphragm is in place by feeling at the center of the dome and around the rim. It is essential to check for snug placement.

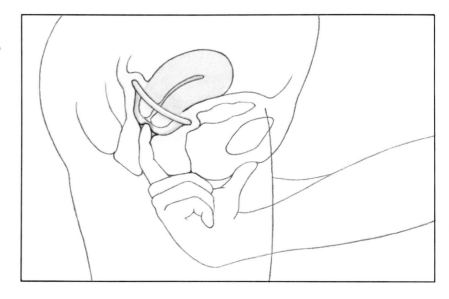

DIAPHRAGM PLACEMENT

The diaphragm is placed correctly. You can check for correct placement by feeling your cervix through the diaphragm.

The diaphragm is placed incorrectly. It has not been pushed up far enough to prevent sperm from entering the cervix.

The diaphragm is placed incorrectly. It has not been pushed up far enough to cover the front of the cervix.

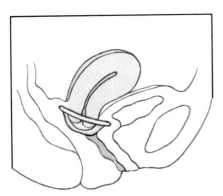 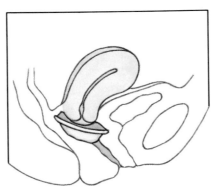 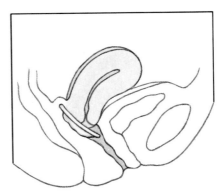

Important tips for diaphragm users.
● Use at least a teaspoonful of spermicidal jelly or cream in the bowl of the diaphragm, and spread a little around the inside of the rim. Jelly and cream are equally effective, but jelly is somewhat more lubricating than cream. *Each time you have intercourse,* insert more jelly or cream. Since you must not remove the diaphragm to do this, it is useful to buy an applicator with your initial purchase of jelly so you can simply "plunge" in more jelly.
● Until you've inserted and removed the diaphragm several times (whether in practice or before sexual intercourse), you should use a backup method of birth control simultaneously. The point is to become thoroughly familiar with the diaphragm before you count on it as your only contraceptive.
● Learn how to feel your cervix through your diaphragm. This is the only way to know whether the diaphragm is properly in place.

The Condom

The condom is a method of birth control used by men. Made of latex rubber or animal membranes, such as the cecum of the lamb, it is one of the barrier methods of birth control, meaning that it serves as a mechanical barrier to keep the man's sperm from reaching the egg. The condom is a sheath that fits over the man's erect penis. It is important that the condom be in place before the penis enters the vagina and that it is quickly and carefully withdrawn by hand immediately after ejaculation. Care should be taken that none of the semen escapes into the vagina or onto the woman's external genitals.

Effectiveness. Used consistently and correctly, the condom has an effectiveness rate of 97 percent. Based on actual user data, however, the effectiveness rate drops to 80 to 90 percent.

HOW THE DIAPHRAGM WORKS

When properly placed, the diaphragm completely covers the mouth of the cervix, holding the spermicidal jelly against the cervical opening. Sperm are prevented from entering the cervix by both a mechanical and a chemical barrier.

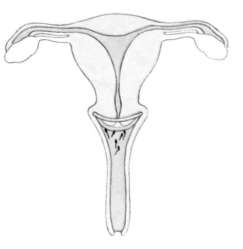

THE CONDOM

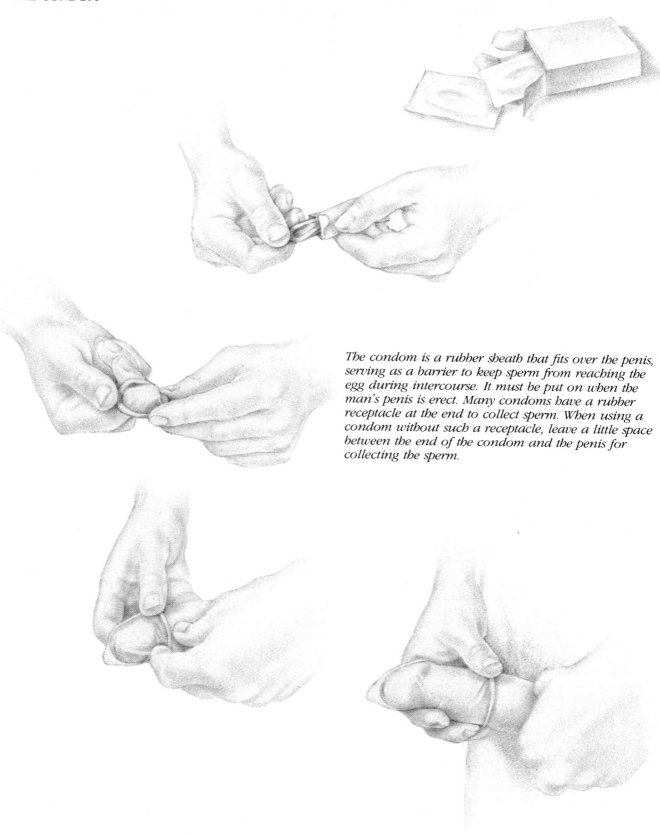

The condom is a rubber sheath that fits over the penis, serving as a barrier to keep sperm from reaching the egg during intercourse. It must be put on when the man's penis is erect. Many condoms have a rubber receptacle at the end to collect sperm. When using a condom without such a receptacle, leave a little space between the end of the condom and the penis for collecting the sperm.

Failures do occur, even when the condom is used consistently and correctly. Condoms may rupture, or rarely, may fail due to a manufacturing defect.

Convenience of use. Because the condom must be put on when the man's penis is erect, it involves a brief interruption of lovemaking. Many couples incorporate this "task" into their foreplay by having the woman place the condom on the man's penis.

Available without a physician's prescription, condoms are inexpensive and may be obtained at drugstores, in vending machines in some restrooms, at VD clinics, and through some mail order houses. Some advance planning is necessary in order to have a condom handy at the time of intercourse, however.

Beneficial side effects. The condom provides protection against venereal disease and sexually transmitted infections.

Protection of the woman from direct contact with the man's sperm diminishes the likelihood of her producing sperm-agglutinating antibodies, which can cause infertility.

Condoms exert a very slight tourniquet effect on the superficial veins of the penis, and thereby may have a beneficial effect for men who have difficulty maintaining an erection, whether from advanced age or because of certain major abdominal operations.

The shielding effect of the condom prolongs the man's plateau phase (see page 139), increasing enjoyment of intercourse for both the woman and the man.

Detrimental side effects. Some few men are not able to maintain an erection after putting on a condom (possibly due to strong negative feelings about having an artificial barrier between the man and the woman).

The woman's vagina and the man's penis are not in direct contact.

The woman is not aware of warm fluid entering her vagina at the time of ejaculation. Considered unimportant or never experienced by some women, for others the sensation is very pleasurable.

The friction of the condom sometimes diminishes clitoral stimulation, making intercourse less pleasurable for the woman. (Lubricated condoms may help to overcome this problem.)

The fact that the man must withdraw his penis from the vagina as soon as his orgasm has occurred may make intercourse less pleasurable for both partners.

Allergic reactions to rubber are rare, but may occur. (One can switch to lamb's-membrane condoms or "skins" in an effort to alleviate or avoid such reactions.)

Important tips for condom users.

● Keep condoms convenient. They're not apt to be used if they aren't handy at the time of intercourse. Since you know where you're most likely to have sexual intercourse, you can make sure your condoms will be there, too.

● The man must withdraw his penis from the vagina as soon as his orgasm has occurred. Otherwise, the condom will rather quickly slide off the penis as erection subsides, letting semen escape into the vagina.

Coitus Interruptus

Coitus interruptus, or withdrawal of the penis from the vagina just prior to ejaculation, is one of the oldest known methods of birth control.

Effectiveness. The total responsibility for withdrawal is with the male. Withdrawal requires a good deal of self-control, and even when practiced consistently, there is an inherent source of error in this method. Some preliminary ejaculatory fluid (stored in the prostate gland, the penile urethra, or the Cowper's glands) can escape into the vagina without the knowledge of either partner. Multiple acts of intercourse in a short period of time increase the likelihood of this happening because the fluid is more potent after a recent ejaculation.

Other causes of failure include the strong desire of the man to achieve deeper penetration at the time of impending orgasm, resulting in the deposition of semen on the female's external genitalia at the time of withdrawal. This semen can cause pregnancy.

Coitus interruptus is 85 percent effective in consistent users, but only 75 to 80 percent effective when errors are taken into consideration.

Couples who use coitus interruptus frequently discover, of necessity, that both the man and the woman can have extremely pleasurable sexual relations without the penis ever entering the vagina. If these alternatives (which we will call close cousins of coitus interruptus) are used, and the penis is never inserted into the vagina, contraceptive effectiveness is obvious.

Convenience of use. Coitus interruptus is always available to any couple, under any circumstances, at no cost, and without physicians or prescriptions.

Some couples, however, will never tolerate sexual intercourse that does not permit the closest physical intimacy at the time of climax, and coitus interruptus is a psychological strain for both partners. A couple may lose a sense of togetherness as the man thinks to himself, "Should I withdraw now?" or as the woman thinks, "Will he withdraw in time?" or "Has he already come?" Sex therapists view such mental activity during intercourse as "focusing on performance or spectatoring," and generally encourage couples to direct their attention elsewhere.

Important tips for using coitus interruptus.

● If you hope to avoid pregnancy, coitus interruptus is a far better method of birth control than none at all.

● Be sure that you trust your partner before you consider using this method of birth control.

● In conjunction with this approach to birth control, you may prefer to find sexual intimacy through relations in which the penis does not enter the vagina.

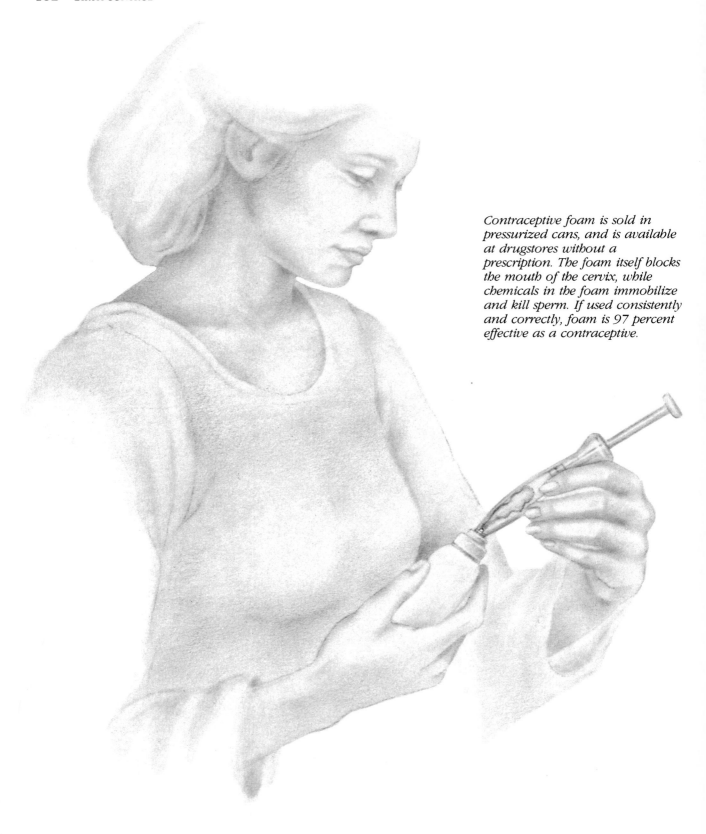

Contraceptive foam is sold in pressurized cans, and is available at drugstores without a prescription. The foam itself blocks the mouth of the cervix, while chemicals in the foam immobilize and kill sperm. If used consistently and correctly, foam is 97 percent effective as a contraceptive.

Contraceptive Foam

The contraceptive foams used today evolved from research into substances that would kill bacteria, and it is of interest that most contraceptive foams also are effective in preventing sexually transmitted infections. Some contraceptive foams currently marketed are Dalkon, Emko, Delfen, and Koromex.

The foam is placed deep in the vagina in the vicinity of the cervix. During coitus, the foam spreads over the cervix, mechanically blocking the cervical opening to prevent entry of the sperm. In addition, the foam exerts a chemical effect through its spermicidal agent, nonyl-phenoxypolyethanol, which immobilizes and kills the sperm.

Recently, the Germans have marketed a vaginal suppository called Patentex. In the United States, the same suppository has been marketed as the Encare Oval. Both of these contraceptive suppositories contain this same spermicidal agent. (For more information on foaming suppositories, see pages 184 and 185.)

Effectiveness. Foam is 97 percent effective if used consistently and correctly. Several errors can be made in using foam, however: not using enough, not shaking the foam sufficiently, or not inserting the foam deep within the vagina. As with any birth control method, errors decrease contraceptive effectiveness. When errors and inconsistent use are taken into account, foam's effectiveness decreases to 80 to 85 percent.

Convenience of use. Foams are available without a physician's prescription and without a physical examination. In addition, they are relatively inexpensive and easy to learn to use. Some women find foam too messy, however, and others complain of leakage of the foam from the vagina. If leakage occurs, a tampon may be used.

Foam must be inserted immediately prior to intercourse. Application can be incorporated into lovemaking by having the man insert the foam. Couples who enjoy oral-genital sexual contact may want to insert the foam after this activity, since it is notoriously bad-tasting.

It is necessary to keep foam readily available in order to ensure consistent use. Because foam comes in an opaque canister, it may be difficult to tell how much remains in the can. For this reason, it's a good idea to have an extra container on hand.

Beneficial side effects. Contraceptive foaming agents also provide lubrication, which may be desirable.

The incidence of sexually transmitted infections is decreased for foam users.

Detrimental side effects. Foams may produce irritation of the vagina or penis.

Allergies to a foam are rare, and usually can be alleviated by changing brands.

Three important tips for foam users.
- Insert foam immediately before intercourse. Additional applications are required before each act of intercourse.
- Shake the container of foam thoroughly, and fill the applicator to capacity.
- Insert the full applicator so that foam is forced deep into the vagina.

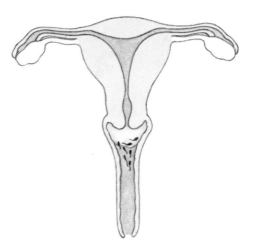

INSERTING CONTRACEPTIVE FOAM

To use contraceptive foam, immediately prior to intercourse fill the applicator full with foam and place it deep in the vagina. A plunger in the applicator "injects" the foam around the cervix.

HOW FOAM WORKS

Contraceptive foam blocks the mouth of the cervix and forms a barrier to sperm entry. Chemicals in the foam also immobilize and kill sperm.

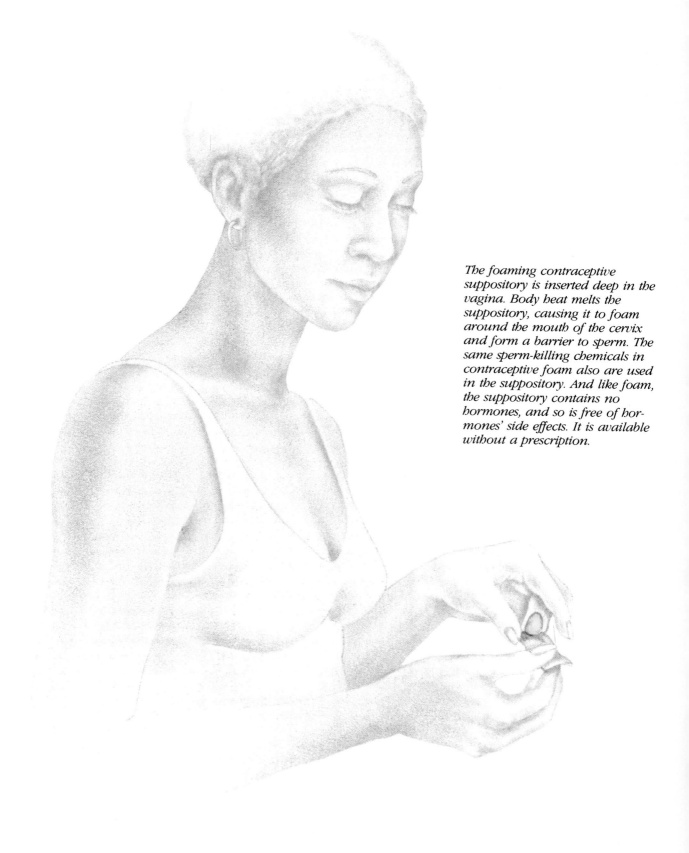

The foaming contraceptive suppository is inserted deep in the vagina. Body heat melts the suppository, causing it to foam around the mouth of the cervix and form a barrier to sperm. The same sperm-killing chemicals in contraceptive foam also are used in the suppository. And like foam, the suppository contains no hormones, and so is free of hormones' side effects. It is available without a prescription.

The Foaming Suppository

The foaming suppository is yet another barrier method of contraception. The small suppository is inserted deep in the vagina with the finger. Body heat causes it to foam, providing a spermicidal barrier at the mouth of the cervix.

As noted earlier, this contraceptive was introduced in the United States in late 1977, when concern about serious complications from IUDs and pills was high.

Effectiveness. The initial drug company claim states that this method is 99 percent effective, but this claim remains to be substantiated. Until there are several controlled studies on women who use foaming suppositories as their only means of birth control, we cannot know how effective it is. We do know it uses the same spermicide as most contraceptive foams, creams, and jellies. Therefore, it is likely that it will prove to be as reliable as those products—about 97 percent effective if used correctly and consistently. As with other spermicides, some women will not use it all the time, and some women will make errors in its use. For these reasons, we might expect the use effectiveness to be between 80 and 90 percent—about the same as with other spermicidal methods.

In order to maximize effectiveness, the foaming suppository should be inserted at least ten minutes but not more than two hours before intercourse. It takes about ten minutes for the suppository to dissolve within the vagina. An additional suppository is required for each act of intercourse.

Convenience of use. As with other barrier methods, the use of the foaming suppository is directly related to the timing of intercourse.

The suppository is small and convenient to carry, in addition to providing a known, pre-measured dose of the contraceptive agent. Heat will cause the suppository to soften within the package, but firmness can be restored by placing the unopened package under a stream of cold water for several minutes.

Suppositories may be obtained without a prescription, and are readily available at drugstores.

As with foam, the suppository has an unpleasant taste should the couple have oral-genital contact after its insertion.

The suppository creates a small amount of heat as it effervesces in the moist vaginal environment. Some women find this flush of heat unpleasant, but others find it pleasant, or at least tolerable. On some occasions, it may not dissolve completely in ten minutes, but this does not seem to impair its effectiveness.

The suppository may feel slightly gritty to a woman who has minimal vaginal moisture, and there may be some leakage following intercourse. Again, leakage can be prevented by wearing a mini-pad or a tampon.

Beneficial side effects. Spermicidal agents in the foaming suppository may slightly decrease the spread of sexually transmitted infections.

Detrimental side effects. The suppository may produce allergic or chemical irritation.

Important tips for suppository users.

● After inserting the suppository, wait ten minutes for it to dissolve, and wait no longer than two hours before having intercourse. An additional suppository is required for each act of intercourse, and a woman should not douche for six to eight hours following intercourse.

● Foaming suppositories are softened by heat, but firmness can be restored by momentarily placing the unopened package under cool water.

● Moistening the suppository with a little water just prior to inserting it into the vagina will speed its foaming action.

INSERTING THE FOAMING SUPPOSITORY

The suppository is inserted deep into the vagina with the index finger. Since it takes about ten minutes for the suppository to dissolve and cover the mouth of the cervix with foam, insert it at least ten minutes but no more than two hours before intercourse.

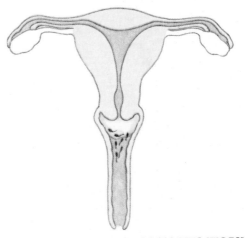

HOW FOAMING SUPPOSITORIES WORK

When a foaming suppository is inserted deep in the vagina, body heat produces a foaming action that acts as a barrier to sperm at the mouth of the cervix.

Natural Family Planning

There are three "natural" methods of family planning: the calendar or rhythm method, the temperature method, and the mucus or Billings method. Basically, each method involves determining the days of ovulation, which differ from one woman to another, so that you can avoid having intercourse during the few days before and after ovulation when you are most fertile.

For some women, a sharp, low abdominal pain about two weeks prior to menstruation signals the release of an egg from the ovary. It is very helpful to be aware of this type of pain as one of the clues to your own ovulatory cycle.

The calendar or rhythm method requires that you record the duration of each menstrual cycle for twelve months. (Days are counted from the first day of bleeding.) The number of days in your *shortest* cycle minus 18 equals the first day of your fertile period, and the number of days in your *longest* cycle minus 11 equals the last day of your fertile period.

If, for example, your menstrual records show that your shortest cycle has been 25 days and your longest cycle 30 days, your first fertile day will be Day 7 of your cycle (25 minus 18 equals 7), and your last fertile day, Day 19 (30 minus 11 equals 19). During this period of time, you should avoid having intercourse.

In addition to being unreliable, this method severely restricts the number of days when intercourse is possible. The two other methods, explained below and on page 189, or a combination of the two, are much better for the prevention of pregnancy.

The temperature method requires that you maintain a daily graph-paper record of your body temperature, using a special basal temperature thermometer, each morning before you get out of bed.

The temperature method is based on the fact that when you are about to ovulate, your temperature drops suddenly. After ovulation, your body temperature then climbs rapidly for three days, and does not return to its pre-ovulation level until the beginning of your period.

With this method of natural family planning, a couple can have sex from three days after the sudden drop in temperature until the woman's period is over. You should *not* have sex from the end of your period until three days after the next drop in temperature.

Not all women have such a sudden rise in temperature after ovulation, however; it may be more steplike. In addition, you should be aware of changes in your life routine, such as illness, vacations, and periods of fatigue or stress—all of which also affect your temperature.

To fully understand your own cycle, you should record your temperature levels for several months before relying exclusively on this method.

The calendar or rhythm method depends on knowing the length of your menstrual cycle so you can stop having intercourse during fertile or unsafe days.

The temperature method depends on taking your temperature every day and keeping a chart of temperature changes. Your temperature will drop just before ovulation, and then rise rapidly for three days after ovulation. You should stop having intercourse from the end of your period until three days after the temperature drop to be most safe.

The mucus method depends on taking a daily sample of mucus from your vagina and checking the stickiness of the mucus with your fingers. Fertile days in which you must avoid intercourse begin when the mucus becomes cloudy and sticky and end when the mucus becomes watery and clear, or when there is no mucus.

Three Natural Family-Planning Methods

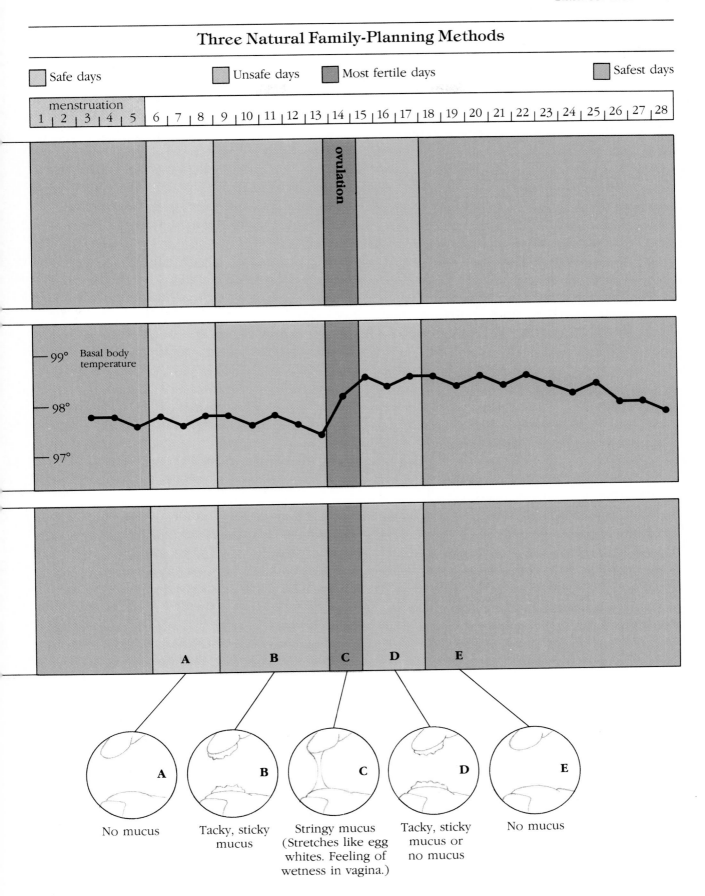

Safe days   Unsafe days   Most fertile days   Safest days

menstruation
1 2 3 4 5 6 7 8 9 10 11 12 13 14 15 16 17 18 19 20 21 22 23 24 25 26 27 28

ovulation

99° Basal body
temperature
98°
97°

A   B   C   D   E

A
No mucus

B
Tacky, sticky
mucus

C
Stringy mucus
(Stretches like egg
whites. Feeling of
wetness in vagina.)

D
Tacky, sticky
mucus or
no mucus

E
No mucus

How to Use the Temperature Method

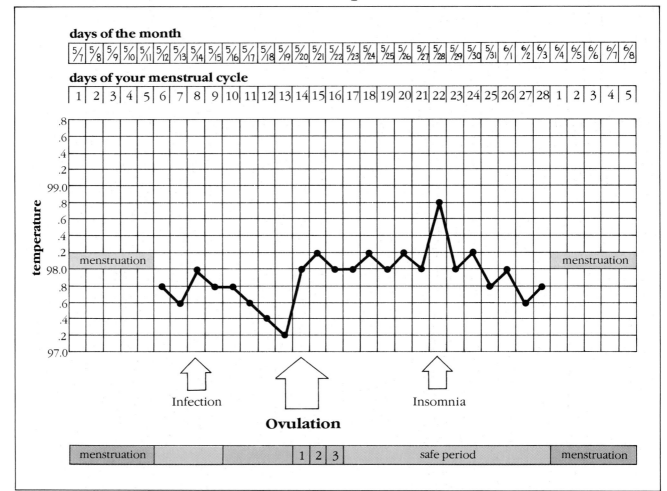

Infection

Ovulation

Insomnia

The basal body thermometer, also known as an ovulation thermometer, only measures temperatures between 96 degrees and 100 degrees F., and can be used orally or rectally. You will want to keep one of these special thermometers at your bedside. You also should have handy graph paper for your temperature chart, and a pencil to record your temperature before getting up.

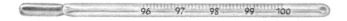

● *In the morning, just after waking and before any activity, take your temperature and record it as a dot on a chart like the one shown.*

● *Note on the chart any event other than ovulation that might make your temperature rise. Insomnia, infections, tension, even using an electric blanket may cause a daily rise in temperature.*

● *Note your menstruation period on the chart.*

● *Keep this chart for six months. Your safe days for intercourse will be from three days after the sudden drop in temperature until three to four days after your period is over.*

For some women, it is difficult to attend to the temperature-taking procedure first thing in the morning. It has been shown that if the temperature is taken regularly at 5:00 p.m., or at bedtime, these temperatures can be charted in the same way as the basal body temperature. Whenever you choose to measure your temperature, accuracy and consistency are of great importance.

The mucus or Billings method shows your time of ovulation by changes in the mucus of the vagina and cervix. Cervical mucus goes through several changes as hormone levels go up and down, and these changes are recorded on a special calendar.

After your period, you may have:
● several *dry* days with no mucus secretion
● several days with a yellow or white, thick, *sticky* discharge
● one or two days when the mucus becomes clear, very *slippery*, and lubricative, with the consistency of unbeaten egg whites
● a sudden change when there is either no mucus or when the mucus becomes *cloudy* and sticky again
● a *watery*, clear mucus immediately before the menstrual period begins.

Ovulation occurs soon after the day of most lubrication, or the peak day, when the mucus is clear and slippery. Fertile days generally begin with the cloudy white or yellow mucus, and continue through the three days after the lubricative mucus ends. If you do not want to become pregnant, you should avoid intercourse on these days.

To examine the cervical mucus, place a clean finger into the vagina, take a bit of mucus near the cervix, and look at it. Place the mucus between your thumb and forefinger to check its consistency. Usually, the mucus does not have a bad odor. If it does, you may have vaginitis and should have a checkup.

Practice charting changes in cervical mucus for at least one or two months before relying on this method. Should you decide to use it, do not ever douche. Douching washes away the mucus in the vagina, leaving you with no way of checking the cyclic changes.

Extensive literature is now available on each of these three natural family planning methods (see page 667). These sources contain detailed instructions for the use of each method.

Effectiveness. It has been difficult to obtain effectiveness rates for the rhythm methods of birth control. Because only 8 percent of women of childbearing age have regular menstrual cycles, we may well expect use effectiveness to vary widely. Rates obtained range from a low of 60 percent effectiveness to a high of 85 percent.

Convenience of use. For many couples, natural family planning begins to feel "unnatural," since there are many days in the cycle when couples are unable to have intercourse. In addition, some women find the record keeping and daily calculations required by these methods inconvenient. These methods do not require the assistance of a physician, however, although counseling of some kind is usually needed to learn how to use them correctly.

How to Record Cervical Mucus Changes

sun	mon	tue	wed	thu	fri	sat
1	2	3	4	5	6 dry	7 dry
8 dry	9 dry	10 sticky white	11 sticky white	12 sticky cloudy	13 sticky cloudy	14 slippery clear
15 sticky cloudy	16 sticky white	17 sticky white	18 dry	19 dry	20 dry	21 dry
22 dry	23 dry	24 dry	25 dry	26 watery clear	27 watery clear	28 watery clear

☐ **days when intercourse might result in pregnancy**
■ **ovulation** ☐ **menstruation**

This chart shows you how to record the changes in cervical mucus in a typical cycle. Keep track of your observations on a similar chart or on a calendar. Mucus characteristics are written in on the day that they are observed, as shown above.

An internal examination for mucus is usually not necessary. You can check for mucus by blotting the vaginal opening with toilet paper before urinating. After keeping track of the changes for about three cycles, your fertile and safe periods will become very obvious to you. On the most fertile days, there is a feeling of wetness and lubrication. The mucus will be slippery, and will form a string when tested between two fingers. It will resemble raw egg white. Its color will be clear or possibly cloudy, yellow, or tinted with pink or brownish blood. This is when ovulation is occurring. Just before and immediately after ovulation, the mucus becomes cloudy and sticky. As it becomes safe to have intercourse without any chance of pregnancy, the amount of mucus will decrease, and it may become clear and watery.

Abstinence is usually necessary for four days before ovulation, and for three days after the peak symptoms of ovulation. The dry days after menstruation are the only definitely infertile days before ovulation. If you have a short cycle, there may be no safe days after menstruation until after ovulation. Any time you notice stretchy, lubricative mucus, you should avoid sexual intercourse for a few days.

This method is sometimes used together with the temperature and calendar methods. Then, if the mucus is obscured by a discharge due to an infection, the other signs of your fertility can be consulted. With all the information combined in one chart, you can be assured of a great deal of accuracy.

Beneficial side effects. Natural family planning methods demand that you learn something about your own body and its reproductive physiology, a useful awareness for women to possess.

Detrimental side effects. Some studies indicate that contraceptive failures among couples who use the various natural methods of birth control have been more likely to produce defective offspring. The reason appears to be that, when fertilization does occur, it occurs with an egg that has survived for a relatively long time, or with a sperm that has survived for a relatively long time. An older egg or sperm is more likely to be defective.

Important tips for rhythm method users.
• Make your own rhythm method calendar, or purchase a printed calendar on which to record physiologic changes during your menstrual cycle.
• You may want to strongly consider using one of these natural methods of family planning along with a second method such as foam, condoms, the diaphragm, or the foaming suppository.
• Consult other women who have used the natural method you are considering so that you can learn from their experiences. In some communities, there are groups of women who discuss natural approaches to birth control.

Lactation

Because fertility is substantially reduced in nursing mothers during the postpartum period when the menstrual flow has not resumed, breast-feeding has been viewed as a period during which a woman is protected from pregnancy. It is true that the hormones released by your body during this time *may* suppress ovulation and thus prevent conception. These hormones are more likely to be released consistently and to suppress ovulation if you feed your baby *only* at the breast, without relying on any supplementary feedings.

However, lactation is *not* a reliable method of birth control, for ovulation can recur during the period of breast-feeding whether or not the woman is supplementing her baby's feeding with other foods. And, ovulation may occur before the return of menstruation; therefore, a woman who continues to have intercourse until the return of her period may be seriously fooled.

Effectiveness. Lactation has an effectiveness rate of 60 to 85 percent. That is, if 100 women use this method of birth control for a year, from 15 to 40 of them will become pregnant unless another method is used simultaneously.

Abstinence

Almost every person, at some time or another, has had to depend upon abstinence (refraining from sexual intercourse) as a method of contraception. Abstinence is obviously the way conception is controlled before men and women become sexually active. Even after men and women become sexually active, and even during marriage, couples often depend on abstinence when they have no other form of contraceptive protection.

Effectiveness. As long as couples refrain from contact between the penis and the vagina, abstinence is undeniably effective.

Convenience of use. Abstinence is always available as a method of birth control. It costs no money and requires no physician intervention.

Beneficial side effects. Abstinence prevents sexually transmitted infections.

Detrimental side effects. Abstinence may cause a great deal of tension and open conflict between partners who disagree about using this approach to birth control.

Important tips for using abstinence.
• Talk with your partner about using abstinence for birth control so you can clarify your own values and better estimate how committed you are to this contraceptive method. Also consider a backup method to ensure against any failure to maintain abstinence.
• Some doctors rather strongly encourage abstinence for the first six weeks after a full-term delivery, since ovulation can occur prior to your six-week postpartum visit. If you do decide to have intercourse prior to this visit, you must use another means of birth control to avoid pregnancy.

Postcoital Contraception

Situations do arise when you will have unprotected intercourse at mid-cycle when ovulation is most likely to occur. Regrettably, sometimes intercourse is forced on a woman. At other times, condoms break. At still other times, a couple may have planned to use a diaphragm, the foaming suppository, or contraceptive foam, and simply fail to do so.

A woman who has unprotected mid-cycle intercourse has several options:
• She may ask her physician to administer high-dose estrogens or progestins as morning-after contraceptives.
• She may have an IUD inserted.
• She may wait to see whether or not her period comes on time. If it is late, she can have menses extraction.
• She may wait until a pregnancy can be detected by test. If the test is positive, she may arrange for a therapeutic abortion.
• She may carry a resulting pregnancy to term.

Obviously, the decision will depend upon whether or not the couple wants to have a child; the cost, convenience, and availability of the options suggested;

and the religious, moral, and ethical values held by those involved. No approach to morning-after contraception is perfect. It goes without saying that using a contraceptive during sexual intercourse is by far the better alternative.

Hormonal approaches. Several hormonal approaches have been used to eliminate the potential consequences of unprotected mid-cycle intercourse. Just how effective these approaches are is not known at the present time.

DES (diethylstilbestrol), ethinyl estradiol, and Premarin are the three most commonly used high-dose estrogen preparations for morning-after contraception.

A great deal has been written about DES recently because of the harmful side effects on female offspring of mothers who were given DES during pregnancy.

It is estimated that somewhere between one and three million males and females were exposed to DES *in utero* from the 1940s through the 1960s when the drug was administered to prevent miscarriage. One in 10,000 of the females exposed *in utero* during the first trimester has developed adenocarcinoma of the vagina during her teens and early twenties.

No definite carcinogenic effect has been demonstrated among women who took DES either to prevent miscarriage or as a morning-after contraceptive. But women should be told that if they take DES as a morning-after contraceptive and still retain the pregnancy, they should obtain a therapeutic abortion. In fact, many clinicians will not provide DES as a morning-after contraceptive to women who find it impossible to accept the idea of an abortion, should they still become pregnant.

The IUD. If a woman chooses to have an IUD inserted at mid-cycle following unprotected intercourse, it is important to realize that the conceptus is still in the fallopian tube at this time, and IUD insertion will *not* be dislodging an already-implanted, fertilized egg from the lining of the uterus.

An IUD inserted the morning after unprotected mid-cycle intercourse operates very much as it would if inserted several months or years previously. Once the fertilized egg comes down through the fallopian tube into the uterus, the presence of the IUD prevents implantation in the uterine lining.

For a woman who has strongly considered using an IUD anyway, it is probably the ideal approach to unprotected mid-cycle intercourse. On the other hand, not all women are good candidates for the IUD, and this factor must be considered at this time (for more information, see page 175).

The alternative of menses extraction and abortion are discussed on page 215 and page 212.

Cooperative Decisions

Until now, women have assumed most of the responsibility for contraceptive protection and family planning. However, there are many opportunities for men and women to cooperate as partners in making decisions, not only about birth control, but about when to have sexual intercourse, when to have children, when to consider abortion, vasectomy, sterilization, and the myriad concerns of two people who are in a committed sexual relationship.

Of course, people differ in their background, their views about contraception, and their ability to trust another. Still, their are specific ways in which men and women can cooperate in the area of family planning, and we suggest them to you.

Discuss together when you will become sexually active.

Discuss whether or not you want to have children. If you do wish to have children, discuss when you hope to have them, how many you hope to have, and how you ideally would like to space your children.

Because of the safety and effectiveness of sterilization, most couples now can consider it as an option when both are certain they want no children, or no more children. Perhaps surprisingly, sterilization is the method of birth control most commonly used by married couples in the United States today.

Discuss together the situations when you will *not* be having sexual intercourse. This may be because of problems, such as the termination of a recent pregnancy, infections, natural or rhythm birth control schedules, or a variety of medical problems for which your physician may recommend that either you or your partner refrain from sexual intercourse.

A man can help his partner remember to take birth control pills daily.

Discuss together what would happen should a contraceptive failure result in a pregnancy. Would it be acceptable to have a child at this time? Could you consider abortion as a backup approach were a pregnancy to occur?

Couples can go together to the physician's office at the time of IUD insertion. Women often need help after an IUD insertion because of pain or nausea, and some women find it difficult to drive home from the physician's office. Likewise, a woman can accompany her husband at the time of a vasectomy; partners often support each other through the physical routine of sterilization (see page 194).

Couples may go together to any routine physical examination. Some physicians will permit others in the examining room; some women like to have their partners present during a pelvic examination, others do not. There is obviously a range of opinion in this area.

A woman can put a condom on for her partner, or a man can insert a diaphragm, foam, or a foaming suppository for his partner. Often these contraceptives can be included in foreplay if the couple is innovative.

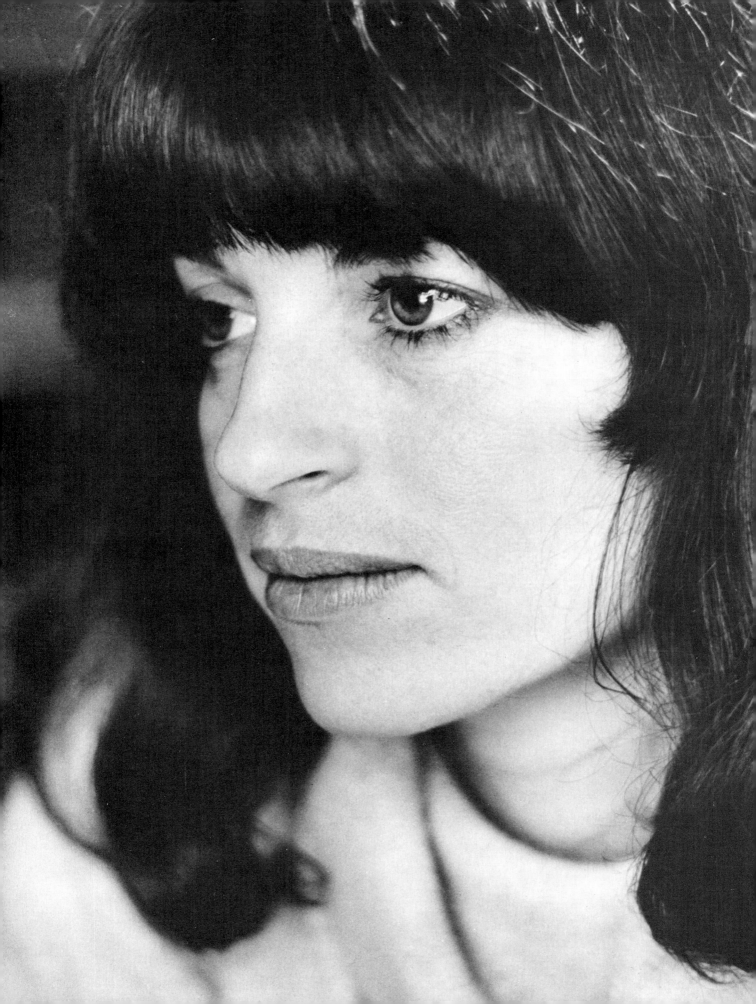

CHAPTER 11

STERILIZATION

LOUISE B. TYRER, M.D., F.A.C.O.G.

For couples who have been married ten or more years, voluntary sterilization is currently the most popular method of birth control. Are sterilization operations reversible at a later date? Is sterilization safe? How does sterilization affect health and sexuality? If you and your partner are considering sterilization, you will want answers to these important questions.

Sterilization

Voluntary sterilization is an elective method of birth control that is intended to be permanent—and almost always is. Every year, about 500,000 men and 700,000 women elect sterilization, which is now the most popular method of contraception for couples who have been married ten or more years.

For a woman, sterilization usually means having an operation to block the fallopian tubes, where the sperm meets the egg and fertilization occurs. The operation, called tubal occlusion, leaves all the organs intact and does not interrupt the normal functions of ovulation or menstruation.

If you are considering sterilization, you may be wondering:
- *How safe is it?*
- *Will it change my sex life?*
- *How will it affect my future health and well-being?*
- *What if I wish the sterilization reversed?*

This chapter will answer your questions and help you make an informed, reasoned decision.

The Important Decisions

Voluntary sterilization means deciding to forever give up the capacity to reproduce. Any woman who seeks this operation must view her decision with this understanding, and hopefully has given the matter long and careful thought. Perhaps she now has one or more children, and feels that her family is now complete. Or, even if childless, she may seek sterilization as a safeguard against transmitting birth defects or inherited diseases. Or, she simply may wish to remain childless.

Whatever the reason, even after a woman has made that first, crucial decision to "turn off" her reproductive potential, she still faces several important questions:
- Who should have the sterilization operation—she or her partner?
- When is the best time for the operation?
- Where will it be performed?
- Who is best qualified to perform the operation?
- Which operative procedure is best?

Many women, in their anxiety to "get it done," fail to consider that sterilization for the male is safer, far easier to perform, involves less risk, and is less expensive. Communication between partners is vital, and if the male partner elects sterilization, it must be without coercion from the woman. Some women feel more comfortable knowing that they will undergo the operation themselves. They perceive themselves as the one who bears the child—and, not infrequently, the one ultimately responsible for its rearing. Therefore, the remainder of this chapter will focus on voluntary sterilization for women.

A woman must never allow herself to be sterilized under pressure or coercion from another person. Nor should she consider the operation if she has any lingering doubts or unanswered questions about the procedure. By the time she goes to surgery, she should have a clear understanding of what she is doing and what the outcome will be, and should have considered each step in the decision making process.

Deciding on sterilization is something you must do alone. However, discussing it with your partner, a counselor, and your physician is important. You need to resolve how you would feel if your life situation changed drastically. Would you want more children if you lost the ones you now have in a tragedy? Would you want to have a baby if in the future you had a different partner who wanted children? If you are ambivalent, the answer is *"Don't do it"*—there are very effective, reversible methods of contraception you can use until you are sure.

Deciding when. Many women don't consider sterilization as an option until they are faced with the dilemma of an unplanned pregnancy. This represents poor planning of one's reproductive life, which certainly deserves more thought than deciding which career to follow or which house to buy. "Sterilization regret," which is really very low, is often higher when a woman makes her decision under such duress.

But assuming you and your partner have decided on the number and spacing of your children and your plan is on target, you can schedule your sterilization at the conclusion of your last planned pregnancy—the easiest and safest time. Don't, however, rush into an after-pregnancy sterilization just because it may be more convenient. If you're the least bit unsure that the time is right, wait. You can always arrange for an interval tubal operation at a later date. The timing of this safe and relatively simple procedure is unrelated to pregnancy.

In some cases, laws or government regulations specify that a woman must wait 30 days from the time she makes a written declaration of her desire for voluntary sterilization before she can have the actual operation. Therefore, if you want the operation done in conjunction with the delivery of your last child, you should make the arrangements with your doctor early in your pregnancy.

Deciding where. Although most sterilizations are performed in a hospital, with the advent of simpler procedures, independent surgical facilities now provide interval sterilization on an outpatient basis, and with all the necessary patient safeguards. After completion of the preliminaries, which must include counseling, informed signed consent, a medical history, a complete physical examination, and certain laboratory tests, a woman may go to the surgical suite in the morning, have her operation—often under sedation and local anesthesia—and go home the same afternoon. Generally, outpatient surgical costs are about half those of inpatient operations.

If you think you would prefer an outpatient procedure but can't locate a facility, contact your local medical society, your nearest Planned Parenthood clinic, or the Association for Voluntary Sterilization, 14 West 44th Street, New York, New York 10036.

Deciding who. Second only to your initial decision to request voluntary sterilization, your choice of doctors is of the utmost importance. Don't be content with the recommendation of a satisfied friend. Although this is significant, even more important are the physician's qualifications and experience.

• Is the doctor qualified in this procedure? He should have taken special training in female sterilization techniques and be able to answer all of your questions about the operation.
• Does the doctor have surgical privileges to perform sterilization procedures in a hospital? This is particularly important if the proposed operation is to use the new laparoscopic technique. And if the procedure is to be done in an outpatient setting, hospital privileges allow the doctor to transfer patients to a hospital in the rare event that a complication develops.

• Does the doctor personally make sure that all your questions and concerns are thoughtfully addressed before you go to surgery? The physician may depend on a specially trained staff for most of the counseling, but a good doctor takes the time to be sure all your questions are answered.
• Does the doctor do a thorough medical history and physical examination, and obtain pertinent laboratory tests, such as one for anemia?

Benefits and Risks

As with any method of contraception, you must list and weigh the benefits and risks of voluntary sterilization as part of your decision making process.

As you study this list of potential benefits, you'll want to rank or weigh each one according to your individual circumstances.

Freedom from unwanted pregnancy and its associated anxiety. Many women report that this freedom lifts a great burden from their minds, and allows them fuller freedom for sexual fulfillment.

The potential for improved health. Scientific data clearly documents that repeated childbearing with short intervals between births is definitely damaging to a woman's health.

Averting the problems of reversible methods. Aside from having to remember to use them regularly, the two most effective reversible methods, the birth control pill and the IUD, have some rare, inherent risks to which a user is continually exposed. Oral contraceptives in particular may not be advisable for women who are 35 years of age or older, particularly if they smoke or have certain medical conditions such as high blood pressure.

Potential risks you should consider are:

The risk of serious complications. Even with today's simplified techniques, sterilization for the female is a major surgical procedure, and, as such, has certain inherent risks. The greatest risk with any operation, including tubal sterilization, involves the use of general or spinal anesthesia. This is why more women are requesting that the procedure be done under sedation and local anesthesia. Even the sophisticated technique of laparoscopy can be performed under local anesthesia.

Serious complications related to the surgical procedure of tubal sterilization are rare— approximately 2 to 3 percent—and usually relate to bleeding or infection. When symptoms are reported promptly to the doctor and are adequately treated, these risks are further reduced.

The mortality rate for tubal sterilization is extremely low—about two deaths per 100,000 women. Additionally, a woman only faces this risk once—at the time of her operation—while the risks related to other forms of contraception are continuous. A woman may experience some discomfort for a few days, but postoperative oral pain medication usually is sufficient to control it. She generally can return to work in two to five days, and can resume sexual activity as soon as the discomfort subsides (except in cases where a vaginal incision is present).

Although sterilization is not known to leave any long-term adverse effects on the body, there is one possible exception. Some women seem to develop abnormal bleeding patterns as a result of tubal sterilization. These may be the result of interrupting some of the blood and nerve supply to the tube and ovary during the operation, or they simply may be inherent problems the woman would have developed anyway with age.

The risk of later regret. If a woman follows the decision making process outlined here, she should avoid the possibility of regretting her choice later. The highest incidence of regret occurs when a woman makes her decision hastily, and is poorly informed about its long-term significance for her future fertility, or when the procedure is combined with abortion. In the latter case, when a woman is under unusually stressful conditions, she may have difficulty making an objective decision about something as important as her entire reproductive future.

Sterilization Techniques

Techniques of Tubal Occlusion

Operating surgeons use several techniques to interrupt the fallopian tube so that the sperm and egg can't meet. One of the most common is to tie the tube with a suture. A modification of this tubal ligation technique is to remove a segment of tube and send it to the laboratory for confirmation.

Another common technique for blocking the tubes—used particularly with laparoscopy—is cautery. It employs an electrical current to produce scar tissue, and is done with or without removal of a piece of the tube. Tubal bands, clips, or rings also may be applied to the tube. Cautery appears to result in the least failures (pregnancies), but also has the least potential for later reversal if a woman experiences sterilization regret.

Interval Tubal Sterilization

More and more women who do not combine a preplanned tubal sterilization with the delivery of their last child are opting for one of the techniques of interval tubal occlusion. The choices for interval tubal sterilization are:

Laparoscopy. This technique is commonly called the "band aid" operation, as it can be performed through a small incision near the navel that is covered by a very small dressing. It takes about 20 to 30 minutes, including the time required for anesthesia.

There are two general types of laparoscopy—closed and open—that both utilize a long magnifying scope with its own cold light source to illuminate the pelvis and help the surgeon identify and block the tubes. The closed technique is more common—as more surgeons generally have been trained in its use—but it presents certain disadvantages over the open technique. The needle used to introduce the expanding gas into the abdomen to provide visibility and mobility must be inserted blindly, as must the sharp trocar that carries the viewing instruments. There are inherent risks of perforating vital organs with the closed technique that are not present with the open technique. In open laparoscopy, the surgeon makes a small incision at the navel and visually inserts the instruments. This method should continue to gain popularity as more women become aware of its inherent benefits.

Mini-laparotomy. This sterilization technique was perfected in less-developed countries where requests for sterilization are high and sophisticated equipment, such as the laparoscope, is generally unavailable. Because of its simplicity, it can be performed in out-of-hospital surgical facilities at less cost and without the potential risks of other techniques, particularly closed laparoscopy.

In this technique, the doctor makes a tiny incision in the lower abdomen just above the pubic bone. With the abdomen opened, he then manipulates each tube into view by moving the uterus up under the incision using instruments previously placed in the uterus through the vagina and attached to the cervix. After the tubes are occluded, the abdomen is closed.

Vaginal Tubal Sterilization

Tubal sterilization also can be performed through a vaginal incision—either by direct visual inspection or with the aid of a Culdoscope (an instrument similar to the laparoscope). Since vaginal tubal sterilization introduces a higher risk of infection, it is not favored by many physicians.

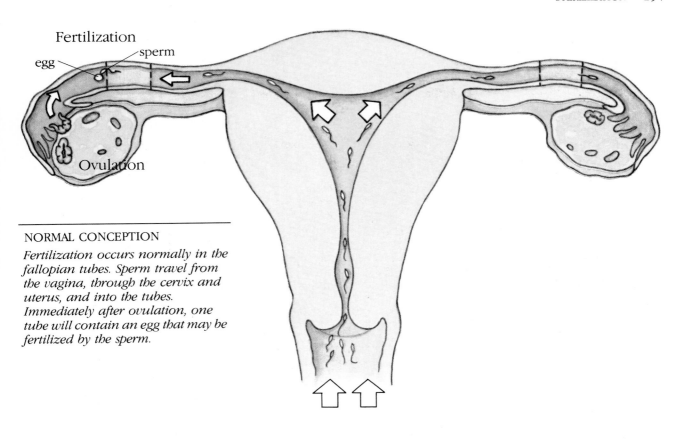

Fertilization

egg   sperm

Ovulation

NORMAL CONCEPTION

Fertilization occurs normally in the fallopian tubes. Sperm travel from the vagina, through the cervix and uterus, and into the tubes. Immediately after ovulation, one tube will contain an egg that may be fertilized by the sperm.

TUBAL OCCLUSION (STERILIZATION) BY LIGATION AND EXCISION

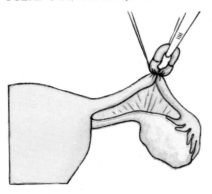
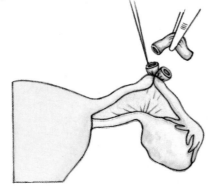
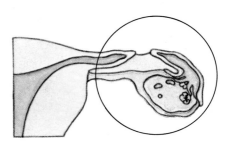
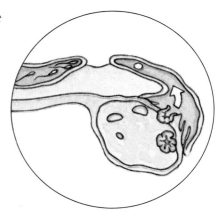

TUBAL LIGATION *Fertilization is prevented by blocking (occluding) the fallopian tube so that sperm cannot pass from the upper tube to the egg. One blocking technique is to tie the tube with a suture. The tied-off pieces then are surgically removed. The cut ends of the fallopian tubes heal, forming blind pockets and ensuring that sperm and egg cannot meet. The adjacent enlargement shows how egg and sperm are effectively separated by this operation. Once performed, tubal ligation is difficult and costly to reverse, and reversal surgery is successful in only 30 percent of cases attempted.*

LAPAROSCOPIC STERILIZATION

Ask your doctor to explain his or her procedure for laparoscopic sterilization so you are prepared for the details of the surgery. The position you assume is similar to that for a pelvic examination. Your legs are raised in stirrups, and the table is tilted to position the head lower than the abdomen. After administration of an anesthetic, the laparoscope is placed in the abdomen through an incision at the navel (see below). If the two-incision method is used, the doctor will make another incision in the lower abdomen.

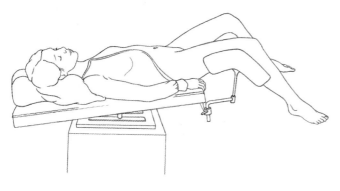

What Is a Laparoscope?

A laparoscope is an instrument that can be inserted into the abdominal cavity to inspect its contents. It consists of a long, slim tube about the diameter of a pencil, and contains a light source for illuminating the cavity. Attached instruments enable the performance of surgical procedures in the abdominal pelvic cavity.

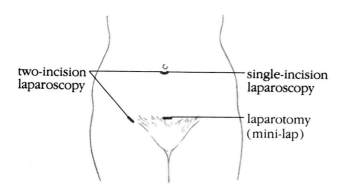

two-incision laparoscopy

single-incision laparoscopy

laparotomy (mini-lap)

SINGLE-INCISION LAPAROSCOPY *In the technique of single-incision laparoscopy, the following sterilization procedure is used:*

● *The doctor will clean and sterilize your abdomen and navel with an antiseptic wash.*

● *He will then strap a metal plate to your thigh to "ground" the cautery machine, which is used to seal and sever the fallopian tubes.*

● *An instrument called a cannula is firmly attached to your cervix so that the doctor can move the cervix around, allowing an unobstructed view of the tubes and ovaries.*

● *After the doctor administers an anesthetic, he makes an incision just below the navel (see below left) and places a long needle into the abdomen. Carbon dioxide gas is pumped through this tube into the abdomen, distending it and allowing better visualization and movement of instruments during the operation.*

● *Then, through the same tiny slit in the abdomen, the doctor inserts a tube through which he passes the laparoscope with tiny light source, more carbon dioxide gas, and the electrical forceps that will cauterize and seal off the fallopian tubes.*

● *The physician views the procedure through the laparoscope, an ocular device that allows him to see internal structures.*

● *After the tubes are coagulated, the doctor removes the instruments from the abdomen and the cervix, closes the incision with a stitch, and applies a bandage. You may then rest in the same room or a recovery room until you feel well enough to go home, usually within two to four hours after the operation.*

INSET *Cauterization effectively seals the tube ends so that egg and sperm cannot meet. Ovulation continues, as does the normal hormonal and menstrual cycle; there is simply a mechanical block to keep the egg from moving down the fallopian tube.*

DOUBLE-INCISION LAPAROSCOPY *This procedure is identical to a single-incision laparoscopy, except that the doctor makes a second incision in the lower abdomen through which he inserts the forceps that will coagulate the tube.*

SINGLE-INCISION LAPAROSCOPY WITH CAUTERIZATION

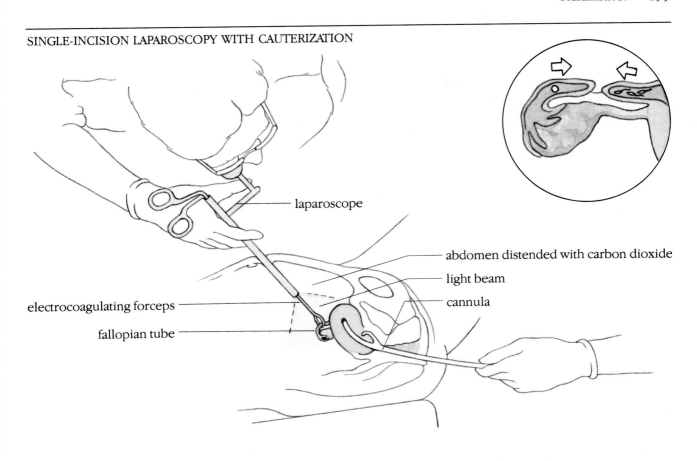

laparoscope

abdomen distended with carbon dioxide

light beam

cannula

electrocoagulating forceps

fallopian tube

DOUBLE-INCISION LAPAROSCOPY WITH CAUTERIZATION

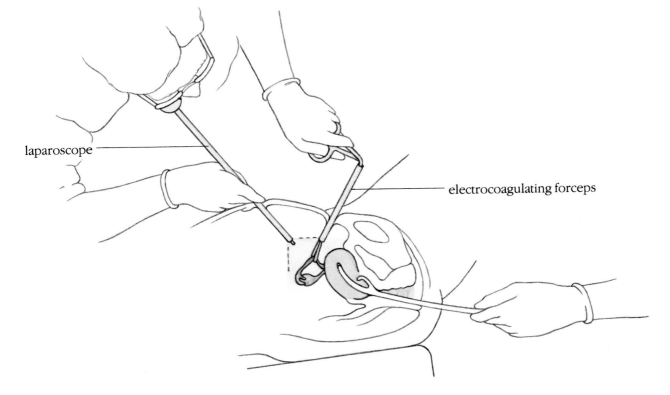

laparoscope

electrocoagulating forceps

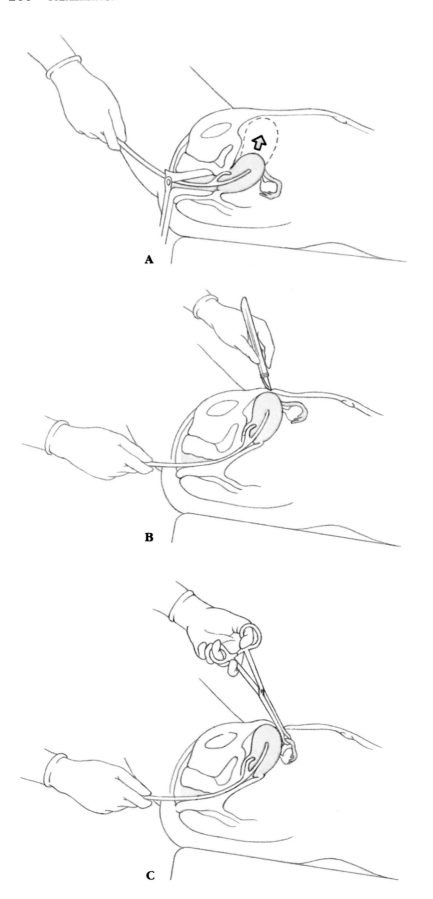

A

B

C

MINI-LAPAROTOMY

This simpler version of female sterilizaton does not use a laparo-scope at all. In a mini-laparotomy, the doctor makes a tiny incision in the lower abdomen just above the pubic bone through which the tubes can be reached. A cannula previously placed in the uterus (A) is manipulated to push the fallopian tubes closer to the surface for easy access. After administering anesthesia, which may be a local anesthetic, the doctor makes a small incision (B) through which he grasps the tube with forceps (C). Instead of sealing the tube by cauterization, the doctor may place a ring or clip over the tube to close it off. Clip and ring techniques are relatively new, and may allow for more ease in reversibility of the operation should it be required. This operation can be done in a surgical clinic in about 30 minutes, and is followed by several hours' rest before going home.

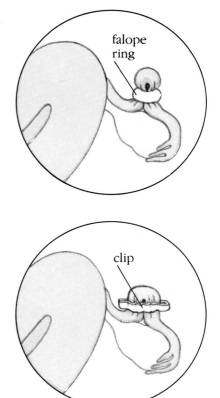

falope ring

clip

VAGINAL TUBAL LIGATION

Another approach for sterilization involves inserting the Culdoscope or surgical tools into the pelvis through a cut in the vaginal wall. Today these techniques are largely replaced by laparoscopy through the abdomen. The complication rate is higher with these techniques due to infection.

COLPOTOMY   *In colpotomy, the uterus is manipulated out of the way by forceps (A) so the doctor can make an incision through the vagina into the pelvic cavity (B). He then brings the tubes out through the incision and ties them (C). The patient must be on her knees with the chest and head resting on the operation table, a position that may be uncomfortable. The only advantage to colpotomy seems to be that it eliminates the small abdominal scar of laparoscopy.*

CULDOSCOPY   *The Culdoscope is another instrument with a light source that allows the physician to see into the pelvic cavity. An older technique than laparoscopy, culdoscopy is now rarely used for sterilization. For this operation, a woman is placed in the "knee-chest" position as for colpotomy. Local anesthesia is used in the vaginal wall before inserting the Culdoscope.*

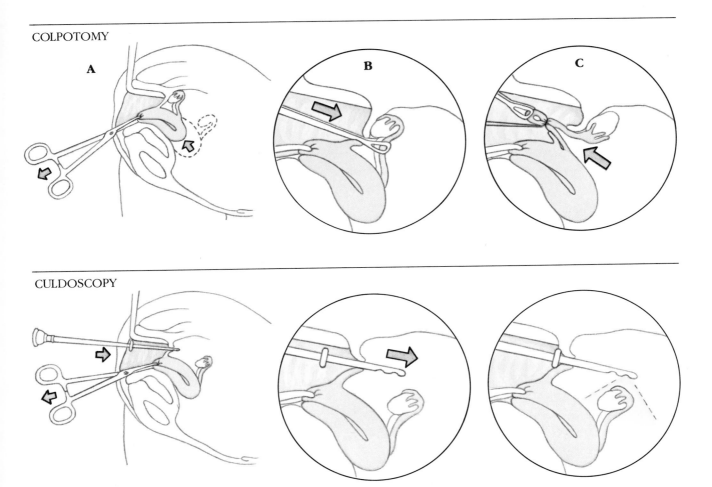

COLPOTOMY

A   B   C

CULDOSCOPY

Pregnancy-Related Tubal Sterilization

Postpartum tubal sterilization. Until the advent of laparoscopy, postpartum tubal ligation was the only procedure generally utilized for voluntary sterilization. It is still widely used, is simple to do, and is appropriate for a woman who has made a prior, considered decision to terminate her reproduction. The operation is performed shortly after a normal delivery or in conjunction with a cesarean birth. After a normal delivery, most doctors suggest at least a 24-hour wait before the sterilization so that the newborn's condition can stabilize and the doctor can give the woman a reading on the infant's health and likelihood of survival.

The operation may be done under local or general anesthesia, and requires only a small incision in the midline of the abdomen near the enlarged uterus. The tubes are then occluded, usually by tubal ligation.

Post-abortal sterilization. When a woman terminates an unwanted pregnancy, she may not be in a state of mind to give thoughtful consideration to her ultimate reproductive goals. This is why regret is higher for women who combine sterilization with abortion, unless, however, they know that they already have reached their optimum family size. When sterilization is combined with termination in the first three months of pregnancy, laparoscopy is the usual technique. When combined with termination in the second trimester, the same approach as for postpartum tubal sterilization is used, but without the 24-hour waiting period.

Hysterectomy for voluntary sterilization. Since the risk of serious complications, including death, is higher for hysterectomy than for tubal sterilization, hysterectomy is rarely performed as an elective procedure. It may be advisable, however, if pelvic disease is identified when the woman considering sterilization has her preliminary gynecologic examination. If the examination uncovers fibroid tumors, for example, a hysterectomy is preferable to tubal sterilization, which would leave the underlying disease unresolved. For more information on hysterectomy and tumors, see the chapter on "Adult Reproductive Problems."

If you have any doubts about the advice you receive from your doctor, ask for and obtain a second medical opinion through consultation. You may select your own consultant or request a referral from your doctor.

Sterilization Reversal

A woman must never decide on voluntary sterilization on the premise that, someday, she may have the procedure reversed and be able to have a baby. Although surgical techniques exist that may successfully rejoin the tubes in about 30 percent of the women who undergo reversal surgery (particularly when reversal surgery is performed under the operating microscope), not all of these women can carry a successful pregnancy to term. Reversal surgery is performed only in a few university medical centers, carries with it the risks of major surgery, and is very expensive—usually between $4,000 and $5,000. In addition, there is no way to know in advance whether your reversal will be successful or unsuccessful.

The risk of tubal pregnancy also is greater after successful surgery for reversal. This occurs when the fertilized egg remains in the fallopian tube—a condition that can endanger a woman's life and requires another surgical procedure to correct. But the largest obstacle to successful reversal operations is that only a select few women are candidates for this delicate procedure, as sufficient undamaged tube must remain to be rejoined. Women who have had their tubes occluded by electric cautery generally cannot even attempt to have a reversal, as too much of the tubes has been damaged.

However, a new door to future conception appears to be opening for women with occluded tubes who cannot or did not have a successful reversal operation. Recent successful research with *in vitro* (outside the body) fertilization offers a unique approach to achieving a pregnancy following tubal occlusion. In *in vitro* fertilization, a ripe egg is removed from the mother's ovary by minor surgery. The egg is fertilized with sperm outside the body in a special fluid-containing dish (see page 526). Although the techniques are not now widely available, they certainly will be in the near future. This may be the breakthrough of the future for women who have had a voluntary sterilization but, because of changes in their life circumstances, feel that they now must have children.

MALE STERILIZATION BY VASECTOMY

Vasectomy is the simple operation for male sterilization. After injection of a local anesthesia, the whole procedure takes less than 30 minutes in a doctor's office or a clinic. The doctor makes a scrotal incision, usually less than one inch long, in both of the scrotal sacs in order to reach the two vas deferens, the tubes that carry sperm from the testicles to the penis (A). The two vas deferens are pulled out through the incisions (B) and are cut (C), and a portion of the tube may be removed. The cut ends of each vas then may be sutured, cauterized, or clipped with a special clip (C), and the incision in each scrotal sac is closed (D).

A man who has been sterilized experiences no change in sexual functioning. Ejaculation still occurs, and the sex glands continue to function normally to produce male sex hormones. The seminal fluid is still of the same volume, but it contains no sperm. Immediately after the operation, however, sperm still may be found in the tubes between the site of the vasectomy and the penis. For this reason, contraception must be continued until no more sperm are present in the seminal fluid, as determined by a semen analysis. Although some vasectomies can be successfully reversed, the procedure is delicate, expensive, and not always successful. The man who chooses to have a vasectomy must be prepared to give up fathering children permanently. Vasectomy is intended to be 100 percent effective as a means of contraception.

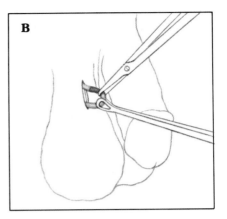

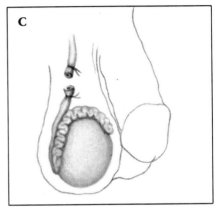

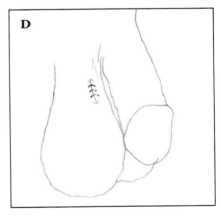

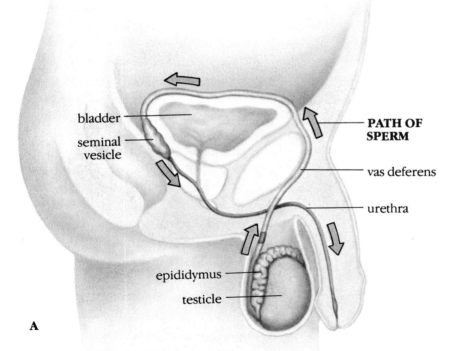

bladder

seminal vesicle

PATH OF SPERM

vas deferens

urethra

epididymus

testicle

A

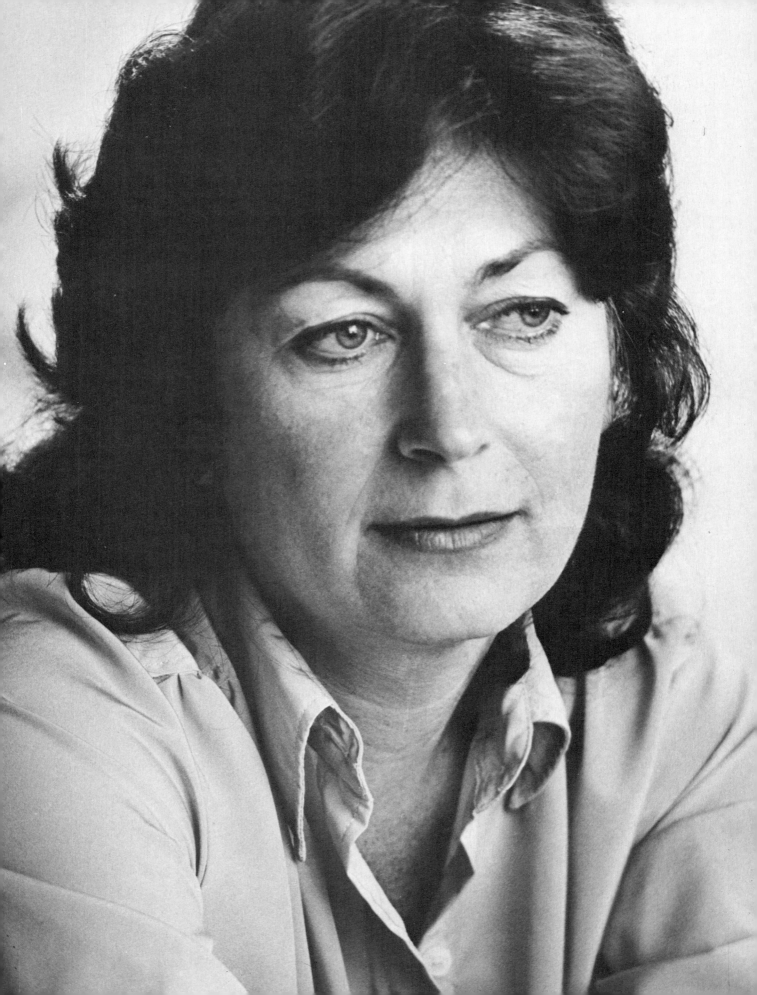

CHAPTER 12

ABORTION

MARJORY SKOWRONSKI LOZEN

Your decision to bear a child has far-reaching consequences, not only for you but for your child as well. There are many factors that you will take into consideration before making a decision to continue a pregnancy or to have an abortion. Abortion continues to be one of the most serious and controversial events in a woman's life, and so it is most important that each woman base her decision on full knowledge of the options open to her, and on her own feelings and needs.

Abortion

Abortion continues to be one of the most controversial issues in the private lives of women, as well as in the public arenas of politics and lawmaking. Men and women both may hold strong opinions about abortion, but women alone actually confront the need for this operation. When faced with an unplanned pregnancy, many women find that their position on the abortion issue moves very quickly from the abstract to the practical—and personal. One solution to an unplanned pregnancy is an abortion, and it is most important that a woman make her choice based on correct information and knowledge of her options.

Time is a crucial factor in deciding whether to continue or to terminate a pregnancy. Early abortions are both physically and emotionally easier for a woman. In addition, if a woman chooses to continue the pregnancy, the sooner she resolves her feelings about it, the better it is for her own well-being and for that of the coming child.

The questions most often asked by women facing the possibility of an abortion are:
- *Is abortion safe?*
- *Will the procedure be painful?*
- *Where can I receive the best care at a reasonable price?*
- *Who can I turn to for help if I'm having difficulty trying to decide?*
- *Will an abortion affect my chances for future pregnancies?*
- *Which medical procedure is best for me?*
- *How long does it take to recuperate?*
- *What are the psychological effects of abortion?*
- *Will I feel guilty or regret it afterward?*
- *Will anyone find out?*

Answers to these questions give information you need to decide if the abortion option is right for you.

The Historical Perspective

Abortion—the induced termination of a pregnancy—has been practiced throughout time and in many cultures. Most of the ancient methods for aborting a fetus — whether medicinal or mechanical — were indirect; that is, such methods upset the physiology of the pregnant woman so much that a miscarriage was one result (among many) of the treatment. These primitive practices were painful, often unsafe, and sometimes fatal. Even so, abortion was sanctioned in most pre-industrial societies where limiting the population held some value. Other common reasons for sanctioning abortion were illegitimacy, economics, and safeguarding the physical health of the woman.

At any time in history, a woman faced with the choice of continuing her pregnancy or aborting has always made her choice within the context of her culture's value system. A thorough study of the relationship between the history of abortion and the history of woman's status in culture and society is beyond the scope of this chapter, but is well documented in other books (see page 667). It is reasonable to suppose, however, that despite a woman's individual concerns, if the culture and society in which she lives condemns, bans, or discourages her from obtaining a legal and safe abortion, there will be some stress associated with her choice to have an abortion.

The historical view of abortion practices shows that abortion has always been part of woman's heritage. Often women risked their lives and health at the hands of illicit abortionists. The first anti-abortion law, passed in Connecticut in 1821, sought to protect women from the hazardous methods of abortion in practice at the time. In the 1920s, first-trimester abortions (those obtained in the first three months of pregnancy) became safe medical operations, but fifty years passed before abortion became legal.

On January 22, 1973, the United States Supreme Court announced their seven-to-two decision on the *Rowe vs. Wade* and *Doe vs. Bolton* cases: a state cannot regulate abortion performed during the first trimester of pregnancy; a state can regulate abortion procedures during the second trimester only to preserve and protect a woman's life or health. This ruling applies to all women regardless of marital status or age. As a result of a later Supreme Court ruling (June, 1977), the states are not required by federal law to provide funding for abortions through Medicaid.

Determining Pregnancy

There are many factors women must take into consideration before making the decision to continue a pregnancy or to have an abortion. But knowing if you are pregnant (and understanding the details of that medical procedure) may relieve one of the biggest anxieties a woman experiences—the fear of the unknown.

Most women don't suspect that they are pregnant until they've missed a period. Women who have irregular or long cycles may be six (or more) weeks pregnant before they suspect pregnancy. And many of the early signs of pregnancy are very subjective (see page 220). There are only two tests that will confirm or reject the possibility of a pregnancy.

The Urine Analysis

Most public health clinics, Planned Parenthood clinics, feminist health collectives, and private gynecologists perform pregnancy testing, and there are several laboratory tests that determine pregnancy. The most widely used laboratory test is a urine analysis that checks for the hormone, human chorionic gonadotropin (HCG), which is produced after conception.

Counting from the first day of the last menstrual period (LMP), it takes 42 days before HCG reaches levels high enough to show a positive result by urine analysis. Though HCG continues to be produced throughout the pregnancy, it reaches its peak level at about 12 weeks after the LMP. After this time, HCG is produced in much smaller amounts, and its level in the urine drops slightly. But the pregnancy test using urine analysis is not as accurate as one might wish. At present, more than 25 percent of women who have abortions prior to the seventh day after the missed period are not actually pregnant.

A pregnancy blood test still under development may put an end to unnecessary abortions. This test, called the radioreceptor assay, appears to be 100 percent accurate six to eight days after conception. That is, you could obtain an absolutely accurate "yes" or "no" answer about your pregnancy as early as the first day after missing a period. The test requires only the blood drawn from a finger prick; the blood is then analyzed, not for human chorionic gonadotropin, but for a HCG-like substance that can be detected soon after the egg is fertilized.

Until the radioreceptor assay test is widely available, the first thing you should do when you want to determine pregnancy is to take a urine specimen to a clinic, a laboratory, or a private physician, making sure that a sufficient number of days has elapsed for the test to produce a reading. Human chorionic gonadotropin cannot be detected in the urine until approximately 40 days from your last menstrual period.

There are some important preparations you must make to ensure that the test is accurate:
- Do not eat or drink anything after dinner the night before. Prepare, in advance, a very clean, dry jar that can hold about one-half cup of liquid.
- Collect the first urine of the morning. (For those who have to go to the bathroom immediately upon arising, be prepared. Forgetting to prepare a jar in advance can result in a mad scramble to find and clean one before it's too late.)
- Keep the urine specimen refrigerated until it's time to take it to the clinic.

The results of the test usually can be obtained within 24 hours. If a pregnancy test comes back "positive," it usually means you are pregnant. However, it could be a "false positive," meaning that you are not pregnant even though the test is positive. Even if it comes back "negative," it's still possible that you are pregnant. The urine analysis pregnancy test can give a "false negative" result because of several factors: the urine was contaminated, too warm, or too dilute (which is likely if you got thirsty at midnight and didn't think it would matter if you drank a glass of water).

If it is too early in the pregnancy, the urine analysis will not be valid because the HCG secreted at the onset of pregnancy may not have built up sufficiently to register a positive result. You must be at least three weeks pregnant, which means that approximately ten days have elapsed since the beginning of your last period. If your results come back negative and your period still has not come in another week, go back for another test. Caution: because of their particular body chemistry, some women never receive a positive test result from urine analysis.

There is now available at your drugstore, without prescription, a do-it-yourself early pregnancy test in kit form (see page 221). This test is 97 percent accurate for a positive pregnancy; negative results are only 80 percent accurate.

The Pelvic Examination

If your period still does not begin after two lab tests, you should go to a doctor for a second type of pregnancy test—a pelvic examination. However, a doctor cannot see or feel characteristic cervical changes until approximately six to eight weeks after the LMP. When a woman is pregnant, her uterus begins to swell from the size of an orange (at about eight weeks after the last menstrual period) to the size of a grapefruit (at about twelve weeks). The uterus also becomes softer.

For a complete description of the pelvic examination procedure, see page 400 of "Choosing a Doctor." If you are tense, the doctor will have a harder time feeling the uterus through your tightened muscles. So, as with many procedures on the body, you will feel better if you can relax as much as possible. Nevertheless, if the doctor is hurting you, speak up. The pelvic examination takes only a few seconds. If the examination is conclusive, the doctor can then determine how long you have been pregnant based on the last menstrual period. If the examination is inconclusive, the doctor may suggest that you wait another week before undergoing another test.

Abortion Counseling

Once pregnancy is determined, you will confront the decision of whether to continue or terminate it.

The role of an abortion counselor is to provide information and advice to women about various abortion procedures, aftercare, and birth control, as well as to offer emotional support. Trained abortion counselors deserve the respect and pay of other health care professionals. Ideally, your counselor and your doctor will continue to support you if you change your mind at the last minute. A counselor may encourage, but should not force you to share any of your emotional feelings concerning the abortion. A good counselor adapts to the needs of each woman.

The presence of a counselor adds dignity and emotional support to the abortion experience. Part of the counselor's job is to inform and prepare you for a procedure that someone else will be performing on you. Knowing what to expect helps dissolve the feelings of helplessness that often arise during any procedure we do not fully understand. If the only available abortion facility does not offer counseling, suggest that they do so in the future.

You also may want to contact a feminist health collective to ask whether or not a "patient advocate" can accompany you, especially if you feel uncomfortable about the facility. A patient advocate is trained not only to give a woman support, but to look out for her well-being during the procedure as well. Above all, trust your own feelings and intuitions: if you are really uncomfortable with the facility, it's best to find another one.

Future Childbearing

A woman's fertility is usually unaffected by an abortion. Most of the fears about abortion and infertility come from past years when all abortions were done sub rosa by unqualified practitioners. In fact, a woman can become pregnant immediately after an abortion and should be very careful to use some form of birth control as soon as she resumes sexual activity.

One British study concluded that although women who had had previous legal abortions tended to have slightly shorter pregnancies, 74 percent of the group studied carried their pregnancies to term. No evidence was found that these infants were smaller or weighed less than normal at birth.

Teen-Age Pregnancy

If you are eighteen years old or younger, are pregnant, and don't want to be, you're not alone. You are in the company of hundreds of thousands of young women. Each year 300,000 teen-age women choose abortions as their "way out" of an unplanned pregnancy. Many thousands more continue their pregnancies and either give up their babies for adoption or raise them, with or without a mate. Regardless of your age, you must make a decision regarding your pregnancy.

How to Tell Your Parents

You may be worried about your parents finding out, and you may be afraid to tell them. Ideally, we should be able to share all of our joys, sorrows, anxieties, and confusions with our parents, but realistically speaking, this is not always possible. A minor has the legal right to obtain an abortion without the consent of her parents, and each young woman must decide for herself if, when, and how she wants to involve them.

You may wish to seek your parents' counsel immediately. Another possibility is to make your decision and then tell your parents about your pregnancy and what you're going to do about it. Another option is to have the abortion or leave town to have the baby, and not tell your parents until it's over. Finally, you may choose not to tell them at all. You'll be encouraged to know that parents are often more understanding and supportive of their daughters during this crisis than you might expect.

You may feel that everyone knows you're pregnant. Actually, no one can know unless you tell them. You do have the option and a certain amount of time to make a decision in private. Pregnancy rarely "shows" during the first three months. But, you must make a decision about what you want to do during this first trimester. There is no running away from the pregnancy. To not decide is to allow the pregnancy to continue. Facing this crisis may be the first time you have had to take on a major decision all by yourself. You may be scared and confused, but the maturity that comes from facing your situation is most valuable.

After thoughtful consideration, you may realize that you would like to talk with someone about making this decision. There are pregnancy counselors available at most Planned Parenthood clinics and at many women's centers. Or you may want to talk to a teacher, an older sister, or a friend whom you already know and trust. If you're confused about what to do, it's best to find someone who will respect your need to come to your own conclusion and who won't try to pressure you one way or the other.

Both having an abortion and continuing your pregnancy are experiences that, once accepted and integrated, can be sources for your further growth toward womanhood. But remember—the worst thing you can do is to delay decision-making so long that your only recourse, should you decide on abortion, is a second-trimester abortion. The procedures used at this stage of pregnancy are very difficult physically, emotionally, and mentally—and should be avoided. A first-trimester abortion, no later than the twelfth week from the beginning of your last menstrual period, is a far simpler procedure.

Making a Decision

One of the most essential issues that a woman must confront is her own moral view of abortion. The Supreme Court decision gives each woman the right to freedom of conscience in this matter:

"When those trained in medicine, philosophy, and theology are unable to arrive at any consensus, the Judiciary at this point in the development of man's knowledge is not in a position to speculate as to the answer.

A woman may opt to accept the thinking of her religious or social group as the final guidance in her decision. Many women, however, are not closely aligned with any system of thought. In any case, each woman should question whether the thinking and advice of others about abortion seriously conflicts with her own needs, intuition, feelings, and life's goals. Sometimes an unplanned pregnancy reveals many inconsistencies in a woman's own thinking that she must clarify before making a decision.

Your feelings about abortion. The answers you give to the following questions may help clarify your thoughts about the morality of abortion:
● At what point between conception and birth do I believe that a fetus becomes a person?
● If I regard the contents of my uterus as only the potential for a human person and not a human person per se, can I accept the choice to terminate my pregnancy, and if so, what are my reasons?
● If I do regard the contents of my uterus as a human person, can I accept the termination of my pregnancy, and why?

There is growing support among religious groups and leaders for a woman's right to make her own choice in the matter of abortion.

Your feelings about childbearing. The decision to bear a child has far-reaching consequences, not only for you, but for the child as well. Deciding whether to have an abortion forces you to think about the quality of life you'll be able to provide your child. For instance, you must consider the commitment in time, energy, and money necessary to raise your child under the best possible conditions.

These questions may help you decide which option is best for you now:
● Am I happy about this pregnancy?
● Do I really want a child now?
● Do I feel ready for all the responsibilities that are involved in child-rearing?
● What are my plans, goals, and hopes for my own future? How does having a baby fit in with the kind of life I want to live?
● How will the continuation or termination of this pregnancy affect my own self-development, health, education, economic status, relationships with others, professional goals, and self-concept?
● If I do continue this pregnancy, what is the quality of life that I could offer my child?
● If I do continue this pregnancy, how will it affect the time I spend with my other children?

Use your imagination to create images of how your life would change if you were to continue or terminate your pregnancy. Often, indecisiveness melts with the realization that your life would change so drastically from the kind you want for yourself that a course of action becomes clear.

Talking with a sympathetic friend is not always enough. A professional pregnancy counselor, one who is able to reflect a woman's own feelings in a non-judgmental way, can be enormously helpful. Pregnancy counseling is offered through Planned Parenthood clinics, women's centers, and health collectives, as well as through private abortion clinics.

Other Options

Although abortion continues to be a very popular solution for unwanted pregnancy, many women prefer other alternatives. A woman may choose to make room for a new addition to her already-existing family, she may decide to keep the child and become a single parent, or she may bring her pregnancy to term and then give the child up for adoption.

Keeping the Child in the Family

Women who already have families have more than half of all unplanned pregnancies. Choosing to make room for one more child requires a reassessment of priorities and resources. Refer to the above list of questions to help you assess your position about adding another child to the family.

Single Parenting

Increasing numbers of women are accepting the challenge of single parenting, especially where the surrounding community offers support for single parents. Even if a woman does not maintain a relationship with the father of her child, it's often possible to share some child-rearing responsibilities with him. If the father of the child is not in the picture, a woman may still choose to keep a child from an unplanned pregnancy. Talking with women who are already single parents is one of the best ways to answer your questions about whether or not to become a single parent. Seeking professional counseling is also advisable, especially for young women considering single parenthood.

Young women who have not yet developed their own skills may be tempted to become mothers rather than to trust using their creative energies in other pursuits that hold some risk or fear for them. If you choose to raise a child alone, remember that you must find ways of fulfilling your own needs for development as well as those of your child. Children flourish when those closest to them are happy and fulfilled persons.

Adoption

Many women prefer the alternative of adoption to that of abortion. If you plan to have your child adopted, contact an adoption agency as soon as you make the decision. Follow their advice, which will surely include the admonition to take good care of yourself during the pregnancy. The baby then has the best start on life, and speedy placement in an adoptive home is often dependent on the child's health.

The legal right to give up a child for adoption belongs to the natural mother, regardless of her age or financial status. The only exception is when a woman is legally proven to be mentally incompetent. A woman always has the option of not naming the father of her child, but if a woman should name the father on the birth certificate, he must also consent to the adoption. However, if a woman is married, her husband, even if he is not the father of her child, must give his consent for the baby to be put up for adoption. This ruling holds whether a woman has completed divorce proceedings less than 300 days before or has not seen her husband for years. In such instances, a lawyer should be consulted.

Whether the adoption is done through an agency or independently, the mother signs over to the adopting parents all her legal rights and responsibilities as parent of her child. Signing the final papers makes this decision irreversible.

Adoption agencies vary in their practices, but it's always advisable to begin adoption proceedings as soon as you decide on that course of action. Final adoption papers are never signed until after the birth of the child, but a delay in contacting an agency before the birth may postpone the baby's immediate placement in a permanent home. In any case, making application to an adoption agency does *not* obligate you to go through with the proceedings.

How Adoption Agencies Work

Agencies attempt to place children in homes that are similar in cultural background to that of their natural parents. Adoptive parents are meticulously screened, and those willing to go through such proceedings are usually highly motivated to be parents. Both natural and adoptive parents have their privacy protected by the confidential practices of adoptive agencies. Often, the state Department of Social Welfare supervises adoptive agencies. Private agencies may be either religious or non-sectarian.

An independent adoption is the result of a direct agreement between a mother and the adopting parents, or between the mother and an attorney or other intermediary. Because either party may decide at the last minute not to go through with the agreement, leaving a woman with no other alternative for placing her baby, it's wise to choose a lawyer familiar with this field to prepare the papers and guide the process.

The choice to place a child for adoption is not an easy one, and naturally involves a sense of loss. Nine months of preparation for a birth and then the abrupt removal of the child can result in temporary feelings of sadness and depression. A woman should accept the soundness of her decision (made at a less emotional point in the experience) and begin to direct her energy into making new beginnings and continuing her life.

Psychological Consequences

For a woman, assuming the responsibility for choosing abortion is the most important factor in determining the psychological consequences of the operation. One of the best follow-up studies concerning this point was conducted by Martin Ekblad. After studying 479 Swedish women, he said, "Sixty-five percent of the women stated that they were satisfied with their abortion and had no self-reproaches; 10 percent had no self-reproaches but felt the operation itself was unpleasant; 14 percent had mild degrees of self-reproach or regretted having had the operation." The women who felt the most guilt were those who allowed their decision to be influenced by others; those who felt the least guilt were those who were confident that they wanted the abortion themselves.

The social context will influence how a woman feels about her abortion afterwards. A woman will find the experience more upsetting in an environment that condemns abortion as morally wrong, that legally restricts her decision to have an abortion, or that financially prevents her from seeking proper care.

A woman's relationship with her partner also will have an impact on her feelings about abortion. If he is loving and supportive and the decision to abort was a mutual one, a woman's acceptance of the abortion will be greater than if the man refuses to share the responsibility for the abortion and ultimately rejects the woman herself. Conflicts also arise if the man wants the pregnancy to continue and the woman clearly does not.

Religious training that emphasizes the evils of abortion also may crop up to confuse a woman who is attempting to make a decision about terminating her pregnancy. Women choose abortion because they believe it to be the best decision at the time. It is helpful to know that religious laws have been reinterpreted throughout history, and that many women have found it necessary to listen to their own guiding inner voice instead of that of religious authority.

The abortion itself will have an impact on a woman's response to the experience, too. If the procedure is carefully and expertly performed and a woman receives support from her abortion counselor, her dignity will remain intact. But if the attitudes of the doctor or medical staff are judgmental or punitive, a woman (who is naturally more sensitive at this time) may absorb this negativity or become angry and mistrustful.

The physiological changes that occur in a woman's body during the first trimester of pregnancy are distinctively different from the non-pregnant state. After abortion, the abrupt return to the non-pregnant state with its associated hormonal shifts also results in a shift in physical and emotional well-being. Some women report feeling "excellent and euphoric." Feeling relieved that an abortion is over and that the crisis of an unplanned pregnancy has passed is a very common response. On the other hand, it's not uncommon to experience a short period of depression, sadness, or fatigue as a result of abortion.

A word of caution: to have an abortion is to let go of the possibility of bearing a child at this time. Although a woman may be sure that this is the right choice for her, she may feel a sense of loss and sadness in surrendering the option, particularly if her choice is based on practical considerations and if in other circumstances she would have kept the child. If talking with a trusted friend at this point does not help, and strong feelings persist or inhibit your ability to move on with your life, talk with a professional counselor.

For many women, choosing an abortion is a major step toward self-determination. But a major advance in our capacity to take responsibility for the direction of our lives can also be followed by what Dr. Jean Baker Miller describes as the "paradoxical depression."

"Such depression may reflect the fact that the individual is forced to admit that she, herself, is responsible for what happens."

Such depression goes beyond the abortion and has to do with the need to assimilate major shifts in our feeling and thinking patterns, or the breaking of patterns themselves that we outgrow.

Prevention

Learning about and using effective birth control methods are basic to preventing the future need for abortion. But a woman's attitudes about sexuality and pregnancy can begin a pattern of risk-taking that may be difficult to break. If your pregnancy came as a "surprise" to you, answering the following questions may help you understand some hidden attitudes you may not have confronted before:

• Do I understand how conception takes place?
• Did I believe I couldn't get pregnant?
• Why didn't I use birth control?
• Do I feel OK about having sex?
• Do I feel OK about having sex and using birth control?
• Does sex seem less spontaneous when I use birth control?
• Did I think getting pregnant would help my relationship with my partner or induce him to get married?
• Did I really want to have a baby but couldn't admit it until now?
• Am I trying to overcome loneliness by having a baby?
• Why do I want to have a baby?
• Why do I want to be a mother?

For more information about risk-taking and your attitudes, see the books referred to in "Further Reading," beginning on page 667, and the chapter on "Birth Control," beginning on page 164.

Methods of Abortion

The Vacuum Aspiration Abortion

The vacuum aspiration abortion is the method of choice up to 12 weeks after the last menstrual period. As part of the preoperative procedure, you will be asked to fill out a complete medical history to alert the doctor to any possible complications. Blood is taken by needle from the forearm to be tested for the Rh factor (see page 248), anemia, and the sickle-cell trait. Temperature, pulse, and blood pressure are then taken to make sure you are in good health. Some clinics schedule these tests the day before, along with a laminaria insertion.

Laminaria is a stick made of dried seaweed. Once it is inserted into the cervical os (the opening to the womb), it absorbs moisture and slowly expands, gradually causing the cervix to dilate or enlarge. Some doctors believe this method is less painful than manually dilating the cervix immediately before the abortion. Laminaria should never remain in place for more than 12 hours, however.

Medical opinion on the use of laminaria is divided. Some Planned Parenthood counselors warn that laminaria should not be used for women who are confused or uncertain about having an abortion, since they may decide not to return for the procedure, and the laminaria left in place could cause infection. One feminist health collective found that the dilation is often uncomfortable, more extensive than necessary, and can increase the possibilities of infection.

The following description of the vacuum aspiration procedure also should be explained to you in person if you request abortion counseling. You *always* are entitled to ask questions and to be treated with respect and consideration.

Some clinics offer a nervous system relaxant drug that is not usually necessary. If you don't want it, make that very clear, since it is often given as a matter of course. A general anesthesia is not given unless a woman asks for it, since overall relaxation softens the uterine walls, increasing the chance that the uterine wall will be perforated during the procedure.

Sometimes a woman is advised to eat breakfast as usual to ward off weakness, but it is just as common to be told not to eat as a prevention against nausea.

The doctor will repeat the pelvic examination to be sure of the uterine size. A speculum—a device for stretching the vaginal walls and holding them open—is then inserted into the vagina. Careful insertion of the speculum is not painful, but if a woman is tense, it may be slightly uncomfortable (be sure to tell the doctor about any discomfort). If the speculum is made of metal, it can feel quite cool, although some doctors are recognizing the simple comfort that comes from warming the speculum before insertion. The speculum remains in place throughout the abortion procedure, as shown below.

FIRST-TRIMESTER ABORTION

THE VACUUM ASPIRATION METHOD. *A speculum is inserted into the vagina to hold open the vaginal walls, and the cervix is anesthetized. The cervix is then gradually dilated with a rod.*

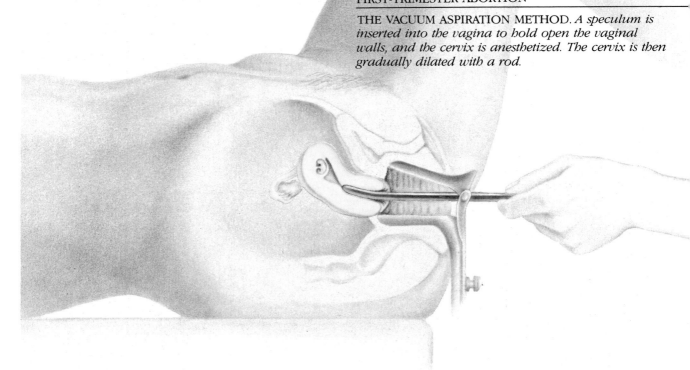

An antibiotic is then swabbed all around the cervix to prevent infection, and a local anesthetic is given. If a woman prefers not to have the local anesthetic because of an aversion to drugs, needles, or because she feels she will not need it, that should be her choice. However, before a decision is made, the doctor should inform her fully as to the level of discomfort she may feel.

Usually 10 cc. of xylocaine, a common local anesthetic, are given. Sometimes as much as 20 cc. are given to ensure minimal pain during dilation, but dizziness or ringing in the ears may result, and the large dose may not be more effective than the smaller dose. There are few nerve endings in the cervix, so the needle should be felt less than a shot of local anesthetic given by a dentist. When pain is felt, it will be felt as a small prickly sensation. A clamp is placed on the cervix to keep it from moving, and this procedure may pinch slightly.

The cervix is dilated gradually by the use of instruments that look like bent rods and that come in varying sizes. The smallest one is inserted first, and then a slightly larger one, and so on, until the cervix is dilated as needed. The length of pregnancy determines how much dilation is necessary; the more advanced the pregnancy, the more contents there will be in the uterus. During dilation, the stretching of the cervical opening can cause cramping sensations.

A flexible or non-flexible plastic cannula (tube) is then passed through the cervix into the uterus, and suction is applied until all the tissue is removed. A flexible cannula guards against uterine perforation, but requires more skill on the part of the physician to remove all the tissue. If the suction pump attached to the cannula is electrical, it will make a loud noise when turned on. Cramping will occur while the tissue is being suctioned from the uterine wall. Even if cramping is painful, it usually lasts only a couple of minutes, although some cramping may continue for a while after the procedure is over.

Some women who are accustomed to having menstrual cramps describe only mild discomfort during an abortion. A number of women report that "it hurts, but it's over very quickly." Each woman responds to the pain differently. Some counselors encourage a woman to breathe deeply and to exert downward pressure into the pelvic area by constricting the abdomen when the cramps occur. This process relaxes tense muscles and reduces pain. Other counselors believe that discomfort, psychological and physical, is alleviated by distracting the woman and encouraging her to think about other things. A third approach encourages the woman to breathe deeply while the counselor explains the procedure itself. This way, the woman knows what to expect before it happens. Some women feel that being able to prepare themselves a few seconds in advance for the next sensation enhances their feeling of being in control. If you know what works best for you, by all means, say so.

A clamp holds the cervix steady while a suction tube is passed through the cervix and into the uterus. Suction is applied until all of the fetus and associated tissue is removed.

The suction tube, clamp, and speculum are removed, and the vagina, cervix, and uterus begin their return to the pre-pregnant state.

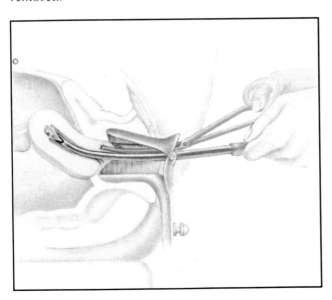

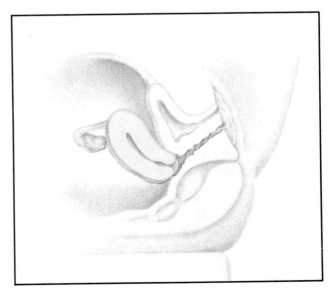

The vacuum aspiration abortion is a very safe medical procedure, almost three times as safe as childbirth. Complications associated with all types of abortion procedures include infection, hemorrhage, perforation of the uterus, and incomplete abortion, but these complications are very rare in the vacuum aspiration method. A skilled and experienced physician seldom faces them. Air emboli (bubbles of air plugging a small vessel) account for some of the rare deaths that occur, but these can be avoided by using pumps equipped with a bypass valve that makes it impossible to push air into the uterus.

A woman is asked to rest for at least a half hour following the procedure. During this time, her blood pressure and pulse are checked. Although some women leave the clinic and continue their day as usual, many prefer to rest for a day or two before resuming their normal activities. Usually it's better to have someone drive you home.

Immediately following an abortion, hormonal changes begin to occur in response to the body's sudden return to its pre-pregnancy state. It's not proven, but it is likely that the "post-abortion blues" may be directly related to this hormonal adjustment. This depression may not occur until 48 hours after the abortion, and may linger for a week or more.

A SUCTION MACHINE

The tube (cannula) is attached to a machine that provides the great degree of suction required. The tube is then attached to the curette, which is inserted into the uterus. The extraction of all tissue takes approximately five minutes.

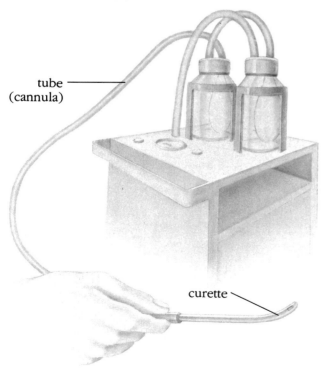

tube ——————
(cannula)

curette

Immediately following the abortion, it is normal to experience some vaginal bleeding. The bleeding is similar to a heavy menstrual flow, lasting from one to three days, and may require three to five pads daily. However, if you thoroughly soak more than four pads, call the doctor or clinic to be sure everything is okay. Some women continue to "spot" on and off for a month, while others experience very little bleeding. The next menstrual period can be expected within four to seven weeks. If it does not come, call the doctor or clinic. Complete aftercare instructions to be followed after a vacuum aspiration abortion are given below and on the next page.

Dilation and Evacuation (D&E)

Prior to the development of vacuum aspiration, dilation and evacuation (D&E) or dilation and curettage (D&C) were the safest and most widely used methods for first-trimester abortions. A D&E can be done up to 15 weeks after the last menstrual period (late D&E), although up to 12 weeks, vacuum aspiration is the preferred procedure. Between 12 and 15 weeks after the LMP, however, the uterus is too soft for a safe vacuum aspiration abortion (perforation can occur too easily), and it is too early for an induction abortion (see page 216). The complications of infection, hemorrhage, and uterine perforation are slightly higher for D&E than for the vacuum aspiration abortion, and more bleeding can be expected following a D&E.

Dilation and evacuation is routinely used to correct other disorders such as infertility, excessive menstrual bleeding, and persistent irregularity of periods. The cervix is dilated as it is preceding the vacuum aspiration abortion, and the uterine lining is carefully loosened with a curette (a metal loop on the end of a long thin handle). The fetal tissue is then removed with forceps. Although the scraping is not painful, you will experience some discomfort and cramping.

Abortion Aftercare

Aftercare instructions for both vacuum aspiration and dilation and evacuation include the following:
● Nothing should be put into the vagina for two to three weeks after an abortion because of the danger of infection. Thus, you cannot use a tampon, have intercourse, or douche. Neither should you take a bath or swim, since infection is also communicated in water. Showering is permissible.
● Activities such as swimming, horseback riding, jogging, and any other strenuous activity that could cause bleeding must be postponed for a couple of weeks.
● After an abortion, a woman is given Methergine or Ergotrate, two drugs that help the uterus contract and return to its original size. The drug must be taken every four hours, day and night.

- For the five days following the abortion, take your temperature morning and evening. Use a good thermometer, and if your temperature goes above 100.4 degrees F. two readings in a row, call the doctor or clinic immediately. An elevated temperature may indicate an infection that needs prompt treatment.
- Cramping may persist for a day or so, and you may find that a heating pad provides relief. Don't take aspirin, though, because aspirin will keep your temperature down, thus disguising one of the most important symptoms of infection. If cramping becomes worse or more prolonged than it was immediately after the abortion, call the clinic or doctor.
- If breasts swell, become tender, or begin to discharge a watery fluid, ice packs may be applied. A well-fitting bra also may relieve the discomfort. The breasts should not be massaged at this time, nor should any discharge be squeezed out. If the discomfort persists, call your doctor or clinic.
- If your blood is Rh negative, be sure to have an Rh (D) immune globulin (RhoGram) shot (see page 248) within 72 hours.
- Because a woman can become pregnant immediately following an abortion, birth control counseling should always be part of abortion aftercare. As we've said, many women worry about the effects of abortion on fertility, and because of that concern, they may unconsciously risk pregnancy again. A woman should realize the risk she takes in not immediately choosing a method of birth control. Even if a woman already has decided on a method, reviewing all of the options can be informative. Birth control pills can be started the same night of the abortion so that when a woman does resume intercourse, she will be protected. Or, a diaphragm can be fitted at the post-abortion checkup.
- Have a medical examination two weeks after the abortion. At the two-week checkup, two conditions, though rare, are looked for: incomplete abortion and ectopic pregnancy, both of which are discussed at right.
- In general, take it easy and be good to yourself after an abortion. Choose a nurturing environment and cheerful company in which to recuperate. Eat nourishing food and be sure you are getting enough vitamins and minerals. Take some leisurely walks in a quiet place, and get as much sleep as your body needs.
- Accept your feelings about the abortion, whatever they are. Should you need someone to talk to, counselors are available in most communities (see page 369).

Complications of Abortion

An incomplete abortion is one in which a portion of the uterine contents is missed and remains. The pregnancy either continues (although invariably damaged), or the remaining tissue begins to cause an infection. Symptoms are a musty, "foul" smell from the vagina, and heavy cramping, discharge, or fever. Any reputable doctor or clinic will perform a second abortion free of charge if the first one proves incomplete. It is not uncommon for an abortion to be incomplete, so be watchful. If you notice any of the above symptoms, call your doctor immediately.

An ectopic pregnancy is one in which the ovum has implanted outside the uterus, usually in the fallopian tube. Since a fallopian tube cannot accommodate pregnancy, the fetus soon will grow large enough to rupture the tube, causing severe internal bleeding and possibly death. If you have an abortion, only the contents of the uterus are aborted, and the ectopic pregnancy remains intact. If you have had an abortion but signs of pregnancy persist, be sure to see a physician immediately. Ectopic pregnancies are rare and usually occur in women with histories of pelvic inflammatory disease or scarring of the fallopian tubes.

Preemptive Abortion

A preemptive abortion (sometimes called menstrual extraction, menstrual regulation, or menstrual aspiration) is a suction aspiration abortion performed with a small, flexible cannula attached to a suction syringe or to a pump. It is very similar to vacuum aspiration, except that the cannula is smaller, and the cervix rarely needs to be dilated. Preemptive abortions usually are given when pregnancy is suspected before laboratory tests can verify it.

Early pregnancy signs are quite variable and may become apparent as early as two to four weeks after conception. Breast swelling and tenderness may occur with a missed menstrual period. Although for many women these occur prior to a normal menstrual period, women who have been pregnant before and know that this is the only time their breasts swell can, and usually do, suspect pregnancy.

For women who keep an accurate basal body temperature chart (see page 188), an elevated post-ovulatory temperature that stays high for longer than two weeks is an excellent indication of pregnancy.

The morning sickness syndrome may simply indicate anxiety, but can also herald a pregnancy. Unusual mood swings, extreme fatigue, and mental haziness can accompany the hormonal changes of early pregnancy (or the onset of the flu). On the other hand, worrying about being pregnant can cause all of these symptoms, and more. A few women "know" as soon as they become pregnant, without any apparent sign—and they are often right.

Another indication of pregnancy is a bluish tint around the cervical os, the opening of the cervix. Your cervical opening can be viewed easily by self-examination with a speculum, mirror, and flashlight. Not all women show this sign, and the only way to be sure that there is any change in color is to be already familiar with your cervix through regular self-examination. Self-help or self-examination can be learned in a self-help class offered by most women's health centers.

A woman who watches and feels her bodily changes, who has missed a period, and who suspects she is pregnant can qualify for this procedure.

Second-Trimester Abortion

Late abortions (after the 15th week) should be avoided. They are more costly, more risky, and more painful, both physiologically and psychologically, than first-trimester abortions. It is also more difficult to obtain a second-trimester abortion than a first-trimester abortion, and second-trimester abortions are subject to state regulations. Some factors that may necessitate a second-trimester abortion are:
• Inability to obtain a first-trimester abortion for reasons of health
• Failure to make an early decision to abort
• Difficulty in ascertaining pregnancy during the first trimester.
Sometimes the decision to terminate the pregnancy develops as the result of amniocentesis (see page 237), a procedure that cannot be done until 14 weeks after the last menstrual period.

Eighty percent of those who seek a second-trimester abortion are teen-age women who do not realize the necessity for making a decision for or against abortion during the first trimester.

Different procedures are used in abortions performed after the 15th week. The induction method and the hysterotomy are discussed below and opposite.

An induction abortion is done from 16 to 24 weeks after the last menstrual period. Until recently, a saline solution was always used to induce expulsion (abortion) of the fetus. Now other substances called prostaglandins are sometimes used as well. In the past, induction abortions using prostaglandins have been felt to be safer than saline induction abortions. Recent literature, however, reveals a higher rate of complications, both major and minor, with the use of prostaglandins. It is important to know the advantages and disadvantages of each so you can choose the one you prefer; your doctor more than likely has a preference as well. Either procedure requires a hospital stay.

Both solutions are used in the same way. A section of the abdomen is cleaned and numbed with a local anesthetic. Then a large needle is inserted in order to draw out some amniotic fluid. Through the same needle, one of the solutions mentioned above is injected into the amniotic sac. Especially with the saline infusion, great care must be taken to avoid getting salt (which could cause shock and death) into the blood vessels. It is common to feel bloated, thirsty, and to have a headache after this procedure, but any feelings of dizziness, backache, or heat waves should be mentioned to the physician immediately.

After the injection comes the waiting. With saline solution, contractions will begin 8 to 24 hours later. With prostaglandins, the contractions will begin sooner. At first the cramping is slight, and then it begins to increase. No general anesthesia is given, since it would inhibit the process; however, pain medication and tranquilizers should be offered. Since the process is like a mini-labor, the breathing techniques used in full-term labor can be helpful.

In most cases, the fetus and placenta will be expelled within 18 to 24 hours with the use of prostaglandins, and within 24 to 36 hours with the use of saline infusion. Your hospital stay will continue for 24 hours. The advantage of prostaglandins is that the interval between induction and abortion is much shorter.

Complications with saline induction include the risk of salt entering the blood vessels, which could be fatal; retention of the placenta, which would necessitate an immediate D&E; hemorrhage at the time of expulsion; or a later infection.

Complications with prostaglandins include: significantly higher rates of nausea and diarrhea, a higher rate of unsuccessful inductions (the solution was injected, but an abortion did not result), excessive bleeding, and retention of the placenta. The cervix may tear due to rapid expulsion, although laminaria insertion may prevent this.

Aftercare procedures are the same as for a vacuum aspiration abortion. The healing process may take longer, and a woman should plan to take it easy for at least a week afterward. The hormonal readjustments may be even more dramatic than those following a first-trimester abortion, and some depression is not unusual.

Hysterotomy. Very rarely, an induction method cannot be performed because of a woman's health, and sometimes the induction method is simply not successful. Major surgery, called hysterotomy (not to be confused with hysterectomy) is the treatment used in such cases. Hysterotomy removes the fetus from the uterus by cesarean section and is used only when other methods have failed or when complications are present. It is not acceptable for routine termination of a mid-trimester pregnancy, and is rarely used today.

Choosing an Abortion Facility

There are certain factors to be considered when choosing a facility for first-trimester and second-trimester abortions. Planned Parenthood has listed the following physical facilities that an abortion clinic must have if it is to be considered acceptable:
- Adequate, private space specifically designated for interviewing, counseling, and pregnancy evaluation
- Conventional gynecologic examining or operating accessories, drapes, and linen
- Approved and electrically safe vacuum aspiration equipment, and conventional instruments for cervical dilation and uterine curettage (an adequate supply to permit individual sterilization for each patient)
- Adequate lighting and ventilation for surgical procedures
- Facilities for sterilization of instruments and linen, and for surgical scrub of all personnel
- Laboratory equipment and personnel (or immediate access to laboratory facilities) for preoperative and emergency determinations and for tissue diagnosis of uterine contents
- A postoperative recovery room, properly supervised, staffed, and equipped
- Adequate supplies of drugs, intravenous solutions, syringes, and needles, including four to six units of plasma volume-expander liquids for emergency use (until blood is available)
- Dressing rooms for staff and patients, and appropriate lavatory facilities
- Ancillary equipment and supplies, including stethoscopes, sphygmomanometers (for taking blood pressure), anesthesia equipment (including oxygen and equipment for artificial ventilation and administration of anesthetic gases), resuscitation equipment, and drugs
- Ability to transfer a patient without delay to a conventional hospital's operating facilities, and a written letter of agreement from a full-service hospital regarding transfer of emergency patients
- Special arrangements for patient emergency contact (on a 24-hour basis) for evaluation and treatment of complications, for postoperative follow-up and examination, and for family planning services.

In addition, check that the procedure suggested is the best for the length of your pregnancy. Ask the doctor whether a flexible rather than a non-flexible cannula will be used if you are having a vacuum aspiration abortion.

Be sure your blood is tested for the Rh factor *before* your abortion. A woman with Rh-negative blood *always* must have an Rh (D) immune globulin (RhoGam) shot within 72 hours of her abortion. Good abortion facilities provide this service, but the cost is in addition to that of the abortion. If no mention is made of your Rh-factor test results, check with the doctor or nurse to be sure you get an Rh (D) immune globulin shot if it is needed.

Inquire about the fees charged, and be sure that they are reasonable for your area of the country. It's better to pay on the day of your abortion and not before, in case you should change your mind. If you plan to use health insurance or Medicaid, check beforehand that these payment methods are acceptable. Despite the Hyde Amendment (see page 206), some states have designated funds for abortions. A minor may apply for this aid regardless of her parents' income.

No facility has the right to maintain consent regulations that require a woman to obtain permission from her husband or parents for an abortion. If such regulations exist, you can take legal action. But first take care of your immediate needs by going elsewhere for the abortion.

Finding a hospital that does late abortions can be difficult, particularly since hospital staffs and boards are opposed to late abortions for medical reasons. A few small hospitals specialize in second-trimester abortions, and there are general hospitals that have a special unit, staff, and counseling for late abortions. It is important to call a hospital and ask about its policies on late abortions.

Woman's Evolving Role

The female role, and indeed, a woman's whole identity, has been interwoven with the ideal of motherhood for hundreds of years. Child-rearing has been accepted as a woman's primary need for fulfillment. Young women who need to assert their independence and feel adult may become pregnant to "prove they are women." This is especially true for teen-agers growing up in an environment where child-rearing seems to be the only option open to them. Women now realize that becoming one's own person is not only satisfying in itself, but is also an excellent preparation for mothering.

Traditional attitudes are slow to yield, but women are beginning to see that those that have confined them to child-rearing roles are not always in their best interests. For women interested in developing a greater awareness of the options available to them, there are women's studies classes, women's centers' programs and libraries, consciousness-raising groups, assertiveness training courses, self-help groups, and meditation training.

Freely and consciously choosing to bear or not to bear children is the right and responsibility of every woman. But the implementation of a woman's right to reproductive freedom is dependent upon society's commitment to creating the necessary educational programs and laws.

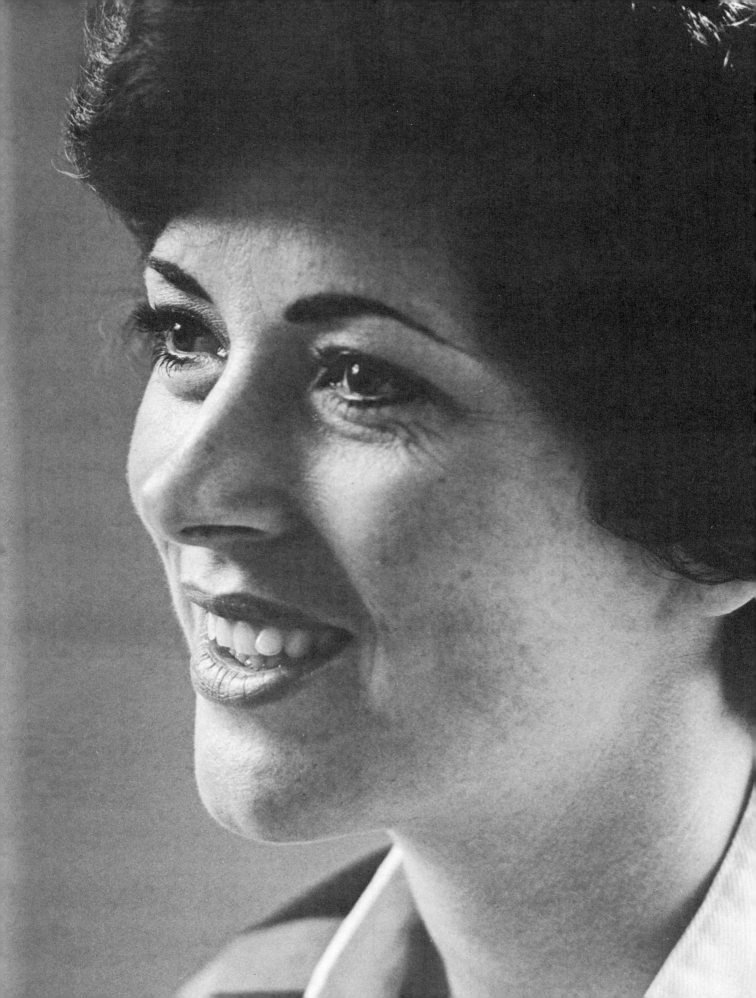

CHAPTER 13

PREGNANCY

MARY GRAY, M.D., F.A.C.O.G.

Pregnancy. It may come to you as a surprise or as part of a well-thought-out plan. You may welcome it or look on it with mixed feelings. And your initial reactions may surprise you.

When you find that you are pregnant, your thoughts and emotions about pregnancy move quickly from the abstract to the very personal. As the fetus grows and your body changes, you will become increasingly aware that you are no longer alone. Your baby is a part of you, yet separate from you.

Pregnancy can cause a radical change in your self-image and life-style, and has the potential to bring great joy and fulfillment. This everyday event that you share with women the world over is a miraculous and deeply personal experience.

Pregnancy

Pregnancy, a sharing in the perpetuation of ourselves and the human race, presents a developmental challenge to both men and women. It can cause a radical change in one's self-image and life circumstances, and has the potential to bring great joy and fulfillment. Women, especially, undergo marked physical and emotional changes during pregnancy. Fortunately, there is much you can do to make the challenge of parenthood add to your personal growth and maturity.

Deciding to Become Pregnant

Knowing about reproductive physiology and the availability of birth control, abortion, and adoption allows couples to make a conscious decision about pregnancy. The choice of having children—and when to do so—is influenced by many social and psychological factors. It's important for a woman to consider her career, the stability of her relationship with the father-to-be, her financial situation, her health, and her emotional needs before deciding that she wants to become pregnant.

If you decide to have a family and are aware of possible health problems you may have, be sure to consult a physician first. You should curtail any use of drugs, alcohol, and cigarettes in anticipation of the pregnancy. If you must take medication for a continuing medical problem, discuss this with your physician. He may prescribe an alternate drug or a decreased dosage of the present drug. When drugs must be continued for health reasons, you should discuss their effects on your potential pregnancy with your doctor and take any appropriate measures. Also be aware that diets for quick weight loss can affect menstrual cycles and fertility, and may leave you in a poor nutritional state to start your pregnancy.

Signs of Pregnancy

Discovering Pregnancy

Suddenly you realize that your period is a week late. Your breasts feel full and slightly tender, and your nipples are sensitive and tingling. You feel so bloated. It's probably just your period getting ready to come . . . but could you possibly be pregnant?

Whether you've carefully planned this pregnancy, or this missed period comes as a complete surprise, you're anxious to know if you really are pregnant. If you have recently consulted a doctor because of an infertility problem (difficulty in becoming pregnant) and are faithfully taking your basal body temperature every morning before getting out of bed (see page 188), you notice that your temperature is remaining elevated. You call your doctor to report that you've had a slight fever of 99.2 for almost three weeks and that your period still hasn't come. Even though you know temperature elevation is an early sign of pregnancy, you're amazed when he tells you that you're probably pregnant.

The following week, about two weeks after your missed period, you bring in a morning specimen of urine for a pregnancy test. "Yes," they say when you call back for results, the test is positive. You're flooded with mixed emotions. You can't quite believe you're really pregnant. You may call your partner to tell him the good news, or you may puzzle over just how to tell him. This tremendous event, the beginning of a unique new individual in which he also shared, is your secret alone, to tell or keep to yourself as you see fit. You may want to spread the news to other family members, friends, and co-workers. Or you may feel a little shy and want to wait awhile.

Signs to Look For

Cessation of menses. Whenever your period is at least ten days late, you can suspect pregnancy. In women with grossly irregular cycles, this sign is less reliable. Occasionally there is a little bleeding when the fertilized egg implants in the wall of the uterus, and this can be mistaken for a menstrual period.

Morning sickness. You may develop symptoms of nausea and vomiting during the first trimester of pregnancy. These symptoms usually are more severe in the morning after the night's fast, but can occur at any time during the day.

Urinary frequency. As the enlarging uterus exerts pressure on your bladder, you'll find that you must void (urinate) more frequently both day and night. This symptom often is confused with a bladder infection.

Breast changes. The premenstrual breast changes of fullness and soreness persist. The nipples become increasingly sensitive, and may tingle.

Constipation and bloating. You may feel an aggravation of the premenstrual symptoms of lower abdominal bloating. Constipation may result from the nausea and vomiting of morning sickness.

Quickening. If this is your first pregnancy, at around 18 weeks' gestation you may experience a peculiar fluttering motion in your abdomen—like a moving gas bubble. Actually, you're feeling the first movements of your baby. You will feel these movements sooner if you've been pregnant before.

Signs and Symptoms of Pregnancy

Approximate time of appearance	Symptoms you will notice	Signs the doctor will look for
2nd week	missed period	HCG in blood or urine (lab tests)
3rd week	breast tenderness and fullness	
4th week	morning sickness	
5th week	frequent urination	
6th week		bluish discoloration of vagina, softening of uterus
7th week		asymmetric uterine enlargement
8th week		softening of the isthmus (area between cervix and uterus)
13th week	abdominal enlargement	fetal heart sounds
18th week	quickening (early fetal movements)	
22nd week	active fetal movements	

Home Pregnancy Tests

Do-it-yourself pregnancy tests are now available and may be purchased at a pharmacy. Be sure to carefully read the instructions that come with these tests. Especially note the time period when the tests can be expected to give reliable results with respect to the date on which you expected your missed period. If you have long cycles, you must take this into consideration in determining how long you are really overdue. Just as with other immunologic tests, home pregnancy tests can give false negative and false positive results. It's possible that you have taken medications that might interfere with the tests. Or you might err in "reading" the results because of unfamiliarity with laboratory tests of this kind.

If your test result is negative but your period still has not come one week later, you should repeat the test or see your doctor or family planning clinic for standard laboratory pregnancy tests. If an ectopic or tubal pregnancy (see page 453) is the cause of your missed period, it may not register on a home pregnancy test. Immediate medical care for this serious condition is extremely important.

Laboratory Pregnancy Tests

All laboratory pregnancy tests work by checking for the presence of the substance human chorionic gonadotropin (HCG), which is secreted by the cells of the developing embryo as it burrows into the uterine lining around nine days after ovulation—even before your period is missed.

The immunologic test. This is the most common test for pregnancy. It is done on a morning sample of urine about 40 days after your last period, and employs test tubes or slides rather than laboratory animals. HCG antibodies are used to check for the presence of HCG.

When this test is performed 10 to 14 days after the expected date of the missed period, a positive result usually means that you are pregnant. But there are times when this test is not accurate. Older women who are approaching menopause, or women with hyperthyroid conditions, may get false positive results. Drugs (especially tranquilizers), protein in the urine, and certain tumors also can cause positive test results when a woman is not really pregnant. False negative reactions can occur if the test is done too soon after the expected date of the missed period, or in the case of a threatened miscarriage or an ectopic pregnancy (see page 453).

Radioimmuno- and radioreceptor assays. The most accurate pregnancy test is the radioimmunoassay, which measures the beta subunit (the unique component of HCG). Since this test is specific, there is almost no possibility of a false result. Also, the test is accurate at extremely low levels of HCG, such as might be present in an ectopic pregnancy. In fact, this test is so sensitive that it can detect a pregnancy even before a period is missed. The only disadvantages of the radioimmunoassay are that it uses highly specialized equipment and requires longer than 24 hours to get results, compared to immunological tests, which require only a few hours.

The radioreceptor assay is a newer test. It is not as sensitive, and can give a false negative result for an ectopic pregnancy, but it can be performed and reported on the same day.

The Physician's Examination

Your doctor will perform the following tests and procedures to determine pregnancy.

Internal pelvic examination. At six to eight weeks' gestation, a doctor will note upon examination with a vaginal speculum that your cervix is bluish instead of the normal pink color. An internal pelvic examination will reveal that the cervix is softened, as is the isthmus (the area between the cervix and the uterus). The uterus will be soft and globular instead of firm and pear-shaped. A repeat examination a few weeks later will reveal progressive enlargement of the uterus.

Ultrasound examination. An ultrasound examination will "picture" the embryonic sac at about six weeks. At around 10 to 12 weeks, the fetal heart can be heard with a doptone. This is a special instrument that works by bouncing constant sound waves off a stationary object. If there is movement, such as a beating fetal heart, the sound wave is reflected back at a slightly different frequency. The fetal heart rate is rapid—120 to 140 beats per minute, compared to the mother's heart rate of about 80 beats per minute. If you are nervous or excited, your heart also may beat faster, and so the examiner may check your pulse at the same time. You and your partner may even be able to listen to the fetal heartbeat along with the doctor if there is a special adaptor on the instrument to amplify the sounds. The ultrasound examination is positive proof of pregnancy, whereas the other signs noted are only presumptive indicators that you may be pregnant.

When you are about 14 weeks pregnant and the fetus is floating in a fluid-filled sac, a doctor sometimes can detect fetal movements during a pelvic examination. By placing two fingers against your upper vagina, the examiner can tap the fetus, causing it to float away and then return with an impulse against the two fingers. The fetal heart may be heard with a special fetoscope at around 18 to 20 weeks.

X rays. Although the fetal skeleton is visible on X rays at mid-trimester, radiation exposure should be avoided as much as possible because of potential harmful effects on the fetus. If you have missed a period or think you might be pregnant and are scheduled to have any X rays, inform your physician or the lab technician before the X ray is taken so that the examination may be postponed. If it is urgent that you have the X ray, your abdomen can be shielded by lead to prevent the rays from reaching your uterus or ovaries. If you had X rays while you were unknowingly pregnant, the chances are that the radiation dose received by the early pregnancy was within "allowable" limits, with no or only very remote risk to the embryo or fetus. You should discuss this with your doctor.

The progesterone hormone withdrawal test is no longer used. In this test, women who missed their periods were given progesterone combined with estrogen. Doctors believed that if the patient were pregnant, she would not bleed, and that there would be no harm to the fetus already exposed to high hormone levels. This test is no longer accepted since the hormones given were synthetic, not natural. In addition, there has been conflicting evidence suggesting that progesterone alone or with estrogen could be implicated in some fetal limb defects of the spinal column.

In the past, progesterone frequently was given to women who seemed predisposed to miscarriage. But recent statistics have shown that progesterone therapy did not improve the outcome of these pregnancies.

The Stages of Pregnancy

The nine months of pregnancy are divided into equal-length trimesters. If you have a 28-day cycle, the expected date of birth is calculated by counting back three months from the date of the first day of your last period and adding a year and a week. Most babies arrive within two weeks of their "due date."

The First Trimester

Different women will exhibit different physical and emotional symptoms during the first three months of pregnancy. Some women psychologically deny or block out the pregnancy, feeling no different than in their non-pregnant state. It's not unusual to have feelings of ambivalence or rejection, and moments of both delight and despair. You may feel guilty for having negative feelings, but be reassured that mixed feelings are normal, especially in the early months of pregnancy. This is a time when you will be absorbed in just accepting the reality of your "pregnant state." Very likely, you'll begin to view your relationships with your own parents, especially your mother, in a new perspective. To prepare for your new role as a mother, you must work through your previous role as a daughter. The happier your own mother-daughter relationship, the easier will be your task.

How you cope with pregnancy will be determined by your own pattern of adjusting to major changes in life, prior family relationships, your individual circumstances, and the support systems you have available. If your family and especially your partner are supportive, your adjustment will be that much easier.

After the initial shock of a positive pregnancy test, the changes of pregnancy are gradual, allowing you to take your time in coming to terms with your pregnant self. As the pregnancy progresses, you'll come to view your baby as a separate individual.

Tiring easily is common. If you work outside the home, you may find that you want to fall into bed as soon as you get home. You may become listless at home, lose outside interests, and have to push yourself to get anything done. Having to get up during the night to urinate because of bladder pressure from the pregnant uterus may only exaggerate your fatigue.

If this is your first pregnancy, you may notice that your nipples and the areolae surrounding them are becoming darker, and the little bumps that appear on the areolae may cause you concern. These are montgomery follicles, and their appearance is a normal response to the increased hormone levels of pregnancy. Another hormone-related symptom is increased skin pigmentation (tanning) on the forehead and upper cheeks, especially in women who frequently are exposed to the sun. This so-called "mask of pregnancy" is more common in brunettes, and will fade after delivery. Using sun screens and avoiding excess exposure to sun will lessen the degree of pigmentation. Women who have this response to pregnancy hormones may experience the same problem with birth control pills, but to a greater degree.

Your appetite may be unaffected by pregnancy, or you may experience anything from a slightly queasy feeling in the morning to extreme nausea and vomiting. Eating frequent small meals and nibbling on crackers, starting as soon as you get out of bed in the morning, often will keep these symptoms under tolerable control. Sometimes anti-nausea medication is needed or, on rare occasions, hospitalization for intravenous feeding.

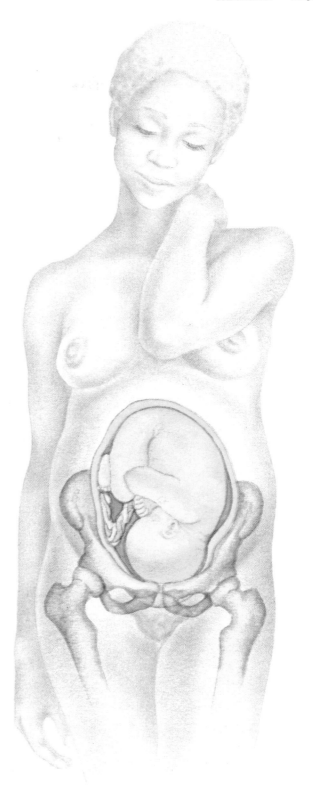

Constipation, a frequent problem throughout pregnancy due to hormonal changes in the gastrointestinal tract, is best controlled by diet and a liberal amount of fluids. Bran cereals, fresh fruits and vegetables, and prune juice help to keep the bowels regular. Dairy products, milk, cheese, and yogurt may aggravate the constipation but still are important to proper diet. Sometimes a stool softener or bulk laxative is necessary, although habitual use of mineral oil or strong laxatives should be avoided.

Most of the two- to four-pound weight gain during the first few months of pregnancy is body fluid. At three months, your uterus is just palpable about your pubic bone. Depending upon the amount of body fluids, you may notice little or great increase in the size of your lower abdomen.

In general, you will experience varying degrees of discomfort in the early months of pregnancy. Summer months are apt to be the most uncomfortable, especially when the weather is hot and humid.

Your partner may complain that "All you want to do is sleep." It's important to remember that he, too, has many adjustments to make. He has shared in creating this new life, and may be thinking about the additional responsibilities involved. Your preoccupations, often accompanied by a decrease in sexual desire, may leave him feeling left out. This is a time that requires increased patience and understanding and, above all, open communication between the two of you.

First Trimester Fetal Growth

During the first three months, the product of conception grows from the just-visible speck of the fertilized ovum to a lively embryo about three inches long and weighing about an ounce

The first week. Conception takes place about two weeks before your expected period in the outer one-third of the fallopian tubes (see page 226). As the fertilized ovum travels down the fallopian tube toward the uterus, it is constantly dividing and subdividing to produce daughter cells, which remain attached to each other. Rarely, the first two daughter cells of the first division completely separate, giving rise to two separate individuals of the same sex (identical twins) who will be carbon copies of each other with the exact same genetic makeup. More commonly, twins are the result of two separate ova being fertilized by two separate spermatozoa (fraternal twins), and will be no more alike than any other family members (see page 229). This type of twinning may be inherited, and is slightly more common among blacks than among Caucasians. Multiple pregnancies also are more common in women who have taken fertility drugs to make them ovulate (produce eggs).

Initially, the dividing cells are all similar, but eventually they begin to form different cell types. The fertilized egg is called a trophoblast at this stage. Some cells will congregate to one side to form the embryonic disk, which will become the embryo.

The second week. Seven to ten days after conception, the trophoblast embeds itself in the endometrium, the lining of the uterus that has been specially prepared to receive this new life. When this happens, vaginal spotting may occur and be mistaken for an early missed period.

The trophoblast sends out sheets of cells that form villi, which are fingerlike projections containing tiny fetal blood vessels. These form the placenta (afterbirth), which is connected to the fetus by an umbilical cord (see page 233).

The third week. At this time, the brain, spinal cord, and entire nervous system are established. The eyes are beginning to form, and premature lungs appear. A tube forms, which will eventually be the heart.

The fourth week. The head and brain have become the largest part of the embryo at this stage. With the beating of the heart tube and the formation of red blood cells, circulation begins. A premature face is forming, including eyes, ears, and mouth. Now there is a recognizable liver and gallbladder, and the gastrointestinal tract begins to develop.

The fifth week. By the fifth week, the embryo measures about one-quarter of an inch. It is bent so that the head is almost touching the "tail." The most important organs are present or have begun to develop during the fifth week. The pituitary gland begins to form, muscles begin to appear, and the upper and lower jaws fuse in midline.

The sixth week. Movements under the control of the brain develop at this time, as do the earliest reflexes. The gonads (ovaries or testes) have differentiated, so the embryo is clearly male or female. The heart now has four chambers. A skeleton is present, and a tail extends from the spinal cord.

The seventh week. The embryo weighs about one-half ounce now. It is recognizable as a human being, having lost its tail, and there are buddings of fingers and toes.

The eighth week. From the eighth week until birth, the unborn child is referred to as a fetus. All the important organs have formed or are beginning to form, so the fetus is less vulnerable to infections from the mother. Facial features are becoming well-formed, fingers and toes are present, and teeth are beginning to form in the fetus' mouth.

The end of the first trimester (twelfth week). The fetus is now a miniature human, measuring about three inches in length and weighing about one ounce. There are movements of the hands and mouth, and the body grows rapidly to catch up with the development of the head.

THE PELVIC OPENING AND THE MUSCLES OF THE PELVIC FLOOR

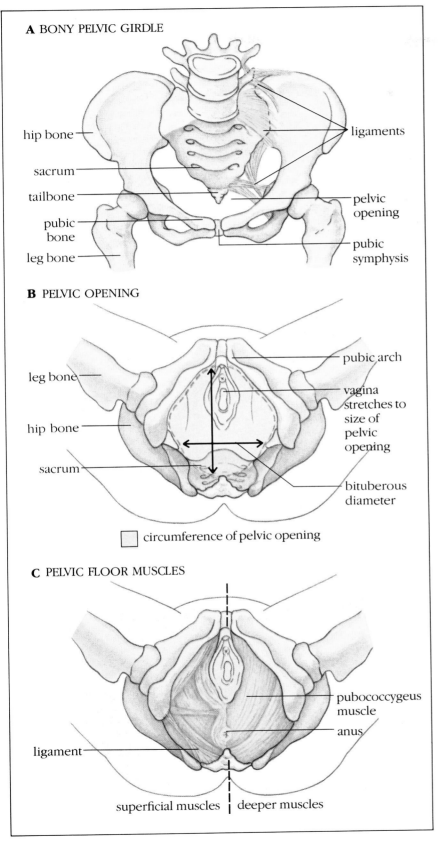

A BONY PELVIC GIRDLE

hip bone

sacrum

tailbone

pubic bone

leg bone

ligaments

pelvic opening

pubic symphysis

B PELVIC OPENING

leg bone

hip bone

sacrum

pubic arch

vagina stretches to size of pelvic opening

bituberous diameter

☐ circumference of pelvic opening

C PELVIC FLOOR MUSCLES

pubococcygeus muscle

anus

ligament

superficial muscles ┊ deeper muscles

A *Shown here from above, the pelvic girdle is a bony ring attached to the spinal column and the leg bones. During delivery, a baby must pass through the pelvic opening; the pelvic girdle contains and protects the reproductive organs.*

B *For a normal delivery, the pelvic opening must be large enough for the infant's head to pass through it. The bituberous diameter, which is the distance between the buttocks bones as shown at left, should be at least eight centimeters. The angle of the pubic arch and the distance between the pubic bone and the sacrum and tailbone also are important measurements. If the fetus is too large to fit through this space, a cesarean section is necessary.*

C *The pelvic floor is a layer of muscles that support the pelvic organs (bladder, uterus, and bowel). The strength and control of these muscles is important during pregnancy and delivery, and to prevent problems after childbirth. It is a good idea to exercise these muscles during pregnancy. See page 297 of the chapter on "Labor and Delivery."*

UTERINE MUSCLE LAYERS

These are the muscles in the uterine walls that contract to push out the baby and placenta during the various stages of labor and delivery.

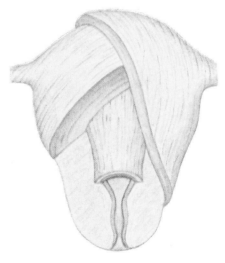

THE BEGINNINGS OF HUMAN LIFE AND GROWTH

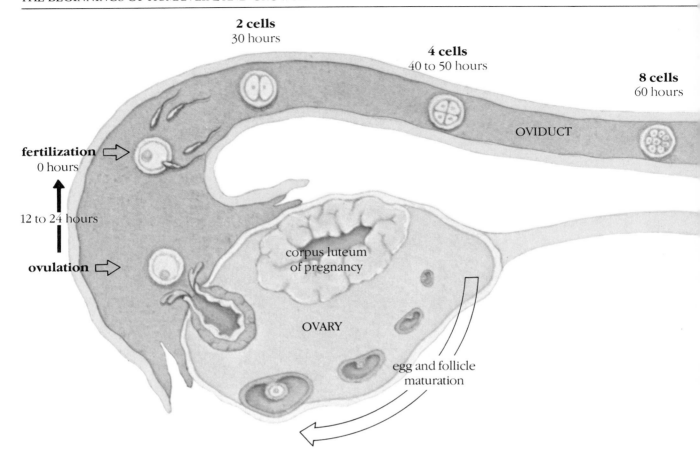

2 cells
30 hours

4 cells
40 to 50 hours

8 cells
60 hours

OVIDUCT

fertilization
0 hours

12 to 24 hours

ovulation

corpus luteum
of pregnancy

OVARY

egg and follicle
maturation

Much of the mystery surrounding the events that begin human life has been dispelled only comparatively recently. It was just a hundred years ago that the human egg was discovered, and only over the last century that the following story has emerged. The ovum, one of thousands that a woman may possess, matures and bursts from its chamber of maturation through the lining of the ovary and into the mouth of the fallopian tube. There, currents created by ciliated cells in the tube lining sweep the tiny egg deep into the lumen of the tube. The egg is surrounded by a corona of cells, beneath which is a layer of gelatinlike material that further protects the egg surface. The sperm must pass through these layers for fertilization to occur.

Approximately 12 to 48 hours after ovulation, the egg has moved some distance down the tube. If intercourse has occurred in this time, sperm are in the tube and will meet the egg. The first sperm to reach and penetrate the coverings around the egg will be the sperm to touch the actual egg-cell membrane. The egg is now fertilized, and only this sperm can enter it.

Fertilization is completed within the egg when the sperm head with its 23 chromosomes fuses with the egg nucleus and its 23 chromosomes. The chromosomes line up in pairs in a very particular way, and the single fertilized cell is now ready to divide into the first two cells of the new individual.

This period of division is called cleavage. The individual changes from a ball of two cells to one of about 100 cells during the first days of development. By day five of development, the embryo has entered the uterine cavity. There is a distinct cavity in the ball of cells now, and the group of acentrically placed cells at one pole will be the cells of the embryo. The surrounding layer of cells forming the outside of the ball will be the cells that form the placenta and the membranes outside the fetus.

At the beginning of the second week of development, the embryo has picked its site for implantation on the uterine wall, and the outer cells are busy burrowing into the lining of the uterus. By the end of the second week of development, the whole vesicle is buried beneath the lining.

From the second week to the fourth week, the cells of the outer layer of the embryo grow rapidly, penetrating deep into the uterine wall, making vital contact with the mother's circulatory system, and beginning to develop a blood system of their own—the future placental and umbilical cord circulation. This system will then join the circulatory system developing within the baby's body, until by the end of the fourth week, about the time a woman may realize she is pregnant, there is a fully established exchange of all life-support substances between the mother and the infant.

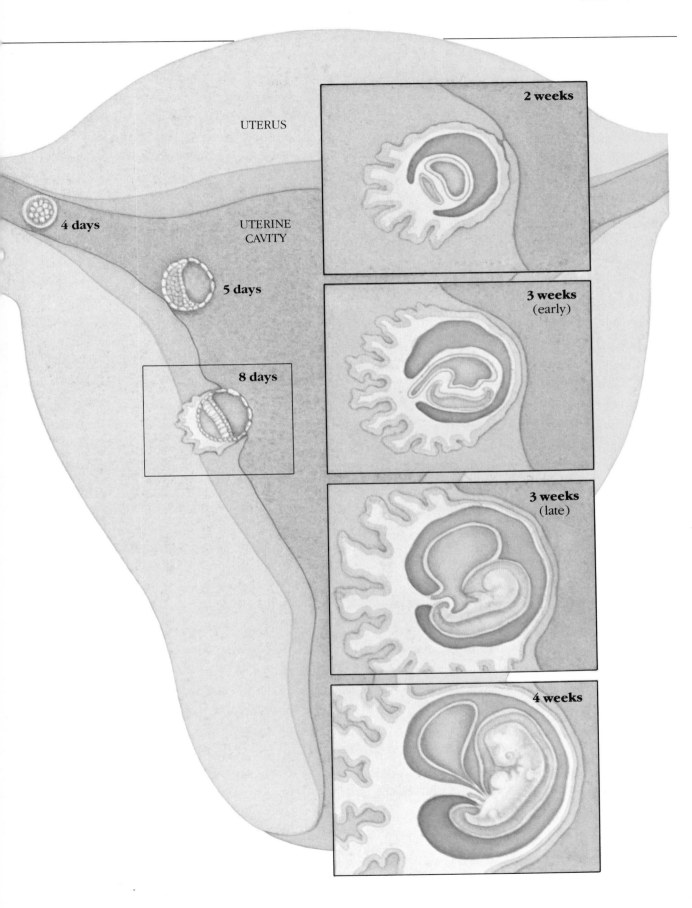

UTERUS

4 days

UTERINE
CAVITY

5 days

8 days

2 weeks

3 weeks
(early)

3 weeks
(late)

4 weeks

The Second Trimester

At the fourth month, your pregnant uterus can be felt midway between your pubic bone and umbilicus. Your appetite is probably improving, and you feel more energetic. You feel so much better that you probably will resume your outside activities if you have interrupted them.

As the pregnancy progresses, you think more in terms of the baby as separate from you. You're thrilled to hear the baby's heartbeat when you go for a routine prenatal checkup. You may even want your partner to accompany you for the next visit to hear the heartbeat. You look forward to when you will feel the first fetal movements, which occur at about 18 weeks if this is your first pregnancy. The first flutterings are a delightful "real" confirmation of pregnancy.

Now your clothes don't fit anymore, and you notice that you are definitely beginning to "show." While some women start wearing maternity clothes as a public announcement, others are a little shy and try to disguise their growing abdomen under bulky sweaters or blouses. You may be proud of the body changes brought about by pregnancy, or you may feel that your increased abdominal size makes you unattractive. Whatever your feelings, many partners are pleased to see the growing changes of pregnancy.

During the second trimester, you may be relieved of much pelvic pressure and bladder irritability, but you may start noticing rectal pain from hemorrhoids or from varicose veins (dilated veins) in your legs. Avoiding constipation and using simple hemorrhoidal ointments are helpful treatments. The tendency to develop varicose veins runs in families, however wearing support hose and taking frequent rests with your legs elevated will relieve pressure on the veins.

By the fifth month, your uterus is at the level of the umbilicus. At this time, your partner may feel the movements of the baby, too. As you become more aware of the growing fetus within you, you will notice neighborhood children more and more, and will want to talk to mothers with young children and babies.

Second Trimester Fetal Growth

The fourth month. This is the month of most rapid growth, due to elongation of the fetal body to almost six inches and a weight increase to about four ounces. The fetus now exhibits stretching movements and reacts to touch. Its skin is red, thin, and loose. In girls, the internal reproductive organs are developing from paired ducts left from the premature kidneys. Two fallopian tubes merge to form a uterus, which empties into the cervix and joins the vagina or birth canal, which is closed by a mass of cells (see page 486).

The fifth month. The fetus is now about ten inches long, weighs one-half to one pound, and has eyebrows and head hair. A white, cheeselike substance, called the vernix, forms to protect the fetus' delicate skin. Its kicking and turning are felt by the mother, as well as by an observer when a hand is placed on the mother's abdomen. Although all the organs are present, the fetus could not survive outside the uterus at this stage.

The sixth month. By the end of the second trimester, the fetus is 12 to 14 inches long, and weighs about 1½ pounds. It now responds to sounds, and the eyes reopen. The skin is red and wrinkled, and the hands have a strong grip. In the male, the testes (male sex glands) start to descend toward the scrotum. Meconium (a waste product of blood and bile) continues to accumulate in the intestines. If born prematurely at this stage, the baby is unlikely to survive due to the immaturity of its respiratory system.

The Third Trimester

During the last months of pregnancy, some of your early anxieties might return. Will labor and delivery be painful? Will the baby be harmed? Will anything happen to me? You find it more and more difficult to be comfortable in any position because of your large abdomen. You become more awkward and may view yourself as clumsy and unattractive.

You may be bothered by edema (collection of fluid in body tissues) or swelling in your legs, especially in the summer heat. Frequent rest periods spent with the legs elevated will give some relief. Sleepless nights may make the pregnancy seem endless.

Childbirth classes during these last months will do much to allay fears you may have concerning the delivery. In the prenatal classes, you can share your feelings with classmates and your partner, while you practice for the coming event and learn what to expect (see page 261).

As term approaches, you will become more and more anxious to "get it over with." You may feel you can't stand it any longer. If this is your first pregnancy, as your delivery date approaches, the baby's head slowly descends to low in your pelvis, giving you more room under your rib cage. This may cause the bladder irritability of early pregnancy to recur. You will be increasingly aware of Braxton-Hicks contractions, periodic painless hardening of the uterus in the last months of pregnancy.

After nine months of waiting, you will more than welcome the onset of labor. Like most couples today, you and your partner will want to be actively involved in the birth of your child.

If you go past your due date, you should see your doctor. Although some pregnancies simply take longer, it may be necessary to induce your labor.

Third Trimester Fetal Growth

The seventh month. The fetus is still skinny with wrinkled skin at this time. There is tremendous development and growth of the brain, and the head is still larger in circumference than the shoulders. The fetus swallows and makes rhythmic breathing attempts. Although the air sacs of the lungs remain collapsed, some amniotic fluid is breathed into the lungs. If born at this stage of development, the baby has an increasingly good chance of survival.

The eighth month. The fetus gains four to five pounds this month. Fat is deposited under the skin, smoothing the wrinkles. This fat also helps to control the infant's body temperature after birth.

The ninth month. Further weight gain occurs during this last month of pregnancy. The head circumference is now the same as the shoulder circumference. There is a slowing down of the rate of the fetus' growth as the time of birth approaches. Because the head is heavier than the feet, and because of the shape of the uterus, the fetus usually assumes an upside-down position.

Meconium, which still is accumulating in the intestine, is being propelled from the small intestine to the large intestine (colon), ready to be passed after birth. Occasionally, the greenish pasty material is passed before delivery, staining the amniotic fluid. This may be a response to fetal stress or a response to aging if the fetus goes much beyond the due date.

Post-term deliveries. Half of all term deliveries occur late or post-term. Although the rate of growth slows down by this point, some fetuses outgrow their placenta and start to lose weight. When this happens, the fetus is considered post-mature, and it often is advisable to induce labor.

THE FORMATION OF TWINS

one egg and one sperm

two different eggs and two different sperm

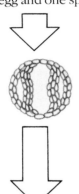

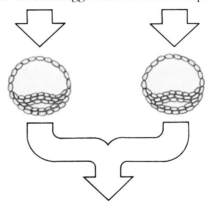

identical twins

- 30 percent of all twins and 3 in 1,000 births
- same sex
- same blood groups
- identical in form and physiology
- usually share some or all fetal membranes

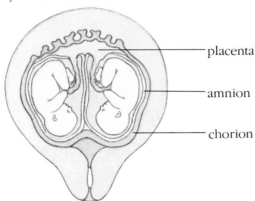

placenta

amnion

chorion

non-identical twins

- 70 percent of all twins and 7 in 1,000 births
- same or different sex
- same or different blood groups
- physically dissimilar
- usually do not share fetal membranes

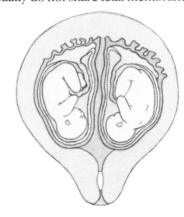

GROWTH OF THE INFANT

Dramatic changes occur in the size and proportions of the infant during prenatal growth. These life-size drawings of an infant from one month until birth let you visualize and compare total body growth as pregnancy progresses.

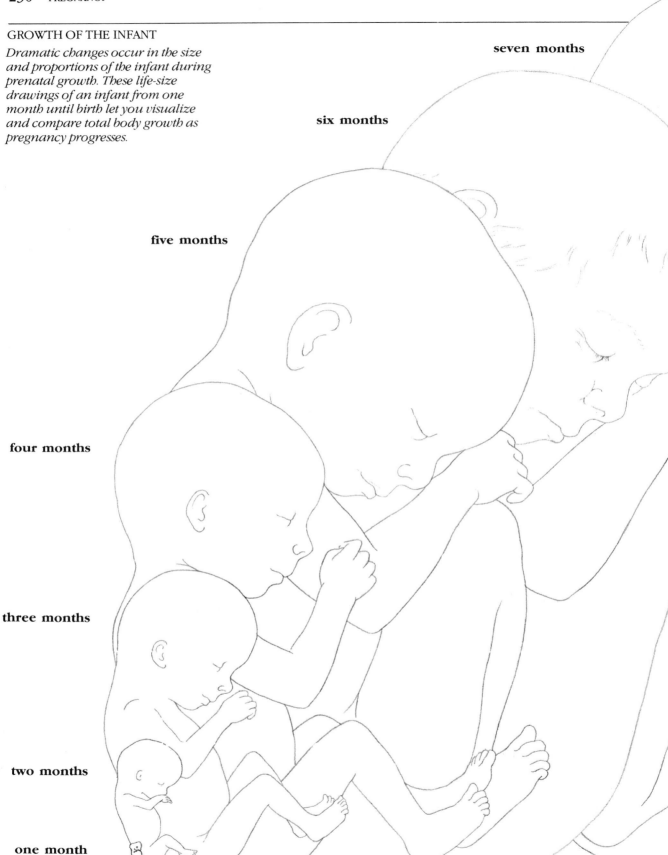

seven months

six months

five months

four months

three months

two months

one month

nine months

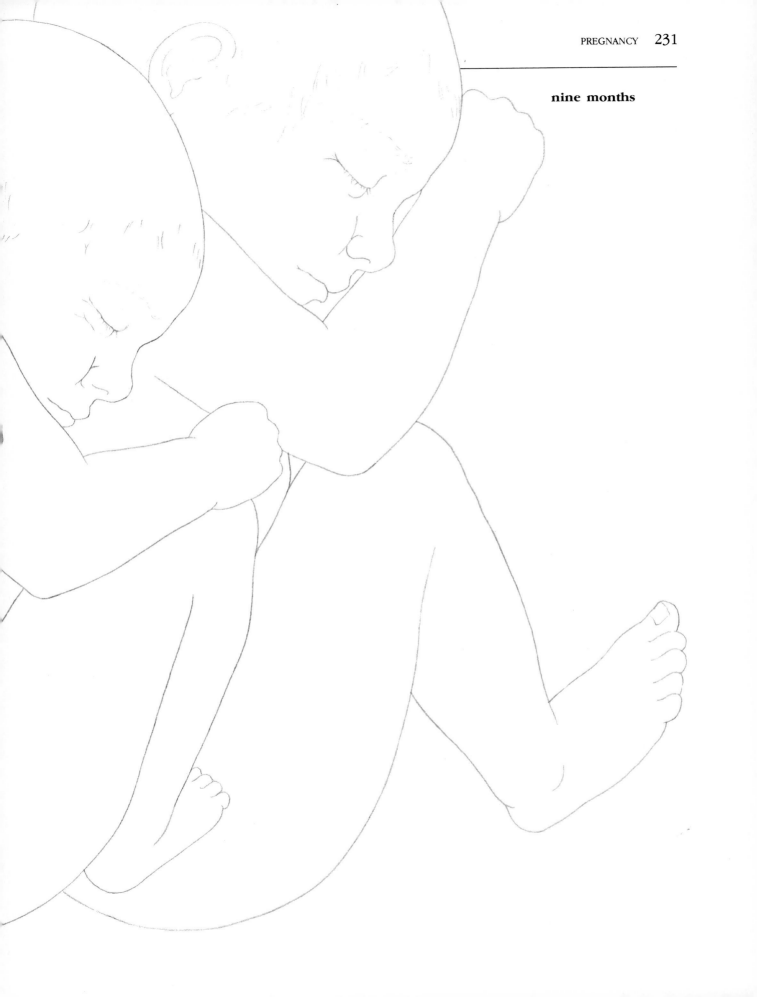

THE PLACENTAL BARRIER AND FETAL-MATERNAL CIRCULATION

Throughout pregnancy, the mother's circulatory system is separated from the fetus' by the placental barrier, a thin layer of cells shown here in highly diagrammatic form. This is where the vital exchange of nutrients and wastes occurs—and where substances that might be harmful to the fetus pass into the infant's body from the mother.

The placental barrier is the crucial bit of tissue standing between the growing infant, the mother, and the outside world. Although it is designed to form an effective barrier to some toxins, it cannot prevent the passage of harmful amounts of nicotine, alcohol, tranquilizers, or other drugs. Given the research evidence to date, a thoughtful woman in her childbearing years should not smoke, drink alcohol, or take drugs, including the over-the-counter variety.

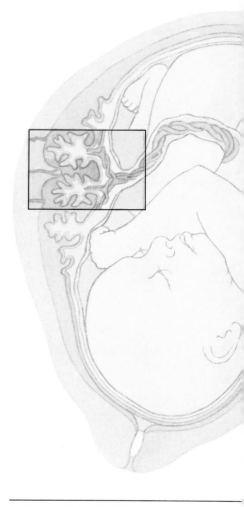

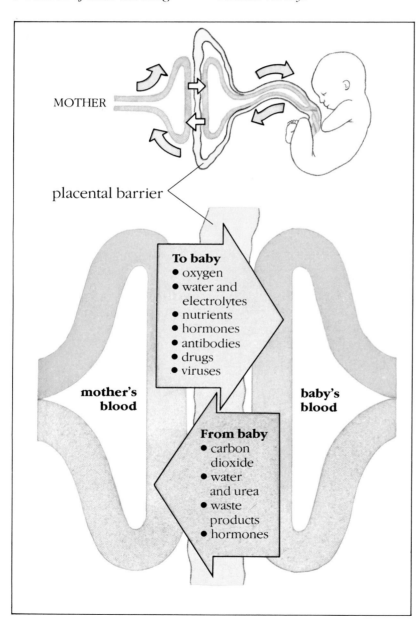

MOTHER

placental barrier

To baby
- oxygen
- water and electrolytes
- nutrients
- hormones
- antibodies
- drugs
- viruses

mother's blood

baby's blood

From baby
- carbon dioxide
- water and urea
- waste products
- hormones

PLACENTAL CIRCULATION

The placenta is an amazing, complex organ that functions throughout fetal life in a variety of jobs, all vital to the infant's life. The placenta acts as a buffer between the infant and the external environment of the mother's body. It allows nourishment to pass from the mother's blood through the "placental barrier" and into the infant's bloodstream. The placenta also forms a protective barrier against some toxins and bacteria; it acts as lungs for the transport of oxygen and carbon dioxide, as a kidney for the infant, and as an endocrine gland for the mother.

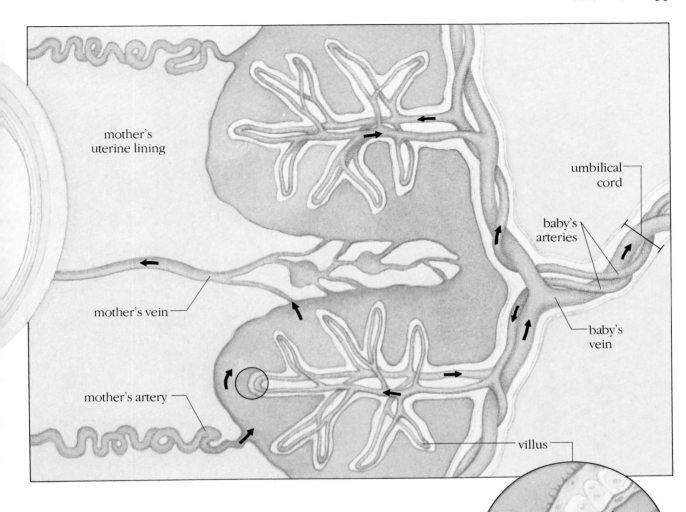

mother's uterine lining

umbilical cord

baby's arteries

mother's vein

baby's vein

mother's artery

villus

A mother's blood
B baby's blood
C placental barrier
D baby's capillary

At full term, the placenta weighs about one pound and is the size of a shallow bowl that would fit neatly in the palms of both hands. The placenta grows to this size from the tiny group of embryonic cells that first burrowed into the uterine wall at seven days of age.

Placental circulation is the communication channel between the infant and mother, and between the infant and the outside environment. Blood enters the mother's uterus through arteries, some of which branch to the region of the uterine wall containing the placenta. At the placental site, the mother's blood, rich in oxygen and nutrients, flows into a space around the treelike branches (villi) of the infant's placenta (arrows). Inside the villi are vessels from the infant.

Blood leaves the infant through the umbilical artery, which, at the placenta, branches into smaller arteries. The blood in these vessels rushes into the villi capillaries pumped by the baby's heart. This blood is low in oxygen and high in waste materials. At the villi, the wastes diffuse out through the placental barrier and into the mother's bloodstream, where they are carried away by the mother's veins. Nourishment and oxygen from the mother flow into the fetal blood and across the placental barrier. This replenished, fresh blood flows out of the villi capillaries of the placenta, into the umbilical vein (enclosed in the umbilical cord), and back into the infant's body, where it is circulated via the baby's own circulatory system.

CHANGES IN A WOMAN'S BODY DURING PREGNANCY

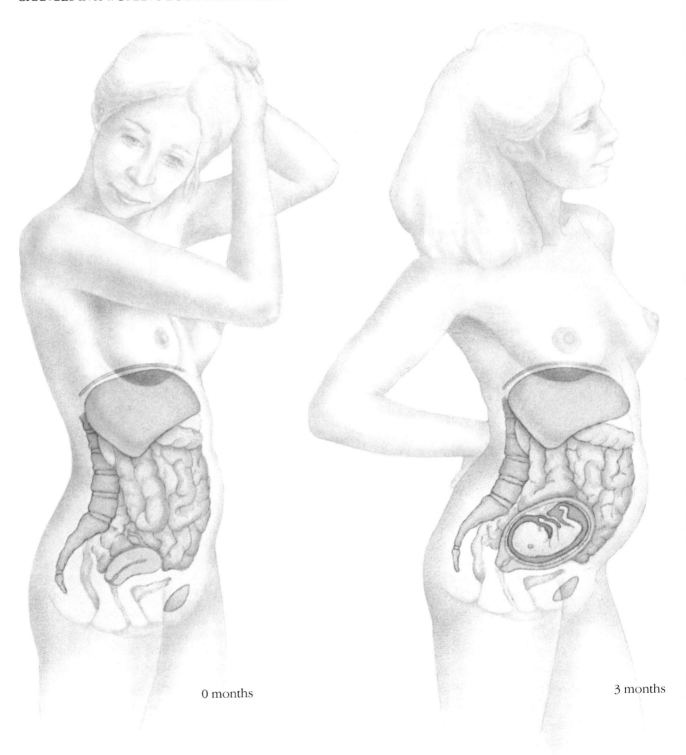

0 months

3 months

These illustrations show the changes in a woman's body shape that occur during pregnancy. Besides the obvious weight gain and abdominal growth, her breasts enlarge and her posture changes.

By the ninth month, the fetus takes up so much area that the mother's vital organs are squeezed up out of place. She will have to eat smaller meals and urinate more frequently, and may not be able to take deep breaths.

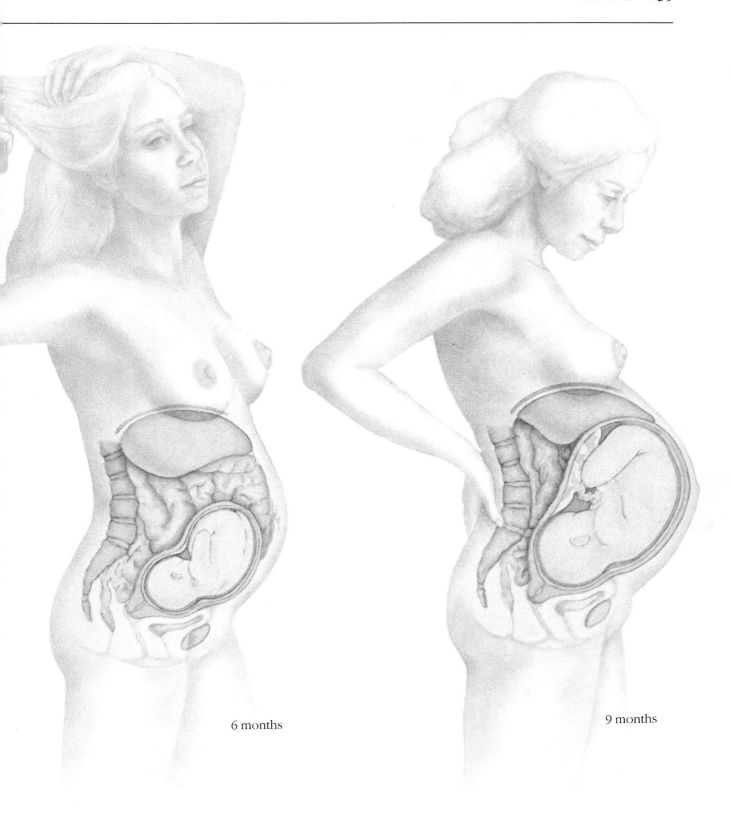

6 months

9 months

Childbirth

How you will respond to the "test" of childbirth depends upon many factors, including the attitude of your mother and the conscious and unconscious lessons you have learned in childhood concerning your femininity. Good preparation, coupled with a supportive partner and supportive birth attendants, will do much to make childbirth a happy experience.

If unforeseen complications arise, or if the course of labor does not meet your expectations, you may be sorely tried and tested. Childbirth isn't meant to be an endurance course. If you feel comfortable with yourself, you will readily accept the help of professionals when needed. Don't allow any increased dependency to make you feel inadequate. When complications prevent a completely natural childbirth, your attitude and cooperation still can contribute a great deal to your experience. The birthing is not an end but a beginning.

For a complete discussion of childbirth, see the chapter on "Labor and Delivery."

Medical Genetics

Pregnant women and women contemplating pregnancy often ask, "Will my child be normal?" No one really can say. Although the outcome of a pregnancy is influenced to some degree by environment, it is largely determined by genetic inheritance.

Birth Defects and Chromosomes

About 3 percent of all live-born infants have some form of birth defect. Some of these are genetic defects that can be passed from one generation to another. Others are acquired because of an isolated accident of development. Still others are caused by intrauterine exposure of the growing embryo to drugs or infection (see page 244).

In normal individuals, all body cells contain 23 pairs of chromosomes, including a pair of X chromosomes for females and an X chromosome paired with a Y chromosome for males. When these cells divide and multiply, they form daughter cells, each with the same 23 pairs of chromosomes. The exceptions are germ cells, which give rise to ova (eggs) in females and spermatozoa (sperm) in males. These germ cells contain only half that number of chromosomes. When they unite to form a new individual, the 23 single chromosomes from the egg cell unite with the 23 single chromosomes from the sperm cell to create 23 complete pairs. The sex of the child, then, is determined by whether the X egg unites with an X or a Y sperm.

All chromosomes carry thousands of paired genes, the carriers of the blueprint for the entire individual. These genes may be dominant (strong) or recessive (weak). The effect of a dominant gene will hide or mask the effect of a recessive gene. If an individual has a dominant defective gene, he or she will manifest the defect and pass it on to the offspring, even if the partner does not have the defective gene.

Most people carry a few defective genes, but most such genes are recessive and, when paired with a normal dominant gene, no genetic disease results. These individuals can be considered "carriers." If both parents are carriers of the same recessive defective gene, the chances are one in four that their children will manifest the disease. The odds are two in four that one child also will be a carrier.

Some recessive defective genes are sex-linked because they are located in the X chromosome. Thus, males, who have only one X chromosome, can be affected by even a single recessive gene on their X chromosome. Females who balance the defective recessive gene with a normal dominant gene on their X chromosome will not be affected, but will be carriers who will transmit the disease to half of their sons. Hemophilia and color blindness are two conditions that are transmitted this way.

Other genetic defects are caused by an abnormal number of chromosomes. Down's syndrome (mongolism) is an example. Ninety-five percent of these individuals will have an extra #21 chromosome, giving a total of 47 chromosomes. For unknown reasons, this disorder increases in frequency as maternal age increases, occurring in one out of 2,000 live births at maternal age 20, but to one in 20 live births at a maternal age over 45 years (see the opposite page).

Certain populations or ethnic groups are more predisposed to particular inherited diseases. For example, about 8 percent of American blacks carry a gene that affects the hemoglobin of red blood cells. If you carry two genes for this trait, called sickle-cell trait, you will have serious anemia and other complications called sickle-cell disease. If you carry a single gene of this recessive trait and your other gene is normal, your general good health will not be interfered with, but you will be a carrier.

If your partner also is a carrier, there is a chance that your child will have sickle-cell disease. You should consult a genetic counselor for professional advice. If you are of Jewish-Ashkenazic descent (Central and Eastern Europe, as are 90 percent of the American Jewish population), you have a 1-in-30 chance of carrying the recessive gene in Tay-Sachs disease, which causes serious illness and eventual death in early infancy. You, as a carrier, will have no obvious effects from this lethal recessive gene. But if your partner also is a carrier, there is a 1-in-4 chance with each pregnancy that your child will be affected. If your partner is not a carrier, none of your children will exhibit the disease.

Now you can take a simple blood test to determine if you are a carrier of Tay-Sachs disease. If your unborn child is at risk because your partner also is a carrier, there are special ways to test if the fetus you are carrying has this fatal disease. This is done at about 16 weeks' gestation by sampling the fluid that surrounds the fetus in a procedure called amniocentesis (see page 238).

Genetic Counseling

Since tests are available that can diagnose certain genetic or inherited biochemical defects, prospective parents who may be carriers of an inherited disease can be tested prior to pregnancy. If problems are indicated, their unborn child can be tested in the fourth month of pregnancy.

In such a screening procedure, the genetic counselor begins by taking a careful history of both prospective parents, with special emphasis on any relatives with possible genetic disorders. Next, appropriate tests and examinations are done. The counselor then can evaluate the risks of your having a child with a genetic disease. Certain carrier states can be identified by examinations of the blood or skin, and decisions can be made accordingly. An amniocentesis (sampling of the fluid that surrounds the fetus) may be suggested to determine if your fetus has a specific defect.

Amniocentesis. This procedure is recommended when the chance that an unborn child has a serious genetic disease is greater than the risk of a serious complication from the amniocentesis procedure itself. The benefits of the procedure always are weighed against the risks. Ultimately, the final course of action is up to you, the prospective mother.

Amniocentesis involves taking a sample from the fluid-filled amniotic sac (the bag of waters) that surrounds the fetus. An ultrasound examination may be done first in order to determine the location of the placenta (afterbirth), the size of the fetus, and the best location to obtain the fluid. Ultrasound waves cannot be heard because they are beyond our hearing range. But they are able to pass through your skin and are reflected off surfaces between two different structures to form a pattern of dots and spaces that can be pictured on a screen.

The amniocentesis itself is a simple procedure. After the abdomen overlying the uterus is cleansed with antiseptic, a small amount of local anesthesia is injected into your skin to make it numb. Then a needle is inserted through your abdominal and uterine wall to reach the amniotic cavity, where about one ounce of fluid is withdrawn. The fluid is sent to a laboratory where the fetal cells are allowed to culture (grow) for two to three weeks. Not all defects can be diagnosed this way. On rare occasions, the fetal cells fail to grow and the test must be repeated. The risk of miscarriage or other serious problems developing from the amniocentesis is very small—less than 1 percent.

Who should be offered genetic counseling? Genetic counseling usually is offered under the following conditions:

- The mother is over 35 years of age. This is probably the most common reason for counseling.
- The mother has a known chromosomal translocation.
- The mother has had a previous infant with a chromosomal abnormality.
- There is a known risk for an inherited disorder that can be diagnosed *in utero,* such as Tay-Sachs disease when both parents are known to be carriers.
- The mother has had a previous infant with a neural tube defect (malformation of the brain and nervous system).

If you fall into one or more of the above categories, the counselor will most likely recommend certain tests, possibly including amniocentesis. If you have had a child with a neural tube defect, such as spina bifida or anencephaly (incomplete brain development), a blood test for a certain chemical (a fetoprotein) is done first. This protein "leaks" from the affected fetus into the bloodstream of the mother. If her blood level of this chemical is above a certain level, amniocentesis may be suggested to measure the chemical's level in the amniotic fluid. Sometimes results are equivocal or borderline, or the defect does not cause leaking of the chemical. In these cases, an ultrasound examination may be useful in "picturing" the defect.

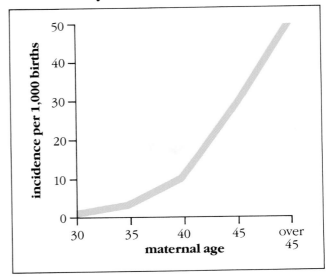

Down's Syndrome and Maternal Age

Down's syndrome (mongolism) increases in frequency as maternal age increases. It occurs in one out of 2,000 live births at maternal age 20, but to one in 20 live births at maternal age over 45.

ULTRASOUND EXAMINATION

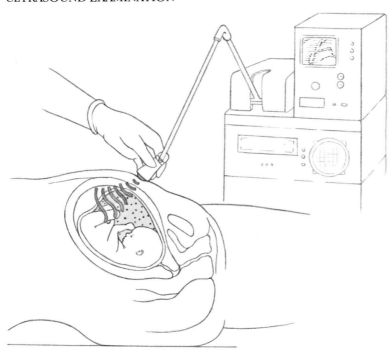

In an ultrasound examination, sound waves generated by the machine on the right are transmitted through a "wand" into the pelvic area. As the sound waves bounce off solid structures, they form a picture on the oscilloscope screen. A technician will move the wand around the surface of the abdomen until the fetus and placenta are localized, allowing the physician to place the needle for amniocentesis very precisely and avoiding damage to the placenta and fetus. Ultrasound visualization also is used to detect twins, and to determine fetal age. The best time for ultrasound scanning is between 16 and 19 weeks of pregnancy.

AMNIOCENTESIS

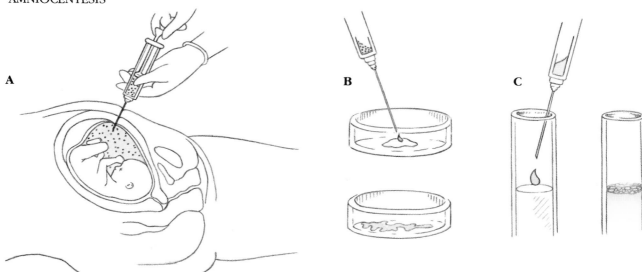

A Amniotic fluid sampled at various stages of pregnancy will reveal the sex of the fetus, allow diagnosis of specific genetic diseases, tell if there is a serious Rh disease, and indicate whether the fetal kidney and lungs are working properly. After anesthetizing the abdominal wall, amniotic fluid is withdrawn with a syringe.
B Cells floating in the fluid are cultured; they multiply and are studied for signs of genetic disease, and the sex of the child.
C The cell-free portion of the fluid is analyzed for other defects, such as failure of the neural tube to close, or lung insufficiency of the fetus.

Normal or negative results can reassure you that your fetus does not have the specific disease tested for. But if tests show the fetus to have a serious defect, it is your choice to continue the pregnancy or to have an abortion.

Effects of Maternal Age

Is it harmful to wait until the thirties to start a family? Physically, the optimal time for childbearing is from your early to mid-twenties, but this may not fit in with your life's plan. You may decide to join the increasing number of women who delay childbearing until their thirties. This allows you time to pursue an education and various career opportunities, as well as to experiment with various life-styles. The increased skills and experience you acquire leave you more options after childbirth as well. In the event that circumstances place you as head of the household or as a single parent, you then will have more marketable skills.

The future father also may want more time to continue his education and develop his career without the responsibilities of raising a family. Deferring childbirth allows you both to get to know each other better and to work out differences that will make being parents that much easier. You can start your family when you are "ready."

What are the disadvantages of delaying childbirth? You probably will not have as much resiliency and energy if you wait to start your family until you are older. As mentioned previously, the older you are, especially after the age of 35, the more likely you are to have a child with a genetic defect, the most common of which is Down's syndrome. Also, your fertility will decline somewhat after age 30, so you may find it more difficult to become pregnant. As you get older, you are more likely to suffer from conditions that can affect the outcome of your pregnancy, such as endometriosis (see page 467), uterine fibromyoma (tumors of the uterine muscle wall), kidney infections, hypertension, diabetes, or obesity. Since most women in their thirties are healthy, they can expect to have a safe and comfortable pregnancy, labor, and delivery. And, the increased risk of bearing a child with Down's syndrome at age 35 or older is controllable by amniocentesis and abortion, if desired by the parents.

If you already know that you have a chronic age-related disease such as the ones mentioned, you should discuss the prospect of future childbearing with your physician so that you can make an informed decision about when and if you want to start a family.

Preparing for Childbirth

Natural Childbirth

More and more women are requesting "natural childbirth" or, to be more accurate, "prepared childbirth," where you and your partner are active participants in the birth process.

The Lamaze method and its various modifications are becoming increasingly popular to help couples prepare for childbirth. Ask your doctor about classes for you and your partner, starting in the later months of pregnancy (see page 371).

Childbirth preparation classes such as the Lamaze method teach concepts concerning childbirth, the control of pain, and what body changes to expect during pregnancy. You also will learn the importance of good posture and appropriate exercise to maintain posture (see page 296 for some examples). The three stages of labor also are discussed in childbirth preparation classes, with emphasis on certain breathing techniques appropriate to the different stages. You will be taught relaxation exercises and will practice with your partner, or whoever you choose to be your labor coach.

The classes will help you to develop a conditioned (automatic) response to contractions by controlled breathing accompanied by a simultaneous relaxing or letting-go of uninvolved muscles. This involves learning a panting or blowing technique to use during the transaction phase when you are almost fully dilated, but should not yet push. This breathing technique also helps facilitate a controlled delivery of your baby's head.

Leboyer "birth without violence" also is increasingly popular. This method emphasizes making the delivery as peaceful as possible, in a quiet, darkened room. Soon after birth, the infant is placed in a bath at room temperature to simulate the environment of the intrauterine bag of waters.

Childbirth classes are available in most communities (see page 261) and usually consist of adaptations or modifications of the classic methods of prepared childbirth. Most women and couples benefit from attending these classes, although some choose not to attend. "Natural childbirth" should be a personal choice of the mother-to-be.

Cesarean Section

For various reasons, sometimes a normal vaginal delivery is not possible and a cesarean section is required. The baby is then delivered through an incision in the abdominal wall and uterus. If you know ahead of time that you will need a cesarean section (for instance, if you have had a previous birth that way), you might inquire about classes and books available to help you and your husband prepare for this operation. Such resources also may be available for emotional support if you have just undergone an unplanned emergency C-section. One such support group is C/SEC (Cesarean/Support, Education, and Concern). For more information on cesarean section, see the chapter on "Labor and Delivery" beginning on page 305.

Becoming Pregnant

Intercourse by the clock or calendar can be stressful. If you are having regular fertile (ovulatory) cycles and have intercourse two to three times weekly, conception ordinarily will take place without a special effort on your part to have intercourse on a specific day of your cycle.

If you have long cycles (35 to 37 days), remember that ovulation, if it occurs, takes place at 12 to 14 days before your expected period. It also is possible to have a period without ovulating. If you have a short 21-day cycle, counting from the first day of one period to the first day of the next period, you may be ovulating as early as day seven to ten of your cycle. This makes it possible for a woman with short cycles to conceive from unprotected intercourse during her period or shortly after. If you frequently skip periods and are very irregular, you should consult a doctor.

Just before ovulation, you may notice your vaginal discharge change from dryness to a clear, watery, stretchy mucus—a sign that you're entering your fertile period. After ovulation, the mucus becomes thick, opaque, and white or yellow (see page 189). Another test of ovulation is to take your temperature every morning before getting out of bed. When this "basal body temperature" drops and then rises to remain elevated, you probably are ovulating (see page 518 of the chapter on "Infertility" and page 188 of the chapter on "Birth Control").

While trying to become pregnant, do not use artificial lubricants of any kind during intercourse. Douches, unless indicated, also should not be used. If you do not conceive within 6 to 12 months of trying, you should consult your doctor. (For further information, see the chapter on "Infertility".)

Intercourse During Pregnancy

As long as you are comfortable during intercourse and your pregnancy is normal, you may continue to have intercourse throughout pregnancy. You may need to try different positions to allow for the increasing size of your abdomen, but orgasm will not harm the baby.

On the other hand, intercourse may be dangerous if you have vaginal bleeding, threatened premature labor, ruptured membranes (bag of waters), or placenta previa (a condition in which the afterbirth covers all or part of the cervix, the opening to the uterus).

You should avoid oral sex during pregnancy because of the possibility of transmitting the oral Herpes Type I virus (the cold sore and fever blister virus, see page 574) to your genitals, which could be harmful to your baby. Most people will have had previous exposure to the virus and therefore have some immunity to it. But the fetus can be infected if you contract the disease, and danger results if you have infected blisters on the membranes of your birth passages when you begin labor. Cesarean section may be necessary to prevent the baby from becoming infected by passing through the birth canal at the time of delivery.

Blowing air into the vagina also can be dangerous in pregnancy because of the possibility that air might enter the congested veins of the pregnant cervix (the opening of the uterus) and cause a fatal air embolism (air bubbles in the blood vessels).

If for any reason intercourse is contraindicated during your pregnancy, consider it an opportunity to explore other means of communication between you and your partner.

Well-Being During Pregnancy

Nutrition and Diet

As mentioned previously, you should avoid rapid weight loss if you are considering pregnancy soon. During pregnancy you can expect to gain 25 to 30 pounds: three to four pounds during the first trimester, and 10 to 12 pounds during each of the second and third trimesters. If you lose weight during pregnancy or fail to gain weight, this can affect your baby's health. But it is important to remember that pregnancy is often a time when women gain weight that they will never lose. It's not necessary to "eat for two" at this time. Instead, you should eat a healthful, balanced diet, and avoid the nutritionless calories of rich desserts and snack foods.

A diet for pregnancy. By your third month of pregnancy, you will require 300 calories more per day than before you were pregnant, and will need extra protein or body-building foods such as milk, eggs, meat, fish, and soy protein. You'll also need extra iron and folic acid, a B-vitamin also known as folacin, to accommodate the extra expansion of your blood cells during pregnancy and to meet the growing needs of your baby. Eggs, meats, raisins, prune juice, and fortified cereals are foods high in folic acid. The extra calcium needed for your growing baby's bones is best supplied by milk and milk products.

At right is a list of foods that should be eaten daily during pregnancy. Also see the "Nutrition" chapter, beginning on page 40, for dietary and vitamin needs during pregnancy.

Daily Food Requirements During Pregnancy

Protein Foods

FOUR SERVINGS EACH DAY

Meats: a serving is 2-3 oz. or 60-90 grams cooked (boneless), unless otherwise noted
● Bacon, 6 slices ● Beef ● Canned tuna, salmon, crab, etc., ½ cup ● Fish ● Frankfurters, 2 ● Lamb ● Luncheon meats, 3 slices ● Organ meats: liver, kidney, sweetbreads, tongue, etc. ● Pork or ham ● Poultry ● Veal

Non-meat protein: a serving is 1 cup, cooked, unless otherwise noted
● Beans ● Lentils ● Nut butters, ¼ cup ● Nuts, ½ cup ● Sunflower seeds, ½ cup ● Tofu (soybean curd) ● Cheese, 1½ oz. ● Eggs, 2

Milk and Milk Products

FOUR SERVINGS EACH DAY

A serving is 8 oz., 1 cup, or 240 cc., unless otherwise noted
● Cow's milk (whole, skim, low-fat, or buttermilk) ● Cheese (except bleu, Camembert, and cream), 1½ oz. ● Cream soups (made with milk), 12 oz. ● Cottage cheese, 1⅓ cups ● Ice cream, 1½ cups ● Yogurt ● Puddings, custard

Grain Products

THREE SERVINGS EACH DAY

Choose whole grain products whenever possible, and look for products made with enriched flours. Amounts listed are for one serving.
● Bread, especially whole or cracked wheat, 1 slice ● Cereals, hot, ½ cup, cooked ● Cereals, cold, ready-to-eat, ¾ cup ● Crackers, 4 ● Noodles, macaroni, spaghetti, etc., ½ cup, cooked ● Muffin, biscuit, dumpling, roll, bagel, 1 ● Rice (preferably brown) ½ cup, cooked ● Corn tortillas, 2 ● Flour tortilla, 1 large ● Pancake or waffle, 1

Fruits and Vegetables

FOUR SERVINGS EACH DAY

Fruits and vegetables rich in Vitamin C
ONE SERVING Canned and frozen products may have lower amounts of vitamin C. Amounts listed are for one serving.
Juices: ● Orange, grapefruit, 4 oz. ● Tomato, pineapple, 12 oz. ● Fruit juices and drinks enriched with vitamin C, 6 oz.
Fruits: ● Cantaloupe, ½ ● Grapefruit, ½ ● Guava, ¼ medium ● Mango, 1 medium ● Orange, 1 medium ● Papaya, ⅓ medium ● Strawberries, ¾ cup ● Tangerines, 2 small
Vegetables: ● Bok choy, ¾ cup ● Broccoli, 1 stalk ● Brussels sprouts, 3-4 ● Cabbage, cooked, 1⅓ cups; raw, ¾ cup ● Cauliflower, raw or cooked, 1 cup ● Greens: collard, kale, mustard, Swiss chard, turnip greens, ¾ cup ● Peppers, chili, ¾ cup ● Peppers, green or red, ½ medium ● Tomatoes, 2 medium ● Watercress, ¾ cup

Leafy green vegetables TWO SERVINGS
Try to use fresh vegetables, and don't overcook them. A serving is 1 cup raw, or ¾ cup cooked.
● Asparagus ● Bok choy ● Broccoli ● Brussels sprouts ● Cabbage ● Dark leafy lettuce ● Greens: beet, collard, mustard, kale, spinach, Swiss chard, or turnip ● Scallions ● Watercress

Other fruits and vegetables ONE SERVING
Fresh fruits and vegetables have the most vitamins, especially when eaten raw. A serving is ½ cup (fresh, frozen, or canned), unless otherwise noted.
Vegetables: ● Artichoke ● Bamboo shoots ● Bean sprouts ● Beets ● Burdock root ● Carrots ● Cauliflower ● Celery ● Corn ● Cucumber ● Eggplant ● Beans, green or wax ● Hominy ● Lettuce, head, boston, or Bibb ● Mushrooms ● Nori seaweed ● Onions ● Parsnips ● Peas ● Pea pods ● Potato ● Radishes ● Summer squash ● Sweet potato ● Winter squash ● Yam ● Zucchini
Fruits: ● Apricot, fresh, 1 large ● Nectarines, 2 medium ● Peach, fresh, 1 medium ● Persimmon, 1 medium ● Prunes, 4 ● Pumpkin, ¼ cup ● Apple, 1 medium ● Banana, 1 small ● Cherries ● Berries ● Dates, 5 ● Figs, 2 large ● Fruit cocktail ● Grapes ● Kumquats, 3 ● Pear, 1 medium ● Pineapple ● Plums, 2 medium ● Raisins ● Watermelon

Pregnancy and Work

As a result of medical knowledge and employment legislation, most women can continue to work during pregnancy and following delivery. Nearly one-half of all women 16 years of age and over in the United States work outside the home. The total female labor force is approximately 40 million, and the majority of these women are of childbearing age. A large percentage are either pregnant or considering pregnancy, and thus are very concerned about occupational hazards affecting their childbearing capacity and the health of their unborn children. Many women workers are exposed to **toxic chemicals** and environmental hazards such as **irritant gases, dusts and fumes, extreme heat, radiation,** and physical and psychological **stress**—in workplaces such as hospitals, textile factories, and laboratories—especially as women increasingly work in what were traditionally male fields.

HEALTH HAZARDS AT WORK

- **Lead**
- **Irritant gases**
- **Radiation**
- **Toxic chemicals**
- **Stress**
- **Dusts and fumes**
- **Extreme heat**
- **Cotton dust**
- **Anesthetic gases**

Toxic chemicals. Excessive exposure to toxic chemicals—added to other environmental hazards such as air pollution, cigarette smoking, and drugs—affect the health of all workers by contributing to diseases such as emphysema, cancer, and heart disease. The hazards often are much greater for pregnant women because many chemicals cross the placental barrier and concentrate in the unborn fetus; these substances also may be transmitted to an infant through breast-feeding. The effects may be minimal or severe, depending upon the particular chemical or toxic substance and:
- the amount and duration of exposure
- the time of exposure (the first trimester is the time of greatest risk to the unborn fetus)
- the genetic makeup of the mother and fetus.

The effects of toxic chemicals on pregnant women include increased fetal mortality (from spontaneous abortion and stillbirths), birth defects from genetic damage in egg or sperm cells that can be passed on to a developing fetus, lowered birth weights, mental retardation, and a variety of physical deformities.

Anesthetic gases. Recent medical studies indicate an above-average incidence of congenital abnormalities in children born of women who were exposed to anesthetic gases (e.g., female anesthesiologists). Studies also suggest an increase of spontaneous abortions.

Lead. Female workers (or their partners) exposed to excessive levels of lead have increased numbers of spontaneous abortions and stillbirths. The children of workers exposed to lead are highly susceptible to neonatal convulsions.

Cotton dust. Excessive exposure to cotton dust may seriously interfere with maternal oxygen consumption and oxygenation of the blood necessary for fetal well-being. Pregnancy involves greater oxygen demands and an increased respiratory rate; a pregnant worker may thus absorb greater amounts of airborne chemical substances than her co-workers, and this may interfere with breathing and increase her susceptibility to infection.

A pregnant woman's tolerance for strenuous physical exertion at home or in the workplace often will be lowered due to postural changes in pregnancy, although this will vary depending on the individual woman's physical fitness and strength.

Most pregnant women are healthy and employable through pregnancy. Current medical knowledge, employment legislation, and equal opportunity programs place little restriction on their continuing to work. All women who are either pregnant or considering pregnancy should discuss their occupational history with their physician. This is necessary to assess potential problems and to make an informed job decision, based on your personal health condition and level of fitness.

Finally, for more information on the health hazards of your particular job, contact the following sources:

The American Occupational Medical Association
150 North Wacker Drive
Chicago, Illinois 60606

The American College of Obstetricians and Gynecologists
One East Wacker Drive
Chicago, Illinois 60601

Be sure to keep an occupational health record, such as the example shown here. Use this as a supplement to your personal health record (see page 396), and always follow company health and safety procedures.

Your Occupational Health Record

Make an occupational health record to supplement your personal medical history. Be sure to include the following kinds of information, and be as specific as possible about your work conditions. It is important to note your exposures at home and in the community as well as your personal habits (such as tobacco, drug, and alcohol use). Finally, be sure to note your husband's or partner's occupational exposures as well.

Place of work
- Office • Factory • Laboratory • Other

Type of work
- Desk work • Sales work • Hospital work
- Assembly line work • Other

Tasks performed
- Physical work • Routine clerical work
- Intellectually stimulating work • Other

Materials handled: intensity and duration of exposure to environmental hazards
- Chemicals • Airborne dusts and fumes
- Noise • Radiation • Excessive heat
- Psychological stress
- Other

Work schedule
- Hours per day and per week • Rest periods
- Shift work and schedule changes

Access to medical care at work
- Physician • Nurse • Other

Pregnant women also should eat at least two tablespoons of butter, margarine, or salad oil a day. Desserts, beverages, gravies, seasonings, and condiments all may be eaten in moderation, but should not replace more nutritious foods. You should not change your usual salt or fluid intake without consulting your doctor. If you are a vegetarian or have other dietary restrictions, you should discuss this with your doctor or with a nutritionist.

Throughout your pregnancy, your doctor may advise vitamins to supplement your diet, especially folic acid and iron in the later months. This is because your body needs more of these nutrients during pregnancy, and they can be hard to get from food sources. But too many vitamins actually can be harmful, and high doses of vitamins should not be taken arbitrarily.

Drugs

Most drugs that you ingest or inhale readily go through the placenta to your baby. Even drugs applied topically to your skin or mucus membranes can affect your baby. The effect on the baby depends upon the nature and action of the drug itself, the amount of the drug you take, and the period of gestation (pregnancy) when it is taken. The drugs may act directly on the fetus, or they may act indirectly by their effects on the mother.

By drugs we mean not only prescription drugs, but non-prescription drugs as well, such as aspirin, cough medicines, nasal sprays, and even some ointments applied to the skin. Also included are alcohol, cigarette smoke, marijuana, and "hard" drugs (see page 244).

The baby is vulnerable to drugs throughout pregnancy, but especially in the first trimester when new organs are being formed and developed. Drugs that produce fetal abnormalities in the first trimester are called teratogens. An example of a potent teratogen is thalidomide, a mild sedative in adults. When given to women between the 28th and 42nd day of pregnancy, it causes serious limb defects in the fetus. Yet when given at term, it produces no ill effect.

Many drugs are weak teratogens that cause damage in only a small percent of cases. Still others, such as diethylstilbestrol (DES), manifest their effects only many years after exposure. Daughters of mothers who had been given DES when they were pregnant developed abnormal cellular changes, including cancer, in their vaginas as they approached adolescence (see page 506 of the chapter "Adolescent Reproductive Problems" and page 482 of the chapter "Adult Reproductive Problems").

Risks of Taking Drugs During Pregnancy

No drugs have been proven to be safe during pregnancy, and most drugs taken during pregnancy can have a harmful effect on your baby. This includes prescription drugs, over-the-counter drugs such as aspirin, and cigarettes and alcohol.

A drug's effects on an unborn child depend on:
- the nature and action of the drug itself
- the amount taken and the duration of use
- the period of gestation when it is taken
- the drug's combination with other environmental hazards, genetic factors, and infectious diseases.

The first trimester is the most critical period of birth defect risks from drugs. However, negative effects from maternal drug use also can occur after the first trimester, when the genitals, teeth, and central nervous system are continuing to mature. In fact, the fetus is "at risk" during the entire nine months of gestation.

Drugs may affect fetal well-being by direct toxicity to the fetus, physiological and nutritional effects on the fetoplacental unit (affecting placental blood flow and depriving the fetus of adequate nutrition), or by metabolic, nutritional, and hormonal effects on the mother. Possible results include congenital malformations that show up at birth, lowered birth weight, increased fetal mortality, fetal kidney malfunction, and behavioral disorders during childhood (see the chart beginning at right).

Avoid drugs—both prescription and over-the-counter—as much as possible during pregnancy. And before you take any drug, ask your doctor how great your need is for that particular medication, and the risks of its use during pregnancy. Also, check the *Physicians' Desk Reference* at your local library for information on adverse effects associated with a drug's use during pregnancy.

The chart at right lists some drugs with known or suspected harmful health effects on the developing fetus, based on available animal and human studies of drug use during pregnancy.

When drugs can cause malformations in the developing fetus

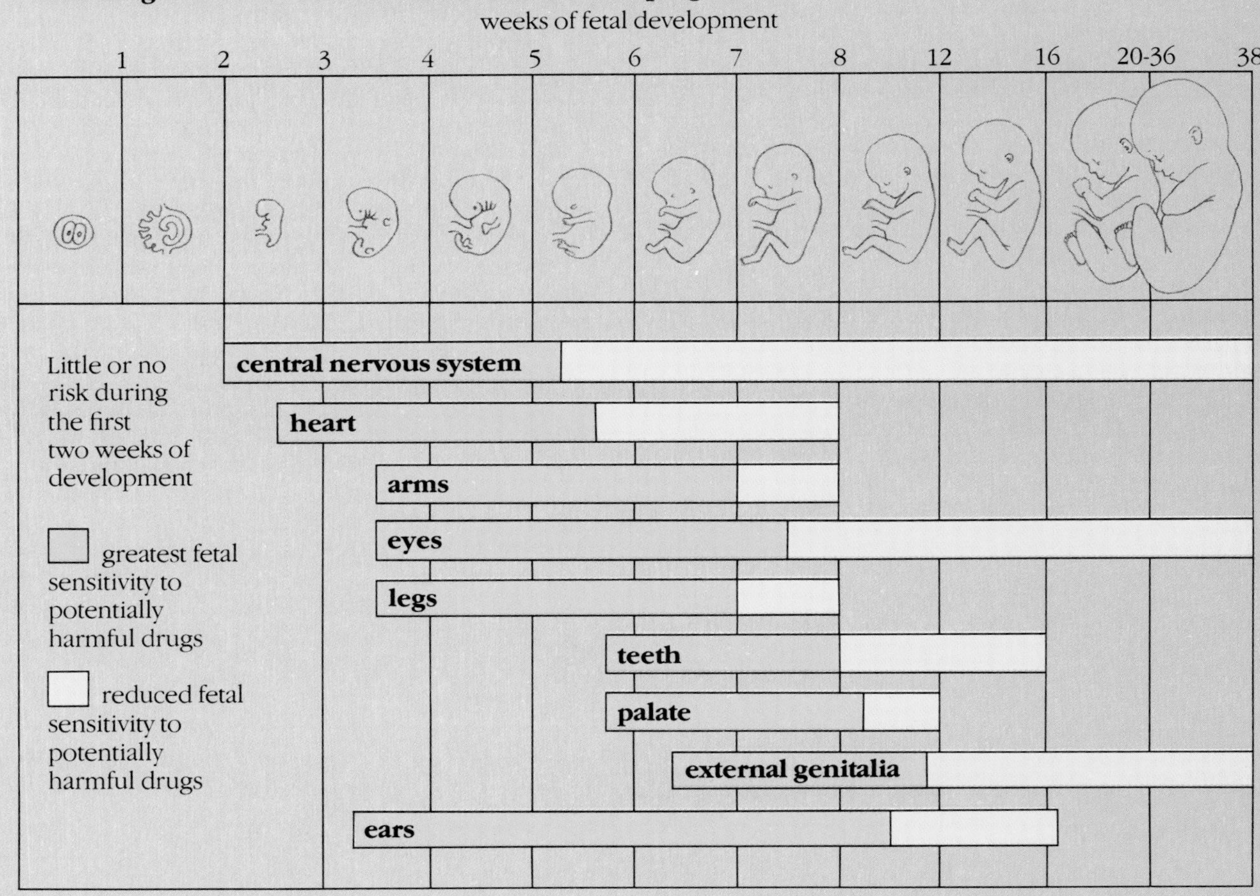

weeks of fetal development

Harmful Health Effects of Taking Drugs During Pregnancy

DRUG AND REASON FOR USE	EFFECT ON FETUS/SPECIAL CONSIDERATIONS
Alcohol Social and psychological factors	Heavy drinking may cause heart defects and facial, arm, and leg malformations. Children born of alcoholic mothers are likely to be addicted at birth and to go through withdrawal.
Cigarette smoke Social and psychological factors	The offspring of women who smoke cigarettes are smaller and are subject to higher perinatal mortality and morbidity. Smoking is related to increased risk of fetal malformations and stunted physical and mental growth. Major birth defects, congenital heart diseases, and cleft lip and palate are more prevalent in children of smoking mothers. • SPECIAL CONSIDERATIONS Cigarette smoking is clearly harmful to your own health as well as to your unborn child's. The more you smoke, the greater the dangers and the higher the risks.

NON-PRESCRIPTION DRUGS

Antacids Upset stomach, heartburn	Possible higher rate of birth defects when mother uses drugs regularly. • SPECIAL CONSIDERATIONS Small occasional doses for extreme discomfort should be safe.
Aspirin Minor aches and pains	Mental retardation, limb abnormalities, fetal death, bleeding in the newborn, and other developmental defects. • SPECIAL CONSIDERATIONS Aspirin is an ingredient in many different medications. Read the label. The effects are increased when taken together with benzoic acid, a common food preservative. Aspirin given within two weeks of delivery may cause serious bleeding in the newborn and mother.
Aspirin substitutes Minor pain and discomfort	It is uncertain what effects acetaminophen (the ingredient in aspirin substitutes) may have on the fetus. Studies have not yet proved its safety.
Cold remedies and sinus medications Itchy eyes and runny nose due to colds **Sleeping medications** Insomnia, nervous tension	Cold remedies, sinus medications, and sleeping medications (non-prescription) often contain aspirin; most use the antihistamines methapyrilene and pyrilamine. Pyrilamine has been shown to produce congenital deformities in animals.

PRESCRIPTION DRUGS

Amphetamines Nervous system stimulation; weight control and psychological dependence	Act as a stimulant on the fetus; heart malformations may occur. • SPECIAL CONSIDERATIONS Amphetamines should never be taken.
Antibiotics Bacterial infections, such as bladder infections.	**Streptomycin** Hearing loss, problems of balance and dizziness, and kidney malfunction. **Tetracyclines** Slows baby's bone and teeth growth; results in discoloration of infant's teeth. These effects are especially noticeable in the second half of pregnancy. **Chloramphenicol** "Gray baby" syndrome; interferes with baby's breathing (especially when given during labor). • SPECIAL CONSIDERATIONS Antibiotics should be taken only if the risk of infection outweighs the drug's risks. For example, women who have untreated bladder infections may develop serious kidney infections that can jeopardize the pregnancy.

Risks of Taking Drugs During Pregnancy continued

Harmful Health Effects of Taking Drugs During Pregnancy

DRUG AND REASON FOR USE **PRESCRIPTION DRUGS**	EFFECT ON FETUS/SPECIAL CONSIDERATIONS
Anticonvulsants For control of epileptic seizures	Rarely cleft lip or palate, cardiac malformations.
Barbiturates and sleeping pills To induce sleep; psychological and physical addiction or dependence	Infant addiction at birth.
Corticosterioids To replace adrenocortical hormones if the body is not producing them; treatment of allergic disease and inflammatory disease	Cleft palate suspected (rare); may lead to other "minor" abnormalities. ● SPECIAL CONSIDERATIONS Use to treat late stages of diseases only with extreme caution and discretion.
Coumarin Anticoagulant or "blood thinner" for treating phlebitis or blood clots in legs	Frequent fetal bleeding when given near time of labor and delivery or birth defects when given in first trimester.
Estrogen: **DES** Was given to women until 1971 to prevent miscarriage (see page 506) **Birth control pill** Contraceptive	Rare vaginal cancer (vaginal adenocarcinoma) in daughters of women who took DES during their pregnancy. Rare but possible anomalies of vertebrae, anus, heart, trachea, esophagus, and limbs of fetus when administered during early pregnancy. ● SPECIAL CONSIDERATIONS Estrogen has many potentially dangerous side effects.
Progestins or progesterone Used in contraceptive pills	Masculinization of female fetus to varying degrees.
Narcotics Severe pain; psychological and physical dependence or addiction	Fetal addiction; may result in need for blood transfusion at birth.
Thalidomide For "nervousness" or nausea; as a mild daytime sedative	An unquestionably teratogenic drug that is no longer in use. Its effects when taken during pregnancy included musculoskeletal defects, such as malformations of limbs, heart, gastrointestinal and urinogenital systems, and sensory organs.
Tranquilizers Anxiety, tension, pain, "nervousness"	Retarded breathing and depression of infant when given at delivery; behavioral disorders; predisposition to birth defects if taken during the first trimester.
Anticancer and antitumor agents To attempt to control growth of cancer cells	Highly teratogenic and capable of producing a wide range of skeletal abnormalities and stunted growth; cleft palate; malformations of the central nervous system; small head; limb malformations; heart and gut malformations. ● SPECIAL CONSIDERATIONS Women undergoing cancer chemotherapy should not become pregnant because of the high possibility of fetal abnormality.

Some drugs—such as heparin, used as an anticoagulant (blood thinner)—do not cross the placenta, so they cannot directly affect the fetus. Others, such as penicillin, do cross the placenta, but have no demonstrable effect on the fetus at any time during pregnancy.

Chronic alcohol abuse causes cumulative damage throughout pregnancy (see page 57). Chronic use of drugs such as heroin can produce an addicted fetus and later an addicted infant who will suffer withdrawal symptoms if suddenly deprived of the drug. The fetus is in danger of dying in the uterus if the pregnant mother is suddenly deprived of drugs and has severe withdrawal symptoms.

Infants born of mothers who smoke more than ten cigarettes daily often are small for their gestational age. This may occur because nicotine causes blood vessels to constrict, and could therefore interfere with the blood flow to the placenta; or, the fetus may not get enough oxygen because of the increased carbon monoxide level in the maternal blood.

Cigarette smoking has also been shown to increase miscarriage rates and the incidence of prematurity. Even though the reasons are not totally understood, it is clear that cigarette smoking is harmful to your unborn baby—as well as to yourself (see page 245).

Many drugs are potentially dangerous to the fetus. When drugs are needed during pregnancy, their benefits must be weighed against their risks. It may be best to leave a problem untreated until after the child is born. Certainly, you should avoid taking unnecessary drugs at all times, but even more so during pregnancy, and especially during the first trimester. If you are taking, or have taken, any drugs while you are pregnant—whether for pregnancy-related conditions (morning sickness, backache, constipation, or hemorrhoids), or to treat a chronic or acute illness— you should discuss this with your doctor.

For information on drugs that may be administered during childbirth, see the chapter "Labor and Delivery."

Exercise

Physical exercise is vital for a healthy pregnancy, birth, and delivery. For a discussion of exercise and sports participation during pregnancy, see the chapter on "Fitness"; also, see the chapter on "Labor and Delivery."

Harmful Effects of Infectious Agents During Pregnancy

A few infections, listed below, are known to cause malformations of human babies. The developing human is especially susceptible to these diseases during the critical first eight weeks of development.

INFECTIOUS AGENT	CAUSE OF INFECTION	EFFECT ON FETUS	PREVENTION
Rubella virus (measles)	From droplet or droplet spray of nose, throat, or mouth of another person with measles	Mental retardation, small brain and head, blindness, deafness, heart defects, death	Avoid people with measles. Have a rubella titer test to determine if you are immune.
Toxoplasma gondii, a single-celled parasite (toxoplasmosis)	Raw meat may be infected; commonly spread when raw meat is fed to a cat, then cat feces are handled or the litter is changed.	Mental retardation, poor development of brain, small head, eye defects	Do not feed your cats raw meat; avoid all possibility of contact with cat feces.
Cytomegalovirus (salivary gland infection)	Direct contact with virus in saliva from infected person	Mental retardation, small head and brain, eye defects	Avoid infection.

Tests and Interventions

Blood Tests

After your pregnancy has been confirmed, your doctor will order the following blood tests:

- **Hemoglobin or hematocrit** to test for anemia.
- **RPR or VDRL or other tests for syphilis,** since this disease can produce serious symptoms and even death in the fetus, while causing only minimal symptoms, such as a painless ulcer, in the mother.
- **Rubella titer** to test for immunity to German measles. This disease can cause very serious birth defects, especially if a pregnant woman acquires it in the first three months of her pregnancy. In adults, German measles is a very mild disease that causes only a slight rash and fever for about three days. But to the unborn child, it can cause mental retardation, blindness, deafness, and death. If this test shows that you are immune, your fetus will be in no danger even if you are exposed to the disease. If the test is negative, you are susceptible to German measles, and if you contract the disease during the first trimester of your pregnancy, you may decide to have an abortion. If you find that you have no immunity, you can be vaccinated against German measles after your baby is born. This is a good time, because you must avoid becoming pregnant during the three months following the vaccination.
- **Your blood type and Rh factor** to determine if you are Rh-negative. Fifteen percent of the population has an Rh-negative blood type. This can be a problem if the baby is Rh-positive. The Rh factor is inherited genetically, with the negative type being recessive. If you are Rh-negative, the baby's father also will be tested. If he, too, is negative, there is no chance of the fetus being Rh-positive.

A problem develops when the mother's body produces antibodies against Rh-positive blood cells. If the mother is Rh-negative, this may happen during childbirth or abortion if any of the fetal Rh-positive blood gets into her bloodstream. This sensitizes the mother, and in future pregnancies her antibodies may attack the baby's blood cells. This can lead to serious anemia and finally intrauterine death of an Rh-positive fetus.

Fortunately, there is a way to prevent this. Rh-negative mothers who have just delivered or had abortions are given a substance called RhoGam. This substance contains Rh antibodies that will attack any Rh-positive fetal cells that have leaked into the mother's bloodstream before she manufactures her own antibodies. Given within three days of delivery, RhoGam can prevent the Rh-negative mother from becoming sensitized.

THE Rh FACTOR IN PREGNANCY

The Rh factor is a chemical complex called a blood group antigen, and it is carried on the surface of red blood cells of about 85 percent of people. If you have it, you are Rh-positive. If you don't have the Rh factor, you are termed Rh-negative, and belong in the other 15 percent. If you are an Rh-negative woman, and you plan to have children, you probably will need to have a RhoGam shot.

Here's why. An Rh− woman pregnant by an Rh+ man usually will be carrying an Rh+ baby. The mother's blood and the baby's blood are incompatible. Under normal circumstances this would make no difference, since their blood would never mix. But if some of the Rh+ blood gets into the mother's bloodstream, as sometimes happens at the end of term, she would make antibodies to it. That is, she would carry a substance capable of destroying red blood cells in her baby. With the first child, this would not matter because the baby would be born before the antibodies had a chance to be made and then recross the placental barrier into the baby's body. But these antibodies are stored in the mother's system and might pass through the placental barrier into the system of her second Rh+ child, destroying its red blood cells.

Fortunately, there is a way to prevent this. An Rh− woman who has just delivered or had an abortion can be given a shot of RhoGam. RhoGam contains antibodies to Rh that will attack any Rh+ fetal cells that have leaked into the mother's bloodstream before she manufactures her own antibodies. The shot must be given within three days to be successful.

Just to be on the safe side, an Rh− woman pregnant by an Rh+ man may have her blood tested for the presence of antibodies. If she has a high antibody count, she and the fetus will be watched carefully for any problems.

There is no complication if the mother is Rh+ and the father Rh−, or if an Rh− mother has an Rh− child.

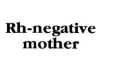

Rh-negative mother

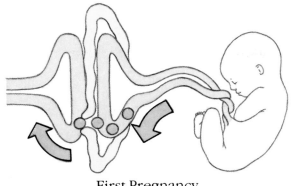

Rh-positive baby

First Pregnancy

Fetal Rh antigen ⬤ may cross the placental
barrier into the Rh-negative mother's bloodstream

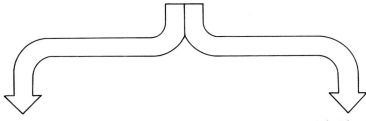

Without RhoGam
Rh-negative mother makes antibodies
to destroy antigen

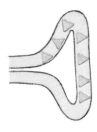

With RhoGam
Antigen destroyed
ANTIBODIES DO NOT FORM

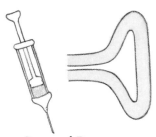

Second Pregnancy

- Maternal antibodies △ enter fetal system
and destroy red blood cells
- Baby in danger of hemolytic disease

Rh-positive baby

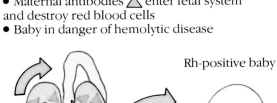

Second Pregnancy

Same conditions are present as
found in first pregnancy, and a healthy
baby is delivered

Rh-positive baby

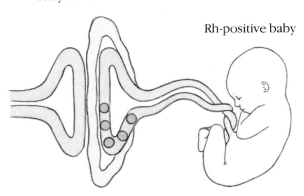

- **Antibody screening tests** are done even if you are not Rh-negative to detect any other antibodies.
- **A sickle-cell test** may be ordered to determine if you have sickle-cell disease or are a carrier of it.
- **Other blood tests** will be done as judged appropriate after the doctor takes your medical history and examines you.

Other Prenatal Tests

A complete urinalysis and screening urine culture will be done to ensure that you do not have asymptomatic bacteria that put you at increased risk for bladder and kidney infections.

At each visit, the doctor will test your urine for sugar and albumin, and will take a detailed history. Then you will have a complete physical examination, including a Pap smear to test for cervical cancer (see page 474) and possibly a cervical culture for gonorrhea. The doctor will assess the size and shape of your bony pelvis by an internal pelvic examination to ensure that there is sufficient room for a normal delivery (see page 225).

What are the points in your medical history that might be of special interest to the obstetrician?

Previous pregnancies. There may have been problems encountered during previous pregnancies that could repeat themselves, such as a premature birth, cesarean section, or a high blood pressure problem.

Your smoking and dietary habits, as well as any drug ingestion during the current pregnancy, can have potentially harmful effects on your fetus.

A family history of diabetes. If a close relative has diabetes, especially if the onset of the disease was during childhood or early adulthood, and you have had a baby weighing nine pounds or more, you are at increased risk of having diabetes or developing gestational (pregnancy) diabetes. In such cases, your doctor will order appropriate blood-sugar tests.

Genetic diseases. If you are over 35 years of age or have a history of possibly being a carrier of an inherited disease, you will be offered genetic counseling, and your doctor will order appropriate tests.

Pet cats. If you have pet cats, you will be advised not to feed them raw meat and to have someone else care for their litter box. Cats may be carriers of toxoplasmosis, a parasitic disease that is spread by eating infected raw meat, and that can cause serious infection in your unborn child. Infected cat feces are very contagious because the fecal bocysts are spread through the air. Contaminated meat is rendered safe by freezing or cooking, but your cat still can become infected by eating wild rodents if it is allowed to run loose.

As your pregnancy progresses, your doctor will ask you to take some of the following tests. It is important for you to understand why these tests may be necessary.

Ultrasound testing may be ordered to more accurately date the pregnancy, or to rule out the possibility of twins if your uterus is increasing in size more quickly than expected. It also is useful if you experience vaginal bleeding in the latter months of pregnancy to determine if the bleeding is caused from placenta previa, where the afterbirth covers all or part of the cervix (the opening to the uterus).

Estriol (E_3) determination. If you develop a complication of pregnancy such as increased blood pressure, or if you are more than two weeks overdue, you may be requested to collect all the urine you pass for a 24-hour period into a single container for an estriol (E_3) determination. Estriol is a hormone found in the urine in increasing amounts during pregnancy. If the fetal adrenal glands and liver are not functioning properly, the placenta cannot produce this hormone, which is a fairly reliable indicator of fetal well-being. This test—the estriol (E_3) determination—is most valuable when it is done several times, so that the results can be compared. A drop of 50 percent or more in the amount of estriol may be an indication that the fetus is in jeopardy, and other methods will be used to further evaluate its status.

The non-stress test or non-contraction test is one of the most reliable indicators of fetal well-being. This is a completely painless procedure that externally monitors the fetal heart. A disklike object is belted on the pregnant abdomen at the point where the heartbeat of the fetus is strongest. This in turn is attached to a machine that records every heartbeat on moving graph paper. A second disk may be attached if there are contractions so that the machine can record the contractions at the same time as the heartbeat.

A normal fetal heartbeat, which is between 120 and 160 beats per minute, is never absolutely regular, although it may sound very regular to our ears. Thus, when we record the fetal heartbeat, we will see that it varies from beat to beat. When the fetus moves, there may be an acceleration or increase in the heart rate, just as when we exercise, our heart beats faster. This is the basis of the non-contraction test.

A normal test will show good beat-to-beat variability, and good acceleration with fetal motion. This is called a reactive pattern, and indicates that the fetus is healthy.

Sometimes when the baby is sleeping or too quiet, the test is nonreactive or questionable. Then a contraction test or oxytocin challenge test may be advised if you are not having contractions on your own. An intravenous drip (IV), which is a needle placed in a vein in your arm, will be started. After about 20 to 30 minutes when a baseline fetal heartbeat is recorded for comparison, very dilute Pitocin (a uterine stimulant) is added to the IV at a slow rate. This rate is increased until you start having uterine contractions that are spaced about three minutes apart. The purpose of the test is to see how the fetal heart responds to contractions. Again, the doctor looks for accelerations or misses in the heartbeat, and decelerations or decreases in the heart rate.

Decelerations may occur at the same time as the contraction, or repeatedly just after the onset of a contraction—late deceleration. The fetus is healthiest if there are no decelerations of the heartbeat at all during regular contractions. Repeated late decelerations may indicate a problem that requires further evaluation. A single abnormal test is not an indication of a severe problem, but it will alert the doctors of this possibility. What the doctor does in the case of a fetus with serious heart decelerations depends on how soon the baby is due and other test results. It is common to monitor high-risk pregnancies with regular estriol collections and fetal heart monitoring tests (see page 303).

If you have had a previous delivery by cesarean section, your doctor will probably advise you to have another before you go into labor. In some cases, it may be possible for a woman to try to have a regular vaginal delivery even though she has had one cesarean, but this is not without risks and must be carefully evaluated. Although it is possible to wait until you go into labor to do the cesarean section, it's always better not to undergo any operation under emergency conditions.

There are several tests that will tell the doctor exactly how mature the fetus is, so that he or she can schedule the cesarean section for just before the time labor would begin. An ultrasound examination is useful because it shows the location of the placenta, and indicates the size and probable maturity of the fetus. Ultrasound findings can be confirmed by amniocentesis. Examining creatinine, bilirubin, and shed fetal fat cells in the amniotic fluid gives many indicators of fetal maturity. Lung maturity, especially important, is checked by examining the lecithin/sphingomyelin ratio (LS ratio) in the amniotic fluid.

The foregoing will give you some idea that you can't always predict what is going to happen during the course of a pregnancy, or what tests will or will not be done. Certain basic examinations and tests are routine; others are done as the need arises.

Complications of Pregnancy

Abortion or "Miscarriage"

Fifteen to 20 percent of pregnancies spontaneously abort in the first trimester. Most of these fetuses are defective and would be incapable of surviving anyway. If you experience slight bleeding with or without mild cramps, this is called a *threatened abortion*. About 85 percent of pregnancies accompanied by slight bleeding go into term with or without treatment. Increased rest and avoidance of strenuous activity and intercourse is usually recommended.

The bleeding and cramping may increase to alarming proportions and be accompanied by the passage of clots (lumps of clotted blood that resemble liver). At this stage, the cervical opening usually has begun to dilate, and nothing will stop the loss of this pregnancy. If this happens, prompt medical assistance should be sought. The administration of drugs and/or a suction aspiration or a D&C (dilation—usually not necessary since it already has taken place—and curettage, or scraping of the inside of the uterus) is necessary to completely empty the uterus and allow control of bleeding.

Frequently, especially after the sixth to eighth week of gestation, the uterus only expels the embryo and/or part of the placenta. The abortion is then incomplete. The bleeding and cramps will continue until all of the pregnancy tissue is expelled. Again, suction aspiration or a D&C will be necessary.

If all the tissue is expelled, as may happen in a very early spontaneous abortion, the bleeding and cramps decrease gradually and the abortion is said to be complete. No specific treatment is needed in this case.

Further examination may reveal the cause of the abortion. Menses usually resume four to six weeks after an abortion, but it is possible to become pregnant again even before the next period comes. If you are Rh-negative, you should have a RhoGam shot anytime you have an abortion.

A missed abortion occurs when a dead fetus is not expelled, but pregnancy symptoms *decrease*. The uterus decreases in size, and often there is a brownish or reddish vaginal discharge. Diagnosis may be confirmed by ultrasound examination or a falling level of the pregnancy hormone, HCG. Treatment is evacuation (emptying) of the uterus by suction or a D&C if spontaneous abortion does not occur within a reasonable time.

Ectopic Pregnancy

A pregnancy that implants outside the uterus is ectopic. The fertilized ovum can implant at many sites, but the most common site for ectopic pregnancies is in the fallopian tubes (especially the outer two-thirds of the tube, although it may implant at any point in the tube or at other sites, including the ovary). Very rarely, it implants in the abdominal cavity.

Cause. Ectopic pregnancies sometimes occur when the fallopian tube is blocked and the egg cannot travel through it to the uterus. This blockage may be the result of infection, but often the cause of an ectopic pregnancy is unknown.

Symptoms. The most common symptom is amenorrhea (a missed period) followed by a one-sided lower abdominal pain and vaginal spotting. In 10 percent of ectopic pregnancies, the symptoms occur before the missed period.

As the size of the pregnancy increases, the narrow, thin-walled tube painfully stretches. Soon it can no longer accommodate the increased size of the embryo. At this time, either the tube ruptures or the contents are pushed out through the tubal opening into the peritoneal cavity. If the tube actually ruptures (bursts open), the woman will experience severe pain, fainting, weakness, cold sweating, and palpitations (rapid heartbeat). These symptoms are caused by the serious internal bleeding.

Diagnosis. Your doctor may suspect an ectopic pregnancy if you have had tubal infections or related problems, or a previous ectopic pregnancy. An internal pelvic examination may reveal tenderness when the cervix is pushed, moving the uterus. There also may be a tender mass (swelling) on one side of the uterus. If the tube has ruptured, there will be signs of decreased blood pressure, cold sweating, and often shoulder pain. The urine test for pregnancy is positive in only about half of all patients.

The more sophisticated radioimmunoassay pregnancy test usually reveals abnormally low levels of pregnancy hormone HCG, but it may take up to three days before test results are known. Ultrasound examination may be helpful by showing that the pregnancy is normal, but it usually cannot detect the extremely rare instances in which an ectopic pregnancy exists with a normal pregnancy.

If the patient's medical history and physical examination indicate that an ectopic pregnancy is likely, the doctor may recommend a diagnostic laparoscopy to look into the peritoneal cavity with a periscopelike instrument.

If there are symptoms that suggest that the ectopic pregnancy has ruptured, the doctor may advise a culdocentesis, in which a needle is inserted through the vagina behind the cervix and into the peritoneal cavity to determine if non-clotting blood is present. If symptoms are severe, emergency laparotomy (surgical exploration through a small incision) usually is advised without delay.

Treatment. An ectopic pregnancy must be removed surgically, since with the exception of the extremely rare abdominal pregnancy, it cannot survive. This may be done by milking or incising the affected tube, or by removing the tube, depending upon the circumstances. If you have had an ectopic pregnancy before, especially if it was your first pregnancy, you are more likely to have another one. For this reason, it is important that you tell your doctor if you have had an ectopic pregnancy so that he or she can carefully watch for any recurring symptoms (also see the "Adult Reproductive Problems" chapter).

Antepartum Hemorrhage

An antepartum hemorrhage is one that occurs before delivery usually sometime in the last trimester.

Causes. About 50 percent of the time, the cause of the bleeding is never determined, although it usually is not severe. Cervical polyps, growths, vaginal or cervical infections, and lacerations (cuts, tears, or varicose vein ruptures) all may cause vaginal bleeding, but usually not in hemorrhagic proportions.

Placenta previa is a condition in which the afterbirth is situated between the fetus and the cervix, so that it partially or totally covers the opening to the uterus, and can cause antepartum hemorrhage.

Symptoms include painless vaginal bleeding during the last trimester.

Diagnosis. Ultrasound examination can be used to locate the placenta, and is almost 100 percent accurate. If placenta previa is diagnosed in the earlier months of pregnancy, the placenta may be "pulled" up as the pregnancy progresses.

Treatment. If the bleeding subsides and the fetus is very premature, it is best to let the pregnancy continue, with no pelvic examinations, except perhaps a gentle speculum examination. If the placenta covers a significant portion of the cervix, cesarean section is advised. This is because, as the cervix dilates during labor, more and more hemorrhaging will occur as the cervix tears away from the placenta. The baby's as well as the mother's health could be seriously threatened if this occurs.

Abruptio Placentae

Also known as accidental hemorrhage, abruptio placentae results when the afterbirth starts to separate from the uterus before delivery. Abruptio placentae is another cause of antepartum hemorrhage, but bleeding is not always apparent because it can be trapped behind the fetus, when it is then called a concealed abruption.

Symptoms include vaginal bleeding, usually in the last trimester, preceded by constant uterine pain. In a concealed abruption, there is constant pain with tenderness in the uterus, but without vaginal bleeding. If the condition is severe, the uterus will remain hard and will contract without relaxing.

Diagnosis. Ultrasound examination is sometimes helpful if a clot has implanted behind the placenta. Frequently, evidence of interference in clotting factors will help confirm the diagnosis. The separating placenta is rich in thromboplastin, a substance that stimulates clotting throughout the body, using up the supply of clotting substances.

Cause. Half of the patients with abruptio placentae have associated hypertension or preeclampsia/eclampsia. In many patients, the cause is unknown.

Treatment. If the symptoms are mild and the fetus is very premature, the pregnancy should continue with careful monitoring of signs and symptoms. If the symptoms are mild and the fetus is mature and ready to be delivered, the doctor will induce labor (if the patient is not already in labor) by rupturing the membranes (bag of waters). The delivery then may proceed normally with careful monitoring. If the symptoms are severe, the baby should be delivered as promptly as possible by cesarean section. If the placenta has separated severely, this may be the only way of saving the baby, even if it is very premature.

Preeclampsia

This disease of the last trimester of pregnancy is manifested by increased blood pressure, proteinuria (increased proteins in the urine), and edema (swelling of tissue due to increased body fluids). Only pregnant women can get this disease.

Symptoms. Initially, this disease is often without noticeable symptoms. The increased blood pressure is usually not noticed by the patient because it causes no symptoms. Some ankle and leg swelling may be noticed, but this is common in normal pregnancies, especially in the hot summer months. Proteinuria causes no symptoms either.

As the disease progresses, blood pressure, swelling, and proteinuria may increase, and there may be sudden excess weight gain. Eventually, the patient will notice more signs of the problem. Hand and facial swelling may occur, accompanied by headache and visual disturbance. Pain just under the breastbone, and vomiting with severe headache and/or blurred vision often precede eclampsic convulsions.

Diagnosis. During regular prenatal checkups, a health professional will check for signs of preeclampsia. This is an easy disease to diagnose when your blood pressure and urine are checked regularly.

Treatment. When the symptoms are mild and the fetus is premature, the doctor may just observe the pregnant woman, sometimes in the hospital, and prescribe bed rest and sedation. The cure for the disease is the delivery of the baby. The symptoms may decrease with rest and sedation, but the disease continues as long as the fetus is present. The more severe the symptoms, the greater the urgency to deliver the baby, since both fetus and mother are at risk.

The fetus is at risk because the disease affects the blood vessels of the placenta, decreasing its nourishment and oxygen supply. Rarely, the placenta may abrupt or separate, as described previously. In addition, the mother is at increased risk of having a stroke or convulsions, as well as heart failure and abruptio placentae.

When the disease is mild, the pregnancy may be prolonged with careful monitoring until the fetus is mature enough to have a good chance of survival. Antihypertensive medication may be necessary to control severe increases in blood pressure, and magnesium sulfate usually is given to decrease the chance of convulsions.

Causes. The cause of preeclampsia is unknown. The disease is more common in the first pregnancy of young mothers, in patients who have preexisting hypertension, and in multiple pregnancies (twins or triplets) with rapid growth of the uterus. The disease has a 25 percent chance of recurring in subsequent pregnancies, although usually in milder form.

Molar Pregnancy

A molar pregnancy is a condition in which the placenta grows totally uncontrolled. Usually there is no fetus at all.

Symptoms. In a molar pregnancy, the normal symptoms of pregnancy often are exaggerated. There is more swelling, and more nausea and vomiting. In half of the patients, the uterus is larger than expected. There also may be signs of preeclampsia, including high blood pressure, edema, and proteinuria. Usually there is prolonged, intermittent slight vaginal bleeding.

Diagnosis. Molar pregnancy is best diagnosed by ultrasound examination. As the molar pregnancy advances, the examiner will not be able to feel fetal movements or hear a fetal heartbeat. (In very exceptional cases, a fetus *is* present.) Often a pelvic examination will show the ovaries to be very large and cystic (filled with fluid).

The pregnancy test is strongly positive, since the HCG reaches very high levels.

Treatment. As soon as the diagnosis is made, emptying the uterus is advised because of the continued rapid growth of the abnormal placenta. On rare occasions, the growth becomes malignant (cancerous). Chemotherapy with powerful anti-cancer drugs may be advised if the growth is larger than a five-month pregnancy, if the HCG hormone level is extremely high, or if the growth is cancerous.

Ordinarily, evacuation of the uterus by drugs to stimulate contractions and/or by suction or D&C will cure the condition. Still, the patient must be monitored carefully for continued disease with repeated pregnancy tests (radioimmunoassay for HCG). After the tests have been negative for six months, the patient may attempt to conceive again.

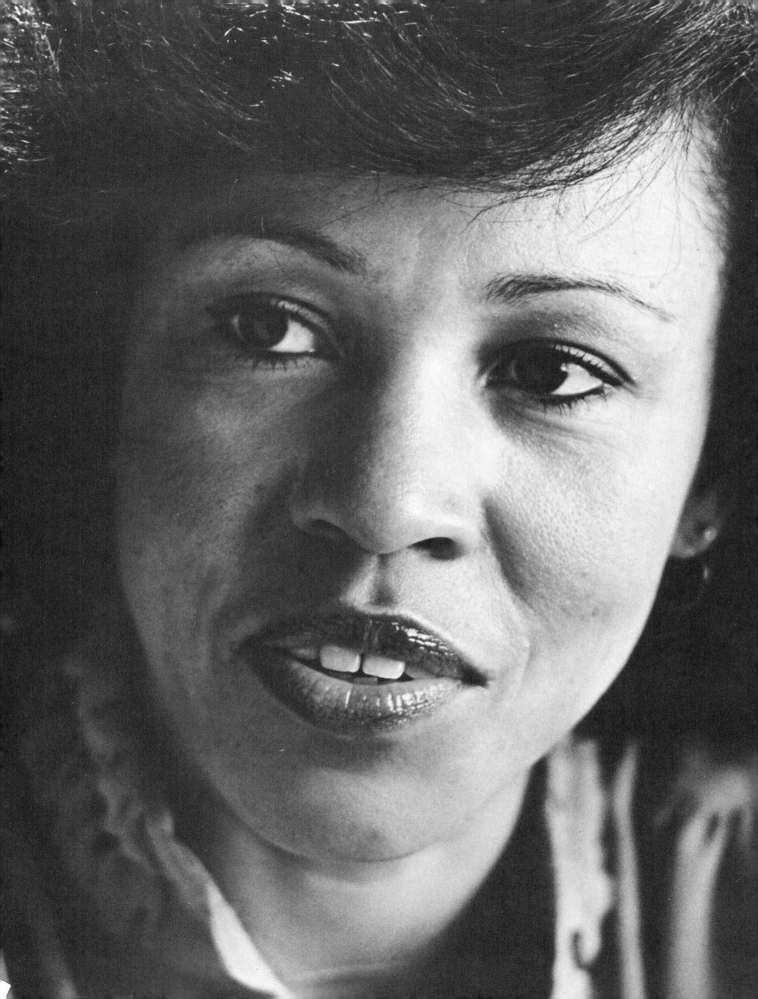

CHAPTER 14

LABOR AND DELIVERY

MADELEINE H. SHEARER, R.P.T.

Labor—aptly named—requires hard work of a woman as at last she delivers her baby into the world. Perhaps at no other time in her life does a woman experience such total involvement. All else fades away as her mind and body focus on the task at hand in what can be the supreme hours of a woman's life.

Preparation for the birth of a baby includes preparation for the labor to come. Women who know what to expect are less likely to approach labor with fear and apprehension. Knowledge also helps you achieve the kind of birth experience you desire for yourself and your baby.

Labor and Delivery

Giving birth is a supreme moment in a woman's life. It is the culmination of hopes and efforts that reach back into childhood, and its outcome affects each woman until the day she dies. In every culture throughout the ages, birth has assumed such importance that we have surrounded it with meticulous rituals and intense care in an effort to assure the birth of a perfect baby.

Usually the rituals and care lavished on an expectant mother express the values of the culture in which she lives. In our present culture, we value any technological and scientific efforts that can assure a normal pregnancy in which both mother and baby survive without harm. Indeed, women today may take it for granted that medical science will enable them and their babies to survive, especially if they enter pregnancy well-nourished and healthy. Now parents expect more than survival. They want the kind of obstetrical care that will enable them to labor and deliver under optimal circumstances—to give birth to a perfect *baby.*

Many of these parents become disappointed when they realize that their aspirations of a "perfect" delivery and child are not always shared by the hospital or

facility in which the mother will give birth. Technologically oriented medicine often simply seeks the quickest and easiest delivery that enables the mother and child to survive without apparent harm. Sometimes the medical procedures used to attain this goal are avoidable and unnecessary. And while no apparent harm results from them at the time of the delivery, we now know that their ill effects can be very subtle, and may be inapparent for years.

Many drugs or procedures are used without real medical need, but simply because they are fashionable, they're profitable for a hospital to administer, or they're part of a convenient hospital routine. Today's parents, having grown up during an era of painful realization that the benefits of science often come with heavy costs, are less willing to leave the responsibility for important health decisions to others. Instead, many now take the trouble to learn about the various kinds of obstetrical care that are available to them—including care outside of hospitals. And instead of merely accepting them without question, they're weighing the risks and benefits of the suggested medical procedures.

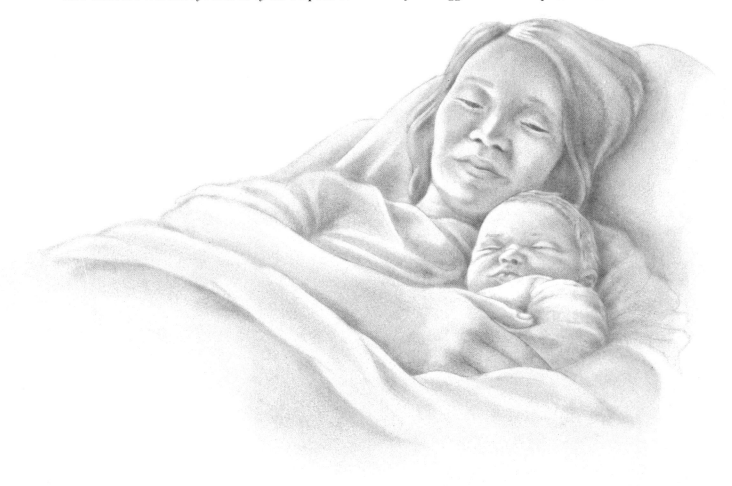

In their search for information, parents may use their physician as one source of expert counsel, but they also should look to community educational services for expectant and new parents, and government and medical publications. Advice frequently conflicts, and often parents must simply decide what they feel is right for them as individuals and as a family. How do they want to have their baby? What kind of care is available in their community? How does the family feel about planning for birth? Are there special factors in this pregnancy that affect planning for care?

Choices for Obstetric Care

Hospital obstetric care. One result of the increasing concern of well-informed expectant parents has been a growth in different types of obstetrical care that are now available. Ten years ago, 98 percent of all American babies were born in hospitals. Today, many small hospitals have closed their maternity units because they were unable to provide the kind of highly technological care that generates income for the maternity service. A hospital that retains its maternity service either does so because it is the only hospital within a large rural area, or if it is an urban hospital, because the maternity service has been able to support itself through a large volume of patients, possibly by offering many different diagnostic and treatment services to childbearing women.

There are now basically two levels of obstetric care as a result of this consolidation. Small rural and suburban hospitals that provide labor and delivery services comprise 80 percent of the hospital maternity units in this country. They have fewer than 500 deliveries per year, and are called Level I hospitals. Most of these hospitals have family practice physicians and general practitioners working in the maternity areas.

In urban areas, however, most of the hospitals have over 1,000 deliveries per year, and many have over 2,000. Although only 20 percent of our maternity units fall into this category of Level II and Level III units, these large services are where over 75 percent of all women deliver their babies. They are staffed almost entirely by obstetricians, and many of the staff have even more specialized training in perinatal medicine. Usually these hospitals have a neonatal (newborn) intensive-care nursery, which is staffed by pediatricians and specialists in the newborn called neonatologists. The Level III hospital offers intensive care for both mothers and newborns, and usually trains young doctors in medical specialties.

This increased volume of maternity patients at Level II and Level III hospitals, brought about by the closing of small urban maternity services, has been accompanied by many technological innovations in obstetrics. During the last decade, literally a hundred new diagnostic procedures have come into use. Among the most widely publicized are prenatal diagnostic tests for inherited diseases of the fetus and congenital malformations, ultrasound scanning of the fetus and placenta, tests of placental function and fetal growth and maturity, tests of fetal reaction to sound and to contractions, and internal and external fetal monitoring of heart rate and contractions. Many of these new procedures require new specialists—ultrasonographers, fetologists, and fetal monitoring specialists. Some tests require an entire section of the hospital for apparatus, such as ultrasound scanning devices, amniocentesis equipment (for drawing and testing amniotic fluid), and fetal stress testing devices.

The response to this remarkable revolution in obstetric practice has been mixed. For the high-risk woman—a very young woman, an older woman, a woman who expects twins, or a woman with premature labor, diabetes, toxemia, or hypertension—chances for the delivery of a healthy baby have greatly improved. Only a decade ago, an infant weighing less than two pounds had only a 50 percent chance of survival, and many of the survivors were mentally retarded or had a serious neurological deficit. Now most of these infants survive, and, in the two-pound weight range, the incidence of long-term handicap is down to only about 10 percent.

For normal childbirth, however, these large hospital maternity services have been less successful, both in providing safer childbirth, and in achieving parents' satisfaction with care. The large volume of patients that must be coordinated and timed to go from labor to delivery and recovery rooms in an orderly fashion virtually requires the hospital to set up routines that save the nursing and medical staff time. On busy days, one woman's labor must be speeded up with hormones, while perhaps another woman's labor must be slowed down with analgesics or regional anesthesia. With several labor rooms busy at one time, and with a shortage of experienced registered nurses, the monitoring of the condition of the mother and fetus must be left to machines. Routines must be followed in order for the department to run well, but this may mean that the individual needs of childbearing families are disregarded.

Where Will You Deliver Your Baby?

You have a choice of where you'll have your baby delivered. Ten years ago, 98 percent of all American babies were born in standard delivery rooms in hospitals. Now there are alternatives to hospital care available to almost any family. Home deliveries are conducted by nurse-midwives, family practitioners, or trained community midwives; the midwife, physician, or assistant comes to the house, bringing all the supplies and medications needed for a normal birth, and any emergency equipment as well. A birth-center birth is conducted like a home delivery, in casual surroundings and with plenty of room and welcome for husband and others. Usually the birth center is in a hospital.

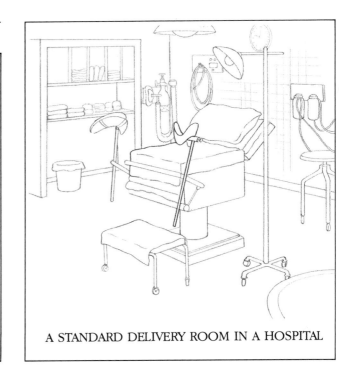

A STANDARD DELIVERY ROOM IN A HOSPITAL

Moreover, for economic reasons, tests and procedures that originally were developed for special pathologic conditions now are used more widely, and have become common among normal women who do not really need them. The hospital's heavy investments in specialty staff and equipment mean that these must be used regularly in order to justify their purchase, and to generate revenue. An example was the purchase of a $100,000 ultrasound scanning device by a suburban Level II hospital in 1975. One of the hospital's radiologists was placed in charge. This radiologist gave noon lectures to obstetricians on the hospital's staff, put an article in the local newspaper, and held two public lectures. Within 17 months, 48 percent of all women delivering at this hospital had been sent by their obstetricians for at least one ultrasound scan. A graph of the increasing utilization of the service was even maintained in the radiology department.

In 1978, some medical publications reported that measurable effects of diagnostic ultrasound scanning on infants could be detected for up to one year of age. These included abnormal neck and grasp reflexes and more serious illnesses in the first year, compared to infants who were not irradiated with ultrasound as fetuses. Also in 1978, the Food and Drug Administration (FDA) held hearings on the effects of diagnostic ultrasound scanning and discovered that in some cases, machinery manufacturers were not disclosing to their hospital customers the energy levels produced by their machines, and that some of the devices sold as having energy levels of 20 milliwatts per square centimeter actually had four times that level. Machines also were found to deteriorate with age so that after three years, they emitted different energy levels than when they were first installed.

Although the outcomes of high-risk pregnancies have been improved by the use of ultrasound scanning and other procedures, normal pregnancy outcomes have not shown improvement. In some instances, as with electronic fetal monitoring, neonatal mortality (from accidents and infections) actually shows a slight increase among low-risk (normal) women. Moreover, in part due to monitoring, the cesarean rate has risen from about 8 to 10 percent to 20 to 30 percent in many hospitals, but without any improvement in infant outcome that could be linked to the cesarean. In one study of 4,000 consecutive cesareans, researchers found that nearly half of the patients experienced one or more complications, some severe enough to jeopardize further childbearing or to be potentially lethal.

Out-of-hospital birth services. A fast-growing alternative to hospital care is home birth, conducted by certified nurse-midwives, family practitioners, and empirically trained community midwives. Home birth services have remained popular in many rural areas, even after women started using hospitals for birth. This is partly because hospitals are located too far from some rural communities, but also because of the excellence of several well-known nurse-midwifery services. The Frontier Nursing Service in Kentucky, the Catholic Nursing Service in Santa Fe, New Mexico, and the Maternity Center Association in New York City still provide maternity services today.

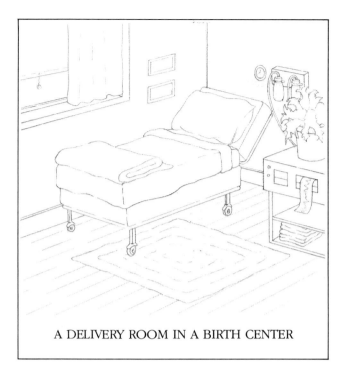

A DELIVERY ROOM IN A BIRTH CENTER

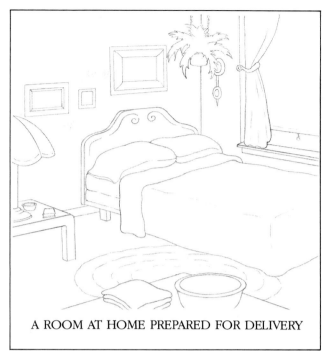

A ROOM AT HOME PREPARED FOR DELIVERY

Midwifery and general practice services like these are reviving to fill the void left by the closure and consolidation of hospital obstetric units. Many states still have great areas that have no obstetric service at all. Massachusetts lost one-half of its maternity services between 1965 and 1975, while California lost one-fourth of its services. Many counties in rural California have no obstetricians and few general practitioners; some are snowbound in the winter, and have impassable roads even in the summer. In urban areas, maternity units can be even harder to reach, especially on public transportation and at odd hours. Many women who expect a normal pregnancy are unwilling or unable to travel long distances for maternity care that is designed for high-risk women, is crowded, unduly expensive, and which they know or suspect carries risks that are unwarranted in a normal pregnancy.

Most large cities now have some kind of home birth service. Usually, these services are operated by groups of nurse-midwives or family physicians who also will tend to patients who need hospitalization at any point during childbirth. Some of these services are designed around a birth center, a place where parents come for prenatal care and delivery, and then leave four to 24 hours later, depending on need. In most home births and birth-center deliveries, the physicians see the mother once or twice during pregnancy, and the nurse-midwife provides all remaining care. Emphasis is placed on education during pregnancy so that the mother can take optimum care of herself and her new baby, and on careful screening for risk. If any suspected deviation from normal occurs, further tests are done as needed in the hospital. If the tests are confirmed, the mother is delivered at a hospital.

During the labor and delivery, a physician and midwife or assistant come to the house, bring all the supplies and medications needed for a normal birth, and any emergency equipment as well. Usually little or no pain medication is required. If problems arise during labor or afterward, the mother is taken to a hospital. A birth-center birth is conducted much like a home delivery, in casual surroundings and with the same general outlook on birth as a normal process. Medical personnel are in constant attendance during labor, and are watchful for any deviation that requires transfer to a hospital. The mother is discharged from a birth center in four to 24 hours, after which the midwife makes a series of home visits for the next several days.

The safety of out-of-hospital birth has been challenged by obstetrical societies and hospital associations, both nationally and in various states. Recently a press release was made by the American College of Obstetricians and Gynecologists stating that out-of-hospital birth carried a two to five times greater chance of mortality for the baby. The statistics were based, however, on mortality figures from 11 states, which later admitted that accidental home births had been included. Miscarriages, precipitous births, accidental taxi cab births, and very premature births had formed the basis for the claim. In contrast, carefully conducted studies by medical schools and health departments have compared planned home births by midwifery services with hospital births, and without exception have supported the safety of midwifery services for home births.

Nurse-Midwifery Services in the United States

A certified nurse-midwife is a nurse who has had special training in maternal-newborn care and normal obstetrics. She is trained to recognize, foster, and support the normal process of pregnancy and birth, including giving prenatal care, delivering babies, and giving gynecological and contraceptive services, with hospital and physician referral, if necessary.

The following is a partial list of nurse-midwifery schools and services in the United States. For information on a service near you, contact the American College of Nurse-Midwives, 1012 Fourteenth Street, N.W., Suite 801, Washington, D.C. 20005, or call (202) 347-5445.

Cincinnati General Hospital
Cincinnati, Ohio 45229

Columbia-Presbyterian Medical Center
Sloane Hospital for Women
168th Street and Broadway
New York, New York 10032

Georgetown University School of Nursing
Nurse-Midwifery Program
Washington, D.C. 20007

Grady Memorial Hospital
80 Butler Street, S.W.
Atlanta, Georgia 30303

Johns Hopkins Hospital
Department of Obstetrics and Gynecology
600 North Broadway
Baltimore, Maryland 21205

Los Angeles County—University of Southern California Medical Center
Women's Hospital
Los Angeles, California 90033

Maternity Center Association
48 East 92nd Street
New York, New York 10028

Medical University of South Carolina
College of Medicine
80 Barre Street
Charleston, South Carolina 29401

New Jersey Medical School
Martland Hospital
Department of Obstetrics and Gynecology
Division of Midwifery
65 Bergen Street
Newark, New Jersey 07101

San Francisco General Hospital
University of California at San Francisco
Potrero Street
San Francisco, California 94110

The University of Illinois at the Medical Center
College of Nursing, Department of Maternal-Child Nursing
Nurse-Midwifery Program
P.O. Box 6998
Chicago, Illinois 60680

University Hospital
655 West 8th Street
Jacksonville, Florida 32209

University of Arizona
College of Medicine
Tucson, Arizona 85724

University of Kentucky
College of Medicine
Albert B. Chandler Medical Center
800 Rose Street
Lexington, Kentucky 40506

University of Pennsylvania
School of Medicine
36th and Hamilton Walk
Philadelphia, Pennsylvania 19174

University of Rochester Medical Center
Rochester, New York 14627

Yale-New Haven Hospital
789 Howard Avenue
New Haven, Connecticut 06510

Hospital birth centers. Starting in 1975, hospital maternity departments began to respond to the loss of families who preferred out-of-hospital births by setting up birth centers. These are usually one or two rooms, located in the maternity area and furnished in a homelike manner, where parents come to labor and deliver and leave in four to 12 hours. A nurse is assigned to give constant supervision, but performs no hospital routines, such as machine monitoring, medications, intravenous solutions, or episiotomy (an incision in the skin below the vagina to widen the birth canal). By 1979, 61 out of 322 California hospitals had some kind of arrangement like this for carefully selected normal women giving birth.

Not all hospitals set aside a special room, however. Some merely allow women to forgo the usual routine procedures and medications, and to deliver in the labor room. These hospitals are usually the large teaching institutions (medical schools or affiliated hospitals where obstetric residents are trained), although other hospitals, which have limited space for a birth center, also convert labor rooms to this use. Generally, using a labor room in this way results in a birth more like a hospital birth. Women are in a labor bed, and nursing may not be constant throughout. Obstetrical residents and medical students still provide care, as in other births. Women usually remain in the maternity section of the hospital for two to three days afterward.

A few very large teaching hospitals also have begun to offer a nurse-midwifery service, although some hospitals only allow nurse-midwives to care for the clinic patients. Kings County Hospital in New York City, San Francisco General Hospital, Cook County Hospital in Chicago, the University of South Carolina Hospital, and Los Angeles County Hospital are a few institutions with nurse-midwifery services.

The success of hospital birth centers is in debate. To be selected to use a birth center, women must satisfy a list of criteria provided by the hospital, as well as the criteria of their own doctors. Only about one-third of pregnant women are able to qualify. Some are eliminated easily; they have premature labor, are diabetic, hypertensive, toxemic, expect twins, or have some other definite problem. Other women are eliminated because they are over 34 or under 18, are too fat or too short, or are just too fearful. Of those who do start labor in a hospital birth room, 25 to 30 percent "risk out"—that is, they are transferred to the regular obstetrics area for treatment of some complication of labor. In most of these cases, labor was too slow and uterine stimulating hormone was given. Because of the risks of uterine stimulation, the women are usually machine-monitored after transfer to the regular labor room.

Some hospital birth centers report that birth-center births result in one-quarter the number of cesarean sections as do births in the regular labor/delivery area. But other birth centers report similar cesarean rates for normal women regardless of where in the hospital they deliver their babies.

Why is there so much difference in outcomes among normal women in hospital birth centers? The answer lies in the fact that, unless the obstetrician is very dedicated to normal childbirth and has sought additional training, the doctors who are pressed into using a birth room are providing care that they were not trained to provide, that most are not comfortable with, and that some actually disapprove of. When labor slows, these doctors may not have the patience or the confidence to try measures such as getting the woman up to walk around the room or to take a bath to stimulate the uterus. If such is the case, the proximity to the hospital obstetrics department makes a technological treatment seem most appropriate to them.

Education for childbirth. Whether parents choose to deliver in a hospital, a home or birth center, or a hospital birth room will depend on many factors, including the parents' own estimate of their medical needs, how comfortable they are with each environment, and the relative costs. However, both the choice of care and the quality of the experience of birth will depend on the parents educating themselves— both before and during pregnancy.

Finding out what type of care is available in the community is the first step, although it may be the most difficult. An active, community-based childbirth education association is one source of information on a variety of maternity services. These groups may be listed in your telephone directory. The person who takes your call should ask what your preferences are for care before giving you names of various types of services. Communities with college campuses often have a student health center or women's health center where referrals will be made. Some of these maintain a file with the names of doctors or clinics, and women's comments about their care. Hospitals often have childbirth education classes, and the teachers are usually nurses or physical therapists. These teachers may be oriented exclusively to the hospital's services and those of local physicians, but most also know what else is available in the area. Finally, you should write to the International Childbirth Education Association, the National Association of Parents and Professionals for Safe Alternatives in Childbirth, the American College of Nurse-Midwives, and the American Society for Psychoprophylaxis in Obstetrics for lists of their members who provide services in your community. Addresses are listed on page 309.

Once you've chosen where you will deliver and who will attend you, the next step is to read in detail about labor and delivery in that particular setting. The number of books published on various types of childbirth care is staggering. For a full catalog of such books, write to the International Childbirth Education Association Book Center, or to the Association for Childbirth at Home Book Store.

Childbirth education classes are extremely encouraging and helpful, *provided they are oriented toward the type of childbirth chosen by the parents.* Frequently, the midwifery service or birth center will conduct its own childbirth education classes. Hospitals usually have their own classes as well. In each case, the philosophy of care, the instructions for calling the doctor or midwife, and the procedures and preferences of the attendants will be described. You will usually be taught ways to relax and control breathing through the contractions of labor, as well as techniques for pushing during delivery of the baby. These classes are good places to meet other parents, who often strike up social relationships and later trade baby-sitting services or start play groups together.

There are two situations in which childbirth education may actually serve parents better if it is *not* oriented toward the type of childbirth the parents have arranged. The first is cesarean childbirth classes. Parents who anticipate a cesarean section may want information on how to effectively *change* the care they receive, rather than what to expect. They may already know too well what to expect. In this case, a consumer-oriented class is needed. These classes are increasingly available now, and a list of such groups may be obtained by writing to C/SEC in Boston.

Another situation in which a consumer-oriented class is best is whenever parents feel forced to accept maternity care that they really do not want. If only hospital care is available when home or birth-center birth is desired, or if very high-technology care is needed for the diabetic or hypertensive mother, parents should seek a class series that presents alternatives to the usual procedures. Quite often, however, parents must be willing to "go in fighting," and this is an uncomfortable way to have a baby.

Parents also need information on breast-feeding and parenting. The La Leche League is a widely known national organization that disseminates information on all aspects of breast-feeding. It has chapters and members in most cities. Classes on breast-feeding begin during pregnancy and continue afterward, and are fine places to meet other mothers and emerge from the loneliness and isolation that many new mothers feel after delivering their babies.

Childbirth education classes provide daytime or evening sessions consisting of two to three hours of discussion and practice during the last two months of pregnancy. Usually, parents can continue on a drop-in basis until they go into labor.

Childbirth education for the older sibling. Many out-of-hospital educational services, as well as some hospital birth-center services, will prepare the parents' older children to participate in childbirth. Children two years and under are led through picture stories and doll enactments of birth, and they find out what to expect when their mommy and daddy have a baby. If the birth is to be at home or in a birth center, the child may be allowed to stay with the parents, and perhaps wakened for the birth. Parents feel that the older child then undergoes the same attachment process with the new baby as the parents themselves, and may be less jealous of the baby. Even if the young child is not wakened for the birth, just being at home with the parents is of benefit.

Older children often get quite involved with the process of labor, and want to bring the mother a cup of tea, or help hold the baby after the birth. A program at Mt. Zion Hospital in San Francisco offers individual sessions with children who will be on hand for deliveries in its birth center.

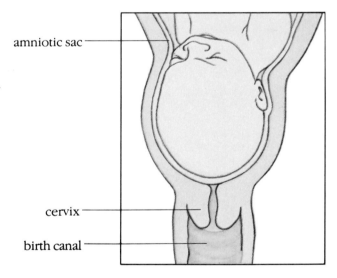

EFFACEMENT AND DILATION

About a month before labor begins, the cervix begins to thin and shorten. This is called effacement of the cervix. Before labor begins, the cervix maintains its original size and shape.

Labor Approaches

Effacement. In a certain sense, labor begins during the month before the actual birth of a baby. In both first and subsequent pregnancies, painless but noticeable contractions of the uterus become more frequent. These are called Braxton-Hicks contractions. They perform the first work of labor by slowly thinning and shortening the cervix, or neck of the uterus, through which the baby must pass before it can be pushed through the vagina and delivered. This thinning and shortening of the cervix is called effacement.

Engagement. In the primipara (the woman having a first baby), effacement of the cervix is often accompanied by "lightening" of the baby. The baby's head, or buttock if it is in a breech position, settles down into the softened, thinned neck of the uterus, making more room for the mother to breathe and to comfortably digest her meals. Some women feel surprisingly less pregnant right before labor begins as a result of this lightening, which is known as engagement into the pelvis of the fetal head, or whatever part of the fetus is presenting (lying against the cervix).

The time of engagement is quite variable. However, most women having first babies note some degree of lightening during the final two weeks of pregnancy. Others may complete effacement and engagement only in early labor. In later pregnancies, the mother, who is now a multipara, usually has a uterus that is softer and thinner due to previous pregnancies, and the lower portion of the uterus accommodates the fetus with no sudden change. In fact, some multiparas actually spend the last weeks of pregnancy with a cervix that is effaced and the fetal head fully engaged.

With engagement of the baby, the lowest part (presenting part) of the baby enters the pelvis, as can be seen on page 270. This descent of the baby is measured in terms of station. The station of the baby is said to be so many centimeters above or below the lowest part of the pubic arch, which is labeled zero in the drawing. When fully engaged, the baby is said to be "at zero station." During labor, the baby descends through plus-1 to plus-5 stations, at which point the head is visible at the vaginal opening.

Bladder pressure. One result of effacement of the cervix and engagement of the fetus in the pelvis is obvious from the drawing on page 270. The baby literally compresses the bladder. Probably the most common complaint of women at the end of pregnancy is that they have to urinate very frequently, both in the daytime and at night.

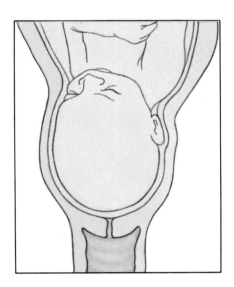

Early effacement begins to occur a month before labor. Women having their first baby will experience a feeling of "lightening" as the baby's head moves into the cervix and away from the diaphragm and stomach.

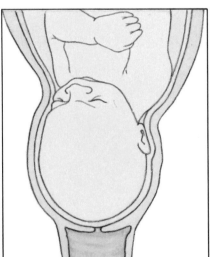

Just before labor begins, the fetal head moves further into the pelvis and the presenting part of the fetus (which is usually the head) is said to be engaged.

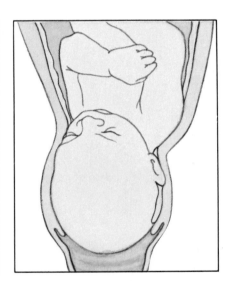

Rupture of the amniotic sac and complete dilation of the cervix occur at the onset of labor.

Aches, discharge, and elation. Some women feel shooting pains or aching in the groin, pelvic floor, or the inside of the thighs in the last weeks of pregnancy as a result of the engaged fetus pressing on sensitive nerves and tissues in the pelvis.

Another result of effacement of the cervix is that the mucus plug, which has protected the uterine interior throughout the months of pregnancy, is gradually loosened. Coupled with this change is an ever-increasing vaginal discharge of clear, thin mucus, which serves the purpose of constantly washing and cleansing the tissues of the vagina.

Some women actually lose a few pounds in the last days of pregnancy. This, along with the lighter feeling of the abdomen and elation at being near term, causes most women to feel a special vigor and enthusiasm for housecleaning or preparing food for the family and space for the new baby. This burst of energy is sometimes called "nesting."

The Onset of Labor

Breaking the bag of water or membranes. In only about 6 percent of women does labor start with a gush, or more commonly, a leak of clear amniotic fluid from the uterus. Although most pregnant women worry about the possibility of their bag of water (membranes) breaking in public places, they should be reassured that only a very small amount of amniotic fluid escapes at this time—the one to three ounces of fluid trapped between the baby's engaged head and the cervix, which is usually thin and about to dilate. After this initial leak or gush of fluid, a trickle may be felt with contractions once in awhile throughout labor. Since the

membranes continue to produce fluid during labor, a "dry labor" is impossible. However, labor may be up to one hour shorter, and contractions may be somewhat stronger after the membranes rupture.

Parents should expect contractions of labor within 12 hours of the breaking of the bag of water. Usually, they have been told to call the doctor, midwife, or clinic when they first notice escaping fluid, and they are often told to come to the hospital or call for the birth attendant within three to six hours, regardless of whether contractions have started. Only rarely are contractions delayed more than 12 hours after rupture of the membranes. In a home birth, the woman may be allowed to wait well beyond that time, and to try to start labor by moving about, bathing, and being active. In a hospital birth, after 12 hours, contractions will be stimulated by a uterine-stimulating hormone, either oxytocin (Pitocin) or prostaglandin.

Until very recently, many obstetricians actually broke the bag of water artificially when they first examined the cervix of the woman in labor. This practice was defended since labor is faster and contractions are more effective after the membranes are ruptured. Also, if any meconium (fetal bowel movement) is seen in the fluid, this indicates that the fetus has been distressed (lacking oxygen) and greater caution and surveillance of the labor is begun.

Today, more obstetricians are aware of new research that has shown the value of intact membranes in protecting the fetal head during contractions, and the value of the bag of water itself in wedging open the cervix as each contraction makes the membranes bulge through the cervix into the birth canal. Although artificial rupture of the membranes does speed up

---

MEASURING THE STATION OF THE BABY IN LABOR

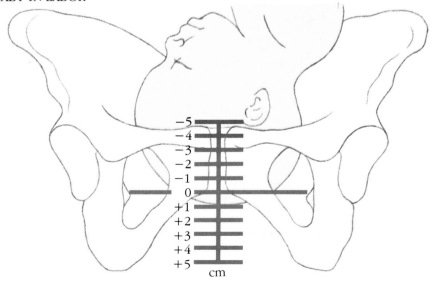

This diagram of the pelvis and the measurement of descent of the infant's head during passage through the birth canal is done during a pelvic examination. The "station" of the baby is the measure of how far the head is above or below the lowest part of the pubic arch (which is called the zero station). *The numbers represent centimeters. When fully engaged, the baby is said to be "at zero station." During labor, the baby descends from plus-one station to plus-five station, at which point the head is visible at the vaginal opening (extension).*

contractions and make them harder, current medical thinking is that such hard contractions and faster labor may unnecessarily stress a fetus, especially if it is already at some risk due to poor intrauterine growth or disease in the mother. Such hard contractions also create more pain for the mother, sometimes requiring pain medication. Speeding up labor can be accomplished more safely and effectively by getting the mother up to walk and sit during labor. In addition, doctors can usually see meconium in the fluid without breaking the bag of water (amniotomy) by using a lighted amnioscope, an instrument that illuminates the transparent membranes. Any dark matter or cloudiness in the fluid that is observed as the membranes bulge through the cervix may indicate meconium.

When can parents expect the membranes to rupture if they are intact at the outset of labor? In about 60 percent of such pregnancies, the membranes ruptured spontaneously at the end of the first stage of labor, when dilation of the cervix was almost complete. About 25 percent ruptured during the pushing or expulsive stage of labor, and 10 percent ruptured during the delivery. Infants whose membranes were intact until late in labor had less molding of the head, higher scores for physical condition at birth (Apgar scores), and a higher acid-base balance of the blood. This means that the blood had been well oxygenated in the babies whose membranes were intact during labor.

Bloody show. Some women notice a bloody-tinged discharge, spotting, or a clot of mucus within 24 hours before the onset of contractions of labor. This blood is due to the thinning of the cervix with effacement, causing the plug to gradually loosen and breaking the small capillaries that serve it. Many women notice no particular change in the discharge or its color prior to the onset of labor.

Changes in contractions. By far, the most common sign of the start of labor is the occurrence of uterine contractions that are distinctive from the Braxton-Hicks contractions that marked the end of pregnancy. What makes these labor contractions different is that they get longer, stronger, and closer together, whereas the warming-up contractions of late pregnancy do not. Labor contractions may never be as regular as clock-work, however.

The contractions of labor may begin as far apart as 30 minutes or as close together as five minutes—but if it is real labor, these contractions will get closer together over the next few hours, as shown by timing the interval between the contractions. The first labor contractions may last only 20 to 30 seconds, but as the next few hours pass, these contractions will last longer and longer, until they are an average of 60 seconds long. Finally, real labor contractions get stronger over a period of hours until they cannot be ignored any longer. The mother is unable to walk or talk through these contractions, but must sit or lie down to cope with their intensity.

If the mother has been to childbirth education classes, she will know how to let all her voluntary muscles relax, including her facial muscles, shoulders, arms, hands, thighs, legs, and feet. The prepared woman may make a mental checklist of each of these sets of muscles, relaxing them in succession while the contraction gathers force, reaches a peak, and then slowly wanes. Afterward, the mother will resume her activities as usual, but she will be alert for the beginning of the next contraction.

Some women feel the first contractions of labor as stomach cramps or a backache that rhythmically comes and goes. Soon, if this is really labor, these sensations feel more like contractions. About 20 percent of women do have backache during middle and late labor, but this backache can be distinguished from uterine contractions, even though it comes at the same time.

False labor. Some women have contractions that mimic real labor by seeming to get longer, stronger, and closer together. However, if these are "false labor" contractions, they will stop if the mother changes her activity—gets up and cooks a meal or takes a bath or a nap. Real labor is likely to be stimulated by activity, while "false labor" will fade.

The First Stage of Labor

The average first labor takes 12 to 14 hours, while subsequent labors take somewhat less—about six to eight hours. However, these averages conceal real differences that are much more meaningful to women who are about to give birth. Many first labors are only four to six hours long, and some second and third labors are longer than first ones. In contrast, some first labors last beyond 24 hours, and if allowed to continue without intervention, might last 36 hours or even longer. Most home and hospital childbirth services will expect the labor to be well advanced after 16 to 20 hours, and if delivery is not imminent by 24 hours, the mother will be considered for operative assistance, either forceps delivery (if the baby is in the birth canal) or most often, cesarean delivery. This is because very long labors are associated with poor outcomes in the newborn infant.

If we look at an average first labor of 14 hours and divide it into the usual three stages, we see that the first 12 or 13 hours will be spent in Stage I—having contractions that dilate the cervix. Stage II, during which the mother may help contractions by pushing the baby through the birth canal, will take from one-half to two hours, and culminates with the birth of the baby. Stage III usually takes only 15 minutes to one-half hour, and involves only one or two contractions to expel the placenta. The typical second labor of six to eight hours is spent with five to seven hours in the dilation stage, also called Stage I, and usually less than an hour in Stage II, during which the baby is born. Stage III is also shorter, usually less than 15 minutes. These time differences are graphed at right. Since nearly all of labor is spent dealing with the contractions of Stage I labor, it is helpful to look at this period in greater detail, examining how contractions feel, what will happen, and the process of birth itself.

The latent phase of Stage I labor. The first stage of labor can be subdivided into three segments, each of which has its own peculiar character. The first phase lasts from the onset of contractions to three centimeters' dilation, and is known as the latent phase of labor. Contractions may or may not be noticeable. They come every three to five minutes, and last 30 to 45 seconds. At the end of this phase of labor, contractions are usually three minutes apart and a minute long—the signal for going to the hospital or the arrival of the doctor or midwife in a home birth. Usually at this point, the mother enters the second phase of Stage I labor, called the active phase of labor. Her cervix is usually two to three centimeters dilated, and medical surveillance of the labor begins.

The latent phase is the most variable of all three phases of Stage I labor. Some women notice contractions for days before they are a minute long and three minutes apart, while other women actually start off labor with contractions this intense.

It helps to keep busy during the day with light activities, and to get a good rest if it is nighttime. A common mistake is to go to bed in early labor in the daytime. This will just slow the labor and each contraction will seem much more noticeable. A nap is fine, of course, and strenuous activity will only tire the mother needlessly. Another common mistake is to get up in the night and time contractions or try to keep busy. Valuable rest is then lost. When contractions really should be timed, they will wake the mother.

Early labor in a home birth. Women who have chosen a home birth are followed very carefully during prenatal visits by their doctor or midwife, who checks for signs that the pregnancy is proceeding normally, without any hint of problems with fetal growth or position, or with the mother's health. During these prenatal visits, the doctor or midwife gives the mother a list of materials to purchase or have on hand during labor, and they agree on when to call for the birth attendant. Most home-birth services request that attendants be telephoned as soon as the woman suspects she is in labor. At that time, decisions are made as to when the doctor or midwife will come to the house. Once these attendants come, they usually plan to stay for the remainder of the labor and delivery. Some doctors send their labor nurse early in labor so the nurse can alert the doctor when labor has become active.

Because more women want to be attended constantly during labor by their chosen medical attendants, and to have family and friends with them if they wish, the popularity of home birth has increased in the last decade. Women enjoy the freedom of being up and about during labor, pausing when they need to deal with contractions and going to bed only when they feel tired. A medication-free birth is usually planned. Some home-birth services will give minor pain relief medication, but most will transfer the mother to a hospital for the administration of anything other than emergency medications. Home-birth services are fully equipped for most emergencies of childbirth, coming to the house with oxygen, blood for transfusions, infant resuscitation equipment, and other necessities.

Upon arrival at the house, the midwife or doctor will examine the mother, listen to the fetal heart sounds during and after contraction, take her blood pressure, pulse, and temperature, and feel the abdomen to sense the strength and quality of uterine action. The midwife may examine the cervix, checking for dilation and for the position and station of the baby. The birth attendant will help the laboring mother to relax and settle into concentration on breathing or whatever the mother finds to be most helpful during contractions. The attendant also gives low-back or abdominal massage and encouragement. When labor is progressing smoothly, the attendant may brew some tea or fix food for the family.

Time Differences Among Stages of Labor

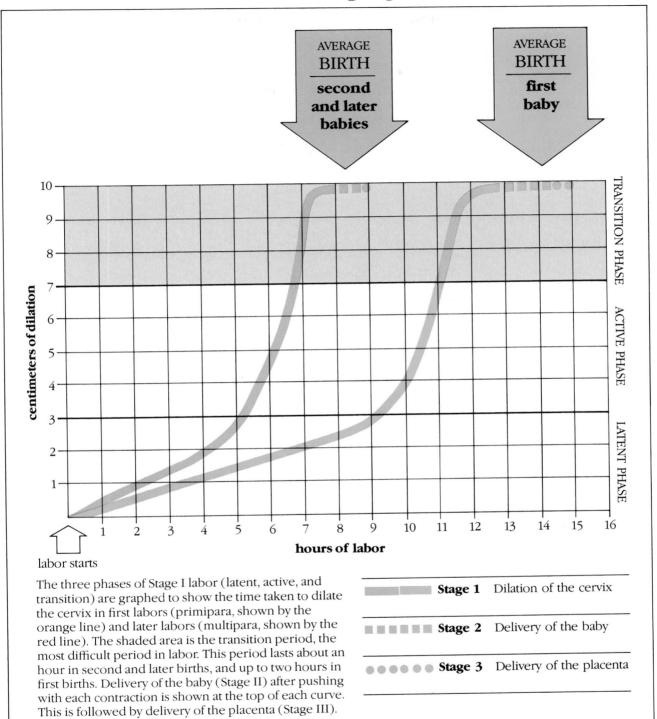

The three phases of Stage I labor (latent, active, and transition) are graphed to show the time taken to dilate the cervix in first labors (primipara, shown by the orange line) and later labors (multipara, shown by the red line). The shaded area is the transition period, the most difficult period in labor. This period lasts about an hour in second and later births, and up to two hours in first births. Delivery of the baby (Stage II) after pushing with each contraction is shown at the top of each curve. This is followed by delivery of the placenta (Stage III).

Stage 1 Dilation of the cervix

Stage 2 Delivery of the baby

Stage 3 Delivery of the placenta

The active phase of Stage I labor. For the doctor or midwife, the active phase begins at three centimeters' dilation of the cervix. For the mother having contractions, it begins when her contractions come every three minutes, last one minute, and are no longer possible to walk or talk through. Unfortunately, this is precisely when women planning a hospital birth will be going to the hospital and getting admitted and examined. It is not surprising that some labors actually stop when women get to the hospital. This may be due to the anxiety of traveling, coping with strangers, answering questions, and undergoing pelvic examinations and other hospital routines while active labor is also taking place. Parents should learn how to deal comfortably with contractions, as well as with admission to the hospital, in their prenatal classes.

The contractions of middle labor begin with a gradual tightening, hardening, and tilting forward of the uterus.

This feeling is familiar to the laboring woman by mid-labor, and she copes best by immediately sitting or lying down and concentrating to relax her voluntary muscles—all the way from her brow down to her feet. As the contraction gathers force, women who have practiced breathing patterns during prenatal classes will begin a slow, regular, quiet breathing in and out. This respiration may not be very noticeable to others, but should be the focus of the mother's utmost attention. Through the peak of the contraction, the mother breathes rhythmically, and she deliberately relaxes, paying attention to nothing else. As the contraction wanes, she slows down her breathing and stops with a relaxing sigh. A few moments later, she is ready to respond to questions from the medical staff, take a sip of ice water, or get up and go to the toilet. She knows that she has only two to three minutes before the next contraction, and is ready when it comes.

What You'll Need for a Home Birth

Good prenatal care

Good food and exercise

Childbirth education classes

Phone numbers of birth attendants

Emergency Childbirth by Gregory White, M.D.

Sterilized Items

- Eight to twelve large, substantial towels (for waters and mucus)
- Two to four washcloths
- Two feet of strong embroidery thread or white shoelace, in a separate envelope.
NOTE: Place these items in a sealed paper bag(s) on the middle rack of your oven, *with a pan of water underneath*. Bake at 250° for two hours. Watch closely!

Mother

- A quiet environment
- Two clean nightgowns—one for during labor and one for afterward
- Sanitary pads (extra large or hospital-size) and a belt
- Bendable straws
- Sweetened liquids, honey, dextrose, and/or sugar
- Ice chips (perhaps sweetened)
- Tea (your favorite, or raspberry leaf)
- Food—something easy to digest, for early labor
- Heating pad (soothes back labor somewhat)
- Cornstarch and a natural oil
NOTE: If you have a child under five years old, it's usually a good idea to provide for someone to care for her/him during your labor. This person should have no other responsibilities during your labor.

Baby

- Four to six receiving blankets
- Diapers and pins
- Newborn clothes
NOTE: You should wash the blankets, diapers, and clothes with a non-irritating soap or detergent.

Labor bed

- Two sets of clean sheets
- One plastic drop cloth that covers the entire bed
- Four to six large pillows for positioning and support
NOTE: Make the bed with one set of sheets, cover it with the plastic drop cloth, then make up the bed with the second set of sheets. You will labor on the second set of sheets. After the birth, these sheets and the drop cloth are removed and your bed is ready to rest in.

Other important items

- A three-ounce ear syringe with a soft rubber tip
- Two dozen sterile 4-inch cotton gauze squares
- One bottle of isopropyl alcohol
- An oral thermometer
- Liquid antiseptic soap
- Two large mixing-type bowls (one for the placenta, and one for washing up)
- One good lamp and/or flashlight
- A telephone
- A car that runs dependably and has a full gas tank—if you need to go to the hospital.

HOME BIRTH WITH PHYSICIAN OR MIDWIFE ATTENDING

LABOR BEGINS

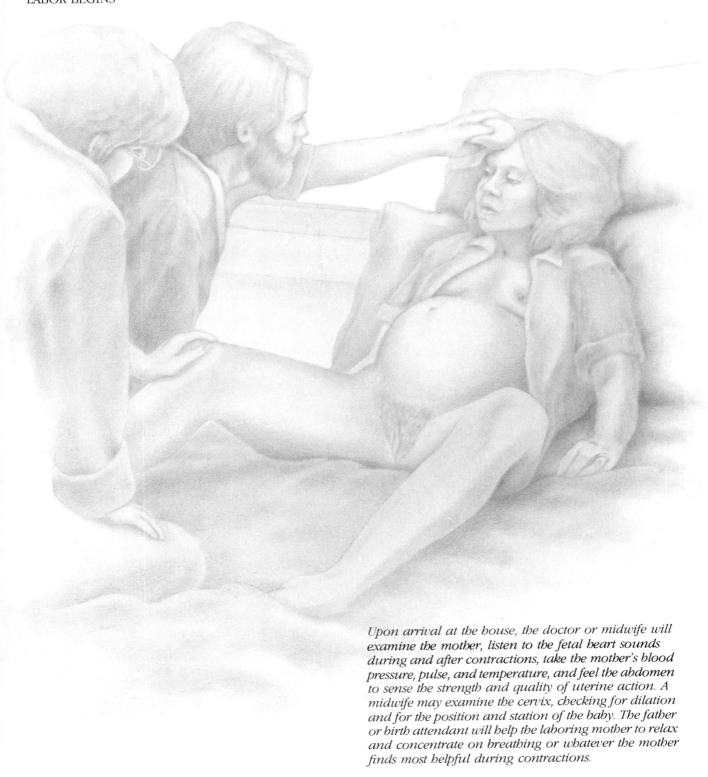

Upon arrival at the house, the doctor or midwife will examine the mother, listen to the fetal heart sounds during and after contractions, take the mother's blood pressure, pulse, and temperature, and feel the abdomen to sense the strength and quality of uterine action. A midwife may examine the cervix, checking for dilation and for the position and station of the baby. The father or birth attendant will help the laboring mother to relax and concentrate on breathing or whatever the mother finds most helpful during contractions.

THE STAGES OF LABOR AND DELIVERY

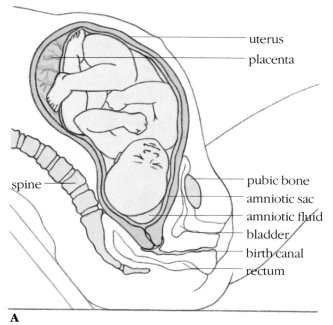

uterus

placenta

spine

pubic bone

amniotic sac

amniotic fluid

bladder

birth canal

rectum

A

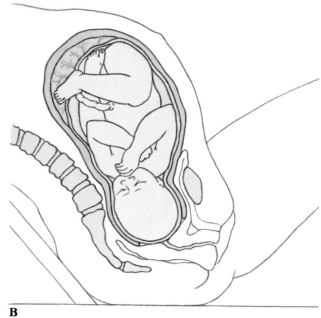

B

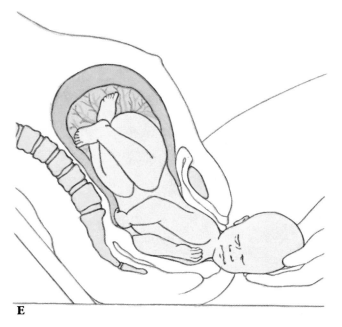

E

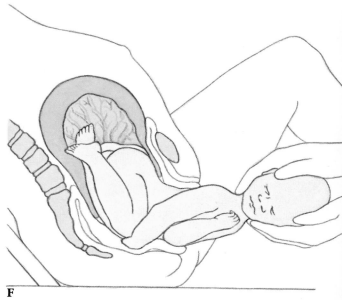

F

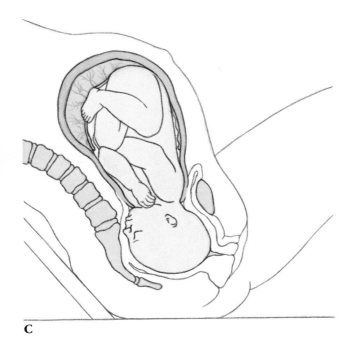

C

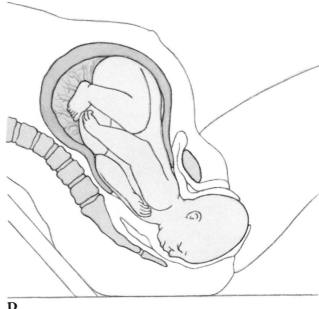

D

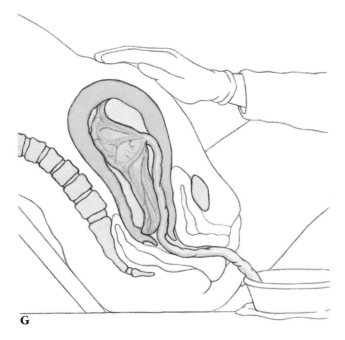

G

These are the major movements of the baby and the mother's pelvic organs during normal labor and delivery.

A *Before labor begins, the head "floats" in amniotic fluid in the womb.*

B ENGAGEMENT, FLEXION, AND DESCENT *The presenting part (usually the head) descends and engages in the mid-pelvic region. The baby's head flexes so that the smallest diameter of the skull passes first into the pelvis.*

C INTERNAL ROTATION *When the head reaches the floor of the pelvis, it rotates in the direction of the least resistance, which is the largest diameter of the pelvic opening.*

D COMPLETE EXTENSION *The extension of the cervix allows the fetal head to pass through, and here the head of the baby negotiates the pelvic curve. As this phase of labor continues, the head passes through the vaginal opening. At the completion of the extension stage, the head is born.*

E EXTERNAL ROTATION *After the head is born, it rotates to realign itself in a normal relationship to the rest of the body.*

F EXPULSION *The birth of the baby involves the upper shoulder pushing its way out of the birth canal, rapidly followed by the lower shoulder. After the shoulders have birthed, the rest of the baby's body (which is smaller) slips out easily.*

G PLACENTA OR AFTERBIRTH *After the baby is born, gentle external massage of the uterus will continue to stimulate contractions of the uterus, and the afterbirth will be delivered.*

THE STAGES OF LABOR AND DELIVERY

These are the stages in which the baby moves out of the vaginal opening.

A *The head appears at the vaginal opening (extension).*
B *As extension is completing, the head emerges from under the pubic bone and is about halfway out of the vaginal opening.*

C and D *After the head is born, the head rotates to realign itself with the body, which is still passing through the birth canal.*
E *The upper shoulder is born first.*
F *The lower shoulder is born next, after which the baby's body slips out.*

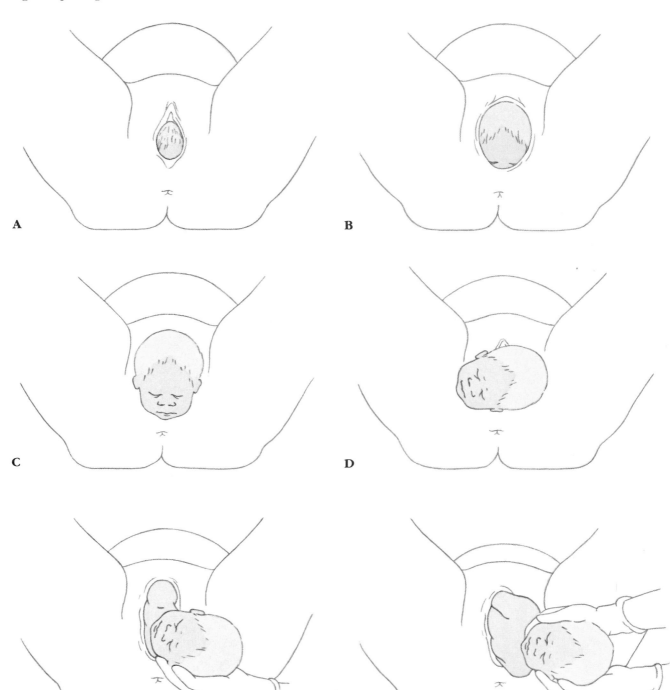

The ride to the hospital or birth center should be planned not to interfere with the mother's comfort and concentration during contractions. A pillow or two to prevent swaying back and forth is often useful. A leisurely pace and preparation beforehand help, too. Touring the maternity service during pregnancy is a good idea, so that the hospital is familiar when the time comes to be admitted in labor. The mother usually will be offered a wheelchair ride to the labor area, but she may decline it and stay with her husband or friends as they sign the admission forms. Upon arrival in the labor area, a nurse will ask the mother to undress, don a short hospital gown, empty her bladder, and get into bed. The nurse then takes the mother's blood pressure, pulse, and temperature, and feels the abdomen to time contractions. A pelvic examination may then be done to see how far the cervix has dilated and to judge the position and station (degree of descent) of the baby.

If the mother is found to be in active labor, two to three centimeters dilated, or otherwise in need of admission to the hospital, the nurse will perform a series of hospital admission routines, each of which is the subject of intense debate and controversy. Parents who object to any of these routines should be certain that their wishes become part of the *hospital* admission record, placed there by the physician when he calls to tell the maternity nurses to expect the parents' arrival in labor. This is a poor time to argue about how labor will be conducted, and advanced planning is essential.

Enemas are often given early in labor to stimulate contractions. Many women find them unpleasant and intrusive, however, and many doctors have ceased ordering them. Contractions usually become very intense when the low bowel is filled with warm water and presses on the uterus in labor, and the value of an enema as a labor stimulant has not been established. Other stimulants for contractions, such as walking around and continuing normal activities, have been shown to effectively shorten labor by at least 25 percent, and to lessen pain.

Shaving the pubic hair is one of the procedures that women occasionally focus on with firm objections. The hair grows back thinner in some cases, and it itches for two to three weeks after birth. Although the purpose of the shave is to reduce the number of bacteria in the area, current research fails to find any direct benefit to the shaving procedure.

An intravenous solution of glucose or saline is installed in an arm vein of most laboring women in hospitals today. This ensures that a vein will be "open" if medication or transfusion is necessary during or after labor. Very rarely, women do hemorrhage during labor or in the hours just afterward. After a certain amount of fluid loss through bleeding (or from failing to drink enough juice and water during labor), the blood volume may be low enough that the blood vessels flatten. At this point, when intravenous blood and fluids might actually save the life of a hemorrhaging woman, it is very difficult to install an intravenous needle into a flattened vessel. Added to this worry on the part of doctors is the concern that women may not keep up their liquid intake during labor, or that if they do and then need general anesthetic, they may vomit the fluid and accidentally take it back into the lungs, where it can cause serious injury or death. The intravenous during labor ensures proper maintenance of liquid intake, along with an adequate blood volume in case of hemorrhage. The IV is already in place in case transfusion is necessary.

But many women object to the IV since hemorrhage occurs so rarely and often can be predicted. Mothers with twin or other multiple pregnancies, women whose labor contractions are being induced with oxytocin (Pitocin), and women with too much amniotic fluid or past bleeding problems are slightly more likely to hemorrhage. Those who object to routine IVs point out that they would rather sip juice, tea, and water in labor to keep up their blood volumes. They also want their hands free, rather than connected to apparatus, so they can be up and about during labor. These women also may remind the doctors that, should a cesarean be necessary, they prefer a regional anesthetic (from the waist down) instead of a general anesthetic, and that they would rather have the anesthesiologist take precautions to prevent the breathing in of fluids during surgery rather than have an IV.

Electronic fetal monitoring is the last routine admission procedure performed on women entering a hospital for labor. This procedure has aroused the most heated debate both in obstetric circles and among parents. The issues are very technical, but they can be summarized by a few general statements. Those obstetricians who require routine fetal monitoring state that continuous tracings of the fetal heart rate are a good replacement for a nurse's constant presence at the bedside of a woman in labor, which hospitals do not have the staff to provide. These tracings give more information about the status of the fetus, and the tracings become a permanent part of the hospital record on file, in case any legal questions arise about the state of the fetus during labor. But most of all, these doctors believe that the technique improves the outcome of the fetus.

Parents who object to electronic fetal monitoring point to the fact that the laboring mother is connected to machinery, which blinks and beeps and produces a paper tape. She is immobilized in a recumbent position and is unable to continue normal activity in labor. The machines are often in disrepair and need adjustments of the belts, wires, and electrodes, and medical personnel may even argue over what the squiggles mean. The belts of the external type of monitor are often tight or itchy, and may cause perspiration. Many parents prefer a nurse by the bedside listening to the fetal heart with a stethoscope, and these parents suspect that the outcome of the fetus is probably as good or better without monitoring.

Since 1976, there have been four randomized, controlled research trials comparing electronic monitoring to nurse monitoring. Three of these trials resulted in a confirmation of the parents' viewpoint. In high-risk women as well as normal laboring women, the electronically monitored infants did no better than the nurse-monitored infants. However, the electronically monitored women had almost three times as many cesarean sections and twice as many postpartum (after birth) infections.

Parents who object to fetal monitoring and other hospital routines but who do not want to have home births can often arrange for a homelike birth in a hospital birth room or birth center. Here a nurse is assigned for the labor to give constant care. Admission to a hospital birth center is a simple process, and the mother may wear her own clothes. Her pulse, blood pressure, temperature, and contractions are examined, and a pelvic examination of the cervix is done. There is no shave, no enema, no IV, and no electronic fetal monitor. The mother is not required to stay in bed, but can sit or walk around as she wishes. Her family and friends can be with her if she desires. Although a hospital birth room is in the labor/delivery area or in the maternity section of the hospital, it looks like an ordinary bedroom. All emergency equipment is out of sight in cabinets, and the room may be equipped with a double bed, a rocking chair, and even a stereo in some cases.

Birth centers have become popular outside of hospitals, as well. Many cities in the United States have birth centers that are operated by doctors or partnerships of doctors and midwives. Birth takes place much as it does at home, but with somewhat more equipment and staff available.

The active phase of labor, from three to seven centimeters' dilation of the cervix, is a long and boring time in some labors, once the doctor or mid-wife has arrived in a home birth, or once the parents have been admitted to the hospital. During active mid-labor, the mother breathes and relaxes with each contraction. She talks or rests or moves about between contractions, and perhaps she uses the toilet or bedpan. Occasionally the nurse or doctor examines the cervix. If contractions are very difficult to manage, pain medication may be offered. Slowly the cervix stretches over the baby's head with each contraction, and imperceptibly labor moves into its most intense phase—the transition phase. In some labors, the pace is so fast that by the time the mother is settled in the hospital, the transition phase or even the expulsion period is ready to begin. In other labors, the pace of the delivery is very slow.

Several factors affect the length of labor, especially at the beginning—the latent phase from onset to about three centimeters of cervical dilation.
● Women who have already had a baby usually have shorter latent and active periods, and sometimes they have shorter transition and expulsion periods.
● Labors with intact membranes are about an hour longer than are labors with ruptured membranes, when all other factors are the same. However, intact membranes protect the fetal head and cord from compression, and protect mother and baby from infection.
● Recumbency lengthens labor. In first labors, women who are up and about, sitting, and walking have 36 percent shorter labors. This means that the average 14-hour first labor may be reduced by as much as 2 to 3 hours by avoiding recumbency. In addition, contractions are more frequent and hurt less when women are up and about in labor.
● Anxiety lengthens labor. The hormone epinephrine, secreted with fear or anxiety, causes diminished blood flow to the uterus, as well as less frequent but more forceful uterine contractions.
● Medications lengthen labor in most cases. If a woman has been extremely fearful, a local or regional anesthetic to reduce pain may actually help labor progress. Oxytocin (Pitocin) causes harder contractions and shorter labors. However, narcotics, tranquilizers, barbiturates, sedatives, and regional anesthetics such as epidurals or spinals generally slow or stop labor if they are given early in the active phase.

The transition phase of Stage I labor. This is the most irregular, tumultuous, and painful time in most labors, but it is also the shortest phase. From seven to ten centimeters is when the cervix stretches its utmost to allow the baby to enter the birth canal. This phase usually lasts less than an hour, and sometimes for fewer than a dozen contractions. The signs are recognizable, and women eagerly await them because they know that soon they will be able to push and the baby will be born. The mother's contractions, which have been coming every two minutes and lasting a minute for several hours, now become irregular. They may come a minute apart, then three minutes apart. They may last 15 seconds, and then 90 seconds. And they may have more than one peak of intensity. Women also get very irritable. They usually tremble, feel cold, or perspire profusely during the last three centimeters of dilation. Some women hiccough between contractions, and some feel nauseated and gag or even vomit. Finally, women feel a distinctive sensation of having a full bowel and the sudden urge to have a bowel movement. Before long, this sensation changes to one of having to push, of involuntarily having to hold one's breath and bear down. This is caused by the baby's head on the rectum and pelvic floor, and signals the passage of the baby into the birth canal.

Contractions of transition are often very difficult to relax and breathe through. Women are taught to use a special type of fast pant-blow breathing to focus their attention and to keep from pushing until the cervix is fully dilated, with the doctor or midwife ready to deliver the baby. In prenatal classes, the mother's husband or friend who will help her during labor is also taught this technique, and will begin it when the mother enters the transition stage of labor. This helps the mother follow the pattern and stay on track. This breathing technique helps most women to refrain from holding their breath, tensing up, and yelling or groaning. However, some women get more relief from yelling at this time than from anything else. If this does not trouble her or those around her, there's no reason not to yell. Otherwise, women are grateful if someone will "pace" them by panting and blowing with them, reminding them to relax. "Pant, pant, pant, BLOW!... relax your brow...good...you're doing great. Soon you can push!"

POSITIONS FOR DELIVERY

A *This is the standard lithotomy position used in hospital delivery rooms.*
B *Most women prefer the semi-upright position during the first stages of labor, and often maintain the position throughout labor.*
C *A reclining position may be comfortable for some stages of labor. Most women prefer the reclining*

position after the baby is delivered and while the placenta is being delivered.
D *During transition, some women prefer an all-fours position; others prefer to squat, stand, or sit upright. When the mother is pushing most actively and is fully participating in the last stages of birth, she should assume any position that feels natural.*

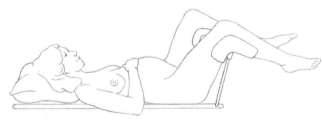

A

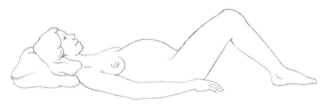

C

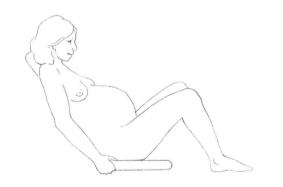

B

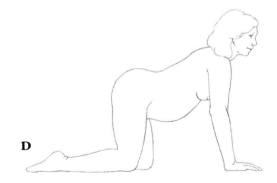

D

Helping the laboring woman may simply entail "being there" to lend moral support and witness the miracle of birth. However, most people who are with a laboring woman are called upon to help in other ways as well.

• Massaging the mother's abdomen is soothing, especially during contractions. A light, fingertip stroking over both sides of the abdomen, or low in the center is often very helpful in reducing pain. This massage is called effleurage, and women may be taught to do it themselves in prenatal classes.

• Breathing with the mother keeps her on track at critical times during labor. It is necessary to breathe audibly so the mother can easily follow, and it often works best if she focuses on the coach's face.

• Reminding the mother to release her tense muscles may be helpful, along with stroking the tense muscles smooth.

• Helping the mother change position is especially necessary if she is connected to an IV and a fetal monitor. She should avoid lying flat on her back, and she should change position at least every half hour, alternating between side-lying, semi-reclining, and sitting propped up. Late in labor, it may be difficult to change positions without assistance.

• About 20 percent of women feel contractions centered low in the back, and experience severe backache during labor. A firm back massage, using talcum powder on the skin to keep from chafing it, can be very soothing. With the mother side-lying, the labor attendant can press the heel of a hand very firmly on the lowest part of her spine near the "tailbone," or on one side. The mother will exclaim with pleasure or pain, depending on whether the place chosen is correct. Constant, firm pressure or slight rotating of the heel of the hand will reduce the backache. Women who are alone can lie semi-reclining on a roll or towel or a tennis ball, forcing the pelvis into a pelvic "tilt" (see page 296). Some women alternately tilt and relax the pelvis to relieve backache.

• Some women breathe too heavily during labor, especially if they have not been to classes to learn and practice specific breathing patterns. These women may react to contractions by gasping, panting, or yelling a great deal, and they sometimes get dizzy, feel numb or tingly in the fingers, or turn blue around the mouth. It is necessary to help the mother slow down her breathing and bring it back to normal depth, not too shallow and not too deep. She should concentrate on each inhalation and exhalation, and release her muscles to become calm. This over-breathing is called hyperventilation. It can be eliminated by breathing into a small paper bag or a small hollow made in the bed sheet. The mother breathes back some of her lost carbon dioxide, and the symptoms of hyperventilation disappear immediately.

The Second and Third Stages of Labor

Delivery of the baby. The reflex urge to bear down with the peak of contractions is triggered by the pressure of the baby's head or buttock on the pelvic floor. Sometimes this urge comes a little before the cervix is fully dilated or stretched around the baby's presenting part. Also, the urge to push may come before the medical attendants are ready to deliver the baby. In either case, the mother will be asked to pant and blow out vigorously to counteract the urge to push. When the cervix is fully dilated, as judged by a vaginal examination, and when the doctor or midwife is ready to deliver the baby, then the mother is told to push with each contraction.

With a first baby, delivery may take well over an hour, especially if the baby is large or the pelvis is small. In first labors, then, pushing may start in the labor room, and only when a little bit of the baby's head is seen at the opening of the birth canal is the mother rolled into the delivery room, helped to slide onto the delivery table, and scrubbed down with disinfectant to make ready for the birth. In the multipara, pushing sometimes produces the baby so fast that she is usually moved straight to the delivery room before being asked to push. In a hospital delivery, the husband or friend chosen by the mother to be with her for the birth will be helped to don a fresh hospital gown, cap, mask, and shoe covers, and this person will be shown where to sit in the delivery room at the mother's shoulder.

It may seem as if the pushing part of labor is the worst time to have to pull oneself onto a rolling cart and be wheeled to another room for delivery. It also may seem ridiculous to have to adjust to a hard delivery table, put your legs into stirrups, and have the vaginal opening scrubbed, along with the pushing of contractions. In fact, very few countries in the world practice obstetrics in this fashion. Instead, women merely use the labor bed, which can easily be fitted with stirrups if needed, and the foot of the bed dropped out of the way.

HOME BIRTH WITH PHYSICIAN OR MIDWIFE ATTENDING

PHYSICIAN CONTROLLING THE CROWNED HEAD

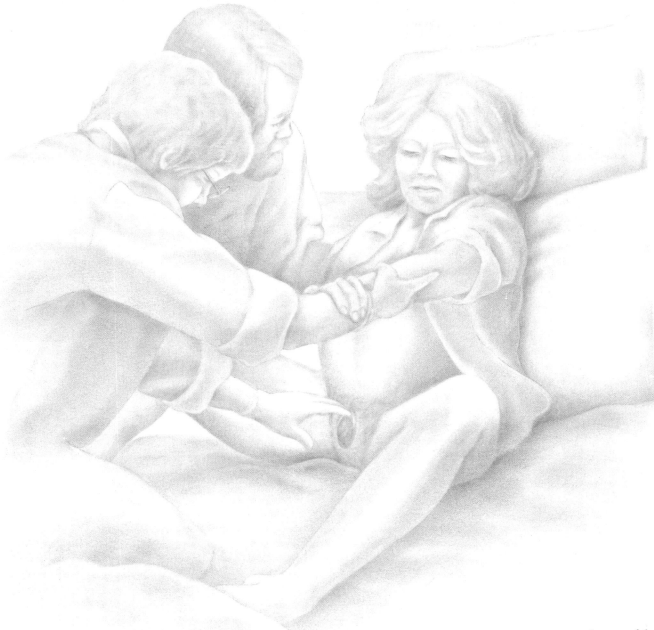

As the baby dilates the skin of the perineum, the top of the head is born, followed by the eyes, nose, mouth, and chin. The head turns to the side with the next contraction, and one of the shoulders is born, followed by the other. The rest of the baby slips out easily.

However, most women find that the pushing part of labor is much easier than the brief transition period that went before. They usually have no trouble listening and following directions, and the contractions of expulsion seem less painful and more purposeful. In contrast to the foggy tumult of transition, the expulsion may seem quite calm.

Pushing during contractions takes some skill, even for mothers who have learned a pushing technique in prenatal classes. Each push must be smooth and gentle rather than violent and prolonged. The peaks of expulsive contractions last about 10 seconds, and this is the period for firm, gentle bearing down. Don't bear down for the major part of the contraction. Studies have shown that this "selective pushing" for only a few seconds at the peaks of contractions puts less stress on the newborn baby. Recent studies also have questioned the wisdom of pushing in a supine (flat on the back) position. Blood flow to the placenta is often slowed or even stopped by the weight of the uterus on the main artery when the mother is in this position. Also, the efficiency of expulsive efforts is considerably reduced. The best expulsive technique, then, is with the mother sitting up or standing, and pushing only during the brief peaks of contractions. Although home and hospital birth-center facilities allow for side-lying, sitting, kneeling, or standing births, hospital delivery rooms usually do not provide these options.

Whether standing, sitting, or lying down to push during delivery of the baby, the same general process is followed during the actual birth. At first, with each bearing-down effort, a little bit of the baby can be seen. The woman who has learned to bulge out her pelvic floor (by practicing the elevator exercise) will make better progress at this time. With each bearing-down effort, the skin just below the vaginal outlet (perineum) bulges and stretches as more and more of the baby shows. Between contractions, the baby may recede somewhat, but with each push, more progress is seen. Finally, the perineum begins to turn white when it is maximally stretched. The doctor or midwife will then massage the perineum with oil, supporting the tissues while the mother is asked to either push very gently or to pant and blow. Slowly, gradually, the baby dilates the skin of the perineum, and after what seems like an eternity, the top of the head is born, followed by the eyes, nose, mouth, and chin. The head turns to the side with the next contraction, and one of the shoulders is born, followed by the other. The rest of the baby's body slips out easily.

HOME BIRTH WITH PHYSICIAN OR MIDWIFE

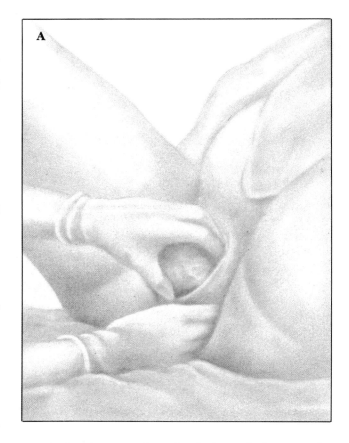

A *The head is extending slowly through the vaginal opening. With each bearing-down effort, the skin just below the vaginal outlet (perineum) bulges and stretches as more and more of the baby shows. The midwife or doctor will assist at this point to help prevent perineal tears.*
B *As the baby slowly dilates the skin of the perineum, the top of the head is followed by the eyes, nose, mouth, and chin, and the head is born.*
C *The baby is being held as it slips out easily.*
D *The umbilical cord is clamped after it has blanched. The cord is clamped near the baby's abdomen, or may be tied off with sterile thread. The cord is then cut and the baby is immediately placed with the mother for cuddling and breast-feeding. Neither the baby nor mother feels the umbilical cord being cut, as the cord has no nerves.*

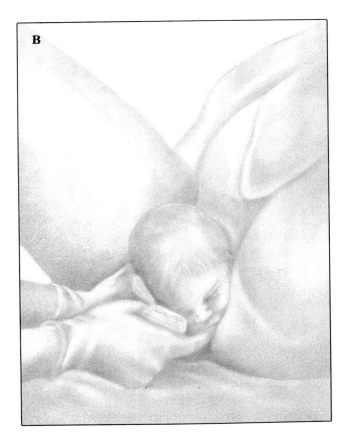

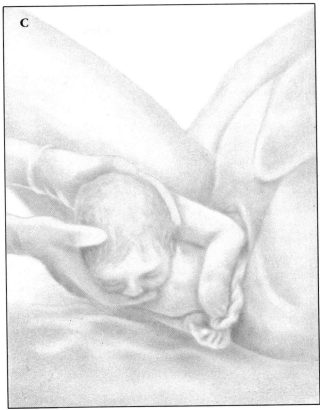

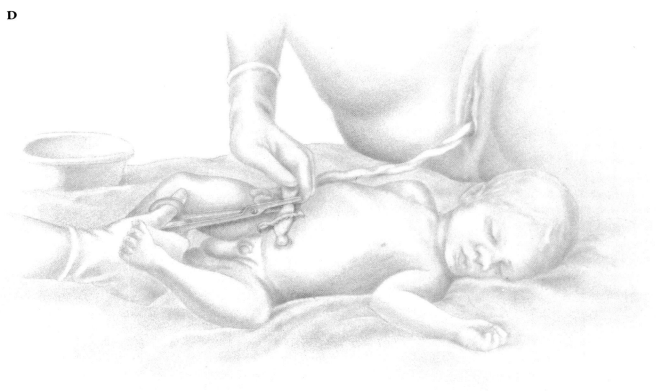

HOME BIRTH WITH PHYSICIAN OR MIDWIFE ATTENDING

DELIVERY AND INSPECTION OF THE PLACENTA

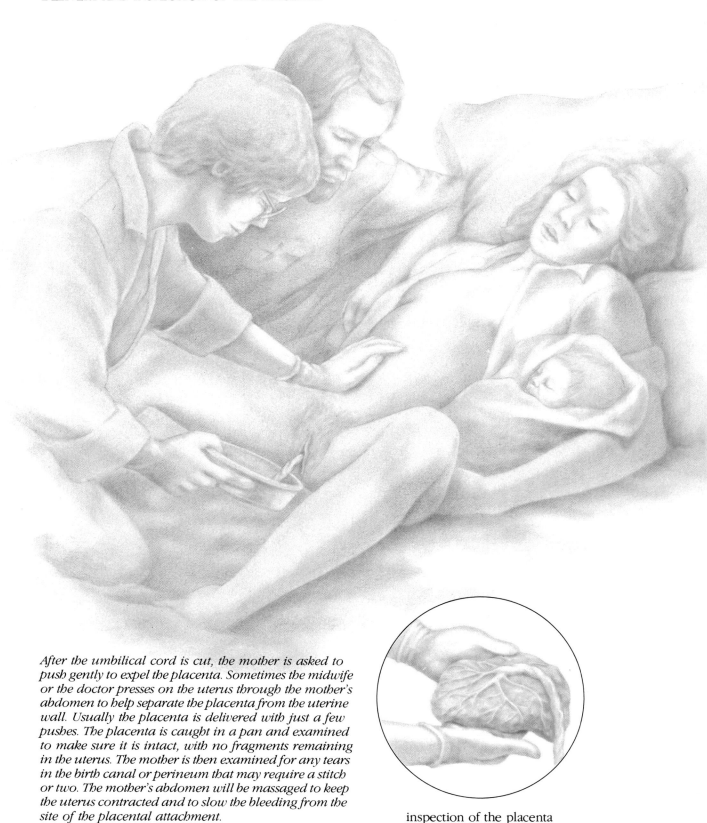

After the umbilical cord is cut, the mother is asked to push gently to expel the placenta. Sometimes the midwife or the doctor presses on the uterus through the mother's abdomen to help separate the placenta from the uterine wall. Usually the placenta is delivered with just a few pushes. The placenta is caught in a pan and examined to make sure it is intact, with no fragments remaining in the uterus. The mother is then examined for any tears in the birth canal or perineum that may require a stitch or two. The mother's abdomen will be massaged to keep the uterus contracted and to slow the bleeding from the site of the placental attachment.

inspection of the placenta

The doctor or midwife uses a small bulb syringe to suction mucus and fluid out of the baby's mouth and allow the first breaths. Some babies simply breathe then, while others make a few wails and then settle into regular breathing. Some babble or cry inconsolably at first, and quiet only after being warmly wrapped and cuddled by their mothers.

Many delivery room practices in the United States are changing. At birth, the baby is no longer suspended by the heels and slapped roughly to make him or her cry. Instead, a gentle massage of the baby's back or chest stimulates breathing. Some people like the idea of a warm bath for the newborn baby, and most prefer to warm up the delivery room so that both family members and the new baby are not chilled by air conditioning. Quiet surroundings and subdued lighting are also requested by some mothers. In choosing a hospital early in pregnancy, parents will need to know what its delivery room practices are, and whether the staff is flexible in allowing the kind of delivery the parents desire.

Delivery of the placenta. The third stage of labor is the delivery of the placenta. As this stage starts, the baby has just been born, and the umbilical cord runs from the abdomen of the baby up into the birth canal, and then to the placenta, which is still in the uterus. Usually, the cord is long enough to allow the baby to lie on the mother's abdomen and be gently massaged to start breathing. After the baby is born, close observation of the cord reveals that it slowly turns pale. It is gradually closing off the vessels that have served the baby during intrauterine life.

When should the cord be cut? There is a controversy in obstetrics as to whether it is better to cut the cord immediately, wait until it turns white in about a minute, to hold the baby down below the birth canal and strip the cord blood into the baby, or simply let placental blood run into the baby for five minutes before cutting the cord. A good rule of thumb is to follow what seems to be the comfortable procedure (probably followed for centuries of human birth). This would be to let the cord blanch and cut it after a minute or so. Studies from Canada and Sweden have shown that letting the placenta drain into the newborn for five minutes causes increased respiratory grunting and irregular breathing in the first few days, along with increased incidence of jaundice. This is a condition in which yellowish pigment colors the newborn's skin and the whites of the eyes (see page 286).

The cord is clamped near the baby's abdomen and one inch further out from the first clamp. Or, sterile thread or string may be used to tie off the cord. The cord is cut between the two clamps. Neither the baby nor the mother feels the cut, as the cord has no nerves. The baby is then handed to the mother to cuddle or breast-feed. The mother is next asked to push gently to expel the placenta. Sometimes the midwife or the doctor presses on the uterus through the mother's abdomen to help separate the placenta from the uterine wall. Usually the placenta is delivered with just a few pushes from the mother.

CHANGES IN THE UTERUS AFTER BIRTH

This figure shows the change in the size of the uterus after birth, a process called involution. It is accompanied by a small amount of bleeding from the vagina for two or three weeks after delivery.

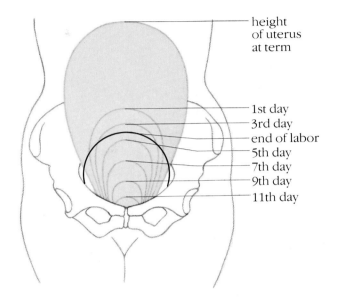

height of uterus at term

1st day
3rd day
end of labor
5th day
7th day
9th day
11th day

The placenta is caught in a pan and examined to make sure it is intact, with no fragments remaining in the uterus. The mother also is examined for any tears in the birth canal or perineum. If they are over one-half inch long or are deep, a stitch or two will help them to heal. The mother's abdomen will be massaged to keep the uterus contracted and thereby slow the bleeding from the site of the placental attachment. The uterus should be about the size and hardness of a grapefruit, and periodic massaging for the first two or three hours after birth will keep the uterus firm. The drawing above shows the change in size of the uterus expected after birth. This process is called involution, and is accompanied by a small amount of bleeding from the vagina for two or three weeks. The amount and type of blood are similar to that seen with a normal menstrual period; this is called lochia. After a few days, the flow turns brownish and ceases.

Your Own Childbirth Record

Dates

Last period:

Calculated date of first
missed period:

Calculated date of conception:

Calculated date of birth:

Doctor Visits

Date	Weight	Tests and Results	Comments

Drugs and Vitamins

Type	Amount	Dates	Comments

Observations

	Date	Comments
Fetal movement:		
Diet:		
Dreams about baby:		
Your emotions and relationship with father-to-be:		

Baby

Weight:

Length:

General appearance:

Labor and Delivery

	Date	Time	Comments
Onset of labor:			
Rupture of membranes:			
Admission to hospital or arrival of midwife:			
Anesthesia:			
Special intervention:			
Delivery:			

You can keep a permanent record of your pregnancy and delivery based on the samples above. Whether it's just a calendar of facts and comments or a detailed journal, you may be glad to have the information available at a later date.

Do Not Diet During Pregnancy

Mother's weight gain during pregnancy

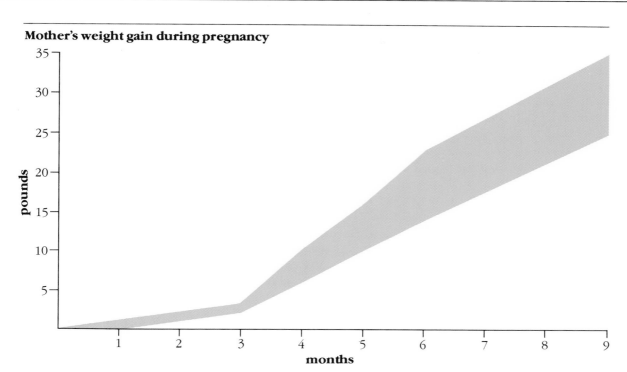

pounds

months

Many tragic outcomes at birth—premature births, growth-retarded infants, toxemia, and other complications—can be traced to poor nutrition during pregnancy.

Calorie needs during pregnancy. Every single day of your pregnancy, you should consume at least 2,200 to 2,600 calories. *Do not diet during pregnancy.* To do so is to risk serious complications. Women who were overweight when they conceived may actually emerge from pregnancy thinner if they stop eating snack foods and gain plenty of weight eating quality foods, such as meat, fish, nuts, beans, milk, eggs, cheese, whole grain cereals and breads, and lots of fresh fruit and vegetables—*every day.*

Weight gain during pregnancy. How much weight should pregnant women gain overall? Several studies have shown that the fewest complications, such as toxemia and low birth-weight babies, occurred among women who gained 30 to 35 pounds during pregnancy. Don't worry about your weight. Instead, *concentrate on eating the very highest quality food at each meal, and eat what you need to satisfy your hunger.* If

you have been told to gain less than 20 to 25 pounds, you probably should seek other opinions from experts. Low weight gains can be harmful, especially if the food consumed is not high quality protein, grains, fruits, vegetables, and dairy products. If you are thin when you conceive, then do your best to *gain* by eating *extra* amounts of the best foods.

Weight loss after pregnancy. If you gain 30 to 35 pounds, will you be left with rolls of fat after you deliver your baby? If you breast-feed your baby, the extra few pounds of fat are actually used in producing breast milk. After several months of breast-feeding (especially if you don't give your baby unnecessary cereal and formula supplements), you will find that most or all of the excess weight has been lost. *Mothers actually need a few extra pounds after childbirth in order to give their babies the best possible start in life, a good birth weight, and adequate breast milk.*

For a further discussion of the special dietary needs of women, see the "Nutrition" chapter. In particular, refer to pages 56 through 57 for information on nutrition during and after pregnancy.

The Newborn Baby

Care of the newborn at delivery. As the baby is being suctioned out and stimulated to begin breathing, the midwife or doctor is assessing his or her physical condition. This assessment is called an Apgar score. If the baby is red and pink, 2 points are given for that, but if he or she is bluish-white, only 1 or 0 is given. If the baby is breathing well, has a strong pulse, a steady pulse, and spreads the toes when the sole of the foot is tickled, then each sign gets 2 points, making a perfect score of 10. At one minute of age, many babies get a score of 7, 8, or 9, but at five minutes, they are usually pinker or breathing better, and the score goes up to 9 or 10.

One of the immediate needs of a newborn is warmth, and cold can actually be quite harmful at this time. Within the last decade, some hospitals have changed their treatment of newborns, not sending them immediately to the nursery to be placed under radiant warmers anymore, but rather letting the baby lie covered skin-to-skin with the mother. She has been "discovered" as the best radiant warmer. If the birth has been in a hospital, the baby will be given an ID bracelet and be weighed in the first few minutes.

State laws require that silver nitrate or antibiotic ointment be put into the newborn's eyes in order to guarantee that the baby will not suffer gonococcal blindness if the mother has gonorrhea at the time of birth. Unfortunately, this treatment causes the baby's eyelids to become red and swollen.

Researchers recently have discovered that the newborn actually focuses his or her eyes in the first hours after birth. Studies of parents' reactions to their newborns revealed that the visual alertness of the baby is a very important element in the baby's attractiveness to its parents. Parents' comments often center around the baby's eyes at birth, and many parents try to bring their faces into alignment with the baby's face and look into the baby's eyes. Studies now have shown that parents who were given this "early contact" with their baby at birth felt much closer to that particular baby for up to two years than did parents who were separated from their newborns. The role of eye contact with the baby was found to be so important that many hospitals delay the silver nitrate treatment in order to foster this delicate bond or attachment process between parents and their baby.

Of course, most parents want to have their new baby with them rather than sending him or her to the nursery. In fact, this is so important to the building of a strong attachment with the baby that when parents find out that a hospital will not allow the baby to stay with the parents after birth, they may go to a different hospital or arrange a birth-center or home birth. This preference has become so widespread that one newborn nursery pediatrician, Marshall Klaus, has recommended that nurseries be abolished for normal newborns. He and many other pediatricians have shown that whatever nursing care the mother and baby need can be given very easily while the mother and baby are together.

In fact, the most sensitive testing of the newborn, the neonatal behavioral assessment, is best done at the mother's bedside. The doctor who developed this scale found that showing the parents all the fascinating talents of their new baby is a useful teaching tool for them, and also increases their awareness of some rather wonderful ways their tiny baby relates to them.

For example, the newborn prefers to stare at a human face over any other pattern offered within his or her range of vision. If presented with various choices, the baby will consistently select the human face. If the baby is spoken to in a delighted, high-pitched voice ("Pretty baby! Pretty baby!"), he or she will move in rhythm to the voice, getting more and more caught up in it, bringing the arms and legs toward the speaker in time to the pitch of the voice. As the voice lowers, so do the baby's arms and legs. On a videotape, this looks like a wonderful "dance" between the parents and the baby as they move in synchrony with each other.

The newborn will focus on a little red ball and turn the head to follow it; will pay attention to a sound for a little while and then accommodate to it and block it out; will cry when given a tiny prick on the foot, but after a few minutes will be able to "contain" the disorganization of behavior, and change to a quiet state. Parents are shown other states that babies have, including the most attentive, quiet, alert, staring state in which the baby is most responsive; a more inattentive, casting-about state; a light slumber; heavy sleep; and the crying state.

Babies born after optimum labors into quiet, gentle hands spend much more time in the quiet, alert state than do babies who have been stressed, whether by medications given the mother during labor, or by the labor and delivery itself. In fact, the differences in neuromuscular functioning and visual attentiveness between babies *with the same Apgar scores* are so stark that many people feel that the Apgar score actually masks our full understanding of the effects of various factors on the newborn. Perhaps the Apgar score should go to 40 or 50 instead of only 10.

Some of the differences between babies are unrelated to labor and delivery, however. There seem to be three distinct tempos of babies: the very sensitive, over-responding baby; the average baby; and the under-responding, satisfied, undemanding baby. One researcher has recommended that parents identify which type of baby they have in the first weeks, and provide quiet containment for the over-responsive baby, with less stimulation, and a more stimulating treatment for the undemanding baby, in order to help them each organize their responses.

One reflex that the newborn is equipped with is the rooting reflex. When the cheek is stroked, the baby will turn the head and open the mouth, searching for the nipple. However, on the delivery table, when first offered the breast, newborns typically lick the nipple at first. Mothers sometimes feel this as a rejection, and nurses sometimes conclude that newborns simply are not ready to nurse. Actually, the explanation is another example of the elegant, reciprocal interplay between mother and newborn. Stimulation of the nipple triggers a complex set of hormonal and reflex responses in the mother, including release of uterine-stimulating hormone, which keeps the uterus firm in the early hours after birth, and a milk-ejection reflex that moves the early milk—colostrum—from the alveoli in the outer breast to the ducts behind the nipple. Later, this "letdown" reflex will be felt by the mother as a tingling of the breasts whenever she thinks about feeding her baby, or whenever a baby cries.

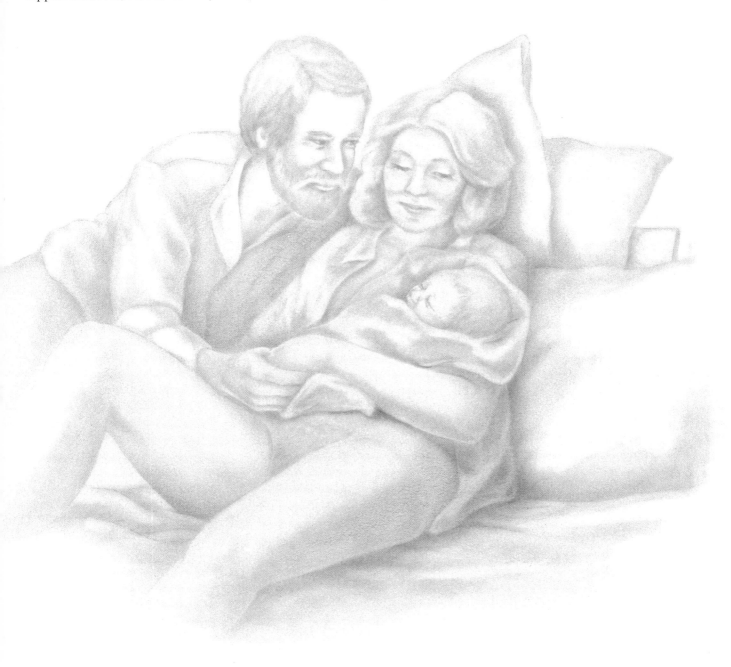

Colostrum is a thick, yellowish-white substance produced by the breast during late pregnancy and for the first 12 to 24 hours after birth. Physicians and researchers have published over three dozen scientific analyses of colostrum in the last few years, and the excitement over the benefits of early feeding of the baby has been remarkable. For years it was recognized that colostrum acted as a laxative for the baby, helping to produce the first bowel movement, meconium. Now it is also known that colostrum is rich in proteins specifically made for human babies, and loaded with antiinfective agents. These lymphocytes, leucocytes, macrophages, and antibodies line the baby's stomach and intestine. They stimulate the development of the baby's intestinal mucosa, increasing the mucosal cells by 70 percent, which in turn produces quantities of digestive enzymes, which play a role in easy, complete absorption of milk. These substances also prevent enteritis and respiratory infections. The normal bacteria in the parent's noses and on their skin populate the baby's respiratory and intestinal tracts, where specific antibodies from the placenta and colostrum prevent infection, and stimulate the infant's own defense mechanisms. Babies removed from their mothers in the first 12 hours develop skin and respiratory infections at much higher rates than do babies who remain with their mothers.

Not only is colostrum important to the baby, but very early feeding prevents most of the signs of engorgement or swelling in the breasts during the first 24 to 36 hours after childbirth. Instead, little engorgement is noted, and the milk "comes in" sooner.

In addition to the many microbiological findings recently reported about early newborn feeding, thirteen different behavioral studies from all over the world indicate that mothers who breast-fed at delivery and were with their babies continuously had, as a group, quite different experiences with the children for as long as four years afterward—experiences that distinguished them from mother-infant pairs who were separated. They breast-fed for longer in infancy; spent more time playing with their babies and less time cleaning them; lined up their face with the baby's face more often; spent more time kissing and talking to their baby; held the baby on the left more often (near the heart, which soothes the baby); spoke to the child with fewer commands and more adjectives; and used twice as many questions as did mothers who were separated from their new babies. At two years of age, these differences in speech were still statistically significant, and at four years of age, children not separated at birth had higher intelligence quotients and more advanced scores on two language tests.

One result of the explosion in knowledge of normal processes in the early newborn period has been the insistence by parents that they keep their babies with them continuously after childbirth. Hospitals have responded to this demand by offering several types of programs. One group of prepaid health plan hospitals offers a "Shared Beginnings" option to parents, whereby they attend classes during late pregnancy and are able to keep the baby with them, supervised by specially trained nurses. Other hospitals simply have what they call "time for bonding"—a few minutes for the mother to hold her baby and nurse. Parents who are fully informed often search out hospitals with birth rooms, in which they can deliver and be discharged home with the baby in 4 to 12 hours if mother and baby are well. Many parents have chosen out-of-hospital birth centers and home births in order to be certain that the mother and baby will not be separated after birth. In early discharge programs, and in the birth-center and home birth programs, a maternity nurse or nurse-midwife visits the home daily in the first postpartum (after-childbirth) days.

At this visit, the mother's uterus is checked, and she reports whether she has had any temperature increase indicating an infection, and whether the normal lochia (bloody discharge) has changed. Her nipples are checked for soreness or cracking, and any treatments she needs are begun. The baby is also examined. The stump of the umbilical cord is watched, first for seepage of blood, and then to be sure it is not infected. It dries and falls off in a few days. The baby's weight and vital signs (heart sounds, pulse, temperature, and reflexes) are examined, and any problems with feeding schedules, fatigue of the mother, or proper nutrition of the mother are dealt with.

For the mother and baby who remain in the hospital for two to three days after childbirth, a number of options are available. The most popular is rooming-in, a system whereby the baby stays in the mother's room in a bassinet from morning until night, or even for 24 hours a day in some cases. New mothers may learn how to care for their babies and start breast-feeding. If they need rest, the baby is cared for in the nursery. Some experienced mothers actually look forward to a good rest for a few days in the hospital, and welcome letting the nurses care for the baby.

Probably the most startling change in newborn care has taken place among infants who are sent to intensive care because they need close supervision after childbirth. These infants are most frequently prematures and infants of high-risk mothers. A few are very sick or have congenital malformations. Recently, there has been a steep rise in the number of infants sent to intensive care for treatment of jaundice. This is a yellow pigment that colors the skin and whites of the eyes of the baby. Some estimates of the incidence of jaundice are as high as 50 percent of all newborn babies. Most jaundice is physiologic—that is, normal. It is usually due to a mild, transient inability of the baby's liver to metabolize drugs or handle the normal breakdown of red blood cells efficiently.

Until recently, there were no quick tests to tell whether the baby's jaundice was serious enough to cause kernicterus (brain damage), and many normal babies were separated from their parents for expensive intensive-care treatment under bright lights known as "bililights." The fluorometric analysis test is now available to pinpoint those few babies who actually need intensive-care treatment.

Intensive-care nurseries now generally welcome parents as part of the intensive-care team. Parents can visit at any time, and can take over some aspects of caring for their sick newborn babies after instruction from the doctors and nurses. We now realize that prolonged separation of sick newborns from their parents may result in long-term or even permanent parent-infant distance or failure on the baby's part to thrive and grow. Mothers are therefore urged to come in anytime, put on a sterile gown, and touch and stroke their tiny premies through the incubator, participate in caring for the baby, and above all, to feed the baby. If he or she is too tiny to be able to suck, the mother learns how to get the baby to take milk. She is encouraged to express her breast milk for this purpose, if she likes, since breast milk is especially valuable for prematures, both as nourishment and for its anti-infective properties. Many hospitals have parent discussion groups and counseling, which can be of critical importance to parents of very sick or malformed infants.

Breast-feeding is regaining its popularity after several decades of being actively discouraged by commercial formula companies, baby equipment manufacturers, and even medical people. Mothers need great support and approval for breast-feeding, because the rushed tenor of life today presents many obstacles to successful lactation. Unfortunately, most doctors and nurses are not sufficiently knowledgeable about breast-feeding to be of help. Women who want to breast-feed may get their most important support from attending group meetings of the La Leche League, an organization with chapters in most towns in the United States. There is a growing body of good reading material about breast-feeding as well. Books and specific information on drugs and illness during breast-feeding can be obtained from the La Leche League or from the International Childbirth Education Association's Book Center.

Several basic facts are necessary in order to breast-feed. First, mothers and fathers need to agree that this is the best way to feed a baby, and that women's breasts are not simply erogenous zones. Next, women should know that the size of the breasts has nothing to do with the amount of milk produced. What controls the amount of milk is the amount of sucking the baby does. Probably the most common mistake that mothers make is to provide their infants with supplemental bottles of water or formula, or supplemental feedings of cereal, often at the urging of the doctor. Babies who receive these supplements do not take as much milk from the breast, and slowly the breast milk dries up.

The last two most common pitfalls of early breast-feeding are feelings of frustration if the baby wants to nurse every hour or two, and sore nipples. Recent research has shown that *the human baby probably should be fed fairly frequently—and every hour or two during periods of growth is not unreasonable.* The composition of human breast milk is more like that of mammals who carry their young with them and feed them rather constantly. Mothers who have adjusted to breast-feeding often carry their babies with them in soft cloth carriers, nursing them while they cook or read, without really noticing when feedings take place. During the night, babies can be taken into bed with the mothers for feedings, and mothers lose very little sleep. Many mothers really cannot remember when their babies started sleeping through the night, because they hardly even notice when they stop being wakened for a feeding.

Mothers used to be advised to limit nursing at first in order to prevent sore nipples, or to rub and brush the nipples during pregnancy to prepare them for breast-feeding. Neither of these measures works for many women. Instead, they simply have a short period of days when their nipples are tender. It's helpful to take the baby off the breast gently—breaking the suction first with a finger—and to air the nipples and not let them stay wet between feedings. Sunlight and an occasional rubbing with lanolin ointment also help, as do nipple shields. These are placed over the nipple, and allow milk to pass through to the baby, who sucks on the shield instead of the sore nipple. This gives the nipple a rest if early soreness or cracked nipples create a problem. Soreness goes away completely in a couple of weeks after starting breast-feeding unless there is cracking of the nipples. In that case, soreness disappears when the cracks heal.

One of the unspoken worries of mothers and fathers concerns the sexual aspects of breast-feeding. Some mothers feel guilty for having an erotic reaction to breast-feeding. This may be especially troublesome if, during the months of breast-feeding, they have less interest in sex in general, as many breast-feeding women do. It helps to talk about these feelings together, and perhaps get reassurance from the doctor that both these reactions are common, normal, and transient.

Working mothers also can breast-feed if they wish. The hours spent away from the baby need not cause a progressive decrease in the amount of breast milk if the mother regularly expresses the milk. Many mothers leave a bottle of expressed milk for the baby to take during her working hours. This milk can be frozen, if needed. Bottles are very easy to draw milk from, however, and babies soon learn that the breast, by comparison, takes more work to drink from.

The breast often will deliver a great deal of milk in the first few minutes of sucking during a feeding, followed by a period during which little milk is let down. A minute or two later, more milk is ejected, and so forth for the typical nursing period. The breast-fed baby learns to suck and wait, often cooing or smiling with the nipple in his or her mouth, dribbling milk out the side of the mouth, playing with the toes, giggling at the mother, and then sucking and swallowing again while milk is being let down.

This cycle may be nature's way of promoting sociable and comforting interactions between mother and baby during the frequent daily feedings.

The milk produced in the last half of each breast-feeding period is whiter and creamier-looking than the "foremilk," which is thin and bluish. During a typical 15- to 20-minute feeding, a perfect nutritional balance is received by the infant, composed of all the fats, carbohydrates, and proteins needed, including—and this is very new data—*all the vitamins and minerals the infant needs for the first full year of life.* Until very recently, mothers were told that breast milk lacks vitamin D and iron in sufficient amounts for babies over six months old. However, researchers were looking for vitamin D in the fat content of the milk, where it exists in other foods. Instead, ample quantities of vitamin D were recently found to exist in the water fraction of the breast milk. No longer do babies have to take added vitamins in order to get sufficient vitamin D if they are breast-fed. Likewise, the breast-fed infant who is otherwise healthy does not need iron supplements or iron-rich cereals after 6 months. Although human milk has been known for years to be low in iron, it contains an enzyme that enhances iron absorption in the baby. We now know that breast-fed infants have as much iron intake as infants fed iron-fortified formulas. Infants on unfortified formulas were iron-deficient, however.

Not only does breast milk have ample vitamins and minerals for the baby's first year, but the fat content of the milk is designed specifically for human absorption and carries several vitally important, newly discovered protective properties for infants, both of which are of lasting benefit throughout the child's life. Fats compose only 3 percent of human breast milk, but are composed of a peculiar chain of triglycerides with lipase, and this peculiarity ensures that the fat is absorbed by the infant with 95 to 98 percent efficiency. Amazingly, this fat is saturated rather than unsaturated, and a large fraction is cholesterol.

In these days of emphasis on low-cholesterol diets and reducing saturated fat intake, one might wonder why human breast milk is not only high in saturated fats,

but is engineered so that virtually all of the fat is absorbed by the infant. Researchers in several parts of the United States have discovered that a high-cholesterol and saturated fat diet in infancy seems to promote the infant's development of enzymes that provide lifetime efficiency in handling saturated fats. Collaborative studies have followed 126 adults from prenatal life to 40 years of age, finding that those men and women who were exclusively breast-fed for more than two months have lower cholesterol levels as adults even if their fat intake is high.

Much publicity has been given to the effect of obesity in infancy on lifelong obesity in adulthood. Formula-fed infants receive a formula high in sugar and carbohydrate and low in saturated fats, but high in unsaturated fat—mostly polyunsaturated vegetable oils. Infants fed on this diet, supplemented with cereals and strained baby foods loaded with starches, gain weight very rapidly. About 20 percent reveal a tendency to remain obese during childhood and adulthood. In contrast, the breast-fed baby gains weight more slowly. The mother cannot "force-feed" the infant, because she is never sure how much the infant already has taken from the breast.

Probably the most compelling benefit of the saturated fat found in breast milk is its function in the maturation of the central nervous system. Myelination (the formation of the fatty protective covering of nerves) continues in infancy from prenatal life, and seems to depend on adequate intake of saturated fats, as well as specific types of proteins—amino acids—that are plentiful in breast milk.

The benefits of breast-feeding without supplement for the first months of infancy, and continued breast-feeding for the first year or two have become so well established that the American Academy of Pediatrics recently sent a memo to the press and to all of its members urging that all mothers be encouraged actively during pregnancy to prepare themselves to breast-feed their infants, and to be given wholehearted support throughout the breast-feeding period. This resounding acclaim for breast-feeding officially replaces the advice of the Academy for the last 20 years, which was that, although breast-feeding had advantages for the baby during the first few months, equal support should be given to the mother who chooses to bottle-feed her baby. Certainly some mothers will find it difficult to breast-feed, or may have an illness that prevents it. However, with encouragement, the majority of mothers are capable of providing all of their baby's nutritional needs through breast milk for the first year.

Medical workers can help at the time of birth by encouraging immediate and constant mother-infant contact and breast-feeding and by not feeding the infant glucose water in the nursery. Doctors also can encourage continued breast-feeding through some mothers' occasional periods of respiratory and breast infections, help the mother cope with sore nipples, and allay any of her doubts that arise.

After the first weeks of the baby's life, breast-feeding continues to have surprising benefits. One is that the mother's body can produce antibodies specifically for various illnesses in the baby, and pass these protective agents to the baby in the breast milk. Another is the social and emotional richness of the breast-feeding period for both the mother and baby. The special closeness and comfort of nursing are felt by both. Researchers timed the amount of contact, talking, and interaction mothers had with their year-old babies, and found that breast-feeding mothers had seven times the contact with their infants that bottle-feeding mothers had. As the infant gets older, the comforting and social aspects of breast-feeding grow. The toddler, who may be rushing around with a play group during the day, may still find breast-feeding before bed the best way to end the day. Weaning takes place very gradually.

In the first days after birth, a test is done on the baby's blood to check for a very rare inborn error of metabolism which causes mental retardation—phenylketonuria. This test is valid only after the baby has taken milk for several days. Babies who were tested on the third day in the hospital before breast-feeding was well established may need retesting. This ailment affects fewer than one baby in 10,000, and a change in diet for the first year or two prevents retardation. Many states require all babies to be tested for phenylketonuria.

Also in the first weeks, the baby will be given routine inoculations for polio, whooping cough (pertussis), diphtheria, and tetanus. Booster shots are given periodically in childhood. Smallpox vaccination is delayed until later in the first year.

Does breast-feeding provide contraception? Women who breast-feed exclusively, providing all their infant's sucking needs and nourishment without supplement, usually experience amenorrhea (lack of menstruation) as well as anovulation (lack of ovulation). These women experience an average of 15 months' spacing between children provided by breast-feeding. When supplemental feedings of mashed fruits and table foods are begun, the breast milk continues to provide the growing infant's liquid needs, and many women continue to have effective contraception. However, they *can* conceive even before a menstrual period has taken place, indicating the resumption of ovulation. A backup system of contraception is usually advised. Oral contraceptives diminish breast milk in most cases, and the mother will pass hormones to the baby via the breast milk. Therefore, a mechanical means of contraception rather than either oral or injected contraception is advised. The condom, diaphragm, or IUD, in combination with spermicidal foam or jelly, is effective when used consistently.

Child spacing is currently recognized as one of the most important determinants of the outcome of pregnancy. An interval of under two years between pregnancies is associated with smaller babies and higher rates of complications. In addition, the onset of a new pregnancy does affect the breast-feeding of the older child. Milk quantity diminishes during early pregnancy and the older child usually must be weaned. A two-year period between pregnancies allows the mother to recover completely, to care for her infant through the first two or three years without interruption, and to provide that infant with the best possible start in life.

Immunizing Your Children

According to the United States Department of Health, Education, and Welfare, many American children are vulnerable to polio, tetanus, diphtheria, whooping cough, measles, mumps, and rubella. Often these diseases may cause only minor discomfort. But they also can kill, and they all may have serious complications that could affect the child for the rest of his or her life.

Immunization against these diseases is safe and inexpensive. Check the calendar below to see whether your child's immunization program is up to date. You should have the information on the yellow card, Permanent Record of Immunizations and Tests, furnished by the health department when you received your child's birth certificate. If you don't have this card, check with your clinic or doctor.

2 months	• Diphtheria, Tetanus, Pertussis (DTP 3-in-1 shot) • The Sabin oral live polio vaccine
4 months	• DTP booster • Polio booster
6 months	• DTP booster
12 months	• Tuberculin test • Smallpox vaccination
15 months	• Measles/Rubella vaccine • Mumps vaccine
18 months	• DTP booster • Polio booster
4 to 6 years	• DTP booster • Polio booster

Pain in Labor and Delivery

Managing pain. About 12 percent of women find labor relatively painless. However, although most women will agree that labor contractions are painful, it is a mistake to assume that the pain of labor is like any other pain, and should be relieved by drugs. Labor pain is peculiar. It is not constant, but is brief and can be relieved by regular periods of rest. Labor pain is not of a single intensity but of varying intensities, and is usually greatest only for a few seconds at the peak of contractions. Labor pain is not the lancing pain of injury, but rather an aching, cramping pain that can be associated with positive functioning, great pressure, or the accomplishing of an important task. Women who have had severe menstrual cramps are often surprised at how easy labor contraction pain was to deal with.

The peculiar qualities of labor pain make it possible to use a number of techniques for relief that are safer—and often more effective—than drugs. In childbirth education classes, women practice techniques such as conscious concentration on muscular release and deliberate respiration patterns. Often, they practice these while their friend or partner simulates a contraction by gradual pressure on a group of thigh muscles, so that they become adept at focusing their attention on their own activity rather than on pain. Women who have a realistic knowledge of what to expect during labor and delivery and who practice these techniques intensively are well prepared for birth. They know that if they sit or walk as they wish, their labors will be faster and less painful.

However, women also need the constant support of an experienced nurse, midwife, or doctor during labor. Without this expert help, many well-prepared women discover that labor is frighteningly intense and that they feel unusually helpless. These mothers suffer needless pain and anxiety, or are easily persuaded to take medications as a substitute for help and encouragement.

Women who are prepared for birth and who have skilled support generally go through normal birth without drugs of any kind. In fact, such normal, unmedicated labors are frequent in most of the civilized world today. In Holland, for example, about 52 percent of women give birth at home, with constant expert help throughout the process, and without drugs.

The need for drugs in labor is clear in many cases, especially if the mother is unprepared or unsupported, if labor is prolonged, if the membranes have ruptured, if the mother is recumbent or immobilized, or if there is fetal malposition. Unfortunately, several of these circumstances are commonly found in hospital obstetrics today. Women are often unprepared—and many are badly frightened of the birth process and have been warned only of its dangers. Women are usually recumbent, and often the membranes have been ruptured in order to affix a screw electrode to the fetus' scalp. A large number of labors are still induced with uterine-stimulating hormones, and these labors are more painful. But the factor most associated with pain in labor is lack of constant expert help, and this is probably the most frequent failure of hospital obstetrics. Rarely is a maternity ward able to assign a nurse for constant support during labor. Not only are there too few nurses on duty, but nursing support in labor is not a money-earning procedure for the hospital, as are fetal monitoring, medications, and surgery. In fact, constant nursing support in labor may be looked upon as a wasteful use of personnel, and may be provided only for low-risk patients who use a hospital birth center.

During the 1960s, most states passed regulations requiring hospitals with more than 500 deliveries per year to provide 24-hour anesthesiology service for labor and delivery. The intent was to provide safer general and regional anesthesia, especially for emergencies in childbirth. However, since these regulations were passed, the number of cesareans has increased two to four times, and at many hospitals, anesthesiologists routinely give epidural anesthesia to all women unless they arrive too late in labor. Thus the added safety of expert anesthesiology has been accompanied by efforts to sell the services of these specialists, and an emphasis on the need for drugs in labor.

Are drugs used in labor and delivery safe? Many parents believe that no drug may be marketed unless it has been proved safe. However, the fact is that *no drug used in obstetrics has been proved safe for the fetus.* Instead, drug manufacturers are required to show only that a drug, when used in the recommended dosage and timing, has not been shown to be harmful to the fetus. The burden of proof falls on consumers and government agencies to show that a drug is harmful to the fetus. Although every drug used in obstetrics can be shown to have harmful side effects in particular instances, past attempts to compel warning labels on these drugs or to control the use of the drugs have met with failure, except in the case of oxytocin (Pitocin), which is used for the elective induction of labor. The usual argument put forth by obstetricians and anesthesiologists is that the benefit of the drug to the mother outweighs any supposed harm to the mother, labor process, or fetus.

This is obviously true in the case of real pathology during labor; women must be anesthetized for a cesarean section, for example. However, there is a growing certainty among parents and government regulatory agencies today that the benefits of many obstetrical drugs are less than advertised, that the risks are greater, and that safer alternatives to certain drugs should be more widely used. In particular, the use of any drug as a substitute for individual nursing and medical support and encouragement throughout labor is being rejected by well-informed parents.

Some parents also believe that certain drugs "do not reach the fetus." *There is no medication used in obstetrics that does not cross the placenta to the fetus.* For example, the five anesthetic agents used in epidurals (lidocaine, bupivacaine, etidocaine, mepivacaine, and prilocaine) each affect the fetus to varying degrees. Neonatal behavioral tests show that affected infants are less responsive for up to eight days after delivery. This is a very sensitive period for the parents to become emotionally attached to the infant, and a less responsive infant may elicit less emotional attachment from parents. In addition, these epidural agents affect the mother and the labor. The mother's blood pressure is lowered, and in 20 percent of these cases, circulation to the fetus is impaired so much that measurable oxygen deprivation is seen. Although the mother's blood pressure can be quickly raised to normal if it should drop, fetal oxygenation is much slower to respond, taking up to 20 minutes to return to normal. Finally, epidural anesthetic relaxes the pelvic floor so much that during the expulsion stage of labor, mothers are rarely able to push the baby through the final rotation under the pubic arch. Forceps are almost always required to assist epidural births.

Although all drugs used in obstetrics cross the placenta and reach the fetus, there are occasions when their use is necessary for medical indications. These should be explained to parents. Parents have a right to refuse any medication or treatment in labor and delivery, as well as afterward. Whether the benefit of a drug is worth the risk is a decision no doctor can make for the parents. This is because the risk is not one that the doctor runs. The parents must assume the risk of drug effects on their baby. Only they can decide whether, for example, pain relief is worth possible impaired attachment with the baby. The parents know, for example, if they may already run a risk of difficulty with attachment, perhaps because the baby was unplanned, or because they had poor parenting themselves. *Such a complex decision is one only parents can make.*

Characteristics of common obstetric drugs.
Probably the most widely used obstetric medication is a form of morphine or synthetic morphine. Demerol (morphine) is a pain medication given to the mother by injection. It is given in doses of from 50 milligrams (mg) to 200 or even 300 mg. This drug takes 20 minutes to work fully as a pain reliever, and at that time the mother usually notices some nausea and may vomit. She usually feels sleepy and disoriented. After about two hours, a 50-mg dose will begin to wear off, but at that point it is at its peak concentration in the fetus. Therefore, it is not advised to take Demerol if the delivery is expected within two hours because the baby may have difficulty breathing vigorously. The mother who has been given 100 mg or more of Demerol will feel definite nausea, and will be so disoriented that the siderails on the labor bed must be raised in order to keep her from falling off. She may scream or writhe at the peak of contractions, but will sleep otherwise. If Demerol is given early in labor, it will stop the contractions.

Women who have been given Demerol in labor generally dislike it. Almost without exception, they report that it made them feel agitated, helpless, and unable to react intelligently to contractions. Many still felt pain, but were simply unable to communicate this or to perform breathing and relaxation exercises to control their pain.

A better drug is Nisentil, a synthetic morphine that is given in smaller amounts, does not cause nausea in these small (30-mg) doses, and causes much less disorientation, sleepiness, and stupor than Demerol. It also is given by injection.

In the 1940s, a popular practice among obstetricians was to give 100 to 300 mg of Demerol with an amnesic agent called Scopolamine. This was known as twilight sleep. Women would be so agitated and disoriented that they were placed in restraints in order to keep from hurting themselves and others who tended them. The medication was repeated throughout labor, and the women woke hours after the birth with only the sense of having lived through a vague nightmare and wondering if they had had their babies yet. Some doctors and hospitals still use this combination of drugs, despite the high number of severely depressed babies born under it who require resuscitation and intensive care after delivery.

Recent studies on children from three days to eight years old have suggested that children whose mothers were given large doses of morphine and morphine with Scopolamine have specific neuromotor and intellectual impairments that persist into the school years. At three days of age, these babies typically were less responsive. They also had difficulty with a certain item on the newborn neuromuscular examination—the ability to stop responding to repetitive stimuli. In the school years, these children also had more reading and concentration difficulties than did children of mothers who did not receive large doses of morphine or morphine with Scopolamine during labor.

One medication technique that was popular during the late 1960s and early 1970s was paracervical block, in which anesthetic is injected around the cervix at several different points. This numbs the cervix immediately, and contractions are felt as mere tightenings in the abdomen. Occasionally, women with great back pain get relief from an extension of the paracervical block to the presacral area. This anesthetic acts locally and lasts about 45 minutes to 2 hours, depending on the drug used. Unfortunately, paracervical blocks are frequently associated with severe slowing of the fetal heart rate and fetal distress.

Another local injection may be given to numb the pudendal nerves that serve the birth canal and pelvic floor. This anesthetic is usually given if forceps delivery or an episiotomy is contemplated, and it is injected between pushes during the expulsion stage of labor. For stitching an episiotomy, a local anesthetic is injected around the incision itself, if no other anesthetic has been given.

Regional anesthesias include spinals, caudals, and epidurals. In each case, anesthetic is injected in or around the nerves in the low spinal area. Within 10 to 20 minutes, women feel numb in the toes up to the hips or waist. These medications can be continuous. The needle is left in place in the low back and a plastic catheter is threaded through it into the caudal or peridural space. This catheter is connected to plastic tubing that is taped to the mother's leg. Anesthetic is injected into the tubing as needed throughout labor.

These anesthetics can stop labor if given before about five centimeters of dilation. They also frequently cause a drop in the mother's blood pressure, which can result in diminished uterine circulation and consequent lack of oxygen to the baby. If the fetus is being electronically monitored, the heart rate pattern frequently loses its bouncy quality, known as "variability." This feature of the fetal heart pattern is the most indicative of fetal condition; loss of variability generally means some degree of fetal distress. There is a higher incidence of fetal malposition after regional anesthesias, especially failure of the fetus to flex the neck and rotate out from under the pubic arch at delivery. This, in turn, requires the use of forceps to assist the delivery. Regional anesthetics can prolong labor, and may have neurobehavioral effects on the newborn as well. These anesthetics generally are administered by an anesthesiologist, resulting in an anesthesia charge of from $50 to $150.

Parents often worry about accidents with regional anesthesia, and should be informed about their possibility as well as the benefits and side effects of anesthesia. Accidents are very rare, especially in well-staffed hospitals; however, most are very serious. For example, accidents reported with epidurals include:
- maternal convulsions, unconsciousness, and possible cardiac (heart) failure
- spinal cord injury
- accidental high segmental (total) spinal anesthesia, resulting in respiratory failure
- delayed recovery of sensation in lower extremities
- infection due to bacterial contamination of the catheter
- inadvertent overdose.

These accidents underscore the points made earlier. One is that no medication has been proven safe in obstetrics. Another is that only parents can make a risk/benefit decision, and routine use of a medication must be avoided. Certainly there is a place for epidural anesthesia in obstetrics. However, it has serious risks and should not be used as a substitute for thorough education and preparation of mothers, with constant expert support, coaching, and encouragement in labor. Many women who inform themselves of the effects of epidural anesthesia on labor, the fetus, and the mother will make a decision that such anesthesia is warranted only in the case of a cesarean section.

For this reason, anesthesiologists and obstetricians have frequently testified at hearings of the Food and Drug Administration that women must not be given "patient package inserts" that describe the drugs and their actions and risks. The information, however, is available in physician package inserts on the various epidural agents, including the statement that "Long-term studies of the effects of this drug have not been carried out in infants and children." In addition, several states have enacted laws requiring physicians to explain in detail each drug and procedure planned for use in labor and delivery, including the risks of each. Women whose states have not enacted such a law are still protected by the doctrine of "informed consent" whereby their requests for information on the risks of any drug or procedure must be fulfilled. One very easy way to find out about any drug is to consult *A Physicians' Desk Reference* or *PDR*. This book is published each year with up-to-date information for physicians on the indications, benefits, and risks of every drug marketed in the United States. A *PDR* is available at medical and public libraries. One may photocopy the material on a specific drug and bring this to the doctor for further explanation.

The last type of drug that is commonly used in labor and delivery is called an "inhalant anesthesia." This term covers any gas that is given to the mother to either "take the edge off the pain" or to provide general anesthesia for cesarean section. In Europe, it is common to provide mothers with hand-held masks through which they may give themselves nitrous oxide during labor contractions. If they get a certain amount of gas, they become dazed or unconscious and the hand holding the mask falls away from the mother's face. In the United States, such gases are available only with the attendance of an anesthesiologist, and usually only in a delivery room. This means that gas is really an expulsion-stage medication, or is used for general anesthesia before operative delivery. These anesthetic gases rapidly cross the placenta and immediately affect the fetus. Some actually concentrate in the fetal tissues. Therefore, care is usually taken to limit the mother's exposure to anesthetic gases. A general anesthetic for cesarean section, for example, may only be in effect 10 or 15 minutes before the baby is delivered through the incision in the abdomen. Whiffs of nitrous oxide in the delivery room between pushes are usually followed within minutes by the delivery of the baby.

Many women feel very strongly that they do not want to have their senses dulled during the delivery.

Probably the most striking change in obstetric anesthesia since women started to use hospitals for childbirth in the 1930s is the reduced use, in the last 15 years, of general anesthesia in obstetrics.

This reduction has taken place not only because of changes in the wishes of mothers, but also because general anesthesia is associated with a very high rate of complications and even deaths. Many women under gas will vomit, and if they have eaten a meal just prior to labor, they may inhale particles of food into their lungs, causing respiratory collapse or pneumonia. This problem can be averted by intubating women under general anesthesia—that is, by passing a tube into their lungs through which anesthetic gas is administered. Even with various precautions, however, the mortality rate from accidents with general anesthesia makes it the most hazardous of obstetric medications. General anesthesia is therefore usually reserved for those cesarean sections in which regional anesthesia is not preferred, either by the doctor or by the mother.

Regional and Local Anesthesia in Labor and Delivery

Many women today give birth with little or no anesthesia. A greater awareness of labor and delivery procedures has led to careful psychological and physical preparation for giving birth. Natural childbirth classes, nutrition and exercise classes, cooperation between the mother and her physician or midwife, access to alternate birth methods, and participation of the father and other loved ones in the birth process have greatly lessened the pain and fear that were a part of modern birth processes. However, for many very good reasons, childbirth for some women is not manageable without pain relief. A crisis in the birth process for the mother or fetus may make anesthesia necessary, or you may feel that you cannot go through labor and delivery without an anesthetic for pain. If so, tell your physician or midwife in advance. You may not use the anesthesia or the anesthesiologist, but you will know that drugs are there if you need them.

Pain in labor comes from two sources: (1) the walls of the uterus and cervix, whose nerves enter the spinal cord at the level of the arrow in the first diagram on page 294 (refer to the illustrated chart on pages 294 and 295 for information on regional and local anesthesia in labor and delivery), and (2) the perineum, which is the area of muscle and tissue between the thighs extending from the tailbone to the pubic arch, and including the lower third of the vagina, the muscles of the pelvic floor, and the external genitalia. The nerve supplying the

perineum is the pudendal nerve, which can be most simply deadened by an injection at the level of the arrow in the pudendal block diagram on page 295.

Anesthetic agents used in labor and delivery are quite varied, but all are members of the "-caine" class of drugs, including procaine, lidocaine, and novocaine. Each drug has its own properties, including its ability to cross the placental barrier and affect the fetus. A great deal is known about the effects of these drugs on the mother, but much less about the effects on the fetus. Generally, the use of drugs may lower the Apgar score of the fetus (see page 284), meaning that the general health of the infant immediately after birth (heart rate, color, cry, muscle tone, and reflexes) is not optimal.

Each anesthetic agent takes effect in from one to ten minutes, lasts for three-quarters to three hours, and is used at a variety of stages of labor and delivery.

Analgesic agents are distinct from anesthetic agents. Analgesics, not illustrated in the chart, are taken by mouth or injection. Analgesics are tranquilizers or narcotics that are given in the first phase of labor to decrease discomfort from uterine contractions. An analgesic usually makes you sleepy and relaxed, and too much analgesic can lengthen the first phase of labor. Analgesic agents affect the fetus much like anesthesia by slowing the heart rate and muscle and reflex response during birth. Again, the exact effects on the fetus are not known.

Regional and Local Anesthesia in Labor and Delivery continued

Also refer to the box on the preceding page.

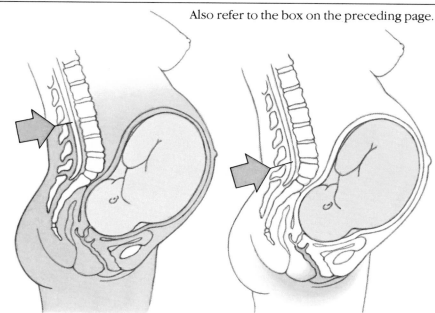
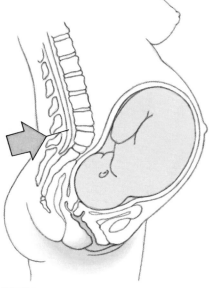
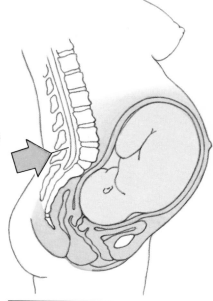

Spinal
(Lumbar sympathetic block)
A regional anesthesia for delivery rather than for the earlier stages of labor. Anesthesia is injected into the spinal fluid or canal.
Area affected Paralysis of the body from the area of injection downward for the duration of the anesthesia.
Advantages Deadens all pain during the delivery phase only. The mother remains conscious (but not active) during delivery.
Disadvantages for the mother
● The mother cannot push or take active part in delivery. ● 8 to 20 percent of women have postpartum headaches. ● Risk of rapid lowering of blood pressure. ● Allergic reactions possible in rare cases. ● Respiratory failure may occur.
Disadvantages for the baby
● Forceps usually are required since the mother cannot push.
● Risk of blood pressure becoming erratic or lowered as the drug is carried across the placental barrier; exact effects on the fetus are not known.

Saddle block
(Subarachnoid block)
A regional anesthesia for delivery rather than for the earlier stages of labor. Anesthesia is injected into the spinal fluid or canal approximately one hour before delivery.
Area affected The buttocks, the perineum, and the inner thighs.
Advantages Excellent relief of pain during the late second stage of labor and delivery. The mother remains conscious during delivery.
Disadvantages for the mother
● Rapid fall in blood pressure may occur. Blood pressure decreases in 20 to 50 percent of women. ● 8 to 20 percent of women have postpartum headaches. ● Allergic reactions to the drug or breathing difficulties occur only rarely.
Disadvantages for the baby
● Forceps delivery may be required because pelvic tissues of the mother are relaxed, not pushing. ● The fetus may have a drop in blood pressure, since the drug crosses the placental barrier; exact effects on the fetus are not known.

Epidural
A regional anesthesia injected into the epidural space near the spinal canal (but not into it) after cervical dilation of 5 cm. Administered by a highly skilled anesthesiologist as multiple injections through a catheter during the latter part of the first stage and all of the second stage of labor, *or* as a single injection just before delivery.
Area affected Numbs the body from the waist down, but movement is still possible.
Advantages Almost complete removal of pain of labor and delivery. No postpartum headaches. The mother is awake throughout delivery.
Disadvantages for the mother
● Danger of a rapid drop in blood pressure, irregular heart rhythm, and convulsions. ● The mother can't bear down and push well.
● Episiotomy frequently is needed.
Disadvantages for the baby
● Because the pelvic floor is relaxed, the baby's head does not rotate, necessitating forceps rotation and delivery. ● The drug crosses the placental barrier; exact effects on the fetus are not known.

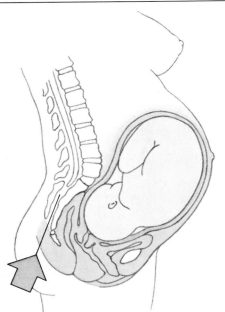

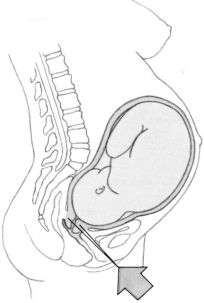

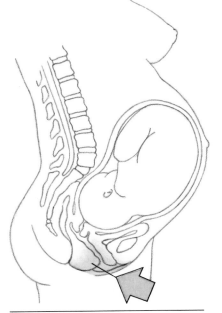

Caudal
A regional anesthetic injected near the end of the spinal canal after the cervix has dilated to 5 cm; requires an experienced anesthesiologist. Sometimes administered in the first, second, and delivery stages of labor.

Area affected Deadens pain in the pelvic area, including the uterus and perineum.

Advantages If administered successfully from early labor through delivery, there is no labor pain at all for 80 percent of women, neither from uterine contraction nor perineum stretching.

Disadvantages for the mother
● Same as for saddle block and epidural, especially the danger of a rapid drop in blood pressure.
● Impairs the length and strength of uterine contractions and thus prolongs labor. ● The danger in giving a caudal early in labor is that it will cease to be effective before the delivery or even a prolonged labor is complete.

Disadvantages for the baby
● Depressed general state from prolonged labor. ● Forceps delivery likely. ● Of all the regional anesthetics, this one seems least harmful to the baby.

Paracervical block
A local anesthetic given in labor or near delivery. An injection is made directly into the cervix during the latter half of labor to relieve the pain of cervical stretching. Additional anesthesia is required for delivery, since a paracervical block does not affect the pudendal nerve.

Area affected The cervix and the uterus.

Advantages Instantaneous relief of pain. Relatively simple to administer.

Disadvantages for the mother
● This is not long-lasting pain relief, and additional anesthesia is required for delivery.

Disadvantages for the baby
● Paracervicals are now under intense investigation since they cause the fetal heartbeat to slow alarmingly. ● Danger of direct injection into the fetal scalp.

Pudendal block
This is a local anesthesia given just before delivery by injections on either side of the vagina that deaden the pudendal nerve. The anesthesia does not relieve the pain of labor.

Area affected All tissues between the tailbone and the pubic arch (the perineum), including the lower third of the vagina and the external genitalia.

Advantages Pain relief for the last stages of delivery and for episiotomy, as well as for a low forceps delivery.

Disadvantages for the mother
● It does not always relieve pain sufficiently.

Disadvantages for the baby
● Very safe; few if any known ill effects for the baby.

Exercises for During and After Pregnancy

Postural Correction

Probably the most common muscular disability among women and men is poor posture. This becomes even more obvious during pregnancy. As weight of the growing fetus increases, such poor posture can result in multiple complications. For example, notice in the slouching woman "A" that the lower back is arched forward in what is known as "lordosis." This is a position of the spine that causes backache. Notice also the locked knees in woman "A." Standing and walking with hyperextended or locked knees is hard on the knee joints, and forces the body into lordosis. Finally, notice the protuberant abdomen in woman "A" with stretched, weakened abdominal muscles. The whole weight of the fetus, uterus, and abdominal contents is leaning out against these abdominal muscles. In contrast, the woman who has corrected her posture, woman "B," has pulled her abdominal muscles in, and the baby and organs are now in proper alignment in the cradle of the pelvis. **How to do the pelvic tilt.** Have a friend place one hand on your abdomen and the other on your low back while you are standing. Feel the area of the low back by moving the hand along the spinal column. Then, tuck your pelvis under and forward, pulling in on your abdominal muscles, and straightening your low back. If you are doing this correctly, you will find that your knees automatically pop forward in an unlocked position, and you also may find that you have some trouble expanding your chest to breathe. So the final step in the pelvic tilt is to hold your good posture while you expand your rib cage in a relaxed, normal breath. If you find your shoulders elevated in the "soldier" position, lower and loosen them comfortably.

Repeat this maneuver, alternately sagging and correcting your posture while your friend feels to make sure that your low back is actually straightening and your abdomen is flattening. Breathe normally, and loosen your shoulders. The last step is to walk around while doing this pelvic tilt. Sit and try this movement, too. You may find that a small pillow in the low back helps because you can press it flat as you do your postural correction. If you have trouble remembering to keep yourself erect in good posture, ask a friend to remind you, or put little signs up around your house where you spend the most time, with reminders to correct your posture and exercise your pelvic floor.

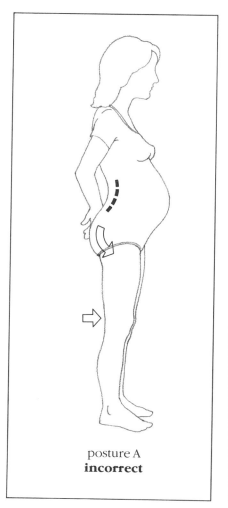

posture A
incorrect

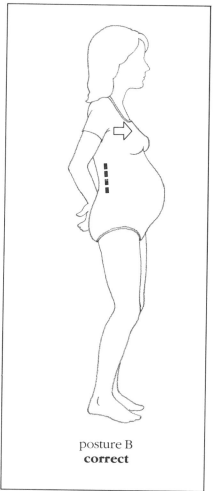

posture B
correct

Exercises for the Pelvic Floor Muscles

Control of the pelvic floor is necessary during pelvic examinations, and during the expulsive stage of birth. Some women also find pelvic floor control prevents accidental escape of urine late in pregnancy. You can recover strength and muscle tone around the vagina and anus by contracting and relaxing the muscles in a pattern known as the "elevator exercise."

The elevator exercise. Sitting on the toilet during urination, stop the flow of urine and then start it again. Start and stop the flow until it becomes easy to do. Now, stop the flow and further contract the muscles as hard and completely as possible. From this maximally contracted position, pretend that your pelvic floor is an elevator in a five-story building, and that you are letting the "elevator" descend slowly, stopping at each floor. When you get to a resting position, that is the "first floor." Finally, hold your breath and push out on the pelvic floor as if the "elevator" is descending to the basement. Hold your breath for a few seconds, and then let your muscles relax again. Do this exercise whenever you think about it during the day. You will gain perfect bladder control, be able to relax the muscles for pelvic examinations, be able to consciously push in the most advantageous way for delivery, and last but not least, you will regain normal muscle tone after delivery.

Regular, Active Sports

Some people enjoy doing a series of exercises each day, but most people forget them or find them boring. In fact, very few exercises are useful for normal people who simply want to keep fit. Instead, vigorous active sports are required to keep fit. This is because all the muscles, the heart, lungs, and organs are stimulated by such activity. So, during pregnancy and as soon as you feel rested afterward, join with friends in yoga or a regular active sport— swimming, running, tennis, or even walking. Studies have shown that a half-hour of vigorous activity that makes you breathe hard four times a week will keep you physically fit into old age.

Exercises to Avoid During and After Pregnancy

A lot of advice is given to pregnant women about exercises by people who are well-meaning, but who do not know kinesiology or therapeutic exercise. There are a few exercises that are not simply useless, but actually carry a potential risk for pregnant and newly delivered women. A basic rule of thumb is: Don't ever do anything that hurts. Don't do exercises that require you to lie flat on your back during late pregnancy, because the heavy uterus can reduce blood flow in the large artery passing through the abdomen, making you feel dizzy and even slowing blood flow to the uterus. *Never do sit-ups to strengthen the abdominal muscles.* This exercise is far too dangerous for the low back and the pregnant abdomen. Even in very strong men who build up their muscles, sit-ups must be done with careful supervision to avoid several common types of muscle strain. Sit-ups are useless for normal abdominal strength, and should be replaced by habitual pelvic-tilt posture correction. Finally, unless you are specifically told to do back-arching exercises by an orthopedist or physical therapist, do not do exercises that involve arching your back. These actually force the back and abdomen into the positions that postural correction is designed to remedy, and are useless and possibly even dangerous.

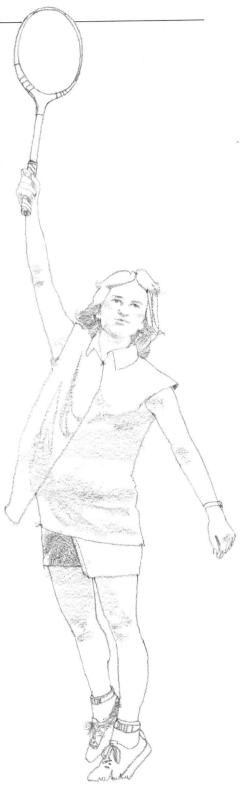

Procedures in Hospital Birth

Episiotomy is a scissors incision made in the skin below the vaginal opening by the obstetrician at the moment of blanching of the skin as the baby is about to emerge. Although the incision is intended to prevent tearing during the delivery, it also speeds up the delivery. After delivery, the incision is sutured; the stitches dissolve in a few days. There may be swelling, burning, and aching at the site of the incision for a few days or a week. Resumption of usual sexual relations is sometimes delayed by an episiotomy. The scar remains as a numb area in the tissues. Episiotomy is done in at least 90 percent of hospital deliveries in the United States, but in only about 10 percent of birth-center and home deliveries, and in only 12 to 15 percent of hospital deliveries in European countries, with a few exceptions. How can these differences in obstetric practice be explained?

• The position of the mother on the delivery table on her back with her legs held apart in stirrups makes over-stretching and tearing of the skin more likely than if the mother delivered with no leg restraints or with full mobility.

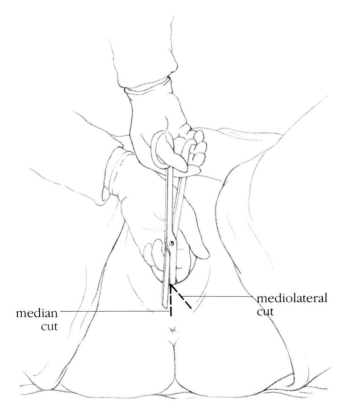

median cut

mediolateral cut

EPISIOTOMY

Episiotomy is a scissors incision made in the skin below the vaginal opening (perineum) by the obstetrician at the moment of blanching of the skin. It is done to prevent tearing during delivery.

• Most obstetricians trained in the United States do not know how to support and massage the intact perineum during delivery and thus assist dilation of the skin without tearing. They have been trained exclusively in delivery-table obstetrics, and may only have seen precipitous deliveries take place without an episiotomy. Since precipitous deliveries often cause tears, obstetricians may decide that delivery without an episiotomy causes tears.

• Obstetricians may prefer a quick delivery. They may associate the second stage of labor with fetal distress. Although expulsion is stressful for the fetus, many authorities say that this stress is necessary to stimulate the baby to breathe actively at birth. Indeed, normal birth without episiotomy is not associated with poor infant outcomes.

• Obstetricians generally feel that episiotomy preserves the tone of the pelvic floor muscles. However, in countries where episiotomy is not routine, no higher incidence of weak pelvic floor muscles is reported.

• Episiotomy may be necessitated by certain regional anesthetics, such as epidural, spinal, and caudal, which often require the use of forceps. Episiotomy also may be required to make enough room to insert and apply the forceps to the baby's head.

How can parents be assured that their wishes for no episiotomy will be respected in a hospital delivery? No one can tell if an episiotomy will be needed until the baby's head crowns or shows at the outlet of the birth canal. Parents can request that an episiotomy be avoided if at all possible, and most doctors will try to respect their wishes.

Beyond this, parents can decrease the chances of needing an episiotomy by making sure that the mother has developed good control over the pelvic floor muscles and knows how to bulge out the area for delivery. Massage of the perineum is thought by some to help the skin distend without tearing, and the use of various vitamin oils is recommended. Parents also can avoid doctors and hospitals with high rates of regional anesthesia use. Choosing a doctor or hospital that is not excessively busy will reduce the chances of an unnecessary episiotomy, as well as other procedures that are designed to save staff time, such as induction and augmentation of labor, medication instead of support in labor, and fetal monitoring. Finally, parents can choose a hospital nurse-midwifery service, a general practitioner, or a foreign-trained or older obstetrician, since these attendants are more likely to know how to deliver a baby without an episiotomy, as well as without a tear.

It is reassuring to know that, if an episiotomy is needed at the last minute, the mother will not feel the incision because the pressure of the fetal head fully numbs the pelvic nerves and the perineum. However, after the birth, when the stitching is to be done, a local anesthetic is injected. In some cases the doctor will inject a local anesthetic prior to the birth between pushes, in order to be ready to suture the incision afterward without further injections. This local anesthetic given between pushes is called a pudendal block, because it numbs the pudendal nerves, which give sensation to the birth canal and the pelvic floor.

Forceps are used in nearly all deliveries in which the mother is given a regional anesthetic, including the most common—epidural. Spinal, caudal, and continuous forms of these three anesthesias also usually necessitate forceps assistance at the end of delivery because the mother is unable to push effectively, and because her pelvic tissues are too relaxed by the anesthetic to rotate the baby as needed for delivery.

The four types of forceps are high, mid-forceps, low, and outlet forceps. High forceps are applied before the cervix is fully dilated. Most obstetricians agree that cesarean delivery is preferable to high-forceps delivery, since surgery is less dangerous to the baby than prolonged forceps traction on the baby's head. Mid-forceps also are usually avoided by most doctors today for the same reason. Mid-forceps are applied after full dilation of the cervix, but before descent of the baby in the birth canal. Low forceps are applied during descent of the baby, and outlet forceps are used during the crowning of the head. The baby's head is simply lifted out from under the pubic arch and delivered. Outlet forceps are the most common type.

Before using forceps, the doctor usually anesthetizes the birth canal, unless regional anesthesia has already been given. A pudendal block is sufficient in most cases to obtain relaxation of the birth canal, along with anesthesia. It is rarely necessary to give the mother inhalant gas to "knock her out" for forceps delivery, nor is it necessary to use a regional anesthetic such as a spinal simply because forceps are being used. The smallest amount of anesthetic that will work is to be preferred, both for the mother and the baby. Most doctors agree on this point, but it is wise for the parents to have a clear understanding of it ahead of time.

FORCEPS DELIVERY

Forceps are shaped like shallow, long-handled spoons. They are inserted one at a time around the baby's head, and, depending on the style of instrument used, they either lock together or are braced against the edge of the delivery table. Gentle traction is then exerted on the baby's head, as well as rotation, if necessary.

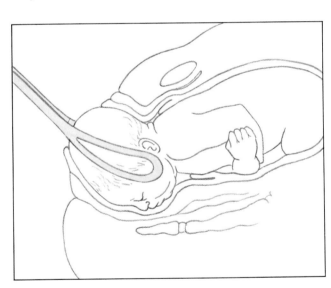

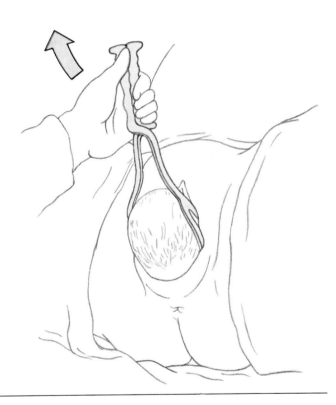

HEAD TRAUMA

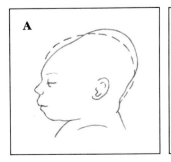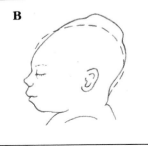

A FORCEPS DELIVERY *Prolonged, forceful application of forceps traction on the baby's head may lead to head molding and forceps injury.*
B VACUUM EXTRACTION DELIVERY *This baby was born after vacuum extraction, and has severe molding of the cranial bones—a common occurrence in this procedure.*

Forceps are shaped like shallow, long-handled spoons. They are inserted one at a time around the baby's head, and, depending on the style of instrument used, they either lock together or are braced against the edge of the delivery table. Gentle traction is then exerted on the baby's head, as well as rotation if necessary. The mother may be asked to push in order to assist this traction.

Do forceps injure the baby? With the advent of more liberal cesarean sections and fewer difficult forceps deliveries, there are fewer forceps injuries. The baby may have small red bruises where the blades pressed, and these may last for one to three days after delivery.

In Europe, vacuum extraction is used more often than forceps. The vacuum extractor is a cuplike device that is inserted as early as seven to eight centimeters' dilation of the cervix, in rare cases. The cup is applied to the fetal head with suction, and the baby is then gently pulled down and rotated as needed for birth. Vacuum extraction is also called ventouse extraction. This technique is associated with less cervical injury, less injury to the vaginal tissues, and less pressure on the baby's head. Vacuum extraction is used very little in the United States, although some doctors are experienced in its use. One reason for its low popularity may be the severe molding of the baby's head caused by the suction cup.

Induction and augmentation of contractions is done by injecting a uterine-stimulating drug called oxytocin (Pitocin) or, as in recent experimental cases, prostaglandin. Induction of labor is so common that some hospitals report that over half of their births are induced. This practice is defended on the grounds that:
• Women want to plan ahead of time for the birth.
• Doctors want to schedule births when they are not having office hours or are not away.
• Births should take place during daytime business hours when all the hospital's laboratories and personnel are available.
• Births can be timed to avoid crowded periods in the maternity unit.
• Induction is harmless.
• Induction avoids post-term deliveries, with their attendant dangers.

However, recent attacks on induction of labor were persuasive enough to cause the Food and Drug Administration (FDA) to ban oxytocin for the elective induction of labor on the following grounds:
• Induction of labor is associated with accidental premature delivery often enough that in several studies, 10 percent of the premature babies in hospital neonatal intensive-care units had been induced.
• Induction of labor is associated with increased episodes of fetal distress due to unduly long, strong uterine contractions.
• Induction occasionally fails, and a cesarean section must be resorted to. Induction occasionally causes uterine rupture or postpartum hemorrhage as well.
• Induction is associated with increased incidence of neonatal jaundice.
• Studies have shown that, although induction rates have increased to over 50 percent in some hospitals, the incidence of post-term delivery has remained the same.
• Exposing the infant to the risks of induction without medical indication or reason is not justified by added convenience to the mother, the doctor, or the hospital.

This action of the FDA may reduce inductions of labor. However, the advantages of induction to the doctor and the hospital are so great that some observers think that doctors will be tempted to simply assign a medical indication or reason for induction when there really is none, or perhaps to use a new substitute for oxytocin, such as prostaglandin. Parents who wish to have their labors induced or augmented only if there is a clear medical indication are entitled to a full explanation of the reasons for this procedure, the alternatives, what drug is planned, and the risks of the drug and the procedure. Parents can get a copy of the physician's package insert, which comes with all drugs and which is published in an annual encyclopedia of drugs called the *Physicians' Desk Reference,* available at public libraries. Parents also may simply refuse to undergo the procedure.

Indications for induction include true postmaturity of the fetus. If definite dates for conception or the last menstrual period can be determined, and if the pregnancy is carried two to three weeks beyond the normal 40-week gestation period, then true postmaturity of the fetus may be suspected. It should be verified by withdrawing a small amount of amniotic fluid (amniocentesis) and examining it for fetal skin and fat cells. An ultrasound scan of the fetus and placenta also may determine postmaturity by showing cystic and fibrous areas in the placenta. If induction of labor is not carried out and the pregnancy is allowed to continue beyond two weeks after the due date, the chances are increased for placental compromise during labor, and for the birth of a baby who has actually lost weight in the final weeks, and has become wizened and stressed in the process.

Induction of labor may be wise in the presence of several other high-risk conditions that affect the baby and placenta, including maternal Rh sensitization, diabetes, hypertension and toxemia, and the small-for-gestational-age fetus. Each of these conditions involves increasing danger for the fetus as it grows, or as the demands on the placenta increase toward the end of pregnancy. The decision must be carefully made as to whether the fetus is better off in the uterus receiving uncertain nourishment and oxygen, or in the intensive-care nursery where he or she can be certain of being well nourished and oxygenated. Several tests of placental functioning are available to pinpoint exactly when the risks of continuing the pregnancy are greater than the risks of induction or cesarean, with subsequent intensive care for the baby.

One such test is of fetal lung maturity. Amniocentesis is the procedure used, and the cells are examined for the ratio of lecithin to sphyngomyelin cells from the fetal lungs. In the mature fetus, there should be at least twice as many lecithin cells as sphyngomyelin cells. This is called the L/S ratio test.

In the presence of a high-risk fetus, induction should be preceded by a test to determine how well the fetus withstands contractions. The mother has an external fetal monitor attached (two belts that encircle her waist). Contractions are stimulated, either by pressing the uterus to the side, or if that fails to elicit enough contractions, by injecting a small amount of uterine-stimulating hormone and waiting for several contractions. The fetus who withstands contractions well will have a heart-rate tracing that is bouncy and shows some speeding up with contractions. The fetus who gets too little oxygen during contractions because of a failing placenta will show a heart-rate tracing that lacks the bouncy quality, or that slows down during and after contractions.

How is induction done? After the usual hospital admission procedures, the cervix is examined to see if it is soft and thin. If so, the doctor may "rim the cervix"—running a finger around the cervix to stimulate it to start dilating. Then the membranes will be broken, because loss of the amniotic fluid often causes the uterus to contract. An IV will be installed in the mother's arm, connected to a constant infusion pump that administers electronically controlled amounts of uterine-stimulating hormone. This pump sits on a bedside stand.

Every effort is made to mimic natural contractions, both in terms of their strength and duration. However, artificially produced contractions do feel quite different to the mother than natural contractions. They come on more suddenly, and the peaks are usually prolonged. Therefore, these contractions may be somewhat harder to handle with the relaxation and breathing techniques learned in prenatal classes. Although many mothers manage quite well, others find it necessary to request pain medication (see page 290).

EXTERNAL FETAL MONITORING

The most commonly used electronic monitoring method is called external because it relies on two elastic belts that are wrapped around the mother's abdomen. One belt holds a device that picks up the fetal heart sounds and electronically transmits them to a printout console beside the bed. The other belt holds a device that records each uterine contraction. The belts with the pickup device are placed directly on the skin. The external monitor belts are confining and the system is not very accurate.

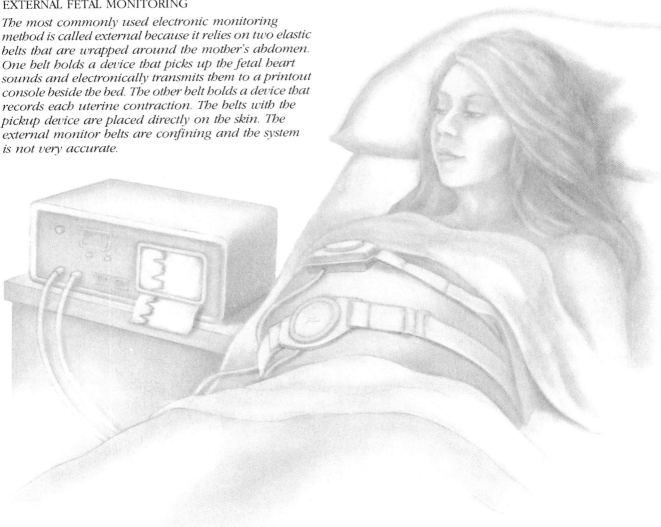

INTERNAL FETAL MONITORING

The internal fetal monitor employs a spiral-shaped needle electrode (A) that is rotated into the skin of the fetal scalp after the cervix has sufficiently dilated (2 to 3 cm) to allow its attachment. This electrode records the fetal heart rate, while a thin plastic hose, threaded past the fetus into the uterus, records the contractions (B). Again, the fetal heart rate and uterine contractions are printed continuously on a paper strip chart that rolls slowly out of the bedside console. This is a more accurate system than external monitoring, but is no better than a skilled nurse with a stethoscope, according to three of four comparative studies.

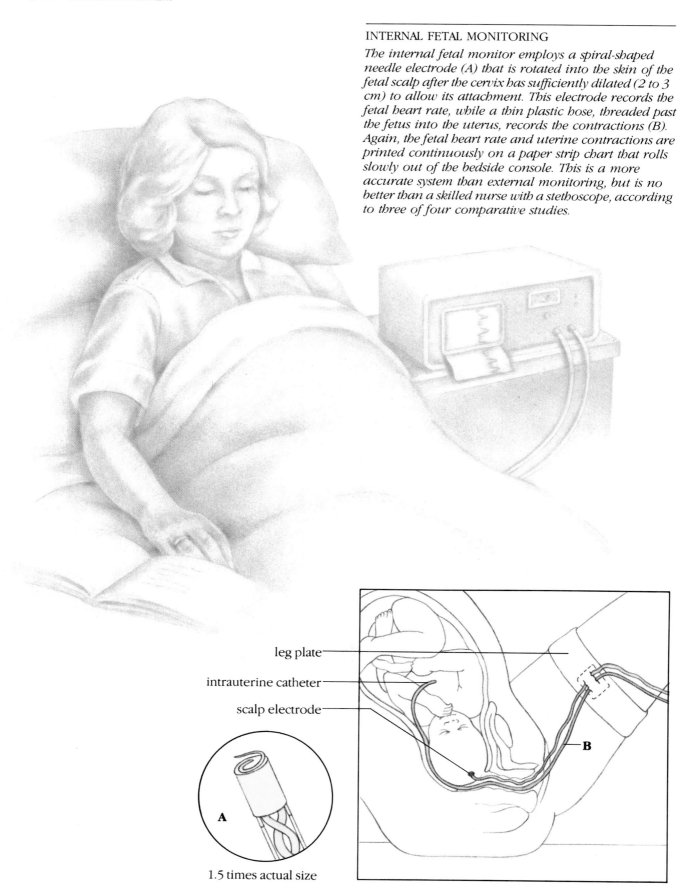

leg plate

intrauterine catheter

scalp electrode

A

1.5 times actual size

B

Fetal monitoring: nurse or machine? One very common procedure in hospital births is electronic fetal monitoring. This is often done routinely in all births, but in any high-risk birth or induced labor, many doctors think electronic monitoring is mandatory. There are two electronic monitoring methods. The most commonly used is called external monitoring because it relies on two elastic belts that are wrapped around the mother's abdomen. One belt holds a device that picks up the fetal heart sounds and electronically transmits them to a printout console beside the bed. The other belt holds a device that records each uterine contraction. This monitor is easy for any nurse's aide to apply, and is often used routinely to screen women in labor. If any problems arise, a more elaborate internal monitor system is used.

Parents generally have mixed feelings about the monitor. The husband may be fascinated by the electronics, and the mother may like being able to actually "see" her contractions begin, peak, and end. Women who have had a problematic or tragic prior labor find the monitor reassuring, while others often find it a nuisance or even frightening. From a technical standpoint, the external monitor is frequently thought of as worse than nothing. This is because it is extremely unreliable, producing illegible tracings about 40 to 60 percent of the time. Even worse, the majority of external monitors employ ultrasound, which can actually reverse the three major signs of fetal distress. Several lawsuits have been brought against monitor manufacturers and hospitals because severely depressed infants were born with "normal" monitor tracings from external monitors.

Added to these technical flaws are a number of practical problems posed by monitors. The machinery frequently sits beside the bed, right where the husband would need to be in order to administer a back rub or help his wife with her breathing and relaxation. The mother is recumbent, and often she cannot even roll over because the monitor may not pick up the fetal heart sounds unless the mother is on her back. Much of the protection and stimulation of being up and about in labor is thus lost. Some researchers have decided that, to a certain extent, electronic monitors actually *cause* some or all of the fetal distress that they are designed to record.

The internal fetal monitor employs a spiral-shaped needle electrode that is rotated into the skin of the fetal scalp after the cervix has dilated enough to allow its attachment (2 to 3 cm). This electrode records the fetal heart rate, while a thin plastic hose, threaded past the fetus into the uterus, records the contractions. Again, the fetal heart rate and uterine contractions are printed continuously on a paper strip chart that rolls slowly out of the bedside console. The internal fetal monitor is reserved for high-risk labors because it is difficult to use. It is very accurate in picking up the fetal heart rate, but there is no agreement among monitor researchers as to exactly what type of tracing warrants what kind of treatment. One study, for example, has shown that 80 percent of the fetal heart patterns that look like fetal distress are really just normal stress patterns. The only way to really tell whether these ominous "squiggles" really indicate fetal distress is to do what is called a fetal scalp blood sampling.

Fetal blood sampling involves a pelvic examination and the insertion of a lighted cone-shaped speculum. This instrument enables the doctor to see the fetal scalp through the dilating cervix, with the spiral electrode in place. The doctor nicks the scalp and draws some of the fetus' blood into a tiny pipette. This blood is then put into a blood-gas analyzer, which tells the doctor whether it is abnormally acid, indicating that the fetus lacks oxygen. Normally, the fetal blood pH (acid-base balance) is about 7.3. If the reading is as low as 7.25, then the doctor must decide whether this is transient stress or progressive distress. *Only a second fetal blood sampling will tell which is the case.* Since each fetal blood sampling takes 10 to 20 minutes, this is a time-consuming procedure. In fact, this procedure takes longer than the average cesarean section.

It is not difficult to understand why cesarean sections have nearly tripled and quadrupled in most hospitals since fetal monitoring began. Of course, not all of these cesareans are due to monitoring. Some are due to medical preference for cesarean over a difficult forceps delivery or a breech delivery. Also, more women with medical problems are attempting childbearing today — and successfully — with the help of cesareans.

However, in about a dozen research centers where monitor tracings are routinely checked with fetal blood sampling if they show distress patterns, cesarean rates for fetal distress have actually gone down. This care to avoid unnecessary cesarean sections is important when one considers that a vaginal birth has many advantages for both the mother and the baby, and a cesarean birth has eight times the mortality rate of a vaginal birth. Cesareans also have considerable added cost and morbidity, such as infections and pain for the mother.

Most hospitals simply do not have the required personnel to do careful fetal monitoring. Most of the researchers who work with monitoring state that nursing and medical staff, as well as repair and maintenance staff, must be *increased* in order to use monitors properly. However, outside of a very few university training centers, monitors are used largely to replace the nursing staff at the mother's bedside.

Parents have a right to refuse to be electronically monitored during labor. This might be a reasonable course if:
• There is no fetal blood-gas analyzer in the labor and delivery unit. (Two floors down in Respiration Therapy is not sufficient.)
• The hospital has a very high cesarean section rate — over 20 percent.
• The hospital has no personnel assigned specifically and exclusively to do fetal monitoring.
• The hospital does mostly external monitoring "as a screening method."

However, any high-risk mother would be wise to go to a large regional perinatal center where maternal and newborn intensive care is practiced on a daily basis. There, she can decide whether she wants to be machine-monitored or nurse-monitored. In a study of over 1,000 high-risk labors, half of which were nurse-monitored and half of which were electronically monitored, the infants were found to be comparable in every way measured, including their physical scores at birth (Apgar scores) and their condition in the nursery.

Since most hospitals do not have enough nurses to assign one to each high-risk woman in labor, parents have recently discovered that they can hire their own private nurse for this purpose. Such a nurse should be chosen very carefully, since the use of the fetal stethoscope is no longer being taught very extensively in most training programs. A certified nurse-midwife, an older nurse with experience in labor and delivery, or a specially trained labor monitress may be skilled enough to monitor a high-risk labor. This nurse should be willing to give constant support, and should be acceptable to the doctor and the hospital staff.

Treatment of fetal distress. Fetal distress during labor is signaled by changes in the fetal heart rate, and is caused by lack of sufficient oxygen. Oxygen is provided to the fetus by transfer from the mother to the placenta, via her bloodsteam, and thence to the fetus through the umbilical cord. Fetal distress is most likely in labors that are "high risk." The most common high-risk condition in labor is the preterm or premature delivery. This accounts for about 7 percent of all deliveries, and for 70 to 75 percent of all high-risk deliveries. The premature fetus withstands the normal stress of labor poorly, both in terms of natural oxygen deficit, which is part of normal labor, and in terms of compression of the head during labor and delivery. In addition, the smaller preterm placenta is more easily compromised by contractions of labor.

Several less common high-risk conditions also affect the placenta or its ability to provide oxygen and nutrients to the fetus. The "small-for-dates" or "small-for-gestational-age" fetus may have intrauterine growth retardation due to a poorly functioning placenta. Labor contractions may decrease the placental functioning further, irreparably damaging the baby. Diabetes in the mother, hypertension, toxemia, and placental malposition in the uterus also affect the function of the placenta, especially during labor. The postmature fetus, one that is two to three weeks overdue, may be stressed by an aging placenta that has less exchange capacity.

Many of the high-risk conditions that are known to exist as a woman nears labor or that arise during labor will be managed by close supervision, prelabor tests, induction of labor, and/or cesarean section.

Although it is relatively unusual, fetal distress can occur without warning in an otherwise low-risk, normal labor. The most common source of this type of fetal distress is compression of the umbilical cord. About 30 percent of fetuses have a loop of umbilical cord wrapped around them one to three times. In these and other labors, the cord may periodically become compressed between the bones of the pelvis and a bony part of the fetus. Normally, the cord is quite stiff with blood flowing through it very fast. It resists compression and knotting, much as a garden hose resists compression when water is flowing through it under great pressure. However, occasionally the mother's blood pressure drops, or the cord becomes compressed for long enough to shut off the flow of blood to the baby and cause well-recognized fetal heart-rate changes that reflect distress.

How common are these cord compression episodes? How are they prevented and managed in labor? Cord compression is very common in the expulsion stage of labor. Between pushes, a nurse listens to the fetal heart to make sure it recovers from its slowing with each contraction. If the birth takes a long time, and if the fetal heart rate remains slow between contractions, the use of forceps may be considered, or perhaps the mother will be asked to push in an upright position.

Transient cord compression patterns are common during normal labor as well as expulsion. Usually the fetus and mother move enough during labor to relieve cord compression if it occurs. In fact, in a series of four studies from Europe, the United States, and Australia, it was found that when women were allowed to walk and sit and generally be ambulant during labor, continuous fetal monitoring tracings revealed *no cord compression patterns*. This is remarkable, since cord compression is a frequent feature of most monitored labors. So, being up and about during labor is the best protection for the fetus against the most common cause of fetal distress in normal labor — cord compression.

How serious is cord compression to the baby? The answer depends on the condition of the baby in general, and on the state of the mother and the labor. Under normal circumstances — when the full-term fetus is of good size and the mother has normal blood pressure — there is plenty of reserve; the fetus withstands the episodes of distress with no trouble and no sequelae. However, if the labor has been long, if contractions have been overstimulated with oxytocin, if the mother has been given a regional anesthetic that lowered her blood pressure (as 20 percent of epidural injections do), if the mother is recumbent, or if the baby is already stressed due to another abnormality, then cord compression can be very serious. It can lead to progressive distress and ultimately, death. Those are many "ifs" and that is why serious problems or death in normal labors is so rare — fewer than one per 1,000 births.

How is fetal distress treated? If the fetal heart does not recover its usual rate after contractions (between 120 and 160 beats per minute) but remains very fast, very slow, or weak and irregular, then immediate treatment is needed. Getting the mother up or rolled over in bed, giving her oxygen with a tight face mask, and preparing for cesarean section are the usual treatments.

Once in a great while the cord slips down past the baby and lies in the birth canal or even slips into view at the opening of the vagina. This prolapse of the umbilical cord also requires immediate action. The birth attendant will help the mother onto her hands and knees and have her lower her chest and raise her hips. In this position, the fetus is lifted away from the cord and pressure is relieved while preparations are made for cesarean section.

Cesarean section. Before choosing a doctor for childbirth, parents are wise to choose a hospital that provides the kind of care they want. One important fact is the cesarean rate. Contrary to what doctors and hospital administrators often claim, cesarean rates do not necessarily reflect higher numbers of high-risk patients. Many suburban community hospitals have 25 to 35 percent cesarean rates, even though they serve predominately well-nourished, middle-class populations. In contrast, some urban hospitals that serve poor neighborhoods with high numbers of women at risk have cesarean rates of around 15 to 20 percent. Parents can find out the cesarean rates of prospective hospitals by calling community childbirth education groups or cesarean education groups. Health department statistics also may be available.

Besides avoiding hospitals with high cesarean rates, parents may reduce the chance of a cesarean by avoiding situations in labor that are associated with cesareans, including recumbency, early rupture of the membranes, induction of labor, regional anesthesia that may cause the mother's blood pressure to drop, fetal drug depression from pain medications given to the mother, and machine monitoring.

If a cesarean is necessary, the doctor should be able to tell the parents exactly why, whether there are alternatives to surgery, and whether a second opinion will be obtained prior to the operation. The physician should discuss what kind of anesthetic is planned and whether the mother's husband or a chosen friend may attend the surgery. Many hospitals will allow the father or a family member to attend cesarean births.

After the decision is made to do a cesarean, the mother's abdomen is shaved, and she is wheeled into an operating room. She is catheterized, a procedure in which a tiny plastic hose is inserted into the urethra to drain off urine during the surgery and right afterward. This helps the bladder stay out of the way of the cesarean, and conveniently deals with the need to urinate. The mother is either given a general or regional anesthetic, depending on her preference and on the available time. When the anesthesia has taken effect, an incision is made, usually along the pubic hairline. This transverse "Pfannenstiel" incision is replacing the weaker longitudinal incision because it virtually never ruptures in later births. Although this incision is only about four inches long, it is sufficient to deliver the baby and the placenta.

Complications of Cesarean Section

To the mother. In a recent study of 4,000 patients from the years 1958 to 1976, almost half of all cesarean patients had one or more complications arising from the operative procedure. These are listed below in approximate order of frequency. Some of these are severe complications that affect future childbearing.

As delivery by cesarean section is on the increase in the United States, it is important for women to be aware that this is a major operative procedure with definite risks. A woman who has had a cesarean should never have labor and delivery outside a hospital.
- Pain and gas (almost all women)
- All future deliveries by cesarean (almost all women)
- Infection (between 20 and 65 percent); intrauterine infection if internally monitored in labor (35 to 65 percent); intrauterine infection if not monitored in labor (20 to 40 percent). Other infections include cystitis, peritonitis, and abscess.
- Hemorrhage
- Adhesions
- Injury to adjacent structures
- Blood transfusion complications
- Respiratory and cardiac complications
- Death

To the infant. Cesarean section is indicated when there is danger to the life of the mother or infant if normal vaginal delivery is allowed. As cesarean frequency is on the rise, it is important for a doctor to tell parents exactly why it is being recommended and whether there are alternatives, for in addition to complications for the mother, the following are complications that arise for the infant. These are listed in approximate order of frequency.
- Jaundice
- Fewer quiet, alert periods after birth
- Respiratory distress due to the procedure
- Drug effects from the anesthesias, causing general depression of neonatal functions.

CESAREAN SECTION

Once used in emergencies to deliver 5 to 10 percent of babies in the population, delivery by cesarean section is increasing rapidly. As there is controversy over whether this procedure is really necessary in many cases, it is important for women to be informed in advance about C-sections, and to participate in decisions regarding this major operation. If it is decided that vaginal delivery is not possible, or would endanger the life of the mother or baby, cesarean section proceeds as follows.

General anesthesia may be used or an epidural or spinal anesthetic (see page 294). A catheter is placed through the urethra and into the bladder to drain urine.
A *An incision is made horizontally in the abdominal wall at the upper edge of the pubic hair. Be sure to specify a horizontal incision since it heals more strongly and leaves an almost-invisible scar.*
B *The incision reveals the sheath covering the rectus muscle. The uterus lies beneath.*
C and D *The physician cuts the rectus sheath and muscle.*
E *The incision into the uterus may be made vertically or horizontally. The cut is made in the lower part of the uterus adjacent to the baby's head. In some cases, the cut is made higher in the uterus. Discuss the operation afterwards with your surgeon to find out where cuts were made in your uterus, and what type of incisions were used.*
F *After opening the amniotic sac, the physician reaches in and removes the baby's head first, except in the case of breech or other unusual presentations. The placenta is then detached and delivered.*
G *The uterine layers are resewn. The bladder is returned to its place over the uterus, and the external cuts are resewn. The complete procedure takes approximately one hour.*

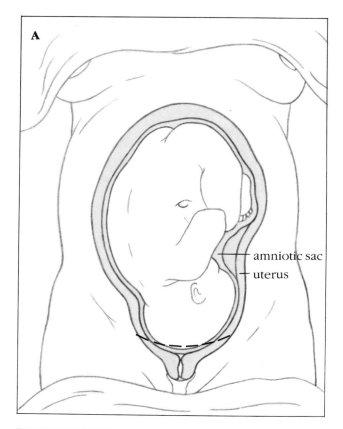

amniotic sac
uterus

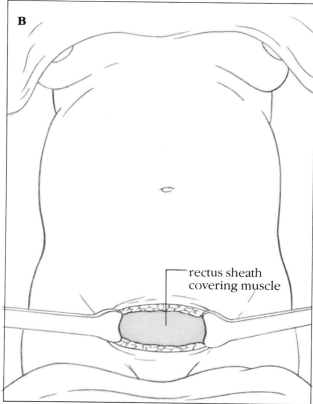

rectus sheath covering muscle

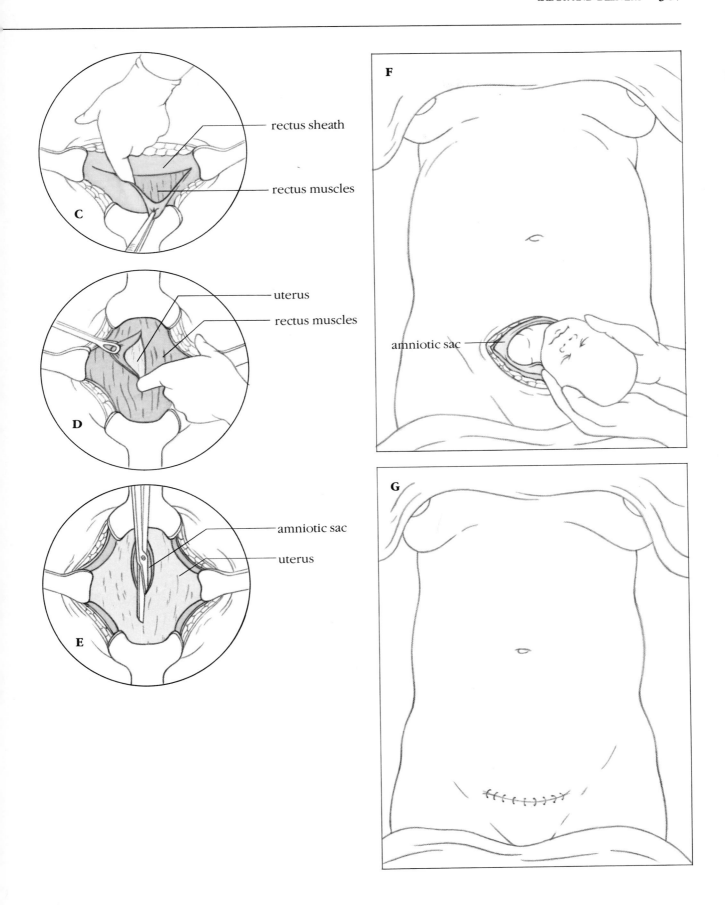

rectus sheath

rectus muscles

C

uterus

rectus muscles

D

amniotic sac

uterus

E

F

amniotic sac

G

Mothers can arrange ahead of time to be able to see the birth, dispensing with the draped screen that separates the mother from the surgical field. The mother may prefer to have a running commentary, describing what is happening as the surgery proceeds. Women generally do not like being totally ignored as if they were not in the room. Some mothers want one arm free from restraints so they can hold the baby on the shoulder while suturing is being done. If the mother must be under general anesthesia and the father outside the operating room, parents can arrange to have a picture of the baby taken as it is born, and to keep the father informed throughout as to how the surgery is going. Otherwise fathers often feel very frightened while they wait for word, especially during an emergency cesarean in what was planned as a vaginal birth.

Expectant parents who have had a previous cesarean often feel angry that they are unable to plan for a vaginal birth. Many will seek doctors who will allow them to try to deliver vaginally the next time. In England, only about 12 percent of women who have had a cesarean are delivered surgically in subsequent births. This is because the reason for the cesarean often does not repeat itself. The cesarean may have been needed because the baby was breech or distress, or because the mother developed hypertension. Unfortunately, in the United States, medical custom is to automatically deliver subsequent babies surgically if there has been a previous cesarean. However, there are doctors who are willing to provide the careful surveillance of the labor that is needed to assure quick action if the old cesarean scar ruptures during contractions. In a recent report of vaginal delivery after cesarean, out of 100 births there were four partial uterine-scar tears with seepage of blood. All four tears were in old-style longitudinal incisions. Two were repaired, and two needed no repair. Of these 100 women, however, only half succeeded in having a vaginal delivery. The other half developed various problems necessitating another cesarean.

Cesarean childbirth classes are good places for parents to share their ideas and experiences with birth. Movies are shown that help them decide what kind of birth they want, and to give them encouragement as they await a repeat cesarean. Many parents arrange with their doctors to be allowed to "go into labor" prior to the planned repeat cesarean, rather than being admitted to the hospital the night before the operation. It is thought that even a little bit of labor gives the baby some of the advantages of uterine contractions in stimulating breathing and assuring maturity.

The first hours after birth are just as important for cesarean parents to be alone with their new baby, rather than having the baby automatically taken to the nursery even though nothing is wrong. Parents want to hold and fondle the baby in the recovery room, and the mother may want to begin breast-feeding. As the anesthetic wears off, pain medications are needed in small amounts so the mother does not feel sick or groggy as she begins to take care of her baby and herself. Medications that do not affect the baby via the breast milk are often discussed ahead of time with the obstetrician.

Finally, many cesarean mothers want to be given the opportunity of earlier discharge from the hospital if they feel fine, perhaps cutting the usual five- to seven-day stay down to four or five days. Older children are being encouraged to visit the new baby and the mother in the hospital more frequently now, as well.

The Rh-negative mother. Until the late 1960s, second and later Rh-positive babies carried by Rh-negative women had a chance of being affected by rhesus hemolytic disease, a serious or fatal disorder in which antibodies from the mother destroy the blood cells of the fetus. The mother who is Rh-negative lacks this factor in her blood. However, blood cells from her Rh-positive fetus enter her bloodstream in trace amounts during pregnancy. These cells with the foreign Rh factor stimulate production of antibodies, which cross the placenta only in second and subsequent pregnancies. These antibodies attack the fetal blood cells as if they were foreign substances to be defended against.

Late in the 1960s, a cure for rhesus hemolytic disease was found. If the mother who is Rh-negative receives an injection of RhoGam after *each* birth, abortion, and miscarriage, her blood will not form antibodies to the Rh factor. As a result of this medical breakthrough, Rh disease is no longer a threat to babies — unless their mothers did not receive the injection of RhoGam after a previous conception. Unfortunately, women who had their first babies before this discovery and are bearing children today will have this problem. Tragically, however, some women who could have had this injection did not get it, either through the ignorance of their doctors or themselves.

For women who do have an Rh-sensitized pregnancy, it is reassuring to know that in the last half of their pregnancy, the fetus is monitored carefully for the effects of maternal antibodies. When tests show that they are present, exchange transfusions of blood can be done while the fetus is still in the uterus. A well-timed cesarean, followed by transfusions, usually prevents damage to the baby.

Organizations with More Information

NAME AND ADDRESS	TYPE OF SERVICE OR INFORMATION
American Academy of Husband-Coached Childbirth P.O. Box 5224 Sherman Oaks, California 91413 (213) 788-6662	Certifying and training agency for childbirth educators in the Bradley Method.
Association for Childbirth at Home International 1675 Monte Cristo Cerritos, California 90701 (714) 994-5880	Instruction on home birth for couples, with or without a birth attendant; trains and certifies teachers.
American College of Nurse-Midwives 1012 14th Street, N.W., Suite 801 Washington, D.C. 20005 (202) 347-5445	Certifying agency for nurse-midwives, both in home and in hospital practice.
American Society for Psychoprophylaxis in Obstetrics 1411 K Street, N.W. Washington, D.C. 20005 (202) 783-7050	Certifying and training agency for childbirth educators in the Lamaze Method. Has chapters in many states and 3,800 childbirth education teachers and interested physician members.
Cesareans/Support, Education and Concern 66 Christopher Road Waltham, Massachusetts 02154 (617) 547-7188	Emotional and educational support for cesarean parents via phone, corrrespondence, literature, audio-visual material, and hospital workshops.
Home Oriented Maternity Experience 511 New York Avenue Takoma Park Washington, D.C. 20012 (301) 587-4664	Instruction on home birth for couples, with emphasis on medically attended birth; trains and certifies leaders.
International Childbirth Education Association P.O. Box 20852 Milwaukee, Wisconsin 53220 (612) 881-9194	All aspects of childbirth education, with emphasis on birth preparation and family-centered hospital care.
Informed Homebirth P.O. Box 788 Boulder, Colorado 80302 (303) 444-0434	Instruction for couples desiring birth at home or in other alternative environments; trains and certifies teachers.
National Association of Parents and Professionals for Safe Alternatives in Childbirth P.O. Box. 267 Marble Hills, Missouri 63764 (314) 238-2010	All aspects of birth, with emphasis on providing coordinated alternatives both in and out of hospital; certifies maternity services.
National Midwives Association P.O. Box 163 Princeton, New Jersey 08540 (915) 533-8142	An association of practicing midwives—largely lay midwives, but nurse-midwives also.
Society for the Protection of the Unborn Through Nutrition 17 North Wabash, Suite 603 Chicago, Illinois 60602 (312) 332-2334	Education in nutrition during pregnancy; provides training seminars and brochures on the benefits and specifics of good diet; trains and certifies nutrition counselors. Has a hot line for nutrition and drug information: (914) 271-6474.

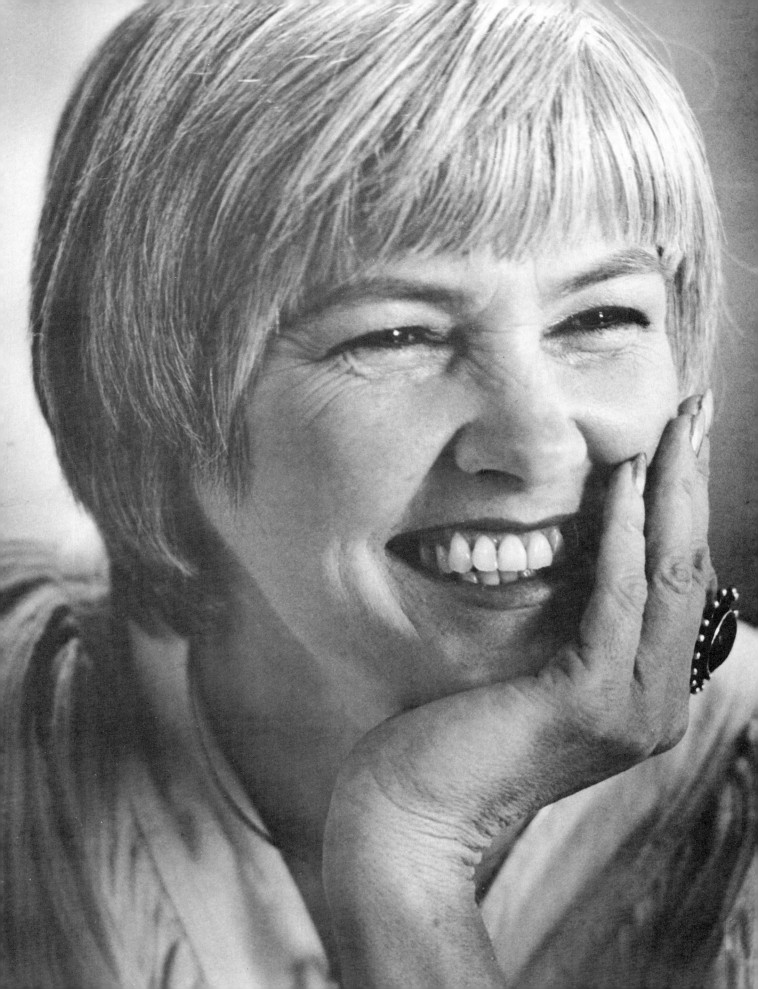

CHAPTER 15

MENOPAUSE

VIDAL S. CLAY, Ed.D.

With menopause, your monthly menstrual cycles come to an end. The years between puberty and menopause, with their periodic hormonal rhythm, give way to a new stage in life. This period of growth can be as tumultuous or as commonplace as that of puberty, depending on how you as an individual are affected.

In the menopause transition, you pass through a year or more of physical symptoms as your body adjusts to changes in hormone levels. Though these symptoms vary from woman to woman, most women cope with them very effectively. After all, at this mature stage of life, women are no strangers to change and physical upheaval.

Many women who are healthy and self-confident pass through this phase in their lives with the same natural composure and competence they exhibited in adolescence. Others experience problems and conflicts. But most women take this major rite of passage in stride —problems, pleasures, and all.

Menopause

The climacteric, or menopause, is a normal developmental phase in the life of a woman. Just as it is biologically appropriate for a girl to begin menstruating in her early teens, so is it normal for a woman to stop menstruating in middle age. However, the normality of this physiological and psychological process has been obscured by societal and cultural myths and taboos—about women generally, about women who do not reproduce, about women who are middle-aged, and about women who are growing older. This chapter takes a different perspective—that menopause is a time for personal growth and rechanneling of energies, and an opportunity for change and renewal.

Menopause is a Rubicon or crossing point, a change or a change of life. The climacteric is only one of a number of important changes a woman faces in mid-life, and in that sense, it can make these years difficult. Of course, your body is affected by the physical process signaling the end of your monthly menstrual periods, but how you deal with this phase in your life is determined in large measure by how you feel about yourself as a woman at this time. To understand why such a natural and inevitable process is often feared and takes on such trauma, it may help to discuss the complex of physical, social, and psychological factors that play a role at this stage in life.

Physical Aspects

Menopause is not an illness. You are not sick when you go through menopause. Most women are in good physical health during middle age and into old age, and go through the climacteric with very little difficulty. Research tells us that about 80 percent of women experience some discomfort or symptoms at this time, most of them minor. Only 25 to 30 percent of women experience complaints that are troublesome enough to bring to a doctor. Despite myths about the trials and tribulations of menopause, most women, especially those who have not confined their lives to the wife and mother roles, will go through this change with very little emotional upset.

Menopause is not the beginning of aging. Human beings age slowly throughout their lives. The only clear distinction between a menopausal woman and a post-menopausal woman is that the former is menstruating

and the latter is not. The climacteric doesn't last long—from two to five years for most women—and is really quite short when compared to the average life-span of women in America today, 76.8 years.

Some women speak of a blossoming after menopause. They feel better physically and have more energy. Others report feeling more self-confident and more certain of themselves. This reaction is common enough around the world that Margaret Mead has used the initials PMZ, "postmenopausal zest," to designate the positive change in women's attitudes and behavior after menopause. The reasons for this response are simple: psychologically, the swings of mood associated with the menstrual cycle have halted, and the fear of becoming pregnant is over. Physically, the problems associated with the menstrual cycle (premenstrual tension, periodic pains or cramps, irregular bleeding, and overstimulation of the uterine walls) have come to an end.

Menopause occurs later than is popularly thought, usually between the ages of 48 and 53, although it is perfectly normal to begin as early as 40 or as late as 55. The idea that early onset of the menstrual period means a later menopause also is a fallacy. The timing of the climacteric depends upon hereditary, constitutional, and environmental factors.

Physical changes. Three distinct physical changes accompany menopause. Menstrual bleeding ceases, the ovaries stop producing eggs, and the body decreases the production of the female hormones, estrogen and progesterone.

Your ovaries already have begun to decrease the production of estrogen some years before menopause. Most women are unaware of these hormonal changes until their late 40s, when there are irregularities in the menstrual flow. Usually, the menstrual period tapers off, both in amount and duration of flow, although flooding occurs in some women. The periods may become more widely or more closely spaced. This irregular phase, before menstrual flow finally ends, lasts from two to three years.

A few women just stop menstruating. One woman said, "I just woke up one morning and it was gone." Such "sudden" menopause frequently coincides with an upset, such as bereavement, moving to a new house or location, or a serious illness. After a women has not had a period for a year, she no longer needs to use a method of birth control.

Even though menstruation ceases, your body continues to produce some estrogen, but not enough to build up the epithelial wall of the uterus, as occurs in menstrual cycles. After menopause, nonestrogenic material produced by the adrenal glands is converted to estrogen at other sites in the body, and occasionally causes postmenopausal bleeding. (Any postmenopausal bleeding should be checked by a physician.) Some women produce significant amounts of estrogen for as long as ten years after menopause, and minor amounts throughout the rest of their lives.

The important point to understand is that menopause does not mean a sudden shutting-off of estrogen. Instead, it is a period when the body must adapt to less estrogen than it had before. Indeed, these changes in hormonal balance are responsible for the distressing effects or symptoms experienced by some women. This period of hormonal disequilibrium can be seen as a withdrawal period, quite similar to the physiological withdrawal process associated with cigarettes, alcohol, or any drug on which the body has become dependent.

Physical Changes and Symptoms

PHYSICAL CHANGES OF MENOPAUSE

- Menstrual bleeding ceases.
- Egg production stops in the ovaries.
- Female hormones decrease as the body slows production of both estrogen and progesterone.

PHYSICAL SYMPTOMS OF MENOPAUSE

- Hot flashes and sweats are vasomotor symptoms that occur when the small blood vessels of the skin periodically dilate.
- Vaginal lubrication is reduced, since the thinning vaginal tissues do not now produce mucus or sweat as readily as they did before menopause.

Estrogen Production Throughout the Life-Span

Infancy Until birth, an abundant supply of estrogen and progesterone is furnished by the mother to her infant.

Childhood Until puberty, girls produce very little estrogen.

Adolescence During adolescence, the ovaries enlarge and active production of estrogen begins. This sex hormone is responsible for the changes in a girl's body at this time, including the start of menstruation.

Adulthood The adult woman produces the most estrogen during her fertile years. This production is cyclical, and the amount of hormone present in each phase of the cycle varies from one individual to the next, and from cycle to cycle.

Menopause At menopause, the levels of estrogen fluctuate and gradually decrease. Some women produce estrogen for as long as ten years after menopause and minor amounts throughout the rest of their lives.

The production of estrogen is cyclical during menstruation, and throughout a woman's life-span and normal sexual development. Physical, emotional, and behavioral changes are tied to this cyclic pattern of sex hormone activity.

There is great variation in the way women experience this process of withdrawal. Some women experience a sudden drop in estrogen that can result in severe symptoms. One woman reported that she felt like "committing mayhem" when she had hot flashes. Other women experience a more gradual withdrawal of estrogen and their bodies are thus better able to adjust. When a woman's ovaries are removed by surgery, she has what is called a surgical menopause. In such cases, the drop in estrogen is precipitous and the resulting symptoms can be severe.

Symptoms of menopause. Surprisingly, there are only two major symptoms that are directly attributable to menopause: vasomotor symptoms that are felt as hot flashes and sweats, and genital atrophy, or thinning of the vaginal walls and reduced vaginal lubrication.

The hot flash or flush occurs when the small blood vessels of the skin periodically dilate. For unknown reasons, the diameter of certain blood vessels increases from time to time, allowing more blood to flow into them. When this happens, you feel a rush of heat to the skin, often followed by sweating, which serves to cool the body and can make you feel chilled. You also may notice temporary shortness of breath and, sometimes, heart palpitations.

Some women never have a single hot flash. In early menopause, perhaps four out of five women have very mild flashes or none at all. For those who do have them, they vary a great deal. In intensity, they range from mild to severe. In location on the body, they most commonly begin on the face, neck, head, and chest, and spread from there, but some women have reported them starting in the ears or on the feet. In duration, they last from 30 seconds to an hour, and in frequency, they vary from a few a day to more than one an hour. Hot flashes occur both during the day and at night.

The overall pattern of hot flashes seems to be cyclic. They come and go. Hot flashes are most common after menstruation has ended, but some women experience them while they are still having periods. In these cases, there are usually corresponding changes occurring in the menstrual flow, such as less volume or more widely spaced periods. Some women report that in the months they are menstruating regularly, they have no hot flashes. When they do have hot flashes, they know they won't be having a period that month.

Hot flashes are described as a vasomotor instability, but what causes them is unknown. Nor is it known why some women have them and others don't. Hot flashes are annoying, they can be very uncomfortable, and they can seriously interfere with sleep. They do respond dramatically to estrogen replacement therapy, however.

In general, hot flashes last from six months to several years, and subside spontaneously even though the hormonal and glandular changes in the body persist. They may return years later at times of emotional stress

Hot flashes are especially unpleasant for the woman who feels self-conscious, exposed, and ashamed when having them. Some women confront these feelings in a direct way by carrying a fan with them and using it whenever they have a hot flash. If anyone should ask what they are doing, they simply smile and reply, "I'm a menopausal woman having a hot flash." In point of fact, the hot flash is not as obvious to other people as it is to you. Most people are very unobservant. Women have described feeling red as a beet and very embarrassed in public as the sweat seems to pour off. They often discover, however, that no one notices—granted that you don't reach for a tissue and mop your brow, or sigh and groan to emphasize your condition. If you check your appearance in a mirror during a hot flash, you may be reassured enough to stop worrying.

The second result of diminished estrogen is reduced lubrication of the vagina, or vaginal atrophy. With age, the tissues of the vagina often become thinner and do not lubricate or sweat as easily as before. This condition can make sexual intercourse uncomfortable or painful, in which case a lubricating jelly or muscle toning exercises may help. ("Elevator" exercises for the pubococcygeus muscle may be especially helpful. See page 297 of the "Labor and Delivery" chapter.)

Vaginal atrophy is always mentioned as one of the results of the climacteric. However, it has not been systematically studied. Most of the available data come from observations of gynecologists. We do not know, for example, what proportion of women experience it, how long after menopause it occurs—five, ten, 25 years —and what differences there are, if any, between sexually active and sexually inactive women. Recent reports that sexual activity continues on into old age and that it is experienced as pleasant and fulfilling indicate that vaginal atrophy is not an insurmountable problem to all older women.

These two symptoms—hot flashes and vaginal atrophy —are the only ones helped by estrogen replacement therapy, or ERT as it is called. These symptoms of menopause and ERT are discussed in greater detail later in this chapter.

Because the physical symptoms and medical treatments are so limited, it's important to take a hard look at the social and psychological aspects of the climacteric if we are to know how to manage menopause, whether as physicians or as women seeking to take care of ourselves through this period of the life cycle.

Child-Rearing Years in a Woman's Life-Span

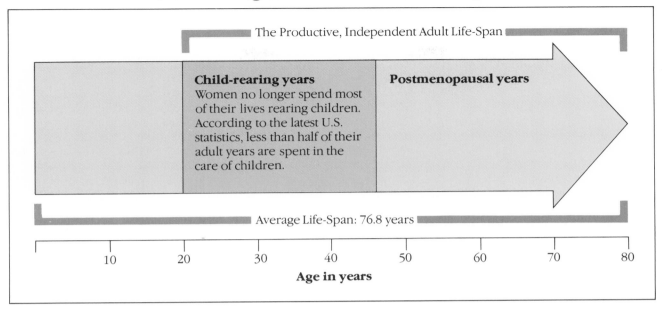

The Productive, Independent Adult Life-Span

Child-rearing years
Women no longer spend most of their lives rearing children. According to the latest U.S. statistics, less than half of their adult years are spent in the care of children.

Postmenopausal years

Average Life-Span: 76.8 years

10   20   30   40   50   60   70   80

Age in years

Social Aspects

Menopause is only one of the issues and concerns of women over 40 today. Before we talk specifically about the social aspects of menopause, we should take a look at the general changes that occur during middle age.

Societal and cultural myths and stereotypes of the older woman—as inactive, asexual, or unhealthy—have contributed to negative images of menopause. The medical profession may even contribute to these stereotypes of the middle-aged woman by focusing only on this one aspect of her life-span (menopause), and by thinking of it in terms of illness or disease instead of a normal change of life. Unfortunately but understandably, women often have accepted society's stereotypes or prejudices about older women and menopause. Frequently they turn to their doctors, who have been better trained to cure and to prescribe than to listen, to understand, and to counsel from the enlightened position the patient expects.

The question of what a middle-aged woman should do with the 25 years of living ahead of her is a relatively new problem. It is due to changes in the life-span, changes in patterns of reproduction, and changes in patterns of work. These changes have affected societal and individual perceptions of the housewife role, and have raised new problems for today's middle-aged woman.

Changes in the life-span. More women are living longer. It is estimated that in the United States today, there are about 27 million women over the age of 50 who can anticipate living an average of 27 years beyond menopause.

Changes in patterns of childbearing. In the past, and in most parts of the non-Western world today, women bore children throughout their reproductive years, and often died before their youngest child was reared. What this means is that the great majority of women in the world have spent their adult lives either pregnant or lactating, and that most have died in the years we now consider to be middle age.

Today, most American women limit their childbearing to a few years in their 20s. Many women believe that smaller rather than larger families are desirable, and with the availability of various methods of birth control, they now can act on that belief. Statistics show that the majority of American women give birth to their last child when they are 27 years old. As a result, by the time they are in their 40s, the children are grown and gone, and the women may be left with no clearly defined, acceptable, or useful work to do—or so they often feel. It is not surprising that many women in this situation feel anxious, hostile, or depressed.

Some women in middle age resolve the problem by moving into a second mothering career. When their daughters go to work, they rear the grandchildren. In the United States today, however, many women reject this role of grandmother except in areas of poverty where it is an economic necessity.

Women who have not developed independent interests nor prepared themselves for this stage may find themselves in a vacuum. These women are not old; they are strong and vigorous, and have a third of their lives ahead of them. Yet to be mothers is all they feel they know.

Changes in patterns of work. Historically, in America as in other cultures, adult women have helped in the fields, mended nets, made cloth, engaged in crafts such as selling lace or pottery in local markets, or worked in factories or in a small family store. With the Industrial Revolution, though, most of the productive labor moved to institutions outside the family. It then became the custom for women to stay at home to keep house and rear children.

Women who are middle-aged today were in their teens and twenties when the Second World War broke out. After finishing high school, most went to work while some continued their education. When the war ended, most women (except for single women, black women, and women married to poor men) left their paid jobs to become fulltime wives and mothers. These were the years of early marriage, large families, and togetherness. The few young, married women who worked outside the home in the 1950s were far from typical of their generation. Instead, most women were busy producing the post-war baby boom. They expected to make a career out of marriage. The prevalent attitude at that time was that a woman was not a complete human being by herself, but needed a man to round-out her existence. Women were taught to live their lives through others, especially their husbands and children. If their marital or love relationship has since faltered, if they were left alone by separation, divorce, or death, and even without separation, when their children grew up and left home, these women who married in the 1940s and 50s may now feel confused and displaced.

Today in the United States, 44 million women work outside their homes. Women comprise 51 percent of the labor force, and make an essential contribution to the economy. Contrary to popular belief, most women are employed because they have to be. Two-thirds of all working women are single, separated, divorced, widowed, or married to men earning less than $7,000 per year. Studies show that most working wives not only work full time but also do most of the housework. Husbands of employed women contribute little more to housework and child-rearing chores than husbands of non-employed women. This pattern holds true for socialist countries where most women work outside the home, as well as for Western Europe and the United States. These facts of life affect the decisions of a middle-aged woman whose children have left home and who is wondering what to do with her life. She knows that staying home and taking care of one husband will not fill her time or satisfy her energies. On the other hand, if she goes out to work, without skills or a working background, she can expect to be poorly paid and, once home again, to be responsible for almost all of the housework.

Volunteer work is an option with something to offer many women. The women's movement has helped to enourage women to use volunteer work as an opportunity to develop skills that can count as work experience. Some women have successfully transferred the managerial skills of running a household and those developed in volunteer work to paying positions. Volunteer work as a choice open to middle-aged women applies only to those women who don't *have* to work for pay. For many single women and for women whose husbands are poor providers, paid employment is essential. For them, the period of the climacteric comes and goes, but the structure of work remains a constant in their lives.

Divorce in middle age also is a new trend. In the 1940s, the divorce rate for marriages of 15 years' duration was 4 percent. Today it is 25 percent. Besides the obvious hardships on the divorced woman with no earning power, the new no-fault divorce laws also have had an impact on her economic status. Alimony is rarely given today, and when it is, it is often terminable or given for a limited period of time. In general, child support ends when the children reach 18.

Psychological Aspects

What does the end of menstruation mean to women on a more personal level? Studies of women in menopause show that those who have ceased menstruation are relieved to be free of it, while women who are in the midst of irregular menstrual cycles feel sad about losing this familiar marker in their lives. A personal fear of aging may surface at this time, since some women say, "I don't mind losing my periods, I just don't want to get old."

The end of menstruation signals the end of reproduction. Just as it is reasonable to want children and to plan pregnancy in the early years of marriage, so is it reasonable to protect against having children in mid-life when pregnancy is more complicated from a biological, social, and psychological point of view. Many women are voluntarily giving up their ability to have children in their 30s (and increasing numbers of men are seeking sterilization through vasectomy). With this new trend toward assuming personal responsibility for one's reproductive life, the end of menstruation and reproductive capacity need not have the same devastating emotional effect on women as in years past.

Menopause and Sexuality

Next to the fact of menopause as the end of reproduction is the long-held myth that menopause marks an end to a woman's sexuality. Happily, we are more enlightened today, and we know sexuality continues to be important in the lives of men and women well into old age. Of course, we experience changes in sexuality with aging. The need for sexual release diminishes, and the time it takes to reach orgasm becomes longer. The *quality* of the sexual communication may improve, however, because the demand for sexual release is less insistent. Many women enjoy sexual relations more after menopause because they no longer are constrained by the fear of pregnancy. Furthermore, the great majority of American women are not worn out from bearing large numbers of children and from doing hard physical work throughout their lives. With proper nutrition and good medical care, for the first time in history, women can easily remain sexually attractive in their postmenopausal years.

Facing Old Age

It is predictable that a woman in middle age will eventually lose her own mother or father through death, see a daughter or son marry, and become a grandmother for the first time. Each of these experiences brings her face-to-face with her own aging and with the fact that she is moving into the next generation and the last stages of her own life. (See the chapter on "Aging.")

One of the psychological burdens of middle age is the responsibility for aging parents. After having adjusted to being free of children and looking forward to an unencumbered life, many people find it hard to have to take care of the parental generation. It *is* hard. It is emotionally painful to switch roles and now take care of the people who once took care of you, and it also can be a burden financially. Women who have devoted their lives to their husbands and children and who resist making a transition in middle age may now seize the opportunity to devote themselves to their aging parents. In reality, this only postpones the task of developing one's own self and finding a meaningful way of life for the years ahead.

Menopause and Drug Therapy

Men and women alike have long searched for a fountain of eternal youth. In the late 1960s, many women began estrogen replacement therapy (ERT) in response to the concept spread by newspapers, women's magazines, and doctors that ERT would make them "feminine forever." Some of the claims, many financially supported by the drug manufacturing companies, were that estrogen replacement therapy would cure hot flashes, sweats, and vaginal atrophy, stop the skin from aging, prevent heart attack and osteoporosis (bone loss), eliminate irritability and depression, and even increase sexual drive.

Facts About Estrogen

Estrogen may be dangerous to women. It now appears that only two of these claims are true: estrogen replacement therapy can help hot flashes and sweats, and reduces vaginal atrophy. The other claims now are known to be questionable or false. The notion that ERT can solve the problems of the climacteric and aging must be rigorously reevaluated.

Recent studies show a relationship between estrogen replacement therapy and the incidence of uterine cancer, and possible breast cancer. Put more specifically, these studies suggest that women who take ERT face a very high risk of uterine cancer. They are about twenty times more likely to get cancer of the uterine lining than are women who do not undergo this therapy. Women who take ERT for five years or more face the greatest risk. But if women stop taking the drug, within six months the risk declines to about the same level as in women who have never used ERT. For women with estrogen-dependent cancers, as in the breasts, uterus, and ovaries, or for women with arteriosclerosis (hardening of the arteries), ERT is life-threatening. In addition, it is contraindicated for women with a family history of cancer and thromboembolic disease (blood clots), or a personal medical history of cancer, high blood pressure, thrombosis, liver disease, or diabetes. And for the remaining women, its use is highly questionable because the short-term benefits may not be worth the suspected long-range risks.

The two menopausal symptoms helped by ERT. As stated earlier, medical opinion holds that the only two menopausal symptoms helped by ERT are hot flashes and sweats, and vaginal atrophy. Estrogen given orally in pill form—it is rarely given by injection today—is effective in stopping hot flashes. The thinning of the vaginal walls that can cause painful intercourse can be helped by local application of estrogen cream.

ERT and heart attacks. It has been thought that estrogen protected women from heart attack and that its decrease after menopause explained the higher incidence of heart problems in postmenopausal women. It was hypothesized that replacing the estrogens no longer produced by the body would solve these problems. This conclusion is now uncertain. Japanese women, black women, and poor women seem not to share in this protection from heart attack.

It is now known that high dosages of estrogen may contribute to heart attack because estrogen has the effect of increasing the fatty deposits in the blood, a predisposing factor to heart attack. High dosages of estrogen also increase the risk of thromboembolic disease, cerebral accidents, and coronary disease in older age groups. Today, women over 40 are urged not to take the birth control pill, which contains synthetic estrogen, because of this increased risk of heart attack.

ERT and bone loss. The bones of both men and women become decalcified with aging, meaning that they are thinner, more fragile, and more subject to breakage. This problem is more severe in women than in men. For example, women have about four times as much spinal osteoporosis as men. Hip fractures are over twice as common in women as in men. Forearm fractures in women begin to increase around age 45; by age 60, women have ten times the number of these breaks as men.

Although in some studies, estrogen or ERT appears somewhat effective in slowing the development of bone loss in older women, the benefit ceases as soon as the drug is discontinued.

ERT and sexuality. There is no evidence that sexual behavior undergoes any radical change after menopause, whether that menopause occurs naturally or is the result of surgery. Nor is there any evidence that hormones, of themselves, increase sexual drive in normal women. In fact, estrogen actually may decrease sexual interest.

ERT and depression. Menopause does not increase the risk of depression for women. Anxiety and depression may occur (or recur) at menopause—not because of the decrease in female hormones, but as a reaction to the woman's total life situation. It appears that women who have coped successfully with other changes in their lives will cope successfully with menopause as well. In general, housewives experience more depression than working women, and middle-class housewives experience more depression than working-class housewives. However, studies of other societies show that middle age per se is not expected to be a difficult time for women.

At the time of the menstrual cycle when women have more estrogen in their systems than after menopause, premenstrual tension and depression are common. We know that estrogen increases the amount of sodium in the body, and that high total body sodium is associated with depression. Indeed, depression is one of the established side effects of the birth control pill. Although the strength of the estrogen in pills given for estrogen replacement therapy is far lower than that used in birth control pills, a depressed menopausal woman who takes ERT may have her mood lowered rather than lifted.

Alternatives to ERT. Many psychiatrists and physicians readily prescribe estrogen for menopausal women. These well-meaning practitioners may be influenced by drug company advertisments, they may not be familiar with the current medical literature on ERT, or they simply may feel that ERT is indicated in the case of a particular woman.

Other doctors share the point of view of Dr. Elizabeth B. Connell, a gynecologist:

"I think one of the most important drugs that you can administer is just plain old-fashioned tender loving care and reassurance....In my days as a general practitioner I discovered that half an hour exploring the life situation of the woman or what was really bugging her was sometimes a lot more helpful than the quarter grain aspirin you gave her as a placebo."

In the absence of severe problems requiring the attention of a gynecologist, women can give each other the "tender loving care" that medical professionals are not trained to provide nor have the time to give. Numerous "menopausal rap groups" have sprung up around the country, and their founders, usually women in menopause themselves, have gone to considerable trouble to research the subject and to dispel the myths and misinformation that abound. Such groups generally can be located through community women's centers or women's health collectives. See the chart on page 321 for some nonmedical therapies for the common problems of menopause.

Health or Disease?

The Myth of Trauma

In point of fact, menopause is not the big trauma it is so often made out to be. Half of the women going through the climacteric don't even go to their physicians. Of course, it isn't known how many of these women, if any, have complaints but think that putting up with discomfort during this change of life is simply woman's lot. Today, medical experts agree that a woman need not take medication if her menopausal symptoms are not severe.

What is a symptom? Symptoms such as hot flashes, muscle aches, or excessive perspiration can be objectively defined, but determining the need for treatment is quite subjective. What may be a serious complaint to one woman may be nothing more than bearable discomfort to another. How disagreeable and troubling a symptom or complaint may be is entirely a subjective matter. For the woman who feels she's got everything going for her, hot flashes may be shrugged off. For the woman who feels her life is in total disarray, hot flashes can be intolerable. Very often, a woman worried about such symptoms as hot flashes can be reassured by a half hour of her doctor's attention and an explanation of what is happening to her body, how long it may last, and what she might expect. The recognition that she is going through a normal process can be extraordinarily helpful, and may reduce or eliminate altogether the need for drug therapy.

The physician's problem. Doctors depend greatly upon a woman's self-report about her symptoms. Unlike a sore throat or a broken arm, the symptoms associated with menopause cannot be examined and verified by clinical tests and observation. Furthermore, physicians know that hot flashes, although they may be very uncomfortable, are not life-threatening symptoms and will go away in time.

By disposition and training, physicians want to make people better. They know that ERT is highly effective in controlling hot flashes and, until recently, was associated with no known risks. In addition, most physicians are not trained to deal with the emotional needs of patients. The supportive counseling given by doctors has been specialized into the field of psychiatry. Finally, as mentioned previously, societal attitudes about the menopausal woman have influenced the medical profession as profoundly as they have the general public.

The woman's problem. Women are afraid of menopause and afraid of aging. They are confused by old wives' tales, they don't always understand their bodies, and they may lack both the knowledge and the confidence that their bodies are self-healing mechanisms. We live in a pill-taking society, and often believe that doctors know what's best for us. Women have heard that ERT pills will solve their climacteric problems and keep them from growing old, so of course they want the medication. And if they don't get it from one doctor, they can easily go to another.

An informed choice. If women are going to take strong hormonal medication for the symptoms of menopause, they should be able to make informed choices. The problem is that, until recently, few clear answers were available.

Evaluating ERT: Benefits vs. Risks

As with any medication, the advantages must be weighed against the risks for each individual. Physicians have generally assumed the decision-making role and, certainly, will help you. On the other hand, the medical profession itself differs in its interpretations of estrogen's risks and benefits.

Until 1975, no long-term epidemiological research had been done on estrogen generally. Women taking the birth control pill and ERT served as subjects in a massive study of the benefits and hazards of taking strong hormones over a long period of time. The subject is complicated medically and chemically, and it is difficult for the lay person to understand and evaluate all of the factors involved. Yet it is extremely important that women participate in these important decisions and that they give up the totally dependent relationships so many of them now have with their gynecologist or regular doctor.

Once you understand your own medical history and that of your family, and understand the basic action of hormones and body processes, the final decision about ERT must be yours. This advice demands a dramatic change in attitude for many women, but the rewards in asserting responsibility for your body—and your life—are many.

Facts About Estrogen Medication

Varieties of estrogen. There is considerable difference between the estrogen used in the birth control pill to prevent conception and that used for replacement at mid-life when normal estrogen levels decline. Contraceptive estrogen is made from an artificial petroleum-type chemical; the estrogen in replacement therapy is either conjugated equine estrogen—a natural substance made from the urine of pregnant horses (thus its name, Pre-mare-ine)—or an artificial estrogen, which comes in various forms. One of these is diethylstilbestrol, also known as DES, which is a coal tar derivative. DES is the drug in the "morning after" pill. It also was formerly used to prevent miscarriage, but is now accepted as the cause of vaginal cancer in the daughters of women who were treated with DES during pregnancy (see page 506 of the chapter on "Adolescent Reproductive Problems").

Synthetic estrogen is much less expensive than conjugated estrogen, but it is associated with more side effects, especially nausea. Although conjugated equine estrogen is a natural product (that is, it comes from another mammal), it is not exactly the same as the estrogen produced by a woman's body.

The most popular ERT pill is Premarin. The names of other ERT pills are Hormonin, Estatab, Evex, Menest, Femogen, and Ogen. The ERT pill, like the birth control pill, is taken cyclically—21 days on and seven days off. As has been shown earlier, physicians disagree about who should take it, about the dosage, and about the number of years it should be taken. Interestingly, however, the FDA has drawn up a set of recommendations that limit the use of estrogens for the treatment of menopausal symptoms. The FDA now requires drug manufacturers to provide a package insert with each package of pills. This warns women that taking the estrogen pills increases the risk of cancer and gallbladder diseases. The pamphlet warns that the risk increases after one year, and suggests reevaluations of the need for the drug every six months.

Contraindications. The contraindications for taking ERT are similar to those for the birth control pill. Women with a history of blood clots and those with a family history of cancer of the breast or cervix, or women who have had cancer themselves, are not good candidates for ERT. Women who have irregular bleeding or benign (noncancerous) tumors of the breast or uterus also should not take ERT.

Regular medical supervision. Women who take ERT, like women on the pill, should go to their doctors every six months for breast, vaginal, and rectal examinations and a Pap smear. All women should examine their own breasts every month (see page 158).

Side effects. Like the birth control pill, ERT has various side effects, including fluid retention and weight gain, headache, skin discoloration, vaginal discharge, breast and pelvic discomfort due to tissue enlargement, and gastrointestinal symptoms, such as abdominal cramps.

One of the main side effects of ERT is so-called "breakthrough bleeding." The problem is in determining whether the bleeding is due to ERT or is a sign of something more serious, such as cancer of the endometrium (lining of the uterus). In other words, the normal "withdrawal" bleeding that occurs in women on ERT (especially high doses) can mask the signs of cancer of the uterus. *Any spotting or bleeding in a postmenopausal woman (one year after all cessation of menses) should be checked by a physician at once.*

After menopause, vaginal bleeding is the most common symptom of cancer of the endometrium (lining of the uterus). When discovered early, such cancers are highly curable by hysterectomy (removal of the uterus) and by radiation therapy (see page 477 of the chapter on "Adult Reproductive Problems").

Does ERT Merely Postpone Symptoms?

Though ERT is effective in relieving some symptoms of menopause, there is serious doubt that it doesn't merely delay the end. Symptoms simply may return when you stop taking ERT, without any significant reduction. If you can get along without the temporary relief that estrogen replacement therapy brings, by all means do so.

If it is true that taking ERT for several years merely postpones the symptoms of estrogen withdrawal, one may well ask what has been gained by taking this drug. Before studies appeared linking ERT with cancer of the endometrium, a leading endocrinologist was asked "What is the point of taking ERT for two years?" His reply was, "No point at all." When pressed further, he stated that the main advantage of ERT is that it promotes better health habits. In other words, he felt ERT was worth taking because it brings a woman to the doctor every six months for a physical checkup.

Estrogen for incapacitating symptoms. It is true that a small percentage of women have a very difficult time in menopause with symptoms that are severe enough to disrupt their normal lives. Some of these women will have had surgical menopause. Their symptoms include not only hot flashes and sweats and occasional heart palpitations, but also mental disequilibrium, such as the inability to remember, to concentrate, or to organize their thoughts.

When the symptoms of menopause are that severe, and estrogen therapy is not contraindicated by personal or family medical history, estrogen replacement therapy should be prescribed.

Dosage per tablet may vary from .02 mg to 6 mg; usually, ERT is given at the lowest dose necessary to control symptoms. After a period of time, the dosage should be lowered further so that medication can be completely discontinued in time. A sudden stopping of ERT will result in an *increase* in symptoms.

Nonmedical Alternatives to ERT

In an effort to help women make their own decisions about menopausal treatment, the chart at right presents nonmedical therapies for the common problems of menopause as alternatives to estrogen replacement therapy.

While the chart covers eight problems of menopause, only the first three—hot flashes and sweats, vaginal atrophy, and urinary stress incontinence—are exclusively related to menopause. The remaining problems are generally related to aging processes at mid-life, and are not restricted to women.

Accepting the symptoms of menopause as tolerable and transient does not mean that you should discontinue regular medical checkups. It is important to learn and practice self-examination of your breasts and to see your physician at least once every six months.

While menopause is often a difficult time, this is changing as societal and cultural attitudes about women change. A significant first step is for women themselves to reject stereotypes of the menopausal woman and to appreciate their own womanhood.

Women in middle age have an opportunity to change the direction of their lives. Menopause is not a sickness; it is the ending of one phase of life and the beginning of another—a time of personal growth and renewal.

Estrogen Replacement Therapy vs. Nonmedical Therapy

Estrogen replacement therapy, in pill or cream form, can be effective in counteracting the uncomfortable symptoms of menopause. But there is evidence to show that this treatment also may be dangerous. Estrogen replacement therapy controls hot flashes, sweats, vaginal atrophy, and urinary stress incontinence, but it may cause cancer of the uterus or breast, and is not recommended for women with a history of blood clots, irregular bleeding, mastitis (non-cancerous tumors of the breast), or a family history of cancer. In many cases, there are nonmedical therapies for these problems of menopause and aging that do not involve the side effects or risks of ERT. Estrogen replacement therapy has not been proved to be effective in the treatment of osteoporosis, heart attack, emotional problems, aging skin, or weight gain.

PROBLEMS	NONMEDICAL THERAPY	EFFECTS
Hot flashes and sweats	Understand and accept the discomfort. It will pass in a year or two. Pay attention to total health care—physical, social, and psychological.	No side effects or risks to health.
Vaginal atrophy (causing painful intercourse)	Maintain regular sexual activity, with or without a partner. Exercise the pubococcygeus muscle (see page 534). Use a lubricating jelly.	May improve vaginal tone and sexual response, without side effects.
Urinary stress incontinence	Exercise the pubococcygeus muscle (see page 534).	Improves vaginal tone, without risk.
Osteoporosis (bone loss, reflected in lower backache, fractures, and dowager's hump)	Exercise daily. Get proper nutrition, especially enough calcium and vitamin D. Limit alcohol and certain antidepressant drugs.	Promotes physical fitness, a healthy appearance, and a sense of well-being, without negative side effects.
Heart attack	Exercise daily. Stop smoking. Control your weight. Avoid foods high in sugar and saturated fat. Eat foods high in protein and vitamins; raw vegetables and fruits.	Promotes physical fitness and improved health, and lowers the chance of heart attack.
Emotional problems	Seek counseling or psychotherapy, or menopausal "rap" groups.	Dispels myths and helps generate self-esteem. Provides a support system.
Aging skin	Avoid too much sun, or use a sunscreen that contains PABA. Good nutrition helps skin, as do moisturizers. Avoid soaps with perfumes and deodorants.	These methods will promote a healthy appearance, but nothing will prevent skin from aging.
Weight gain	Maintain good nutrition while cutting your calorie intake. Eat fruits, nuts, grains, vegetables, and foods low in animal fats. Exercise regularly.	Promotes good physical health, and lowers the chance of heart attack.

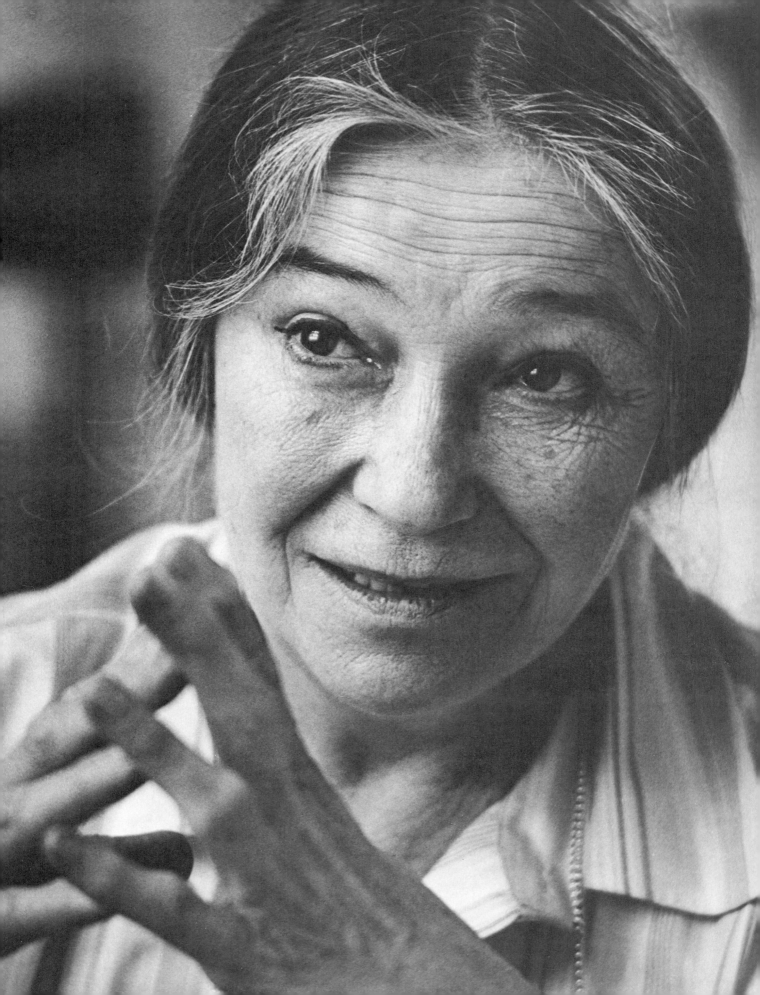

CHAPTER 16

AGING

ANNE HARRIS ROSENFELD

We are all growing older. Some aspects of aging are appealing—the wisdom borne of experience, leisure earned from hard work, freedom from the responsibilities of parenthood, and a broader perspective on life. Other aspects of aging may cause us discomfort— physical change, retirement, the prospect of illness or dependency, and loneliness as others in our generation die.

So in aging, as in other stages of our lives, we can anticipate both rewards and challenges. By looking ahead and planning for our physical and mental health, we are more likely to adapt successfully and maintain satisfying lives.

Aging

Chances are, you're going to lead a long, long life. One hundred years may be too much to expect, but seventy-five or more is not. You're one of the lucky ones. You escaped childhood's once-fatal diseases, steered past the shoals of childbirth, and now face a challenge unknown to many in preceding generations: the prospect of living twenty-five, thirty, or more years past menopause. You may take this modern miracle for granted, or view it with mixed emotions, but it's a miracle nonetheless.

Most of us prefer not to look very far ahead to envision our future selves and lives. We'd rather think about the present and immediate future, where perennial optimistic fantasies can have full play. But look ahead we must, to understand where we're headed and to do justice to our special gift of time. To make the most of our long life-span, we must plan ahead and prepare for the journey as best we can. To be sure, unknowns abound, but it helps to know your general itinerary. We'll explore here the nature of the aging process—and examine some of the ways you can make the most of your later years.

The Challenge of Growing Old

Despite its universality, aging is one of the most mysterious and misunderstood parts of the human life cycle. The mystery may be with us for some time to come, but there's no need for myths and misunderstanding to cloud our vision. Aging is a basic, natural biological process that happens to all living organisms. We all have a finite life-span, whether the mayfly's few days or the redwood's millennia, and all of it is spent aging. In each of us, there is an inborn biological "clock" with its own subtle rhythms that ticks out our fetal development, infancy, childhood, adolescence, maturity, and decline. For the whole of life, cells are born and die, and new ones serve in their stead. (Amazingly, despite this renewal process, we retain a single, recognizable identity. In the early phases of the life cycle, cell growth exceeds cell death; later, this replacement and renewal process is outstripped.) Somewhere in the late 20s or early 30s, there is a biological turning point that starts us past our physiological peak. We might say that that's when aging really begins, although in a sense we've all been aging since the moment of conception.

Your body does not announce the moment when you shift biological gears, but sooner or later you know that you have. To one person, that realization may start at the sight of a gray hair; another may sense it on a tennis court, or the morning after a late-night party. Whatever the signal, and it usually comes relatively early in the life-span, you know you've come of age.

The biological process of aging sets the stage—and some of the limits—for the character and duration of our adult life. But, as you will see, biological aging per se is not the bugaboo it's often made out to be. While no one has yet found a way to reverse the basic biological programming that makes humans age, we are beginning to better understand some of the factors that affect the pace of aging. In time, we may be able to slow it down appreciably so that we'll have more good, full years available to us, even if the basic human life-span remains unaltered. For some people this already seems to be possible. Although the secret of their "success" is still somewhat elusive, there are some basic guidelines that we'll explore shortly.

The physical facts of biological aging are but one small part of what we experience with the passage of time. Strongly coloring our perceptions of ourselves and others are the social meanings we attach to the various phases of the life cycle. The way we humans label others and assign them roles varies considerably from one society to another, and sometimes even within a given social group. Most societies celebrate major transition points in the life cycle—birth, marriage, death—and acknowledge some passage from childhood to adulthood. But they don't necessarily distinguish among their adults as we do; if distinctions are to be made between "elders" and the rest, they are unlikely to be based on chronological age. Indeed, in many primitive societies where no exact birth records are kept, people don't know their age! They become elders gradually, as children and grandchildren are added to the clan. As the years pass and valued experience and wisdom mount, social status rises, too. In some societies where life is short and hard, the life cycle may be so compressed that one becomes an "elder" at an age when our "young" doctors barely finish their specialty training!

In our own complex society, however, there are many contexts and criteria for youth and old age. Our expanded time frame permits us to have an extended period of pre-adulthood, and allows us to delay our assumption of parental and career responsibilities until biological aging is well under way (e.g., the 35-year-old new mother or the comparably aged "new" doctor). Only in the athletic sphere or in certain highly physical occupations do we recognize that by our early 30s we have already passed our physiological peak.

When an "old" athletic champion "retires" at 30 or 35, we wince at the reminder that our own biological clockwork also is winding down, but usually go on about our physically less demanding lives as they shift from locker room to boardroom. One of the most interesting pathways through our social age-role system is that of Byron "Whizzer" White, who passed, over time, from being an "old" man on the football field to a "young man" on the Supreme Court.

Imposed on our informal age-labeling system is a strange formal system bred by the needs of a bureaucratic society. Since numerical cutoff points ease the burdens of administrative decision making, policy makers use them all the time, slicing the world up into groups depending upon, for example, the number of dollars they make, or the number of years they've lived. Our traditional gateway to statistical "old age" and retirement is 65 years of age, the heritage of German administrative policies under Bismarck's late-nineteenth-century leadership. A century ago, 65 was a reasonable, if biologically arbitrary, dividing line. Most people were nearing the end of their lives at that age, and had very few years left as productive workers. Today, with many 65-year-olds quite able to continue for five, ten, or more years as excellent workers, retirement at 65 appears wasteful, and mandatory retirement downright punitive. While our retirement policies are undergoing attack and change, it may be a long while before we truly celebrate older birthdays. No wonder many people lie about their age; they'd prefer to be accepted for what they are, and not judged by the number of years they happen to have lived.

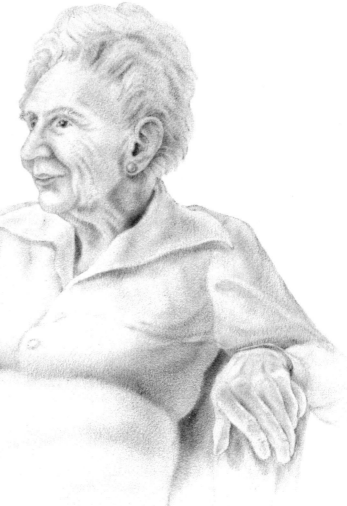

The Aging of America

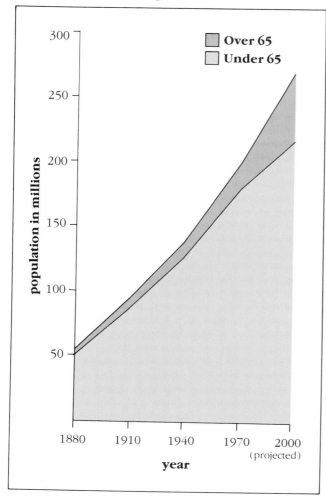

population in millions

year

(projected)

Since 1900, the elderly population of the United States (those 65 and older) has increased from three million to more than 22 million (1975). This seven-fold increase is much greater than that for the United States population as a whole, which almost tripled — from 76 million to 215 million — over this same time period. The proportion of the elderly in the total United States population also has been increasing — from 4 percent in 1900 to 10 percent in 1970 — and will reach an estimated 20 percent by the year 2000.

It's interesting to watch the direction of the lies, because they reveal the underlying values of our society. Teen-agers try to seem older so they can participate in the special privileges of adulthood; adults try to seem younger, afraid of the stigma attached to old age. Were there status attached to the *later* phases of life in our society (as there is in others), Jack Benny might have been a chronic 79, not 39, and silver hairs would buy prestige, not membership in a "Golden Age Club."

The question of why we stigmatize our elders is too complex to examine here, but it's important to remember that we do — so much so that we now have a word for our prejudice: ageism. It's a sad and ironic phenomenon, because all of us, if we live long enough, will join that beleaguered minority we call the elderly. And its ranks are swelling daily. If we accept the 65-year-old designation as old, then 10 percent of our nation is old now, and 20 percent will be old by the year 2000. That's a ridiculous number of people to consign to irrelevance and disparagement. And it's equally cruel to expect anyone to spend ten, twenty, or more years of life —potentially good and productive years — burdened with prejudice, discrimination, and negative expectations.

The fact of the matter is that our society has not quite caught up with itself and its coming of age. There was once a time when its long-term survivors were few, and were often sickly folk. But modern medicine has changed that. Not only do we have more old people, but we have more old and well people. In essence, we have added a new stage to the life cycle — the post-retirement years — but don't know what to do with it. Our old roles and expectations for the elderly no longer fit, and we still don't have good new ones. With our families scattered, it's hard to play the "elder." With our general good health, it's folly to play the dependent fading flower. With our vigor and capabilities intact, it's demeaning to play the acquiescent, passive "Whistler's mother." It's obvious that some new roles and new values are in order. And, it's up to us to start creating them.

Let's consider another aspect of later life: its psychological side. "You're as old as you feel," we say. For some, the feeling never comes, while for others it starts early and never departs. Depression and physical illness can make anyone feel and act ponderously ancient, regardless of age. Conversely, good health and buoyant spirits can keep a person feeling and acting "young" well into the upper limits of the human life-span. Subjective youth or old age may have relatively little relationship to chronological age, the physical aging process, or social criteria for distinguishing the young from the old. But since many factors may conspire to undermine the physical and mental health of older people, it may be harder for some to retain their psychological youthfulness. Nonetheless, many do, and you can as well. There is nothing in the biological aging process per se that can rob you of your youthful spirit.

The passage of time will affect you in many ways, not all of them predictable. You will continue to age, as you have already been doing, with certain consequences for how you look and feel. You will change appearance and lose certain capabilities, but your biological limits are unlikely to be severe. You will be susceptible to more illness, but you will not necessarily confront it until very late in your life, especially if you guard your health. Because you live in a society that arbitrarily decides who is old, and then stigmatizes people for it, you may find yourself deprived of certain social opportunities, unless you fight back. You will need a new kind of toughness and creativity to forge a life for yourself that is fulfilling. But it can be done, and your efforts will help not only yourself, but countless others.

Your subjective experience of your later years will be colored by many factors: your health, your finances, your neighborhood and living conditions, your social life, your personality, your strategies and philosophy of living, and the match between your expectations and the actualities of daily life. While no one can predict the length and quality of your future days any more than you have total control over them, there are ways to increase your chances of having a long and good life. We'll concentrate on some of the key ones related to your mental and physical health. But first, so that you can understand better the nature of health and illness in later life, let's go over some of the basic biological and psychological facts of normal, healthy aging.

The Aging Body

We are all aging every day. Yet, despite the universality of this common biological process, it poses many baffling scientific and philosophical questions. Why do humans rarely survive longer than a century? Why don't they stay at their youthful peak forever? What makes us age? And why can't the process be stopped or reversed?

How We Age—and Why

Considerable research and speculation notwithstanding, we still don't know very much about how and why we age. To many scientists, however, one clue to biological aging and its control lies in our cells, and in the mechanisms governing their reproduction. Our bodies are replacing cells all the time, but according to the "error theory" of aging, over time the genetic material in our cells loses its capacity to create perfect cell replicas. It starts to make small errors that add up to impaired physiological function as increasing numbers of imperfect cells become the basis of our being. Theoretically, if we could prevent these errors, we'd last much longer. However, as yet such victories over aging seem remote. There are many other theories and many other avenues being explored, but if there's a fountain of youth at the end of one, it's presently out of sight.

What Older People Say About Aging

You remain yourself as you age, and there's little to stop you from continuing your usual life-style into old age. Recent studies have shown that in our culture, prejudices against the elderly are reflected in false stereotypes about the physical and social conditions of old age. Throughout this chapter, some of these misconceptions are contrasted with true statements about aging and the health, life-style, and personality of the elderly.

Recent studies conducted with the elderly indicate that there is great diversity among older people, and it is as difficult to talk about a typical 60-, 70-, or 80-year-old as it is to make generalizations about any particular age group. There are large differences in rates of aging from person to person, and even from organ system to organ system in a single individual.

Life-styles, values, and personality vary as much among the elderly as among other age groups. There simply is no one set pattern to describe old people as a group.

An individual's physical change with age depends on individual heredity, on past health practices and past medical history, on the stress of a lifetime, and on socioeconomic factors and family relationships.

Among the majority of the elderly, old people report that old age is a time of satisfying emotional and physical health with a minimum of impairments.

Youth   Young Adulthood   Mid-life

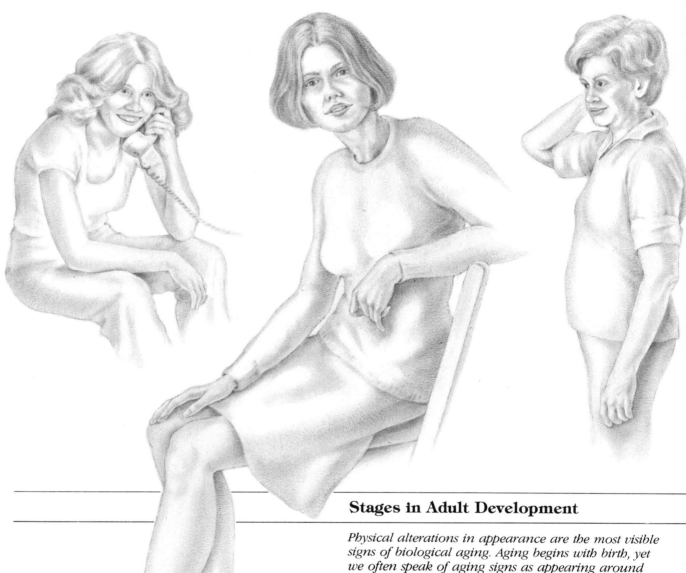

Stages in Adult Development

Physical alterations in appearance are the most visible signs of biological aging. Aging begins with birth, yet we often speak of aging signs as appearing around mid-life. The physical characteristics of youth are flexibility, good muscle tone, and ease of weight control. But in young adulthood, one usually gains some weight, and unless regular exercise becomes a personal routine, there is a slight loss of muscle tone. At mid-life, food intake must be restricted to keep from gaining weight, which takes on a different distribution and causes changes in posture as well. The loss of muscle tone is more marked than earlier, and skin becomes wrinkled.

With further aging, women often find it easier to control weight. As skin and muscle tone slackens, the delicate, bony contours of the body are revealed. Skin wrinkles become pronounced, and unless a daily routine of flexibility exercises is followed, the body becomes quite stiff. Usually some motion restriction occurs by age 70, even in the most athletic women. By age 60, the spine will begin to droop unless regular exercise has retained good strength and flexibility.

Mature Adulthood

Old Age

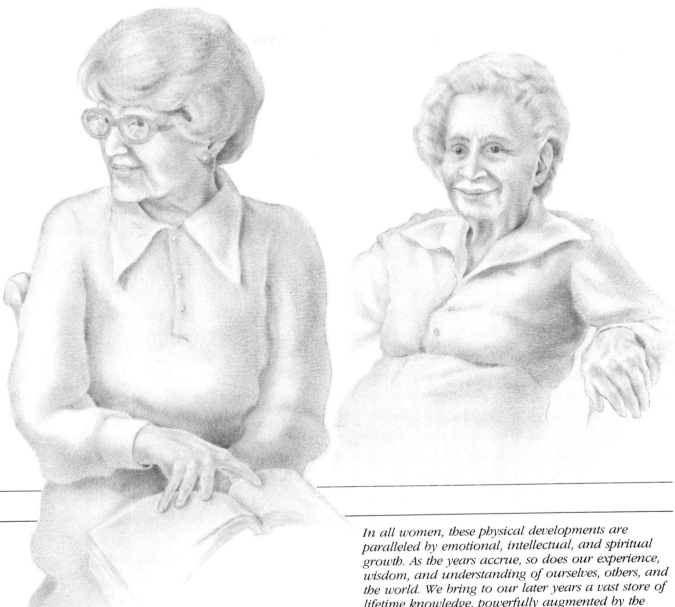

In all women, these physical developments are paralleled by emotional, intellectual, and spiritual growth. As the years accrue, so does our experience, wisdom, and understanding of ourselves, others, and the world. We bring to our later years a vast store of lifetime knowledge, powerfully augmented by the continuing capacity for learning and growth. Small wonder that some of the finest creations of art have been the mature works of truly old masters.

What does seem possible — although unlikely to yield human applications within our lifetimes — is to slow down the pace of biological-aging changes through various types of dietary and environmental manipulations. Experiments with animals have shown that it's possible to defer many aspects of aging for a while, or, to put it another way, to extend the middle years so they last longer. Unfortunately, most of the experimental procedures now being explored require artificial living conditions few of us would or could endure, even if it meant more good times.

As things stand now, there is no magic pill, potion, hormone, or nostrum that will stave off or reverse aging. But there are known ways of upping your chances of living long and well, while aging nonetheless. See "How To Live Long and Well" on the opposite page. Although the fundamental biological aging process still seems to elude control, research scientists are beginning to understand much better the ways in which people age. Descriptive studies of healthy older people have given us a picture of how physical and mental abilities and functions change as we grow older. Among the most valuable of these investigations are the ones that follow individuals over relatively long time spans, so that we learn not only what people are like at various chronological ages, but how they change as individuals over time. Such studies provide some basis for predicting different patterns of aging, and for spotting — and possibly averting — later problems through early treatment.

Myths About Aging

Social Relationships

FALSE STEREOTYPE: Elderly people are grouchy, self-pitying, inflexible, depressed, narrow-minded, and meddlesome. They are old-fashioned, stuffy, and have no interest in sexual relationships.

TRUE STATEMENT: Personality traits of people do not change markedly with old age, according to life-span longitudinal studies. The personality of older people, however, may be affected by social definitions and expectations of how they will behave. Most people develop characteristics of evenness, self-reliance, and strength as they age. Sexual activity is usually possible lifelong, and sexuality remains an important part of relationships throughout the life-span.

Intelligence

FALSE STEREOTYPE: Old age results in senility and a decline in intelligence. Elderly people are confused by simple facts and have poor memories.

TRUE STATEMENT: Only a small percentage of elderly people ever develop serious mental impairments. Mental functioning, intelligence, and the ability to learn usually remain unchanged long after age 80. When senility does occur, it is often the result of depression, brain damage, or medication. While decision-reaction time may slow in some individuals in later years, other skills and intellectual abilities improve with age.

Health

FALSE STATEMENT: Elderly people are usually sick and helpless, and spend a great deal of time in bed because of illness; many are institutionalized in hospitals and nursing homes. Old people have many accidents and often are unable to live successfully by themselves.

TRUE STATEMENT: Ninety-five percent of elderly people live in the community, and the majority are healthy. Household interviews indicate that two-thirds of the elderly judge themselves to be in good or excellent health compared with others of their own age, and over four-fifths of those interviewed reported no hospitalization within the previous year. Persons over age 65 may even have some health advantages over younger people, such as fewer colds, infections, and acute digestive problems.

One of the most striking findings from these longitudinal studies is the great diversity among older people, even within a given age group. Although some generalizations are possible, it's difficult to talk about the "typical" 60-, 70-, or 80-year-old. Time, of course, takes its toll on everyone, but the years add up in quite different ways, with some individuals seemingly breezing through, while others are quite physiologically impaired "beyond their years." On the average, a group of older subjects will perform less well on most physiological measures than a group of young adults, but some individual oldsters may run circles around their juniors, even when it comes to such basic physiological functions as cardiac function and respiration. The same holds true when groups of older people of various ages are compared; on the average, the edge goes to the relatively young, but there are some startlingly vigorous people whose bodies simply refuse to age as others do. See page 327 for "What Older People Say About Aging."

Another interesting finding concerns the rates at which different parts of our bodies age. People seem to have highly individualistic ways of aging, and unique vulnerabilities. Parts of them may stay relatively youthful, while others succumb readily to aging and disease. Heredity may play a strong part in determining these unique patterns. Those with the good fortune to have healthy, youthful circulatory systems are particularly blessed (even if other systems take aging less lightly) since they are likely to live long. As one aging expert put it, "Older women with low blood pressure are practically immortal."

Given the great individuality that marks our aging, it is difficult, if not impossible, to give a "normal" timetable of aging, as we do for childhood development. It's hard to say what you'll be like in ten, 20, or 30 years, although you're likely to have an edge over many of your peers if you're a nonsmoker, on the thin side, generally healthy now, and married. Many other factors could be added to the crystal ball, but your particular future is still unknown.

Nonetheless, it *is* possible to say that you will continue to age, and will undergo, as we all do, certain changes that are a natural part of the life cycle. Their timing is variable, but their appearance sooner or later is predictable. The important point to remember is that we are talking about changes that are part of *healthy* aging. While they do spell some lessened capabilities, for the most part they are quite compatible with continued good and active living. Basically, healthy people have enough physical and psychological resilience and reserves to take time's wearing-down processes in stride and still function well. Dr. Alex Comfort, one of this country's leading gerontologists, describes the terrain before you:

"You need not count on illness or decrepitude. Your memory, sexuality, activity, capacity for relationships, and zest should normally last as long as you do, and do last in the majority of people. When they do not, it is for the same cause as in earlier years, namely, illness."

How To Live Long and Well

Loss of vigor and attractiveness does not have to naturally accompany old age. There are no specific diseases caused by old age or the aging process; diseases prevalent in older groups are frequently the result of chronic disorders that occurred years earlier, often having their beginnings between the ages of 30 and 40.

Numerous studies indicate that daily habits and individual life-style play significant roles in longevity and health, and that prevention is the key to living long and well. Many conditions of the elderly—hypertension, incipient diabetes, cancer, and heart disease—can be prevented or halted through early detection and/or treatment, as well as modified by individual behavior and life-style. The following guidelines are especially important in this respect.

- EXERCISE REGULARLY

- EAT A SENSIBLE AND BALANCED DIET

- DON'T SMOKE

- LIMIT EXPOSURE TO THE SUN

- SEEK PROPER DENTAL CARE REGULARLY

- HAVE AN ANNUAL PHYSICAL EXAMINATION (INCLUDING AN EYE EXAMINATION)

Sensory Changes

Aging dulls the senses somewhat, particularly vision, hearing, and taste. The muscles that help eyes to focus become less elastic, and many by their mid-40s need glasses to help them focus on nearby things, especially for reading. Aging also increases susceptibility to certain eye diseases, particularly glaucoma and cataracts — two serious eye problems that require early detection and treatment. Thus, it's important to have your eyes checked regularly to help them retain their best function.

Hearing losses, which start at around age 30, often go unnoticed, although sensitivity to high tones diminishes appreciably over time. Men seem to suffer more hearing loss than women, but it's well to know that these losses can happen to you, too, particularly during the later years. Fortunately, tiny hearing aids can compensate for many types of hearing loss, so one need not miss the joys of music or conversation. You may never need a hearing aid, but if you do, it should be prescribed only by your doctor after careful tests of your hearing. Beware of door-to-door salesmen; peddling hearing aids is a common racket.

Losses in the sense of taste are among the least acknowledged of aging-related sensory changes, but they can affect, unknowingly, the palatability of food, and even dietary habits and nutrition. Many factors contribute to taste loss, particularly fewer and less sensitive taste buds. If you sense that foods don't have the kick and quality they once had, don't blame it all on plastic processing. Eat more slowly and chew well, savor scents (a great part of what we perceive as taste), and use spices judiciously. However, don't oversalt to compensate; salt just adds to potential high-blood-pressure problems.

Hair and Skin Changes

Gray hair — and eventually white hair — is one of those unavoidable and irreversible parts of the aging process. Hair loses its pigment over time, at a pace determined primarily by your genes. Whether you're "prematurely" or "maturely" gray, it's nature's way. You can go along with nature and enjoy the dignity and flattering softness of gray, wear a wig, or fight it with hair dyes. Some caution is in order if you take the latter route, though. There is some evidence of a link between some hair dye ingredients and cancer in animals. Although the matter is far from settled regarding people, why risk your health trying to look younger? Wigs might be a safer choice, if you really want to hide this sign of maturity.

Whatever you decide, if your hair is turning gray, it's also becoming drier and more brittle. Treat it kindly, with a minimum of chemical treatments and excess heat. Hormone supplements may minimize some hair texture changes after menopause, but that's a matter to discuss with your doctor. If you're feeling blue about the grays, just contemplate what aging does to many men: at least you've got hair!

Another of the more visible aspects of aging is increasing dryness and inelasticity of the skin. Your face takes more of a beating than the less frequently exposed parts of your body, with wind, sun, and weather adding to ongoing aging changes in the composition of facial skin and muscle cells. Some lines, wrinkles, bags, and sags are part of the inevitable picture, and unless you're a makeup wizard, they're going to show.

There's little that can be done to get rid of wrinkles and lines you already have, save plastic surgery (see pages 657 and 658). But there are a few things you can do to prevent things from proceeding unduly fast. First, stay out of the sun, unless you love leathery lined skin. (This also may save you from some skin cancer risks.) If you do sunbathe, be sure to use a sunscreen lotion or wear a hat. Second, don't smoke. There are lots of reasons for not smoking, but wrinkles should be added to the list: women who smoke are more susceptible to wrinkles than those who don't. Third, use moistening creams if you don't already. They don't have to have fancy names or fancy prices: the point is simply to make up for some of the moisture your skin has lost.

Most of the high-priced techniques and products sold to aid aging skin are ineffective but harmless to all but your pocketbook. (If it makes you happy to slog in mud, cucumbers, or queen-bee jelly, enjoy. But don't expect more than a momentary happy glow.) Most hormone creams have too few active ingredients to do you much good. If you're past menopause and need hormone supplementation, your doctor should be the one to supply it, not your beautician.

Let's face it. Probably the healthiest approach to wrinkles is to enjoy them, or at least to ignore them and pursue loftier issues. On the positive side, ponder these comments from some wise women in their 80s who have learned to see the bright side of wrinkles: "Wrinkles are beautiful.... When younger people get old, they'll understand exactly why wrinkles are beautiful, 'cause then they'll have more sense." "Wrinkles are from heaven. They show that God let the person grow older. He let them live to see the beauty of wrinkles."

Changes in Muscles and Fat

Aging affects not only the skin and muscles on the face, but on the rest of the body as well. As we grow older, muscles lose their elasticity and power. Fibrous tissue in the muscles increases, and muscular contractions become less powerful. These changes start gradually in our late 20s, increasing in pace after our 50s. In addition, body muscle is replaced by fat. All of these changes spell greater difficulty in maintaining our figures, our physical stamina, and our athletic ability. Derrieres tend to slump and spread, waistlines expand, bellies bulge, necks and arms get crepey, breasts tend to sag, and we become generally softer and less firm all over.

Although the years may seem to be out to rob us of our fine form and function, there's considerable room here to fight back. You cannot and should not expect to sustain the body of a 20-year-old. But you can keep your body in good shape for your age. Most of us lead lives far more sedentary than nature ever intended, and consequently go to pot far sooner than we ought. We drive and droop, sit and sag, and then fret that we're frumpy, dumpy, and fat.

The keys to staying in shape are well known to all of us: regular exercise and a sensible diet. You are never too old to get in better shape. Whatever your age, your muscles thrive on use, and your body can firm up and become more limber with exercise. Check pages 334 to 341 for some exercises to help you tone up. You don't have to do exercises to get exercise, though. If you're the type who'd rather jog, swim, play tennis, or go bike riding, by all means do. But do it regularly — say, twice a week — and vigorously enough to get nearly breathless. If you've been away from these activities for a while, don't try to make up for years of inactivity with sporadic weekend athleticism. Check with your doctor first, and ease in gradually. Otherwise, you'll simply be asking for trouble, and your body will tell you so. If you think exercise can't help at *your* age, consider this: one study of 70-year-olds in a one-year exercise program revealed that by the end, they had the bodily reactions of 40-year-olds. Now that's something to work for!

Although, as we've noted, aging tends to pad you out with fat (even if you're in good condition), much of what passes for "middle-age spread" has nothing to do with biological aging — just overindulgence, and perhaps ignorance. The battle of the bulge often starts visibly in middle age (although the stage may have been set in childhood), with former skinnies, shocked to find size eights much smaller this year, skulking into size tens or twelves. They've probably lost sight of the fact that they're less physically active than in their hectic youth, and no longer need — or burn up — as many calories as they once did. As you grow older, your caloric needs diminish. An "average" young woman of 18 to 35 might require 2,000 calories a day. But between 35 and 55 this drops to 1,850, and from 55 on it's even less — 1,700 calories daily. Anyone who, at 55, eats as she did at 20, and hasn't stepped up her physical activity since then is probably in for some unwanted poundage (see page 47).

Your best bet is prevention: reining in your appetite just a notch to cut out the extras and the nibbling, and making those choices in your daily life that mean expending more energy — particularly walking instead of taking a car or an elevator. The added exercise can benefit your overall health and physical condition, too.

If you're the kind who has already launched on a "large is lovely" campaign, convinced that fat is fabulous, it's time to reconsider. The issue is not simply one of fashion; it's a matter of survival. Excess fat is a killer when it mounts up, adding to your chances of heart disease, diabetes, kidney and liver diseases, and accidents. It also can complicate medical problems often found in later life, such as diabetes and arthritis. If you want to live long and well, stay on the skinny side of average. On pages 47 to 50, there are suggestions for sensible eating that may add years to your life.

Skeletal Changes

Make no bones about it, aging is not particularly kind to the skeletal system. Joints move less freely as their cartilage cushions wear thin and joint fluids lessen, and backs shrink up a bit as the disks between the vertebrae atrophy. When these changes are combined with muscular alterations, the result is often less flexibility, occasional stiffness, and discomfort. These are normal changes, and not to be confused with the joint diseases often found among older people. We're not talking about the kinds of joint pain severe and frequent enough to warrant regular use of aspirin (see pages 630 to 639). For these, you should see your doctor. Although none of these normal aging changes can be prevented, there are several ways to minimize their effects. First, make sure your shoes permit easy, comfortable walking. Foot joints take an incredible beating, and deserve to be treated with respect; they're all you've got for walking, and they support all the rest of you. You don't have to become a "little old lady in tennis shoes," but comfort, not fashion, should rule. Second, treat your body to some regular exercises that maintain overall flexibility (see pages 336 to 338). Third, help out your back with a reasonably firm mattress, good posture, and careful, efficient stooping and lifting.

Another skeletal aging change that particularly affects us later in life is bone brittleness. It can be minimized somewhat through estrogen replacement therapy, if you're past menopause and your doctor thinks it's warranted. But some brittleness is bound to increase over time, and can cause problems if you're not careful. Brittle bones are easily broken if you fall hard, and may mend slowly. Your best strategy, whatever your age, is to prevent accidents before they happen. Since falls frequently occur at home, make sure your domestic scene doesn't easily trip you up. Get rid of skiddy carpets, keep a rubber mat in tub and shower, and watch your step. You don't have to totter around like you're made of eggshells, but a broken hip is no picnic, and a little precaution can go a long way.

Exercises for Life

The exercises that follow are as vital to your health and well-being as the air you breathe and the food you eat. Exercise can literally save your life while adding a quality of vitality that allows you to live each day to its fullest. No one is too old to begin exercising. New exercise studies show that people 70 years of age who follow a daily exercise program for one year can recapture the endurance and flexibility of people 40 years of age.

- **Start gradually without strain.** Begin exercising very slowly. Everyone has a different capacity for exercise, depending on their body condition, physical capabilities, and general health. It may only be a few minutes before you begin to breathe hard. If so, try exercising for only two minutes a day for the first few weeks. If at any time you find exercising to be painful or exhausting, sit down and relax. Don't expect that it will be a completely painless effort, though — especially if you haven't exercised for years.
- **Warm up before exercise.** Always begin exercising with a warm-up to loosen your body for more fatiguing activity. Your warm-up may be as simple as walking around the room for five minutes. Continue to move and stretch until you feel slightly warm and noticeably more flexible.
- **Wear comfortable, loose-fitting clothing.**
- **Exercise at any time of the day — except after eating.**

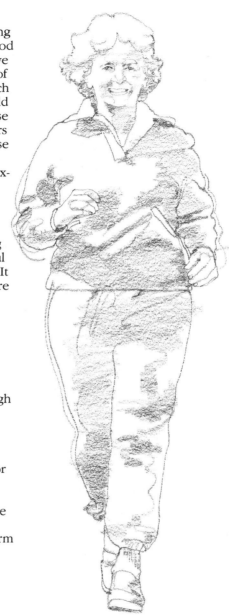

Circulation Exercises

Running, jogging, or fast walking. Running is a natural human movement, and the best exercise for cardiovascular fitness. Begin to develop your running habit with short walks, then longer fast walks, then easy jogging. Alternate all these forms and you'll find yourself running from time to time. The point is to keep moving for a distance of one mile a day. Even in old age, beginning joggers make remarkable adaptations toward fitness and health. No matter what your age or how fat, awkward, or lazy you are, put on some running shoes, go out the front door, and keep moving. Don't worry about how you look or whether you'll make it around the block — just begin. Once on the move, concentrate on how your body feels, and you'll soon find yourself fast-walking, running, or jogging one mile a day — and enjoying it.

Exercise dances. Put a lively, fast piece of music on the stereo, and perform these exercises standing or sitting and in time to the music. Alternate the following movements in any way that feels comfortable to you.

- (A) Lift one leg and then the other, stepping or marching in time to the music. Change the step into a lively bounce, first on one leg and then the other. When you need a change of pace, skip in place, or hop first on one foot and then the other.
- (B) Snap your fingers in time to the music.
- (C) Push your arms straight out in front of you, as though boxing. Alternate right and left arm pushes straight over your head. Put your whole body into these punches.
- (D) Kick your right leg, then your left leg out in front of you. Kick your right leg, then your left leg to the side.

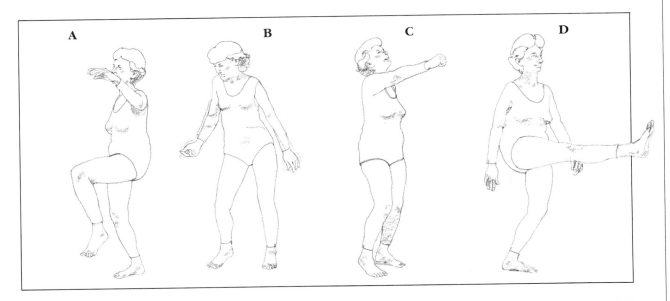

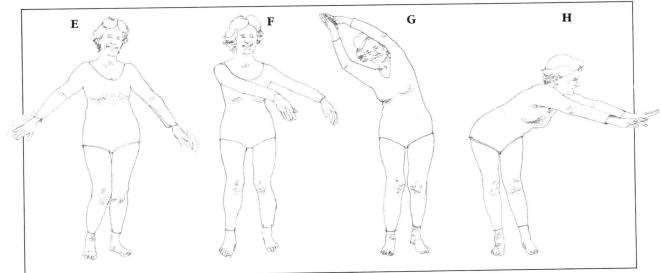

- (E) Holding your arms straight out from your shoulders, rotate your hands in a circle, forward and then backward.
- (F) Stretch your arms straight out in front of you, and rotate your hands in time to the music.
- (G) Clap your hands in front of you, overhead, and behind your body in time to the music.
- (H) Bending from the waist, stretch out your arms—first the left, then the right, as if picking apples from a tree.

Dancing. Put on a favorite record and begin to move in time to the music. Just let go and move your body in any way that feels good. If you are in a slow mood, put on slow, soft music. In a lively mood? Put on a fast tune with a steady beat. Dance alone or dance with friends. Your body receives nearly the same benefits as with running. See the "Fitness" chapter for what you need to know to measure the effect of jogging or dancing on your body, heart, and circulation.

Exercises for Life continued

Flexibility Exercises

Hands. (A) Hold your hands in front of you. Make fists and hold for a count of five, squeezing them tightly together. Open your hands and extend your fingers; hold for another count of five. Repeat five times. Drop your hands to your sides and shake your hands briskly, letting them dangle loosely at the wrist. Clap your hands and massage them.

Press the fingers of your hand tightly against your thumb, forming a shape like a bird's beak. Hold for a count of ten. Release and stretch out your fingers as wide as possible. Hold for another count of ten. Repeat this exercise five times. Drop your hands to your sides, and shake and rotate them from the wrist. Now hold your hands in front of you and shake them briskly from the wrist. Finally, clap your hands together and massage them.

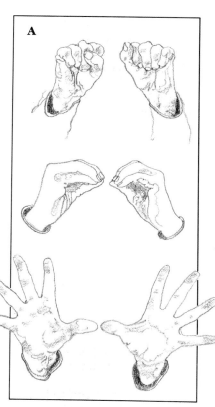

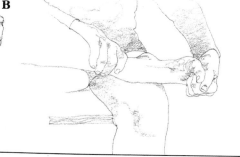

Feet. (B) Sitting, hold your bare foot in your lap and gently knead and rotate each toe. Grasping all the toes with one hand, bend them forward and backward. Knead, press, and stroke the soles and sides of your feet. Repeat this foot massage daily.

● (C) Standing erect with arms at your sides, slowly rise up on your toes. Leave your right foot on the ground and flex your knee; as your knee moves forward, roll your foot out over your toes. Repeat with the left knee and toes. Alternate until you are in the rhythm of a slow walk while standing in place.

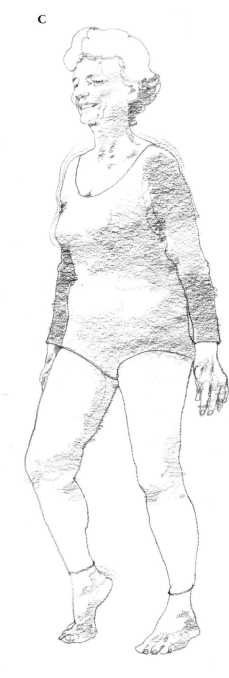

C

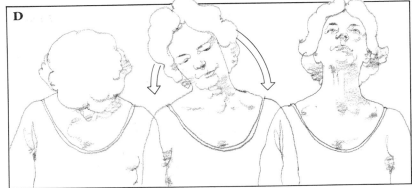

D

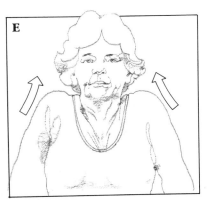

E

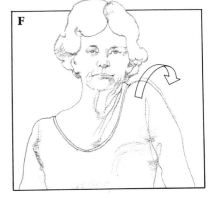

F

Neck and shoulders. (D) To improve the flexibility and function of the neck and upper spine, sitting or standing, lower your head gently forward so that your chin touches your chest. Let the weight of your head naturally respond to gravity. Returning your head to a centered, upright position, slowly move your head to the right as though you were trying to touch your right ear to your right shoulder. Repeat that movement to the left, again letting the weight of your head naturally respond to gravity. Return your head to an upright position. Moving very slowly and gently, lift your chin to the ceiling, letting your head drop backward. Move *slowly* and *gently*.

● (E) To increase flexibility of the shoulders and to ease tension in this area, shrug your shoulders deeply as follows: Facing forward with your head centered, lift both shoulders up in an attempt to touch them to your earlobes. Hold for a count of twelve, then drop your shoulders and relax them for a count of twelve. Repeat this sequence five times.

● (F) Rotate your right shoulder forward, then up to your earlobe, then back as far as it will go, and finally down. Now rotate your left shoulder in the same movement. Repeat this sequence five times on each side.

Exercises for Life continued

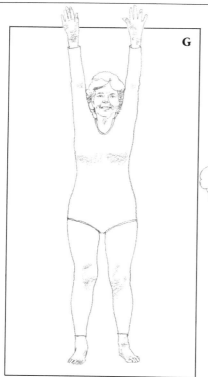

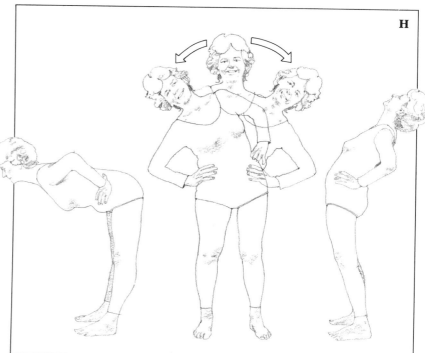

Flexibility Exercises
continued

Spinal column. (G) Standing erect or sitting on a stool, imagine a string attached to the top of your head, pulling your spinal column straight up and erect. Stretch the upper part of your body toward the ceiling. Then raise your hands over your head and, using your arms and fingers, reach for the ceiling, feeling the stretch all the way up your spinal column as it lengthens upward.

● (H) Standing erect or sitting on a stool, gently bend from the waist forward, stretching your spinal column and feeling it lengthen between each vertebra. Return to an upright position. Gradually stretch your body first to the right and then to the left, returning to an upright position after each movement. Now move backward from the waist only, one or two inches. Keep your gaze straight forward to avoid becoming dizzy.

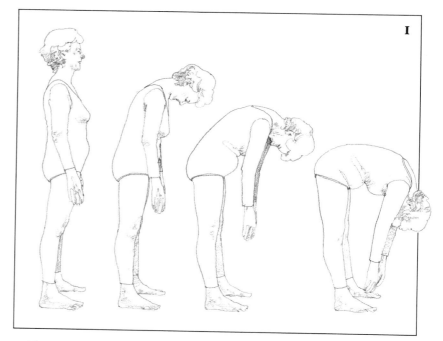

● (I) Standing erect with your feet slightly apart, lower your head, then your shoulders, and finally your body from the waist. Keeping your head between your arms and hands, allow gravity to pull the top of your head toward the floor in front of you. Feel the lengthening and stretching in your spine. Slowly return upright.

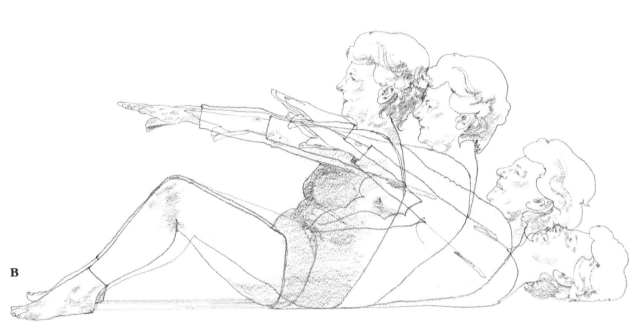

B

Strength and Endurance Exercises

Upper and lower back. (A) Kneel on your hands and knees, with your arms straight. Keep your back straight and parallel to the floor. Lower your chin to touch your chest, and arch your back as a cat arches its back (the common name for this exercise is the cat stretch). Pull your abdominal muscles up toward your backbone and hold for a count of five. Relax and resume your starting position. Repeat this sequence five times. Starting in the first position, repeat the cat stretch of the second position. Add the motion of bringing your left knee to your chest. In a slow motion, extend your left leg behind you as you make your back concave and lift your chin toward the ceiling. Hold for a count of five. Relax and resume your starting position. Alternate right and left legs for a total of three times each.

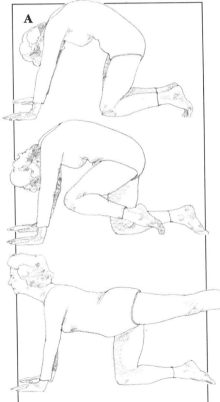

A

Abdominal muscles. (B) Sit on the floor with your legs bent and your back straight; place both arms straight out in front of you, palms facing. Lean backward slowly, keeping your back straight. When you feel a pull on your abdominal muscles, stop and hold the position for a count of ten. Lean back a little farther and hold for a count of five. Lean back until your head is only a foot off the floor, and hold for a count of five. Lower your body all the way to the floor and relax totally. Remember to breathe while doing this exercise. It's easier to "hold" when the breath is exhaled.

Exercises for Life continued

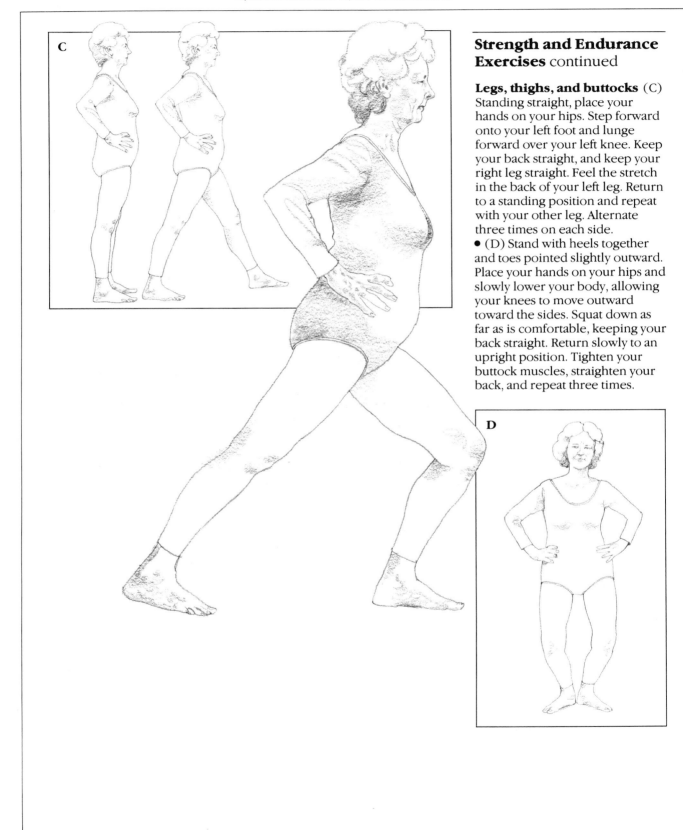

Strength and Endurance Exercises continued

Legs, thighs, and buttocks (C) Standing straight, place your hands on your hips. Step forward onto your left foot and lunge forward over your left knee. Keep your back straight, and keep your right leg straight. Feel the stretch in the back of your left leg. Return to a standing position and repeat with your other leg. Alternate three times on each side.

● (D) Stand with heels together and toes pointed slightly outward. Place your hands on your hips and slowly lower your body, allowing your knees to move outward toward the sides. Squat down as far as is comfortable, keeping your back straight. Return slowly to an upright position. Tighten your buttock muscles, straighten your back, and repeat three times.

E

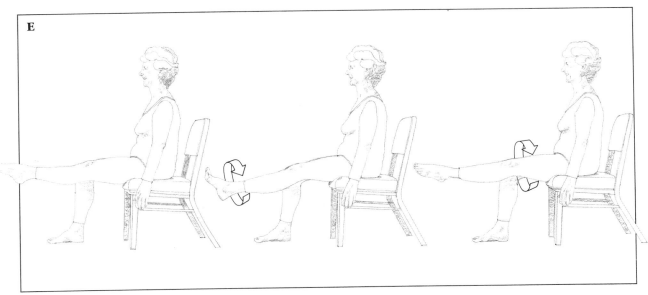

● (E) Sitting in a chair with your back straight, stretch your left leg straight out in front of you. Move your foot in a circular motion from the ankle. Circle the foot five times to the left and five to the right. Repeat with the right foot. Now lift your left leg off the floor and stretch it out in front of you with the knee straight and the toes pointed. Turn your whole leg as far as you can to the right and then to the left in a smooth, slow motion. Repeat with the right leg. Alternate legs five times.

Relaxation Exercise

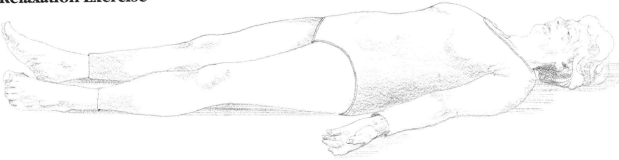

Lie on your back on a comfortable rug or bed. Place your feet apart so that they feel totally comfortable. Place your arms at your sides, palms turned upward. Center your head by turning it gently from side to side and returning it to the center. Close your eyes. Now bend your knees slightly and tilt the small of your back flat against the floor. Press down with the small of your back and hold it against the floor for a count of five. Relax and release your legs. Go limp all over, and breathe in a normal rhythm. Talking to yourself (silently), instruct each part of your body to relax, beginning with the scalp and moving to the toes. Sink into the bed or rug. Totally let go, and notice how tension drains from each part of your body as you give it instructions to relax. Repeat this relaxation technique at the end of your exercise period, once in the morning and once in the evening.

Changes in Circulation and Respiration

Your heart, lungs, and circulatory system work for you day and night, getting oxygen and other essential ingredients to all your body's cells, and carrying away waste materials they generate. No matter how healthy you are, this fine machinery becomes less efficient with age. Lungs hold and expel less air, the heart muscle thickens and becomes more rigid, arteries become less flexible and accommodating (and often clogged with fatty deposits), and blood pressure usually rises somewhat to help pump blood through narrowed passageways. The result is that you work harder to keep those body cells well nourished.

Functionally, these changes can mean somewhat lessened stamina and energy for you, and greater susceptibility to many circulatory diseases. Women seem to have an advantage over men in their resistance to circulatory disease, but may be losing this edge as more smoke and join the stressful workaday world. Given the fact that normal aging changes already make it harder for your respiratory and circulatory systems to work at peak efficiency, it's folly to give them an even harder time by abusing them. After all, you owe your life to them.

There is considerable scientific controversy about the best ways to ward off the major circulatory and respiratory diseases that kill and cripple millions of Americans yearly. But there is little disagreement that one key step is to stop smoking. Heavy smokers may lop as much as eight years off their potential life-span. Smoking also is an invitation to three major diseases: lung cancer, respiratory disease (chronic bronchitis and pulmonary emphysema), and coronary heart disease. Women between 45 and 54 who are heavy smokers have double the coronary heart disease death rate of nonsmokers. Smokers risk lessening not only their length of life, but the quality of their life. Living with a chronic disease like emphysema can leave you quite literally breathless, and chronic heart disease is equally debilitating.

If you think it's too late to change your smoking behavior, ponder this: your lungs are particularly forgiving and prone to recover from years of abuse. No matter how long you've been smoking, or how heavily, you can add years to your life if you stop. If you've tried and failed alone, give a smoke-ending group a try. If that doesn't work, try a visit to your local hospital's cancer ward. If all else fails, at least cut back, switch to the lowest-tar brand you can tolerate, or cultivate using a pipe. If you're already a non-smoker or a convert, congratulations; you've saved money and years. But don't be smug — there's more you, too, can do to help your cells live and breathe.

Regular exercise is a boon to your heart, lungs, and circulation, and one major key to long life and good health. The kinds of exercise needed to keep your circulatory system fit are outlined on pages 334 and 335. They're of two types: one to get your heart and lungs to work as efficiently as they can, and another to teach you how to relax and breathe properly. The latter type can take the edge off the stress, and may help to keep your blood pressure low.

The right type of exercise, regularly maintained, can help keep your circulatory system fit — and may even reverse some circulatory problems. One extraordinary example is Eula Weaver of Santa Monica, California. At 73, she had heart trouble and circulation so poor she needed gloves even in summer. Although at first she could barely walk, she took up running, on her doctor's advice, and by age 80 she held Senior Olympic medals for the mile and half-mile.

One of the most controversial areas of preventive medicine concerns the effects of diet on circulatory health, particularly the contribution of dietary cholesterol to heart attacks. As things now stand, it's clear that cholesterol, a white, waxy solid substance, collects in the arteries as we age, especially if we're inactive. When cholesterol deposits get too thick, they can completely block our arteries so blood can't flow through. While cholesterol is manufactured in the body, it is also found in foods, such as eggs. We all have cholesterol in our blood; its level depends, in part, on the amount and kind of fats we eat; saturated fats, such as animal fat, raise the blood cholesterol level, while polyunsaturated fats, such as those in many vegetable oils, lower it. The case against excess saturated fats in the diet seems fairly strong, but it's still not clear whether they actually cause cholesterol to be deposited in the arteries.

In the face of strong but still debatable evidence, it seems wise to follow the advice of the American Heart Association, which recommends a diet low in cholesterol and modest in fats, particularly animal fats. Key items to watch are egg yolks (only three a week, even in cooking); whole milk products (keep them to a minimum); commercial cakes, pies, cookies, and mixes (solid fats and shortenings), and certain types of animal fats (avoid or use sparingly duck and goose, heavily fatty meats, and organ meats). Shellfish, although low in fat, are also high in cholesterol, so also should be taken sparingly. A key switch in your cooking and eating habits should be from butter and shortening to margarines and liquid oils containing corn oil, cottonseed oil, safflower oil, sesame seed oil, soybean oil, or sunflower seed oil. The shift can spell the difference between raising or lowering your blood cholesterol.

If you think that long, good life requires a spartan existence, then read on. True, you've been advised to give up smoking, start exercising, and watch your diet. On the other hand, not all of life's pleasures are bad for your health. For example, *modest* drinking, such as an occasional glass of wine or beer, especially with others at mealtime, may be downright good for you, pepping up circulation and lowering blood pressure. However, it's well to remember that aging diminishes alcohol tolerance, so a little goes a long way.

Another pleasure that's good for you is sex. Unless you're just recovering from a coronary or another major illness, lovemaking can be a decided boon to your physical and mental health. As exercise, it's excellent and rarely risky. And, of course, it has other rewards as well.

Sleep Changes

Sleep patterns and needs change throughout the life cycle. As we age, we seem to require less sleep than in young adulthood. There's nothing holy about eight hours of sleep a night, and our bodies may well tell us so. If life is quiet and undemanding, one might nap in the daytime and lop off additional time from nighttime sleep needs.

Many older people complain about sleep problems, not realizing that their behavior is quite normal for their life stage, even if it represents a shift from prior sleep patterns. By middle life, some people may already have some difficulty getting to sleep, may sleep less soundly, and may not be able to return to sleep once awakened. Don't get in the vicious cycle of causing sleep problems by worrying about lack of sleep. Your body's pretty wise, and if it needs sleep, it will grab it. You don't necessarily need to dope it up with sleeping pills. Just enjoy your hours awake — in night or day.

Many people find that they wake very early in the morning and then are unable to go back to sleep. If you repeatedly wake early with grim thoughts and a sense of doom and gloom, it may be a sign that you're depressed; you should talk over these symptoms with your doctor. If you simply arise at 4 a.m. or so, happy and ready to start the day but feeling it's premature, don't worry about losing sleep. You're up at a fine time for contemplating, meditating, and enjoying the majesty of a new day's birth.

Aging, Stress, and Disease

Having read this far, you know that it's quite possible for you to be a healthy, vigorous woman well into later life. You have what appears to be a biological advantage over men that delays many of the leading health problems of later life, such as heart disease and arthritis. You, as a woman, also seem to be less vulnerable to many of the diseases that deprive men of their full life-span.

Nonetheless, it's well to understand some of the aging changes that make good health more difficult to maintain as the years roll on. Our bodies are subjected to many types of stress all the time: accidents, injury, infection, polluted air, and the pressures of daily living, to name just a few. When we're young, we are exquisitely structured to roll with these threats to our physical and psychological integrity. The pituitary gland and adrenal glands send out hormone messengers to many parts of the body, commanding them to make adjustments to help us cope with whatever might disturb our equilibrium. If a bacterial infection arises in a particular part of your body, the blood supply to that part of your body will increase. While the inflammation you experience may be annoying, it's the body's way of fighting, and it usually works. If you cut yourself, your hormone messengers will marshal the troops to minimize blood pressure to stop the bleeding, beef up clotting mechanisms, and give you more energy through increased blood sugar.

Aging changes make our stress response system function less effectively. Thus, insults and injuries that the body might have tossed off lightly when we were younger become more difficult to handle as we age. We are more susceptible to certain types of acute illnesses, and also to chronic degenerative diseases such as arthritis, high blood pressure, and arteriosclerosis. We heal less rapidly when illness strikes, and have less energy reserves. As in so many other aspects of aging, the pace of these tendencies varies considerably from one individual to another, and depends on how much wear and tear you've already encountered. You may be blessed with a super constitution that will serve you in good stead even if you lose some of your disease resistance and recuperative powers. But what the general trend means is that you will have decreasing resilience and reserve, and that your body is less likely to be forgiving if it's pushed too hard. And the pushes need not be purely physical; psychological stress also can tax our bodies to the limit.

On the plus side of aging is the fact that we — and our bodies — have learned a few things as we've gone along. We've weathered and become immune to many infectious diseases — and been inoculated against others — so that many do not pose the same hazards they might for the very young. Also, we have learned, if we're wise, how to cope with many of life's problems and stresses, and to take them in stride. Further, if we're lucky and have planned well for our later years, we may be free of many of the domestic pressures that can make the middle years so harried.

On the negative side, we may be called upon to cope with multiple problems at a time when we have lessened biological coping ability. It's easy to get involved in a vicious cycle in which one kind of loss precipitates many others. This is particularly true in advanced old age. People in their 80s and above are regarded by many geriatric experts as particularly vulnerable, both physically and psychologically. Good mental and physical health may well last into the 80s, but both may topple in the face of illness or situational problems that might not have been serious in younger years. If a young child breaks a hip, recovery is likely to be relatively swift and uncomplicated. If an 80-year-old undergoes the same stress, a fatal chain of events may be set off: healing may be slow, prolonged bed rest may undermine general physical and mental well-being, and the person may decline precipitously.

Aging well obviously requires adopting a strategy of living that makes best use of the resources you have, and avoids undue threats to your biological and psychological well-being. This does not mean sealing yourself off hermetically from the rough-and-tumble of life — that's tantamount to a living death — but it does mean making the wisest choices you can that can keep undue stresses to a minimum. And it means getting yourself in the best possible physical and mental condition so that you have the odds of living long and well in your favor.

You're likely to be in the strongest position to handle the challenges of later life if you maintain your basic physical health, have sufficient income to assure that securing the basic necessities of life is no problem (adequate food, clothing, housing, etc.), and have a social support system that really works for you. It helps to be married, but good friends, neighbors, and relatives can go a long way to give you a sense of mutual help and support. You'll also need to develop the kinds of psychological coping strategies that allow you to handle the inevitable stresses of living most efficiently and effectively.

The point to remember is this: most of these strategic advantages can't be conjured up overnight. Good health, post-retirement financial security, a good social support system, and sound coping strategies are best developed and maintained long before you reach later life. If you enter your later years without them, it's going to be tough. Not that your hands are tied if you're already silver-haired, sick, and struggling — but it takes more guts, and it's likely to take more out of you. There are a startling number of older people who manage quite well in the face of incredible hardships. But if you can avoid some of them, why not?

The Aging Mind

One of the ironies of aging — or perhaps its saving grace — is that all the while our bodies are declining, our psyches are growing and expanding. As the years accrue, so does our experience, wisdom, and understanding of ourselves, others, and the world. We bring to our later years a vast store of lifetime knowledge, powerfully augmented by the continuing capacity for learning and growth. Small wonder that some of the finest creations of art have been the mature works of truly old masters.

The Myth of Senility

One of the most pernicious myths perpetrated about the elderly is that "senility" is a natural consequence of aging. So common is our expectation that older minds will crumble away, that we still note with some surprise any person past 70 or so who's still on the ball, saying with some shock and admiration that he or she is still "keen" or "spry." The facts of the matter simply don't bear out our expectations. *Most* healthy older people retain their intellectual faculties in fine form throughout their lives; they never enter that "second childhood" we all dread. One of the cruel consequences of our mythology about aging and senility is that older people are often treated as if they're witless — despite the fact that their faculties are fully intact. After a while, some people actually believe this hype. They become anxious about minor memory slips, thinking that they're evidence of senility, while in fact their mind is as good — or as bad — as it ever was. Because there's so much misunderstanding about the nature of aging and how it affects mental ability, let's set the record straight.

Old dogs may have problems learning new tricks, but old people do not. Your IQ and learning ability remain remarkably intact through the years, and sometimes even improve with age. Older people do, however, differ from younger people in their ability to perform mental tasks fast. Reaction time does slow down over the years (e.g., the time it takes to press the brake pedal when you see a red light), a factor that should be taken into account by older drivers. In addition, a barrage of new and complex information may be hard to assimilate in a hurry. Usually, this latter change can be handled simply by asking people to slow down when explaining things. This is particularly important in your transactions with doctors. Ask them to explain things slowly and clearly, and, if necessary, write down what they advise, particularly regarding medication. There's no need to go home muttering: "Did he say two pinks every three hours, or three pinks every two hours?"

Minor memory slips are a part of life at all ages, and should be dealt with accordingly. If you have trouble remembering phone numbers or appointments, keep a note pad and write them down. But if you really perceive a downward trend in your ability to remember things, it's best to check with your doctor; chances are, there's nothing seriously wrong. Mental abilities are affected by many factors, however, and key among them is our emotional state. Anxiety and depression can alter our ways of perceiving ourselves and our abilities, and may sometimes make us inattentive and confused. Medications also can alter mental faculties, as can some non-neurological diseases.

The chances are very slight that you will ever become "senile." Only a small proportion of older people ever develop serious mental impairment —perhaps less than 10 percent — and of these, an estimated half have conditions that are entirely reversible if diagnosed and treated correctly. The kind of progressive, debilitating senility that ultimately means irreversible and severe brain damage is quite rare. It seems to be the result of a brain disease —perhaps a virus — that one day may be prevented. Although there is progressive brain cell loss with normal aging (brain cells aren't replaced as others are), most of us seem to be magnificently overendowed to begin with, so we can function perfectly fine despite our losses.

Sad to say, some doctors know less than they should about the psychology and physiology of aging, and share the layman's view that any older person who shows signs of mental confusion and memory loss is the victim of irreversible brain deterioration. They may overlook many other possible causes of "senile" behavior, such as alcoholism, the effects of medication, or the presence of heart disease or diabetes. Frequently missed is one of the biggest causes of apparent "senility": depression. Given this state of affairs, some older people with treatable, reversible conditions are summarily written off as doomed and are sent to nursing homes where, unhappy and unstimulated, they fulfill everyone's dire prophecies.

While medical educators are beginning to remedy this flaw in physician training, it's well to be on your guard. If your doctor is the type to write everything off with a jaunty "well, you're not getting any younger," you may not be getting the best medical care possible. And if you should develop any mental problems in your later years, you may miss out on a treatment that could restore your peace — and

alertness — of mind. If you have any doubts about the appropriate diagnosis of mental problems in yourself or loved ones, be sure to get a second opinion —preferably from someone who specializes in treating the problems of older people.

Coping with Depression

Depression is a common problem among older people. Often it arises in response to real losses, not only the physical changes we have already discussed, but losses in income, status, work opportunities, companions, and loved ones. Coping well with these challenges is by no means easy. We tend to underestimate the courage and fortitude of many older people who manage exceedingly well in the face of serious life problems. Most older people seem to have the flexibility and resilience to handle some of the most difficult problems life can bring: the death of a spouse or other loved one, the end of a meaningful career, or the presence of serious and sometimes debilitating illness. They become appropriately grieved and unhappy, then somehow pick up the threads of life and carry on as best they can. But there are others who find it all too much to bear and who fall into a pattern of depressed living.

Unfortunately, many behavioral patterns of depression resemble the behavior expected of older people: slowness of thought and action; passivity; loss of libido, appetite, and sleep; and general lack of energy. Thus, a treatable mental illness goes unrecognized and untreated. Since, to boot, we have brainwashed old and young alike into thinking that old people can't change or get better, many older people who recognize that they're depressed simply accept their state in silence instead of seeking help.

You, like everyone else, will have your ups and downs. There will be difficult times. But if you're lucky, you'll have friends and relatives to help you through. Most older people do. If you sense that you've lost your zest for living, however, and have any of the symptoms described above for a protracted period — it's worthwhile checking with your doctor to see if you need help. There are many effective ways of coping with depression, including drugs, counseling, and even such old-fashioned remedies as travel or involvement in a new type of work or volunteer activity (see page 349). You should be able to find a treatment that's right for you, and have every right to expect to recover your old *joie de vivre*.

One word of caution, though. If your doctor is fond of prescribing pills for problems, make sure that pills are what you need, and that you get only the amount you need. Some doctors tend to overprescribe psychoactive drugs for their patients, forgetting that older bodies metabolize them differently from younger ones, and usually require smaller doses.

Also, be sure to let your doctor know what other medications you're taking. Sometimes various medications don't mix well and can themselves even cause depression. If you get in a deeply depressed state for no apparent situational reason, make sure your doctor does a thorough physical. Sometimes depression can arise as a symptom of physical illness. Whatever the cause, there's no need to accept depression as the price of growing older. It's not!

There's a final point to remember. Aging per se is unlikely to rob you of your mental agility and abilities. But the mind, like the body, thrives on exercise and variety in its diet. Even young children, deprived of stimulation and challenge, can lose their potential brightness and ability. And so can older people. If you lead a highly routine, dull, and isolated life, you're going to be under-challenged, underexercised, and under par mentally. To retain your fullest mental abilities, give your mind the exercise it loves: read newspapers and good books, take classes, share in discussion groups, do puzzles, hone your creative skills, and open yourself to new environments, experiences, and people. And if you can find work or volunteer activities that please and stimulate you, participate. Not all of us are bustly and sociable, nor need we be, but each of us knows when we're bored and understimulated. If you prefer largely solitary activities, you can structure in some new challenges, too; try exploring a new museum, learn to identify birds in your neighborhood, take up Chinese cooking, take a neighbor's child to the zoo, or switch from oil painting to graphics. One group of researchers on aging in Minneapolis has a fine phrase for what's needed: "maintaining the growing edge."

The Social Side of Aging

"No man is an island," Donne said, and no woman is, either. Most of us thrive best when we can share our lives with others. One of our abiding nightmares is of spending our old age utterly alone. Fortunately, very few people actually do. Almost two-thirds (66 percent) of those now over 65 live with a spouse or other relatives, and another 2 percent live with non-relatives. The tiny proportion (5 percent) who live in institutions are also not alone. Thus, only about one-quarter live by themselves. Even then, they may hardly be isolated. Most are in contact with relatives (on the average of once a week), and they have friends and neighbors to support them. The presumably lonely oldsters we sometimes see on the streets by themselves may in fact be neither alone nor lonely. The chances are quite good that you'll have many companions in your later years, whatever your marital status.

Husbands and Lovers

One of the difficult facts of later life, however, is that even if you are now married, you are far more likely than your husband to face widowhood. Better than half (52 percent) of women over 65 are widowed, while only 14 percent of older men have lost their spouses. The differential longevity of men and women, combined with the fact that women usually marry men older than themselves, has created this imbalance.

If you are now married, you and your husband may nonetheless beat the odds and remain together and well for many years to come. His chances of survival may be helped if you encourage him to follow the same health maintenance measures you do: cut out smoking, get adequate exercise, stick to a diet that is not excessively caloric or high in saturated fats, and get regular checkups. Your understanding also may help him handle the stresses of the later years, such as retirement and some physical impairments, with emotional honesty and wisdom.

Preserving marriage into the later years requires more than good health. Although divorce is uncommon among today's older Americans, unhappy marriages are not. Some couples, although basically compatible, flounder in the face of some common stresses of later life. When you're in the throes of rocky times, it's well to know that some marital problems are largely situational and will be overcome once you've gotten through certain critical passage points. Let's look at a few.

One potentially difficult time may be around the age of menopause. Some women's largely biologically induced emotional volatility may well collide with their husband's non-biological but equally difficult "male menopause." When both are confronting the "empty nest syndrome" as well, with lessened child-rearing responsibilities to distract them from themselves and their relationship, hard times may follow.

Another tough passage point may be the period surrounding retirement. Retirement is often made out to be a protracted vacation of leisure, travel, and the realization of long-held self-indulgent fantasies. There is, indeed, often a "honeymoon" phase. But all too often couples come back to earth with a thud, unsure of how to conduct the rest of their lives, and unused to the loss of long-accustomed roles and life-styles. Again, under such pressures and with little other distraction, it's easy for some couples to pick one another and their marriage apart.

If one can weather these crisis points, the later years together are likely to be good ones. And surprisingly, they may yield not only the traditional rewards of comfortable companionship and mutual support, but also greater sexual pleasure. You may need more patience — both with yourself and your spouse — because as in other aspects of later life, responses may be slower. But if you are on good emotional terms with one another, there's nothing to stop you from having a rewarding sex life as long as you live. Many older couples find their greatest satisfaction in simply holding and being held. Others remain quite athletically and adventurously sexual. Whatever suits both of you is fine. There's no right amount or kind of lovemaking at any age. If you and your partner are satisfied with the way things are, that's great. If there is a mismatch in desires and expectations, it's time for an open discussion. Remember, though, if for reasons of illness, alienation, or depression you've been sexually inactive for an extended period of time, both men's and women's bodies are likely to "forget" how to function well sexually. Masturbation is one way of staying in sexual shape, although it's no match for making love.

A good marriage is unquestionably a boon in later life. But what if you're widowed? There was once a time when a widow — whatever her age — was expected to remain single. Remarriage was considered a form of disloyalty, both to her husband and her children. Those days are rapidly waning. Although barriers to remarriage still remain — especially in the financial realm — it is becoming far more acceptable, and grown children are increasingly likely to accept the right and need of a widowed parent to enjoy love and companionship at any age. Because our pension and Social Security laws still may make it difficult for some to retain a decent income if they remarry, some older couples prefer to live together unmarried. While this can be socially awkward, they feel it beats living alone and celibate. The near future may see revisions in our pension policies that make this dodge unnecessary.

Some women adjust well to single living and don't want to change. Others find it hard to live without a man, but sense the odds are against them. The disproportion of older men and women does pose its own problems. Nonetheless, if you want to recouple, your best bet is to get out and socialize. Don't get caught up in a round of self-pity, staying home, or playing cards all the time with other women. Join an organization or social group, take classes, get a job; in short, boost your chances of meeting new people. Second, keep your body in good shape and sexual practice. Third, don't let unrealistic expectations or conventional wisdom cut you out of potential relationships. Your best prospects are recently widowed men. Although social conventions might decree that they wait at least a year before socializing again, some widowed men seem to have a harder time than women adjusting, and frequently remarry sooner. Don't be surprised if a bereaved male friend wants to be more than a friend. And keep your mind open about who's "eligible." The key issue is whether you're basically comfortable and compatible.

Friends and Relatives

Most women, married or not, have multiple social resources: family, friends, and neighbors. They're all important parts of our social milieu, and they can become increasingly important with the passage of time. We all need sharing, caring, relationships, and a network of mutual support. When one part of the network is weakened, there's a natural tendency to shift to other parts for more intense relationships.

Many older, healthy women living alone, particularly if they're recently widowed or divorced, try to establish closer ties with their families. But if you're tempted to move in with your children or other relatives, think twice. First, given the geographical dispersal of most families, this may require uprooting yourself from familiar surroundings. Second, even if you mutually feel it's a good idea, it can turn out later to cramp everyone's life-style. Sometimes it works, but often it doesn't. The most frequently successful arrangement is to live close to your family, but physically separate. You can share as much as you like, and still be free to maintain your own life. (If you become seriously disabled or ill, however, that's another story. If your family is willing and able to have you join them, you'll probably be a lot better off than in a nursing home or trying to manage alone.)

If you're thinking for whatever reason of moving, it's wise to keep a close eye on the kinds of social and work opportunities your new locale is likely to offer. Some older women feel most comfortable in the company of age peers, and thrive in a setting where most people are like themselves. High-rise or garden apartments or other settings that cater to older people offer many advantages and leisure opportunities. However, unless they're in an urban location, they can cut you off from the rest of the age spectrum. Suburban locales sometimes can be isolating, offering fewer age mates and leisure activities, with greater transportation problems than urban settings. Whatever your choice, it involves more than physical surroundings, and should be made with an eye toward the types of people and activities that best suit you. In general, older women gravitate toward cities, where, despite the problems of crime, resources of every kind are relatively plentiful and diverse: doctors and hospitals, colleges and universities, museums, senior centers, concerts, special support programs for older people, and a variety of helping agencies.

Community Programs for the Elderly

	COMMUNITY PROGRAMS	WHERE TO FIND THEM
HEALTH INSURANCE	Medicare (public health insurance for retired Social Security recipients)	Local Social Security office
	Medicaid (public health insurance for the low-income elderly)	Local Social Security office
MEDICAL CARE	Senior citizens' health clinic	Mayor's office or Area Office on Aging
NUTRITION	Group lunch programs Home delivery of meals	Area Office on Aging or senior citizens' center
	Food stamps	County food stamp office
EXERCISE AND RECREATION	Special exercise classes for older women	Local YWCA or yoga class
EDUCATION	Free or reduced tuition programs in local colleges and high school adult education programs	Local school district or community college
	Elderhostel (a one-week live-in study program for elderly men and women on over 100 U.S. college campuses)	Elderhostel, Newton, Massachusetts 02158
INCOME AND SOCIAL SERVICES	Housing aid, legal services, employment programs, transportation (including Dial-a-Ride and reduced bus and train fare programs), homemakers' and volunteer programs (such as Foster Grandparents)	Area Office on Aging or mayor's office

A number of community programs (both public and private) provide free or low-cost services to the elderly. This chart lists some of these resources; to contact them, check your phone book, local senior citizens' center, mayor's office, or Area Office on Aging.

Wherever you choose to live, you may never need to go beyond your immediate circle of friends, relatives, and neighbors for help in times of trouble, but should you find you need services they can't provide, it's nice to know there's usually a backup system available. It's often clumsy, uncoordinated, and hard to get your hands on, but it's there if you need it. Don't be afraid or ashamed to ask; there are times when it can come in very handy. Say you're coming home after an operation and need someone to help you with shopping, cleaning, and cooking for a week or so until you can handle it yourself. There are home aid services that can serve you well. Say you need help with your income tax. Again, there are public services — often free — to give you legal aid (see opposite).

There's an increasing amount of public money being spent to help older people, and it's high time. If you qualify for their services (it usually requires being 65, but sometimes 55 will do), why not take advantage of them? There aren't many social advantages to being a senior citizen, but whatever privileges come your way are worth exploiting. A good way to find out more about services in your community is to contact your Area Office on Aging (see opposite).

Working Past Retirement

A critical factor in the quality of your life-style in later life — socially, psychologically, economically, and possibly even medically — may be you and/or your husband's decision to continue to work past the "normal" retirement age. Even if faced with mandatory retirement on one job, there are many other opportunities for continued work if you seek them, especially if you're self-employed. For some people, retirement is a boon and a blessing, and they're only too glad to quit. Others itch to keep working, particularly if they have made a heavy emotional investment in their work and don't have well-developed leisure activities. In general, women adjust better to their own retirement than men, but there are many individual factors to consider. It's a matter of understanding yourself, your sources of gratification, and your likely need to supplement a fixed retirement income.

If you're now working but approaching retirement age and you sense that you're unlikely to want to quit working, it's a good time to start thinking about alternate careers or work. You may decide to go back to school and develop some new and marketable career skills in relative shortage areas, say in the human services. Or you may want to start researching the possibilities of setting up your own business to turn a long-loved hobby into possible income. Interior decoration, writing, and running antique shops are businesses that can lend themselves nicely to post-retirement living. But they also can be risky financial ventures, and warrant some sound business advice before you plunge.

One thing to consider as you contemplate alternatives to retirement is the meaning of work to you. If work has largely been a means of getting out of the house and being with others, you may find similar satisfactions in volunteer activities. If you need and/or want to be paid for your efforts, a new career is a better choice. If you're forced to retire from a professional, high-status job, it may be somewhat difficult to find gratifying alternatives. One possibility is to share your expertise with your community as a paid or unpaid consultant or teacher.

If anticipating or finding your post-retirement niche is a problem, your community may well offer several sources of help. One good resource may be your local community college. In addition to a raft of arts and crafts courses, many offer programs designed to help older people keep fit, understand aging, protect their rights as consumers, handle the financial and psychological aspects of retirement, and prepare for potential second careers. And if you're already well-versed in a particular craft or hobby, consider volunteering to teach a community college course in it yourself.

Our society still has a long way to go in liberalizing its retirement policies, but with some initiative and creativity, you should be able to forge a life-style that's fulfilling. As things stand now, you may not be permitted to stay on your old job, but there's nothing to stop you from a new career — if you want it.

A Plan for Successful Aging

Living long and well requires a touch of the poet, the shrewd investor, and the alley cat. Creativity, wise planning, and an instinct for survival can go a long way toward helping you make of your later years what you want them to be. To be sure, there's an element of luck, too. But that's just another way of saying that there are limits to how much of our lives we can control — at any stage. Nonetheless, once you understand the nature of aging, you realize that there's enormous room to shape your life the way it feels best to you — and feels good. There *are* constraints — but no more than any artist faces from his or her chosen medium. The trick is to understand them, work around them, and come up with a creative solution that satisfies.

Biological aging per se, and some of the social problems that plague older people in our society, may make some aspects of your life more difficult, but by the time you have to confront these challenges, you've also acquired a great store of wisdom and experience that will serve you in good stead. No one reaches later life without a certain psychological strength borne of having confronted and mastered innumerable problems. Indeed, many people find that later life is infinitely easier and pleasanter than their supposedly joyous youth. Many who dreaded growing older have found that *experiencing* it is far different from *anticipating* it, and far better. They're surprised to find that while their appearance is changed, their essential identity is not. And most healthy older people simply don't feel "old." Indeed, each passing year requires some readjustment in our notion of who is "old," since it's obviously not us and our peer group; we just don't fit the stereotypes.

Our heads have been filled with all kinds of nonsense about the nature of aging—most of it negative. It's hard, with this kind of brainwashing, to develop a realistic notion of what we can—and ought to—expect from ourselves. We have notions of "successful parenting," "successful careers," and all kinds of implicit and explicit developmental timetables and role models, but there's precious little available to suggest how we might age successfully. Here's where the creativity comes in. Since there are relatively few guidelines, you can shape your later years your own way, and you can create your own criteria for successful aging. If you're strong enough to resist playing the few clear roles society mistakenly provides for older people as powerless —passive, irrelevant has-beens—you've already won a good part of the battle.

Think of a few of the older women you've admired. Maybe your list includes such women as Golda Meir, Margaret Mead, Georgia O'Keeffe, Louise Nevelson, Maggie Kuhn, Martha Graham, Grandma Moses, Mae West, Moms Mabley—each one an individual, creative and productive, who refused to bow down and become stereotypically "old." Or perhaps you've known someone in your community—less famous, but no less vivid—who has forged her own definition of later life and its potential. These people are important to think about, because they suggest that there are many more blueprints for later life than most of us imagine. You don't have to recapitulate the style of your parents' older years; you're of another generation, part of a vanguard blessed with far more freedom, good health, and potential than they ever had.

These are interesting times in which to be growing older, changing times. There are many barriers, but if you appreciate and use your own power and potential, they're surmountable. The biggest barrier is the brainwashing you've undergone that makes you expect —and fear—the worst, and act accordingly. Once you realize that you have the capability for sustained enjoyment of life, you will demand your due. This doesn't mean that problems won't arise. No stage is free of them, and later life can sometimes bring more than its share. But you won't take them lying down, assuming that they're simply the price you pay for living long.

Those who find aging depressing often do so because they sense that their fate is out of control: they are being swept along on the current of life and feel frustratingly helpless. It's true that there are some biological aging changes we can do little or nothing about, save accept them gracefully and try to avoid their premature onset. But, as we have emphasized, there's been a lot of misunderstanding about what is and isn't an inevitable and unavoidable part of aging. Many lay people—and, sad to say, professionals, too—have been unduly pessimistic about aging, and have stood by going "tsk, tsk" when they should be out there seeking change. Now that you understand how little biological aging need constrain you, you also see how much potential control you actually have, and how much room there is for growth, change, and improvement. The trick is in accepting what must be accepted, but fighting like the devil that which must not.

We can view aging as a game in which you win some and lose some, but the point is to keep your win-to-lose ratio as high as possible. It's like having a stock market portfolio, or managing a highly diversified corporation. You know you'll take some losses, but you try to keep them to a minimum while maximizing your gains. If we look realistically at the aging process, it's bound to yield some losses. But that's hardly the whole story. There's nothing to stop you from counterbalancing them with tremendous psychological gains. Your big ace in the hole is that magnificent, growing mind of yours. Or, in the narrow intellectual sense, perhaps a better word is your selfhood.

Again, looking somewhat rationally, the only thing that can keep you from growing and developing fully throughout your life is illness—mental and/or physical. Although we have no way of guaranteeing that we can stave off illness indefinitely, there are ways to up your chances of staying mentally and physically well. We've talked about a lot of them throughout this chapter:

• Start planning for and investing in your later years as early as you can, building up your financial, health, social, and psychological resources so they'll serve you in good stead later.

• Build into your life-style some basic strategies for good health: exercise regularly, don't smoke, keep your weight under control, eat well-balanced meals that skimp on saturated fats, and get regular checkups.

• Keep your social support system in good working order, building and developing the relationships you have, and remaining open to new ones.

• Prevent and avoid unnecessary stresses where you can. This applies across the board to all aspects of life: e.g., throw out a skiddy rug to prevent a nasty fall; live in an apartment if it will save you the hassles of managing an ailing house; get shots to ward off infections; pace your day so it's not overscheduled and overpressured.

• Keep your mind in shape with exercise, whether it's through reading, taking courses, doing puzzles, talking with intelligent company, or pursuing challenging hobbies. Maintain the "growing edge."

• Find a social niche that makes you feel useful and worthwhile. Working may be one route, but there are many others—immerse yourself in helping family and friends, do community volunteer work, develop a creative ability, etc.

• Feed your senses: sunrises, snowflakes, flower scents, good meals, candlelight, concerts, and the loving touch of others are all meant to be enjoyed—at all ages.

• Don't grin and bear it—unless you have to. We all have worries and troubles, and they're usually easier to take if you share them with someone who cares: a mate, a friend, a family member, a minister, or a professional counselor. If the worries and troubles are about your body and its functioning, let your doctor know. No one can read your mind, and most people don't know when you need help unless you ask for it. Don't be afraid to ask. There are health problems and problems of living for which there is no satisfactory solution, but don't automatically assume you're confronting one until you've sought help.

Finally, let's consider the alley cat, a scrappy survivor in a world that makes survival tough. Sad to say, our society expects you to act like a pussy cat, but it may relegate you to its ignored back alleys. It's hard to retain your dignity and self-worth when you're pushed aside and treated like a non-person. You can protect yourself against many potential problems and indignities if you know your rights and have the courage to assert them. You also can help to create a better social environment for yourself and many others through your active support of and participation in organizations working to better the lives of older people.

One of the best investments you might make is membership in the nonprofit American Association of Retired Persons, 1909 K Street, N.W., Washington, D.C. 20006. This powerful advocacy group, some 11 million members strong, performs many vital lobbying, educational, and service activities on behalf of older Americans. It is concerned with bettering the whole spectrum of conditions that affect the quality of our later years. It puts out many publications to keep you up to date on your rights and potentialities as an older person, including a bimonthly magazine, a monthly news bulletin, and other special publications on issues of particular concern to older people. The AARP also has local chapters you can join.

You might also check to see if your community has a local chapter of the Gray Panthers. This rather militant advocacy group, started by Maggie Kuhn, is small but tough, and is vocal on issues pertaining to the rights of older people.

National Organizations for the Elderly

National Council of Senior Citizens
1511 K Street, N.W.
Washington, D.C. 20005

American Association of Retired Persons
1909 K Street, N.W.
Washington, D.C. 20006

The Gray Panthers
3700 Chestnut Street
Philadelphia, Pennsylvania 19104

National Council on the Aging
1828 L Street, N.W.
Washington, D.C. 20036

U.S. Administration on Aging
U.S. Department of Health, Education, and Welfare
Social and Rehabilitation Services
Washington, D.C. 20201

This box lists some of the national organizations of special interest to the elderly. Among the services offered by these organizations are: information and referral services, monthly newsletters, group health insurance plans, prescription drug programs, and group travel arrangements.

Another useful touchstone on the local front is your federally funded Area Office on Aging. It is designed as an information and referral resource. Although its primary function is to give out information on government programs, it also may provide other types of information on local nongovernmental activities and programs relevant to older people.

Finally, an often overlooked resource is your public library. It's a good spot to find notices about local educational opportunities and service programs, and is likely to have many books available on aging. Two books by straight-talking gerontologists that might be particularly recommended are "A Good Age," by Alex Comfort and "Why Survive?: Growing Old in America," by Robert Butler.

After all is said and done, there's still much truth in the familiar cliché, "You're not getting older, you're getting better."

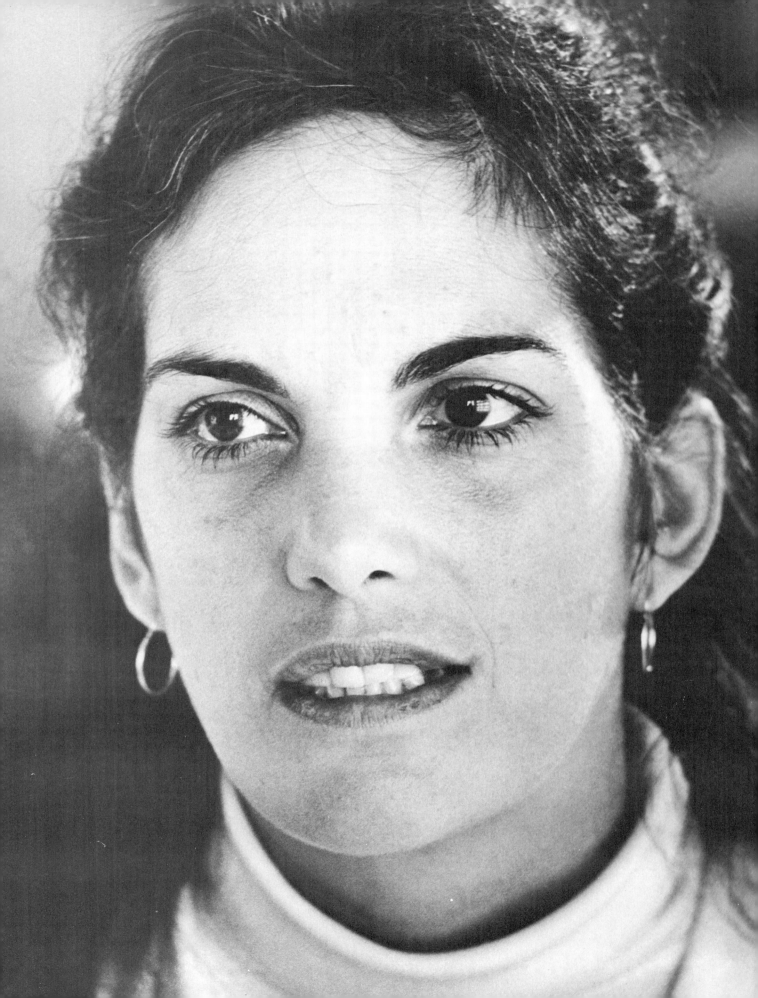

CHAPTER 17

DEATH AND DYING

JEANNE BUNDERSON EWING, Ph.D.

Death is a necessary part of life, and as such, deserves our respect and attention. Many of the fervent goals of our lives would be trivial without the personal knowledge of our own eventual deaths. The simple yet awesome awareness that our time is limited helps us to order priorities, to sort out our most valuable efforts, and just to appreciate the wonderful gift of life.

Death and Dying

Since prehistory we have steadily increased our ability to manipulate and control the environment. As a result, life expectancy has increased dramatically, especially since the turn of the century. The average female child, born in 1900, could expect to live about 40 years. The average woman born today can expect to live almost 80 years. Some gerontologists predict that many of the children born today will live to be 120 to 130 years old! Women no longer die routinely from childbirth in America. Death rates of infants, too, have been reduced to a very low level. Dreaded diseases, such as cholera, smallpox, and diphtheria, which formerly killed people by the thousands, have been nearly eradicated in this country. Whereas other animal species are becoming extinct, the human species has become very successful at survival—largely because of our ability to understand and control the natural world.

On the other hand, much of our human progress since the Industrial Revolution can be seen in mercantilism, B-52s, DDT, napalm, and atomic holocausts. War in the twentieth century has annihilated millions; automobile accidents kill thousands of Americans daily; our suicide rate is one of the highest in the world; in our cities, thousands die each day from drug addiction; and the threat of nuclear global death continually reminds us that we really control very little.

Human ingenuity has reached out into space and the unknown; first to the Moon and Mars, and next to Jupiter and Saturn. Death, however, is still the universal mystery, the terror of millions. Newscasters can tell us of thousands of deaths by war, earthquakes, floods, and other disasters all over the globe, but we don't really comprehend their meaning in our lives. We are caught in a peculiar tension between the awareness of death's presence on one hand, and its denial on the other. Death seems so un-American. The deaths of our friends and the members of our families seem to us somehow outrageous, unfair, and unnatural. But death does happen; it will happen; it must.

Death: The National Taboo

Most of us are afraid of death, but our awareness of death is widely repressed. One of the ways we express this repression is in our contemporary preoccupation with sex. We have some strange notions of power and strength in America—that physical weakness is

somehow disgusting. Despite our apparent progress in many areas of social life, we may be becoming more primitive by substituting death, instead of sex, for our national taboo. Modern America is obsessed with intense materialism and loss of personalization. We have become a youth-oriented and power-conscious nation. Meanwhile, our appreciation for the earth and for human relationships has suffered from lack of attention. Americans worship youth, good health, and science. We greatly admire astonishing medical feats to save and prolong life. Yet death—the symbol of weakness—still comes to all of us.

Remarkable heart and kidney transplants in recent years, along with modern life-support systems, can keep people "alive" for a very long time. For the very rich, a system of "cryonics" has been developed, whereby the body (immediately following death) is stored at very low temperatures until some late date when scientific genius, it is hoped, will be able to bring the person back to life. Yet, despite such grand hopes, the truth is that the myth of modern science is not really that comforting, and most Americans continue to hold a deep and often secret fear of death. In fact, Americans resist the mere mention of the subject, which keeps large numbers of people from even thinking about it.

The condition in modern America is in sharp contrast to that found in Samoa many years ago by Margaret Mead. Dr. Mead found no fear of death there; since childhood, the Samoan people came into daily contact with it. In America, however, we no longer bury our own. Instead we are confronted by brutal violence, mass death, concentration camps, terrorism, and other modern horrors. To be sure, there is a great deal of joking about death and corpses in our society. But terrifying "creature features" that portray modern-day Frankensteins are but macabre fantasies—grotesque attempts to avoid the reality of death. Western culture no longer treats death as the collective destiny of the human race, but instead develops ways to avoid and deny it, in effect placing it in that category of forbidden topics formerly reserved for sex. Ironically, violent death may play to mass audiences, but natural death usually remains hidden in secrecy.

Preparing for Death

During our entire lifetimes, we play a succession of roles. Death, too, is a stage we must pass through—a role we all must play. We *can* prepare for it—if there is time, if we start soon enough. Ideally, people should have time to prepare for death—by living their lives so that they have real meaning, and also perhaps by taking care of the arrangements for their own deaths in practical ways.

Once we accept death as our inevitable destiny, it makes good sense to be concerned about our surviving loved ones. Making one's own arrangements before death, and making those arrangements known to one's loved ones, may well be one of the most human and worthwhile acts of one's entire lifetime. This is especially true when there are financial considerations involved, or when simplicity is desired. Funeral (or memorial) societies in major cities all over the country are nonprofit, nonsectarian agencies that provide information on low-cost and simple burial and cremation.

There seems to be a wide variety in preferences these days—from crematoriums to crypts, from recycled body parts to cryonics, from traditional funerals to very simple memorial services. Thinking a little about some of these preparations as soon as possible is a good deal more realistic and psychologically healthy than pretending that death isn't going to happen.

The quality of our lives may be a good deal improved if we begin to recognize the reality of our own deaths quite early in life. Strangely enough, school curriculums offer courses in human biology that deal with birth and reproduction, but seldom is the death of an organism considered a suitable topic of learning. Yet, an enlightened and sensitive teacher often can alleviate many fears of death that students have, and can contribute greatly to the meaning of people's lives. Most people, however, learn about death just as they did about sex—from "other" sources. Just as the popular literature about sex is usually crude and pornographic, much of the popular literature dealing with death portrays it in gruesome, ugly, and fearful terms.

In fact, as a society we seem to find death such a morbid topic that we usually avoid it even when people want to talk about it. The common fears of adults are passed on to their children, who learn quickly from even the most subtle clues that some topics are not talked about—especially at home. Meanwhile, they continue to play with toys of destruction, playing "bang-bang-you're-dead" or other games of fantasy.

We are beginning, albeit slowly, to recognize the mentally therapeutic aspects of discussing questions about birth and sex, and we should do the same for death. Truth can be cold and cruel, but it also can be gentle, merciful, and full of hope. Death education is not intended to encourage a preoccupation with death nor to develop hedonistic attitudes so that people won't care how they live. Rather it seeks to make the love of life more plain. From experiments with people who have been immobilized, immersed in water, or deprived of sound, we have learned that they "lose their minds." People need the touch of other people; we need sights, sounds, and sensory stimulation of all kinds; we need the movement and activity of life.

Most of all, this chapter is intended to point out that death deserves our respect, attention, and honesty because it is a necessary part of life. Many of the fervent goals of our lives would be trivial without the knowledge of our personal, eventual deaths. Our time is limited. The knowledge of this helps us to order priorities—to sort out the most valuable efforts in life to pursue. Sometimes as people age naturally, the realization of personal impending death appears to give them permission, even freedom, to be themselves. Another very important aspect of realizing one's death is that a sort of miracle occurs: you get "grabbed" by things—by sunsets, delicate flowers, smiling faces, puppies, clouds full of rain—by all the beauty of life.

> Let go, let go. . .go forward into the light. Let yourself be carried into the light. No memories, no regrets, no looking backwards, no apprehensive thoughts about your own or anyone else's future. Only light. Only this pure being, this love, this joy.
>
> ALDOUS HUXLEY

Psychologists have been telling us for a long time that the greatest of all human goals is the development of the self. This can be accomplished only in relationships with other human beings. To this we must add the old reminder that "life is short." We do not have time for casualness, for selfishness, for thoughtlessness, or for pettiness. If we can learn to live daily with the awesome knowledge that we are dying, death loses its power over us, and we are free to become dedicated to life. Then we will seek friendships, love, truth—all of the eternal qualities that endure beyond death.

To live and to understand life, we must deal with death and put it in proper perspective. Yet despite our brave words, our wisdom, and our experience, we most likely will cry out in pain when death touches us—simply because we're human. There is an old saying that if you visit the gates of the grave, you will not fear them when it is your time to pass through. We all know some people who seem to have "visited" these gates. They appear as though they are totally ready to meet their moment—and they bring all they are into that moment to sum up in an instant the meaning of their lives. So it is that dying people are such wonderful teachers; they have put aside all their masks. Finally, all any of us can hope for is to see that our lives have real meaning, and to face the moment of death when it comes, with honesty and without fear.

The Fear of Death

But we have been taught to fear death. In our time-precious, power-conscious culture, the stopping of all being is a state of reality that is impossible for us to comprehend. In death, time has no meaning, and so we try to run away from the reality of our own eventual deaths.

It has not always been this easy to avoid death. At one time in America, there was little need for death education because death was a routine part of life. In rural America in the early decades of this century, people died at home, surrounded by their extended families. Women often died in childbirth, as did their infants; young children frequently died from disease and epidemics; parlors at home contained deathbeds or coffins; and people walked past the headstones of their relatives' graves on their way down the path each Sunday to the country church. Remnants of frontier burial practices still remain in the family plots and public cemeteries of scattered communities across the United States. In rural America, children were not protected from the reality of death, but were socialized to accept it. Death was experienced as natural, as human, and as inevitable.

Whereas in the past, societies found it necessary to organize around patterns of recurring death, modern societies provide structures for continuity, particularly in social roles, despite losses by death. Death is not permitted to disrupt modern societies. The old become separated by mandatory retirement from work and community roles to permit the "efficient" changeover of personnel. Replacing a community leader who retires can be arranged quite smoothly because the society has advance notice, but replacing a community leader who dies suddenly creates difficulties of adjustment and disruption.

Modern societies also make efforts to disguise death—we cosmetically dress up the dead in order to allow the living to pretend that the deceased person is merely sleeping. The practice of embalming—purely an American invention—is another example. The professional handling of death, rather than by family members, also makes avoiding it all the more possible. The one remaining vestige of active family participation is in the role of the pallbearer. Morgues and cemeteries are located, too, so as to render death invisible. Whereas a person used to die from a stroke, today it is the result of a cerebral "accident," as though it were not really meant to happen. Modern hospitals isolate the very ill; funeral directors and other nonrelatives of the deceased not only accept, but encourage the rather impersonal and routine handling of death through systems of isolation and out-of-sight procedures. Much of this isolation is furthered by doctors and nurses (trained to save life), who often feel great despair when a patient

dies. Commitment of the aged and infirm to institutions is a frequent alternative to accepting death or to living with it. Because of fewer deaths among the young, death is associated with old age; consequently, when we try to separate death from society, we tend to separate the aged as well.

The degree of death fear may vary from that of sheer terror in some individuals to only a mild concern or even anticipation in others. Furthermore, some people do not seem to have much fear at all. Nor is the problem of death the same for everyone. Death fears depend on the dispositions and destinies of individuals and their development within a sociocultural context. Individual differences in death attitudes vary by age, ethnic affiliation, gender, religion, church attendance, personal experiences, and the like. One study found that regular churchgoers have less fear and anxiety of death and dying than do those who attend less frequently. Other writers, whose social perspectives differ, believe that traditional religion contributes to fears of death. Our social class, philosophical orientation, age, relationship with parents, prior experiences with death, and a number of other variables probably contribute to our psychological attitudes toward death.

Psychologically, it's unhealthy for people persistently to avoid dealing with reality, and so a realistic attitude toward death becomes important to mental health. Yet health care professionals frequently see this avoidance of reality in patients who exhibit maladaptive responses to stress in the form of psychosomatic illnesses.

The basic human motivation, sometimes called the "survival instinct," is to preserve oneself, to preserve one's life. The term "self-preservation" implies making an effort against some force of disintegration. A normal aspect of this effort is fear of death. That is to say, we don't want to die; we want to live. This is why we are so impressed by acts of heroism and bravery, and by daredevils who "play" with death. But not even the most courageous is entirely free of the fear of death. In studies of soldiers suffering from combat fatigue during the two world wars, the fear of death was always found to be lurking partly hidden.

Fear and the Need for Security

Fears of death during childhood and those of adulthood are often closely related. Adult death fears are similar to childhood insecurity and intolerance for separation, and vary according to the person's prior experiences and the degree of security or insecurity developed as a child.

Psychologists have come to see human growth in terms of conflicts, noticing that throughout the life cycle there seem to be stages of human development, each marked by crises that must be successfully resolved. In adulthood, just as in childhood, there are stages of development when a person is particularly vulnerable to life events. Erik H. Erikson has described human development as having a proper *rate* of growth and a proper *sequence* of stages, according to "laws" of psychological development. The healthy personality, according to this theory, must pass through these stages in order to be capable of mastering the environment and to have a correct perception of self.

The desired outcome of healthy personality development is a sort of understanding of oneself as well as an acceptance of oneself as a person. This is sometimes referred to as a balance between identity and self-esteem. One's identity is one's sense of who one is. Self-esteem is how one feels about oneself. When favorable self-esteem or identity are lacking, a person often feels despair and, frequently, an unconscious fear of death. Such fears of death vary with periods in the life cycle and with conditions of stress. Sometimes during an especially stressful period, people express a longing for death ("I wish I were dead"), or possibly even attempt suicide. Fears of death that begin in childhood may either diminish or increase in adulthood, depending to a great extent on the experiences a person has while growing up.

Death Fears of Children

On the whole, children are willing to talk about death. One psychologist found that children mentioned death spontaneously, often at bath time. Only a few children avoided the word "dead" in vocabulary lists. Very young children think only of separation, or sometimes of mutilation; children between the ages of five and nine often personify death as a frightening figure. Most children do not recognize death as final before the age of five. After age nine, however, most children begin to accept that life ends in death. But some children continue to think that the dead "live" in another place.

One of the most important influences in a child's attitude toward death is that of the child's relationship to his or her parents. Children may fear that a parent who leaves them temporarily may not return. When the parent promptly returns at the promised time, this reassures the child that separation is only temporary. The child is not only influenced by parental example and training, but also by the degree of emotional security felt. Children are not only curious about where they came from, but also about where people go. But since many adults cannot cope with children's fears about death, children are left to meet death in fairy tales, on television, and from pets that get run over by trucks. Adults tend to teach children what they themselves learned—fear, doubt, and repression.

Sudden death is difficult to handle at any age. For a child, *any* death is sudden. Children should be prepared for the eventuality of death in their lives, and not be "protected" from normal biological death. But just as sex education on the day of the wedding is not very helpful, neither is death education on the deathbed. Both sex and death have been considered "adults only" topics for too long, instead of normal life processes. The child who is strongly dependent upon the adults in his or her life for security and self-esteem is able to accept the notion of "not being" if those adults show that they can accept it, too.

> The last enemy that shall be destroyed is Death.
>
> 1 CORINTHIANS

Even for a child with well-developed self-esteem, the death of a parent may seem like a deliberate abandonment—or like a hostile act for which the child is to blame. To a child, death never is seen to occur by chance, but is believed to be caused. Thus, the child also may feel guilt when someone dies, as if he or she were the secret killer. When a death occurs, children also may develop evasive behavior—avoiding significant adults—because they don't know that it's normal for them to be afraid and confused. Death cannot be locked away in the closet until children reach adulthood. But talking with children openly and honestly about their feelings about death helps them to deal with their fears. Many children are very afraid of pain and should be reassured, for example, that the state of death is not painful. Sometimes a suitable book read to the child can help an adult explain death and dying as a part of life.

Death Fears of Adults

Naturally, there is a much greater tendency for older people to think about death. Preparation for death, such as writing wills and arranging for one's burial, is more common among older people, too, and among the better educated. The most common fears of death in adults are associated with violence or suffering. Adults frequently have given up the desire to live forever. It is also obvious in everyday life that adults often avoid the mention of death, particularly when the subject has a personal connotation.

It is very rare to talk of another's death in that person's presence. This tendency is usually more evident if the death would bring about personal gain. One reason people often die without making preparations may be that they hesitate to talk of death with their loved ones. Whether or not one talks about death, however, is not really an accurate indication of the degree of one's fears of death. A hidden fear of death may arise in a disguised form without the real source of the fear even being recognized.

> The moon is so high it is
> Almost in the Great Bear.
> I walk out of the city
> Along the road to the West.
> The damp wind ruffles my coat.
> Dewy grass soaks my sandals.
> Fishermen are singing
> On the distant river.
> Fox fires dance on the ruined tombs.
> A chill wind rises and fills
> Me with melancholy. I
> Try to think of words that will
> Capture the uncanny solitude.
> I come home late. The night
> Is half spent. I stand for a
> Long while in the doorway.
> My young son is still up, reading.
> Suddenly he bursts out laughing,
> And all the sadness of the
> Twilight of my life is gone.
>
> LU YU

As already indicated, fear of death does not affect only older adults, but those of all ages. Every American family, it has been said, lives with the knowledge that a beloved family member may die at any time, even though they may continue to behave as though they don't worry about it. This is an unspeakable terror for many families. In fact, probably the greatest fear of all is that of losing a deeply loved family member. Such fear is frequently made obvious by the absence of manifested concern where concern is definitely in order. But pretending it won't happen won't stop it from happening. Death will come. We must learn to deal with it. Whether it is self-taught or received in groups of other people, death education often can be very beneficial in alleviating fears of death. Community colleges across the country are beginning to offer such courses to the public, often free of charge.

Fear and Social Stress

Social stress and "signs of the times," too, can heighten fears of death and affect family mental health. In the 1890s, death was a frequent visitor, but families lived nearer to one another than they do now and could share their grief. Whereas death came often, it may have caused less actual anxiety because people were impelled to face it realistically. Fear of death ran high during the 1930s, heightened by the intense economic insecurity felt during the depression. Fears of death also were heightened during World War II in Europe. Yet in London during the severe bombing and bombardment by German artillery, even though many people were terrified, others remained quite calm. Children apparently responded to the emotional attitudes of their mothers. If the mothers were terrified, the children were, too. During periods of severe economic hardship, war, social upheaval, or when people doubt the validity of their social order, large numbers can be expected to exhibit a fear of death.

In recent years we have experienced widespread loss of faith in our political leaders and in our social institutions. As a result, a feeling of dislocation and uncertainty can be seen in large numbers of people who seek treatment for stress-related illnesses. Young adults today, we might think, have little reason to think of death. Yet, it is precisely the young people of recent generations—the youth shaken by city riots, assassinations, nuclear fallout, and the non-heroes of the Vietnam war—who may have suffered most from death anxiety in recent decades. The acceptability of death depends upon the psychological context in which it occurs. Death today is unacceptable to us because it is associated with holocausts and meaningless annihilation, and because it disconnects our lives.

Of course, from time to time most people will experience "normal" fears about death that stem from the basic need to survive. There is no easy distinction between "normal" and "abnormal" fears of death. Certainly death fears are somewhat closely linked with most aspects of growing older, and as we age may be discovered to be the secret to the meaning of life. That is, life is what it is—sacred, precious, and unique—just because it is limited. If we were to live forever, life would lose its meaning because it would never be renewed. It is difficult to comprehend our not being, our total disappearance. But we can try to understand the role death plays in our lives. Gaining an understanding of the purpose of death can bring new meaning to life. In fact, planning ahead for one's death is a part of healthy living.

Fears of the Dying

The experience of dying itself may be a time of real fear. Death means traveling into the unknown. Any new role we play—motherhood, adolescence, marriage, or occupational roles—requires time and preparation.

Those who realize they are dying have some time to prepare for it. Even though people also are influenced by their previous attitudes and fears, it does not necessarily mean that as one lies dying only unpleasant thoughts of death arise. Dying people often reach a courageous serenity in accepting the inevitable, and often their fears of death leave them.

Dr. Elisabeth Kübler-Ross has studied the several stages of dying with perhaps thousands of dying patients. She found that the final stage for the dying person is one of acceptance of the inevitable and is a state of increasing self-reliance. She found, too, that the process of dying is not one of sorrow and fear, but is a process of recommitment to life and the lives of others. One learns to live life as a dying person; it is similar to the learning that takes place when the life of any important person is separated from our own.

Dealing with Grief

Grief brings confusion. We ask "Why? Why did death take this person?" Bereaved people also feel anger and guilt when they are left alone to mourn. When someone dearly loved dies, those who grieve feel helplessness and a sense of overpowering weakness by their inability to do anything about it. Death cannot be recalled. We cannot "buy" someone back; no amount of physical strength can help us; and pleading with God will be to no avail.

The fear, confusion, and sorrow following the death of a loved one can bring suspicion of others' motives, too. Feelings of powerlessness and a total loss of control are sometimes known to overwhelm bereaved people. These feelings are intensified when the grieving person tries not to show the true feelings of the heart. Grieving people should be allowed to weep, to talk about their loved one, and to express their sorrow. Failure to express pent-up emotions can have seriously damaging effects. People who mourn need the love and concern of others. They need to remember the deceased person—to recall the good times, to express their feelings of guilt and anger, and to face the reality of the loss.

Grief is painful, and unwanted feelings of guilt frequently are part of the pain. Somehow we believe that there might have been something we could have done either to prevent the death or to have made that person happier during life. Such mourning is a necessary process. It is not a "matter of time" or a process of forgetting.

Friends may have difficulty in knowing what to do and what to say to the grieving family. They even may be afraid to mention the name of the deceased, thinking that they will create pain for the bereaved family members. Instead, a barrier may be created for the family, who desperately may need to talk about their loss. Loving friends are usually a great source of comfort during periods of sorrow. If there is one thing people can't take during a period of grief, however, it is deception or evasion. The truth about death is almost always best. It is better to talk about it, to express the tears that are felt, and to remember the person you mourn.

Sometimes family counselors or members of the clergy can provide ways in which people can focus their grief. Some people handle grief by buying the most expensive casket they can find. Others light candles, place flowers, or simply meditate. The New Orleans brass band funeral is "slow to the burial" but "boogieing on back" to celebrate both death and life. The important thing is that grief needs to be expressed. Of course, that does not mean that it should be exaggerated, but simply that by expressing grief, people come to realize that they can handle the difficulties of bereavement.

Much of the grief and helplessness comes from making "arrangements" for someone who has died. How a funeral is conducted, too, can contribute to feelings of frustration, especially if the deceased has made no preparations and the grieving person does not know for sure how the deceased person "would have wanted it." Some people are more elaborate in dealing with death; others prefer simplicity. In our culture, funerals and memorial services are not usually set up for the person who died, but for those who survive and for those who grieve.

Grief frequently accompanies—but is not restricted to—old age. Deaths of lifetime friends and relatives may be survived quite well. But after the initial shock and sadness wear off, a feeling of emptiness and apathy often sets in. Grief also comes at the time when older adults are taking stock of themselves, reviewing their lives, trying to determine where they've been and what they will do with the remaining time they have, and deciding whatever psychological or material legacies they may leave to others.

An important but little-realized fact is that grief can kill. Dr. Robert Butler, Director of the National Institute on Aging, recently stated, "Grief kills one-half as many people as highway accidents." Grief can be a fatal condition—probably by lowering the body's resistance to other illnesses, and certainly, too, by precipitating suicide. Failing to work through grief and the bereavement process also can manifest itself in psychosomatic symptoms.

Widowhood

Bereavement for anyone is a major crisis. But for people who have lived together and survived together for many years, widowhood is especially difficult because it forces the survivor to make drastic adjustments at a time when change is not easily made. Widowhood is associated with high death rates. It is hard to prove that the death of a spouse actually causes the death of the survivor, but spouses do share a common environment, and some of the forces that contributed to the death of one may act equally on the other. Illness, mental and physical, also is associated with widowhood. Bereavement can be compounded when the survivor is left dependent on others for material needs.

Of the 16 million widowed persons in America today, 12 million are widows. Because women tend to marry men older than they are (and because they tend to live longer), the *majority* of women who marry ultimately will become widows. And because of the close relationship between grief and suicide, widows' bereavement deserves special attention.

Suicide

Suicide is the act of voluntary, intentional self-destruction—death at one's own hand. Suicide has been both condemned and honored. The Koran regards suicide as a grave sin worse than murder. The Talmud emphasizes the sacredness of life and also condemns suicide as a sin. Christians generally have opposed suicide, too, although for a time in history a Christian woman was excused for suicide if she did it to avoid rape. On the other hand, the Brahmans of India honored the person who voluntarily "became free from the body" and highly praised the Hindu widow who perished on her husband's funeral pyre. The ancient Vikings, worshipers of the god Odin, also held such women in high esteem. In ancient Japan, noblemen were given the privilege of *hara-kiri* (self-destruction by the sword) to punish themselves for a wrong, or to demonstrate their loyalty to the emperor. During World War II, Japanese soldiers and pilots were known to commit acts of suicide *(banzai* and *kamikaze)* to further the Japanese war cause. And Buddhist monks and nuns have sacrificed themselves by burning themselves alive in acts of social protest.

But our culture does not find suicide acceptable, thus there is the assumption that people who commit suicide are mentally ill. Of course, sometimes they are, but a direct correspondence between suicide and known forms of mental illness has not been demonstrated. Karl

Menninger suggested that suicide has three elements: the wish to kill, the wish to be killed, and the wish to die. According to one theory, an individual's aggression is turned inward against the self instead of outward against another (homicide). No psychological theory explains suicide, however, because of the numerous extraneous factors in individuals' lives: religious and societal beliefs vary greatly, as do the conditions surrounding suicide.

Conditions Surrounding Suicide

While every instance of suicide is different, some generalizations still can be made. Urban suicide rates are higher than rates for rural areas. Suicide rates tend to rise during times of economic depression, with a greater percentage among higher-status men; rates decrease during periods of prosperity. There seems to be no accurate relationship between war and suicide, although men in the military tend to have higher rates of suicide than do civilians.

There is a close relationship between suicide and prolonged and severe depression. In older people, suicide is invariably associated with the suffering of vital losses. Loss of loved ones, loss of income or prosperity, and loss of health head the list of reasons. Whereas just one of these factors taken by itself may not push a person to self-destruction, a combination of them might very well do so.

Persons in higher-status occupations are more prone to commit suicide than are those of lower-status occupations. The traditional Christmas holiday season and long periods of rain have been associated with increases in suicide rates. Suicide is a serious problem in all industrialized societies. Suicide also is the second highest cause of death among college-age students. Rarely, even young children have committed suicide. There also is a high rate of delinquency associated with the wish to commit suicide. This behavior is revealed in certain self-destructive tendencies such as drug abuse and extreme risk-taking. There also is a marked *increase* in actual suicides among adolescents in recent decades. Some researchers believe that increased stress in their lives, lack of job opportunities, fears about the stability of the world, the threat of nuclear war, loss of confidence in political leaders, and other signs of insecurity are all possible reasons.

Who Commits Suicide?

Suicide is more frequent among the widowed and divorced than among the married. People who have children seem to commit suicide less frequently than do those who are childless. Also, even though statistics say that more men than women actually *succeed* in suicide attempts, a shocking 85 percent of the people who *try* to commit suicide are women. The differences in the success rates are most likely due to the more violent and sudden means employed by men as opposed to the less violent and less sudden means usually attempted by women. If access to firearms increases for women, female suicide may tend to be an even more serious problem. The incidence of suicide for men also seems to increase dramatically as they grow older, whereas suicide is more frequent in women at younger ages. Roman Catholics have lower rates of suicide than do Protestants. Jews' rates tend to be very low, but fluctuate according to historical trends.

Suicide Prevention

Most major cities have suicide prevention centers staffed by psychologists and trained lay people where a person contemplating suicide can call for help. Suicide prevention personnel do not try to keep the person who really desires to die from doing so, but rather they focus on the human problems that make people want to end their lives. That is to say, the person who wants to commit suicide believes strongly that he or she has excellent reasons for doing so. The suicide prevention workers try to find out why the person is suffering so and try to help resolve some of those problems. When people "cry out" for help by announcing their intention to kill themselves, it should be regarded as a genuine distress signal. Many suicides have been prevented because early warnings were recognized and heeded.

Beliefs About Death

People have held many beliefs about death and what happens when people die. These beliefs have been passed on (gradually changed over time) to succeeding generations since early times. There seems to be a universal human desire for life after death (immortality) that expresses the human fear of disappearing into nothingness. Historically, the belief or desire for immortality has been sustained primarily by religions. In its primary usage, immortality means a continuation of spiritual, rather than bodily, existence after death.

A belief in life after death was widespread even among primitive cultures. Legends have told of people who have been granted immortality both as a reward and as a punishment. Most religious tradition surrounds the idea that humankind is both body and spirit. The body passes away at death, but the spirit (or soul) is believed to be immortal; that is, the soul never dies.

The idea of immortality is usually associated, too, with concepts of an afterlife in another world. Hell as described by St. Augustine was a dark and terrible place of "fire and brimstone" where the damned would be tormented forever. Heaven is usually described as a paradise where no evil exists, a place of bountiful goodness, joy, and peace.

The Persian followers of Zoroaster accepted the notion of a bridge to be crossed after death—a bridge that was broad for the righteous, but narrow for the wicked who fell from it into hell. The Cheyennes of the Great Plains believed that when a person's soul (the *tasoom*) leaves the body, death comes and the *tasoom* then travels to heaven. All the Cheyennes of the past are believed to live in heaven just as they did on earth. There is no hell for the Cheyennes because sins are expiated for here and now. Only the souls of those who commit suicide are barred from heaven. The fundamental belief for most religions of India— Hinduism and Buddhism—revolves around the notion of a series of reincarnations, or multiple lives, based on one's performance in past lives. By living properly, a person could look forward to increasingly better lives in the future.

The Christian faith, however, believes in a literal resurrection of the body after the Last Judgment, as well as the soul's separate existence after death. Christian beliefs are invariably versions of the Last Judgment, when the good or evil nature of a person would be discovered at or after death. In early Christianity, the wicked did not awaken after death; they were merely abandoned to a state of nonexistence. But the saintly population, after a long sleep, would awaken when Christ returned at the Second Coming and join together in a glorious afterlife. Many Christian cemeteries still place bodies at burial so that they face toward the east—the direction from which Christ is expected to come again. The Roman Catholic tradition, however, holds that all souls live after death. They rest until the Judgment, then live eternally either in hell or in heaven. Whatever a person's attitude toward death, it invariably reflects their attitude toward life as well.

> Who says the dead do not think of us?
> Whenever I travel, she goes with me.
> She was uneasy when I was on a journey.
> She always wanted to accompany me.
> While I dream, everything is as it used to be.
> When I wake up, I am stabbed with sorrow.
> The living are often parted and never
>   meet again.
> The dead are together as pure souls.
>
> MEI YAO CH'EN

In more modern times, space travel, computerized knowledge, and automation have altered religious attitudes. For many Americans, the Scriptures no longer reassure them that there is a "time to be born" and a "time to die." Today, awareness of the presence of death by nuclear war cannot be seen as an act of God, nor can automobile accidents, suicides, and homicides. We have clearly witnessed the role played by humans in these events. Thus, religion does not seem to be as helpful to people as it once was.

Freud believed that people should be educated to accept reality; religion, he thought, was primary among humanity's illusions. Spiritual comfort, Freud believed, was a false dependency of immaturity—whereas genuine maturity would face reality squarely with no false hopes. While there is much in society to support this position, there also is much evidence to support the view that it is the absence of religious belief that is at the root of many of our fears of death.

At one time in this country, religion reassured most people by providing a belief in continuation after death that not only made death meaningful, but the miseries and injustices of day-to-day life tolerable. In modern societies, however, humanity is only temporary; it is the corporations and the bureaucracies that seem immortal.

On the other hand, there are people who accept death as a part of life. In simple societies, people are able to live with death and to surmount periods of grief because of more meaningful belief systems and strong ties of kinship. The power of belief in simple societies lies in their ability to bring the dead "back to life" in ancestor worship, in ghosts, or through other concepts of power. Thus, it is comforting for people to believe that the dead loved ones are still "living."

In societies like ours with very low death rates, a mental association is made between the aged and death, even though we know that death can come at any age. A rejection or avoidance of old people by the young may be due to this unconscious association and the fear of death.

Because of the extent of scientific knowledge and the rapidity of social change, traditional religious thought no longer provides a belief in immortality for many people. But this does not necessarily mean that hope or belief should be abandoned. If we stop believing in things unseen, we would hardly accept molecular motion, wind velocity, or hundreds of other valid beliefs. Rather, more meaningful language may need to be substituted for some of us in order to develop beliefs.

The Question of Time

Beliefs about life and death focus primarily on the concept of *time*—the time that extends beyond one's mortal life. The key to a sense of immortality is belief in the human ability to rise above earthly existence. Beliefs in life after death (immortality) are ways to master fears of death: belief provides a link between one's sense of the present and the unknown future.

One way we can envision life after death is through symbols, such as images of angels strumming harps, beautiful gardens with waterfalls, or paintings such as Michelangelo's Sistine Chapel ceiling. There also are notions of immortality that can be compared to the spiritual rebirth one may experience several times throughout life as we resolve crises, or "turn over a new leaf." In death, time has no meaning, but we know that life goes on in the physical world even after people die. Another way to believe we are part of life even after death can be discovered in nature. That is to say, humans, like other animals, are comprised of the natural elements—created from "dust" and returned to dust—and are part of all enduring life—in the oceans, in the trees and flowers, and in the daily cycle of the moon and the planets.

> You would know the secret of death.
> But how shall you find it unless you seek it
>   in the heart of life?
> …If you would indeed behold the spirit
>   of death,
> Open your heart wide unto the body
>   of life.
> For life and death are one, even as the
>   river and the sea are one.
>   KAHLIL GIBRAN, *THE PROPHET*

Furthermore, one can believe in an ongoing life without denying the finality of death. Once one accepts the finality of death as having meaning in one's life, it becomes easier to develop a sense of historical connection beyond the individual life. People can believe in life after death in the biological sense, too, through one's children and in the ability to reproduce oneself. This idea can be confined to the notion of family or group, or it can be extended to all of humanity who share a common future. Acquiring knowledge of one's family history and keeping a family album are other ways for people to express and recognize their biological significance.

There also is a belief in life after death in the creative sense, through one's works, healing, teaching, art or poetry, inventions, occupational contributions, or lasting influences on the world from what one has done. A belief in life after death also comes from one's ideas and philosophy that are passed on to others. We see the eternal, too, just in being part of the never-ending cosmic universe and in the vast storehouse of knowledge accumulated over time.

When a person develops such a belief or sense of life after death, the concern for the physical life diminishes. Something similar occurs during adulthood when a person becomes resigned to one's maturity, thus gaining serenity for life and work. During this middle stage of life, the principal task is in achieving mature and independent adulthood.

Death: A Stage of Life

Death, too, can be seen as a stage of life we must all pass through. Dr. Elisabeth Kübler-Ross, in writing about her experiences with the terminally ill, has contributed greatly to our understanding of the dying process. She speaks of life having direction even for the dying, in achieving the final stage—that of acceptance, when a person's life is more complete and is more self-sufficient. We all have a wide range of possibilities for experiencing the joys and problems of being human, she says, and we have a seemingly endless capacity for creative change. Within the realm of the mind's power, she believes, lies the ability to achieve transcendence.

By "transcendence" we mean the ability to rise above or to exceed that which is expected to be possible. We transcend reality in our minds when we dream. We fly, we fight dragons, we escape our realities in unique and marvelous ways. We can sing in our dreams, or dance, skip, climb trees, become like a bird, or like children again. We can create oceans, flowers, and butterflies in our mind's eye. We can travel to outer space and "feel" the exhilaration of rising above—of *transcending*—our realities.

Close your eyes for a moment and imagine yourself being transported to the Moon. Now you are looking at the earth from a lunar vantage point. The night sky is clear and full of stars. Do you get the feeling of transcendence? Or imagine you are on top of a mountain looking down into the valleys below. You can see tiny rivers, tiny farms, and tiny cities. Perhaps you can recall a time when you were lying on your back in the middle of a grassy field. You were looking up at the clouds gently moving or at the millions of tiny stars twinkling at night. Your sense of time and space was temporarily altered because your imagination was set free. These are all examples of transcendence.

Transcendence also has to do with issues of self-identity, of self-actualization, and of one's perception of one's role as part of the universe. Recognizing the ability to transcend, yet remaining aware of the present reality, is self-objectivity—the ability to be reflective and insightful about oneself. It is a time when one loses confusion about oneself—rather like "growing up." Individuals with such insight can see themselves in a cosmic (or universal) perspective—in a confident knowledge of themselves. It can be described as having a healthy wholeness of oneself, which simply means having the ability to fit one's present situation, whatever it is, into some meaningful life pattern. In the psychological sense, "wholeness" means that the human will takes control and creates its own reality and its own immortality.

We cannot ignore the role of death in our lives; the best we can do is to stall it awhile. All of our role changes have to do with loss and separation, and each one is like a rite of passage that requires preparation and understanding. A necessary aspect of such preparation must be devoted to death—the final stage of development.

The Hospice Movement

From the Latin, *hospes* means either host, guest, or mutual caring. In England in the Medieval Period, there were 750 hospices; 40 were in Paris alone. The ancient hospice was a welcoming place to all in need—the sick, the dying, the poor—who were all treated alike in a caring place for human pilgrims traveling on the journey of life. The attitude of the hospice today as then is to treat death as a part of life. Spiritual and personal growth, it is believed, continue throughout the dying process despite the physical decline. The hospice connotes a positive attitude toward the meaning of life and the significance of death. This is an opposite approach to that of most hospital staffs who sorrowfully avoid dying patients—perhaps because it is a sign of their failure to heal, and perhaps because it is a reminder that death is inescapable.

The hospice movement is growing rapidly. St. Christopher's Hospice in London was established in 1967. The Hospice, Inc. in New Haven, Connecticut, established in 1974, was the first in this country. The Hospice of Marin in northern California was founded in November, 1975 by William M. Lamers, Jr., M.D. with a group of professionals offering their services free of charge. The National Cancer Institute has recently awarded three-year contracts to Riverside Hospice in New Jersey, Hill Haven Hospice in Tucson, and Kaiser Permanente Hospice near Los Angeles. There also are teams of hospice workers at hospitals such as St. Luke's in New York. At the present time, there are about 200 hospice programs in various stages of development in about 40 states.

The Hospice of Marin is at present a home-care agency. One important part of the hospice plan is to help every dying person who so desires to die at home. People who are dying often want to go home. They want to have life around them, to be surrounded by familiar things, and to receive spiritual and emotional support from people they know and trust to care for them. There are many who would like to help people and their families in this manner but who don't know how to begin. This includes relatives and friends as well as nurses and other members of the medical profession. We frequently hear people say "I feel so helpless," or the sad comment, "I was afraid, so I ran away." A hospice, with its large numbers of caring volunteers, can help people to help others, and help them to recognize that dying is a part of living. Too many dying persons have made the lonely journey alone because others did not know how to help.

In order for the family to have its rightful place in caring for their loved ones, they may need support, to have someone say, "I'll be there with you, because I care." The hospice philosophy recognizes that a terminal illness affects every member of the family. Hospice staffs make regularly scheduled visits, but also are available around the clock to make house calls when their help is especially needed.

Family members often worry whether they have sufficient information and knowledge about caring for their loved one. The hospice staff helps people provide care if they want to do so. They teach family members how to care for patients, how to give medications, how to prepare tasty and nutritious foods, and other practical things. They also help to educate the family about the progression of the illness so that no one will be surprised about new developments. Sometimes hospice volunteers take a patient fishing, do the ironing, care for children, and perform other day-to-day tasks.

Whether it is perceived as religious caring or simply humanitarian, the hospice force is eternal. The early Christians cared for lepers, the pariahs of the ancient world, exhibiting the highest in human love. But in every religion there are the saints who see the value of all human life. And the "places of welcome" profoundly remind us that we are all part of one human family whose destinies are linked together.

Referrals to hospice programs are made by physicians. Hospice workers become involved only in cases where an attending physician is involved, and only when there is a limited life expectancy accompanied by considerable pain. The hospice is more than a hospital; it is a human community. It furnishes not only medical care, but care for someone as a person, to stand by that person to the end, and to honor that person for what her or his life has been.

The hospice philosophy believes that decision-making should not be taken away from dying patients. It is important that patients be asked to decide for themselves what they want to eat, what they want to wear, and be encouraged to plan their days. They also need to be included in family problems. The effort to spare patients only creates more isolation from the living. Reorganizing their lives to accommodate the limitations that are part of illness requires much understanding and support. The hospice philosophy includes the dying person in all aspects of living for as long as possible, while it also helps to ease the awesome burdens on the bereaved family. A hospice is thus both a hospital and a home. It provides comfort, patient support, help for the family, education, total care, grief counseling, and most important, it helps people to bear the truth.

The hospice plan controls pain with drugs so that the life left is bearable. The drugs do not attempt to create a false euphoria, but seek to make the pain bearable and to bring the suffering individual as nearly as possible to a normal conscious state. Pain is *avoided* before it occurs by use of a comfort chart, so that patients remain alert, yet relieved of discomfort. After accidents, surgery, and so forth, PRN (medication as needed) may be suitable. But terminal care that involves severe or chronic pain requires different demands. It makes no sense to worry about drug addiction when a person is going to be dead in a few weeks. The *fear* of pain increases the intensity of pain. Patients in severe pain, if they are permitted to suffer, can unnecessarily enter a world of horror and hopelessness. Knowing that the pain will not come is part of the comfort offered not only to the patients, but to their families.

Other symptoms, too, are dealt with in the same careful humane manner. These often include combinations of discomforts such as nausea, bladder or bowel incontinence, and headaches. In addition to medical and drug care, hospices provide such comforts as gentle massage, soft pillows, changes in diet, quiet listening, concerned and loving companionship, and music or other familiar pleasures of the ill person—all aimed at recognizing the human worth of the dying individual.

Hospice care is both old and new. More and more, we are coming to realize that we must treat death with respect as a natural part of living. Dying, after all, is a role like any other that we all must one day play. But everywhere there have always been individuals who knew this, who for their own private reasons continue to work quietly to care for their fellow human beings through selfless action and loving choice. Not surprisingly, women have been a significant force in the hospice movement.

What the Dying Can Teach Us

To be with a dying person—to provide human caring—and to offer comfort and companionship is one of the highest of all human roles. The ancient Christians knew this and treated the sick and dying with great love because they believed they were at the doors of heaven. But in our society children do not play in the sickroom of a dying person. Even doctors avoid the terminally ill, preferring instead to deal with patients who get well. And all of us too often avoid places like "nursing" homes. There are strong expectations of death in nursing homes, but they are not openly expressed. Because of our hypocrisy, many of us are suffering from emotional poverty and spiritual starvation.

The Task of Dying

Dying is hard work—but a task to be faced. Exceptions are instances when people die suddenly; then the mourners suffer most. Dying, like birth, is more than a biological event; it is a psychological and social role. We give assistance to the woman who is giving birth. There are medical teams, months of preparation, exercises, diet, and the moral support of a husband and/or family—even if a birth is initially unwanted. Rarely does a person come into the world unassisted. But dying, too, requires assistance.

The dying need care—and the caring need the dying. We need to learn from the terminally ill, not so that we might escape their fate, but so we can better share and participate in our own fates. The dying can be seen as other human beings who have progressed before us on the journey of life. They have learned that the mind and the spirit are as important as the body.

To love and to comfort the dying is to live, just as to die is to live. Most of us don't realize that if we were born, we, too, are dying. The dying need what the living need—comfort in an atmosphere of love. That is why dying people long to go home or to a place where they feel at home, to familiar surroundings, to be surrounded by life and love. The dying, after all, still live, and they often feel a strong responsibility for the living. They have a sense of generational belonging, and long to participate in intergenerational sharing because their time is running out.

When a woman first learns that her illness is terminal, there is a tremendous feeling of loss—just like the grief and mourning the family feels. Knowledge of approaching death is not accepted readily. There seems to be a cyclic pattern of discovery. First, there is denial—a refusal to believe that this could happen to her—then anger that fate has selected her to die, and later despondency and a genuine sorrow at the loss of her precious life. But finally there comes a recommitment to life and to the lives of others. At this stage, the dying person wants to make living and dying easier for those remaining behind. Finally, there is a feeling of love for the world and a total acceptance of the reality of death.

Euthanasia

Euthanasia, which literally means "good death," may be defined as "a mode or act of inducing or permitting death painlessly as a relief from suffering." It is an effort to make possible a "gentle and easy death" for those afflicted with an incurable disease or injury in its terminal stages. It is beneficent euthanasia if, and only if, it results in a painless and quick death, and if the act as a whole is beneficial to the recipient.

Our first commitment as human beings is to preserve and enhance life. Sometimes, under certain conditions, this may not be possible. It is natural for people to hope that when their time comes, they will be able to die peacefully and with dignity. When there is great distress and the end is inevitable, people sometimes elect to ease the suffering without moral or legal ramifications.

Individuals who believe in voluntary euthanasia may sign a "living will," similar to the one shown, preferably when they are in good health, that requests unequivocally that the person's right to die with dignity be respected. The individual's physician should be informed of the living will and be given a copy of it. One's family and close friends also should have copies, or at least be aware of the person's desire in the event that at the terminal stage of an illness, the person is not capable of communicating with others.

The Living Will

TO MY FAMILY, MY PHYSICIAN,
MY CLERGYMAN, MY LAWYER—

If the time comes when I can no longer take part in decisions for my own future, let this statement stand as the testament of my wishes:

If there is no reasonable expectation of my recovery from physical or mental disability, I, _____ , request that I be allowed to die and not be kept alive by artificial means or heroic measures. Death is as much a reality as birth, growth, maturity, and old age—it is the one certainty. I do not fear death as much as I fear the indignity of deterioration, dependence and hopeless pain. I ask that medication be mercifully administered to me for terminal suffering even if it hastens the moment of death.

This request is made after careful consideration. Although this document is not legally binding, you who care for me will, I hope, feel morally bound to follow its mandate. I recognize that it places a heavy burden of responsibility upon you, and it is with the intention of sharing that responsibility and of mitigating any feelings of guilt that this statement is made.

Signed_____ Date_____
Witnessed by: _____

CHAPTER 18

HEALTH RESOURCES

PETER L. ANDRUS, M.D., F.A.C.P.

SHARON N. ANDRUS, R.N.

Health care professionals are trained to serve you. Your health and well-being are their primary concerns. Every woman in America, regardless of her age or income, can learn to use the health care services in her community. Often we may not know which facilities are best for the needs we have, especially as our lives and needs keep changing. Because of this, it is wise to become familiar with a variety of different health resources.

Whether you live in a city, a small town, or a rural area, you can find family counseling centers, hospitals, birth control clinics, exercise classes, and food and nutrition services to assist you in evaluating your health needs, treating your symptoms, or making health care decisions. Take the time to research the options open to you and assemble the components of your own personal health care system.

Health Resources

When we think of health care, we tend to think of hospitals, with their operating rooms, emergency centers, and ultramodern equipment. But the fact is, for most people most of the time, health care does not involve hospitalization, and takes place in a variety of other facilities, including the home. For a discussion of hospitals, see "Hospitals and Hospital Care," beginning on page 384.

Health care services exist to serve every member of the community in a number of ways. These services should be used not only when one is ill, but also when one is enjoying good health. And women can utilize health care services to maintain the best health throughout their lives, provided only that they know what they need and how to find out what is available.

To help you accomplish these goals, we will explore the broad spectrum of services that are a part of comprehensive health care. Then we will suggest sources of information regarding health care services in your own community. And finally, we will describe in some detail the specific services that may be of use to you as a woman at some time in your life.

Comprehensive Health Care

Most women are familiar with the "traditional" type of health care that involves a direct physician-patient interaction. An appointment is made for a regular checkup or due to a specific complaint. The doctor then examines the patient and prescribes treatment.

By now, however, you also may have been involved in what is called *comprehensive health care*. This term has come into use to describe a more extensive range of services than those prescribed by "traditional" medical care. These services take into account the wider variety of factors that contribute to the health of an individual. For example, we know that the quality of an environment plays a part in the health of the individuals who live in it, and that health education can contribute to the prevention of disease. Thus, environmental health services and health education services are components of comprehensive health care.

Specialized health professionals have joined the doctor in providing health services. These professionals form *health teams* that coordinate their services in an effort to ensure the health and well-being of the individual. So, in addition to seeing your doctor, you also may see a nutritionist for a special diet, a physical therapist for an exercise program tailored to a specific disability, or a social worker for aid in making financial arrangements to meet medical expenses. All of these, too, are components of comprehensive health care.

Comprehensive Services

Health-education and -promotion services provide the public with information about health and illness. These services are intended to help patients remain healthy, to follow a treatment program to regain health, or to control a disease to the best of their ability. A wide variety of approaches to public health education and patient education are currently used. Organized counseling programs help patients —singly or in special groups — with such problems as hypertension and overweight. In addition, TV and radio "spots," brochures, audio-visual programs, and health-care books provide valuable public health education.

Environmental health services are those related to noise abatement; maintaining clean, safe water and air; providing sanitary sewage and waste disposal; and other services directed toward improving and maintaining the health of our environment. Typically, such activities are undertaken by agencies of the government. These services do not fall under the category of personal health services since they are applied on a population-wide basis, but their contribution to the personal health of individuals should not be minimized.

Preventive personal health services include services in two broadly defined areas. *Primary prevention* focuses on measures that prevent disease before it occurs. The classic example is childhood immunization ("baby shots"), which offers protection against severe infectious diseases such as diphtheria, whooping cough, and polio. *Secondary prevention* focuses on measures that detect a disease process in its early or symptom-free stage when the likelihood of cure or prevention of eventual death or disability is greatest. A good example is the periodic Papanicolau (Pap) smear, used to screen for cancer of the uterine cervix (neck of the womb).

Diagnostic and treatment services focus on identifying a specific illness problem as presented to a physician by an individual patient, and then prescribing appropriate therapy (such as drug therapy, surgery, or a special diet) to resolve the problem.

Doctors refer to illness as *acute* (usually rapid in onset and short in duration) or *chronic* (slower in onset and longer in duration). Cure is the outcome usually sought for acute illnesses such as pneumonia or strep throat, whereas ongoing care and control of the disease process often is the best that can be expected in chronic illnesses, such as diabetes or high blood pressure.

Rehabilitation services include a wide range of services directed toward minimizing the degree of disability or deformity left by illness or injury. Among the services offered are: *physical therapy,* which directs its efforts toward restoring full use of the voluntary muscle (motor) functions of the arms, legs, and trunk; *occupational therapy,* which attempts to restore full ability to perform the fine motor skills necessary for satisfactory performance of one's occupation or the activities of daily living; and *speech therapy,* which attempts to restore full capacity for meaningful speech in patients who have completely or partially lost this ability through injury or illness.

Social services provide various non-medical services for individual patients. For example, social service workers frequently arrange transportation to and from medical appointments for home-bound patients, aid in making financial arrangements for medical costs or living expenses, provide home health services or medical appliances, and refer patients to appropriate sources for family counseling when necessary. The social service department in your community hospital or voluntary health agency is an excellent source of information when you need to know where to go for a specific kind of help.

Mental health services also are available in most communities, and in an astonishing variety. Services may range from an informal group of women (which you may organize yourself) who meet to support one another through personal or family crises (see page 104) to the myriad mental health services provided by large urban mental health institutes (see page 377).

Finding Health Services

Knowing what you need is the first step toward finding what you need.

Allow your imagination free rein to create a health care system that contains all of the elements and services you require. Think about it; make a list. Chances are, everything on your list is available in your community, but probably not all in one place. For a sample list of personal health care needs, see the box at right.

We will list a number of resources for you to consider. Some will be more reliable than others, but all have the potential for providing needed information. Use the following suggestions to start you on your way. And remember that it's important to evaluate information from any source with an objective appraisal as well as one that is personal and subjective.

A Sample List of Health Care Needs

SERVICES AND WHERE TO FIND THEM

Breast Examination
- Women's Health Clinic
- City or County Health Department

Pregnancy Test
- Planned Parenthood
- City or County Family Planning Clinic

Dental Examination
- Community Dental Clinic
- County Dental Society

Individual Diet and Nutrition Information
- City or County Health Department
- Local Department of Consumer Health

Weight Loss Program
- Local YWCA
- Weight Watchers International, Inc.

Counseling About Personal Problems
- Community Mental Health Center
- Local Family Service Agency
- Suicide Prevention Center

Hypertension Screening and Blood Pressure Examination
- City or County Health Clinic
- YWCA
- Local chapter of National Heart Association

Abortion and Abortion Counseling
- Abortion Counseling Center
- Women's Health Clinic

Venereal Disease Screening
- City or County Health Clinic
- National VD Hot Line (Operation Venus)

Create a list of your personal health care needs using this sample as a guide. You'll want to add or omit items to meet your individual needs.
Information on all of these services also can be provided by a private physician as well as a variety of other organizations (see page 372).

Community Health Resources

THESE SERVICES ARE AVAILABLE NATIONWIDE

150,000	physicians' offices and medical group practices
90,000	dentists' offices and dental group practices
65,000	pharmacies
22,000	nursing care and related homes
18,000	eye care establishments (opticians and optometrists)
15,000	chiropractors' offices
7,000	hospitals
6,000	hospital or community blood banks
5,300	family planning clinics
5,000	other inpatient health facilities
2,300	Medicare-approved home health agencies
1,200	psychiatric outpatient clinics
600	poison control centers
600	community mental health centers
200	suicide prevention centers
200	women's health clinics and counseling centers
200	neighborhood health centers

• Other community facilities: telephone "hot lines," college health centers and counseling services, and voluntary and public health agencies.
• Business: health facilities within business establishments and manufacturing plants.
• Your home.

Friends and neighbors may be a ready source of information about the health resources available in your community. Personal acquaintances are often willing to offer advice (solicited or not) about physicians they have known or have heard about. The counsel of a trusted friend regarding how she related to a physician may be extremely valuable to you in judging whether or not that physician also would suit your needs.

On the other hand, your friend or neighbor may not be able to shed much light on the professional credentials or competence of a given physician, and may not be able to advise you of the full range of health services available in the community.

Church offices and auxiliary organizations generally are willing and able to help newcomers to the community locate a physician or other health services. If it is important to you to use a practitioner or health care organization with religious convictions similar to your own, begin by seeking guidance through your church or synagogue.

Civic or community associations often maintain rosters of available services or physicians and will provide you with names on request. *Service clubs* may provide more specific information. The Lion's Clubs, for example, have a special interest in the problem of blindness and can offer guidance in that area. The Chamber of Commerce also may be helpful. The American Red Cross directly sponsors a number of activities, and it can refer you to many others.

Voluntary health agencies such as heart, lung, cancer, arthritis, and other societies or foundations offer direct programs, advice, counseling, and referral in their individual areas of interest and expertise.

Voluntary health agencies will be listed in your telephone directory in the white pages. Some examples of such listings are: American Cancer Society, Planned Parenthood, Arthritis Foundation, Women's Health Center, Breast Screening Clinic, and American Heart Association. If you do not find the voluntary agency for your needs listed in the directory for your area, phone your local county medical society for information. See the chart on page 372 for a list of services and addresses of national voluntary health agencies.

Your local county medical society, listed under county offices, can be an excellent source of objective information about the physicians practicing in your community. They're able to provide you with factual information about a physician, such as year of graduation from medical school, hospital affiliations, specialty training, and professional society memberships. This information provides a good basis for the objective aspect of your decision. Also, see the chapter on "Choosing a Doctor," page 392.

Hospital social service departments are excellent sources of detailed information on a wide range of health and health-related services. The staff should be glad to answer your questions, and will provide information directly or will refer you to a reliable source.

Your city or county government generally can provide accurate information on a wide range of topics. The city or county health department is the best general resource, although a special "mayor's hot line" may be available in your area as a supplemental source of information.

Your local telephone directory lists the numbers of the resources described above. In addition, the yellow pages list physicians and dentists (both alphabetically and by specialty), hospitals, medical supply houses, nursing homes, and other related organizations.

Your family physician is frequently the best source of referral for specialty care when you have a specific medical problem. Your own physician or the physician's office staff also can provide accurate information regarding other services available to you.

Again, it's important to determine clearly in your own mind what you are looking for—that is, what services you want—before beginning to make your initial contacts. Formulate specific questions ahead of time so that you acquire all the information you need. Your questions and the answers you get should allow you to objectively evaluate each facility and its personnel.

Your personal evaluation is most important, so make sure the services offered are those that *you* require. Learn as much as possible about the potential biases or goals of the practitioner or agency you plan to contact, and be sure that yours and theirs are not at cross-purposes. As a specific example, if you plan to seek information about an abortion, organizations opposed to abortion are not the best places to seek the objective information you need.

Types of Community Services

At this point, you may have a clear idea of the types of health services you need, and you also may have information about the ones that are available in your community. Still, it may be helpful to have more information about specific services and what they have to offer.

A wide variety of specific health resources are available to women in community settings. It will, of course, be necessary for us to remain general in our remarks since the specific organizations available in your particular community will vary from those in others. However, we hope that the general information provided will help you find your way through the sometimes bewildering maze of health services available to you.

Self-Care and Self-Help Groups

In recent years there has been a ground swell of activity in the self-care or self-help movement. And the underlying theme of this movement—to demystify medical and health care and to reassert individual responsibility for maintaining personal health and well-being—is a healthy one. At its best, the self-help movement is functioning effectively to reestablish a more reasonable balance between what one can and should expect from health professionals, and what one can manage for oneself. At its worst, it may encourage the tendency of some people to reject *all* professional aid, even that which represents a significant advance forward.

A wide range of philosophical and political points of view are represented in the self-help/self-care movement; local women's clubs, the National Organization for Women (NOW), and women's health collectives all represent different vantage points and positions in this area. So you, as an individual woman, probably can find an organization whose views are consistent with your own.

Finally, self-care/self-help groups are publishing various books and manuals. The material covered in these books differs widely, both topically and in quality. They may be general in nature, disease-specific (for example, high blood pressure), or they may focus on prevention and health maintenance. There is a rapidly growing market of books related to mental or emotional health, and to human sexuality. While some of these books are well-balanced, well-written treatments of their subjects, prepared by authorities or lay people, others are biased and clearly propagandizing unproven theories or remedies. In general, if an individual volume claims to have "the answer" to a major health problem, you should be skeptical.

Special Interest Organizations

These organizations focus on the needs of particular groups of women. The special interest may involve a particular philosophy of health management, a preferred method of dealing with a natural phenomenon such as childbirth, or a particular health problem or disease. For the national headquarters of some special interest organizations for women, see the chart that begins on page 378.

The La Leche League, for example, encourages breast-feeding and provides support and educational programs to women who are breast-feeding their infants.

Lamaze classes, and other groups involved in natural childbirth methods, emphasize pregnancy, labor, and delivery as natural processes, and encourage self-management and active participation by both mother and father in the labor and delivery process.

Major Voluntary and Professional National Health Organizations

Al-Anon Family Group Headquarters, Inc.
P.O. Box 182 — Madison Square Station
New York, New York 10010

Provides literature on alcoholism and arranges local meetings to relieve anxieties and frustrations of families with an alcoholic member.

Alcoholics Anonymous World Services, Inc.
Box 459 — Grand Central Station
New York, New York 10017

Aids willing alcoholics to achieve and maintain sobriety through meetings, group help, and literature.

Allergy Foundation of America
801 Second Avenue
New York, New York 10017

Answers specific questions about allergy; provides a regional list of allergists, clinics, hospitals, and extended-care facilities; provides educational pamphlets.

American Academy of Pediatrics
1801 Hinman Avenue
Evanston, Illinois 60204

Provides publications on health care problems and needs of children (including accident prevention and nutrition), as well as literature on abortion, adoption, and day care.

American Cancer Society
777 Third Avenue
New York, New York 10017

Provides health education services that emphasize ways in which individuals can protect themselves against cancer; breast cancer programs to teach women breast self-examination; anti-smoking campaigns; and cancer-detection programs. The ACS also sponsors special programs for persons who have undergone ostomy, laryngectomy, or mastectomy. Volunteers visit these patients while they are still in the hospital, giving them practical advice and emotional support.

American Chiropractic Association
2200 Grand Avenue
Des Moines, Iowa 50312

Provides educational literature on chiropractic medicine.

American Dental Association
211 E. Chicago Avenue
Chicago, Illinois 60611

Provides literature on dental-health education, including nutrition, smoking, gum diseases, and tooth decay.

American Diabetes Association
600 Fifth Avenue
New York, New York 10020

Provides literature on diabetes mellitus; publishes a cookbook for diabetics; provides diabetes detection and education services; provides physician references.

American Dietetic Association
430 North Michigan Avenue
Chicago, Illinois 60611

Publishes pamphlets and books on a wide variety of subjects related to nutrition and diet.

American Foundation for the Blind
15 West 16th Street
New York, New York 10011

Provides information and referral services for blind and visually handicapped persons.

American Heart Association
7320 Greenville Avenue
Dallas, Texas 75231

Provides: educational literature on cardiovascular diseases, heart attack, and stroke; counseling on special diets such as low-cholesterol or sodium-restricted diets; smoking withdrawal programs; stroke clubs (mutual aid organizations for persons who have had a stroke); screening programs for high blood pressure and rheumatic fever; and cardiopulmonary resuscitation training.

American Lung Association
1740 Broadway
New York, New York 10019

Provides educational literature on lung disease and anti-smoking programs.

American Medical Association
535 North Dearborn Street
Chicago, Illinois 60610

Distributes literature and serves as a clearinghouse for information on health or health-related topics such as hypertension, diabetes, nutrition, physical fitness, cancer, and kidney disease.

American Osteopathic Association
212 East Ohio Street
Chicago, Illinois 60611

Provides training programs in emergency lifesaving procedures such as mouth-to-mouth resuscitation, and written materials on venereal disease, first aid, cancer, and nutrition.

American Podiatry Association
20 Chevy Chase Circle, N.W.
Washington, D.C. 20015

Provides information and literature on health-education programs that deal with foot care.

American Red Cross
18th and D Streets, N.W.
Washington, D.C. 20009

Operates first-aid programs at local schools, churches, and many Red Cross chapters. These programs provide basic first aid, emergency care, and cardiopulmonary resuscitation. Teaches water safety, swimming, and lifesaving courses; provides nursing and health programs (including preparation for parenthood); provides screening for hypertension, sickle-cell anemia, glaucoma, and diabetes.

American Social Health Association
1740 Broadway
New York, New York 10019

Provides information and referral sources for venereal disease.

American Society for Psychoprophylaxis in Obstetrics
Suite 410
1523 L Street, N.W.
Washington, D.C. 20005

Promotes the development and acceptance of the Lamaze method of childbirth in classes taught in hospitals, clinics, schools, and other settings. Provides literature on the Lamaze method of childbirth.

Consumer Federation of America
1012 14th Street, N.W.
Suite 901
Washington, D.C. 20005

Provides literature (such as prescription drug prices) to assist individual decision-making in health and medical care.

Consumer's Union
256 Washington Street
Mount Vernon, New York 10550

Publishes books and pamphlets on health problems, finding a doctor, health insurance, and dental care.

Cystic Fibrosis Association
3379 Peachtree Road, N.E.
Atlanta, Georgia 30326

Provides literature on cystic fibrosis; conducts local health-education programs; publishes a listing of over 100 cystic fibrosis centers across the nation.

Epilepsy Foundation of America
1828 L Street, N.W.
Washington, D.C. 20036

Provides educational literature, emergency information, and medical referral services concerning epilepsy; arranges mutual-aid groups for persons with epilepsy and their parents; provides employment counseling.

Major Voluntary and Professional National Health Organizations continued

La Leche League International, Inc.
9616 Minneapolis Avenue
Franklin Park, Illinois 60131

Provides information on prenatal care and practical and psychological aspects of childbirth; provides personal instruction to mothers who want to nurse their babies; arranges monthly meetings at which small groups of mothers discuss breast-feeding and related aspects of bearing and caring for children.

Maternity Center Association
48 East 92nd Street
New York, New York 10028

Provides information and classes on pregnancy and childbearing that focus on various aspects of the childbearing cycle.

National Association for Mental Health
1800 North Kent Street
Arlington, Virginia 22209

Produces and distributes educational materials on mental illness, good mental health practices, and aging.

National Foundation—March of Dimes
1275 Mamaroneck Avenue
White Plains, New York 10605

Provides information on birth defects and their prevention through prenatal care, good nutrition, and good health habits; and arranges genetic counseling and screening for birth defects.

National Kidney Foundation
116 East 27th Street
New York, New York 10016

Provides educational brochures on kidney disease and the organ-donor program.

National Retired Teachers' Association/ American Association of Retired Persons
1909 K Street, N.W.
Washington, D.C. 20049

Assists persons age 55 or older through health-education programs on specific health care needs of this age group.

National Society for the Prevention of Blindness, Inc.
79 Madison Avenue
New York, New York 10016

Distributes literature on the care, protection, and use of eyes; provides glaucoma screening programs; makes referrals to facilities or local eye-care professionals.

Planned Parenthood Federation of America, Inc.
810 Seventh Avenue
New York, New York 10019

Distributes a wide variety of literature on family planning and birth control methods. Planned Parenthood clinic programs provide pregnancy testing, counseling on contraception and birth, and referral services for abortion, VD testing, voluntary sterilization, breast- and cervical-cancer detection, and adoption referral.

Society for Nutrition Education
2140 Shattuck Avenue
Suite 1110
Berkeley, California 94704

Publishes and distributes literature and serves as a clearinghouse for nutrition education materials, including dental health, special diets, nutrition and pregnancy, nutrition for different age groups, and weight control.

United Cerebral Palsy Association
66 East 34th Street
New York, New York 10016

Provides literature on causes of CP, its effects, and appropriate services available—including diagnosis, physical therapy, and vocational counseling.

Many of the agencies listed here will have a local chapter in your area. For this information, as well as available publications, contact the address listed.

The Reach to Recovery Program and other groups of post-mastectomy patients provides psychological support and practical guidance for women who need to readjust to life following breast surgery.

Ostomy clubs provide help to patients who have undergone bowel surgery necessitating the creation of a stoma (artificial opening) in the abdominal wall for the evacuation of feces. Among their services are emotional support, practical advice regarding use of appliances for sanitary disposal of feces, and stoma care. In addition, these groups provide assistance in helping patients reestablish normal family life as well as a normal social and sexual life.

Alcoholics Anonymous (AA), available to both men and women, is perhaps the best known of the self-help groups that employ a peer-group approach to helping members recognize and deal with major health-related problems.

General Medical Services

In most instances, an adult will find that primary health care services are best served through an ongoing relationship with a family practitioner, general practitioner, or general internist. By "primary care," we refer to a) the level of care given at the patient's first contact with the health care system; b) an implicit agreement between physician and patient for continuous, long-term health care; and c) care that integrates preventive and curative measures and offers a comprehensive, coherent plan for you as a patient to follow.

Such a doctor/patient relationship, whether obtained through a physician in private practice or at a public clinic, will adequately see you through about 80 to 90 percent of the health care needs you're likely to have.

Most hospitalizations not requiring extensive diagnostic evaluations or major surgery will be managed or overseen by your primary physician. When you have a very complex or unusual health or medical problem, your primary physician will refer you to a specialist or subspecialist. In general, the primary physician will remain in contact with any consulting specialist and will resume ongoing professional responsibility for you as soon as that illness, acute phase, or surgical procedure is over. For further details regarding how to choose a doctor and how to participate effectively in a physician/patient relationship, see pages 392 and 395.

Reproductivity and Sexuality Services

Family planning services are provided by private physicians, city and county family planning departments, and voluntary health agencies.

Private physicians, mainly obstetrician/gynecologists and family physicians, represent the major source of family planning advice and care for the American population as a whole. In a private practitioner's office, information and assistance in choosing a method of birth control generally will be given by the doctor or by a member of the office staff. The physician will take your medical history and give you a physical examination prior to making recommendations of birth control methods. In some instances, a particular type of contraception may be considered unwise or unsafe for you, based on your medical history. If a diaphragm or IUD is selected, you will be fitted in the office. Birth control pills (oral contraceptives), foam, or condoms are prescribed by the doctor and then purchased at a pharmacy.

Most city or county departments provide family planning services to all residents. Generally, such services offer educational programs to help you choose a suitable method of birth control, a physical examination by a physician or specially trained nurses, and provision of the contraceptive method you choose. Such clinics generally provide follow-up services at periodic intervals. Because they are supported by local, state, or federal funds, these services generally are provided free of charge.

In many communities, a voluntary health agency such as Planned Parenthood may provide family planning services at a somewhat lower cost than a private physician's office. These voluntary health agencies usually offer the same range of services as those described above.

Venereal disease treatment may be obtained at the city or county health department, at college health services, or at the office of a private physician.

All city and county health departments provide services for the diagnosis and treatment of venereal diseases at no charge to the individual. The anonymity the patient may feel in this setting is a positive factor and may account for the heavy utilization of these services. Because of the highly communicable nature of VD, health departments, within their limited resources, need to locate the sexual contacts of the patients they treat in order to halt the spread of disease. In the case of syphilis, the most devastating venereal disease when left untreated, their efforts will be strenuous. Thus, if you have occasion to use the health department for care of a sexually transmitted disease, you should cooperate in referring contacts for treatment. Of course, your need for privacy will be respected.

Venereal diseases are most common in the young-adult population, and college health services see a significant proportion of cases. They are sensitive to issues of confidentiality, and also will urge you to refer contacts for treatment.

But the vast majority of cases of venereal disease are treated in private physicians' offices. Some individuals are hesitant to reveal to their own primary physician (who also may treat other family members) that they suspect venereal disease, and will seek care elsewhere. Private physicians will respect a patient's desire for confidentiality and will try to work through the difficult matter of informing and treating a marital partner.

Maternity care includes pregnancy testing as well as care before the baby is born, during the delivery, and after the delivery.

Prenatal care (care before the baby is born) includes periodic physical examinations and laboratory tests as well as nutrition counseling. In addition, a woman can seek advice about the delivery, breast-feeding, and infant care.

There are a number of resources a woman can use for prenatal care. Among private practitioners, obstetrician/gynecologists and family physicians are most often the providers of prenatal care. City and county health departments usually operate free maternity clinics on an outpatient basis, but have arrangements with local public hospitals or voluntary (private) hospitals for delivery and inpatient services.

The role of Lamaze Groups and other organizations interested in prepared childbirth has been mentioned. Women interested in breast-feeding their infants can receive information, guidance, and support from the La Leche League. Private physicians and local health departments can refer you to these and other organizations.

The delivery itself is a vital part of maternity care. Most deliveries in this country take place in hospitals. Recently, however, home delivery has been gaining new popularity among some women. Home delivery lets you enjoy the supportive environment of family and friends, and may even avoid hospital infections. But in the event of complications during delivery, special facilities and equipment are unavailable. Whether or not the supposed benefits of home delivery outweigh the potential disadvantages is still debated heatedly. If you wish to have your baby at home, you should put much time into the decision and carefully carry out certain preparations. Discuss all aspects of home delivery with your obstetrician and find out the extent to which he or she will cooperate with your plans. If you choose to deliver at home with the aid of an obstetrician, you will need one who is supportive and cooperative.

Another interesting development in recent years has been the reemergence of the midwife. While the midwife has always been used in some geographical areas and by some groups of the population, it is only recently that nurse-midwives have been trained and registered as a new type of health professional. Licensed nurses interested in midwifery can enter training programs designed to teach additional skills in prenatal care; medical history-taking and physical examinations; management of normal labor and delivery; and immediate postnatal care of the infant, including learning how to identify neonatal (newborn) complications. Nurse-midwives must undergo special examinations for licensure in those localities where they have been accepted, and must work in cooperation with and under the supervision of physicians. For more information on these topics, see the "Pregnancy" and "Labor and Delivery" chapters.

The termination of a pregnancy may be the medical service you seek. Among the issues that a woman must confront in choosing to obtain an abortion are the following: her own philosophic and emotional views regarding abortion, assurance of medical competence and safety in obtaining the procedure, and the cost involved. These issues are dealt with in depth in the chapter on "Abortion," beginning on page 206.

Although a woman now can find many competent obstetrician/gynecologists willing to perform an abortion, there remain many who will not. Your primary physician, the local health department, or Planned Parenthood can be contacted for information and referral. The method of therapeutic abortion used depends upon the individual patient and the stage of her pregnancy. Hospitalization may or may not be required.

Recently, women's health collectives (or centers focusing their efforts on gynecological problems, menopause, and abortion) have sprung up in many cities. Generally, these centers are staffed by licensed physicians who specialize in obstetrics/gynecology and provide information and outpatient services. For early abortions, the expense of hospitalization is avoided: the client is admitted in the early morning, she receives a physical examination and laboratory tests, and the abortion is performed the same day. After a suitable recovery period, she generally is released.

Clearly, the quality of medical service varies, and it is wise to investigate carefully the reputation of the center by consulting reputable sources before choosing a facility (see pages 217 and 379).

Health care services for children are provided through health departments, special interest organizations, child development centers, and school health services, as well as through private physicians.

Virtually all health departments offer immunizations to the public, and most provide "well-baby clinics" where parents can check the normal growth and development of their infants and young children. One of the major efforts of such facilities is to educate parents in the care and feeding of infants and children. These services usually are provided free of charge.

General medical care for children also can be obtained through a private pediatrician or family physician. Typically, immunizations, preventively oriented checkups, and variable amounts of parent education can be obtained from a private physician.

There are a variety of special interest organizations that focus wholly or largely on medical problems related to children. Organizations dealing with problems such as cystic fibrosis or sickle-cell anemia can provide specific information in their particular area of interest. Your physician, the social service department of your local hospital, or the community health department can refer you to an appropriate agency or organization in this category.

Child development centers offer a wide range of diagnostic and treatment services for children who are failing to develop at a normal rate because of physical or emotional problems. Examples of the types of problems evaluated in these centers are nervous system disorders (such as cerebral palsy and epilepsy), learning disabilities, and behavior problems. These facilities commonly employ a team of health professionals from medicine, psychology, nursing, and social work who carefully review your child's medical history, conduct physical and neurological examinations and appropriate laboratory tests, and administer a battery of psychological tests. The findings provide a basis for evaluating various aspects of intellectual, psychomotor, and emotional development in your child. From this "work-up," a program may be prescribed involving various treatments, alone or in combination. Depending on the circumstances of the individual child, this program may involve medication, physical or speech therapy, prosthetic devices, special educational programs, or emotional counseling.

School health services vary widely from community to community. Some offer minimal services, while others have well-developed health education programs and diagnostic screening services designed to pick up a variety of conditions to which children are prone.

Most school districts offer a dispensary or first-aid room in each school, staffed on a full- or part-time basis by a nurse or nurse's aide. An ill or injured child usually is kept there until he is picked up by parents.

Most school nurses are permitted to administer medication to children requiring it, as long as the parents make special arrangements with the school. For your child's protection, however, school nurses will not provide even simple medications without first obtaining parental consent.

Mental Health Services

Mental health services are provided through community mental health centers, private mental health professionals, special programs developed for specific problems, and crisis centers.

Community mental health centers continue to develop in response to federal legislation enacted in the mid-1960s mandating that local communities provide a broad range of mental health services, including diagnostic facilities, day-hospital (outpatient) treatment, facilities for alcohol and drug addiction problems, and other services.

Once again, a team approach is emphasized in these settings, where psychiatrists, nurses, psychologists, mental health social workers, and others work together to provide appropriate and needed services. Fees usually are charged on a sliding scale, ranging from no charge to full charge, depending on family size and income.

Private mental health professionals, who are licensed to work in the mental health field, include psychiatrists, psychologists, and family or marital counselors. Psychiatrists are those who hold an M.D. degree and have received special training in the diagnosis and treatment of mental disorders. Psychologists are non-physicians who have specific training in various aspects of professional psychology at either the master's degree level or the doctoral degree level. Family and marital counselors include a wide range of individuals—from the very well-trained to self-styled practitioners.

While each of these professionals brings a different perspective to his or her work, they still may share common goals and attitudes. As in other areas of health care, it is wise to evaluate the credentials and professional reputations of a practitioner before committing yourself to his or her care.

Fees for mental health care obtained from private practitioners vary, but usually are set on an hourly basis.

A Selected List of Special Interest Organizations for Women

AGING

Grey Panthers National Health Service Task Force
3700 Chestnut Street
Philadelphia, Pennsylvania 19004

National Council on the Aging
1828 L Street, N.W.
Washington, D.C. 20036

American Association of Retired Persons
1909 K Street, N.W.
Washington, D.C. 20049

These organizations provide literature and information on health care problems and other needs of persons age 55 or older.

BREASTS

La Leche League International
9616 Minneapolis Ave.
Franklin Park, Illinois 60131

Through monthly meetings of small groups of mothers, the La Leche League provides personal instruction to women who want to nurse their babies. Also provides information on the practical and psychological aspects of breast-feeding.

Reach to Recovery Program
American Cancer Society
777 Third Avenue
New York, New York 10017

Part of the American Cancer Society, the Reach to Recovery Program includes women who have undergone partial or complete mastectomies. Volunteers visit mastectomy patients while they are still in the hospital, giving them practical advice and emotional support.

CONTRACEPTION AND BIRTH CONTROL

Planned Parenthood Federation of America
810 7th Avenue
New York, New York 10019

Clinic programs provide pregnancy testing, counseling on birth control, and referral sources for abortion, VD testing, and voluntary sterilization.

Association for Voluntary Sterilization
708 Third Avenue
New York, New York 10017

Provides referral services for individuals seeking this permanent form of birth control.

DISABILITIES

National Information Center for the Handicapped
Box 1492
Washington, D.C. 20013

Provides information and referral services for disabled persons.

United Cerebral Palsy Association of America
66 East 34th Street
New York, New York 10016

Provides literature on causes and effects of cerebral palsy and appropriate services available, including diagnosis, physical therapy, and vocational counseling.

Epilepsy Foundation of America
1828 L Street, N.W.
Washington, D.C. 20036

Provides information, referral services, and counseling for epileptics; arranges mutual aid groups for persons with epilepsy.

EXERCISE
President's Council on Physical Fitness and Sports
7th and D Streets S.W.
Washington, D.C. 20202

Promotes home and school exercise programs.

PREGNANCY AND CHILDBIRTH
Lamaze Classes
American Society for Psychoprophylaxis in Obstetrics
Suite 410
1523 L Street, N.W.
Washington, D.C. 20005

Classes in this natural method of childbirth are taught in hospitals, clinics, schools, and other settings.

National Abortion Council
120 West 57th Street
New York, New York 10019

These organizations provide abortion counseling and referrals as well as information on political programs to repeal restrictive abortion laws.

National Abortion Rights Action League
706 7th Street, S.E.
Washington, D.C. 20003

MENOPAUSE
Women In Midstream
University of Washington YWCA
4224 Union Way, N.E.
Seattle, Washington 98105

Provides literature on menopause, and guidelines for developing menopause support groups.

NUTRITION AND WEIGHT LOSS
U.S. Department of Agriculture
USDA, Office of Information
Washington, D.C. 20250

Provides literature on nutrition and diet.

Overeaters Anonymous
1246 LaCienega Blvd.
Suite 200
Los Angeles, California 90035

Diet-club organization with local chapters.

TOPS
4575 South 5th Street
P.O. Box 4489
Milwaukee, Wisconsin 53207

Diet-club organization with local chapters.

Weight Watchers International, Inc.
175 East Shore Road
Great Neck, New York 11023

Diet-club organization with local chapters.

SEX COUNSELING
SIECUS— (Sex Information and Education Council of the United States)
1855 Broadway
New York, New York 10019

Works with physicians, educators, clergymen, and social scientists to develop sex education programs for all ages.

Special programs have been developed for people who have difficulty with drug or alcohol abuse. Perhaps the best known of these is Alcoholics Anonymous (AA) for those with drinking problems. AA also operates a closely associated program for family members of alcoholics known as Al-Anon. These programs emphasize the necessity for the individual to make a decision to change his or her drinking behavior. Group support, based on a set of principles or "steps," serves as the major mechanism for bringing about changes in drinking behavior.

The Al-Anon program for spouses, children, and friends of alcoholics is designed to help these individuals separate the alcoholic's problems from their own, to receive information about alcoholism, and to gain emotional support from each other.

Drug abuse programs frequently are offered through community mental health centers and through psychiatric clinics associated with hospitals.

Both alcohol and drug abuse programs have experimented with various psychiatric and medical approaches, and both offer individual and group therapy on a regular basis. In addition, drug addicts may be maintained on methadone, and alcoholics may be given antabuse as medical intervention. An essential part of the treatment in acute cases is detoxification, which generally involves hospitalization. When the patient is drug-free, intensive outpatient therapy of various sorts can be initiated.

Crisis centers are available in many areas, sometimes as a telephone "hot line" or storefront operation, ready to respond on a 24-hour basis to a request for help. Crisis centers receive calls from abused wives, alcoholics, or individuals undergoing major emotional stress at home or at work. Some centers focus on a single problem, such as rape. Crisis centers generally function to provide immediate supportive care and counsel, and usually make subsequent referrals to other resources designed to provide continuing or long-term help.

Home Health Services

Home health services enable a person who has been incapacitated as the result of illness, injury, or advancing age to be cared for at home rather than in a hospital or other institution. For some, care may be required only on a short-term basis; for others, care may be required over a longer period of time. The level of care needed also varies. Nursing care may be necessary for some, while others may need help only with household tasks.

The Visiting Nurse Association is an extremely useful complement to a community's health care system. Organized as a voluntary health agency, this organization provides nursing services in the home. In addition to routine bedside nursing services for elderly or bedridden patients and for those who cannot leave their homes to visit a physician's office, visiting nurses offer patient education in a number of areas, such as diet, exercise, and self-care. In general, the Visiting Nurse Association is called in by attending physicians who determine whether or not such services are required. The fees for the nursing service vary, depending on the income status of the individual recipient.

Public health nurses operate as an outreach arm of the city or county health department, and their services are similar to those of the Visiting Nurse Association. By training, however, public health nurses hold a community health perspective and emphasize screening programs, prenatal care, and preventive measures, such as immunizations. Frequently, they investigate potential outbreaks of communicable disease, or spot environmental health problems that require further action by the health department. Although public health nurses work in close association with private practitioners in the community, their affiliation still is with the public health department.

Homemaker's organizations are available in many communities to provide basic housekeeping and house-maintenance services to homebound individuals not capable of carrying out such activities themselves. They provide a valuable service by making it possible for these people, who do not require hospitalization, to remain in their homes. Once again, you should obtain references and credentials on any homemaker's organization you may be considering.

Dental Services

Until recently, dental care had not developed the high degree of specialization characteristic of medicine. A general dentist provided preventive dental services, removed teeth, performed various restorative procedures, and provided periodontal care (care related to the gums and supporting structures of the teeth). Recently, however, dentists have begun to specialize. Some major specialty areas in dentistry are the following: pediodontics, dealing with the dental problems of children; periodontics, dealing with the maintenance of supporting structures in older patients; and orthodontics, dealing with the alignment of teeth to ensure appropriate bite and satisfactory cosmetic appearance.

Changes in dental practice have resulted in changes in dental office staffing. Typically, dentists now employ such health professionals as dental hygienists and dental technicians to provide basic services under the supervision of the dentist. As a group, dentists have strongly endorsed the concept of the health team and have used it effectively.

The increase in the number of dentists has not paralleled the increase in the number of physicians over the last several decades; thus, dental care remains a luxury for many Americans. Yet, dental disease in its various forms — tooth decay and periodontal disease, especially — is probably the most prevalent disease in any human population and is significantly related to general health. Furthermore, the resources available through the public sector are fewer than those available privately. Local health departments generally offer dental programs for children, but nationally, coverage remains inadequate for the population as a whole.

Weight Control Services

Probably more has been written about the problem of controlling excess weight than any other single topic in the health care field. In addition, since physical attractiveness as well as health is involved in the problem of weight control, the public is exposed to a great deal of misinformation.

A number of physicians now specialize in weight control and do so within the bounds of good medical practice and current scientific knowledge. In general, a family practitioner, pediatrician, or general internist evaluates each patient for any underlying disease process that may be causing the problem and can provide sound, individualized advice.

Another potential source of aid to the overweight or obese person is a nutritionist or dietician. Physicians frequently will refer patients to a nutritionist who is trained to devise appropriate diets that emphasize a balance among the three major food types (protein, carbohydrates, and fats) and that also regulate caloric intake. Whenever possible, the nutritionist also will modify a diet to satisfy the particular likes and dislikes of an individual patient. For more information on nutrition and weight control, see the "Nutrition" chapter, beginning on page 40.

Health food stores, appearing in ever-increasing numbers on the American scene, also are potential sources of information on weight control. A great deal of useful information can be obtained from health food stores by an intelligent and well-informed consumer. On the other hand, health food stores remain in business by selling their products, and the information they provide is not always unbiased. The consumer always should guard against slanted or misinformed recommendations.

Two additional sources of information regarding weight control programs are the numerous health spas available to the public today, and the seemingly infinite number of books on the subject of weight control. Again, the consumer must balance what she is told by spa personnel or what she reads in books with her own commonsense understanding of good health, exercise, and sound nutritional practices. When all is said and done, an individual's appropriate weight rests upon a sensible balance between the calories consumed in food and the calories expended through daily activity and physical exercise. Any quick weight loss program that ignores these basic principles is hazardous to the individual's health.

Voluntary health agencies such as the American Heart Association and the American Diabetes Association have a particular interest in the problem of weight control and appropriate nutritional practices. If you are concerned about dietary cholesterol or the appropriate nutrition for diabetics, excellent advice regarding an appropriate diet can be obtained from the local affiliates of either of these organizations.

Behavior modification is an approach that holds great promise for achieving sound weight control habits. However, behavior modification techniques are still in an early stage of development, and much further work must be done before fully satisfactory results can be guaranteed. Nevertheless, psychologists already have used behavior modification techniques effectively to help patients better structure their eating habits. For instance, one technique might be to restrict your eating to just one place in the house, such as the dining room table, so that snacking at the refrigerator ceases to be automatic. When these techniques are combined with a sound program of nutritional information and appropriate exercise, many individuals who previously had been unsuccessful in dealing with their weight problems are now having success.

Services for Specific Disabilities

There are a number of diseases associated with prolonged disability or physical disfigurement after medical or surgical treatment. Two examples are mastectomy for breast cancer and intestinal surgery that results in the formation of a stoma. In both instances, the surgery—performed as a lifesaving or life-prolonging measure—leaves the patient with significant physical and emotional disabilities.

Special interest organizations such as the *Reach to Recovery Program* (formed to aid post-mastectomy patients) and *ostomy clubs* (organized to aid post-intestinal-surgery patients) are designed to serve these people. These organizations help patients deal more effectively with the problems that begin when they leave the hospital by offering practical advice regarding self-care as well as emotional support. Often patients are drawn into the activities of the group and themselves become helpers for others in the same situation.

Physical or occupational therapy is vital in many types of orthopedic disabilities and in post-stroke disabilities to enable the patient to regain the fullest possible body function. In most cases, the patient's physician will refer her to a physical therapist or to an occupational therapist, usually in the rehabilitation department of the hospital. Rehabilitation clinics also are available in most communities.

Community Health Information

We all can become better-informed consumers of health services by utilizing the general and specific information resources available to us.

The neighborhood pharmacy represents a valuable resource. Most pharmacists are prepared and willing to provide you with general advice related to health problems and specifically to the use of over-the-counter drugs (those drugs that do not require a prescription) in the treatment of minor ailments. Generally, pharmacists also can be trusted to refer you to a doctor if the symptoms described suggest a more serious illness than you suspect. Many physicians regard the pharmacist as a source of information for their patients and expect them to discuss the drugs prescribed, how they are to be used, and what side effects may occur.

Food stores and supermarkets sometimes provide general information. In particular, with new legislation requiring that nutritional information be provided on the labels of many foods, the consumer can become better informed about dietary and nutritional needs.

Spas and health clubs already have been mentioned, and more people are using such facilities as a means of disciplining themselves to regular exercise. However, it's advisable to double-check their advice if you have specific health problems, since these facilities generally do not have extensive background in health care.

Chiropractors and naturopaths are additional resources that some people may use. While these health practitioners may not be held in the highest regard by physicians, they can provide significant relief in many cases. We would only emphasize that both the practitioner and the patient understand clearly the limits of their practice. The major concern about these forms of health care is that a problem may remain undiagnosed and untreated for a prolonged period of time, so that when a diagnosis finally is made, little can be done. If you have been thoroughly examined by a physician first, you can be more assured that this situation will not occur.

Other health professionals operating in specialized areas are recognized as legitimate by the physician community. These include podiatrists, who specialize in disorders of the feet; optometrists, who are specifically trained to examine the eyes and prescribe eyeglasses to correct defective vision; and opticians, who are licensed to fabricate eyeglasses on prescriptions from an optometrist or an ophthalmologist.

Financing Medical Care

There are several basic ways that health services and medical care are paid for and provided:
- *Direct out-of-pocket payment* (e.g., for prescription drugs, a general checkup, or other services that may not be covered by an individual's health insurance).
- *Provision of service* (e.g., by a city hospital or county clinic that may provide free care for a specific health care problem, such as screening for venereal disease).
- *Insurance and prepayment* (Individuals make a contractual agreement, either singly or in groups, with an insurer who promises to pay for an agreed-upon range of services under specified conditions).

Most people's medical care is financed totally or in part by health insurance. The section that follows describes various kinds of health insurance and what to consider when choosing a particular plan.

Health Insurance

There are three basic categories of health insurance:
- *Hospital coverage.*
- *Hospital plus surgical coverage.* Commonly called "Basic Protection," this generally covers hospital care, surgery, and physicians' services.
- *Major medical coverage.* This usually is sold as a supplement to basic coverage and may cover a variety of services that are either not covered or are covered only partially under basic hospital and surgical policies (e.g., dental and optical care, or catastrophes).

Choosing among the many different types of health insurance available often is difficult and depends on the particular health care needs of a woman and her family. Several government agencies provide information to help you make decisions about health insurance. These include state departments of insurance and state and local departments of consumer health. Private organizations such as the Health Insurance Institute (277 Park Avenue, New York, New York 10017) and the Blue Cross Association (Box 4389, Chicago, Illinois 60680) also are good sources of information on health insurance. Finally, if you're choosing among health insurance policies at work, don't hesitate to ask your personnel officer to explain the different plans.

There are essentially three ways for an individual to obtain health insurance:
● By qualifying for a federal or state health insurance program such as:

Medicare (for elderly and disabled Social Security recipients).

Medicaid (for the low-income aged, blind, and disabled, and for families with dependent children).
● Through groups such as companies, unions, professional organizations, or employers (who usually share premium costs with the worker). The following options usually are offered:

Blue Cross/Blue Shield (contracts with providers).

A prepaid plan or health maintenance organization (provides medical services directly).

Other private plan (provides insurance).
● By individual purchase from an insurance company. Individuals who are unemployed, self-employed, or who want more coverage than their company may provide can purchase insurance directly from a private insurance company.

All types of health insurance have: deductibles (the amount a consumer must pay for a medical service before the insurance company takes over); uncovered or partially covered care (such as dental care or prescription drugs); and maximum benefits for services.

Personal Expenditures by Category

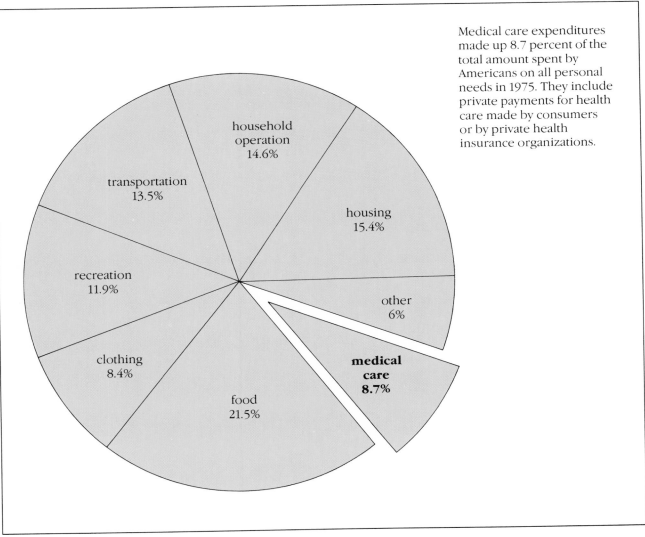

Medical care expenditures made up 8.7 percent of the total amount spent by Americans on all personal needs in 1975. They include private payments for health care made by consumers or by private health insurance organizations.

household operation 14.6%

transportation 13.5%

housing 15.4%

recreation 11.9%

other 6%

clothing 8.4%

medical care 8.7%

food 21.5%

Hospitals and Hospital Care

MARCIA STEWART

While most women receive medical care in a private physician's office (for diagnosis and treatment of routine health problems), the best known medical facility for the care of people who are sick or injured is the hospital. Here we will describe different types of hospitals and provide information that will assist you in selecting and evaluating hospital care.

Most of us use hospitals for the following services:
- *Surgery—whether it be a required operation, such as gallbladder surgery, or elective cosmetic surgery, such as a face-lift*
- *Delivery of your baby*
- *Medical emergencies, such as fractures or burns.*

Types of Hospitals

All hospitals have an organized medical staff and permanent facilities that include inpatient beds. They provide a variety of diagnostic, therapeutic, and rehabilitative services, both surgical and non-surgical, by bringing together many different health professionals, including physicians, nurses, medical technologists, nutritionists, and X-ray technicians, and a variety of technological and laboratory equipment (such as a blood bank, and equipment for cobalt therapy and renal-dialysis services).

Hospitals are usually divided into categories by their type of service, size, and ownership or sponsorship.

The most common type of hospital is the *general medical and surgical hospital,* which primarily takes care of patients with acute illnesses or with flare-ups of chronic conditions. The average length of stay is usually short—less than two weeks. General medical hospitals vary in size and may be privately or publicly owned. *Specialty hospitals* are usually affiliated with a medical school or research foundation; they are designed for the diagnosis and treatment of patients who have specific medical conditions and diseases such as cancer, bone and joint diseases, or burns. Both the general medical and surgical and the specialty hospitals are short-term facilities, with the average length of stay usually less than thirty days.

Another type of hospital is the *chronic disease or long-term hospital,* which cares for patients who require long-term (over thirty days) medical care for a variety of chronic health conditions such as orthopedic or neurological illnesses. Nursing homes, rehabilitation facilities, and psychiatric institutions all fall into this category. Long-term hospitals are not the focus of this chapter; for further information and reading (for example, on how to choose a nursing home), see the list of references that begins on page 667.

Hospitals also vary as to size and extent of facilities; they may contain anywhere from 20 to 2,000 beds, and have simple or sophisticated technological and laboratory equipment. The average community hospital has 150 to 160 beds. The largest hospitals (with over 400 beds) are those affiliated with medical schools or research foundations; these are called *teaching hospitals* and have interns, residents, and medical students on the hospital wards. They usually have excellent technical facilities and a specialized staff for open-heart surgery, kidney transplants, etc.

Finally, administratively and financially there are three types of hospitals.

Private proprietary hospitals are owned and operated for profit by individuals or stockholders in a partnership or corporation. Many of these owners may be the same physicians who admit their own patients to the hospital. Proprietary hospitals tend to be small, having less than 100 beds, and generally focus on patients with simple maladies. Hospitals operated for profit are less likely to provide community services, such as outpatient care and emergency room services, that are often found in nonprofit hospitals.

Private nonprofit hospitals are the most common hospital facilities in the United States. They operate under a wide variety of sectarian and nonsectarian auspices, and are usually run by a board of trustees. A variety of hospitals fall into this category, including small community hospitals, big teaching centers, and religious-affiliated institutions. Private nonprofit hospitals may range in size from 25 to 2,000 or more beds, although the majority have fewer than 200 beds. Nonprofit hospitals are eligible for various state and federal funds (such as through bond issues for hospital construction); other sources of financial support include private contributions, church support, and patient fees.

Public hospitals also are nonprofit, and include city, county, state, and federal hospitals. Federal hospitals usually provide services to one particular group, the best known example of which is veterans. State hospitals are usually psychiatric hospitals. Other types of public hospitals include general medical, city, and county hospitals. Public hospitals are usually large, with from 500 to 1,000 beds. They are tax-supported and often provide free medical care to eligible individuals, charging fees to others.

A Hospital's Staff and Services

A hospital's staff usually includes a permanent full-time house staff as well as physicians from the community who admit their private patients. Patient care in hospitals may be the responsibility of an *attending physician,* who is either a member of the hospital staff or has admitting privileges, or a *resident,* who, with *interns,* makes up the *house staff.* A resident is a house officer who has completed medical school and a one-year internship. Interns are in their first year after medical school. Consultants, usually specialists from outside the hospital, may also provide patient care. In addition to physicians, hospital services are provided by a variety of other health professionals, including nurses, medical technologists, and X-ray technicians.

Inpatient Hospital Care

Hospitals today provide a variety of inpatient and outpatient services. Most people associate hospitals with overnight stays for surgery or maternity care, although both these types of care are increasingly provided in physicians' offices or in non-hospital settings. Among the types of inpatient medical care generally requiring an overnight hospital stay are *surgery,* either for the complete removal of an organ, tissue, or body part (such as the gallbladder, kidney, tonsils, uterus, or appendix), or for the removal of an abnormal or diseased part with preservation of the rest (such as cysts or tumors on the ovaries, kidney stones, varicose veins, or rhinoplasty or biopsy surgery). *Delivery and maternity care* usually require inpatient care.

Outpatient Hospital Care

Hospitals today may also provide a variety of ambulatory services or outpatient care that do not require an overnight stay. These include the following:

Emergency room services. Most general hospitals have emergency rooms (ERs) that are equipped to handle all kinds of problems, from the flu to a heart attack. While emergency rooms were originally established to handle medical emergencies, they now are often used by patients in other circumstances — such as when they cannot find a physician at night or do not know where else to go for care, as when traveling in a strange city, for example. In general, it's best to avoid the use of ER services for minor and chronic illnesses that can be treated in a physician's office or in other facilities; this will help prevent delayed treatment of truly urgent cases by emergency room staff and also is more economical. Emergency rooms often charge higher fees, and ER services are not always covered by health insurance.

If you need emergency medical care in a foreign country, it's best to check with your hotel or the American Embassy for a referral; an American airline or cruise ship line also may be helpful. In addition, before you travel you may want to purchase one of the publications that lists physicians and hospitals in cities throughout the world. The list of references that begins on page 668 includes titles and addresses of such publications.

Hospital clinics. Hospitals are increasingly providing primary or specialty care in outpatient departments; these are especially common in large urban hospitals and include general checkup as well as X-ray and abortion services. These medical services may be available by appointment, walk-in, or referral (as from an emergency room staff).

Social services. Hospitals also may include social service departments that provide counseling (such as family planning) and make referrals to community health care and social welfare agencies for such services as nutrition counseling and home health care programs.

Hospital Care at Home

As an alternative to full-scale hospital care for some convalescing patients and those with prolonged or chronic illnesses, several different kinds of health care programs are available to the patient at home. Some hospitals have developed excellent home care programs to provide equipment in the home, periodic visits by medical personnel (including doctors, nurses, social workers, and physical therapists), or even volunteer aides as needed. At-home patients then may return to hospital outpatient clinics at regular intervals for necessary hospital services.

In addition to hospitals, a number of other professional sources provide home health care programs. An example is the community-sponsored Visiting Nurse Association, which provides a specialized nursing staff as well as home health aids to help with cleaning, shopping, or meal preparation. Also, private assistance is available in many forms; in most cities there are companies that rent hospital beds, wheelchairs, and other home care equipment. Private-duty nurses are also available to assist with patient care at home. When home health care is feasible, it can be less expensive, more convenient, and more comforting to a patient and her family than hospitalization. For more information on hospital care at home, check with your doctor or a local hospital.

Choosing a Hospital

In most cases requiring hospital care (surgery and delivery), people don't choose their hospital but go where their doctor sends them. This depends on several factors, including where their physician has admitting privileges and where an empty bed exists, as well as the particular type of medical care needed. Thus, physician choice requires careful thought and consideration, as discussed in the chapter, "Choosing a Doctor." There is more individual choice of hospitals for emergency room services, except in life-threatening situations when it may be necessary to go to the closest hospital.

There are no absolute rules concerning which credentials are necessary for a hospital, or which type is best. The type of medical care you need is one determining factor. Routine surgery may be done as well (and at less cost) in a small community hospital as in a large teaching center where the presence of interns and medical students may pose some minor

inconveniences to you as a patient. In fact, if you don't need a specialized medical staff and equipment, a small community hospital may be your best choice; it may offer more floor care and attention, as well as closer proximity to your home. When you do need sophisticated surgical procedures, such as open-heart surgery or treatment for cancer, a specialized medical center will be necessary.

While there are no absolute rules by which to choose and judge hospital care, the following list may be used as a guide in evaluating hospitals.

Accreditation. All hospitals must be licensed under state legislation and public health law; this licensing is primarily related to hospital buildings and construction. In addition, hospitals may be accredited by the Joint Commission on the Accreditation of Hospitals, which is an independent nonprofit organization composed of representatives from the American Colleges of Physicians and Surgeons, the American Hospital Association, and the American Medical Association. Accreditation requires conformity with certain

Nationally Renowned Hospitals and General Clinics

Barnes Hospital
Barnes Hospital Plaza
St. Louis, Missouri 63110

**Baylor University
Medical Center**
3500 Gaston Avenue
Dallas, Texas 75246

Cedars-Sinai Medical Center
8700 Beverly Boulevard
Box 48750
Los Angeles, California 90048

**Columbia-Presbyterian
Medical Center**
622 West 168th Street
New York, New York 10032

Duke University Hospital
Box 3708
Durham, North Carolina 27710

Emory University Hospital
1364 Clifton Road N.E.
Atlanta, Georgia 30322

**Hospital of the University of
Pennsylvania**
3400 Spruce Street
Philadelphia, Pennsylvania 19104

Kaiser Foundation Hospital
280 West MacArthur Boulevard
Oakland, California 94611

Lovelace-Bataan Medical Center
5400 Gibson Boulevard S.E.
Albuquerque, New Mexico 87108

Ochsner Foundation Hospital
1516 Jefferson Highway
New Orleans, Louisiana 70121

The Cleveland Clinic Hospital
9500 Euclid Avenue
Cleveland, Ohio 44106

The Lahey Clinic
605 Commonwealth Avenue
Boston, Massachusetts 02215

The Mayo Clinic
Rochester, Minnesota 55901

Massachusetts General Hospital
32 Fruit Street
Boston, Massachusetts 02114

Mount Sinai Hospital
One Gustave L. Levy Place
New York, New York 10029

**Northwestern
Memorial Hospital**
Superior Street and Fairbanks Court
Chicago, Illinois 60611

Peter Bent Brigham Hospital
721 Huntington Avenue
Boston, Massachusetts 02115

The Johns Hopkins Hospital
601 North Broadway
Baltimore, Maryland 21205

University of Utah Hospital
50 North Medical Drive
Salt Lake City, Utah 84132

Vanderbilt University Hospital
1161 21st Avenue South
Nashville, Tennessee 37232

Yale-New Haven Hospital
789 Howard Avenue
New Haven, Connecticut 06504

University Hospital of Jacksonville
655 West Eighth Street
Jacksonville, Florida 32209

University Hospital of Seattle
1959 N.E. Pacific Street
Seattle, Washington 98195

UCLA Medical Center
10833 Le Conte Avenue
Los Angeles, California 90024

**University of California at
San Francisco—Medical Center**
San Francisco, California 94143

University of Chicago Hospital
950 East 59th Street
Chicago, Illinois 60637

standards regarding hospital facilities, staff, and functioning; these are considered minimum standards that hospitals must meet to provide an acceptable level of care. Certification by the Joint Commission on the Accreditation of Hospitals is voluntary, although necessary if the hospital is to receive Medicare funds and other government support. About 75 percent of the 7,000 hospitals in the United States are accredited.

Staff. The training and caliber of physicians who practice in a particular hospital are important indicators of the quality of a hospital. Among the questions that you may want answered are:
• What kinds of doctors are on the hospital staff?
• How many board-certified specialists are on the house staff or have admitting privileges?
• Is there always a doctor on duty?
• What is the percentage of doctors who are foreign medical school graduates?

You also may want information on the nurse staff-patient ratio and on any other types of hospital staff available, such as physical therapists and blood-bank technologists.

Services and facilities. Depending on your particular medical needs, you'll also want to know:
• What technological and laboratory facilities are available?
• Is emergency care available?
• Does the hospital have an intensive care unit to provide care for life-threatening illnesses such as heart attack or kidney failure?

Regarding hospital maternity care, you should know:
• What intensive care facilities are available for premature babies?
• How are babies cared for after they arrive?
• Does the hospital have a central nursery system?
• Are babies allowed in their mother's room?
• Are fathers allowed in the labor and delivery rooms?

Administration, policies, and financing.
• Is the hospital affiliated with a medical school?
• What are hospital policies on visitors?
• May a parent stay overnight with a hospitalized child?
• Does the hospital have a consumer advisory board or a physician peer review committee?
• What are fees and payment arrangements, and how will you be billed?
• What hospital services are covered by your health insurance?

The best way to choose and judge a hospital is to inquire. Ask your physician, friends, neighbors, and relatives. Also check your public library for a copy of the *American Hospital Association Guide to the Health Care Field;* this is the best reference source on individual hospitals throughout the country, including information about accreditation status, staff, and facilities. Finally, visit the hospitals in your area and ask for a copy of the hospital's annual report or for a staff list.

For more information on choosing and evaluating hospital care, refer to the chapter "Choosing a Doctor." Also, see the boxed material opposite and on the following two pages, which lists some of the top hospitals in the United States for general and specialized medical care. It was developed through conversations with leading medical experts, physicians, and consumer-health advocates, and from statistical information in the *American Hospital Association Guide to the Health Care Field.* Most of these hospitals are affiliated with a medical school and have highly specialized staffs, equipment, and facilities. For more information on specific hospitals or specialized medical services, see the list of community resources and national voluntary health organizations on page 372.

Entering a hospital for surgery or other medical care can be a very emotional and anxiety-provoking experience, no matter how minor the procedure. Don't hesitate to express your concerns to your physician or to seek a second opinion from another doctor if you question the advisability of the surgery. Try to get as much information as possible prior to admission regarding what to expect of your hospital stay.

Your Rights as a Patient

It's important to remember that a hospital's first responsibility is to its patients. The American Hospital Association has developed a *Patient's Bill of Rights* that outlines hospital responsibilities and patient rights while under hospital care. These rights include the following:
• Considerate and respectful care, including a reasonable amount of time and attention, and confidentiality of health records
• Full information about your condition, care, or treatment, as well as medical alternatives necessary to give informed consent or to refuse treatment prior to the start of any procedure and/or treatment
• Continuity of care
• Explanation of medical costs.

For further information on the rights of hospital patients, refer to the Further Reading references that begin on page 667. Also, for a discussion of your responsibilities as a patient, refer to page 395 of "Choosing a Doctor."

Some Leading Hospitals and Clinics for Specialized Care

EYE AND EAR PROBLEMS

Bascom Palmer Eye Institute
University of Miami School of
Medicine
P.O. Box 520875 Biscayne Annex
Miami, Florida 33152

Case Western Reserve University
School of Medicine
Department of Surgery
Division of Ophthalmology
2119 Abington Road
Cleveland, Ohio 44106

Johns Hopkins University
School of Medicine
Wilmer Ophthalmological Institute
720 Rutland Avenue
Baltimore, Maryland 21205

Massachusetts Eye and Ear
Infirmary
243 Charles Street
Boston, Massachusetts 02114

University of California
School of Medicine
Jules Stein Eye Institute
Los Angeles, California 90024

University of Pennsylvania
School of Medicine
Scheie Eye Institute
51 North 39th Street
Philadelphia, Pennsylvania 19104

University of Texas Medical School
Department of Surgery
Division of Ophthalmology
7703 Floyd Curl Drive
San Antonio, Texas 78284

FERTILITY PROBLEMS

Boston Hospital for Women
221 Longwood Avenue
Boston, Massachusetts 02115

New York Fertility Research
Foundation
123 East 89th Street
New York, New York 10028

Tyler Clinic Research Foundation
921 Westwood Boulevard
East Los Angeles, California 90024

Yale-New Haven Hospital
Fertility Clinic
789 Howard Avenue
New Haven, Connecticut 06504

PAIN

City of Hope Medical Center
Pain Clinic
1500 East Duarte Road
Duarte, California 91010

Emanuel Hospital
Portland Pain
Rehabilitation Center
3001 North Gantenbein Avenue
Portland, Oregon 97227

Emory University Pain Clinic
1364 Clifton Road, N.E.
Atlanta, Georgia 30322

Johns Hopkins University School
of Medicine — Pain Clinic
725 North Wolfe
Baltimore, Maryland 21205

Massachusetts Rehabilitation
Hospital — Pain Unit
125 Nashua Street
Boston, Massachusetts 02114

Mayo Clinic-St. Mary's Hospital
of Rochester — Pain Clinic
Rochester, Minnesota 55901

Mount Sinai Medical Center
Pain Consultation Center
4300 Alton Road
Miami Beach, Florida 33140

Mount Zion Hospital and Medical
Center — Pain Center
1600 Divisadero Street
San Francisco, California 94115

Rush-Presbyterian-St. Luke's
Medical Center — Pain Center
1725 West Harrison Street
Chicago, Illinois 60612

The Pain and Health
Rehabilitation Center
615 South 10th Street
LaCrosse, Wisconsin 54601

UCLA School of Medicine
UCLA Pain Management Clinic
10833 Le Conte Avenue
Los Angeles, California 90024

University of Washington
School of Medicine — Pain Clinic
Seattle, Washington 98195

ASTHMA AND ALLERGIES

Duke University Medical Center
Division of Immunology,
Allergy, and Pulmonary Diseases
Box 3708
Durham, North Carolina 27710

Mayo Clinic and Foundation
Allergy Unit
200 First Street, S.W.
Rochester, Minnesota 55901

National Institute of Allergy
and Infectious Disease, NIH
Allergic Diseases Section
Room 11 N. 246 — Building 10
Bethesda, Maryland 20014

Tulane University School
of Medicine
Department of Clinical
Immunology
1700 Perdido Street
New Orleans, Louisiana 70112

University of Colorado
School of Medicine
Department of Clinical
Immunology
4200 East Ninth Street
Denver, Colorado 80220

University of Kansas Medical Center
Department of Allergy and
Immunology
39th and Rainbow Boulevard
Kansas City, Kansas 66103

University of Wisconsin
Medical School
Center for Health Sciences
Allergy Division
504 North Walnut Street
Madison, Wisconsin 53705

Washington University
Medical Center
Division of Immunology and
Connective Tissues Diseases
660 South Euclid Avenue
St. Louis, Missouri 63110

PSYCHIATRIC PROBLEMS

Columbia University College of
Physicians and Surgeons
Presbyterian Hospital
722 West 168th Street
New York, New York 10032

Langley Porter Institute
401 Parnassus Avenue
San Francisco, California 94143

Massachusetts Mental Health Center
74 Finwood Drive
Roxbury, Massachusetts 02119

PRENATAL SCREENING

Children's Hospital Medical Center
300 Longwood Avenue
Boston, Massachusetts 02115

Johns Hopkins Hospital
601 North Broadway Street
Baltimore, Maryland 21205

University Hospital
1959 N.E. Pacific Street
Seattle, Washington 98195

**University of California
Medical Center**
225 West Dickinson Street
San Diego, California 92103

**University of California
Medical School**
San Francisco, California 94143

UCLA Hospital
10833 Le Conte Avenue
Los Angeles, California 90024

Yale-New Haven Hospital
789 Howard Avenue
New Haven, Connecticut 06504

CARDIOVASCULAR PROBLEMS

**Baylor College of Medicine
Texas Medical Center**
1200 Moursund Avenue
Houston, Texas 77025

Duke University Medical Center
Box 3708
Durham, North Carolina 27710

Massachusetts General Hospital
32 Fruit Street
Boston, Massachusetts 02115

**New York University
Medical Center**
560 First Avenue
New York, New York 10016

Stanford University Hospital
300 Pasteur Drive
Stanford, California 94305

Texas Heart Institute
6621 Fannin Street
Houston, Texas 77025

**University of Michigan
Medical School**
1335 Catherine Street
Ann Arbor, Michigan 48104

**University of Virginia
School of Medicine**
Jefferson Park Avenue
Charlottesville, Virginia 22901

ARTHRITIS AND RHEUMATISM

**Hospital for Special Surgery
Rheumatology Department**
535 East 70th Street
New York, New York 10021

**Massachusetts General Hospital
Arthritis Unit**
32 Fruit Street
Boston, Massachusetts 02114

**Mayo Clinic
Rheumatology Research
Laboratory**
Rochester, Minnesota 55901

**UCLA Hospital
Division of Rheumatology**
10833 Le Conte Avenue
Los Angeles, California 90024

**University of Chicago
Pritzker School of Medicine**
950 East 59th Street
Chicago, Illinois 60637

**University of Colorado
Medical Center**
4200 East 9th Avenue
Denver, Colorado 80220

**University of Tennessee Memorial
Research Center and Hospital**
1924 Alcoa Highway
Knoxville, Tennessee 37920

CANCER

Colorado Regional Cancer Center
935 Colorado Boulevard, B127
Denver, Colorado 80220

**Comprehensive Cancer Center
of the State of Florida
University of Miami School of
Medicine**
P.O. Box 520875
Biscayne Annex
Miami, Florida 33152

**Fred Hutchinson
Cancer Research Center
University of Washington**
1124 Columbia Street
Seattle, Washington 98104

**Johns Hopkins Oncology Center
Johns Hopkins Hospital**
550 North Broadway
Baltimore, Maryland 21205

CANCER

**Georgetown University-
Howard University
Comprehensive Cancer Center:
Vincent T. Lombardi
Cancer Research Center
Georgetown University
Medical Center**
3800 Reservoir Road, N.W.
Washington, D.C. 20007
Howard University Cancer Center
2041 Georgia Avenue, N.W.
Washington, D.C. 20060

**Mayo Comprehensive
Cancer Center
Mayo Clinic and Foundation**
200 First Street, S.W.
Rochester, Minnesota 55901

**Ohio State University
Comprehensive Cancer Center**
1580 Cannon Drive
Columbus, Ohio 43210

**Sidney Farber
Comprehensive Cancer Center
Harvard University School
of Medicine**
44 Binney Street
Boston, Massachusetts 02115

**Sloan-Kettering Institute
for Cancer**
410 East 68th Street
New York, New York 10021

**University of Alabama
Comprehensive Cancer Center**
619 South 19th Street
Birmingham, Alabama 35233

**UCLA Comprehensive Cancer
Center**
924 Westwood Boulevard
Los Angeles, California 90024

**University of Chicago
Cancer Research Center**
905 East 59th Street
Chicago, Illinois 60637

**University of Texas—
M.D. Anderson
Hospital and Tumor Institute**
6723 Bertner Avenue
Houston, Texas 77030

**University of Wisconsin
Clinical Cancer Center**
1300 University Avenue
Madison, Wisconsin 53706

**Yale University
Comprehensive Cancer Center**
333 Cedar Street
New Haven, Connecticut 06510

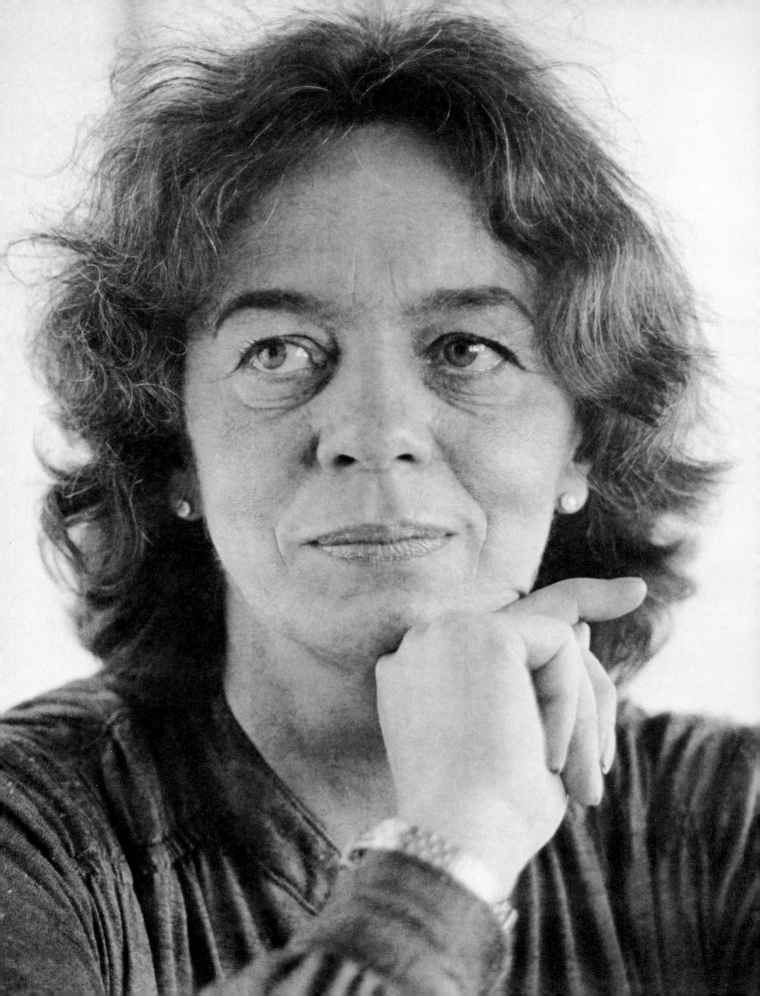

CHAPTER 19

CHOOSING A DOCTOR

SHARON N. ANDRUS, R.N.
PETER L. ANDRUS, M.D., F.A.C.P.

As adults, we have full responsibility for choosing the physicians who will assist in our health care. A friend may suggest a good doctor, or one physician may refer us to another or to a health service agency, but the ultimate choice is still our own.

Choice involves asking questions of ourselves. What do we expect from a doctor? What are the symptoms that bring us to a doctor? What do we want to understand about our treatment? Choice also involves asking questions of our doctors. To make an informed choice, we need to know about physicians' credentials and training, the hospitals they use, their fee schedules, their hours of availability, and their procedures for handling emergencies.

As a patient, you have specific rights—including the right to consent to treatment or to refuse treatment. By being aware of these rights and understanding your own body, you can help ensure a cooperative, effective relationship with your physician.

Choosing a Doctor

As a child, the medical assistance a woman receives is, of course, determined by others—notably, her parents. But with the passage of time, a woman must use her own judgment in choosing a doctor.

A wise woman will choose a doctor before a crisis arises. By doing so, she can best see to regular preventive needs, enable her doctor to acquire normal or base-line measurements (such as normal weight, blood pressure, and chest X ray), and maintain a healthy "health" status. A doctor who is well acquainted with a woman when she is in good health is obviously in a better position to make appropriate diagnoses and treatment decisions when an illness arises. More commonly, though, a woman seeks care—either for herself or others—after an illness has begun. But whenever medical assistance is sought, certain selection criteria are always involved. And of course, care should be taken that the qualities a woman looks for in her physician are the ones best suited to maintaining her health.

Ways to Choose a Doctor

There are a variety of ways to choose a doctor—with a variety of results. Here are four of the most common ones:

Referral by a friend or neighbor. If a friend's or neighbor's idea of a good physician is similar to your own, the results generally will be good. However, this process does not always consider the physician's actual qualifications.

Referral from another physician. This method is used when general practitioners need to refer their patients to a specialist, as well as when specialists refer their patients to general practitioners. Frequently, physician referrals are requested by women who are moving to other locales. Having a physician select a doctor for you should mean, at least, that the new doctor is respected by his peers. But you cannot be assured that your relationship with the new doctor will be a comfortable one, as physicians may not take individual personalities into account when making referrals.

Referral by the county medical society. Acquisition during an emergency room visit.

These methods all have been used to obtain medical assistance—often with successful results—but they are not without potential pitfalls.

This chapter will:
• Give you information that will aid you in selecting a physician who can meet your needs
• Give you the confidence and the knowledge you need to become a more active participant in your own medical care
• Help you formulate more clearly what your own expectations are in regard to medical care
• Tell you what most doctors expect of their patients.

The Doctor's Credentials

A doctor begins professional training in medical school after having earned a bachelor's degree. Depending on where your doctor studied, medical school consisted of either a three- or a four-year curriculum, and included both course work and practical experience with patients. During this time, student physicians usually decide what type of practice they are interested in. Then, following medical school, a doctor generally pursues specialty training, which is called a residency. Residency training may add three to seven years to a doctor's professional education, during which time the doctor gains practical experience in his or her chosen area.

But some doctors go directly into practice following medical school. Several states allow doctors to practice with no additional training, but most require at least one additional year, called an internship. Whatever the state requirements, doctors must acquire a license to practice by passing a medical examination and by making application to the state in which they intend to work.

One further indication of a physician's competence is specialty board certification. Most doctors who have completed a residency in a special area of medicine will take additional examinations in that area. The passage of these examinations is not necessary in order to practice medicine or to call oneself a specialist, but it does certify that the doctor has been evaluated by other specialists as being competent in this specific area. Board certification is available in over twenty specialty fields.

Despite the titles given to specialists (see page 394), absolute boundaries between them seldom exist and their duties often overlap. Moreover, many general surgeons, general internists, and family practitioners are well qualified to treat patients with disorders that might otherwise be treated by a specialist. And some specialists are more specialized than others; they may require referral from another physician rather than make appointments directly. The best way to learn about an individual specialist's style is to inquire.

Professional society affiliations are also part of a doctor's credentials. Thus, it's possible for your doctor to belong not only to the county, state, and national medical associations, but also to specialty societies on the local, state, and national level. Most county medical societies will supply on request the name of your doctor's medical school and year of graduation, as well as information about board certification and professional affiliations. You also may consult medical directories in researching your doctor's credentials. *The American College of Surgeons Yearbook, The Directory of Medical Specialties,* and *The American Medical Directory of the American Medical Association* are good reference books that are available in many libraries and hospitals.

It's also important that your prospective doctor have hospital privileges. A doctor obviously needs a hospital where he or she can admit patients who need special care. And since hospital medical staffs screen each doctor's qualifications before they grant admission privileges, hospital affiliation is another way of assuring that your doctor meets the standards of the local medical community.

Hospitals differ in their regulations about such matters as visiting hours, whether the delivery room is open to expectant fathers, and whether one may stay overnight with a hospitalized child. So if you know which hospital a doctor uses, you're in a better position to know whether this doctor also can meet your expectations in case hospitalization is necessary.

Keep in mind that a lengthy list of credentials is not always necessary in order to obtain good care from a physician, nor do such credentials guarantee good care. Situations occur in which a doctor has received excellent training, is obviously skilled, and yet is unable to communicate effectively with patients. On the other hand, there are physicians who have received a minimum of training but who possess innate skills at effectively evaluating, diagnosing, and treating patients. These individuals, aware of their own limitations, make referrals when appropriate.

There are no absolute rules concerning which credentials are necessary for a physician. Minimum qualifications, however, are graduation from an accredited medical school and state licensure. And, if the physician labels himself or herself as a specialist, there should be evidence of additional training and board certification. Generally, these diplomas and certificates are displayed on the walls of a doctor's office. But if you have any question concerning a doctor's education and training, ask the physician or office staff directly, or contact the county medical society for information.

Knowing What You Want

A woman must have a clear idea about what she expects and wants from her dealings with a physician. She should try to decide prior to her first visit what she would like the doctor to do for her, what questions she needs answered, and what areas of her health she feels she can and wants to control for herself. Otherwise, no matter how adept the physician is at treating her, she'll have no way of evaluating how successful her visit to the doctor has been.

Reasons to Go to a Doctor

PREVENTIVE NEEDS

- You wish to have annual checkups.
- You wish base-line measures such as weight, blood pressure, and chest X ray to be on permanent file with a doctor whom you have chosen.
- You wish to establish a good relationship with one primary care physician, even though you are well and may not need a doctor in the foreseeable future.

CURATIVE NEEDS

- You get an illness and diagnose it yourself, but your body does not get well at the rate you think it should. This worries you enough to go to a doctor for help.
- You get an illness, diagnose it yourself, but instead of getting better, you get worse. So you go to a doctor for help.
- You get an illness but are completely unable to diagnose what you have. You go to a doctor for help in diagnosis and treatment.
- You get an illness and know that you need the resources of a doctor or hospital to treat it: X ray, cultures, surgery, etc.
- You are in an accident or a medical crisis and must go to a doctor or hospital, or you're taken there by others.

The first step in establishing what you desire from your doctor is to decide who is to be in charge of your health. Is it yourself alone, the physician, or some combination of the two? There are some women who wish to place themselves totally in the doctor's hands where their health is concerned. At the other extreme are women who wish to remain completely in control themselves, who will consult a physician but not necessarily take his advice, and who feel, many times, that they are better able to handle their own health problems. The ideal approach for most women, however, is probably somewhere between the two styles.

A patient's attitude toward this issue of control may shift, depending on the nature of the problem. When a woman consults a physician for help in deciding which method of birth control to use, she may simply prefer that the physician give her all the facts and then allow her to make up her mind. The same woman, if she were experiencing a great deal of stress in her life, might consult her physician for help in dealing with her nervousness and headaches. Under these circumstances, she might want her physician to be supportive, reassuring, and more assertive—to prescribe a course of action.

Your Rights as a Patient

The responsible patient should be fully aware of her rights. A so-called "Patient's Bill of Rights" has been developed by Marvin Belsky, M.D. and Leonard Gross in their book *How to Choose and Use Your Doctor,* and is reprinted here in the hope that it will make you a better-informed and assertive consumer of personal health care services.

A Glossary of Common Medical Specialists

- An ALLERGIST diagnoses and non-surgically manages patients with allergic diseases.
- An ANESTHESIOLOGIST administers drugs that produce loss of consciousness, operates heart/lung machines, and monitors a patient's physiological responses during surgery.
- A CARDIOLOGIST non-surgically manages patients with heart disease.
- A CARDIOVASCULAR SURGEON performs surgery to correct heart and blood vessel malfunctions.
- A COLON AND RECTAL SURGEON performs surgery to correct conditions and diseases of the colon or rectum.
- A DERMATOLOGIST non-surgically treats diseases of the skin and scalp.
- An ENDOCRINOLOGIST non-surgically treats diseases related to glandular disease and hormonal imbalance.
- A FAMILY PRACTITIONER non-surgically treats both adults and children (ideally, within the context of the family unit) and does not focus on any one body system. Rather, this specialist treats general illnesses and assists in maintaining the patient's overall health.
- A GASTROENTEROLOGIST non-surgically treats diseases and disorders of the digestive system.
- A GASTRIC SURGEON performs surgery to correct malfunctions and diseases of the digestive system.
- A GENERAL INTERNIST non-surgically treats diseases and illnesses of adults without limitation to a specific body system.
- A GENERAL SURGEON performs surgery to correct malfunctions and diseases of the body that are not limited to a specific area or system.
- A GERONTOLOGIST non-surgically treats the elderly.
- A GYNECOLOGIST surgically and non-surgically treats female malfunctions and diseases, especially those of the reproductive system.
- A HEMATOLOGIST non-surgically treats diseases and disorders of the blood.
- A NEPHROLOGIST non-surgically treats diseases and malfunctions of the kidneys.
- A NEUROLOGIST non-surgically treats diseases and disorders of the brain and nervous system.
- A NEUROSURGEON performs surgery to correct disorders and malfunctions of the brain and nervous system.
- An OBSTETRICIAN manages pregnancy and assists with childbirth.
- An ONCOLOGIST non-surgically treats patients with tumors.
- An OPHTHALMOLOGIST surgically and non-surgically treats diseases and disorders of the eye.
- An ORTHOPEDIST surgically and non-surgically treats deformities, disorders, diseases, and traumas of the bones and joints.
- An OTORHINOLARYNGOLOGIST surgically and non-surgically treats disorders and diseases of the ears, nose, and throat.
- A PATHOLOGIST identifies disease through examination and analysis of body fluid and tissue.
- A PEDIATRICIAN non-surgically treats patients from birth through their teens.
- A PHYSICAL MEDICINE PHYSICIAN (PHYSIATRIST) non-surgically treats patients who are physically handicapped.
- A PLASTIC SURGEON performs surgery to repair or correct body disfigurement or irregularity.
- A PROCTOLOGIST diagnoses and non-surgically treats diseases and disorders of the colon and rectum.

A Patient's Responsibilities

It is vital to establish an ongoing relationship with your physician if you are to become a responsible and effective patient. Part of this relationship involves not contacting the doctor just for emergencies and problems, but also for regular physical examinations and other health maintenance procedures. By establishing a relationship with a doctor who sees you not only in times of illness and stress, but also in times of well-being, you ensure yourself of better care. This also provides your doctor with many baseline (normal) measurements on which to base future diagnostic and therapeutic decisions. The physician is then able to make comparisons between this healthy picture of you and the view that is presented in situations where medical attention is needed.

An ongoing relationship helps your physician to know you better. And the better you are known to your doctor, not only by body systems but also as a total person, the more likely it is that his or her recommendations will be appropriate for you.

Being a responsible patient also involves the type and quality of the information you supply to your physician. Most doctors will say that they wish patients would bring to their initial visit information concerning their past medical history (either from past medical records, immunization records, baby books, or memory) as well as the known results of laboratory tests and previous X rays that are pertinent to your evaluation. Physicians also would like patients to be able to tell them about medications that are presently being taken, known allergies, and their family and social history. And, of course, the patient should be prepared to discuss any present complaints, including the onset of the problem, its duration, and the types of discomfort experienced.

It's a good idea to write down ahead of time anything about yourself and your health status that you feel would be helpful, as well as questions you want to ask during your visit. In this way, you'll be sure that you and your doctor can talk about all of your concerns. And you might even want to take notes during your discussion with the physician so that information and instructions are not forgotten after your visit.

In addition, a responsible patient is an observant and accurate reporter about her body. As such, she will not only become a valuable resource to her doctor, but also an active participant in her own care.

Being a responsible patient also means being a considerate one. As such, you should be on time for your appointments and report appointment cancellations to the physician's office as much ahead of time as possible.

A Patient's Bill of Rights

- You have a right to be fully informed; you should learn from your doctor anything he finds out about you. This information should be given to you in a manner and with a vocabulary that you can understand, without jargon or lingo.
- You have a right to the doctor's time. He should be available and accessible to you. If for some reason he can't be, he should arrange for a suitable substitute.
- You have a right to the doctor's continuing professional competence.
- You have a right to be treated with compassion.
- You have a right to confidentiality.
- You have a right to know everything about a physician that is relevant to your treatment.
- You have a right to be educated.
- You have a right to question the doctor, to make suggestions, and to be critical when appropriate.
- If you change doctors, you have a right to have your records sent to a doctor of your choice.

Information to Take to Your Physician

ON AN INITIAL VISIT

- Your personal health record
- Your family health history
- A list of your occupational health hazards
- Samples of drugs you are taking
- A written list of drugs to which you are allergic
- A list of the names and addresses of doctors you have visited so that your medical records may be sent for
- Previous X rays pertinent to your examination
- A written list of questions that you intend to ask the doctor concerning your present condition

ON SUBSEQUENT VISITS

- An accurate and observant report on your body conditions since the last visit
- A written list of questions that you intend to ask the doctor
- Any new information on your family health history or occupational health hazards that will bring your records up to date

Your Health History: A Life-Span Record

General Information

Name:

Date of birth:

Blood type:

Allergies:

Major physical abnormalities:

Health Insurance Company:
Policy No.:
Medicare No.:
Medicaid No.:

Social Security No.:

Inoculations

Type	Date	Doctor or Clinic
DPT (Diphtheria, Whooping Cough— Pertussis, Tetanus)	#1 #2 #3 Boosters	
Polio	#1 #2 #3 Boosters	
Measles		
German Measles		
Smallpox		
Mumps		
TB Skin Test		
Other		

Childhood Diseases

Type	Date	Place	Treatment	Remarks
Chicken Pox				
German Measles (Rubella)				
Measles				
Mumps				
Whooping Cough				
Flu				
Colds				
Scarlet Fever (Scarlatina)				
Other				

Disease and Illnesses

Type	Date	Place	Treatment	Remarks

Surgery and Broken Bones

Reason	Dates	Physician Name and Address	Hospital Name and Address	Healing Record

Record all information about your health and illnesses in a notebook, using these forms as examples. Then take the record with you on your initial visit to a physician or hospital for ready reference. You may adapt the charts and records to your personal needs. For example, you might also wish to include a record of breast self-examinations, or a personal diary of each pregnancy.

Hospitalizations

Reason	Dates	Hospital Name and Address	Attending Physician Name and Address	Remarks

Drugs and Medications Taken

Drug Name	Dates Taken	Taken For	Prescribed By	My Reaction
	Began: Stopped:			

Blood Pressure Record

Date	Blood Pressure	Place	Remarks

Laboratory Procedures

Date	Lab Test	Reason	Results	Hospital or Clinic Name and Address

X Ray, Mammogram, Thermogram, and Other Radiation Record

Dates	Reason	Hospital or Clinic Name Address	Results

Your Health History: A Life-Span Record continued

Menstruation Record

Onset of menstruation:

Remarks on cycle length and regularity:

Menstrual complications:

Date   Description   Treatment   Remarks
of Complication

Menstruation record pertaining to pregnancy and nursing:

Menstruation record during menopause:

End of menstruation:

Birth Control Record

Method   Dates   Physician   or   Remarks
Organization
Consulted

Pregnancy Record

Date of first missed period:

Calculated date of conception:

Calculated date of birth:

Persons assisting with pregnancy:
Name   Address   Phone   Remarks

Hospital:
Name   Address   Phone

Hospital procedures or special permissions:

Personal Diary of Pregnancy. You may wish to keep a daily or weekly record of the progress of your pregnancy, describing your own experiences and the results of visits to your doctor, and including notes from classes in childbirth preparation, childbirth methods, and your own preparation for birth.

Family Health History

Parents:

Brothers and sisters:

Grandparents, aunts, and uncles:

Your children:

Family Health History. Use this form as a guide to record your family health history. Write down birth and death dates, the time when major disease occurred in each person's life, and the general health of each person you include. From a medical point of view, the important diseases that are passed down from generation to generation are: heart attacks, high blood pressure, strokes, allergies, diabetes mellitus, cancer, and mental disorders. In addition, there are important behavioral traits that we learn in a family setting, such as eating and drinking habits, reactions to stress in general, relaxation habits, personal hygiene, exercise, and self-care. Note these as well.

Over the years, more and more information will collect on the pages of your family health record, forming a valuable family history.

Be sure to mention your emotional reactions to the events you record, and your feelings about how your family history affects your health.

The Physical Examination

After you have selected and arranged an appointment with a physician, a physical examination will probably be the first part of your initial visit. Physicians utilize four basic techniques in conducting a physical examination: inspection, palpation, percussion, and auscultation.

Inspection is the visual observation of a patient, with or without the aid of various types of lighted instruments (for example, an otoscope to examine the ears, or an ophthalmoscope to examine the eyes).

Palpation takes place when a doctor touches various parts of a patient's body to acquire clinical evidence.

Percussion is a tapping maneuver, utilizing both the physician's hands. This tapping produces various sounds that can be differentiated, depending on whether the maneuver is carried out on skin that overlies air, fluid, or solid tissue.

Auscultation is the use of a stethoscope to amplify sounds within the body (for example, breathing, heartbeat, or digestive sounds).

A physician correlates and interprets the results of these techniques in conjunction with other data in drawing conclusions about bodily structure and function.

The initial step in a complete physical examination is to obtain *vital-sign* measurements, including measurements of height, weight, body temperature, pulse rate, respiratory rate, and blood pressure. These measurements generally are taken by a staff member and are then reviewed by the doctor before he or she begins the actual general examination.

Usually, a doctor will start by examining the head of a patient and then work down the body. (This order often is reversed in examining children; it may be less threatening to a child if the doctor begins at the feet and works toward the head.)

Examination of the head, ears, eyes, nose, and throat is typically the first part of the examination.

Head. A physician will examine the head by inspecting the shape of the skull, palpating or feeling the scalp for any lumps or bumps, and looking for any abnormalities of the skin.

Ears. Examination of the ears includes inspection of the appearance of the outer ears, and otoscopic examination (using an instrument called an otoscope) of the ear canals and eardrums for signs of abnormality or infection. A doctor may measure hearing ability in a more or less unscientific manner by asking a patient to listen for a whisper, the ticking of a watch, or the sound of a tuning fork.

Eyes. Examination of each eye includes inspection of the sclera (the whites of the eyes), the iris, and the pupil. The physician looks for equality of pupil size, regularity of contour, and specifically checks for the pupil's reactions to light and accommodation (adjustment of the eye for various distances). By shining a light in the pupil of each eye, the physician observes pupil contraction. By asking the patient to focus alternately on near and far objects, the physician checks for the ability of the eye to see objects at various distances. The physician also will guide the patient's gaze to either side and up and down to evaluate function of the muscles that control eye movement. Finally, the physician will use the ophthalmoscope to look through the pupil into the inner portion of the eyeball, inspecting the lens, the substance filling the interior of the eyeball behind the lens (viscous humor), blood vessels, and the retinal surface at the back of the eyeball for signs of disease.

Nose. The doctor examines the nose to see if there is an open airway on both sides, looking at the inner structures by means of ordinary lighting. If necessary, the physician will use a nasal speculum (an instrument used to enlarge the nostril opening) in order to see further into the nostril.

Mouth. Examination of the mouth includes looking at the teeth, gums, tongue, inner cheeks and lips, and the roof of the mouth. The physician will note the condition of the tonsils and the back of the throat, which can be seen with ordinary lighting. Asking the patient to say "ahhh" helps to check the function of the nerves and muscles that raise the roof of the mouth. A tongue depressor is used to check the gag reflex and to keep the tongue out of the physician's line of sight.

Neck. The neck is examined by having the patient demonstrate a variety of movements. Then the physician will check that the trachea (windpipe) is aligned properly down the center of the neck. Palpation is the technique used to examine the lymph nodes in the neck, as well as the thyroid gland, located at the base of the neck just above the upper rib cage and breastbone. The carotid arteries are examined by means of palpation and auscultation.

Chest and lungs. The physician then will examine the chest and lungs, looking for asymmetry and equality of chest movements when breathing. Palpation is used to check respiratory movements; percussion provides differing sounds in response to tapping over various portions of the chest that overlie air, solid tissue, or fluid. Percussion generally is done over both the posterior (back) and anterior (front) of the chest. The final maneuver in evaluating the chest and lungs consists of auscultation over all major segments of the lung fields.

Breasts. Breast examination is an important device for early detection of breast cancer in women. The physician observes the breasts while the patient is both sitting and lying, with hands held at the waist or over her head. In this way, the physician can check for any abnormalities in breast contour that might suggest an underlying tumor. The physician then palpates each breast, moving in a circular fashion and working from the outer portion of the breast toward the nipple. This is done with the doctor's fingers held together, compressing tissue between the fingers and the rib cage. The physician also compresses the nipple to see whether fluid can be expressed, and palpates for lymph nodes in each armpit.

Heart and cardiovascular system. Examination of the heart and cardiovascular system includes measurement of blood pressure. In some cases of particular concern about a patient's blood pressure, measurements may be taken from each arm and leg, with the patient in various positions. Usually, though, the pressure is measured only once, using either the left arm (closest to the heart) or the right arm while the patient is seated. The physician probably will check various pulses, including those in the neck, wrist, groin, and feet to determine the strength and quality of the pulse beat at each location.

Examination of the heart proper actually includes inspection as well as palpation, percussion, and auscultation. The physician looks for the normal small movements on the anterior chest wall that are associated with the heartbeat. Perception of these movements depends on the size of the patient's breasts and the patient's weight. The physician also will use the flat of the hand to feel the heartbeat and to palpate over the anterior chest for a vibratory sensation; this sensation is called a *thrill* and is sometimes present with heart murmurs. By percussing over the heart, the physician tries to get an estimate of heart size. This may be supplemented by chest X rays when indicated. The final maneuver of heart examination includes auscultation, which is carried out by placing the head of the stethoscope at different positions on the chest wall and listening while the patient assumes various positions (sitting, leaning forward, sitting straight up, lying on her back, or lying on her left side). The extent of the use of the stethoscope depends on the initial observations.

Abdomen. The physician then examines the abdomen, inspecting its contours for surgical scars or abnormalities. The physician palpates the abdomen, gently at first, and then more firmly once the abdominal wall is relaxed. This maneuver is carried out in all four quadrants of the abdomen in order to check for any abnormally large organs or unusual masses. Auscultation of the abdomen also is carried out in the four quadrants by listening with a stethoscope for the normal sounds of intestinal action and for sounds of blood flow in the liver, kidneys, and the abdominal aorta. In addition, percussion of the abdomen may be performed in cases where a specific abdominal abnormality is suspected.

Extremities. Evaluation of the four extremities usually consists of a general survey of the patient's ability to move arms and legs through the full range of motion expected at each joint, checking for general symmetry and the quality of muscle bulk on both sides of the body. Further evaluation may be undertaken in cases where the patient has a specific complaint.

Skin and nails. The skin and nails are evaluated either as a separate maneuver before or after other portions of the examination, or as part of the physician's examination of different body parts.

Lymphatic system. Evaluation of the lymphatic system generally is carried out as the physician progresses through the examination of different regions of the body, since the lymphatic system extends throughout the body. The physician will check for any abnormalities in the size and consistency of lymph nodes in the neck, armpits, and groin.

A complete neurologic examination generally is not performed as part of the usual physical examination. However, a neurologic screening evaluation often is part of a routine physical examination and includes evaluation of the twelve cranial nerves (the nerves to the head and neck); a rough evaluation of motor muscle and sensory nerve status; an evaluation of the reflexes at the elbows, wrists, knees, and ankles; and a general evaluation of the patient's gait and mental status.

A pelvic examination also is included in a general physical examination for a woman in order to evaluate the female genitourinary system. The pelvic examination usually is performed with the patient lying on her back on the examining table with her feet in stirrups on either side of the foot of the table, and her knees spread apart. The examination has four steps. The first is visual inspection of the external genital organs and anal area. The physician notes hair distribution, size and symmetry of the labia (lips of the vagina), and size and position of the clitoris and urinary urethra (opening), as well as the vaginal introitus (entrance) and anus (rectum).

The second portion of the examination involves placing a metal or plastic speculum into the vagina. This device allows the physician to see the vaginal walls and the cervix of the uterus. At this point in the examination, a Pap smear and, optionally, a culture for gonorrhea will be taken. Following completion of the Pap smear, the speculum is slowly withdrawn from the vagina, allowing the physician to inspect other parts of the vaginal walls as it is removed.

The third portion of the pelvic examination consists of a bimanual (two-handed) palpation of the pelvic contents. First, two fingers of one of the physician's gloved hands are inserted into the vagina. By exerting general pressure with these fingers against the other hand, which is placed on the patient's abdomen, the size, shape, and consistency of the uterus, ovaries, and fallopian tubes can be evaluated.

The fourth portion of the pelvic examination is a variation of this bimanual technique. The index finger of the examiner's hand is inserted into the vagina and the middle finger into the anus, and manual palpation between these fingers and the hand on the anterior abdominal wall is carried out. This portion of the examination allows a better evaluation of the back portion of the cervix.

In some instances, additional examination procedures or maneuvers may be carried out when warranted by a specific situation. Likewise, a briefer physical examination, omitting some of what has been described, may be justifiably performed in the case of a patient who is frequently examined for specific reasons and is thus well known to her physician. Since it is difficult to specify what a physical examination would consist of under all possible circumstances, the preceding description should be taken as a guideline on which to base your expectations. If a portion of an examination that is important to you has been left out by your physician, feel free to call this fact to his or her attention. Your doctor should either explain the reason for the omission, or complete those portions you feel to be important.

Common Medical Tests

Here are brief descriptions of some of the tests your physician might perform as part of a general medical evaluation.

Complete blood count (CBC). This is a blood test commonly used for diagnostic purposes. It helps the physician to diagnose blood loss, anemia, viral infections, dehydration, bacterial infections, bleeding tendency, and allergic responses. The complete group of tests under this heading includes a red-cell count; white-cell count; hemoglobin, hematocrit, and platelet count; and differential blood count. Usually, the CBC is done by drawing blood from a vein in the patient's arm, but it also can be done by taking blood from a "finger stick" (a small puncture made in a patient's finger). Both methods are relatively painless.

THE PELVIC EXAMINATION

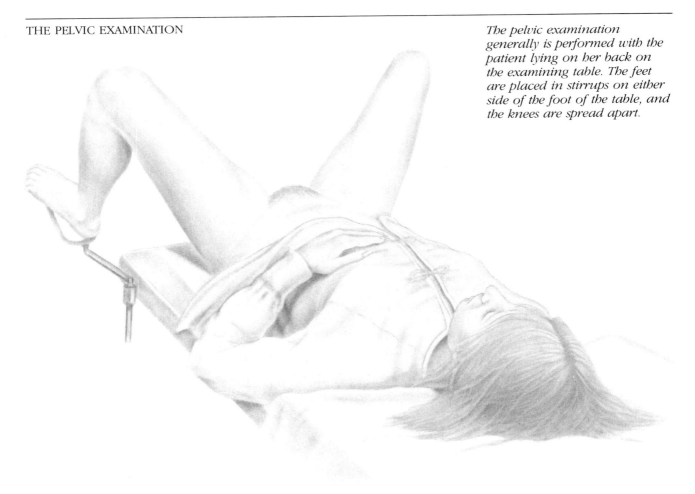

The pelvic examination generally is performed with the patient lying on her back on the examining table. The feet are placed in stirrups on either side of the foot of the table, and the knees are spread apart.

THE FIRST STEP OF A PELVIC EXAMINATION

The physician notes hair distribution, the size and symmetry of the labia (lips of the vagina), and the size and position of the clitoris and urinary opening, as well as the vaginal opening and the anus.

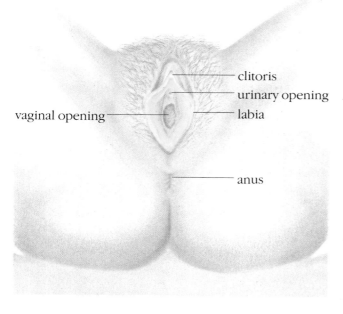

clitoris
urinary opening
vaginal opening
labia
anus

THE SECOND STEP OF A PELVIC EXAMINATION

A metal or plastic speculum is inserted into the vaginal opening, allowing a view of the vaginal walls and the cervix, or opening into the uterus.

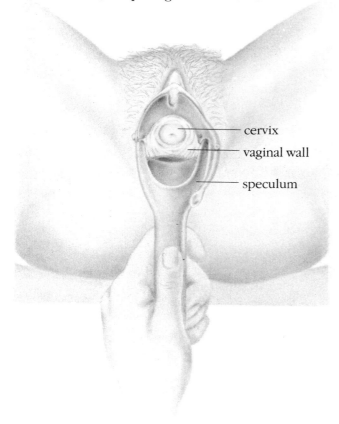

cervix
vaginal wall
speculum

Sometimes, only a few parts of the complete blood count are done when the doctor has a specific diagnosis in mind and is looking for laboratory confirmation. For instance, only a hemoglobin and hematocrit may be done to confirm blood loss or anemia, and only a white and differential blood count may be done to confirm the presence of both viral and bacterial infections. The CBC is probably the most common screening or base-line laboratory test performed as part of a routine general medical examination.

Urinalysis (UA). This is a group of tests performed on a patient's urine. Although no single test provides conclusive proof of a specific disorder or disease, tests taken in combination with each other as well as with the physical examination and the patient's history, usually give the doctor a good indication of what is wrong. This is especially true with urinalysis. Urinalysis can help the physician diagnose kidney disease; kidney stones; bladder obstruction; jaundice; bleeding from the kidney, ureter, bladder, or urethra; dehydration; diabetes; or infection within the genitourinary tract.

The specific studies that make up a complete urinalysis are: urine color; specific gravity; pH; protein content; sugar content; presence or absence of ketones, bilirubin, and blood; red blood-cell count; white blood-cell count; and the presence or absence of bacteria. Frequently, the patient may be asked to bring a urine specimen with her to the doctor's office; any clean bottle may be used. The specimen often may be produced in the doctor's restroom. If you are menstruating, be sure to tell the doctor, since there may be red blood cells in your urine that might otherwise be interpreted as abnormal. If you need to urinate at the doctor's office anyway, you might check beforehand to see whether a urine specimen will be expected of you later.

Chest X ray. This common X-ray procedure may be done by your physician for screening or diagnostic purposes. As a screening technique, the chest X ray can be used to look for lung or heart disease, including tuberculosis, emphysema, or heart enlargement. As a diagnostic test, it can be an invaluable tool in the diagnosis of lung tumors, pneumonia, asthma, bronchitis, congestive heart failure, and congenital anomalies, as well as many other conditions. The chest X ray is painless and can be done in the doctor's office. The patient usually is asked to disrobe to the waist and to put on a gown for the X-ray procedure.

Electrocardiogram (ECG or EKG). Also called heart tracing, this test is usually done on adults over 35 as a screening procedure. But it also is done as a diagnostic procedure on patients of all ages who now have or are suspected of having a heart disorder. Again, although the ECG is not conclusive in and of itself, it is helpful in diagnosing heart disease. It shows the amplitude and direction of electrical current generated by the heart, thus providing graphic information related to heart function.

THE THIRD STEP OF A PELVIC EXAMINATION

Two fingers of the physician's hand are inserted into the vagina. By feeling and exerting pressure with these fingers against the other hand, which is pressing on the outside of the abdominal wall, the physician evaluates the size, shape, and consistency of the uterus, ovaries, and fallopian tubes.

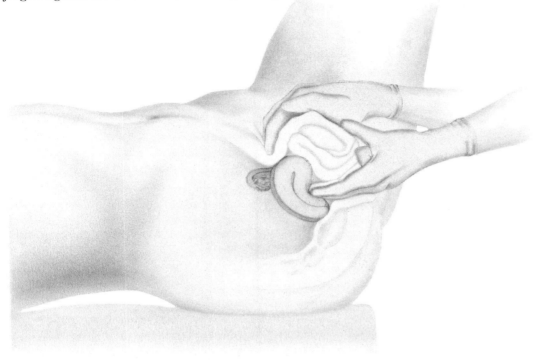

THE FOURTH STEP OF A PELVIC EXAMINATION

The index finger of the examiner's hand is inserted into the vagina, and the middle finger into the anus. The examiner feels the organs and tissues between these fingers and the hand pressing on the abdominal wall, allowing an evaluation of the back portion of the cervix, or the lower end of the uterus.

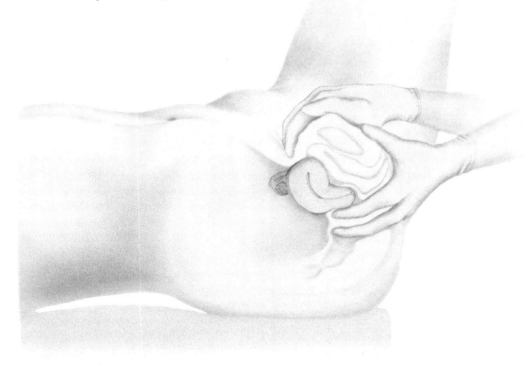

The ECG is painless. It is done by connecting electrodes (metal discs) to the patient's wrists, ankles, and chest by means of rubber straps or suction cups. To make a good electrical contact between the electrode and the skin, electrode paste (an ointment) is applied. Patients usually recline for the test, although an "exercise ECG" or "stress test" also may be done with the heart being monitored during and after moderately vigorous exercise, such as step-climbing, walking on a treadmill, or bicycle pedaling.

Papanicolaou (Pap) smear. This test is very helpful in the early detection of cervical cancer. Most doctors recommend that a Pap smear be performed every year from the onset of sexual activity. Specifically, the test is a microscopic examination of cells that have been collected by scraping the cervix with a wooden stick. The test is painless and is performed as part of a pelvic examination. A doctor can do the Pap smear either before or after your menstrual period, but not during it; so don't schedule an appointment for the same time as your expected menstrual period. Usually the doctor also will want to know the date of onset of your last period.

Skin test for tuberculosis (PPD or Tine Test). This test is used to screen for tuberculosis, and is relatively painless, inexpensive, and requires no special preparation. It is commonly administered by injecting a purified protein derivative just beneath the skin on the forearm. Two days later, the test is "read"—that is, the arm is observed. If the area is not swollen, the test is negative, indicating that the patient is assumed not to have been exposed to the tuberculosis bacterium. Children frequently will be given this test during a visit to the doctor, after which the mother reads the test two days later and reports the results. Usually, the patient can read her own or her children's test, so an extra trip to the doctor is unnecessary as long as the result is reported. The rate of administration of PPD and Tine Tests varies depending on whether or not the locale or socioeconomic group in question is one that is known to have a high incidence of TB. Many school systems have an ongoing TB screening program.

Venereal disease screening. Two types of venereal disease, syphilis and gonorrhea, are commonly diagnosed by specific tests. Since syphilis is the more serious of the two, screening tests for the disease are routinely done upon hospital admission, as well as when a marriage license is applied for. A blood specimen is taken from the arm, and the test is almost painless. If the results are positive, the patient may be asked to reveal all sexual partners to the health department so that they may be notified and treated; this is usually done in as confidential a manner as possible.

For gonorrhea, a different procedure is used. The usual testing method involves collecting vaginal secretions with a swab and placing them on a slide for microscopic examination. This test also is painless. A gonorrhea (GC) culture is not always a routine screening procedure. Moreover, following up on sexual contacts is not as aggressively pursued as in the case of syphilis, although most doctors will recommend that the patient advise her sexual partners so that they also can be treated. This also safeguards the woman against reinfection. No special arrangements are needed for a GC culture, although the patient will have to disrobe and assume the same position as for a pelvic examination in order for the secretions to be collected. If you suspect you may have been exposed to gonorrhea, you should specifically request that this test be done.

There are many more tests that could be discussed here, but those listed are the ones most likely to be encountered in the course of normal, outpatient care. Again, most laboratory and radiographic tests alone do not supply the doctor with a diagnosis. The results must be considered along with other information—such as past medical history, the patient's symptoms, and physical examination—before the doctor can arrive at a diagnosis or evaluation. Physicians vary in their use of such tests, and there are no strict definitions as to what is appropriate. A doctor who relies too heavily on laboratory and radiographic studies should be suspected just as much as one who uses them very infrequently.

Since many tests are relatively expensive, physicians should carefully consider the patient's economic situation when ordering them. However, the individual patient also should remind her physician of the cost factor so that only necessary tests are performed and the expense does not become an economic burden for her.

Evaluating Your Medical Care

Medical care is more than simple diagnosis and treatment. There are many subtle environmental, financial, and interpersonal issues that also are part of the doctor-patient relationship. Many of these considerations can be evaluated before the initial visit by asking the appropriate questions of the doctor's appointment secretary or receptionist or by talking directly with the doctor, either over the telephone or in person. Shopping for a doctor—a popular term for this technique—assists the patient in examining the doctor's style of practice before an actual commitment is made via a formal appointment.

During and after the first appointment, many more aspects of the physician's practice can be noted.
• Is the doctor's office clean and attractive?
• Does the waiting area increase or decrease your initial apprehension?
• Is the doctor's office staff easy to deal with, and are they helpful in relaying messages to the doctor?

- Does the staff appear to care about you?
- Is the physician available after regular office hours?
- Does the physician return your calls?
- Does the physician have associates? If so, who will respond to calls and emergencies at times other than regular office hours—the physician or an associate?
- When one of your doctor's associates talks with you or sees you after hours, is this information relayed back to your own physician?
- Do you feel that your doctor spends enough time with you during a visit?
- Is the time sufficient for all of your questions to be answered?
- Do you feel rushed?

The financial aspect of your doctor's practice is another important consideration.

- Do you feel the doctor's fees are reasonable?
- Do you have to remit for services at the time of your visit?
- How often are you billed, and how soon is payment expected?
- Can your bill be paid in installments?
- What insurance programs are accepted?
- Once a diagnosis is made, does your doctor give you an estimate of the cost of treatment?
- Can you get an approximate cost for a complete physical examination, laboratory studies, immunizations, etc. prior to your initial visit?

Finally, the physician's style should be considered—especially in relation to your feelings about who is responsible for your own health.

- Does your doctor agree with you about who is responsible for your health care?
- Is he or she willing to share the responsibility for your care with you?
- How do you think your doctor would react if you disagreed with aspects of his or her evaluation, or if you expressed an inability to totally comply with any proposed treatment regimen?
- Do you feel your doctor treats you with respect?
- Are you comfortable with your physician's interpersonal style?
- Can you talk easily and frankly with your doctor?
- Does your doctor seem non-judgmental and accepting of what you tell him or her?
- Do you feel your doctor knows his or her limitations and would refer you to another physician for a second opinion?

As a woman seeking medical attention, you are entitled to answers to these questions, and you should expect the majority of the answers to be favorable. If they're not, it's time to reflect on what is amiss and to evaluate just how important these aspects of the physician's style are to you. Often, just a few words to the doctor or the staff can resolve the difficulty.

There are two other major points relevant to the evaluation of your medical care. The first is that you should not be afraid to get a second opinion. It will allay many qualms you might have concerning the appropriateness of the treatment, and most doctors prefer that their patients obtain another opinion if they have any misgivings. For the doctor, patient confidence in the prescribed treatment reduces the likelihood of a patient-physician misunderstanding developing, and thus prevents patient dissatisfaction and even a potential malpractice suit. A good relationship also enhances the effectiveness of the treatment.

The other point involves the issue of patient consent. Is it permissible to say "no" to your physician? Many women assume that it's not, especially if a doctor asks for treatment consent in a manner that makes it seem difficult to refuse. A woman should be aware that, ultimately, she is in control. She can accept or reject her doctor's advice at any time during the course of medical treatment, and she should keep this fact in mind once treatment has begun.

Many patients feel that once initial consent has been given, there is no turning back. This is simply not the case. Every time the treatment regimen is changed, a woman should be consulted for her consent. And with each change in treatment, the decision to continue should be a joint one between the physician and the patient, with the patient making the final choice.

Dr. Donald Hayes, in his book *Between Doctor and Patient,* has raised many of the same concerns. "It has been my experience that many patients are anxious to please their physician. Thus, presented with a question of whether they will undergo a particular treatment, test, or procedure, these patients will make the choice their physician wants them to make. These patients, then, do not truly have a chance to decide."

Regarding the patient's involvement in making specific health-care decisions, Dr. Hayes says: "The patient should be consulted at each of these decision-making points. Unfortunately, this is not always the case.

More often, however, the patient is ostensibly consulted, but with certain reservations or qualifications. These are (1) She may not be given all the information needed to make an intelligent decision. (2) She may be swept along on a tide of professional furor that simply assumes she will be agreeable. (3) She may allow things to be done to her or for her simply to avoid disrupting 'the system.'"

Perhaps the best way to avoid such problems is to realize that alternatives always exist and that you needn't be intimidated by your physician. You should realize, too, that as the purchaser of your physician's services, you have the right to expect and receive medical care that includes your physician's willingness to discuss, thoroughly and openly, your health status and all intended medical procedures.

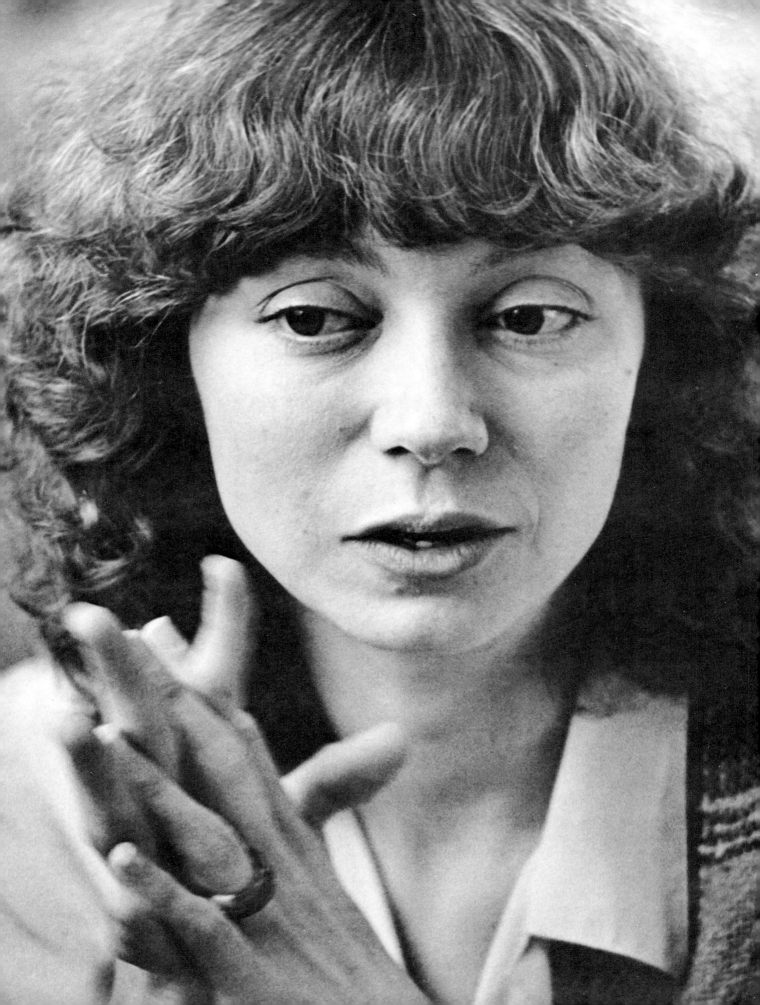

CHAPTER 20

DEPRESSION

MYRNA M. WEISSMAN, Ph.D.

Depression as a normal, transitory mood is something we've all experienced. It is part of being human and is a signal that something is not quite right in our lives. By contrast, a deeper, longer-lasting depression may be a clinical condition that requires counseling and treatment. This clinical syndrome of depression is of special concern to women: it is the mental complaint most often reported by women to their physicians. This kind of depression is consistently found to be more common in women than in men, and is not confined to any one age group. Understanding the syndrome of depression and its common symptoms is the first step in recognizing and treating this important condition.

Depression

Sadness and disappointment are normal life experiences that no one escapes. By contrast, the syndrome of depression is a clinical condition that seriously impairs one's life, family, and friendships, and often requires treatment.

Depression, or melancholia as it was originally termed, has been recognized as a condition for over 2,000 years. Detailed clinical accounts can be found throughout recorded history and in many different cultures. In modern times, the clinical syndrome of depression is of special importance to women. Depression is consistently found to be more common in women than in men. It is the mental complaint most often reported by women in physicians' offices and in outpatient psychiatric clinics, as well as by women who may not be receiving any medical or psychiatric treatment. While the incidence of depression may be increasing, it is no longer confined to the middle-aged and the elderly, and it seldom leads to hospitalization. Today, the typical depressed patient is apt to be a young woman in her most productive years, often married and rearing children. The disorder can have a serious impact on her capacity to enjoy life.

What Is Depression?

The term depression has multiple meanings and covers a range of moods and behaviors, from the disappointments and sadness of normal life to the suicidal acts of the severe melancholic. There are at least three meanings to the word—a mood, a symptom, and a syndrome. Depression as a normal mood is a universal phenomenon that no one escapes. It is part of being human, and it alerts us that something is not quite right in our life. These transient moods are normal. They pass quickly and nudge us to reappraise aspects of our life that are not going well. To the extent that they lead to personal reassessment, these mood states are constructive. They do not impair functioning and do not require treatment.

Depression as a symptom, or an abnormal mood, also is common, although there is a fine line between what is normal and what is pathological. Sadness that is unduly persistent, pervasive, or inappropriate to one's life circumstances generally is considered pathological. The symptom of sadness or depression, again, is a common one experienced by most psychiatric patients, including many for whom the depression may be secondary to another illness, such as alcoholism or schizophrenia. Depressive symptoms also can be experienced by persons who are medically but not psychiatrically ill.

Beyond the symptom, a more specific and limited psychiatric meaning to depression is that of the syndrome. A syndrome refers to a group of symptoms that occur together, even though they may have different causes. These symptoms occur in the absence of other conditions that might explain the presence of the symptoms. This is the clinical depression that will be described here.

The Syndrome of Depression

The cluster of symptoms that make up the depressive syndrome include, but are not limited to: dysphoric mood; loss of energy; appetite and sleep difficulties; loss of interest; feelings of worthlessness, helplessness, and guilt; agitation or retardation; difficulty in thinking; bodily complaints; and thoughts of death.

Dysphoric mood is described as feeling sad, blue, unhappy, gloomy, or down in the dumps. Crying often occurs, although there are some depressives who say they are "beyond tears." The depressed person not only experiences these inner feelings of unhappiness, but will appear sad as well.

Loss of energy (anergia) may be expressed as a feeling of fatigue or heaviness, of being "run down," or an inability to get out of bed or to get through the day. The depressed person may describe herself as overworked, vitamin-deficient, and less able to carry on with the usual daily activities because of these feelings of fatigue.

Appetite disturbances include a loss of interest in food resulting in weight loss, which at times may be considerable. Alternately, although there is no enjoyment of food, there may be increased appetite and weight gain. Instances of appetite increase are more likely to occur at night as a compensation for loneliness and unhappiness.

Sleep disturbances are quite common and include difficulty getting to sleep at night, disturbed and restless sleep with frequent awakening and troubled dreams, or waking early in the morning and being unable to get back to sleep. The early morning wakening is often accompanied by intense worrying and fear, and a review of life failures and imagined—and often unrealistic—unfulfilled obligations.

Loss of interest and pleasure in activities and friendships that used to bring pleasure also is reported. Neglect of personal grooming and work can accompany this loss of interest. There is a loss of zest for life and a loss in interest in sex. For women, the loss of sexual interest does not necessarily mean reduced frequency of intercourse. But the woman who continues sexual relations out of feelings of obligation, rather than out of interest and pleasure, usually develops considerable resentment toward her partner.

Feeling worthless, helpless, and guilty. Additional disturbances include feelings described as helplessness, hopelessness, worthlessness, and incompetence, ranging from a vague sense of feeling worthless, as if the person had never accomplished anything, to intense feelings of failure. Guilt over past failures may become paramount and entirely out of proportion to what is appropriate. For example, the depressed woman may become guilty over premarital sex that occurred 20 years ago, or may label herself a bad mother because she missed some P.T.A. meetings.

These feelings of helplessness and worthlessness may not be a reflection of actual performance. The woman may be an extremely competent housekeeper, a loving mother and wife, an accomplished gardener, and a success professionally, but still may feel that she doesn't live up to some imagined or unrealistic expectation of herself. She may anticipate misfortune and gloom, early death, a serious illness, or financial disaster. Pessimism about the future is characteristic and is often unrelated to the actual life situation.

Feeling retarded or agitated. Many depressives show psychomotor retardation—a slowing in the speed of thoughts, speech, and movement, and a general lethargy. In rare cases, this may extend to virtual immobility and absence of speech.

The opposite state, overactivity or agitation, may also occur. This is experienced as feeling "jittery," being unable to sit still or to relax, and being "high-strung" or tense.

Decreased ability to concentrate. A "blank mind" or poor memory, difficulties in concentration, and "slowed down" thoughts are other symptoms. They can lead to difficulty in making even simple decisions, such as what to wear or what to have for dinner, as well as difficulty in carrying on a conversation or completing a work project that requires concentration.

Thoughts of death or suicide may occur, ranging from the feeling that life is not worth living, to wishing one were dead, to thoughts of taking one's life, to unsuccessful or successful attempts at suicide. Suicide has been called the mortality of depression.

Bodily complaints. There may be vague bodily complaints—headaches, backaches, or stomach pain—in the absence of any physical abnormalities.

Not all depressed persons show all of the above symptoms. However, a person is considered to be clinically depressed and to require treatment if she has a depressive mood, sleep and appetite disturbances, at least one or two of the other symptoms listed, persistence of symptoms for at least two weeks, and symptoms pervasive enough to impair her usual daily activities at home or at work.

Periods of "Highs"—Mania

A small number of persons who experience depressive disorders also have periods of "highs" or elation during which they feel very good—in fact, "too good." During these "highs," they report feeling more active than usual, more talkative, restless, or distractable, and irritable. Their thoughts race, they feel less need to sleep, and they dream up grand and inappropriate schemes. They may go on shopping or travel sprees, become sexually indiscreet, or engage in activities without realizing possible painful consequences for themselves or others.

Bipolar Disorder

Persons who experience both the "lows" of depression and the "highs" of mania are said to be suffering from bipolar disorder. Fortunately, the bipolar disorder is not common, as it has a devastating impact on social and family life, and can involve the person in destructive situations. Moreover, the suicide rate among persons with bipolar disorder is higher than that for those with other types of depression.

How Common Is Depression?

There is little doubt that depression is a common disorder. It is the most common psychiatric disorder in outpatient clinics, physicians' offices, and among the general public. Anywhere from 10 to 30 percent of adults experience depression at some point in their lives, and the risk for women is even higher.

Hospital admissions reflect rates for the most severely ill depressive. In the United States, the most recent figures for the annual rate of first admissions to a psychiatric hospital for the treatment of depressive disorders is about 11 per 100,000 persons in the adult population.

Outpatient figures reflect the rates for the mild-to-moderately-ill depressive. A recent report from the National Institute of Mental Health notes that well over 200,000 persons annually receive outpatient treatment for depression in the United States. This figure does not include the depressed outpatients who attend public mental health centers.

Untreated depression is considerably more common. It is believed that most individuals with depressive illness never see a physician. Only an estimated 20 to 30 percent of depressed persons receive any treatment from any professional for depression.

In a recent survey of an urban community in the northeast United States, it was found that on the day of the interview, about 3 or 4 out of every 100 persons interviewed were in the midst of a depressive syndrome, and that only about one-third had received any treatment for their depression.

Causes of Depression

The causes of clinical depression are certainly complex and not yet fully understood. Thus far, theories and research have involved genetic predisposition, neuropharmacologic abnormalities, vulnerability to stress based on personality or early learning experiences, or an excess of stressful life events. Depression in any single person probably results from a convergence of causes.

Parents, siblings, and children of depressed persons have a higher chance of becoming depressed than persons in the general population. About two-thirds of identical twins are concordant for depression (i.e., both become depressed), and this concordance rate for depression is higher than is found in fraternal twins. This evidence suggests a genetic factor in depression, but the mode of inheritance, if any, is not known.

There have been many studies examining a host of other biological factors that may cause depression. Currently, evidence suggests that depression may result from a change in the chemistry of the nerve cells at central nervous system transmission sites in the brain.

It is a common observation that a variety of stressful life events precede depression, as well as many other psychiatric and physical disorders. The evidence for an association of life stress and depression has been reasonably well established in several studies. Events such as separations from loved ones and other losses, as well as interpersonal difficulties with loved ones, may cause depression. However, some depressions occur in the absence of any obvious life stress. And most persons who experience separations and losses do not become clinically depressed.

Personality characteristics of depression-prone persons include an inability to overtly express anger, low self-esteem, dependency on others, obsessionality, and excessive guilt. While many depressed persons may have these personality attributes, it is unclear if they are unique to persons who become depressed, or if they are to some degree a consequence of being depressed.

Who Is Vulnerable?

No one is immune to depression. Everyone is vulnerable. Depression affects people from all walks of life, all races, religions, ages, and occupational groups. It is found in all climates and in all parts of the world.

Although depression can affect anyone, with few exceptions, it is considerably more common in women than in men. The increased vulnerability of women to depression has been noted in writings that date back more than 200 years, and in almost every country. The period of greatest risk for depression in women coincides with the reproductive years, ages 25 to 44.

Why Are Women More Vulnerable?

There is considerable debate as to why women are more vulnerable to depression than men. While the reasons have not been fully decided (and certainly no one reason will be the exclusive answer), there are some leads. These leads include observations about factors in a woman's biology, psychology, and social situation that make her more vulnerable.

Biological explanations. Among the biological explanations for women's vulnerability are genetic explanations that depression could be a dominant X-linked gene that would affect women twice as often as men, since women have two X chromosomes. Researchers also theorize that it could be the consequence of the differing hormones of the two sexes, which are genetically transmitted. As yet, however, there is no reasonable scientific evidence to suggest that sex-linked genes can explain the excess of depression among women. The hormonal theory is a suggestive but by no means conclusive explanation for some of the preponderance of depression among women.

Psychological explanations. The psychological explanations for women's vulnerability to depression have been related to childhood training in which women are encouraged to appear and to behave as if they are helpless. The traditional feminine ideal has been described as a form of "learned helplessness." Such training, in fact, can lead to a woman actually believing that she is helpless so that, as she matures and is faced with the usual stresses of life such as loss, moves, and disappointments, she may be less able to cope and may truly be helpless. The classic notion of "femininity" may be a form of helplessness that is not adaptive to the pace of life in the 1980s.

Social explanations. The social explanations for women's increased rates of depression have to do with long-standing social and economic disadvantages, including discrimination of women in work, finances, and other areas. These real discriminations can make it difficult for a woman to achieve mastery of her own actions or to be in charge of her own destiny. In fact, socially, women more often than men may be legally and economically helpless and dependent on others, a situation that could contribute to feelings of helplessness, pessimism, and possibly clinical depression. The economic dependency becomes more serious if there is a divorce or early death of the husband, two situations that are occurring with increasing frequency. The marked increase in marital breakup has been well documented, and its impact on emotional well-being is appreciated by most women.

Perhaps less appreciated, however, is the increasing gap in life expectancy between men and women. Today, women live 4 to 7 years longer than men. And most women are younger than the men they marry. Therefore, the majority of women who marry, even if the marriage does not end in divorce, can expect to spend nearly ten years alone as a widow. The woman who is neither emotionally nor economically prepared for this situation is vulnerable to depression beyond normal grief.

It is certainly a possibility that social inequities can lead to economic helplessness, dependency on others, chronic low self-esteem, and low aspirations, any or all of which can be final catalysts of clinical depression.

While there is no question that women have more depressions than men, scientists consider it unlikely that any one explanation—biological, psychological, or social—will account for all the differences. Moreover, it is not certain that these sex differences are found in non-Western countries. Understanding why women are more vulnerable to depression is currently of scientific interest and activity.

Vulnerable Periods In Life

Certain periods and situations in life may carry a higher risk for developing depression. These times include some periods in the woman's reproductive cycle, as well as periods of transition in which there are losses or disruptions of emotional bonds and attachments—for example, following the death of a loved one, a divorce, or a geographic move.

The Premenstrual Period

Premenstrual tension includes feeling irritable, bloated, tense, and blue during the three to five days before the onset of menses. Although they are reported by many women, these feelings usually do not occur with regularity, do not seem to affect a woman's performance at work or in the home, and are not particularly apparent to others.

There is no evidence to suggest that women are more vulnerable to the syndrome of depression during the premenstrual period. The blue feelings reported by some women in the premenstrual phase seem to be transitory and not related to clinical depression.

Oral Contraceptive Use

While there is widespread belief that oral contraceptive medication "causes depression," there is little scientific evidence to support that belief. If a relationship exists between the use of oral contraceptives and the onset of depression, it may be associated with the psychological conflicts over preventing pregnancy or unwanted exposure to sexual relationships rather than the pharmacologic ingredients of the "pill." Whereas a small number of women may be sensitive to the steroid hormones in oral contraceptives, it has been difficult for scientists to untangle just what may be the cause, if any, of mood changes associated with taking oral contraceptives. As yet, there is little evidence that oral contraceptives cause depression.

The Postpartum Period

The "new baby blues," mild and transitory feelings of sadness and tearfulness, are so common in the first few weeks following childbirth that they are considered "normal" and rarely require treatment. Reassurance, emotional support, comfort from the husband and doctor, and help in caring for the baby are all that the mother of a newborn usually requires. However, for a small number of women, a longer postpartum period of up to six months does carry a risk of more serious clinical depression. Moreover, women who have previously become clinically depressed (not just mildly blue) in the postpartum period are at much greater risk of another recurrence with subsequent pregnancies and deliveries. Therefore, future pregnancies in women who have already experienced a postpartum depression should be considered with caution. If a woman with such a history decides to become pregnant, the postpartum period should be planned so that she is not subjected to undue emotional stress and fatigue.

The Menopause

Despite conventional wisdom and popular folklore, women in the menopausal period are not at an increased risk of depression. Depressions that happen to occur in the menopausal period are not more severe and are not different from those that occur in other periods, and do not require special treatment. Recent studies show that most women who are in the menopause or who have passed it do not view it as a particularly stressful period in their life. In fact, many women whose children are leaving home—an event that often coincides with the menopause—do not view the "empty nest" as stressful. Rather, they see it as an opportunity to rest, recover, and undertake new ventures with renewed freedom.

The gradual decrease of the menopausal depression, called "involutional melancholia," may be a recent trend in the United States, and one that is also reported in the United Kingdom and Scandinavia. This decrease may have to do with woman's increased life-span and the opportunities for personal fulfillment as she ages. As a result, the child-rearing role is only one of a range of options now open to women. The woman whose children have left home now can look forward to nearly 30 more years to explore other opportunities. Thus, the menopausal period is not a period of increased risk for depression.

Deaths

Grief is a normal reaction to the death of a loved one, but it usually resolves within two to four months. Abnormal grief is a specific problem that arises from an inability to go through the usual process of mourning. Factors contributing to abnormal grief reactions leading to depression include loneliness and the unavailability of family and social supports at the time of the death; conflicted and unresolved angry feelings toward the dead person; guilt over the circumstances of the death; and failure to acknowledge grief at the time of the death, such as an inability to cry at the funeral or to talk about the dead person. Persons who have lost a loved one and who do not go through a normal grieving reaction nor allow themselves an opportunity for rest, recovery, and reconstitution of their life are vulnerable to depressive reactions in the future.

Transitions

Any transition period during which one must adapt to a separation from familiar surroundings, life patterns, and friends is a vulnerable period for depression. Such transition periods occur during geographic moves, a divorce, retirement, or a job change. Depression can occur even if the transition is a favorable one, involving a better job, a bigger house, or leaving an unhappy marriage. Transitions can challenge one's adaptive capacity, leaving the person feeling uncertain, alone, and in unfamiliar experiences.

Marital Disputes

Marital disputes are highly associated with the onset of depression in women. Marital disruption and increased arguments with a spouse are the most commonly reported problems in the six months prior to the onset of depressive symptoms. The absence of an intimate, confiding relationship with the spouse can lead to depression in women in the face of common life stress. Alternately, the availability of an intimate, confiding relationship with a man can protect a woman from depression in the face of adversity. Marital disputes are the most common problem discussed by patients being treated for depression.

Depressive symptoms often represent an acknowledgment of frustration, failure, hopelessness, and unmet needs in the marriage, where there is either an impasse or an overt conflict. The astute clinician should be alert for opportunities to engage the spouse in the treatment of the depressed woman to see if renegotiation and resolution of the dispute is possible.

Who Is Most Vulnerable?

Certain family histories or social experiences may contribute to an increased risk of depression. But it must be remembered that all or even most people who have these characteristics do not become depressed.

Persons who have been deprived of the love and warmth of a parent as children are more susceptible to depression as adults than are children who have had love and parental care. Parental deprivation can occur if a parent is absent through death or geographic separation, if the parent has been abusive, rejecting, or disinterested in the child, or if the childhood home has been a hotbed of parental discord.

Similarly, persons who have a strong family history of depression, particularly severe depressions in their parents, are more open to developing a depression themselves. However, since the number of persons who become depressed at some point in their life is high, the chance that any person has a family member who has been depressed also is high. Therefore, a strong family history implies that at least several close family members have been depressed.

It has been shown convincingly that the lack of an intimate confiding partner, usually a spouse, can contribute to increasing the chance of depression in the face of life stress. The presence of someone a woman can openly trust and to whom she can talk about her feelings, fears, and disappointments, especially when she is faced with adversity, can be an important buffer to despair. The absence of such an emotional resource is reflected in the fact that many depressed women who seek treatment report marital disputes as a serious problem in their lives.

The Impact of Depression

Women who suffer from acute depression are considerably impaired in their daily lives. When acutely depressed women were compared with normal women who have never been depressed, it was found that the impairments were most marked in work and in the intimate relationships of marriage and parenthood. Although depressed persons may remain at outside employment during the acute episode, actual comfort and satisfaction with their work and their general level of performance generally diminish.

Marriage

The marital relationships of depressed persons, in contrast to relationships with co-workers, distant colleagues, and family, are characterized by open warfare. There is often a lack of affection between husband and wife, coupled with feelings of guilt and resentment. Sexual relationships and communication are either diminished or absent.

Parenthood

Depression has a serious impact on being a parent. The typical depressed person is sad, apathetic, and listless, and is not fully able to meet the demands of parenthood, which require energy, interest, emotional involvement, and affection. Depressed mothers are only moderately able to be involved in their children's lives, and have difficulty communicating with them; they express a loss of affection and considerable anger toward their children. These mothers feel guilty about their inadequacy but are unable to control their feelings or to change their behavior. There is anger and resentment at the entire family for making what are interpreted as unfair demands.

Involvement and interest. Acute depression impairs the parents' ability to be involved in their children's lives. For younger children, this includes participation in their play and genuine concern for their physical care and development; for older children, it involves taking an active interest in their school progress, social activities and friends, and the dispensing of discipline.

Irritability, self-preoccupation, and low energy levels (anergia) prevent depressed parents from meeting their children's normal demands for attention. Involvement is limited either by the emotional or physical distancing of the parent or by overcontrol. For example, one mother went shopping to avoid answering her children's questions; another went to bed when the children came home from school. Still another regimented household activities, allowing the children only specified times for snacks, meals, or homework; any deviation from the schedule was met by her harsh reprisal.

In some families, especially where there are younger children, household chaos can become the norm. Younger children look physically uncared for and can suffer more than the usual accidents as a result of parental inattentiveness and disinterest.

Communication. Children become less inclined to talk over daily events or problems and deeper feelings with the depressed parent, whose own troubled feelings and self-preoccupation convey disinterest and unwillingness or inability to listen, and hopelessness about a solution.

Children either take their problems elsewhere or allow them to build up inside of them. One thirteen-year-old youngster abruptly stopped attending school during the height of her mother's illness. She had been having academic difficulties, felt her teacher was unsympathetic to her, and was embarrassed by her own poor performance in the class. She had not discussed the problem at home because she didn't wish to overburden her mother, nor did she feel that her mother would understand. The mother was totally perplexed by her daughter's sudden refusal to attend school, yet didn't have the energy or direction to sensitively question her. Moreover, as part of the mother's own depressive state of mind, she saw her daughter's behavior as another reflection of the hopelessness of life.

Affection. Depressed parents report a lack of affection for their children, which in turn produces feelings of guilt and inadequacy. This is particularly true for the mothers of small children and infants who worry about not being able to love their children or to spontaneously feel tender emotions. Some mothers worried about doing pyschological harm, and others became frightened about their own hostile feelings toward all of their children or, at times, toward one child who was singled out as particularly difficult to handle.

Hostility. Contrary to earlier writings about depression as a state of anger turned upon oneself, acutely depressed patients show increased irritability, anger, and hostility that is directed more toward family members (especially spouse and children) and much less toward casual acquaintances or the professionals who are carrying out their treatment. The patient who is compliant and obsequious to her physician can be quite hostile at home.

While most of the hostility toward the children takes the form of irritability, overtly intense conflicts and physical violence sometimes are reported. The conflicts could become quite serious with an adolescent child, especially if the child exploits the parent's helpless state and becomes rebellious and demanding.

Some children themselves become withdrawn and sad when the parent is depressed. For example, one youngster was afraid to make any comments that would disturb his mother. His mother had spoken so openly of the hopelessness of her life that he was afraid she might kill herself.

At times, the depressed parent's intense range toward the children can be frightening to both the parent and the child. When one patient came for her weekly appointment, she could barely speak. With a trembling voice, she described an incident that happened the previous evening. Her daughter had been deliberately defiant and challenging and the mother couldn't take it any longer. In a fit of rage, she held a pot to her daughter's head, ready to hit her. But when she considered the impact of what she had done, the mother felt weak, terrified, and full of remorse.

In general terms, the acute symptoms of depression conflict with the demands of being a parent. Depression signals the need for nurturance, help, and care. These are the very demands made on parents by their children. At the simplest level, apathetic, sad, and anergic depressed parents are put in the untenable position of having demands made upon them by their children for the help, care, and affection that they themselves require.

The Impact on Children

Does parental depression have a short-term impact on children, and are there long-term consequences? Intense human emotions can arise during the formation, disruption, and renewal of affectional bonds within the family, and many forms of psychiatric disorders result from a person's incapacity to make and keep warm, close emotional bonds.

This is significant because for a child, depression in a parent can be experienced as a disruption of close emotional bonds.

For the young child, the parent's withdrawal is felt as a loss of love, care, and protection, and for the older child, as a loss of guidance, boundaries, and a model of behavior. Depending on the pervasiveness, severity, and recurring nature of these symptoms and on the availability of alternate caretakers, the impact on the child's development could be short-term, subsiding with the parent's recovery, or it could have long-term serious impact that is resistant to change.

Most of the social dysfunctioning described is a consequence of depression; when the depression lifts, the patient returns to a normal family social life. This return may be less rapid than the recovery from the symptomatic state, and may take several months.

For many patients, psychotherapy to deal with social and interpersonal problems that preceded the depression is most helpful (see opposite page).

The Chance of Suicide

Suicide is a real possibility in all depressed patients. Recent estimates are that approximately 15 percent of the most severely depressed patients (especially bipolar patients) will end their life by suicide. In assessing suicidal risk, patients are asked such questions as "Have you felt that life is not worth living?" "Have you wished you were dead?" "Have you made a suicidal plan?" and "Are you thinking of suicide now?". The patient's positive answer to these questions must be taken seriously. It is just not true that a patient who talks about suicide will not commit suicide. A substantial number of persons who do commit suicide have seen a physician in the week prior to their death.

Factors that increase suicide risk include being over the age of 40, having a family history of suicide, making previous suicide attempts, having a chronic physical illness, the recent loss of a loved one, alcoholism or drug addiction, severe depression, severe insomnia, and social isolation or living alone. A combination of suicidal feelings with any of the above factors would constitute a serious increased risk, requiring psychiatric consultation and sometimes hospitalization.

Treatments for Depression

"The duty of those that take care of distressed, melancholy persons…is of two sorts: 1) In prudent carriage to them; 2) In medicine and diet; a little of both..Choose for them a skillful, prudent minister…for their secret counsel and public audience; one that is skilled in such cases, and one that is peaceable, and not contentious, erroneous or fond of odd opinions…neglect not psychic, and though they will be adverse to it, as believing that the disease is only in the mind, they must be persuaded to it…Medicinal remedies and theological uses not to be given together by the same hand; but in this case of perfect complication of the maladies of mind and body, I think it not unfit…for the soul and body are wonderfully co-partners in their diseases and cures…" (Reverend Richard Baxter, 1615-1691).

There are now available a variety of effective treatments for depression, both pharmacotherapy and psychotherapy. In practice, moderately depressed patients often receive a combination of an antidepressant and psychotherapy.

When to Seek Treatment

Transitory depressive symptoms are so common as to be considered normal. These usually resolve on their own or with the aid of advice and support from trusted friends and family.

Question arises as to when these symptoms are no longer normal and require professional help. Three aspects should be taken into account—the persistence and pervasiveness of the symptoms, and their impact on daily functioning. Any person who has several of the symptoms listed on page 408 should seek help. If these symptoms are less pervasive but are accompanied by suicidal thoughts, then professional help should be sought. Where a person seeks help depends on their own preferences and on the resources of their local community. Help can be obtained in a local mental health center, from a family physician, a private psychiatrist, or from another mental health professional.

When to Seek Psychiatric Consultation

Most depressives are treated by nonpsychiatric physicians, or by nonmedical mental health professionals. A psychiatrist definitely should be consulted if the person is actively thinking of suicide or is so severely ill that hospitalization may be necessary; if there are complicated psychological and social problems requiring long-term or specialized psychological intervention; if there are concurrent medical problems in which the use of psychotropic medication may be contraindicated or must be closely monitored; if there is a history of recurrent depression that may require long-term management; or if there is evidence of manic behavior (past or current) suggestive of bipolar disease.

Prognosis

Acute depression carries an excellent prognosis. Nearly all patients recover, and social functioning between episodes is usually unimpaired. Formerly depressed patients return to their normal life, resuming their accustomed work, child care, and social life. While most acute symptoms resolve rapidly, especially with modern treatment, there is a tendency for depression to recur in some patients. About one-third of all patients who had initially recovered from an acute depression remain completely asymptomatic and never have a recurrence. About 10 percent return with mild chronic symptoms, and about half have mild recurring symptoms at some point in their lives, including disturbances of mood, sleep, and appetite. These periods of symptom recurrence are usually accompanied by difficulties in participating fully in family and social life. Since persons who have had an acute depressive episode have an increased likelihood of a recurrence, they should learn to detect the early signs of depression and to seek treatment promptly. They also should learn to identify those aspects of their social and interpersonal lives that are associated with the onset of their symptoms.

Medications for Depression

One of the promising advances in the treatment of depression has been the availability of a range of drugs that elevate moods, making a person feel happier.

There are now a number of widely available antidepressant medications or mood elevators that are relatively safe and can be administered by most physicians.

Antidepressant medication. Antidepressants are *not* tranquilizers. They are a completely separate group of chemical compounds technically referred to as tricyclic compounds and monoamine-oxidase compounds (see the chart at right). These drugs, used specifically for the treatment of the *depressive syndrome* as described in this chapter (see page 408) were discovered in the 1940s, and came into wide and effective use in the 1950s.

Seventy to 80 percent of acutely depressed patients receiving antidepressants experience symptom relief within one to four weeks. Sleep and appetite usually return to normal within one to two weeks; improvement in mood may take two to four weeks. As a result of this time lag in response, patients often need considerable reassurance that their symptoms eventually will diminish.

The most common side effects of these drugs include dry mouth, blurred vision, dizziness, increased appetite, and gastrointestinal symptoms. Hypertension, cardiac arrhythmia, and myocardial infarction (heart attack) have been reported, and these drugs should not be used in the presence of heart disease. Patients over 45 years of age should have an EKG before commencing treatment. Elderly patients may require smaller doses and always should receive careful monitoring by their physicians.

People suffering depression usually stay on tricyclic antidepressants for four to eight months after the acute symptoms of depression have subsided in order to prevent a relapse and return of symptoms. Maintenance medication for four to eight months has been shown to reduce the chance of relapse by about one-half. Patients who have had a mild depression and no previous history of symptoms have a low chance of relapse, even

ANTIDEPRESSANT DRUGS

General Class	Generic Name	Trade Name
Tricyclic Compounds	Imipramine	Tofranil
	Desipramine	Norpramin
		Pertofrane
	Amitriptyline	Elavil, Endep
	Nortriptyline	Aventyl
	Doxepin	Sinequan
		Adapin
	Protriptyline	Vivactil
Monoamine-Oxidase Inhibitors	Phenelzine	Nardil
	Isocarboxazid	Marplan
	Tranylcypro-mine	Parnate
	Pargyline	Eutonyl

without medication. In such cases, the physician may want to withdraw medication and just be available to the patients if symptoms begin to reappear.

Lithium carbonate is a drug that has recently received attention because of its use in persons with the severe form of depression called bipolar disorder (see page 409). Lithium is a chemical element originally used in Europe as a dietary salt substitute for the treatment of a variety of medical complaints. In 1949, an Australian investigator noted its usefulness in ending a manic attack. Since then, considerable research has shown convincingly that it is a useful drug in the treatment of persons with bipolar disorders. Like all medications, however, it does not work for all bipolars. Persons who are receiving lithium must undergo controlled monitoring of their blood levels and must be under the close supervision of their physician because of the narrow margin of safety between therapeutic and toxic dosages.

Psychotherapy

Antidepressant drugs have by no means replaced psychotherapy as a treatment for depression. In fact, prior to the advent of antidepressant drugs, psychotherapy was the main treatment.

While antidepressants have been found to reduce symptoms of depression—such as sleep and appetite problems, and anxiety—and to prevent the return of symptoms, they do not have any major impact on the patient's social and personal life. Medication does not repair marriages and improve parent/child relationships. It only has an impact on these problems to the extent that a person who is feeling poorly cannot devote herself to the task of improving the impaired relationships. In practice, some form of psychological assistance in dealing with problems in living is usually combined with medication, although either treatment may be used independently.

There is a wide range of psychological treatments that are effective in depression. Some of the treatments include interpersonal, cognitive, behavioral, marital, and group therapies. Psychological treatments differ widely in their aim, intensity, duration, and in the training of the therapists who administer them. See the chapter on "Mental Illness" for an extensive discussion of the therapies available. Generally, the purpose of psychotherapy is to provide emotional support and the opportunity for talking, to help the patient deal with the consequences of being depressed, and to provide an understanding of the patterns of behavior, interpersonal disputes, or losses that may have contributed to the depression. Depression rarely occurs in a vacuum, and it is important to understand the social and inter-personal context in which the depression occurred.

The patient who needs psychological treatment should see a qualified and fully trained specialist in these treatments, a psychiatrist, psychologist, or psychiatric social worker.

Women's Self-Help Groups

Self-help groups have been suggested as an alternative to traditional treatment for dealing with female depression. This suggestion rests partially on the premise that the traditional feminine role leads to helplessness, and that depression is a state of helplessness. "Self-help" has been suggested as a treatment in cases of learned helplessness. The concept of self-help for learned helplessness has an intuitive appeal. However, self-help groups, as the sole therapy for the full-blown syndrome of depression, are not as specific as psychotherapy.

Self-help groups may be useful supplements but are not necessary alternatives to traditional therapies for the clinically depressed. By their very nature, self-help groups require energy, engagement, and optimism, which may be more than someone with moderate-to-severe clinical depression can muster. While some women attending these groups may have mild depressive symptoms, few probably have the full-blown depressive syndrome.

On the other hand, self-help groups may help to prevent more serious symptoms in dissatisfied, unhappy, and lonely women. They also may be useful as

an adjunct to traditional therapy following symptom reduction. A deeper understanding of nontraditional therapies such as women's self-help groups, and an evaluation of their role in preventing depression and in providing support and emotional bonds to women, is both timely and warranted. In the absence of such evidence, the depressed woman can rely on the traditional therapies, drugs and psychotherapy, for the alleviation of clinical depression.

Family Involvement in Treatment

The successful treatment of a depressed outpatient can depend in part on the quality of the family's involvement and on their understanding of the treatment. Even when overt interpersonal problems between patient and family do not exist, families of outpatients may become intolerant of the patient's decreased activity, her diminished communication, and hopeless affect. Daily confrontations with the patient's gloomy affect, as well as the necessity for the family to assume some of the caretaking, may create additional conflicts.

Families often have questions about medication. The most common inquiries refer to the possible addictive qualities of the drugs used and whether the patient will have to take these medications indefinitely. The physician may have to stress to the the family the patient's need to continue taking medication even after improvement is evident. In cases of potentially suicidal patients, it may be necessary to ask a responsible relative to dispense the drug. In outpatient treatment, it is critical to gain the patient's and family's confidence and cooperation. It is not unusual for the patient and the family to be discouraged by a lack of immediate improvement in a patient who is receiving an antidepressant drug. This is often interpreted by the patient as further proof of the hopelessness of the condition. Alternately, when improvement does occur, the patient and family may assume that the depression has been cured and may not want to continue medication, fearing a possible drug dependency. In either case, the expected course of events should be discussed. The patient and family should be reassured about delayed effects of the medication, the side effects, and the necessity of continuing the medication for the prescribed course of treatment.

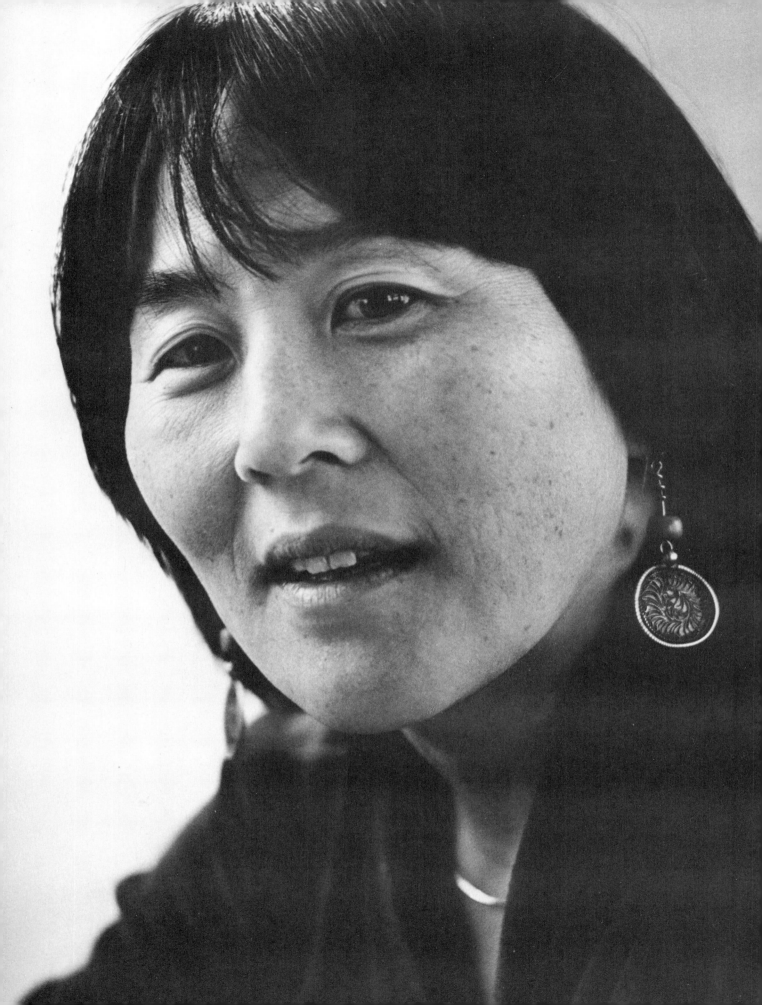

CHAPTER 21

MENTAL ILLNESS

MADELEINE REICHERT, D.M.H.

Mental illness can be very difficult to define or assess, especially since there is no general agreement on what constitutes mental health. Still, we can consider a mental disorder to be any psychological or behavioral state that is felt by you or by others to be painful, unpleasant, or disruptive of your normal day-to-day functioning.

Today more women than ever before are seeking professional guidance when they are suffering from emotional or psychological distress. An awareness of the definitions of common mental illnesses will give you a sense of confidence in choosing psychological assistance for yourself or for others.

Mental Illness

How do we define a mentally healthy woman? Traditionally, women have relied on others (parents, husbands, and professionals) to define and control their physical and emotional health. And although today women are exercising far more control over maintaining their physical health, unfortunately they are not exercising such independence when defining and regulating their psychological health.

Women today are less willing to relinquish control of their physical well-being to health professionals than they were a generation ago. A dramatic example of this trend is the change in birthing procedures. Thirty years ago, many women gave total control to their obstetrician (usually male), trusting his judgment about how to deliver, what kind and how much anesthesia to use, and how to handle the baby during its first minutes and hours of life. Today, women are more often seeking an obstetrician or midwife who will respect their wishes as to how to deliver, whether or not to use anesthetics, and how to handle their newborns.

This change is largely due to women feeling greater trust in their own judgment about what is right for them and their families. It also is based on greater knowledge and understanding of pregnancy, the birth process, and the first minutes of life. Nowhere is this type of self-trust and increased understanding more important than in the field of mental health.

Often the same women who have become more inclined to exercise control over their physical health are not inclined to do so with their psychological and emotional well-being, preferring instead to delegate this responsibility to professionals. More women today than ever before turn to professional guidance when suffering from emotional or psychological distress. In this age of free-flying psychiatric jargon, everyone is "neurotic," "uptight," "hung up," "messed up," or just "out of touch with their feelings." A popular line today is "There is no such thing as normal. Find someone too normal and chances are, they're sick." In such an era, it's tempting for women who are suffering to assume that it is due to an internal flaw or weakness, and that only a professional can tell them what is wrong and what to do about it. Sometimes both assumptions are true; sometimes neither one is.

Before we can discuss psychological disorders in women, we must define a few terms as they will be used here. Abnormal *means different than the norm. In this chapter, it will carry no positive or negative connotations, but will merely indicate something out of the normal range.* Maladaptive *refers to a response or manner of coping with an internal or external problem that is unhelpful, unhealthy, and disturbing to the person or to others. A* mental disorder *is any psychological or behavioral state (not just one response) that is felt by someone or by others to be painful, unpleasant, or disruptive of normal functioning. These disorders may have symptoms that range from mild to incapacitating; they may be largely due to a particular individual's response to external stress, or to a combination of a biological predisposition and a response to external stresses. They may be acute (sudden), chronic (ongoing), or episodic (from time to time). The term* mental illness *will be reserved for those disorders that involve actual neurological problems or damage, or where personality disorganization is so severe that hospitalization, medical treatment, and/or removal from the community become necessary.*

Although women are not unique in the types of mental disorders they develop, the frequency of some disorders, as well as their etiology (causes), diagnosis, and treatment, are often very different than in men. These differences are due to many factors, including biological differences between the sexes, different cultural expectations of the sexes, different socialization practices with male and female children, and the different social stresses experienced by men and women in our society.

A woman evaluates her psychological health in a social context. Thus, before we can discuss the types of mental disorders women encounter, we must first ask: What is considered mentally healthy for women in our society? How did this view evolve? If we live in a society in which women are still second-class citizens, how does this affect our perception of mental disorders in women? How does it affect the diagnosis and treatment of women? What are the signs of mental disorders, and to which disorders are women more vulnerable? What are the common precipitating stresses of mental disorders? What kinds of treatment are available, and who provides them?

As we learn more answers to these questions, we will grow more confident in taking control over our psychological as well as our physical health.

A Historical Perspective

Today more people are seeking help from mental health professionals such as social workers, psychologists, psychiatrists, and counselors than ever before. Women, far more than men, have increased their use of mental health facilities. Why? Certainly there is greater acceptance and knowledge of psychiatry today than in the past. (Only 200 years ago, mentally ill women who were considered "bewitched" were burned at the stake.) Many professionals also cite the rising degree of stress and conflict in the lives of today's women.

Regardless of the reasons, more women are openly complaining of psychological distress today than in the past. In addition, women tend to experience certain types of disorders far more than other types. In order to understand why women are experiencing or at least are reporting more mental disorders and what happens to them when they seek assistance, we first must understand how our society defines mental health and illness in women, and how this cultural view evolved.

In any society, people who obey the rules and adopt culturally expected roles are considered mentally healthy, while those who break the rules, who cannot or will not adopt those culturally expected roles, are defined as abnormal, mentally disordered, or criminal. However, not everyone who is abnormal (i.e., who fails to comply with social norms) is mentally ill or disordered. Many healthy individuals prefer to live in a manner deemed inappropriate by the majority of people in their culture. The culture may respond by labeling these individuals "deranged" as a punitive social control. Still other individuals who may wish to adopt socially acceptable work and relationship roles are unable to do so because of a mental illness or disorder.

Our society, like any other, has generally accepted roles based on an individual's age, sex, social status, and profession. Let's take a look at the generally accepted role of the American woman.

Outwardly, this is the age of women's awareness. As we see the amount of media coverage devoted to women's issues and concerns, it is tempting to see ourselves as living in an enlightened era in regard to women. Unfortunately, this is largely a myth. As the 1970s came to a close, controversy raged over whether to ratify an Equal Rights Amendment for women, and, in fact, such legislation may very well fail. As we applaud the increased number of women who are gaining economic and political power, how many of us realize that in the early 1970s, *proportionately fewer* of the nation's masters and doctoral degrees were awarded to women than in 1930!

Generally, women still are expected to place top priority on marriage, a home, and children. They are expected to depend on their spouse for both economic and social support, while developing most fully their own capacities as nurturant caretakers who are loving, compassionate, and sympathetic. Thus, it's not surprising that, outside of the roles of wife and mother,

the most socially acceptable career roles are nursing and teaching, especially teaching in elementary and secondary schools. Most women are encouraged to live vicariously, sharing the triumphs and sorrows of their husband and children. They are allowed and encouraged to focus intensely on their physical charms, clothing, makeup, and other adornments. Few women want to age in this culture, which emphasizes the delights of being 20 forever, and millions of dollars are spent yearly by women who try to alter their skin, hair, shape, and size in order to appear younger. Finally, women are encouraged to be passive and dependent. Aggression, assertiveness, and attempts to achieve power are often frowned upon or rejected, unless they occur in the home or in dealing with children.

If anything, the roles of women today are less equal and *less valued* by our society than they were a century ago. Contrary to popular belief, the preoccupation of today's women with marriage and motherhood is not an age-old inheritance. Until the industrial revolution forced a separation between the home and workplace, there was far less division of work between the sexes. Women enjoyed important economic and productive, as well as reproductive, roles. Far more often than today, men and women worked side by side building and maintaining the home, raising and harvesting crops, and producing and preserving food. In addition, women made clothing and other essential items.

The industrial revolution had a profound effect on women's roles. Men took on the role of worker and "breadwinner," while women were assigned primarily domestic roles, which were now greatly reduced. As urban areas developed, food production occurred elsewhere. Women now needed only to shop for groceries and to cook. Food preservation became unnecessary with refrigeration and mass production. Clothes were ready-made, and soap and dairy products were mass-produced. Public school systems took on the job of educating children, and hospitals and medical practitioners tended the ill. The women hardest hit by these changes were in the middle classes. Whereas the salaries of working-class women were still needed for the family's survival, middle-class women were often overeducated for domesticity, but were insufficiently educated and/or barred from more rewarding work outside the home.

It was in this social context, the Victorian era, that Sigmund Freud grew up, and introduced the most influential theory of human psychology and personality development in the Western world. Although there have been many revisions of his theory, and many different and opposing views have evolved in the past 50 years, none have had as much power and widespread influence as Freud's original formulations. In fact, some Freudian terms ("ego," "unconscious," and "Oedipal complex") have become so widely used that people often are unaware of their origin. No single theorist has contributed as much to our understanding of the human mind.

Although Freud's brilliance is unrefutable, he was seriously limited in three major ways: his method, his era, and his knowledge of physiology. Nowhere did these limitations hamper him more than in his theory of female psychology. Freud employed a *clinical method.* He saw women who sought his help because they suffered from emotional disturbances, but he relied on his clinical findings with such women for his theory of normal, as well as pathological, female development. Since these were adult women, he was forced to rely on their retrospection and memory to piece together their developmental histories. At no time did he directly observe young children as they developed. (This is a serious general criticism of Freud's theory, and not just of his model of female development.) Second, Freud lived in the *Victorian era,* which we have just described as a time of tremendous inhibition and devaluation of women, socially and sexually. The middle- and upper-class women seen by Freud were neither highly valued nor essential figures at home or in the work force. Finally, by today's standards, Freud operated with very *limited medical and physiological knowledge.* Today we know that Freud's understanding of female genitalia, in particular his theory of differential vaginal and clitoral orgasms, was simply wrong.

As we examine Freud's statements about female development, we will quickly agree with at least one of his observations—that he understood very little about female psychology. His work in this area is fraught with clinical and theoretical contradictions, and with factual errors. Let's examine four of Freud's theories and their flaws. First, he believed that *biology is destiny,* and that the anatomical differences between the sexes shape their different natures in a fixed, irrevocable fashion. He stated that the personality structure of the female is forever shaped by her discovery that she has no penis. Freud's second theory, the notion of *penis envy* in women, asserted that it is normal and universal for a girl to want a penis. She perceives her own external sexual equipment as inferior, believing not only that she once had a penis, but also that she was castrated.

According to Freud, the discovery of this "castration" is a turning point in a young girl's life. She turns away from her mother, whom she blames for her castrated

state, and toward her father, from whom she hopes to obtain a penis. Soon this wish for a penis is replaced by a wish for a child from the father. This is the stage commonly referred to as the "Oedipal" stage of psychosexual development. Freud believed that a girl remains in this stage for an indefinite period, and in fact often never abandons it.

The girl's alleged difficulty in resolving her Oedipal attachment to her father led Freud to his third theory, the view of *faulty superego development in females.* According to Freud, boys fear castration by the father if they do not give up a desire for the mother. Consequently, they abandon these desires. They identify with the feared father in order to grow up like him and possess a woman like the loved mother. As they identify with this loved and feared father, boys incorporate the adult male's superego and sense of justice. In contrast, girls believe that they have already been castrated and blame their mothers for this. Thus, they turn away from their mothers and take longer to resolve the Oedipal conflict, if in fact they ever do. Freudian theory emphasizes that the development of a sound superego (conscience) depends on the resolution of this Oedipal attachment. Therefore, Freud postulated that women have weaker superegos and social interests, less capacity to sublimate their impulses, and, in general, a lesser sense of justice than men.

Freud's fourth theory maintains that there is an *anatomical basis for passivity* in women. Women are physically built to receive the penis into their vagina. Based on these observations, Freud asserted that women are constitutionally equipped to be receptive and passive. Whereas aggression and assertiveness are characteristic of normal men, Freud viewed submissiveness and passivity as normal female traits.

The flaws in these four theories, which have so powerfully influenced the twentieth century's view of women, are numerous. Of course anatomical differences undoubtedly contribute to personality differences between the sexes. Feminine body image, endocrine function, menstruation, pregnancy, childbirth, and menopause play major roles in shaping the female personality. However, Freud himself realized that he had forgotten a major part of the picture. Women are human beings apart from their sexual function! To develop a theory of female psychology based on biological differences between the sexes and without examining the cultural reaction to those differences is to develop only half a theory.

Still, Freud operated within this limited view. He assumed that penis envy was a universal, inevitable phenomenon rather than a product of a society in which girls were devalued and restricted, while boys were valued and granted freedom. At no time did he address a phenomenon widely discussed in folklore, namely womb-, breast-, and woman-envy. Men, unable to bear and nurse infants, often envy women these capacities. Undoubtedly, had Freud noticed such a phenomenon, he would have viewed it as highly pathological and not as the normal occurrence that it is now thought to be.

Nowhere are Freud's cultural biases more flagrant than in his theory of a faulty female superego. Today no social scientist would claim that women inherently have weaker impulse controls, lesser social interests, less capacity for objective reasoning and social justice, or are more disposed to envy. The evidence indicates that, in fact, girls are socialized in our culture to be better behaved than boys, and therefore, at least in the early years, demonstrate a *stronger* superego development.

As for the view that submissiveness and passivity are based on physical differences between the sexes, we now know that this is simply not the case. As women are granted greater permission to initiate sexual activity, it is becoming clear that a male can be a relatively passive penetrator with a female as a relatively assertive, dominant recipient. In fact, increasingly, sexual research is demonstrating the extreme activity of the female genitalia during sexual intercourse. If we want to explain submissiveness and passivity as "normal" female characteristics, we need to look at our cultural definitions of "normality."

Freud, living in a male-dominated society and perceiving the penis as the major source of power, developed a model of the "normal" female as passive, weak, and envious. In reaction to such an unflattering description of women, it became popular among some theorists to attribute Freud's theory to masculine jealousy of woman's reproductive function. Such a theory could explain the historical, political, and economic dominance by men as their attempt to compensate for their perceived sense of inadequacy. For example, a man who cannot produce a child compensates by constructing a building. A third theory, particularly popular today with the feminist movement, states that, in fact, there are no significant inherent differences between the sexes. Woman's second-class position is due merely to the oppression of a male-dominated society.

Probably most of us will find some truth and fallacy in all three of these theories. It is hard to believe that throughout life, women and men are primarily motivated by a desire for the genitalia they do not possess. Equally hard to accept is the notion that there are virtually no differences between the sexes, other than actual anatomical ones. As we examine the social and cultural influences that affect mental disorders in women, we will retain the perspective that, in fact, there are basic psychological differences between men and women, and that some are based on anatomical differences.

Thus, as we define mental health and mental illness in women, we must at all times understand that such definitions reflect our political, economic, and social conditions, as much as the state of our mental health science. Furthermore, such definitions always reflect personal viewpoints and ideologies as well.

Social/Cultural Influences

The National Institute of Mental Health has collected data from general and mental hospitals, outpatient psychiatric clinics, and private clinicians that indicate that more women than men are being diagnosed and treated for mental disorders. In addition, certain disorders are becoming increasingly "feminine" psychiatric disorders. These include the neuroses, the affective psychoses, and schizophrenia. In recent studies of general practitioners (not psychiatrists), it was found that two out of three patients are women, and that, in almost every age group, women were perceived as twice as likely to suffer from psychological problems as men. We can understand these figures in two ways. First, women are in a socially disadvantaged position. This places them under greater stress, making them more vulnerable to mental disorders. Second, we live in a male-dominated society in which the female "norms" described by Freud are still a major influence. In essence, maleness is considered healthy and femaleness unhealthy.

Historically, women have had fewer rights and a lower social status than men. As a result, they have suffered from lower self-esteem, a sense of helplessness and lack of control over their lives, and economic hardship when they attempted to function independently of men. We now understand the connection between these conditions and mental disorders. During the past decade, studies have shown that people with low self-esteem are far more vulnerable to depression and all mental disorders that involve depression. (As we will discuss later, depression is the most common mental disorder in American women, and it plays a major role in most of the disorders to which women are particularly vulnerable.) We also have learned that major life changes, particularly changes over which we often lack control, are important precipitants of mental disorders. Such stresses include illness, the death of a loved one, changes in marital status, job losses or changes, changes in place of residence, pregnancy, the birth of a child, and menopause. We have recently learned that women, especially those who are heads of households (which many women are now becoming), report significantly more life stresses than men.

When rates of mental disorders are compared between the sexes, an interesting picture emerges. When single, divorced, and widowed women are compared to men in equivalent social positions, these women possess superior mental health, despite the greater stresses just described. In our society, it is married women who account for the greater number of mental disorders in females than in males. Whereas marriage appears to enhance the mental health of men, it is far less advantageous to the mental health of women. Of course, one explanation for these figures is that seriously disturbed males are less likely to marry. For example, male schizophrenics marry less often than do female schizophrenics.

Another explanation states that the married state is less conducive to sound mental health in women than in men. Why? When a couple marries, both partners give up a number of freedoms, but the wife usually loses far more independence and autonomy than her spouse. In our society, women usually take on major housekeeping chores even if both partners work. In one study, men and women agreed that wives make more concessions to preserve harmony in a marriage than do their husbands. Nonworking wives suffer from greater psychological distress than do working wives. Research indicates that when women play a variety of roles (such as career woman, wife, and mother), their mental health is enhanced. This makes sense. When women feel less successful in one arena but can compensate in another, their outlook remains happier and healthier.

Motherhood itself embodies significant stresses as well as delights. Even without children, married women report decreased freedom in self-expression. For those women who become mothers, there is an even greater loss of freedom. Motherhood, especially when children are young, requires the ultimate in patience and sacrifice of one's needs, and often entails isolation from satisfying adult contact. The emphasis by mental health professionals on the importance of a child's early years in shaping future behaviors further increases the pressure on young mothers to be "perfect."

At one time, the roles of wife and mother were revered. To some extent they still are, as evidenced by the observation that most girls are raised to believe that they should become wives and mothers. However, in the past 30 years, since the decline of the post-World War II "baby boom," there has been a subsequent demand for smaller families. With fewer children, there is a decrease in the time devoted to motherhood, and in the status associated with the role of mother. Many children are in nursery school or day-care as soon as they are out of diapers (or before). Once in school, increased numbers of activities pull children away from the home and into the community. Although many women retire from the work force to devote themselves to the roles of wife and mother, within a relatively short period they are no longer needed full time. Many respond by returning to work or school. Others, particularly those in the middle class, feel devalued, worthless, and suffer a loss of self-esteem. This devalued social position of women, particularly married women, may help explain their increased risk of mental disorders. However, there is also another important explanation for these statistics.

If a woman has classically "feminine" traits, she embodies just those traits deemed less "healthy" by most mental health professionals. In a classic study, it was shown that, because masculine traits are viewed as both more desirable and "healthy" in our society, women are placed in a no-win situation. To be described as "normal," a woman must embody characteristically feminine traits. Yet these same traits that make her a healthy female are deemed less healthy than more "masculine" traits. The clinicians interviewed in this study described "healthy" women as more submissive, excitable, easily influenced by others, emotional, and conceited, while being less independent, adventurous, competitive, objective, and scientific than men. In contrast, clinicians' views of a "healthy adult" and a "healthy male" were almost synonymous. Thus, there is a double standard of mental health. The ideal adult standard of health is applied only to men. "Normal" women (that is, women who exhibit the traditional "feminine" traits) are judged significantly less healthy by these same "adult" standards. How does such a cultural bias affect the diagnosis and treatment of mental disorders in women?

A number of mental health practitioners perceive their role as clarifiers—as people who help others to better understand their thoughts, feelings, and desires. They deny that they have a view of how people should be, what they should want, or the paths they should follow. In reality, however, most mental health professionals operate within an "adjustment" model that is influenced by their stereotypes of "normality." We live in a society with certain norms and requirements. Individuals must adapt and adjust to these structures. Even when an external situation is viewed by a clinician as disruptive and unhealthy, pathology still is often viewed as being within the individual in treatment. Clinicians often purposefully or inadvertently assist clients to behave in a more "normal," socially acceptable way.

Research findings indicate that clinicians, both male and female, are strongly influenced by our cultural stereotypes of men and women. How are these stereotypes and values transmitted in treatment? Many clinicians view marriage and maternity as the normal, healthy female role. When female clients choose these paths, such clinicians will view both choices as positive, without challenging these decisions. However, if the same clients prefer careers to marriage and mother-hood, such clinicians may view this as a defensively motivated choice. They would be concerned that these women were avoiding more traditional female roles out of fear or anxiety. Such decisions are far more likely to be questioned and challenged.

Many mental health professionals feel that this type of bias occurs only in shoddy practice. Others state that this problem occurs only in certain types of psychotherapy, especially psychoanalytic or other nondirective therapies in which attempts are made to uncover unconscious feelings and to enhance psychological insight. However, the psychoanalytic followers of Freud have no corner on the market of cultural stereotypes. Clinicians of all theoretical persuasions are members of our culture, which is imbued with a bias against women. This does not mean, as some women have suggested, that psychotherapy can serve no helpful role for today's troubled woman. Yet it certainly does call for a serious reexamination of values among mental health professionals.

The mental health professions are beginning to take just such a look at themselves. Recently, the American Psychological Association investigated sex bias and sex-role stereotyping in psychotherapy. They questioned women psychologists about sexism in psychotherapy, and found five areas of major concern: fostering traditional sex roles, bias in expectations and devaluation of women, sexist use of psychoanalytic concepts, viewing women as sex objects, and actual sexual exploitation of women. A set of guidelines was then published that urged psychologists to reassess their values and therapeutic techniques. Clinicians were asked to rethink their own sex-role stereotypes, to aid clients' awareness of sex discrimination in our society, and to become more knowledgeable about research findings on sex roles and sexism. More specifically, they were urged to avoid the use of sexist language, and to avoid seeing clients as the source of problems when such problems are the result of situational and/or cultural factors. Further, they were told to respect the client's autonomy in the therapy relationship, to avoid authoritarian techniques that reinforce stereotypic dependency in women, and to respect the client's assertiveness, to aid clients in their recognition of physical and sexual abuse when they have been victimized, and to refrain from having sexual relations with clients or treating clients as sexual objects.

Changes are slow but they are occurring. A new type of feminist therapy is evolving, focused on helping female clients become aware of the social and political context of their psychological problems (see page 439). In addition, many therapists who would not describe themselves as "feminist" therapists are increasingly more sensitive to these concerns.

We have just taken a look at the social context within which women are treated by the mental health profession. Regardless of its flaws and inequities, many women will find in the course of their lives a need or a desire for assistance from the mental health profession. Let us now turn our attention to some of the real-life situations in which women find themselves in need of professional assistance.

Warning Signs

As we have discussed, not everyone who is abnormal is mentally disordered. In fact, in a culture in which "normal" feminine behavior is less healthy than "normal" masculine behavior, a sign of superior mental health for women may be abnormality. With such a confusing state of affairs, how do we ever decide if we or someone close to us is in psychological trouble?

Let us define mental health as the ability to enjoy life and to experience satisfying, meaningful relationships, the capacity to give and receive love, the capacity to work, the possession of adequate self-respect and self-love, the ability to accept losses and rewards, and some acceptance of one's strengths, weaknesses, and limitations. With such a framework, it becomes easier to spot warning signs of mental disorder. Such signs include:

• Chronic unhappiness or depression as manifested by apathy, fatigue, loss of appetite or overeating, and problems in sleeping.
• Withdrawal from normally close, satisfying relationships, a sense of isolation, inability to sustain friendships or love relationships, and sexual disorders, such as frigidity.
• Inability to hold onto a job.
• Temper tantrums or inexplicable rages.
• Unreasonable fears or feelings of persecution.
• Suicidal thoughts or attempts; self-destructive behaviors such as alcoholism, drug addiction, compulsive gambling, or excessive risk-taking.
• Dramatic, unexplained shifts in self-esteem and affect (i.e., from feeling all-powerful and "on the top of the world" to feeling hopeless, helpless, and despondent).

Again, we must always retain a perspective of a mental health continuum. All of us have been subject to the types of problems listed above. The *intensity* of such symptoms, the *regularity* with which they occur, their *duration,* the extent to which they are not under *control,* the degree to which they *disrupt* normal functioning, and the degree to which they cause us or others *pain* determine whether or not we should seek professional assistance.

Let us explore the types of stresses that occur in the lives of women that may precipitate mental disorders. Then we will take a look at the various types of mental disorders, focusing primarily on those most prevalent among women.

Precipitants of Disorder

What are the typical stresses women face in life? Let us first employ a developmental perspective, and focus on the stresses most likely to occur at each stage of a woman's life.

Leaving home. Whether a young woman goes to work, to college, or to marriage, the late teens and early twenties usher in the time when most women leave their parents' home for good. Some women find this an exciting, relatively easy transition, while others experience panic and a sense of loss and abandonment. This is a time when many women attempt to resolve their uncertainty by entering marriage, hoping to find a new caretaker and source of security. It is not surprising that so many marriages among adolescents and young adults fail under these conditions.

Remaining single. Well over 90 percent of American women have been married at least once by age 40. What happens to the few who remain single? There are a number of social, economic, and sometimes emotional problems associated with remaining single. Our culture defines the "normal" female roles as those of wife and mother. Women who remain single often face censure, curiosity, sympathy, and discrimination from their communities. Once single women reach their late 20s, people who are normally polite and circumspect often begin to ask: "Why isn't a nice girl like you married?" "Don't you want a family?" "Don't you think perhaps you're too choosy?" Whether a woman elects to remain single, has not met "the right man," or has "never been asked," such prying questions are often embarrassing and annoying.

Many women, spared such intrusions by friends, relatives, and acquaintances, still encounter various social situations in which being alone feels awkward. Career women who travel often find themselves barred from enjoying the same pleasures as their male colleagues. Going alone to a restaurant and particularly a bar may invite stares or unwelcome advances. Married friends often exclude single women from guest lists at parties "where an even number is a must," or else pair them off with single men whom they have never met.

Single women often face a number of economic hardships. They frequently are paid less than men in equivalent positions. They may be denied managerial positions because "workers just don't relate well to women bosses." Credit is often denied them, and loans and mortgages are hard to secure. Although there is increasing legislation that bars discrimination against women, inequality still prevails. Married women faced with a similar bias in their jobs may rely on their husband's salary as well as their own, and thereby reduce the impact of this economic discrimination.

When women decide that marriage is not for them, they face a number of profound personal questions. Do I want children? If so, how do I feel about having them out of marriage? (For single childless women in their 30s, these questions may be of pressing, imminent concern.) If I decide against both marriage and children, what will my advanced years be like? Will I regret my decision when it is too late? The decision to remain single or to marry is difficult for many women. Once a woman opts for remaining single, she may find her status quite satisfying or very stress-laden, largely depending on her inner resources, needs, and desires, as well as her social support system.

To work, to marry, or both. For those women who delay marriage to go to school or to work, the 20s often bring a new series of concerns and sometimes crises. Depending on a woman's social, economic, religious, and educational background, her questions may

include: Why aren't I married? Why don't I have children? Why isn't my education completed by now? Why can't I combine it all? Some women allow themselves time to resolve these issues while others are thrown into an identity crisis.

Marriage. As we have already discussed, there are a number of stresses attached to marriage. These stresses often include a loss of autonomy and freedom, a reduction in the number of roles married women play in the world, stresses associated with motherhood, and a loss of status currently attached to the roles of wife and mother.

Pregnancy. For many women, pregnancy is a time of contentment, excitement, and wonderment. However, it also is a time of upheaval. The first pregnancy, in particular, marks a woman's passage from "daughter" to "mother." Thus, in addition to the phenomenal physical and endocrine changes a pregnant woman experiences, she often revives many old longings, concerns, and conflicts with her own mother. Many young women are beset with panic: How will I handle the responsibility? What if I hate being a mother? What if something is wrong with my child? How tied down will I be? All these "future" concerns occur at a time when women often are feeling fat, unattractive, tired, unfeminine, and unsexy. For those women who have supportive spouses or mates and contact with other women "who have been there too," these concerns often are easily resolved. For single mothers, women with husbands who feel uneasy and unsure about fatherhood, or women whose own childhoods were unhappy, pregnancy may be experienced as a crisis.

Abortion. An entire chapter is devoted to this subject (see page 206), so it will not be considered in detail here. However, no discussion about stress in the life of today's woman is complete without reference to abortion. The decision to terminate a pregnancy is stressful for any woman. For a woman raised without strong religious proscriptions against abortion, who has thought out her decision carefully, and who feels supported in her decision by her lover or husband, the problem still is not an easy one. If a woman feels that abortion is morally wrong, or feels alone, rejected, or uncertain of her decision, she may face a very serious crisis. Long after an abortion, women may suffer feelings of guilt, loss, and mourning. The healthiest of women may need some professional guidance at such a time. In fact, many physicians now require counseling for any woman for whom they perform an abortion.

Motherhood. We have already discussed some of the stresses as well as the pleasures associated with motherhood. For many women, mothering young children is the most fulfilling, exciting time of their lives. For others it is a time of frustration, disillusionment, longing for escape, and drudgery. Economics and education play major roles here. For women who are mothers within a marriage, whose children are spread out in ages, who are emotionally supported by husbands, who can afford assistance in the form of nursery school, day-care, or baby-sitters, and who retain outside friendships and/or employment, these years may be particularly enriching. At the same time, they may be hectic and often exhausting. For women raising children without a partner or with several preschoolers and no access to outside assistance, life may become unbearable.

Living in a society that glorifies the joys of motherhood and defines the normal mother as loving, patient, all-giving, and self-sacrificing, an unhappy mother may fear censorship and disapproval if she shares her feelings. Her problems then become compounded by an even greater isolation. Unfortunately, all too often mental health professionals have done little to assist women in this regard, because they do in fact censure dissatisfied mothers. This is largely due to another inheritance from Freud. Many clinicians view the primary cause of most mental disorders in their clients as the product of unhappy, inefficient, and unloving mothers. Textbooks are filled with descriptions of "schizophrenogenic" mothers— mothers who are viewed as inducing schizophrenia in their children. Similarly, homosexuality, promiscuity, criminality, and neuroses also are often laid at the door of the mother. Very rarely do we read of "schizophrenogenic" fathers or of any disorder being largely attributed to poor fathering.

Conflicts between motherhood and career.
For women who must work to help support a family, the decision to return to work is not a dilemma. While it may be viewed as unpleasant, a burden, or a relief, it is nonetheless essential. However, women in the middle classes who return to work voluntarily may find the decision conflictual.

Most parents are very concerned about the development of their children. Many are aware of the psychological theory that stresses the importance of the first years of a child's life as a basis for healthy emotional development. This theory has emphasized the importance of the mother's role far more than the father's, and has led many mothers to believe they should devote themselves full time to motherhood. Although we know from clinical work that a consistent loving relationship is crucial to a child's early development, there is no evidence to suggest that the mother's full-time attendance is necessary. However, women often feel guilty or are made to feel guilty by husbands, parents, in-laws, and children who reproach them for leaving home.

Women who bow-under to guilt and remain at home may present themselves to a mental health professional suffering from such problems as depression, isolation, and fears of abusing their children. Those who retain their careers but feel intense guilt may present different types of complaints. Conflicted about their decision, such women often feel guilty for succeeding in their work. Others find their marriages "on the rocks."

The empty nest. Women who retire from the work force to become wives and mothers experience an upheaval when their last child enters school. At this time, some women return to work or school, or become involved in community activities. Others suffer from depression and isolation, and turn to alcohol for comfort (see page 433).

Like many other life stresses, the outcome of this event depends as much on the support system in a woman's life as on her own inner resources. For a woman with marketable skills and a husband who recognizes and supports her need to reenter the work world, this transition may be far easier than for a woman who lacks such skills and support. After a 10- to 15-year absence from jobs or careers, women may find they are unable to compete successfully in today's tight job market.

Divorce. As we have mentioned, women often fare far better than do their ex-husbands after a divorce. However, the stress of ending a marriage is tremendous and often precipitates a major crisis in a woman's life. A woman with young children may face serious economic hardship, especially if her husband was the primary breadwinner or if he is irresponsible in his support payments. Even when an ex-husband is well-intentioned and makes alimony and/or child care payments promptly and regularly, running two households on one salary stresses everyone concerned. In addition, a woman with a family often worries about finding another man who will want her—family and all. This usually compounds the concerns a divorcing woman already has regarding her attractiveness, her ability to sustain a relationship, and her guilt.

In our society, relationships between older men and younger women are tolerated and often encouraged. For younger women, an older, "mature" man may provide economic and social security. An older man, worried about aging, may feel rejuvenated and proud of his capacity to attract a young woman. However, our society has strong proscriptions against relationships between older women and younger men. A "Mrs. Robinson" stereotype prevails in which the older woman is seen as an immoral seductress of the innocent younger male, who is searching for a mother figure. Thus, divorced women in their middle years often accurately perceive a shortage of men whom they find attractive, and who are both available for marriage and attracted to them.

Menopause. The cessation of menstruation is caused by a decrease in sex-hormone production, particularly estrogen output. These changes are often accompanied by both physical and psychological symptoms. Many menopausal women experience breast pains, hot flashes, headaches, and heart pounding, as well as depression, irritability, crying spells, and an inability to concentrate. There is tremendous variation among menopausal women, but most experience some symptoms. In addition to the psychological stress suffered by some women in the realization that they are aging and are no longer able to bear children, research indicates at least some correlation between high estrogen levels and positive mood, versus low estrogen levels and depression. Many women now take estrogen during and after menopause and feel significant relief from the symptoms previously described. However, recent research findings that tentatively link estrogen supplements with a higher incidence of uterine cancer must be considered by any woman who contemplates this form of treatment.

Widowhood. Three times as many women become widowed as men. The death of one's husband is perhaps the greatest psychological stress in the lives of most aging women. The process of mourning and bereavement occurs during the time a woman may be called upon to make a number of practical decisions about settling her husband's estate, where to live, and what to do with the family home and belongings. Often women at first feel numb, and later experience intense sorrow and depression. They may suffer weight loss, insomnia, and irritability. Healthy widows with families and friends who can assist with practical details, listen compassionately, and help shore-up confidence are the ones who make it through this tragedy most successfully. Others who are alone, unhealthy, or without a practical and emotional support system may suffer severe and debilitating depression and a decline in physical health.

These are by no means the only stresses faced by many of today's women, but they are some of the more important ones. In our review of these events, we see more clearly how the same event may cause one woman psychological stress with which she can cope, while precipitating a psychological disorder in another woman with different inner and environmental resources.

Let us turn our attention now to the various types of mental disorders. We will first define and describe the major diagnostic categories and then focus on those disorders most prevalent among women.

Classifying Mental Disorders

Mental health professionals differ widely in their classification of psychological disorders. Some even oppose the attempts to develop standard diagnoses on the grounds that such terminology fails to capture the complexity and uniqueness of each human being. Most professionals, however, believe that some standard diagnostic procedure is necessary, both to treat disorders and to further our knowledge through research. As a result, the American Psychiatric Association adopted a standard classification of mental disorders in 1917. This classification was broadened and

extended with advancing knowledge, and culminated in a Diagnostic and Statistical Manual (DSM) in 1952. A revised DSM II, printed in 1968, is now widely used, although a third edition is being developed. These revised manuals reflect the rapid change in our thinking about mental disorders.

As our classification of mental disorders is modified, so is our understanding of their etiology or causes. For example, schizophrenia is defined as a "functional" psychosis, an illness caused primarily by psychological rather than physiological determinants. Some research now indicates an inherent biological predisposition to schizophrenia, and may in fact ultimately show schizophrenia to be primarily a biochemical, organic illness. Conversely, senile dementia (senility) was once believed to be the sole result of organic degeneration in the central nervous system with age. Recent research indicates that senility is also largely a psychological problem. When "senile" elders are returned to environments where demands are made of them, social contacts increased, and responsibilities restored, we often see remarkable decreases in "senility." Because our understanding of many mental disorders is tentative and rapidly changing, we will primarily describe these mental disorders rather than focus on their underlying causes.

Despite the rapid shifts in the mental health field, the following categories of disorders continue to be widely recognized.

Transient Situational Disturbances

This category is reserved for any relatively brief disorder, regardless of its severity, that occurs in a person who appears to have no underlying mental disorder, and who is reacting to an overwhelming environmental stress. When the stress diminishes, so do the symptoms. As we have mentioned already, women report far more life stresses than do men. Therefore, we might well expect greater numbers of transient situational disturbances in women. In fact, approximately 35 percent more women than men are treated for these disorders. In addition, with the bias toward seeing women as less healthy than men, many women who seek help in the face of acute environmental stress may be misdiagnosed as having more serious underlying disorders.

Neuroses

It is popular today to describe anyone whom we find peculiar as "neurotic." Neurosis, however, is a specific psychiatric diagnosis used to describe a class of disorders characterized by anxiety. People are said to be neurotic if they misperceive the actual demands and problems of everyday living, feel threatened and anxious in situations others would define as nonthreatening, and attempt to cope with this anxiety in disruptive, maladaptive ways. It should be stressed that often the coping mechanisms of neurotic individuals do, in fact, ward off anxiety so well that they do not feel anxious. However, when prevented from using the coping mechanisms they have developed, these individuals quickly feel overwhelming anxiety. Usually, however, it is the coping mechanisms themselves that motivate neurotic individuals to seek professional help. Such mechanisms are often very disruptive and create a whole new set of problems. Individuals with neuroses, unlike individuals with psychoses, are in contact with reality. They often feel unhappy and realize that their coping mechanisms are maladaptive and their fears irrational. Since women are diagnosed as neurotic about 70 percent more often than men, we must take a hard look at these disorders, especially those most often assigned to women.

Anxiety neurosis is characterized by such severe anxiety that it may reach panic proportions. It is often associated with somatic symptoms such as heart pounding, shortness of breath, and nausea. This anxiety appears to be "free-floating" or without specific cause. This must be distinguished from the normal apprehension or fear that all of us experience in realistically dangerous situations.

Hysterical neurosis. There are two types of hysterical neuroses: *conversion type* and *dissociative type*. Both are characterized by an involuntary loss or disorder of a physical function. Symptoms often begin and end quickly in highly emotional situations, and often symbolize the underlying conflicts. For example, a young man has an impulse to stab his father and suddenly his arm becomes paralyzed. If there is no physical explanation for this paralysis, we might diagnose it as a symptom of a *conversion type* of hysterical neurosis. Other typical symptoms include blindness, deafness, and loss of other senses. Often these individuals show an inappropriate lack of concern about their symptoms. This type of disorder must be distinguished from malingering—conscious faking of symptoms. In the *dissociative type* of hysterical neurosis, people experience alterations in consciousness, such as amnesia, sleepwalking, and multiple personalities. The last of these, though common in soap operas, is in fact exceedingly rare.

Phobic neurosis is characterized by extreme fear and avoidance of an object or situation that the person recognizes as harmless. A person may experience faintness, a pounding heart, perspiration, nausea, trembling, and panic when encountering the phobic object or situation. Phobias are viewed by psychoanalytic theorists as fears displaced from an underlying conflict (of which one is unaware) onto the phobic object. For example, a woman harboring an unconscious hostility toward her husband, including a fantasy of drowning him, may suddenly develop a phobia of water. Phobias are viewed by behavioral theorists as faulty learning—generalizing from one frightening experience onto a neutral object or situation. Thus, if a woman presented herself to a behavioral therapist with a phobia of water, the therapist would probably inquire about earlier traumatic experiences involving water or near drownings.

Obsessive-compulsive neurosis is characterized by persistent intrusions of unwanted and uncontrollable thoughts, urges, or actions. A person may continually think about a particular word, idea, or train of thought, often perceived as nonsensical. Uncontrollable actions may vary from simple movements to rituals such as handwashing, counting, and the like. When prevented from performing these acts, the person often feels tremendously anxious, confirming the belief that the purpose of such symptoms is the warding-off of anxiety.

Depressive neurosis. This diagnosis, and all other diagnoses involving depression, are the most commonly applied to women. Women are diagnosed with depressive disorders more than twice as often as men. Symptoms of depression include feelings of extreme sadness, anxiety, sleep disturbances, eating disturbances (under- or overeating), fatigue, irritability, crying spells, a feeling of hopelessness, and often suicidal ideas or attempts. Depressive neurosis is diagnosed when this symptom picture is in reaction, at least in part, to a specific event.

Why is this disorder so much more evident in women than in men? There are two major explanations. First, depression is traditionally viewed as a response to loss. The loss may be of a loved person, a crucial role one has played, one's self-esteem, or loss of meaning in one's life. The point is often made that women are encouraged to invest most of their time and energies into the wife-mother role. Therefore, they suffer a major role loss if their marriages end or if their children leave home. This theory is supported by the fact that depression so often occurs in middle-aged women whose children are leaving home or who have been recently widowed. A second important explanation for the high rates of depression in women involves a hypothesized relationship between depression and anger. According to this view, a normal response to loss involves rage as well as sorrow. In our society, men are more likely to express this rage through antisocial acts, such as aggression, criminality, and alcoholism or drug abuse. Women, on the other hand, are more likely to turn their rage and hostility against themselves, responding to loss or disappointment with depression rather than aggression.

Other neuroses. There are several other less-common neuroses. *Neurasthenic neurosis* is characterized by chronic weakness, fatigue, and exhaustion. *Depersonalization neurosis* is characterized by lasting feelings of unreality, and estrangement from the self, body, or environment (not just one dissociative episode). *Hypochondriacal neurosis* is characterized by a preoccupation with imagined illnesses and diseases. However, there is no actual loss or distortion of physical function as is found in hysterical neurosis.

Personality Disorders

This is a broad diagnostic category used to describe individuals with character disorders, sociopathic disorders, sexual disorders, and addictions to alcohol or drugs. These disorders are grouped together because it is believed that all are characterized by deeply ingrained maladaptive behavior patterns, and that such patterns are "ego-syntonic" to the individual. This means that, unlike neurotics who feel acutely uncomfortable with their symptoms, those individuals diagnosed as having personality disorders have incorporated their symptoms into their total personalities and "styles." This does not mean that these symptoms are unproblematic to these individuals, but rather that they are far more difficult to "cure" because they have become so ingrained in the personality.

As we describe these disorders, we must again remind ourselves that mental health is a continuum. Each of us will recognize aspects of ourselves in the styles of every personality disorder. Such disorders are, in fact, exaggerations of traits that all of us have. However, it is just this exaggeration of traits, *not* the traits themselves, that differentiates individuals with personality disorders from mentally healthy individuals. Although men are diagnosed as having personality disorders more often than women, there is one personality disorder diagnosed far more often in women.

Hysterical personality is probably one of the most overused and misused diagnoses with women. One experienced clinician summed up the situation by commenting, "Hysteria is a diagnosis used by most young male therapists for any reasonably attractive female client." This diagnosis is applied to individuals who are excitable, emotionally unstable, overreactive, and dramatic. It is believed that these symptoms are performed in an attempt to seek attention and to seduce (whether or not the individual recognizes the purposes). Such individuals are described as immature, vain, self-centered, and overly dependent on others. Their style of thinking is often global, diffuse, and impressionistic. They lack the capacity for intense intellectual concentration and are often lacking in intellectual curiosity. Unfortunately, this diagnosis is too often used as a label for any female client who suffers from physical complaints and/or is animated or vivacious. Because this diagnosis is used so loosely, it has lost much meaning and is frequently used inaccurately, divorced from its original intent.

Paranoid personality is characterized by extreme sensitivity, rigidity, and unwarranted suspicion, envy, and jealousy of others. Some individuals diagnosed in this category appear clearly furtive, suspicious, and rigid, while others are more aggressively suspicious, rigidly arrogant, and seem possessed with an excessive sense of self-importance. This is perhaps one of the more serious and certainly painful character disorders, since paranoid characters find it so hard to trust others. They often have poor relationships with family, and very few friends. We must stop for a moment to consider how difficult life with other people becomes if we lack the capacity to trust.

Chronic suspiciousness affects one's entire cognitive style because often this suspicion reflects unrealistic thinking. At the same time, suspiciousness may make an individual extremely perceptive, but only to slights, threats, and other attacks. People suffering from a paranoid disorder are often hyperalert, scrutinizing anything new or unexpected, and seizing only those facts that confirm their suspicions. Often such individuals project onto other people the angry, hostile feelings they cannot tolerate in themselves. This makes it difficult to feel tender, sentimental feelings toward those they now see as hostile and threatening.

Obsessive-compulsive personality is another of the more painful character disorders for both the afflicted individuals and those with whom they live, work, and socialize. Such individuals are noted for excessive concern over conforming to rules and standards, being overly inhibited, overdutiful, conscientious, and rigid. Not surprisingly, they find it extremely difficult to relax. In fact, a famous clinician once described obsessive-compulsive characters as "living machines." Often they are extremely rigid in body posture, social manner, and most of all in their mode of thinking. They appear incapable of seeing things from a different point of view. Whereas most of us can pay attention to what we choose, often obsessive-compulsive individuals seem unable to shift their attention from one aspect of a situation or task to another. They concentrate with great intensity, often on small details. Because of this narrow, intense focus, they often miss many more-obvious aspects of social situations, making them appear insensitive or very unperceptive. Typically such individuals feel compelled to work continuously, often on routine or technical tasks. They seem driven, as if they are pushed by a force other than real interest or enthusiasm. They frequently are motivated by intense feelings of moral responsibility.

Not surprisingly, obsessive characters do not feel free; they feel burdened. In fact, when faced with freedom, especially in the form of choices or decisions, such individuals are unable to cope. They stew incessantly, exhausting themselves as they ponder every aspect of the decision. In general, individuals with obsessive-compulsive character disorders get little enjoyment out of life because it feels unsafe to relax. In addition, there are some important but less common character disorders.

Labile personality is characterized by alternating periods of elation and depression, which appear unrelated to external events. Although such individuals do not suffer as severe a loss of reality as individuals diagnosed as manic-depressive psychotics (to be discussed later), they do experience very disruptive, often painful, frightening mood shifts. When elated, they may feel great warmth, optimism, ambition, and high energy; but when depressed, their moods are dominated by feelings of sadness, worry, pessimism, and low energy.

Schizoid personality is characterized by painful shyness, oversensitivity, avoidance of close relationships, and an apparent lack of interest in people. Often such individuals retreat into a world of daydreaming and fantasy. However, unlike those diagnosed as schizophrenic, schizoid characters can differentiate fantasy from reality. But under environmental stress, these individuals are vulnerable to psychotic episodes.

Dependent personality, often referred to as an "oral-dependent personality," is characterized by excessive reliance on other people. Often such individuals become very anxious when left alone to make decisions, experiencing a sense of abandonment and terror. They appear to lack judgment and resourcefulness, often seeming immature and demanding, as they rely on others for support and guidance.

Narcissistic personality is another diagnostic category that has become so loosely applied that it has lost a great deal of meaning and utility. It has become such a catchall diagnosis that one author described our current culture as a "narcissistic society." This diagnostic category is intended to describe individuals who primarily view all others as need-gratifiers. They are intensely preoccupied with themselves and worry that others will be unable to meet their needs. Because such individuals are so needy, their concerns over abandonment are often borne out, as friends and relatives flee their tremendous demands. This triggers strong criticism and rage from narcissistic characters who are so self-absorbed that they fail to see their own inability to meet the needs of others. Often they appear vain, selfish, egotistical, and sometimes cruel, as they anxiously attempt to fill a void in themselves by using others.

Sociopathic character. In this era of growing violence and cold-blooded, senseless criminality, this disorder is of increasing interest and concern. Although the number of sociopaths (psychopaths) is small, they are of great concern because of the disruption and pain they inflict on others. Unlike most individuals suffering from neuroses and character disorders, these individuals appear totally unperturbed and undistressed by their antisocial behavior. Their total lack of concern for others, their inability to feel loyalty and affection, and their apparent lack of conscience often raise questions about their sanity. Yet they show none of the traditional signs of psychosis. Although they may often be irresponsible, dishonest, and callous, they are in contact with reality, fully oriented, and often emotionally appropriate. Not all sociopaths are violent. Often this tendency is related to upbringing. Those raised in violent homes have an increased tendency to be assaultive, while others from less violent homes perform less violent crimes.

This disorder remains one of the most puzzling to the mental health professions. Sociopaths are often regarded as untreatable. While appearing to progress satisfactorily in therapy, they may nonetheless continue their antisocial activities. They frequently appear friendly, sincere, intelligent, insightful, and quick to instill confidence in others. They often rationalize their behavior by describing their disordered family life and hardships, assert their repentance, and then continue their illegal activities. Despite the amount of media attention focused on such sociopathic characters, they play only a small role in the huge crime problem our nation experiences today.

Sexual disorders. Every culture sanctions certain sexual patterns while labeling others as "deviant." In our society, we are witnessing a widespread challenge to traditional sexual mores. Extramarital and particularly premarital sex are becoming increasingly common. There is decreasing concern over the type of sexual gratification any couple chooses to seek in privacy. Whereas oral-genital contact (oral sex) is still technically illegal in many states, it is no longer viewed within the mental health professions as deviant or disordered. Many other sexual patterns once considered "immoral" or "perverse" are now accepted, or at least are tolerated. Whether to define bisexual and homosexual activity as permissible alternatives to heterosexuality is still debated among the general public as well as in political and mental health circles.

It is difficult to define sexual disorders in such a brief discussion as this. We will not include patterns that may be atypical or morally frowned upon in our society, but that are not inherently maladaptive. For example, depending on our particular religious and moral values, we might define any of the following as perfectly acceptable or as immoral and perverse: premarital sex, extramarital sex, group sex, oral sex, masturbation, bisexuality, and homosexuality. None of these patterns will be defined here as sexual disorders, although many in our society would view them as "deviant." For our purposes, we will examine only two classes of sexual disorders—sexual inadequacy and sexual perversions.

Sexual inadequacy refers to sexual behaviors experienced by an individual as maladaptive and distressing. Feelings of sexual inadequacy are common, but can be very distressing and disruptive to individuals and their sexual partners. This type of sexual disorder often impairs one's desire for sexual contact or one's ability to achieve sexual fulfillment. Typical complaints for women include the following:

• *Orgasmic dysfunction* is a condition in which women cannot achieve orgasm, or can do so only in particular situations. Although "frigidity," a total lack of sexual feelings and responsiveness, is fairly rare, difficulty achieving orgasm is the most common female sexual problem.

• *Dyspareunia* (painful coitus) is a condition that may occur in males as well as females. It is usually due to infections or structural problems of the sex organs, but it often has a psychological base. This is particularly true in women who have been taught that sexual intercourse is frightening, distasteful, or immoral. Dyspareunia is relatively rare.

• *Vaginismus* is an involuntary spasm of the vaginal muscles that prevents penetration and sexual intercourse. This condition is sometimes found in women who are frigid, possibly due to a previous traumatic sexual experience such as rape. However, it also may be found in women who are sexually responsive. Vaginismus, too, is a relatively rare disorder.

Sexual perversions are behaviors that are viewed as pathological by mental health professionals, as well as by the general public. These include patterns that are deviant because of the choice of sex object and/or the mode of gratification.

Sexual perversions that involve *inappropriate sexual objects* include the following:

• *Rape* is defined as sexual intercourse with an unwilling partner. This crime has increased more rapidly than any other violent crime, and is primarily committed by young men in their teens and early 20s. In our society, women have often suffered not only the trauma of being raped, but the subsequent insinuations by police (and all too often by mental health professionals) that they invited the assault. (This notion has evolved primarily from the theory that the normal female is masochistic, which shall be discussed later.)

• *Incest* is defined as sexual relations between parent and child, or between brother and sister. The incest taboo has existed, with only a few exceptions, throughout history and throughout all cultures. There are great risks of infant death, mental retardation, and other birth defects when offspring are produced through incest. However, evidence now indicates that incest in our society is far more common than was once believed.

• *Pedophilia* (child molestation) refers to sexual activity in which the sexual object is a child, male or female. Often this involves manipulation of the genitals, but sometimes with female children, partial or total vaginal penetration occurs. Occasionally, children are forced to manipulate the pedophiliac's sexual organ, or to engage in oral-genital contact. Most pedophiliacs are men, but occasionally women engage in this sexual offense. Girls are sought out as victims about twice as often as boys.

Sexual perversions also may involve *maladaptive modes of gratification.*

• *Exhibitionism* (indecent exposure) involves the intentional exposure of the genitals to members of the opposite sex, in public or under inappropriate circumstances.

• *Voyeurism* (scotophilia) involves seeking sexual gratification through secretly viewing the sexual organs or sexual activities of others. "Peeping Toms" usually focus on females undressing, or on couples engaged in sexual activity, and often masturbate while they watch.

• *Fetishism* involves focusing one's sexual interest on a specific body part or on an inanimate object, such as a piece of clothing. Often the fetishist who is obsessed with the latter will commit crimes such as burglary, robbery, or assault in order to obtain the desired article. Fetishists frequently masturbate in the presence of the fetishistic object.

• *Sadism* involves the obtainment of sexual gratification by inflicting pain, restriction, or humiliation on a sexual partner. The severity of this disorder may vary from relatively harmless biting, pinching, or tying a partner up, to severe whippings, mutilations, and murder.

• *Masochism.* All of the previous sexual disorders occur almost exclusively in men. Masochism is found in both sexes, and involves the obtainment of sexual gratification through suffering pain, restriction, or humiliation. Because sadistic individuals often have masochistic fantasies and vice versa, these disorders are frequently discussed in combination as sado-masochism. Today, sadism is used outside of its sexual connotation to refer to cruelty, while masochism now refers more generally to self-derogation and self-denial. Ever since Freud described the normal female as receptive and passive, masochism has frequently been viewed as "normal" female submission. Too often, the term has been used to explain a female victim's role in rape and sexual abuse. "She asked for it" or "She clearly gets *something* out of it" are not uncommon explanations for the sexual and physical abuse of women.

Here the difference between fantasy and reality cannot be emphasized too strongly! Many women are in fact sexually aroused by masochistic fantasies. Often such fantasies involve being an unwilling or uninvolved sexual partner, such as a slave, prisoner, or prostitute. We live in a society in which women have often been taught that to desire sex is unfeminine or immoral.

Therefore, by fantasizing that one is an unwilling partner, a woman may free a number of sexual restrictions that normally inhibit her sexual gratification. However, though many women enjoy masochistic fantasies, this in no way implies that they enjoy or invite masochistic realities. For mental health professionals, law enforcement officials, and most important, for women themselves, to blur the boundaries between masochistic fantasy and reality is to invite further abuse of women.

Addiction to alcohol and drugs is an ever-increasing problem, and therefore is receiving more and more attention from social scientists, physicians, mental health practitioners, and the media. In the past, dependence on alcohol or drugs (particularly heroin) was viewed as a "moral flaw" or a "sign of weakness." Little attempt was made to treat these problems in any way but legally. In recent years, particularly through the efforts of Alcoholics Anonymous, addictions are now widely viewed as illnesses and/or maladaptive adjustment reactions to stressful life events. With this modern view, we have learned more about the underlying causes of addiction as well as potential treatments. Yet we are far from having systematic, highly successful treatment approaches.

Drug or alcohol "abuse" is defined as excessive use of either substance irregardless of whether one is dependent on it. Drug or alcohol "dependence" is defined as psychological and often physiological dependence. "Addiction" specifically refers to *physiological* dependence.

The most frequently abused drugs are alcohol, barbiturates, heroin, and amphetamines. We will focus here only on the first of these, alcohol, since alcoholism is a rapidly growing problem for American women. Alcoholics are defined by the World Health Organization as excessive drinkers whose dependence on alcohol has reached such extremes that mental and physical health, interpersonal relations, and social and economic functioning are all impaired.

Once considered to be primarily a male disorder, alcoholism is increasingly occurring in women. Since many women, particularly married women, do not work outside the home, their alcoholism is often far better concealed than it is in men. However, some visible signs of a drinking housewife include weight loss, an unkempt appearance, an inability to physically care for her children or to function as a homemaker, and greater susceptibility to physical illnesses, particularly of a urologic or gynecologic nature. Often, a female alcoholic may neglect or abuse her children, or the children's school attendance or grades may suffer.

Alcoholism in the single, working woman may be spotted far more quickly if she is fired. Often women cannot turn to lower-level manual jobs when they are fired from positions of greater authority, as men frequently do. Physical symptoms associated with alcoholism include high blood pressure, ulcers, and diabetes. Of course, such disorders also have other causes besides excessive alcohol consumption.

What causes alcoholism and, in particular, why is it on the rise in women? One suggested explanation involves *low self-esteem.* Many female alcoholics feel inept, inadequate, and futile about their female roles. Studies have shown that women alcoholics feel alienated, socially isolated, anxious, and depressed. (These traits characterize women undergoing treatment for other psychiatric disorders as well.) Most mental health professionals agree that a fairly high level of self-esteem is necessary for adequate functioning. Female alcoholics who suffer from low self-esteem do seem to respond to therapy focused on raising self-esteem.

Some early warning signs of alcoholism include:
● *Increased desire* for alcohol, such as eager anticipation of a drink after work or an increased monitoring of the liquor cabinet supply.
● *Increased consumption,* which may be gradual over a period of months.
● *Memory losses* surrounding drinking binges.
● *Extreme behavior* when under the influence of alcohol, which leaves the drinker feeling embarrassed or guilty.
● *Morning drinking.* This is a crucial indicator of alcoholism, whether the drinker is attempting to "cure" a hangover or "brace" herself for the day to come.

Psychosomatic Disorders

In these disorders, a person responds to anxiety, stress, guilt, anger, and the like with physical illness or disease. These psychosomatic disorders are not imaginary. They are very real and often lead to irreversible organ or tissue damage, even though their origin was emotional rather than organic. It is easy for all of us to understand this class of disorders when we stop to recall the times we have experienced queasy stomachs when upset, headaches when tense, or a shortness of breath when frightened.

Illnesses often viewed as emotional in origin include:
● *Gastrointestinal disorders*—stomach ulcers, colitis, diarrhea, and constipation.
● *Headaches*
● *Respiratory disorders*—bronchial asthma, recurring bronchitis, and hyperventilation syndromes.
● *Skin disorders*—rashes, mouth ulcers, and cold sores.
● *Cardiovascular disorders*—hypertension, irregular heartbeat, heart pain, poor coordination, and migraine headaches.

It is crucial to understand that all of these disorders may be primarily physical in origin rather than emotional. Even when such disorders are based mainly on emotional factors, they often can and should be treated by physical means. However, medical intervention without psychotherapeutic intervention is unlikely to produce lasting benefit in such cases.

A psychosomatic disorder that occurs almost exclusively in women is *anorexia nervosa*. The chief symptom is severe starvation that leads to life-threatening weight loss. In fact, there is a 10 to 15 percent mortality rate associated with this disorder. Anorexia nervosa usually occurs in middle- and upper-class females, who are often bright, attractive adolescents. It also may begin in preadolescence and adulthood. Physical symptoms include amenorrhea (cessation of menstruation), increased activity, and a lowered body temperature. Psychological symptoms include a loss or denial of appetite, an obsessional pursuit of thinness and a terror of gaining weight, a distorted body image (a 75-pound adolescent may see herself as obese), a struggle for control, and a sense of powerlessness.

Although the cause of anorexia nervosa continues to baffle mental health practitioners, some theories have been developed. One theory asserts that anorexia follows childhood obesity. A young girl goes from one extreme to another as a result of being ridiculed for her fatness. Another theory connects sexual fears with anorexia nervosa. A young adolescent female, who is newly menstruating, unconsciously links eating with impregnation. She stops eating, loses weight, and ceases to menstruate. Thus, the budding young woman soon looks like a much younger child. A third theory associates anorexia with overintrusive, dominating parents. The young girl, who previously has been obedient and compliant, asserts her independence in this masochistic fashion. These are only a few of the many explanations currently being considered.

Often anorexia progresses to the point where the young girl must be hospitalized and fed intravenously. In addition to medical care, intensive psychotherapy usually is required. Often such psychotherapy involves family members as well as the young girl.

Our society focuses a great deal of attention on the young female figure. Magazines feature skinny models in clothes that look wonderful only on stick figures. Ads claim that, if the young woman will only drink the right diet drink, attend the right weight clinic, buy the correct exercise gadget, she, too, will develop the perfect shape. Busy adolescent girls with big appetites often find that dieting becomes a major concern. They may attempt fad diets, including starvation and rigorous exercise programs. Others may decide to enjoy food without paying the price of weight gain by inducing vomiting after eating.

Although these behaviors may concern parents and young women themselves, they should not be confused with anorexia nervosa. These crash diets, exercise programs, and splurge-vomiting binges are usually under control. A girl will cease when she has achieved the weight or size she wishes to be, or when she tires of the whole process. However, when a girl's perception becomes so distorted that she feels obese when she is in fact underweight, this is cause for greater concern.

Psychoses

People are described as psychotic when their psychological functioning is so impaired that their daily-life coping capacities are grossly affected. Their impairment may involve a serious distortion of reality. Hallucinations (the perception of voices, objects, people, and events that are not present) and delusions (beliefs maintained despite their logical absurdity or their lack of foundation in reality) are two primary examples of perceptual distortion. Psychotic impairment also may be manifested by inexplicable and dramatic mood alterations that prevent a person from responding appropriately to social stimuli. Other psychotic symptoms include language and memory deficits, a blunting of emotions, disorientation, a lack of insight, poor judgment, and impaired social relationships.

Traditionally, two classes of psychoses have been defined. *"Organic"* psychoses are those mental disorders for which physical cause has been firmly established. Alcoholism, drug addiction, injuries, brain tumors, hardening of the arteries, and thyroid and kidney disease all may cause serious psychological disorders. The second class of psychoses, the *"functional"* psychoses, are those disorders for which physical causes have not yet been firmly established. In the past, these disorders were said to be psychologically determined. Today, however, with advancing knowledge, many professionals believe that a number of the so-called "functional" psychoses may well have organic, biochemical causes that simply are not yet fully understood. Let us first discuss this latter category, which includes schizophrenia and the major affective disorders (mania, depression, manic-depressive illness, and involutional melancholia.)

Schizophrenia is the diagnosis used to describe a large group of psychotic disorders with a number of shared characteristics, including: withdrawal from social interaction; fragmented and disorganized thought, emotion, and perception; a blunted affect; and very little insight. A classic symptom of schizophrenia is "thought broadcasting"—the belief that one's thoughts are being transmitted and heard by others. Other diagnostic signs include a depressed or bland facial expression, poor rapport with people, incoherent speech, bizarre and often destructive delusions (such as the belief that one's body is dissolving), trouble sleeping (particularly early waking), and hallucinations (usually auditory).

Although schizophrenia sometimes occurs in childhood, a large majority of first-time hospital admissions for this disorder are in people ages 15 to 45. Statistics from the 1960s indicated that slightly more women than men develop schizophrenic disorders, of which there are many types.

In *paranoid schizophrenia,* people may be governed by illogical, often absurd delusions of persecution. Such individuals often feel that they are being watched, followed, talked about, poisoned, or plotted against. Frequently, they explain these persecutions by developing delusions of grandeur: "I am being followed because I am the unrecognized ruler of the world." Such delusions are sometimes accompanied by vivid hallucinations. In general, there is less extreme social withdrawal than in other types of schizophrenia, although social functioning is obviously impaired.

In *hebephrenic schizophrenia,* people may be inappropriately silly, develop peculiar mannerisms, and behave in a bizarre and often obscene fashion. This more serious type of schizophrenia often develops at an earlier age than other types.

There are two subtypes of *catatonic schizophrenia: excited catatonia,* characterized by excessive and often violent motor activity, and *withdrawn catatonia,* characterized by sudden loss of all movement and animation, and by periods of stupor lasting for moments, hours, or even days.

In *simple schizophrenia,* people appear isolated, uninteresting, colorless, and inaccessible. This type comes to the attention of mental health practitioners less often than other types because there is less personality disorganization and some superficial contact with reality. Frequently, such individuals will live as vagabonds and hermits with minimal social contact.

The causes of schizophrenia are still unclear, but theories have emphasized three possible explanations:
- *Psychological factors*—focused on pathological family patterns, early deprivation, and excessive life stresses.
- *Sociocultural factors*—focused on the role of pathological social conditions.
- *Biological factors*—focused on the genetic, biochemical, and neurophysiological predispositions to schizophrenia.

Affective psychoses are those disorders characterized by extreme, inappropriate emotional responses and mood swings. Extreme depression, excitement (mania), or alternation between the two are the most common affective disorders within this class. Far more women than men are diagnosed with affective psychoses.

Manic-depressive psychosis—manic type is frequently characterized by a euphoric, elated mood, great sociability, and tremendous impatience when criticized or restrained. Individuals in extreme manic states may appear hyperactive and indefatigable, with a decreased need for sleep, an increased interest in sex, and a variable appetite. Often they have grandiose delusions about themselves, are unable to concentrate because their thoughts race so quickly, and are impulsive and extremely talkative.

Manic-depressive psychosis—depressive type is characterized by social withdrawal, irritability, and feelings of hopelessness and despondency. Depressed individuals experience decreased physical activity,

fatigue, insomnia, a loss of appetite, and a decreased sex drive. Often they suffer from delusions that they are incurably ill, have greatly sinned, or are headed for a major disaster. They may exaggerate personal and world problems, worrying excessively and blaming themselves irrationally.

Manic-depressive psychosis—circular type is characterized by at least one episode of both depression and mania.

Like schizophrenia, the causes of manic-depressive disorders are largely unknown. Research has demonstrated that psychological, sociocultural, and biological factors all play some role. However, it is unclear which causes are primary and which are secondary.

Involutional melancholia is differentiated from other depressive reactions by its time of origin—during the climacteric (change of life). Professionals debate whether to maintain this as a separate diagnosis from the other depressive disorders because its symptoms are so similar.

Involutional melancholia is diagnosed over three times more often in women than in men. The onset is gradual. Individuals begin to feel irritable, pessimistic, and restless. Often they have trouble falling asleep. They may worry excessively or cry for no apparent reason. A great sense of hopelessness prevails. As the disorder worsens, individuals become increasingly anxious, depressed, and guilt-ridden. They may begin to complain of somatic problems and delusions ("My insides are drying up." "My brain is dissolving."). Without treatment, this disorder often runs a long course.

Women who develop involutional melancholia sometimes do so during menopause. However, the type of menopausal depression described earlier is quite different from involutional melancholia. The latter is far more serious and does not respond to estrogen treatment as menopausal depression so often does.

Organic brain syndrome. Now let us turn our attention to those psychoses in which organic causes have been well established. Injuries, disease, and certain chemicals may affect the brain, causing abnormal thinking and behavior. Approximately one-fourth of psychiatric hospital admissions are due to disorders associated with brain pathology. Such disorders may stem from infection, brain tumors, head injuries, endocrine disorders, postpartum reactions, alcohol or drug toxicity, reactions to surgery, and finally, deterioration of the central nervous system with advancing age.

Brain infections. A number of psychological disorders are associated with *infections of the brain* that destroy neural tissue. Such infections may be bacterial or viral, and include cerebral syphilis and encephalitis.

Brain tumors. A tumor involves an abnormal growth or enlargement of body tissue. Often tumors appear in the G.I. tract, the breast, and the uterus. Sometimes they appear in the central nervous system. Benign brain tumors disrupt functioning only by virtue of causing increased pressure within the skull. Malignant tumors destroy the neural tissue in which they grow. The psychological and physical effects of a brain tumor depend on its location, size, and rate of growth.

Head injuries often occur as a result of auto and other accidents, falls, or blows to the head. Usually they do not result in serious brain damage. However, in severe injuries in which there is a great deal of bleeding, more serious, permanent damage may result. As with brain tumors, the psychological and physical effects of a head injury depend on the site of the injury, its severity, and the amount of time before treatment can be administered.

Endocrine disorders. Endocrine glands produce hormones that are necessary for normal physiological and psychological functioning. Under- or overactivity of any endocrine gland may disturb psychological well-being. The most common endocrine disorders that affect psychological health are thyroid and adrenal disorders.

The thyroid gland regulates body metabolism. It influences one's growth rate and the development of intelligence. Thyroid dysfunction may involve the underproduction or overproduction of the thyroid hormone thyroxine. Underproduction or hypothyroidism is usually associated with an iodine deficiency. In infancy, it may cause *cretinism* — with physical dwarfing and mental retardation of the child. In adults, hypothyroidism causes *myxedema* — in which a slowed metabolism causes weight gain and sluggishness. Psychotic depression may result, as well as slowed physical and mental functioning.

Hyperthyroidism, the oversecretion of thyroxin, accelerates body metabolism, resulting in insomnia, emotional excitability, and decreased concentration, as well as weight loss and tremors. When psychotic symptoms occur, they often include transitory delusions and hallucinations, as well as severe agitation and anxiety.

The adrenal glands, located over the kidneys, are paired glands with two major parts. The *adrenal medulla* secretes adrenaline and noradrenaline, which affect neural functioning and emotion. The *adrenal* cortex secretes steroid hormones called *corticoids,* which affect body metabolism and activity and secondary sexual characteristics. Undersecretion of the adrenal cortex may cause *Addison's disease,* involving many metabolic as well as psychological disturbances. A person with Addison's disease suffers lower blood pressure and body temperature, and skin darkening, as well as fatigue, anemia, irritability, a decreased appetite, and general listlessness. Hypersecretion of the adrenal cortex may cause a variety of disturbances, including: *Cushing's syndrome* — excessive cortisone causes muscle weakness, fatigue, obesity, and spinal curvatures. *Feminism* — an excessive corticoid production in men causes an increased estrogen output and subsequent development of female characteristics. *Virilism* — an excessive corticoid production in women causes an increased androgen output and subsequent development of male characteristics (breast shrinking, voice deepening, increased body hair, etc.). Hypersecretion of corticoids in children may cause *puberty praecox* — early sexual maturation.

With all of these adrenal disturbances, psychotic symptoms also may result. Severe mental disturbances are rare in Addison's disease but common in Cushing's syndrome. As in other endocrine disturbances, the psychiatric symptoms may not subside once the adrenal disturbance is medically treated. Additional psychotherapy often is needed.

Postpartum disorders. Pregnancy and childbirth bear a relationship to psychological disturbances. Some research indicates a lower risk of psychosis in pregnant women. After childbirth, however, there is a significantly increased risk of psychosis. In approximately one out of every 360 births, mothers suffer a postpartum psychosis. A majority of such psychotic reactions occur in the first postpartum month. Many women suffer postpartum "blues," a mild depression after birth. Such "blues" are easily distinguished from postpartum psychosis, which is characterized by deep depression, physical inactivity, listlessness, and dejection. A mother may appear disinterested in her new infant or hostile toward both spouse and infant. Often such disinterest and hostility mask tremendous fears of unworthiness and inadequacy as a mother. Such severe depression may result in suicide, infanticide, or both, and must be taken very seriously.

Traditionally, postpartum psychosis has been described as resulting from psychological and sociocultural factors. Such theories have emphasized the role of immaturity, an unstable marriage, a rejection of feminine and maternal roles, financial crisis, and physical illness of mother or baby. Often postpartum depression has been defined as a severe guilt reaction by a mother who feels ambivalent about her marriage and child.

Recently, however, more attention is being given to physiological explanations. Childbirth is accompanied by extreme, sudden changes in estrogen and progesterone levels. Such changes may trigger brief psychotic depressions that occur soon after delivery and are of short duration. This theory is supported by the fact that most postpartum psychoses are self-limiting. With some assistance, over 90 percent of women recover in very short periods.

Toxic psychoses are disorders caused by various toxins (poisons), metabolic disorders, or nutritive deficiencies that adversely affect the brain. A common toxic psychosis is *delirium* accompanying various diseases such as diphtheria, uremia, and pneumonia. Deliria may also result from severe exhaustion, as well as ingestion of certain drugs, metals, and alcohol.

Alcoholic *delirium tremens* (dt's) are fairly common in chronic heavy drinkers who are unable to obtain alcohol or who receive head injuries or develop infections. Symptoms include disorientation of time and place; acute fear; tremors of hands, tongue, and lips; fever; rapid and weak heartbeat; coated tongue; and vivid hallucinations. Often these hallucinations are of small fast-moving creatures such as roaches or bugs scurrying over one's body.

Another common psychosis associated with alcoholism is *Korsakoff's syndrome,* characterized by a memory deficit for recent events. Sufferers may be unable to recognize people, objects, and places they have just seen. Often people with Korsakoff's syndrome attempt to mask this deficit by falsification. Such individuals fill in their memory gaps by weaving fanciful tales. Korsakoff's syndrome is due to deficiencies in Vitamin B and other dietary inadequacies. Even when a healthy diet is restored, however, frequently there is permanent memory and intellectual impairment.

Postoperative psychosis is a class of disorders that arise after surgery. Symptoms often include depression, anxiety, delusions, hallucinations, and bizarre behavior. Various theories explain this type of psychosis as the result of psychological stress, medication, biological trauma, or a combination of all three. Increased pre- and postsurgical psychotherapy, along with improved surgical techniques, have decreased the incidence of this disorder. However, elderly people are more susceptible than others to postsurgical psychosis.

Psychoses of the elderly include *senile dementia* and *psychosis with cerebral arteriosclerosis.*

Senile dementia is associated with atrophy and degeneration of the brain. More women than men are diagnosed with this disorder, primarily because women are outliving men. The onset of senile dementia is gradual, and symptoms vary tremendously from one individual to the next. Typical symptoms include social withdrawal, narrowed interests, preoccupation with bodily functioning (eating, excretion, etc.), decreased mental alertness, and decreased tolerance of change in daily routine.

There are five types of senile dementia. The *simple type* involves a gradual loss of contact with reality, memory loss, disorientation, restlessness, insomnia, and poor judgment. This is by far the most common type of senile dementia. The *paranoid type* involves delusions of persecution. Often individuals with this type of senile dementia remain more alert and oriented. The *depressed, agitated type* often involves hypochondriacal delusions, as well as delusions of impending disaster and poverty. Such individuals frequently feel they are terrible sinners and will be punished. The *delirious, confused type* often involves extreme mental disorientation, confusion, incoherence, and restlessness. Such delirious states are often precipitated by accidents or illness. The *presbyophrenic type* often involves marked memory loss with subsequent fabrication; a jovial, amiable mood; rambling discourse; and restless activity.

Although senile dementia is largely based on organic deterioration, a growing body of research indicates that psychological and sociocultural factors play important roles. When the elderly remain active, in positions of control and responsibility, senile dementia is greatly reduced.

Psychoses with cerebral arteriosclerosis are similar to senile dementia, with several important anatomical and behavioral differences. A "hardening" of the brain's arteries involves an accumulation of fatty materials in cerebral blood vessels. These interfere with circulation, and often cause one of the following: *cerebral thrombosis* (blood clots that block blood vessels); *cerebral embolism* (fragments of hardened material that block blood flow); or *narrowing of vessels* (with accumulation of deposits).

Such conditions may cause an inadequate blood supply to the brain, or the rupturing of a small blood vessel and a cerebral hemorrhage, often called a *small stroke.* When individuals suffer a series of small strokes, frequently there is cumulative damage and gradual personality change.

If a large blood vessel ruptures, an individual suffers a *major stroke* or a cardiovascular accident (CVA). Those who survive such massive strokes often have at least some residual brain damage.

In cerebral arteriosclerosis, psychosis symptoms often appear rapidly and include disorientation, incoherence, a clouded consciousness, and often hemiplegia (paralysis of one side of the body). Confusion may last for a long time.

When symptoms evolve more gradually, they often begin with weakness, fatigue, depression, memory defects, headaches, and periods of confusion. Later, individuals become irritable and emotionally unstable. They also may become paranoid.

We have just explored a wide range of mental disorders. The mental health professions encompass an equally broad range of practitioners and facilities with which to treat psychologically disturbed individuals. As already pointed out, there are a variety of treatment approaches and philosophies within the mental health profession. Let us examine *who* provides mental health services, the *settings* in which they are provided, and the *philosophies of treatment.*

Treatment of Disorders

Mental Health Professionals

Mental health practitioners come from a variety of educational and clinical training backgrounds.

Psychiatric social workers complete a two-year master's degree program, receiving M.S.W. degrees. They usually receive far more training than other mental health professionals in community work. They are most familiar with community resources and social agencies. In addition, many M.S.W.s are psychotherapists who see individuals, families, and groups.

Clinical psychologists usually obtain Ph.D. degrees that necessitate at least four to five years of graduate training, culminating in a major piece of original research in the field. Many clinical psychologists are experts in psychological diagnosis and assessment, as well as psychotherapy. In addition, many become professors of clinical psychology at the university level.

Psychiatrists first obtain M.D. degrees by completing four years of medical training. After completing an internship year, doctors who wish to become psychiatrists must complete another three years of psychiatric specialization. Psychiatrists are usually less knowledgeable than M.S.W.s about community resources, and are far less knowledgeable than Ph.D.s about assessment and research techniques. However, as M.D.s, they are best equipped to diagnose medical problems that are often intermingled with psychological problems. They are the only mental health practitioners who may prescribe drugs.

Psychoanalysts are usually psychiatrists (M.D.s), though some are psychologists (Ph.D.s) who have trained at a Psychoanalytic Institute.

In recent years, there has been increasing experimentation in training mental health professionals. Several schools now produce Doctors of Psychology (Psy.D.) who receive more clinical training and less research training than Ph.D.s.

A new mental health profession, a Doctor of Mental Health (D.M.H.) is tbe most recent newcomer to the field. Doctor of Mental Health training is a composite of psychiatric, psychological, and social work training, borrowing relevant portions of each to produce a new breed of mental health professional.

Many other professionals work in the mental health field. Psychiatric nurses have R.N. degrees with a specialty in psychiatry. School, vocational, and rehabilitation counselors always have B.A. and usually M.A. degrees in psychology, education, or counseling. Generally, their focus is on helping clients to adjust socially, academically, or vocationally. Psychiatric occupational therapists (O.T.s) have professional degrees and usually work in hospital settings, helping people to recover from and adjust to illnesses, accidents, and life stresses. Many ministers and community religious leaders also provide counseling. Dance, drama, art, and music therapists treat people through artistic expression. Their knowledge of psychology and mental health varies.

In this era of paraprofessionalism, psychiatric aides, who have high school degrees and often some college education, are trained to perform specific tasks within mental health facilities. They may assist therapists in community settings, inpatient units, rehabilitation programs, or crisis clinics.

Mental Health Facilities

There are three major classes of mental health facilities: inpatient hospital settings, nonhospital residential treatment programs, and outpatient facilities.

Inpatient hospital units include publicly funded local and state hospitals as well as private hospitals. Usually, locally funded general hospitals provide psychiatric care only on a short-term basis. When individuals need long-term hospitalization, they are usually admitted to private or state psychiatric facilities, depending on their financial resources.

Residential programs are available in many areas for people who, although ready to leave a hospital, are not ready to function independently. Such programs, often called "halfway houses," provide people with a place to stay, regular meals, and often social programs while they readjust to the community, look for work, or continue their vocational training. These programs often serve ex-drug addicts and alcoholics.

Outpatient services are provided by public and private hospitals, community mental health clinics, and private therapists. In recent years, many clinics have been established to deal specifically with drug addicts, alcoholics, and people suffering from sexual problems. High schools and universities have traditionally provided counseling for confused or troubled students. Now there are increasing numbers of counseling centers for women, often (but not necessarily) providing a feminist perspective. Counseling centers for homosexuals also are becoming more popular.

To locate a mental health professional or facility, one can call a local Mental Health Association, Family Service Agency, or the family physician.

Treatment Philosophies and Modes

There are as many types of mental health treatments as there are mental health practitioners. Let us examine a few of the major types of psychological intervention and treatment that are available.

Counseling. Whether in a school, rehabilitation center, clinic, or the like, counseling usually offers a mixture of education, advice, reassurance, and support. Often intervention is focused on particular issues and concerns, and frequently is time-limited.

Behavior therapy is based on the idea that abnormal as well as normal behavior is *learned.* Behavior therapists believe all nonorganic psychological disorders are the result of maladaptive learning. Treatment is focused on the *present,* not on the past. Insight and awareness of one's internal state are often considered irrelevant. Therapists using this model define a client's problems in terms of overt behaviors, not internal feelings. For example, behavior therapists would not treat a person for "depression," but would ask for the behavioral manifestations of this depression (insomnia, loss of appetite, or crying spells) and would treat these.

Exploratory therapies, including psychoanalytic, Jungian, humanistic, and existential techniques, are all derived from Freudian psychoanalytic theory. All these psychotherapies utilize patient-therapist dialogue as the basis for treatment. Some therapists see couples, families, and groups; but since internal exploration is a major goal, individual therapy is often preferred by these therapists. They share a number of therapeutic goals. These include increased insight and understanding of one's mental and emotional life, changing maladaptive behavior patterns, resolving disabling inner conflicts, altering inaccurate assumptions about oneself and one's world, and—hopefully—the alleviation of psychological distress. Psychoanalysts, in particular, place top priority on enhancing insight, believing that ultimately greater self-understanding will lead to improved functioning.

Interpersonal techniques, such as group, family, and marital therapies, focus on interaction and relationships between people. These therapists define pathology not within individuals but within social systems. By addressing faulty communication patterns, such practitioners assist clients in their interpersonal, family, and marital relationships. The majority of people receiving professional psychological assistance are in some form of group therapy.

Experiential techniques such as dance, drama, art, and music therapies are becoming increasingly popular, particularly in this era of holistic health. Our society is just beginning to take interest in the relationship of body, mind, and spirit, unlike Eastern cultures that traditionally have viewed people more holistically. Experiential therapies are based on the idea that by improving one's sense of physical well-being and by employing one's creative, artistic spirit, psychological well-being is enhanced.

Gestalt therapy bridges the gap between traditional verbal therapies and more physical, experiential techniques. The word "gestalt" means "whole," and gestalt therapy emphasizes the unity of mind and body, stressing integration of feeling, thought, and action. Although gestalt therapy is usually done in a group, focus remains on individual awareness. Members may be asked to act out fantasies, feelings, and conflicts with one another, switching roles from time to time.

Physical (somatic) therapies most commonly include chemotherapy (drug treatment) and electroconvulsive therapy (ECT).

The most commonly used drugs for psychological disorders are antipsychotics (major tranquilizers), antianxiety drugs (minor tranquilizers), and antidepressants. These drugs, particularly the antipsychotics, have made it possible for many individuals who once would have been permanently hospitalized, to function in the community. However, there are many limitations and complications, including a variety of possible side effects, associated with most psychiatric drugs.

Recently, the wide misuse and overuse of minor tranquilizers has received national attention. Antianxiety medications have been prescribed at such a high rate that the United States government has placed restrictions and controls on some of these minor tranquilizers.

Electroconvulsive therapy involves the use of electroshock to treat seriously depressed individuals. No one knows why or how ECT works, but it does. It is particularly helpful for quick alleviation of depression in suicidal individuals. Antidepressant drugs take far longer to work. In addition, taken in an overdose they can be lethal. Therefore, suicidal individuals cannot be given anitdepressants except in a controlled hospital setting.

It seems fitting to conclude this chapter with a description of a new type of psychotherapy relevant to women, *feminist therapy.* Feminist therapists often direct their attention to social and political action, alleviating sexism in the mental health professions, and educating women about the role of sex bias in their lives. Many such therapists allocate maximum power to their female clients within therapy, in order to enhance self-determination. For example, some feminist therapists offer "leaderless groups" in which they do not take an active, dominant role.

The feminist therapy movement has an important message for all women, whether they choose to define themselves as feminists, traditionalists, or somewhere in between. Just as women are taking more control over the many facets of their physical health, they can and *should* exercise more control over their psychological and emotional well-being.

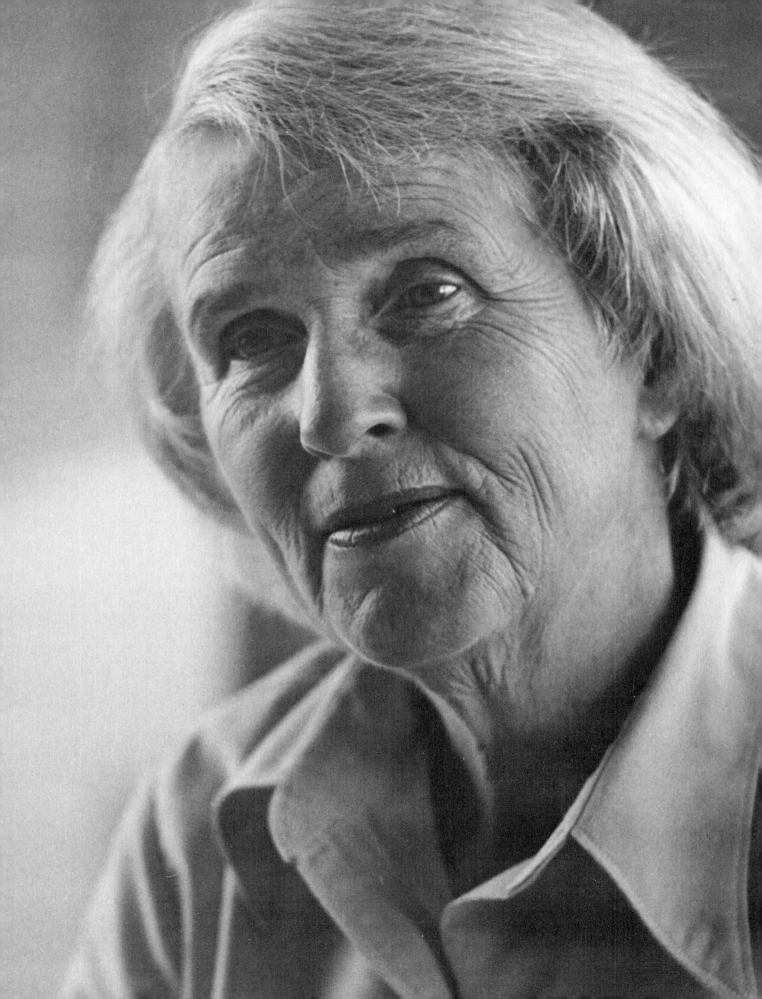

CHAPTER 22

ADULT REPRODUCTIVE PROBLEMS

LUCIENNE T. LANSON, M.D., F.A.C.O.G.

At some point in her life, almost every woman consults a gynecologist about a reproductive system problem. For this reason, it is wise to understand how the reproductive system functions in health and disease, and to distinguish between normal conditions and those that require professional care. Such a knowledge will help you discuss this important body system with your physician with accuracy and confidence.

Irritations and Infections

All women are bothered at some time in their lives with irritations and infections of the genital organs. While most of these problems are relatively harmless, they almost inevitably are embarrassing to women, and therefore quite often are not treated. To help you recognize these conditions and feel comfortable discussing them with your doctor, this section presents some typical examples—beginning first with the vulva, and then proceeding to the vagina, cervix, uterus, tubes, and ovaries.

The Vulva

Skin Disturbances

Itching of the vulva no doubt is one of the most common female complaints. The cause is frequently traced to an irritating vaginal discharge, but there are other reasons for vulvar itching, too.

Contact or allergic dermatitis, for example, is a condition seen by doctors with increasing frequency. Initially, symptoms of contact dermatitis may be mild—nothing more than a slight itching and redness of the vulvar skin. Severe reactions could include marked swelling of the labial lips with an eruption of tiny blisters that eventually drain and crust over.

If you have sensitive skin (or if you are an allergic person), exposure to any number of substances may trigger acute vulvar irritation. For example, washing with a strongly alkaline and antibacterial soap is a common cause. Soap can hide between labial folds and lead to irritation and itching. Bubble bath products, particularly when used by young girls, have been responsible for acute inflammations of the vulva. Other products capable of causing dermatitis include nail polishes, perfumes, hygiene spray deodorants, douche ingredients, vaginal foams, condoms, sanitary napkins, and synthetic fibers in underwear. Even the use of colored toilet paper can evoke an allergic reaction in women sensitive to the dye. Common medications also can occasionally cause acute vulvitis. Some known culprits are aspirin, phenacitin, sulfa drugs, and phenolphthalein (an ingredient in many laxative preparations).

Correcting the problem depends on identifying the irritant or allergen and then avoiding it. In the meantime, don't use soap and hot water because they only aggravate the condition. For temporary relief of contact dermatitis, use cool compresses of boric acid (one tablespoon per quart of water) three or four times a day. Also, you could try soaking in a cornstarch bath (two cups of cornstarch in half a tub of lukewarm water) twice a day. Afterwards, be sure to gently pat yourself dry (no rubbing). Also, you should avoid wearing nylon underwear and pantyhose. Instead, slip into some loose-fitting white cotton underwear. If additional relief is needed, your doctor could prescribe a soothing cortisone ointment or cream to apply locally. In severe cases, antihistamines (as well as cortisone) taken orally for a few days may be necessary.

If the itching seems to be more confined to the rectal area, the possibility of hemorrhoids, rectal polyps, or even infestation by pinworms should be considered. Anal itching also can be caused by traces of fecal material trapped within one of the anal folds. Washing the area with a cotton ball soaked with cool water (or preferably witch hazel) after each bowel movement usually will solve the problem.

Chronic vulvar itching, particularly in older women, deserves special attention. Estrogen withdrawal at menopause ultimately thins the vulvar and vaginal tissues, making them more susceptible to trauma and infection. Any irritation (especially itching) should be treated promptly to avoid a chronic debilitating problem. Itching leads to scratching. Scratching causes breaks in the skin that can lead to more inflammation and infection. If the vulvar skin loses pigmentation or if white patches appear, it is a sign of chronic vulvar irritation. The fact is, cancer of the vulva frequently is preceded by a history of chronic vulvar itching, so this symptom should not be ignored. Local treatment for relief of these symptoms can be helpful if the condition is diagnosed early. Sometimes the application of estrogenic creams can control the symptoms and eliminate the itching. Skin lesions or sores that fail to heal promptly should, of course, be biopsied and examined for cancer.

Pediculosis pubis, infestation of the hair of the vulva with crabs, is another frequent cause of itching. Although this six-legged louse also can infest axillary hair and eyebrows, it is irresistibly drawn to pubic hair. Most cases of crabs are acquired through sexual intercourse with a person harboring the parasite. Less commonly, physical contact with contaminated articles such as sheets, blankets, sleeping bags, and toilets may invite a louse invasion. Indeed, some women have acquired the culprit from trying on swimsuits at their favorite apparel shop.

The first symptom of crabs is a maddening itch over the affected area. The itching is worse at night and is apparently caused by a noxious substance excreted into the skin by this mini-vampire. Since the crab louse requires human blood for survival, it latches on by piercing the skin and burying its head inside a pubic hair follicle. At times, the bite can result in an inflammatory skin reaction (bluish gray in color).

Diagnosis is made by spotting one of the crabs. An average infestation has about six or seven adult crabs. Each crab louse measures only about 1.2 mm in diameter, so you may need a magnifying glass for identification. Other telltale signs are eggs or nits, seen as tiny white oval specks usually attached to the base of the hair near the skin.

Fortunately, pubic lice are not carriers of disease. They can be easily eliminated without resorting to shaving or the use of questionable (and potentially irritating) local medications. The best treatment for crabs is the prescription drug Kwell, which is available as a shampoo or as a lotion or cream. A four-minute shampoo of pubic hair with Kwell, followed by a thorough drying, will eliminate most infestations. The crabs die and the nits can be removed by a fine-tooth comb. If you use Kwell cream or lotion, liberally apply it over the pubic area and leave it on for 24 hours. The cream or lotion has the added advantage of being able to kill lice on clothing. If a repeat treatment of Kwell is necessary, it's best to wait four days before reapplying.

If you are embarrassed about visiting your doctor because you suspect you have crabs, your doctor most likely will phone a prescription in to a drugstore for you. Or, you can visit your local public health or venereal disease clinic.

Be careful that you don't immediately become reinfected with lice. Your toilet seat should be carefully scrubbed, and your sexual partner also should be treated with Kwell. All clothing, bedding, or anything that might have been contaminated with crabs or nits should be laundered (in boiling water) or dry-cleaned.

THE FEMALE REPRODUCTIVE SYSTEM

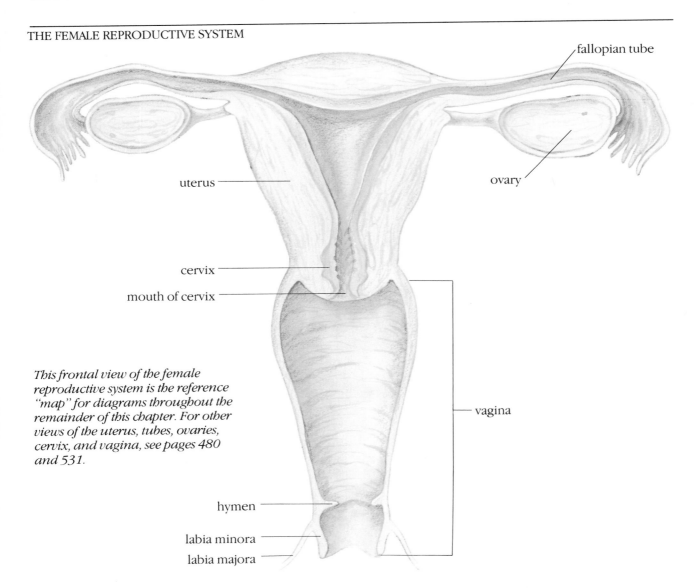

This frontal view of the female reproductive system is the reference "map" for diagrams throughout the remainder of this chapter. For other views of the uterus, tubes, ovaries, cervix, and vagina, see pages 480 and 531.

fallopian tube

ovary

uterus

cervix

mouth of cervix

vagina

hymen

labia minora

labia majora

If you can't afford a large cleaning bill, there is an alternative. Since the nits hatch in ten days and adult crabs die within 24 hours if deprived of human blood, all articles will become crab-free if left undisturbed and free from human contact for at least two weeks.

Cysts of the Vulva

A sebaceous cyst of the vulva is a cystic tumor of the skin. The cyst usually forms because a duct or outlet of an oil (sebaceous) gland (see page 564) is blocked. As a consequence, the oily material within the gland accumulates and forms into a rounded, non-tender swelling of varying size. Most vulvar sebaceous cysts grow slowly, tend to remain small, and usually appear along the inner margins of the labia majora. Sometimes they may disappear spontaneously or, more commonly, remain in place without ever causing problems. If one of these cysts is drained or squeezed, a grayish white, frequently malodorous, cheesy material is extruded. These cysts do not become malignant, but they can become infected and form into a painful abscess. Incision and drainage provide temporary relief, but a permanent cure would require surgical removal of the entire cyst and its surrounding sac.

Epidermal cysts are also cystic tumors of the skin. They are even more common than sebaceous cysts and are frequently mistaken for them. Since epidermal cysts

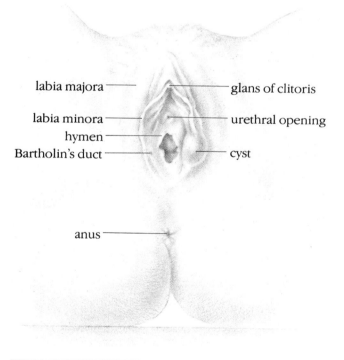

labia majora — glans of clitoris
labia minora — urethral opening
hymen
Bartholin's duct — cyst
anus

WHERE VULVAR CYSTS MAY FORM

Cysts of the vulva may form along the margins of the labia majora due to blockage of an oil gland (sebaceous cyst) or blockage of a mucus gland (Bartholin's duct cyst). A third type of cyst, and the most common, is an epidermal cyst.

usually remain asymptomatic, treatment is rarely required. However, if they should cause problems or become infected, they, too, require surgical excision.

Bartholin's duct cyst. Bartholin's glands are two mucus-producing glands that help lubricate the lower vagina. The main duct of each gland empties just outside the vaginal opening. Ordinarily, the glands are too small to be seen or felt on a routine pelvic examination. Cysts form when a duct becomes plugged, causing mucus secretions to accumulate and creating a non-tender swelling that can be as small as a marble or as large as a hen's egg. In extreme cases, a Bartholin's duct cyst may be large enough to block the vaginal opening. Why these ducts become blocked frequently is unknown, but infection, trauma, and even congenital narrowing of the duct have been implicated.

If a cyst remains small and isn't causing problems, most doctors advise leaving it alone. Some cysts require surgical treatment, however—especially those that cause pressure because of size, interfere with intercourse, or become a source of recurrent abscess formation. Simple drainage isn't very effective, because the cyst could promptly return. Good-sized cysts are best treated by a procedure called *marsupialization.* This procedure creates a small, permanent opening into the cyst wall that allows mucus secretions adequate drainage. Marsupialization is a relatively simple, short procedure that can sometimes be done under local anesthetic in a doctor's office. Postoperative pain is minimal; healing is usually complete within three to four weeks. Surgical removal of the entire cyst is another form of treatment, but it is seldom done.

Bartholin's abscess. The formation of an abscess in a Bartholin's gland usually starts when bacteria enter the gland by way of the duct. Although gonorrhea was once blamed for many of these infections, other bacteria, such as E. coli, are frequently responsible. Abscess formation invariably produces a swelling that is acutely hot, sensitive, and painful. If the bacteria are particularly virulent, the abscess can become full-blown within two to three days. Such an abscess quickly becomes an emergency because any pressure against the vulva causes excruciating pain. Normal activities such as walking, or even sitting, become almost impossible. At times, the application of heat or sitz baths may help localize the infection and precipitate spontaneous drainage. Yet even spontaneous drainage won't give complete relief because the site of the rupture typically is too small to provide adequate drainage and promptly closes. The best treatment is immediate surgical incision and complete drainage of the abscess. This usually can be done under a local anesthetic in a doctor's office. Once the abscess is properly drained, relief from pain is dramatic. A small wick of iodoform gauze temporarily placed in the abscess cavity helps maintain drainage and facilitates healing. Antibiotics sometimes are used, but they are seldom necessary if there is adequate drainage. For women who have recurrent abscesses, the marsupialization procedure described for the Bartholin's duct cyst provides permanent relief.

Genital Warts

Genital warts (condyloma accuminatum) are a prevalent viral disease among sexually active women. They commonly are found on the vulva, vagina, or cervix.

Genital warts have been plaguing men and women for centuries. Until recently, they often were called venereal warts because of their frequent association with gonorrhea, plus the common belief that the wart virus was transmitted exclusively by sexual intercourse. It's now known that the wart virus can be acquired without close intimate contact, but how it is transmitted remains obscure. Even the incubation period is unknown.

Genital warts first appear as discrete, tiny, pinkish-tan, papillary growths, not much bigger than a grain of rice. Initially, there may be only two or three warts clustered around the vaginal opening or along the labial lips. There are no symptoms at this stage. In fact, warts frequently are discovered inadvertently by a woman when washing or touching the vulvar area. However, if conditions are favorable to their existence, genital warts can flourish.

Vaginal discharge and excessive vulvar moisture contribute to the growth of genital warts. Vaginal infections or increased vaginal secretions (during pregnancy or from taking birth control pills) can cause genital warts to thrive and spread. Once the warts gain a foothold, scratching (due to itching or minor irritation) can seed the virus to other parts of the vulva, causing more warts to develop. Genital warts also tend to coalesce, with several small warts fusing together to form a larger cauliflowerlike growth. If neglected, large warts can become infected from scratching. In extreme cases, they can grow to cover the entire vulva. Extensive growth of warts along the vagina and cervix has even been known to block the birth canal during pregnancy, necessitating cesarean section for delivery.

Treatment. As long as excessive vaginal secretions or discharge continues to bathe the vulva, genital warts are tough to eradicate. Small warts will disappear suddenly if the vaginal infection is cleared or the vaginal secretion is minimized. For women taking birth control pills, this may mean interrupting medication temporarily. Clothing that tends to trap moisture (such as nylon underwear, pantyhose, and tight jeans or pants) also should be avoided.

Otherwise, specific treatment varies with the size and extent of the warts. Small warts usually are treated with topical applications of podophyllin, a caustic substance that causes the warts to slough off in two to four days. Since podophyllin can irritate the surrounding healthy skin, it should be carefully applied to the warts and the entire area should be washed with soap and water four to six hours after treatment. Furthermore, only a few lesions should be treated at any one time. Podophyllin is toxic and can be absorbed through the skin and mucous membranes. During pregnancy, in particular, excessive absorption of podophyllin has caused abortion and fetal death. In fact, vigorous treatment of warts during pregnancy may have to wait until after delivery. Interestingly, genital warts may spontaneously disappear during the postpartum period.

Larger warts should be treated by electrocautery, cryosurgery (freezing), or surgical excision. Although most of these treatments can be done under a local anesthetic in the doctor's office, a woman with extensive warts of the vulva or vagina may require hospitalization for their removal. Regardless of the treatment selected, the vulva, because of its rich blood supply, usually heals quickly with little or no scarring.

The Vagina

Vaginal Discharge

Many women assume that a vaginal discharge means an infection, but that's not necessarily so. Under normal and healthy conditions, cervical glands produce a clear mucus secretion. As this mucus drains downward and mixes with discarded vaginal cells, normal bacteria, and Bartholin's gland secretions, it assumes a white color (leukorrhea). Furthermore, when this normal white vaginal secretion comes into contact with underwear, it gradually changes in color to pale yellow as the result of oxidation (exposure to air). The discharge can be considered normal if it is not excessive, does not cause itching, irritation, or swelling, and does not have an unpleasant odor.

In young girls, the appearance of this normal, physiological discharge usually coincides with breast development, as a result of increased estrogen output by the ovaries. In addition, the vaginal mucosa thicken at this time, and the secretions become relatively acidic due to the growth of certain normal bacteria (lactobacilli).

With the advent of menstruation, the volume of secretions and the acidity of the vagina vary depending upon the phase of the menstrual cycle. Just after a menstrual period, for example, estrogen output is relatively low and the amount of cervical mucus is scant. As ovulation approaches, increased estrogen output causes a profuse outpouring of mucus from the cervical glands. At this time, many women will clearly notice a discharge or increased moisture around the vaginal opening. In fact, the recognition of this increased "wetness" as a sign of approaching ovulation is used by some women to practice natural birth control methods (see page 189). Prior to menstruation, the vaginal secretions once again diminish as estrogen levels drop. Vaginal acidity normally decreases around the time of menstruation, too, fluctuating in response to estrogen output.

With menopause and advancing age, the vaginal walls become relatively thin, dry, and smooth. Cervical secretions diminish, and the lactobacilli indirectly responsible for maintaining a normal vaginal acidity become scarce. As a result, vaginal secretions become scanty and relatively alkaline. All of these changes make the postmenopausal vagina more susceptible to trauma, irritation, and infection.

Sexual excitement (and emotional stress) also are associated with an obvious but temporary vaginal discharge. During sexual excitation, the vagina is lubricated from vasocongestion of the vaginal blood vessels. Engorgement of these veins causes a mucoid-like fluid to seep through the walls and coat the entire vaginal canal. Within moments of erotic stimulation, the entire vagina and introitus can be bathed with this profuse, clear, mucoidlike secretion. Older women also produce considerable vaginal lubrication when properly stimulated. Factors such as age, relative lack of estrogen, or even a previous hysterectomy operation do not significantly affect this normal response in women.

Abnormal discharges are usually caused by vaginal or cervical infections. Occasionally, abnormal discharges are the result of chronic cervical irritation, hormonal imbalances, or even the retention of a forgotten tampon or diaphragm. Yet the three primary organisms responsible for almost all vaginal infections and abnormal discharges are: Trichomonas vaginalis (a protozoan), Candida albicans (a fungus), and Hemophilus vaginalis (a bacteria). (Gonorrhea also causes an abnormal vaginal discharge, and is discussed on page 457.)

Infections of the Vagina

Trichomonas (TV) vaginitis is caused by a microscopic protozoan. Although an estimated one out of five women harbors this organism without signs or symptoms, the TV organism is not a normal inhabitant of the vagina (or any part of the human body). The infection is considered a venereal disease because most cases are acquired through contact of sexual organs or coitus with an infected partner. Furthermore, the TV protozoan, unlike other disease-causing organisms, cannot survive in the mouth or rectum. Even if TV organisms were to be introduced into these areas by a variety of sexual play, they would not survive long enough to ultimately become a source of vaginal reinfection. The infection, therefore, is specifically acquired by penis-to-vagina intercourse or close vulva-

ORGANISMS RESPONSIBLE FOR VAGINAL DISCHARGE

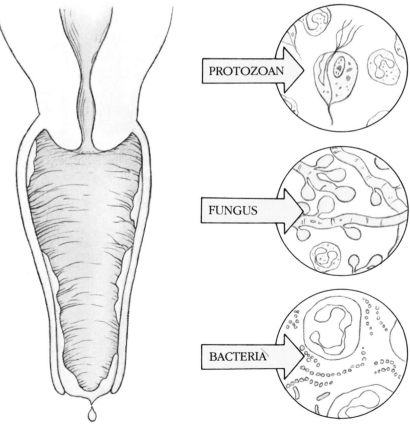

Most abnormal discharges from the vagina are caused by vaginal infections. Infection of the vagina by a protozoan, Trichomonas vaginalis or Trich for short, causes a copious, watery discharge. The fungus Candida albicans causes the intense itching commonly known as yeast infection. Bacterial infections of the vagina result in a slight discharge and milder symptoms than from Trich or yeast infections. Each organism is shown at right as it appears in the field of a microscope.

PROTOZOAN

FUNGUS

BACTERIA

to-vulva contact with an infected partner. Men acquire the infection only from infected women. Women can acquire the infection from both men and women.

Occasionally, cases of TV vaginitis have been attributed to the sharing of a moist washcloth or bathing suit (or to sitting on that infamous toilet seat), but these are uncommon sources of the infection. Sharing a swimming pool with a group of TV carriers is another unlikely mode of transmission. Most TV organisms would rapidly die in chlorinated water.

Symptoms. The most common symptom of TV vaginitis is a heavy watery discharge, green-white or yellow in color. Most women also are aware of a very disagreeable odor. In a severe infection, the discharge is so excessive that it causes marked irritation of the vulva and upper thighs. Another symptom is itching and pain on intercourse because of a mucous membrane inflammation of the lower vagina and introitus. Sometimes urinary frequency increases (with painful urination) if the TV organisms gain access to the urethra and bladder. Although the majority of men with TV vaginitis do not have symptoms, a few may notice slight burning after urination or ejaculation. In rare cases, TV organisms can cause a prostatic infection.

Diagnosis of TV vaginitis usually is made by examining a drop of vaginal discharge under a microscope. The protozoan is readily identified by its pear-shaped body and long whiplike tail. The presence of TV organisms also can be detected by a Pap smear and reported as an incidental finding.

Treatment. The most effective anti-TV drug currently available is the prescription drug Flagyl (metronidazole). In 95 percent of women with TV vaginitis, a single course of treatment with this medication eradicates the infection promptly. It is necessary, however, that the sexual partner also be treated, or recurrence is only a matter of time. Since it is virtually impossible to find the TV organisms in men, most doctors simply order treatment for men without any laboratory tests. The medication is taken in divided doses over a five- to seven-day period. During treatment, both partners should avoid drinking alcoholic beverages because the combination of the drug and alcohol could cause abdominal pain, nausea, vomiting, and headache. Flagyl also should be avoided during the early months of pregnancy. Flagyl's safety during early pregnancy has not been adequately studied. It is known, however, that Flagyl can cause cancer in certain strains of mice.

Local treatment for TV vaginitis includes creams, suppositories, and vinegar douches. At best, local therapy brings only temporary relief by decreasing the vaginal TV population. It would have no effect on possible TV organisms in the urinary tract, which would escape treatment and remain potential sources of self-reinfection. Occasionally, however, doctors prescribe local vaginal therapy, in conjunction with Flagyl, to reduce excessive vaginal discharge and make the patient more comfortable.

Candidiasis

Candidiasis is currently the most prevalent vaginal infection and the most stubborn to treat. Also known as moniliasis, vaginal thrush, or just plain yeast, candidiasis is caused by the fungus Candida albicans. This fungus is a normal vaginal inhabitant in 40 percent of all women. It is frequently harbored in the mouth and intestines of both sexes without any apparent signs or symptoms. In healthy individuals, this fungus also has been recovered from urine, seminal fluid, and between folds of opposing skin surfaces (i.e., beneath the foreskin or between the buttocks). All of these areas can be potential sources of vaginal infection or reinfection.

If a woman doesn't harbor Candida as a normal vaginal inhabitant, the fungus can be acquired by fecal contamination of the vagina, or less commonly, by oral-genital sex or coitus with a partner who harbors the organism. But unless certain conditions favorable to its growth and propagation also occur, the fungus usually will remain quietly unobtrusive.

There are factors that predispose a woman to the development of a vaginal fungus infection. They include pregnancy, use of oral contraceptives, increased blood sugar levels, antibiotics, and perhaps even stress— plus various unknowns. Fungus infections during pregnancy are quite common because of the relatively high levels of estrogen present at this time. Estrogen causes an increase in the glycogen content (carbohydrate) of vaginal cells, which creates the perfect environment for the growth and nourishment of the fungus. Under these circumstances, a woman whose vagina was previously unreceptive to Candida may now experience her first real vaginal infection. Similarly, the use of birth control pills with a high estrogen content may precipitate fungus infections in susceptible women. Antibiotics (particularly tetracycline) appear to cause these vaginal infections because they destroy or suppress the growth of protective vaginal bacteria that normally exert an antifungal effect.

Symptoms. The most notable symptom is an intense itching. Itching is invariably followed by scratching. The more persistent the itch-scratch cycle, the greater the irritation and inflammation around the vaginal introitus and labia. Breaks in the skin from scratching also can start a bacterial infection. Frequently, just voiding causes a burning sensation as the urine contacts the raw and irritated tissues. Obviously, intercourse may become impossible because of pain.

The discharge itself can vary from woman to woman. Some may notice only a slight watery, white drainage. Others might complain that the vagina actually feels dry and irritated. More commonly, thick curdlike chunks of a white cheesy substance mixed with a watery discharge appear at the vaginal opening. In severe cases, the entire vulva may be red and inflamed.

Diagnosis of moniliasis usually is made by simple inspection or by examining a drop of the discharge under a microscope. Sometimes a culture is taken.

Treatment. There is no oral medication that cures vaginal fungus infections. Vaginal creams or suppositories are the treatments of choice. Currently, the prescription drug Monistat, a vaginal cream, probably is one of the most effective. One intravaginal application at bedtime for a two-week period will clear the infection for most women. Other treatments may include nystatin vaginal suppositories for a two- to three-week period. In severe infections, some doctors paint the vagina with a solution of gentian violet, an old and reliable anti-fungal medication. Such topical applications can bring fast relief, but be aware that the stubborn purple stains on underwear will challenge any enzyme detergent. In sensitive women, gentian violet also can cause a form of contact dermatitis if overused.

Recurrences of vaginal fungus infections usually are the result of inadequate treatment or self-reinfection. This means that unless the treatment eradicates the fungus lurking around the vagina and in unsuspected areas, such as between labial folds and beneath the foreskin of the clitoris, recurrences are possible. It's important to recognize and eliminate any predisposing factors wherever possible to control flare-ups.

For women with persistent vaginal reinfections, many doctors recommend daily use of a vaginal cream or suppository for at least four to five weeks, and the application of an anti-fungal ointment between the labial folds. The same treatment is then repeated just prior to and during menstruation for an additional three to four months. Women also should make it a habit to wipe only from front to back after each bowel movement. This will help prevent vaginal contamination by bowel fungi, another source of self-reinfection. A doctor may prescribe Mycostatin tablets to suppress the growth of bowel fungi. Adding unpasteurized yogurt to your diet may help in the same way. But neither oral Mycostatin nor yogurt will have any effect on Candida organisms already present in the vagina.

Substituting showers for tub baths and avoiding soaps that contain hexachlorophene may decrease the number of recurrent fungus infections. Deodorant soaps that kill bacteria actually may promote fungus infections by destroying protective bacteria normally found on the skin and mucous membranes.

Since increased blood glucose levels also can precipitate fungus infections, cutting down on sweets and carbohydrates (and that includes wine and alcoholic beverages) may be beneficial. If you should require antibiotics, simultaneously using an anti-fungal vaginal cream during and after treatment is advisable. It's also a good idea to avoid nylon underwear, pantyhose, and tight-fitting jeans or slacks—all of which aggravate fungal problems by keeping the vulva warm and moist. And lastly, don't forget that fungus infections occasionally can be acquired from a sexual partner.

Hemophilus Vaginalis

Hemophilus vaginalis infections of the vagina are caused by a bacteria. Symptoms frequently are mild and may be nothing more than a scant grayish white malodorous discharge. For the affected woman, treatment with oral antibiotics for five or six days is usually curative. Since transmission of this bacteria can and frequently does occur during coitus, the sexual partner also should be treated. Most other vaginal bacterial infections (E. coli, etc.,) will similarly respond to oral antibiotics. At times, a vaginal antibacterial cream also can be applied locally.

Atrophic Vaginitis

Atrophic vaginitis is any irritation or inflammation of the vagina as a result of thinning and shrinking of the vaginal tissues from lack of estrogen. Although this condition usually occurs in women over fifty, it also appears in younger women following surgical removal of the ovaries. The most common symptoms are a slight vaginal discharge, burning on urination, tenderness around the vaginal introitus, and pain with intercourse. Often there is no specific infection, but rather a localized tissue reaction to normal bacteria and their metabolic products. Treatment with estrogen—taken orally or, when not contraindicated, applied locally— is usually effective in overcoming the problem.

The Cervix

Because the vagina provides a warm, dark, moist environment, chronic irritations and infections of the cervix are not at all uncommon. The presence of bacteria (both normal and abnormal), menstrual blood, and tissue trauma from childbirth all contribute to the problem. In fact, cervicitis or an infection of the cervix is probably the most common gynecological problem.

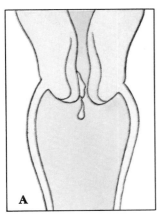
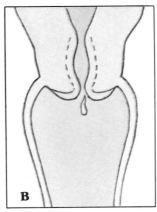
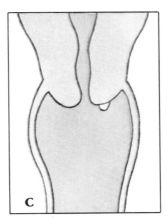
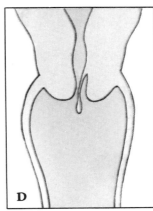

BENIGN DISEASES OF THE CERVIX

A CERVICITIS *or infection of the cervix can be caused by a variety of organisms. Symptoms are a heavy discharge and pain.*
B CERVICAL EROSION *is also the result of infection, and causes a clear mucus discharge.*

C CERVICAL CYSTS *occur when the duct of a cervical gland is blocked.*
D CERVICAL POLYPS *are outgrowths of tissue from the wall of the cervix. They originate from the tissue lining the cervical canal and may be caused by infection.*

Acute Cervicitis

Acute cervicitis is an acute infection and inflammation of the cervix. Although many cases are the result of gonorrhea, any organism can affect the cervix, including staphylococcus, streptococcus, and so forth. Cervicitis also can be associated with a vaginal infection such as trichomoniasis or moniliasis. Symptoms usually include a yellowish and often heavy discharge and a sense of pelvic pressure or heaviness. The cervix is red and swollen and the vaginal walls may be inflamed from the infected discharge. During a pelvic examination, pressure against the cervix may be painful. Since the infection can spread upward to involve the uterus, prompt treatment with appropriate antibiotics is essential. Most cases respond favorably in a few days.

Chronic Cervicitis

Chronic cervicitis is a long-standing low-grade infection of the cervix. Although there is usually a dis-charge, pain is absent, and the infection tends to remain localized. If a Pap smear is negative and there is no suspicion of malignancy, chronic cervicitis can be effectively treated in the doctor's office by electrocauterization or cryosurgery. Electrocautery destroys the infected tissue by heat application; cryosurgery destroys infected tissue by the application of extreme cold. Since the cervix is remarkably insensitive to painful stimuli, these treatments usually require no anesthesia and cause minimal discomfort. Following treatment by either method, the cervix will heal within six to eight weeks and revert to its normal pink and healthy state.

Prompt treatment of chronic cervicitis is important, since there is evidence that a woman with a chronically infected cervix may be more predisposed to subsequently develop cervical cancer. Among women anxious to conceive, a thick purulent mucus discharge may prevent sperm from passing through the cervical canal and therefore be a factor in sterility. Women often conceive following treatment for a cervical infection. In addition, chronic cervicitis can be a focus of infection and theoretically spread bacteria to other parts of the body.

Cervical Erosion

Cervical erosion is a term frequently and incorrectly applied to any red or irritated-looking cervix. It also is used to describe a cervix with an obvious ulceration due to infection or mechanical irritation (as from wearing a pessary). In actuality, a cervical erosion is the replacement of normal cervical tissue on the surface of the cervix by tissue from within the cervical canal. Since this endocervical tissue is normally red and granular, it gives the cervix a red, eroded, and inflamed appearance. Most cases are the result of infection, and are accompanied by a clear mucus discharge. The treatment of choice is cauterization.

Cervical Cysts

Cervical cysts, also known as Nabothian cysts, are mucus-filled cervical glands whose ducts or outlets are obstructed. Cervical cysts can occur singly or in groups. They appear as white pimplelike elevations on the surface of the cervix, and are rarely larger than a small pea. They are not a threat to health nor do they ever become malignant. Their presence, however, does indicate some past or recent infection or irritation of the cervix. Unless treated, cervical cysts do not spontaneously clear. They are easily cured by electrocautery in the doctor's office.

Cervical Polyps

Cervical polyps are small, fragile, tear-shaped growths that dangle on a stalk and protrude through the cervical os. They originate from the tissue lining the cervical canal and are usually the result of infection. Since they bleed easily on touch, intercourse or douching may provoke painless spotting or bleeding. Less frequently, cervical polyps may be responsible for irregular bleeding at other times. In most cases, they can be easily and painlessly removed by a gentle twisting motion. Although they are almost always benign, cervical polyps are routinely submitted to a pathologist for microscopic examination. On occasion, the successful removal of polyps located well within the cervical canal may require hospitalization.

The Uterus

Infection of the Uterus

The most prevalent uterine infection is endometritis, an inflammation of the uterine lining. It can occur as part of a generalized pelvic infection or, more commonly, as a complication of pregnancy, either after childbirth or abortion. Women who have had induced abortions or long, hard labors with ruptured membranes are particularly susceptible to endometritis. The raw lining of the postpartum uterus is a perfect breeding ground for vaginal bacteria that invariably invade the uterus shortly after delivery. Fortunately, most uterine infections are mild and are readily overcome by the body's own defense mechanisms. In more severe cases, uterine tenderness, fever, and a foul-smelling discharge are the usual symptoms. Appropriate antibiotics and good drainage of infected material from the uterine cavity will usually clear most cases promptly.

Endometrial polyps are fleshy, tear-shaped growths that sprout from the uterine (endometrial) lining. They are not the result of infection, but rather are discrete and usually benign overgrowths of normal endometrial tissue caused by continuous estrogen stimulation. They are frequently multiple and can either spread out within the uterine cavity as broad, flat projections of tissue or dangle from small stalks. Occasionally, if one of these stalks is long enough, an endometrial polyp can prolapse through the cervical os. Under ordinary circumstances, however, endometrial polyps can neither be felt nor seen. Unless they cause symptoms—usually bleeding between periods, prolonged postmenstrual spotting or staining, or heavy prolonged periods—their presence may be completely unsuspected.

Diagnosis is readily made by scraping the uterine lining (dilatation and curettage). In a good percentage of women, a D and C also may be curative.

Adenomyosis, also known as "internal endometriosis," most commonly affects women between the ages of 40 and 50. It is a condition wherein fragments of endometrial tissue (uterine lining) become embedded within the muscular walls of the uterus. How or why this happens remains unclear, but the end result is an enlarged, soft, and boggy uterus. Periods become increasingly long and profuse, and are associated with cramping and pelvic pressure. Other symptoms can include more frequent bleeding, premenstrual staining, and pain during intercourse. Unfortunately, adenomyosis does not respond to hormonal medication nor can the symptoms be relieved by dilatation and curettage. The best treatment is therefore hysterectomy. The ovaries need not be removed in this procedure.

Fibroid Tumors

Fibroid tumors of the uterus, also known as leiomyomas or myomas, are benign tumors of muscle and connective tissue. They are the most common pelvic tumor, and probably occur in 25 to 30 percent of women over 30. Although they can occur singly, fibroid tumors usually are multiple and begin as small seedlings scattered throughout the muscular walls of the uterus. As they progressively enlarge and become more nodular, they can encroach upon the uterine cavity and/or grow outward and project beyond the normal contours of the uterus. In extreme cases, a fibroid can even dangle from a long stalk attached to the outside wall of the uterus, the so-called pedunculated fibroid.

The growth of fibroids seems to depend on regular estrogen stimulation. They rarely appear before the age of 20, and tend to shrink after the menopause. As long as a woman is having menstrual periods, fibroid tumors probably will continue to enlarge. Birth control pills with a high estrogen content can accelerate their growth. As a general rule, however, most fibroids grow slowly even among women using oral contraceptives. With regard to their size, some fibroids can be microscopic whereas others can weigh several pounds.

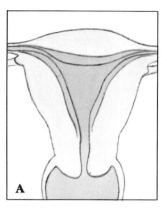 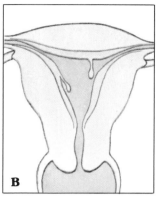 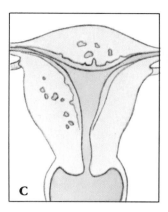 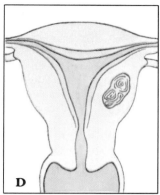

BENIGN DISEASES OF THE UTERUS

A ENDOMETRITIS *is an infection of the lining of the uterus. It occurs most commonly after childbirth or abortion when the raw lining of the uterus is susceptible to any bacteria that might be in the vagina.*
B ENDOMETRIAL POLYPS *are outgrowths of uterine tissue that may remain undetected unless they cause bleeding between periods.*
C ADENOMYOSIS *is caused by fragments of the uterine*

lining becoming embedded within the muscular walls of the uterus, resulting in a soft, spongy uterus. The symptoms are heavy periods with cramping and pelvic pressure.
D FIBROID TUMORS *of the uterus are benign growths in muscle and connective tissue. Most small fibroids go undiscovered, but as they enlarge, they may cause symptoms of pressure and excessive menstrual bleeding.*

Symptoms. Surprisingly enough, many fibroids never cause problems and are inadvertently discovered on routine pelvic examination. Others, because of size or location within the uterus, give rise to a variety of symptoms.

Large fibroids can cause a sensation of pelvic fullness or discomfort. At times, a fibroid may press against the urinary bladder and thereby limit the amount of urine the bladder can effectively hold. Although this is rarely serious, it can create annoying urinary frequency. Less commonly, a fibroid may aggravate constipation or interfere with normal stool evacuation by impinging against the rectal walls. Even small tumors can cause nagging backaches if they happen to press against pelvic nerve fibers.

Bleeding between periods or after the menopause is rarely caused by fibroid tumors. However, if the tumor or tumors bulge into the uterine cavity, heavy and long periods with the passage of blood clots can occur. In effect, tumors that in any way distort the normal contours of the uterine cavity can cause heavy menstrual blood loss by increasing the bleeding surface of the uterine lining. Such bleeding can occur in gushes and be unexpectedly profuse—even to the extent of causing anemia and chronic fatigue. In contrast, tumors that are located in the outer walls of the uterus and away from the uterine cavity rarely provoke bleeding problems.

Pain is not normally a symptom of fibroid tumors unless there is a complication involving the tumor. Tenderness over a fibroid or dull abdominal pain with fever may indicate infection of the fibroid or perhaps degenerative changes. A fibroid that hangs on a

stalk may twist or turn in such a way that the blood vessels feeding the tumor become kinked. In these instances, pain can be sudden and severe, requiring hospitalization and even surgery to correct the situation.

Fibroid tumors and cancer. Malignant changes within a fibroid tumor are fortunately rare and occur predominantly in postmenopausal women. Although the most common warning sign is rapid enlargement of the fibroid, there is little else in the history or physical examination that helps distinguish a malignancy from an ordinary benign fibroid. Diagnosis is usually made at the time of surgery.

Fibroid tumors and pregnancy. As a rule, fibroid tumors do not interfere with fertility. The one possible exception is where the tumors block the fallopian tubes and prevent the sperm from fertilizing the egg. However, once pregnancy is established, previously small and asymptomatic fibroids do enlarge because of higher estrogen levels, greater blood flow to the uterus, and increasing uterine size. Although many women with fibroid tumors can successfully deliver a full-term baby, a few may have problems. If, for example, the fibroids bulge or jut into the uterine cavity, the baby may not have enough room to grow properly. Thus, premature labor and delivery—sometimes as early as the second trimester—are not uncommon. In women who do carry to term, normal vaginal delivery may not always be possible. If tumors block the birth canal and/or cause

FIBROID TUMORS OF THE UTERUS

COMPLICATIONS OF FIBROID TUMOR ENLARGEMENT

Benign fibroid tumors of the uterus are the most common pelvic tumors, occurring in approximately 25 percent of women over 30. Fibroid tumors may enlarge to block fallopian tubes (1), crowd the uterus so that a baby cannot grow properly (2), or block the birth canal (3).

TREATMENT OF FIBROID TUMORS

A *Tumors may shrink on their own, especially after menopause when estrogen production decreases. The growth of fibroid tumors depends on regular estrogen secretion.*
B *Myomectomy, removal of the fibroid tumors, may be the treatment suggested for young women whose fibroids interfere with pregnancy.*
C *Hysterectomy may be the most reasonable treatment in women over 40, particularly if large fibroids are causing many problems.*

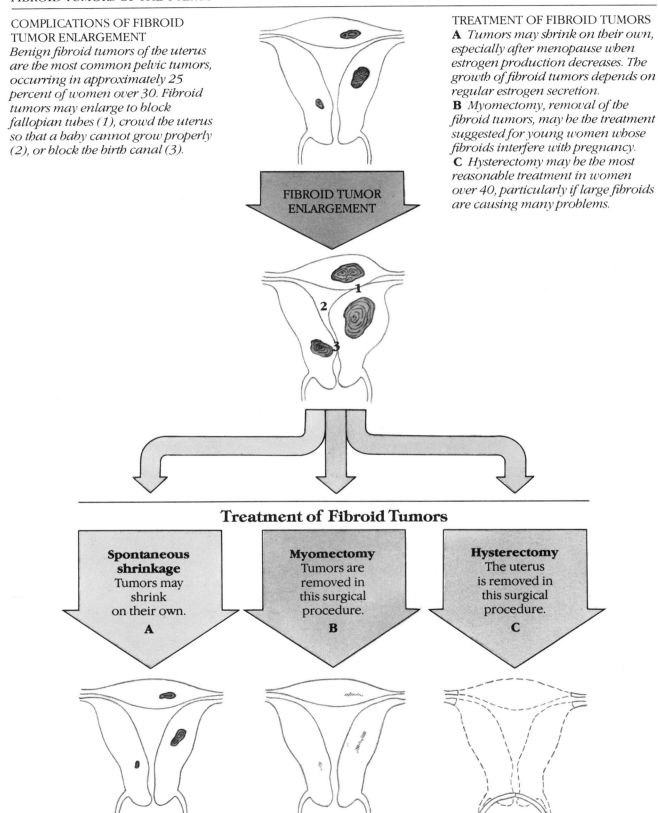

FIBROID TUMOR ENLARGEMENT

Treatment of Fibroid Tumors

Spontaneous shrinkage
Tumors may shrink on their own.
A

Myomectomy
Tumors are removed in this surgical procedure.
B

Hysterectomy
The uterus is removed in this surgical procedure.
C

the baby to lie in an abnormal position, cesarean section may be necessary. Following delivery, fibroid tumors usually return to their size before pregnancy.

Diagnosis. Since most fibroids distort and enlarge the uterus, they usually are detected by feeling the uterus on routine pelvic examination. Nevertheless, it is possible for a uterus to seem normal in size and shape and yet have its cavity distorted by a single small fibroid. Suspicion that such a fibroid exists may be aroused by repeatedly heavy menstrual periods. Under these circumstances, a special X ray of the uterine cavity or a dilatation and curettage (D & C) may be required to confirm the diagnosis. Where the uterus is markedly enlarged by fibroids, a woman herself may notice a lump in her lower abdomen.

At times, however, diagnosis of fibroid tumors by physical examination alone can be difficult, particularly in an obese woman. Fibroids have been mistaken for ovarian tumors, inflammatory processes of the tubes, and even pregnancy. In these cases, further studies may be necessary to establish the true diagnosis.

Treatment depends on the size of the tumors, the problems they are causing, the age of the woman, and whether she wants children. Since many fibroids remain small and asymptomatic, doctors frequently advise "watchful waiting." Regular pelvic examination every six to twelve months usually will be sufficient to keep track of any changes. The fact that fibroids do stop growing after the menopause and even shrink warrants this conservative approach in many women. Where the tumors are large, however, hysterectomy or removal of the uterus is usually the treatment of choice in an older woman. Fibroids that cause pelvic discomfort or consistently heavy menstrual bleeding also are best handled by removal of the uterus.

An alternate method of treatment is myomectomy or removal of the fibroid tumors without sacrificing the uterus. Although this procedure is usually reserved for the younger woman with symptomatic fibroids or for the woman whose fibroids interfere with pregnancy, myomectomy can be done on any woman providing that the uterus is not too extensively involved. As effective as myomectomy can be, it is not generally advisable in older women, in whom there is a good chance that a new crop of fibroids may develop. Then, too, if fibroids are really causing problems, most women (particularly if they are over 40) would just as soon have the problem permanently resolved. Furthermore, myomectomy as a surgical procedure can be more difficult and involve greater blood loss than a hysterectomy. Apart from these considerations, fibroid tumors are frequently found in association with other pelvic conditions such as endometriosis or chronic pelvic inflammatory disease. Under these circumstances, and especially in older women, hysterectomy may be indicated on the basis of these coexisting female problems.

The Fallopian Tubes

Infection. Most tubal infections (salpingitis) are the result of gonorrhea, but as many as 20 percent can be caused by other bacteria. Since the fallopian tubes are continuous with the uterine cavity, it's not surprising that infections initially localized at the cervix or uterus may ascend and ultimately involve the tubal lining. Septic abortions, postpartum uterine infections, and even the insertion of an intrauterine device have all been responsible for acute infections of the tubes. Some uterine infections also can spread by the lymphatics and blood vessels to involve the outside walls of the tubes rather than the lining. But regardless of the specific cause or mode of infection, the symptoms are the same—abdominal pain, tenderness, and fever. The pain usually begins as a dull aching discomfort on one side of the pelvis with subsequent involvement of the other side within 24 to 48 hours. Fever is usually low grade and may be accompanied by chills. A vaginal discharge and perhaps irregular bleeding also may be present.

Prompt medical treatment with appropriate antibiotics and supportive care are extremely important in preventing serious complications. Otherwise, abscess formation and peritonitis can become real threats necessitating possible surgical intervention. Despite adequate care, however, infertility because of partial or complete occlusion of the tubes still is possible.

Women with recurrent tubal infection run an increased risk of developing chronic pelvic pain, irregular bleeding problems, and ectopic pregnancy (see below).

Tubal ectopic pregnancy currently accounts for 2 percent of maternal deaths in this country. It is a pregnancy that implants and develops within the tubal passageway rather than in the uterine cavity. Most cases are the result of previous tubal infection, but a few can be traced to congenital tubal abnormalities, endometriosis, tubal scarring and kinking from a ruptured appendix, and various other conditions. Since the tube has relatively thin walls and little space to accommodate a growing embryo, rupture usually occurs six to ten weeks after the first missed period.

The typical symptoms of an ectopic pregnancy are a slight reddish brown vaginal discharge two to four weeks after a missed period. There may also be a mild cramping pain on one side of the pelvis. Examination at this time may or may not reveal swelling and tenderness of the tube. Diagnosing an ectopic pregnancy prior to rupture sometimes can be difficult, as the signs and symptoms are frequently subtle and misleading. Once the tube ruptures and hemorrhages into the abdomen, however, the pain is usually severe, sharp, and sudden. Shock from excess blood loss as well as shoulder pain from irritation of the diaphragm by free blood within the abdomen are common.

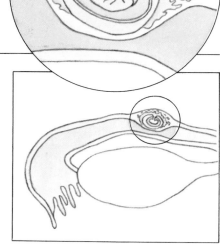

FALLOPIAN TUBE DISORDERS

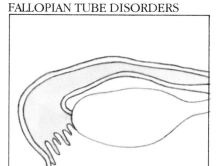

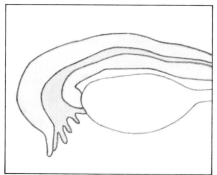

NORMAL FALLOPIAN TUBE

TUBAL INFECTION
Infections of the fallopian tube may begin when bacteria from a uterine infection spread upward through the common cavity shared by the uterus and fallopian tubes. The infected tube becomes inflamed and swollen, resulting in abdominal pain, tenderness, and fever.

TUBAL ECTOPIC PREGNANCY
Tubal ectopic pregnancy occurs when an embryo implants in the tube wall rather than in the uterine wall. Because the tube is small and thin walled, the growing embryo usually ruptures the tube six to ten weeks after the first missed period. It is important to diagnose a tubal pregnancy before the tube ruptures for prompt surgical treatment.

COMMON SITES OF ECTOPIC PREGNANCY
During the early crucial stages of pregnancy, an embryo may implant itself outside the normal site of implantation in the uterus. This abnormal condition is called ectopic pregnancy. Since fertilization occurs in the fallopian tube (see page 226), the most common site for extrauterine implantation is in the tube. This occurs about once in every 100 births. Sites (3) and (4) are the most common for ectopic pregnancy. Sites (2) and (5) are rather rare. Ovarian (1) and abdominal (8) implantations are rare, as are low uterine sites (6) and (7). The embryo's normal site of implantation is high on the back wall of the uterus.

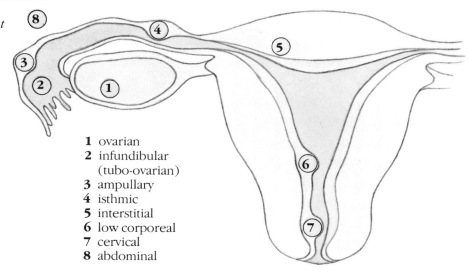

1 ovarian
2 infundibular (tubo-ovarian)
3 ampullary
4 isthmic
5 interstitial
6 low corporeal
7 cervical
8 abdominal

Treatment is immediate surgery with removal of the involved tube and replacement of blood loss. Among women who subsequently become pregnant after an ectopic pregnancy, less than 40 percent will have a normal full-term pregnancy. Approximately 30 percent will have another ectopic pregnancy, and another 30 percent will spontaneously abort during the first trimester.

The Ovary

The ovary normally undergoes changes in size, shape, and weight, depending upon age and hormone stimulation. It also can be the site of more than twenty different types of cysts and tumors, both benign and malignant. The discovery of an enlarged ovary during a pelvic examination can therefore pose a problem in diagnosis. To make the matter of ovarian growths even more complicated, some can spontaneously disappear, whereas others can grow to enormous size if left unattended. Only a few of the more common cysts and tumors are discussed here.

Physiological or Functional Cysts

Physiological or functional cysts of the ovary arise from normal ovarian tissue and are usually the result of hormonal or circulatory disturbances. They are not true ovarian tumors, but rather represent physiological enlargements of the ovary. Two such cysts are the follicle cyst and corpus luteum cyst.

Follicle cyst. All normal functioning ovaries contain cystic structures (follicles) in various stages of growth and degeneration. These follicles not only produce estrogen but each one of them contains an immature egg or ovum. On a selective basis during every menstrual cycle, some of these follicles will begin to grow. But in order for one follicle to mature and release its egg (ovulation), countless other follicles fail in the attempt and ultimately disintegrate into microscopic specks of scar tissue within the ovary. Ordinarily this process is very orderly, with none of the follicles ever exceeding the size of a small pea. Occasionally, however, and usually for some unknown reason, the chosen follicle may fail to release its egg, or one of the competing follicles may refuse to disintegrate. In either case, the disturbed follicle may continue to enlarge and fill with clear fluid, thus becoming a follicle cyst.

Follicle cysts rarely cause problems, and are usually discovered during a routine pelvic examination. Since they usually disappear within two or three menstrual cycles—either through absorption of the cyst fluid or spontaneous drainage of the cyst—most doctors will merely advise a repeat pelvic examination in three months. If, however, the cyst should remain and increase in size or begin to cause pain or menstrual disturbances, surgery may be indicated.

A corpus luteum cyst also is a physiological cyst, but in this case it arises from the remnant of the ruptured follicle after the release of the egg. Corpus luteum cysts are usually larger than follicle cysts, and tend to cause menstrual disturbances, such as irregular spotting. They may even cause a period to be delayed for several weeks. Although corpus luteum cysts can regress spontaneously, they also can persist and rupture, causing internal bleeding sufficiently heavy to necessitate immediate surgical removal of the cyst.

Other Ovarian Cysts and Tumors

In contrast to physiological cysts, other ovarian growths—whether they are solid or cystic or a combination of both—will usually continue to grow and ultimately will cause problems.

A dermoid cyst of the ovary is a common ovarian tumor. Although it can occur at any age, it is more prevalent among adolescents and young women between 20 and 30. The cyst itself is unusual in that it frequently contains oily material as well as hair, teeth, bone, or cartilage. The presence of these radiopaque substances makes it one of the few ovarian growths that can sometimes be diagnosed by X-ray examination. Because the oily material is highly irritating to pelvic tissues, rupture of such a cyst can cause serious chemical peritonitis.

The mucinous cystadenoma is another common ovarian tumor. It is usually filled with gelatinous straw-colored fluid and can attain enormous size. Some mucinous cystadenomas have weighed more than 30 pounds.

Symptoms from these cysts (as well as from other ovarian growths) are surprisingly few at first. Although some benign ovarian growths may cause pelvic discomfort or pressure, it is amazing how large they can become before their presence is even suspected. Furthermore, menstruation is frequently normal and pain is uncommon as long as the cyst or tumor has room to expand. But continuing growth of a dermoid cyst, mucinous cystadenoma, or any other ovarian mass gradually can constrict and press against the surrounding normal ovarian tissue and reduce its blood supply. Thus, with less blood flow and nourishment reaching the otherwise normal and uninvolved portion of the ovary, it may eventually atrophy, shrink, and cease to function. In young women, the diagnosis and correction of this condition is of the utmost importance, not only from the standpoint of reproduction but in terms of preserving hormonal function. Since some of these tumors may also involve both ovaries, there is even greater risk of compromising or losing ovarian function by unnecessarily delaying treatment.

Ovarian masses also demand prompt attention because there is no way of determining whether they are benign or malignant by a pelvic examination alone. Shape, size, and feel of the mass may be helpful in this regard, but physical findings can be deceptive. Laboratory studies, Pap smears, and X-ray examinations are usually of little value in most cases. In addition, malignant ovarian tumors do not have specific signs or symptoms. Fortunately, few ovarian growths prove to be malignant. But even assuming one could be certain that a particular ovarian mass was benign, prompt treatment still would be advisable. Ovarian tumors and cysts can rupture, bleed, become infected, twist, become gangrenous, and cause pelvic havoc in general.

Treatment. Most doctors advise surgical exploration when dealing with an ovarian mass not considered to be a physiological enlargement. Only by removing the growth and examining the tissue under a microscope can an accurate diagnosis be made. In young women, the treatment of choice is cystectomy, or simple removal of the cyst with preservation of normal ovarian tissue wherever possible. Ovarian tumors in women past menopause have a greater potential to become malignant. They are therefore best treated by removal of the entire ovary, or more commonly by hysterectomy and removal of both ovaries.

BENIGN OVARIAN GROWTHS
The common cysts and tumors of the ovary shown below are usually discovered because the ovary feels large to a physician during a routine pelvic examination. Prompt treatment involves surgically removing the growth and carefully examining the tissue under a microscope to accurately diagnose the growth as benign or malignant.
FOLLICLE CYSTS *Follicle cysts develop in the structure that normally houses a mature egg. The cyst is filled with a clear fluid and may enlarge enough to cause pain or menstrual disturbances.*
CORPUS LUTEUM CYSTS *Corpus luteum cysts arise after the follicle ruptures and releases the egg. This cyst also is*
filled with fluid, and like the follicle cyst, may disappear spontaneously in one to three months.
DERMOID CYSTS *Dermoid cysts vary in size and may become as large as an orange. They are fairly common ovarian growths or tumors, and are thought to be caused by the development of an egg parthenogenetically, or without fertilization by a sperm. The cysts contain hair, skin tissue, bone, muscle, and even teeth.*
MUCINOUS CYSTADENOMAS *Mucinous cystadenomas are gelatinous-filled sacs that may become quite large, causing much damage to the ovary before they are discovered and treated.*

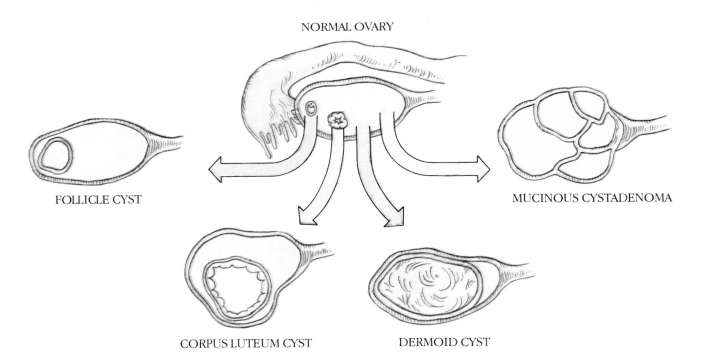

NORMAL OVARY

FOLLICLE CYST

MUCINOUS CYSTADENOMA

CORPUS LUTEUM CYST

DERMOID CYST

Venereal Disease

A venereal disease is transmitted or acquired by sexual intercourse or close, intimate contact with an infected individual. Traditionally, medical science recognized only five venereal diseases: gonorrhea, syphilis, the less commonly known lymphopathia venereum, chancroids, and granuloma inguinale. Today we know of at least 25 other diseases and infections that can be sexually transmitted. And the list keeps growing.

Venereal disease is not limited to the sexually promiscuous or confined to the economically disadvantaged. Regardless of social background, education, or age, more and more women, including those who limit their sexual activity to one partner, are no longer safe from possible infection.

Gonorrhea

Next to the common cold, gonorrhea is the most prevalent communicable disease in the United States. In 1977, there were over a million verified cases, and an estimated three million that never came to the attention of public health officials. Slang terms for the infection include GC, drip, strain, dose, and clap.

Gonorrhea is a highly infectious disease caused by the bacteria Neisseria gonorrhoeae. The gonococcal organisms require a moist mucosal surface for survival; exposure to air, heat, or drying causes them to die rapidly. In the majority of cases, the gonococcus enters the body through the genital tract. The disease, therefore, is almost exclusively transmitted or acquired by sexual intercourse or other intimate contact with the genital organs of an infected person. Other sites of initial infection are the rectum and pharynx (throat).

Gonorrhea sometimes can be spread by indirect means. Infection of a newborn baby at the time of delivery is a well-known example. Children, however, can acquire gonorrhea by being touched by an infected adult, or less commonly, by contacting freshly contaminated articles such as bed linens. Among adults, one sometimes hears the story of acquiring the disease by sitting on an infected toilet seat, but this is by far the most improbable mode of transmission.

Once the gonococcus establishes a foothold, the infection can take one of several courses:
- It can remain localized until treated or spontaneously cured by the body's own defense mechanisms.
- It can spread to involve other organs of the genital tract.
- It can gain entrance to the bloodstream and set up disease elsewhere in the body.
- It can remain hidden and unsuspected in the genital tissues and produce the so-called carrier state.

Localized Gonorrhea

The usual incubation period for gonorrhea is two to seven days following sexual contact with an infected person. Some men, however, may harbor the GC organisms for as long as six weeks before symptoms appear. In women, the incubation period may vary even more—from one week to several months. Furthermore, 30 percent of men and 60 to 90 percent of women with gonorrhea may never develop symptoms. Some of these individuals will overcome their infection without treatment. Others can become carriers and harbor the organism without symptoms. Thus, they unknowingly become a source of continuing infection to all of their sexual contacts.

Symptoms. Among women who do develop symptoms, gonococcal infections are initially localized in the lower genital tract and adjacent structures. Because of its vulnerable position near the vagina, the urethra (urinary channel) is usually the first site attacked by the gonococcus. Inflammation of the urethral lining causes a purulent (pus-laden) discharge with burning, stinging pain and frequent urination. Since these initial symptoms of gonorrhea can at times be mild and fleeting, they may be mistaken for a passing bladder irritation.

Subsequent involvement of the cervix and specifically the endocervical canal usually provokes a thick, yellowish, profuse discharge. Only specialized tests can distinguish between a gonorrheal infection and one caused by other organisms. With more severe infections, the gonococcus can invade the deep cervical glands, thereby making a cure more difficult. It is within these deep cervical glands that the organisms are frequently harbored by unsuspecting carriers.

The Bartholin's glands are another area of possible involvement in localized gonorrhea. They are two small mucus-producing glands whose ducts are located just outside the vaginal opening. Gonococcal infection can cause one or both glands to swell painfully and form abscesses. A Bartholin's gland cyst or abscess, however, is not necessarily the result of gonorrhea. Various other bacteria can cause similar problems.

In the adult, the rectum and pharynx (throat) also can be sites of early localized gonorrhea. Women usually acquire rectal gonorrhea by anal intercourse with an infected partner or by contamination of the anal orifice by a copious gonococcal vaginal discharge. A woman with gonorrhea of the cervix can transmit her infection to the rectum by engaging in anal coitus following vaginal intercourse.

An estimated 60 percent of individuals with rectal gonorrhea do not have symptoms. A few may notice mild anal itching, burning, or perhaps increased mucus discharge with the stools. In severe cases, painful rectal spasms, bloody stools, and drainage of pus may be prominent complaints. But even in severe cases, the infection usually remains localized in the anus and rectum. In about 5 percent of women with gonorrhea, infection may be entirely limited to the rectum. Men and women with asymptomatic rectal gonorrhea also may be unsuspected carriers of the infection.

Gonococcal infections of the pharynx are acquired by oral-genital sex or oral copulation. Most cases in men and women result from fellatio or mouth-to-penis copulation with an infected partner. Cunnilingus or mouth-to-vulva stimulation is a less frequent source of pharyngeal infection. Symptoms are usually absent, but there occasionally can be a mild sore throat or tonsillitis. Although the tongue, gums, and buccal mucosa are usually resistant to the gonococcus, there have been cases of multiple ulcerations of these areas following oral copulation. Infection of the mouth and pharynx also can occur without genital involvement. In these instances, an individual with oral gonorrhea could theoretically transmit the infection to the mouth or genital organs of another person.

Diagnosis. Since there are no reliable blood tests for gonorrhea, the infection must be diagnosed by identifying the gonococcus either by smear or culture. In the smear method, the discharge is spread onto a glass slide, stained with a special dye, and examined under the microscope for the presence of the

---

HOW GONORRHEA TRAVELS THROUGH THE BODY

Gonorrhea usually enters the body through the genital tract, and is almost exclusively transmitted by contact with the genital organs of an infected person. Other sites of beginning infection are the throat and rectum, shown in brown. Once the gonococcal organism is established, it may spread to the upper genital tract (orange); to the uterus, fallopian tubes, and ovaries (yellow); and through the bloodstream to the skin, joints, heart, brain, and spinal cord (pink).

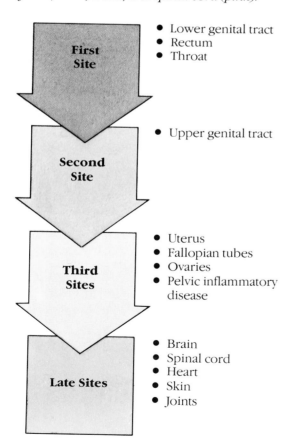

First Site
- Lower genital tract
- Rectum
- Throat

Second Site
- Upper genital tract

Third Sites
- Uterus
- Fallopian tubes
- Ovaries
- Pelvic inflammatory disease

Late Sites
- Brain
- Spinal cord
- Heart
- Skin
- Joints

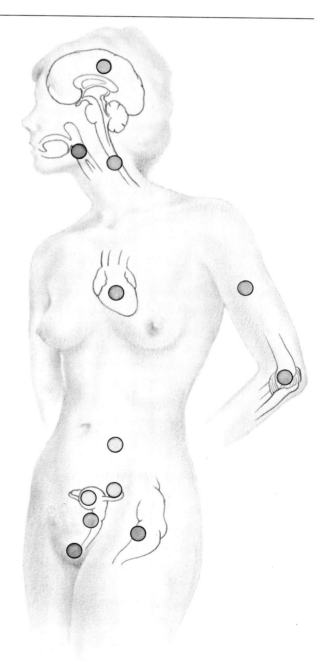

gonococcus. Although smear tests are accurate in diagnosing urethral gonorrhea in men, they are notoriously unreliable when applied to women. For this reason, most doctors depend on the culture method. This involves taking a sample of the secretion or discharge and combining it with a specific nutritive medium. If the gonococcus is present in the material tested, the medium will stimulate sufficient growth of the organism to make definite laboratory diagnosis within 24 to 48 hours.

Where there is a strong suspicion of gonorrhea, an accurate diagnosis can be made in 95 percent of cases by taking cultures from the cervix, urethra, and rectum. In routine screening procedures, most doctors will simply take a single culture from the cervix (endocervix). In women harboring the gonococcus without apparent symptoms, the vulva, vagina, and cervix may appear completely normal. In these cases, detection may well depend on a routine screening or on a history of probable recent exposure.

To diagnose pharyngeal and rectal gonorrhea in both men and women, the doctor will swab these areas with a cotton-tipped applicator and culture the material. With the increased prevalence of anal coitus and oral-genital sex, many venereal disease clinics now take routine cultures from these extragenital sites.

Treatment. Despite the increasing resistance of the gonococcus to various antibiotics over the past twenty years, penicillin is still the drug used to treat most uncomplicated gonococcal infections. When it was first introduced in 1943, a single dose of 300,000 units of this wonder drug completely eradicated an early GC infection. Today the recommended treatment for localized gonorrhea in individuals not allergic to penicillin is 4.8 million units of aqueous procaine penicillin G (APPG) given at one time in two deep intramuscular injections (at the buttocks). In addition, one gram of probenecid (Benemid) is given by mouth. This drug allows the penicillin to remain at higher and more effective concentrations in the body for a longer period of time. At these dosage levels, penicillin, unlike other antibiotics, has the unique advantage of being able to abort incubating syphilis should it also be present. In other words, if syphilis and gonorrhea were contracted from the same sexual encounter, penicillin would eradicate the syphilis before signs and symptoms of the disease ever became apparent.

At times, Ampicillin (an oral form of penicillin) has been substituted for injected penicillin, but treatment failures have been much more frequent. Ampicillin is also ineffective against pharyngeal gonorrhea, and is considerably less capable of aborting incubating syphilis. Therefore, it should not be regarded as equivalent therapy.

For individuals allergic to penicillin, the second most effective drug is tetracycline. The total oral dose is 9.0 grams: 1.5 grams initially, followed by 0.5 grams every six hours for four days. When tetracycline is taken as directed, treatment cures compare favorably with those obtained by penicillin injection. In a pregnant woman, however, tetracycline may have toxic effects on fetal tissue and cause yellow discoloration and mottling of the newborn's permanent teeth. Therefore, in cases where a pregnant woman is allergic to penicillin, oral doses of Erythromycin are substituted for tetracycline. Unfortunately, cure failures with Erythromycin can approach 25 percent.

Recently, a drug-resistant form of gonorrhea that apparently originated in Southeast Asia has appeared in scattered areas throughout the United States. This so-called penicillinase strain of gonococcus produces an enzyme that in effect protects it from penicillin, Ampicillin, and tetracycline. When this gonococcus was first isolated in this country, public health officials feared an epidemic. Fortunately, however, all cases to date have responded to intramuscular injections of the drug spectinomycin HCL (Trobicin). At the moment, this drug is strictly reserved for resistant cases of gonorrhea or treatment failures following other antibiotic therapy. Spectinomycin does not abort incubating syphilis nor is it effective against pharyngeal gonorrhea. Its safety for pregnant women has not yet been established.

Treatment follow-up. Regardless of the antibiotic used to treat localized gonorrhea, proof of cure depends on repeated negative cultures. The first culture should be taken about a week after treatment. Even if negative, the culture should be repeated in two weeks as a safety precaution. Individuals who have been treated and cured of gonorrhea do not develop immunity to the disease. They are as vulnerable to repeat infections as if they had never before contracted the disease.

Pelvic Inflammatory Disease

In 15 percent of women with gonorrhea, infection will ultimately spread to other genital organs and produce pelvic inflammatory disease (P.I.D.). This upward extension of the gonococcus to involve the uterus, fallopian tubes, and ovaries usually happens during the first menstrual period following exposure. Menstruation, in fact, encourages the spread of infection in the pelvis: the cervix softens, the endocervical canal dilates, and menstrual blood stimulates the growth of the gonococcus by providing the perfect nutritive medium. As a result, the GC organisms readily pass into the uterine cavity where their presence frequently causes a longer and heavier period. Inflammation of the uterine lining, however, is short-lived. The gonococci rapidly move on into the fallopian tubes to cause inflammation, swelling, and pus formation within the tubal passageways.

Even if signs of early gonorrhea were absent or minimal, infection that spreads to the fallopian tubes almost invariably causes symptoms. Lower abdominal tenderness, increased vaginal discharge, fever, chills, and the aggravation of pelvic pain on sexual intercourse are common complaints. When pus actually spills from the tubes onto the delicate tissues within the pelvis, pain can become severe and unremitting, and may be felt over the entire abdomen. From the fallopian tubes, the infection can spread to the nearby ovaries, causing the formation of large tubo-ovarian abscesses. In such severe infections, nausea, vomiting, abdominal distention, high fever, and peritonitis are common.

Treatment. Women with an early and mild tubal infection can be treated on an outpatient basis with adequate amounts of antibiotics (penicillin), analgesics for pain relief, and bed rest. They should avoid sexual intercourse for six to eight weeks; premature resumption of sexual activity could cause flare-ups and recurrences of infection by introducing other unwanted bacteria into the healing but still inflamed tissues. It is well known that the gonococci may do the initial damage but other bacteria (E. coli, Strep., etc.) can contribute to permanent tissue damage with long-term consequences. Chronic pelvic pain, abnormal uterine bleeding, increased risk of ectopic or tubal pregnancies, and sterility because of blocked tubes are a few of these consequences. In one particular study, 13 percent of the women had blocked tubes after only one tubal infection. After two infections, 36 percent had blocked tubes, and after three infections, 75 percent of the women were sterile due to blocked tubes.

SITES OF GONORRHEAL INFECTION IN THE PELVIS

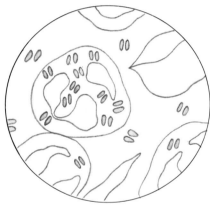

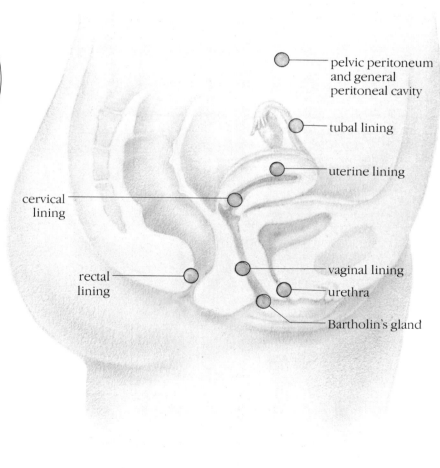

Gonorrhea is caused by the bacteria Neisseria gonorrhoeae, shown in the inset microscopic enlargement. Gonorrhea is highly infectious, and next to the common cold, is the most common communicable disease in the United States today.

Early sites of pelvic infection are shown in this diagram. The first symptom is a white discharge from the vagina and urethra that produces cloudy urine. Urination becomes frequent and painful. If untreated, the infection will spread to the other reproductive organs and the pelvic peritoneum, producing pelvic inflammatory disease. The symptoms are lower abdominal pain, fever and chills, and increased vaginal discharge.

Gonorrhea is usually curable with large doses of penicillin or other selected antibiotics (see page 459).

In more severe gonococcal infections, hospitalization is necessary. Treatment usually includes large doses of antibiotics given by injection until improvement occurs, after which oral medication can be substituted. For critical, life-threatening situations, such as the rupture of a large tubo-ovarian abscess, surgery may be necessary. In extreme cases, only removal of the uterus, tubes, and ovaries may save a woman's life.

Other Complications of Gonorrhea

In 1 to 3 percent of individuals with gonorrhea, the infection can spread by the bloodstream to involve the skin, joints, and other body areas. Women are more susceptible than men to such disseminated infections—particularly when pregnant. Furthermore, some of these women may be unaware that they have gonorrhea until they suddenly develop one of these complications.

Gonococcal arthritis is one such complication and occurs in about 90 percent of blood-borne GC infections. It is a septic arthritis that commonly involves the knees, wrists, and ankles. Symptoms range from pain to acute arthritis with swelling and fluid formation within the joint. If the disease progresses, it can lead to permanent joint damage and deformity. Prompt diagnosis and treatment with penicillin in non-allergic individuals readily clears the problem in the majority of cases.

At other times, blood-borne gonococcal infections can cause endocarditis (damage to the heart) and meningitis, but these complications are very rare.

Gonorrhea and pregnancy. If gonorrhea is acquired during the early weeks of pregnancy, there is a possibility of a spontaneous abortion and tubal infection. Contracting the disease after the third month of pregnancy tends to confine the gonococcus to the lower genital tract. The cervical plug, a thick, tenacious blob of mucus, seems to afford protection against the upward extension of the organism. Symptoms, if present, are therefore localized until after delivery. If undiagnosed and untreated, spread of the infection can then occur in the postpartum period.

Gonorrhea and the newborn. The eyes of the newborn are particularly vulnerable to the ravages of the gonococci. Contamination of the delicate ocular tissues by GC causes a violent inflammatory reaction that can rapidly progress to corneal ulceration, scarring, and blindness. Although most of these neonatal eye infections occur at the time of delivery, they can be acquired beforehand with premature rupture of the membranes. Because gonorrhea was once a common cause of blindness in the newborn, hospitals require that the eyes of every newborn be treated with a prophylactic instillation of either silver nitrate or penicillin solution immediately after delivery. On rare occasions, gonococcal conjunctivitis also can affect adults with similar end results if not promptly treated.

Syphilis

Of all sexually transmitted diseases, syphilis is potentially the most destructive. Early symptoms disappear spontaneously and yet, years later, the disease can return with devastating consequences. Syphilis is a highly infectious disease caused by the spirochete Treponema pallidum. This organism is shaped like a corkscrew and can twist and burrow its way through tiny breaks in the skin and mucosal tissue. Even the slightest scratch on any skin surface or mucous membrane can provide a portal of entry for this spirochete. The disease is acquired by sexual intercourse or intimate contact with an individual who has an open syphilitic sore. If the disease is present during pregnancy, the spirochetes can cross the placenta and infect the fetus. On rare occasions, medical personnel have acquired the disease by careless handling of infected patients or contaminated laboratory material.

Syphilis is divided into four stages: the primary and secondary stages of early syphilis, the latent stage of syphilis, and the late stage of syphilis (formerly known as tertiary syphilis).

The Primary Stage of Early Syphilis

The first sign of syphilis is the chancre, a painless red swelling about the size of a small pea. Within a week's time, it enlarges, erodes, and forms a non-tender ulcer with firm, sharply defined edges. The chancre marks the place where the spirochetes originally entered the body, and usually appears 10 to 90 days after contact with an infected person. The length of the incubation period depends on the number of active spirochetes that entered the body at the time of exposure; generally, the greater the number of spirochetes, the shorter the incubation period. On the average, the incubation period is three weeks.

In 95 percent of cases, the chancre is located near or around the penis or vulva. At times, it may be found on the lips, tongue, or breast, and occasionally a chancre located on the cervix or inside the vagina can escape notice by the woman. As a rule, there is only one chancre, but there can be more. Since each of these lesions is teeming with spirochetes, an individual is highly infectious at this time. In association with the chancre, there is usually a painless swelling of the regional lymph nodes on one or both sides, usually the groin or inguinal nodes. Whether treated or untreated, the chancre will gradually heal and the lymph node swelling will subside within four to ten weeks.

The Secondary Stage of Early Syphilis

If untreated, the secondary stage of early syphilis begins when the spirochetes invade the bloodstream and are disseminated throughout the body, usually six to eight weeks after the appearance of the chancre. In some instances, the secondary stage may begin even earlier or be postponed for several months.

The most characteristic sign of secondary syphilis is a skin rash. Skin lesions typically appear as a generalized non-itchy rash or as multiple skin or mucous membrane eruptions—anywhere from the scalp down to and including the soles of the feet and the palms of the hands. Occasionally the rash is so transient and indistinct that it goes virtually unnoticed. Other times, an individual may develop flat wartlike growths in the genital area. These syphilitic warts are called condyloma lata and are not to be confused with the common venereal or genital wart. Other symptoms of secondary syphilis may be nonspecific such as sore throat with hoarseness, headache, general malaise, aching muscles, and patchy loss of scalp hair. Some individuals may even pass through the secondary stage of syphilis with few if any of these symptoms.

The skin lesions of the secondary stage, like the chancre, are teeming with active spirochetes. It is during these stages of early syphilis (primary and secondary) that an individual can transmit the infection to a close contact. If untreated, the skin lesions of secondary syphilis spontaneously heal within three to six weeks, and the disease evolves into latent syphilis.

Diagnosis. There are two reliable methods of diagnosing early syphilis: identification of the spirochete in a skin lesion, or serological testing (a blood test). In primary syphilis, the chancre is usually scraped and the material is examined for the presence of spirochetes under a special dark-field microscope. Otherwise a blood test can be taken. In primary syphilis, however, the blood test is not usually reactive (positive) until one to four weeks *after* the appearance of the chancre. Since a chancre can sometimes go unobserved, any woman worried about the possibility of having contracted syphilis should have an initial blood test. If negative, the test should be repeated in six weeks and again in three months (90 days). A negative blood test for syphilis three months after possible exposure would be virtual assurance that there had been no contact with the disease. In secondary syphilis, the blood test is *always* positive.

The most common blood test for syphilis is the serological screening test VDRL (Venereal Disease Research Laboratory). It is accurate in detecting syphilis, but it also can be positive in the presence of other diseases not related to syphilis. Such so-called biological false-positive reactions can occur in a variety of illnesses. For example, patients with infectious mononucleosis, measles, chicken pox, hepatitis, and collagen diseases have at times shown false-positive tests for syphilis. In fact, any illness with a fever or any immunization such as a smallpox vaccination can result in a temporary (usually six months or less) false-positive VDRL test for syphilis. For this reason, a positive VDRL test may require confirmation. A specific and sensitive test for syphilis, the FTA-ABS test (Fluorescent Treponemal Antibody Absorption Test), can provide this confirmation. However, this test is not routinely used for the simple reason that it is complicated and expensive. At the present time, routine testing for syphilis with the VDRL is almost standard procedure in all hospital admissions, during pregnancy, and for individuals applying for a marriage license (premarital blood test).

Treatment. Once the diagnosis is confirmed, the treatment of choice is penicillin. Unlike the gonococcus, the spirochete has not developed any resistance to penicillin. Consequently, control and cure of the disease in the early stages can be obtained with relatively low doses. In individuals allergic to penicillin, tetracycline is used, except of course during pregnancy, when Erythromycin may be substituted.

Following adequate treatment, repeat blood tests should revert to normal and register negative. This means that if an individual has been successfully treated for early syphilis, subsequent VDRL blood tests such as that required for a marriage license would show no evidence of previous contact with the disease. Should the infection be diagnosed and treated at a later stage (for example, during latent syphilis), the blood test in certain individuals may always remain weakly positive despite successful treatment and eradication of the infection. Again, prompt and adequate treatment of early syphilis does not confer immunity; reinfection is possible.

Latent Syphilis

In about 25 percent of untreated individuals, relapses with recurrences of infectious skin lesions may occur during the early months of the latent phase. Thereafter, however, there are no signs or symptoms of the disease. The latent stage may last three to ten years or even longer. At this point, the disease can be detected by blood test only, and cannot be transmitted. The only exception is the pregnant woman with latent syphilis, who can infect her unborn baby. Interestingly enough, only one out of three untreated individuals with latent syphilis ultimately progresses to late syphilis.

THE PROGRESSIVE STAGES OF SYPHILIS

Syphilis is a highly infectious disease caused by the spirochete Treponema pallidum, shown enlarged in the inset below. If untreated, the disease may pass through the stages shown below.

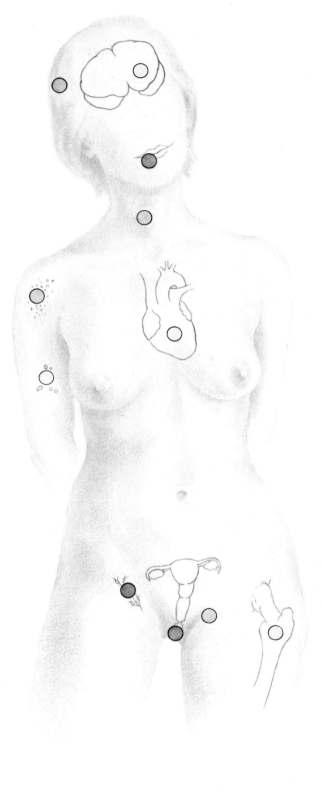

Primary Stage

SYMPTOMS
- Appearance of chancres on lips, tongue, external genitals, or anus
- Inguinal lymph nodes may swell

Secondary Stage

- Appearance of skin rash
- Patches of hair fall out
- Lesions may appear in most areas where skin surfaces meet
- Mucous patches may appear on throat, mouth, and tonsils

Latent Stage

No symptoms apparent

Late Stage

- Lesions appear anywhere on skin or body—even on brain, spinal cord, heart, and bones

enlarged view of spirochetes

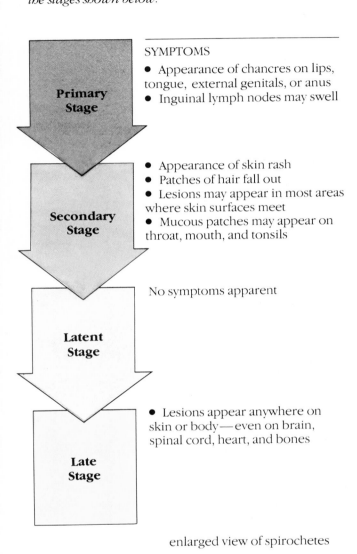

Late Syphilis

Since the spirochete can affect almost any organ or tissue in the body, late syphilis can be responsible for a variety of lesions. Among the most common are destructive lesions of the heart, large arteries, brain, spinal cord, bone, and skin. In this advanced stage, treatment is of little value.

Syphilis and Pregnancy

Early diagnosis and treatment of syphilis in the pregnant woman is essential if the fetus is to be spared. Unborn babies acquire syphilis from an infected mother through the placenta. Since maternal spirochetes do not readily pass the placental barrier until after the sixteenth week of pregnancy, treatment before the fourth month of pregnancy usually will prevent infection of the fetus. Treatment after the fourth month of pregnancy may cure the fetus of infection, but it won't necessarily prevent the symptoms of congenital syphilis such as neural deafness, corneal scarring, and joint deformities. Furthermore, once the fetus is infected, every month that passes without treatment increases the risk of more serious involvement. Where the disease is not diagnosed, the pregnancy can terminate in a spontaneous abortion, a stillborn baby at term, or a live infant with syphilis. Since the spirochetes invade the bloodstream of the fetus directly, there is no primary or chancre stage in congenital syphilis.

Of those affected infants who are born alive, 40 percent may have multiple skin or mucous membrane lesions, pneumonia, and bone, liver, and spleen involvement. Treatment at this stage may or may not

save the child's life. For the other 60 percent, the disease may remain latent and unsuspected for two years and frequently is asymptomatic until just before puberty. Diagnosis in these cases depends on a blood test. Any delay in detecting congenital syphilis can result in corneal scarring with blindness, destruction of the nasal bones (saddle nose deformity), notching of the permanent teeth (upper incisors), sight nerve deafness and/or brain, spinal cord, and bone damage. Treatment of congenital syphilis at this stage will stop progression of the disease, but will not reverse damage already done.

Genital Herpes

In the past ten years, genital herpes has become one of the most commonly seen infections in venereal disease clinics. It is a highly contagious disease caused by the herpes simplex virus.

In contrast to gonorrhea, genital herpes does not have the potential to cause permanent genital damage, but it can be painful and temporarily disabling. More importantly, the herpes virus has been linked with the development of cervical cancer and is a known cause of disseminated infection in the newborn. Recurrences or repeat infections of genital herpes also can occur without close physical contact. In other words, once an individual acquires genital herpes for the first time, there is no currently known way of permanently eradicating the virus. Even after signs and symptoms of the initial infection are gone, the virus (albeit inactive) will remain within the tissues of the body (see page 574).

GENITAL HERPES
The very first sign of a genital herpes infection is the appearance of small vesicles or blisters along the labial lips near the opening of the vagina. These blisters soon rupture and become quite painful.

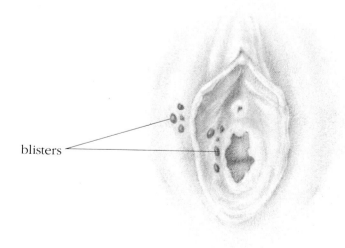

blisters

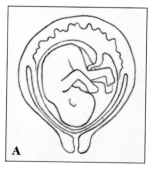
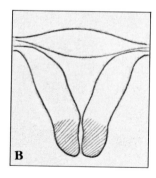

A

B

POSSIBLE COMPLICATIONS OF GENITAL HERPES
A *Newborn babies acquire herpes infection if their mother has herpes when they pass through the birth canal at the time of delivery. Once infected, the newborn has only a 50 percent chance of living.*
B *Women who have had genital herpes should have a routine Pap smear every six months. Studies suggest that women with antibodies to Herpes Simplex Virus Type II are more likely to develop cervical cancer than women with no antibodies.*

Among some women, emotional tension, stress, non-related illnesses with fever, menstruation, and even hormonal imbalances have been implicated as factors responsible for recurrences of this infection. Some experts contend that flare-ups of genital herpes can even be triggered by increased genital warmth from wearing nylon underwear and pantyhose. Fortunately, however, as the body builds up more antibodies against this viral disease, repeat attacks tend to become milder, less frequent, and of shorter duration.

For years it was believed that all genital herpes infections were caused by contact with the Herpes Simplex Virus Type II (HSV 2) during sexual intercourse. We now know that about 12 percent of cases are the result of Herpes Simplex Virus Type I (HSV 1), the virus responsible for the common fever blister or cold sore (see page 575). Furthermore, primary or first infections are acquired by intimate contact with an individual who is shedding the live virus. For practical purposes, this implies having sexual intercourse with an individual who has fresh genital sores or lesions just emerging, or lesions not completely healed. It also implies that an individual with a fever blister or cold sore around the lips or mouth can transmit the virus to his or her partner's genital organs during oral-genital sex. Conversely, herpes of the throat can be acquired by having oral-genital sex with an infected partner. But regardless of whether one is infected with Herpes Simplex Virus Type I or Type II, the symptoms are the same.

Symptoms of genital herpes vary depending on whether it is a woman's first exposure to the disease or a recurrent infection. If a woman has never had a herpes infection (for example, a cold sore, shingles, etc.) and thus no antibodies against this group of viruses, experiencing genital herpes for the first time can be distressing.

Following a two- to seven-day incubation period, the very first sign is usually the appearance of small vesicles or blisterlike eruptions along the labial lips, around the vaginal opening, and even on the cervix. These "blisters" soon rupture and become extremely painful, small, shallow ulcerations. Swelling and irritation around the urethral opening can also make urination very painful. Some women may be unable to pass their urine and thus require temporary catheterization until the edema subsides. Vaginal discharge and spotting can be expected where there is involvement of the cervix. Other symptoms include low-grade fever, general malaise, and swollen and tender groin nodes. In general, primary genital herpes infections will spontaneously clear within three to four weeks with no residual scarring from the vulvar ulcerations.

Recurrent infections are considerably more mild. Itching and slight burning discomfort of the vulva may signal the onset of a flare-up. In contrast to a primary attack, the blisters are smaller and less numerous, and frequently are localized in one area. A recurrent infection localized in the cervix and upper vagina may even go unnoticed because of few or no symptoms. Constitutional symptoms such as fever and swollen lymph nodes do not occur in repeat infections. Most cases will heal within seven to twelve days.

Diagnosis of genital herpes is usually made by the patient's medical history and physical findings. Few diseases can cause such distressing vulvar pain in association with small, shallow labial ulceration. Laboratory diagnosis can be made by taking a special Pap smear in which the bottom of the ulcers is scraped. Although the virus is not seen, the presence of certain multinucleated giant cells is indirect proof that the virus was present and responsible for the lesions. Where facilities are available, the virus can be isolated and grown in special tissue cultures. This method of diagnosis, however, is expensive, time consuming, and rarely necessary.

Treatment. There is currently no available treatment that will permanently eradicate the herpes simplex virus. Therapy for acute genital herpes is still limited to relieving symptoms and preventing secondary infection. Applying cold milk compresses four to six times a day for five to ten minutes—as well as a local anesthetic ointment such as lidocaine—may be helpful. Where pain during urination is extreme, spraying cold water onto the vulva while voiding can minimize the discomfort. For this purpose, a small plastic bottle filled with cold water and equipped with a spray top can be very helpful. In some instances, applying ether-soaked cotton balls directly to the lesions has helped relieve pain and shortened the course of infection. Another technique in which special dyes were applied to the lesions in conjunction with fluorescent lighting provided marked relief within 24 hours. But this photodye technique now has been largely abandoned because animal studies have shown that virus particles so treated may potentially become malignant.

Treatment aimed at reducing the frequency of repeat infections by building up antibodies against virus diseases also has been tried. Smallpox vaccinations, BCG vaccinations, and even polio vaccinations have been used, but to date, none of these treatments has been consistently effective.

There are, however, several new antiviral drugs that appear most promising. As of this writing, their release in this country is being delayed pending the results of clinical trials.

Genital Herpes and Cancer of the Cervix

Although there has been growing concern that genital herpes may predispose a woman to cervical cancer, there is no conclusive evidence of a cause and effect relationship at present. Nevertheless, it is known that the same factors associated with a high risk of cervical cancer also are associated with a high risk of genital herpes—namely, first intercourse at an early age and a history of multiple sex partners. Studies have shown that women with antibodies to Herpes Simplex Virus Type II are up to ten times more likely to develop cervical cancer than women with no antibodies to this virus. Some experts suggest that the virus may make the cervical cells more susceptible to malignant change. Until the issue is clearly settled, women with a known history of genital herpes should have routine Pap smears every six months.

Genital Herpes and Pregnancy

Genital herpes during pregnancy can cause miscarriages and premature labor, but the biggest risk to the baby is at the time of delivery. With few exceptions, babies acquire herpetic infections by being exposed to the virus as they pass through an infected birth canal. Women with no signs of active infection at the time of labor are probably not shedding the virus. This means that women could deliver normally and without fear of infecting the baby if they were not having a flare-up at the time of labor. If, however, there was a repeat infection of genital herpes near term, or obvious genital lesions (blisters or ulcers) at the time of labor, delivery would be by cesarean section. This would help protect the baby from contracting the virus.

Since there is no known effective treatment for disseminated herpes of the newborn, prevention of this disease is of the utmost importance. Once infected (and there is a 40 percent risk if exposed), 50 percent of the newborns will succumb. Among those infants who do survive, 25 percent may have severe neurological damage, and an additional 25 percent may have extensive skin lesions.

The severity of this disease in the newborn makes it imperative that any pregnant woman be alert to the possibility of genital herpes. Primary infections near term can be especially threatening to the newborn. A woman with a past history of genital herpes should be closely followed during pregnancy and particularly as she approaches her due date. She, herself, should be on the lookout for any suggestion of recurrence. Where the diagnosis is uncertain, the doctor may take serial smear tests of the cervix to check for the presence of herpes virus.

Although most herpetic infections of the newborn are the result of exposure to Herpes Simplex Virus Type II at the time of delivery, any contact with herpes virus during the first 48 hours of life is potentially lethal to the newborn. Thus, any individual with any herpetic lesions such as a fever blister or cold sore (Herpes Simplex Virus Type I) on the lips or anywhere on the body should not be allowed to handle or touch the newborn during those critical first two days. For some inexplicable reason, contact with herpes virus after the third day of life is rarely a serious problem. At this time, newborns usually can handle and successfully overcome a herpetic infection.

Other Venereal Diseases

Of the three other diseases traditionally classified as venereal—lymphopathia venereum, chancroids, and granuloma inguinale—infection with any one can cause ulcerative and destructive genital lesions. Fortunately, their overall incidence is less than one affected individual per 100,000 population.

Prevention of VD

For the sexually active woman, there is no foolproof way of avoiding any of these diseases. Nevertheless, a condom worn by the male partner is still the best protection against gonorrhea, syphilis, genital herpes, and other venereal infections. Also of value but less effective in preventing gonorrheal infection are contraceptive creams, vaginal jellies, or foams used prior to intercourse. All of these contain chemical substances that discourage the growth of gonococcal organisms. Douching immediately after intercourse also may help, but is not advised for women using vaginal creams or foams as birth control, as the douching could flush away their contraceptive protection.

If you are concerned that you may have been exposed to any of these venereal diseases, the best advice is to promptly see a doctor or visit a venereal disease clinic. With the epidemic increase in such diseases, more and more women are making appointments for the specific purpose of being checked for venereal disease.

Endometriosis

Ever since endometriosis was first described in 1860, it has been one of the most baffling of all pelvic diseases. Not only can it cause pelvic pain, irregular bleeding, and infertility, but it also can mimic infections and tumors, and certainly can take the joy out of any woman's sex life.

An Elusive Disease

By definition, endometriosis is a condition in which fragments of tissue from the uterine lining are deposited and embedded outside the confines of the uterine cavity, where they then grow. Although the precise cause of this disease is unknown, doctors believe that during menstruation, tiny fragments of endometrial tissue actually "back out" through the fallopian tubes and spill onto adjacent pelvic organs and structures. The ovaries, in particular—as well as the outer walls and ligaments of the uterus—can virtually become peppered with these tissue deposits. Furthermore, endometrial tissue fragments in these unusual locations behave much like the tissue lining the uterine cavity. In other words, they too swell, thicken, and bleed every month in response to hormone stimulation by the ovaries. The amount of bleeding is, of course, minute, but it does cause the surface of these endometrial implants to become sticky and to adhere to adjacent normal tissue. Although non-cancerous, the implants do tend to merge and slowly encroach upon neighboring organs. For example, tissue fragments on the backside of the uterus have been known to gradually invade the wall of the nearby large bowel. In an attempt to protect the surrounding pelvic organs from further involvement, the body covers these areas of endometriosis with scar tissue. In advanced cases of endometriosis, there can be so much scar tissue and so many adhesions that the female pelvic organs (uterus, tubes, and ovaries) are virtually glued to the bladder and bowel.

Symptoms. Strangely enough, the symptoms of endometriosis don't always match the extent of the disease. Women with severe endometriosis can be completely pain-free, while women with just a few tissue implants along the back wall of the uterus may have the most discomfort. One of the earliest and most common complaints is the onset of increasingly painful menstrual periods. Cyclic bleeding from the abnormally located tissue fragments can cause a steady dull-to-severe lower abdominal pain. Initially, the pain may be noticed just before or during the period. But later on, as the endometrial implants accumulate, merge, and press against the confining scar tissue, a nagging soreness in the lower abdomen can precede menstruation by one to two weeks. For some women,

the pain may begin as early as day fourteen of their cycle and reach a peak at mid-period. The pain sometimes can be localized in the low back area or felt along the vulva, rectum, or legs.

Dyspareunia, or pain during intercourse, is another major symptom that prompts women to see a doctor. The pain in this case is a sharp shooting sensation on deep penile penetration—a pain that has been likened to being impaled on a knife. Since endometriosis frequently involves the uterine ligaments, which are richly invested with nerve fibers, even the slightest touch or pressure against these affected ligaments can cause marked discomfort. During sexual intercourse, therefore, each penile thrust against the upper vagina and cervix stretches these ligaments and causes acute pain. In extreme cases, intercourse may only be tolerable for two or three days after menstruation. Partners may attempt different coital positions to limit the depth of penile penetration, but at best, the pain of endometriosis can be a sexual turn-off.

Heavy menstrual periods, more frequent periods, or totally irregular periods are other symptoms of endometriosis. The explanation for some of these bleeding problems has a hormonal basis. If the ovaries are involved with endometriosis, they may fail to function normally. In severe endometriosis, large single or multiple cysts (endometriomas) of both ovaries can occur. Some doctors refer to these cysts as "chocolate cysts" because they are filled with thick, brown, syrup-like fluid as a result of previous bleeding episodes. Ovulation is usually not affected unless there is extensive ovarian involvement.

Infertility or the inability to become pregnant is another problem. In 30 percent of women with endometriosis, this may in fact be their only complaint. Sometimes the cause of the infertility is obvious. Scar tissue and adhesions around the tubes and ovaries may prevent the egg from entering the fallopian tube. Infrequent intercourse because of severe pain during coitus also contributes to a low conception rate. At other times, there doesn't seem to be any reasonable explanation. All known factors necessary for conception seem normal—a fertile, willing partner, good cervical mucus, normal menstrual periods, regular ovulation, and open and functioning tubes. In these cases, some experts theorize that a chemical factor (possibly a prostaglandin) may interfere with the proper transport of the egg down the tube.

Women at risk. Endometriosis affects an estimated 10 percent of women in their prime years. Symptoms usually begin in the early twenties and may persist until menopause. Most cases are diagnosed between the ages of 25 and 35, but the process probably starts shortly after the onset of regular menstruation. Since the reflux of menstrual blood from the tubes seems to initiate endometriosis, women who ovulate and have regular uninterrupted periods over many years are definitely more vulnerable. Pregnancy—with its suppression of menstruation—tends to delay the onset and progression of endometriosis in otherwise susceptible women.

The use of tampons during menstruation does not appear to play a role in the development of endometriosis. Even if a woman should insert two tampons (side by side for heavy flow), it is highly improbable that they could block the cervical canal and allow menstrual blood to "back up." Furthermore, women with heavy menstrual periods do not run a higher risk of endometriosis. Conversely, women with lighter periods aren't necessarily protected from endometriosis. Some experts contend, however, that the long-term use of combination birth control pills (estrogen-progestin) may lessen the risk of developing endometriosis by reducing the amount of menstrual flow.

Diagnosis. The symptoms mentioned previously are usually the first indication of endometriosis. Increasingly painful periods and premenstrual pain are particularly suggestive. Where pain during intercourse is a prominent complaint, the uterine ligaments often can be felt as thick, beaded cords on pelvic examination. The pain experienced during penile thrusting frequently can be duplicated by manually stretching the affected ligaments.

ENDOMETRIOSIS

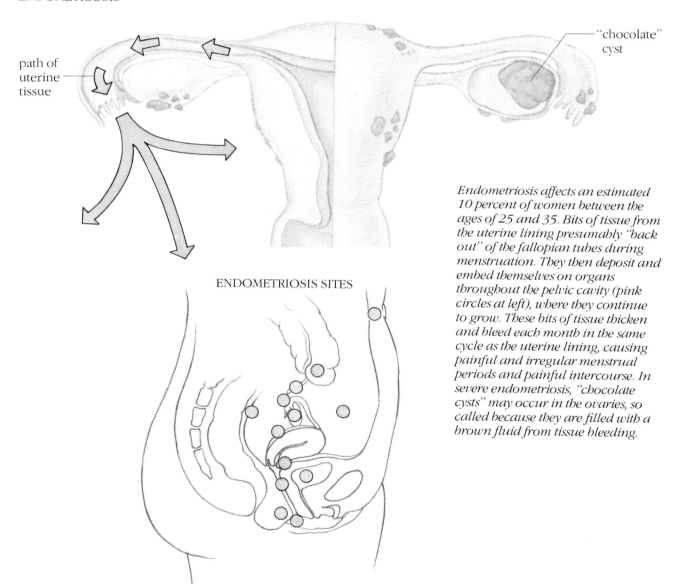

path of uterine tissue

"chocolate" cyst

ENDOMETRIOSIS SITES

Endometriosis affects an estimated 10 percent of women between the ages of 25 and 35. Bits of tissue from the uterine lining presumably "back out" of the fallopian tubes during menstruation. They then deposit and embed themselves on organs throughout the pelvic cavity (pink circles at left), where they continue to grow. These bits of tissue thicken and bleed each month in the same cycle as the uterine lining, causing painful and irregular menstrual periods and painful intercourse. In severe endometriosis, "chocolate cysts" may occur in the ovaries, so called because they are filled with a brown fluid from tissue bleeding.

But a definite diagnosis of endometriosis still depends on actually seeing the disease—examining the pelvic organs by laparoscopy. This can be done in a hospital operating room under general anesthesia. In laparoscopy, a slender telescopelike instrument (laparoscope) is passed into the abdomen through a small puncture wound just below the navel. This technique can verify the presence of endometriosis and evaluate the extent of the disease. In women with infertility problems, laparoscopy is particularly helpful in allowing the doctor to visually inspect the tubes for adhesions or scar tissue. Laparoscopy findings also help determine the best possible individual treatment.

Treatment. Ideally, the treatment of endometriosis should halt the progression of the disease, eliminate active areas of endometriosis, alleviate pain, and increase the fertility potential of the woman who desires pregnancy. Depending upon individual symptoms and physical findings this treatment can take the form of hormone therapy or surgery, either conservative or radical. Sometimes hormone therapy and surgery both are necessary.

Hormone therapy. Unless there are specific reasons for surgery at the time of diagnosis, most doctors initially will treat endometriosis with hormone therapy. This means preventing ovulation and menstruation by creating a pregnancylike state. The fact that pregnancy can cause areas of endometriosis to shrink and virtually melt away is the basis for this treatment concept. In the past several years, birth control pills taken daily and in doses high enough to prevent menstruation as well as ovulation have been a common form of treatment. In other instances, hormone therapy (Depo-provera injected every two weeks) has been substituted. There also are treatment regimens that use oral progesteronelike compounds.

LAPAROSCOPY

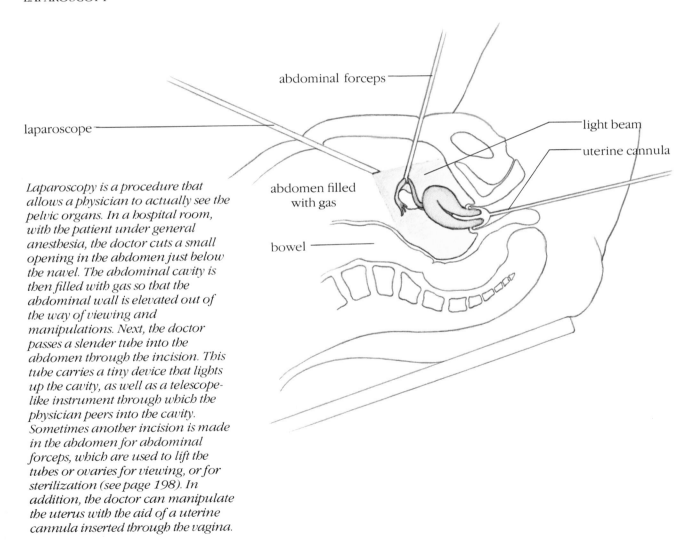

Laparoscopy is a procedure that allows a physician to actually see the pelvic organs. In a hospital room, with the patient under general anesthesia, the doctor cuts a small opening in the abdomen just below the navel. The abdominal cavity is then filled with gas so that the abdominal wall is elevated out of the way of viewing and manipulations. Next, the doctor passes a slender tube into the abdomen through the incision. This tube carries a tiny device that lights up the cavity, as well as a telescope-like instrument through which the physician peers into the cavity. Sometimes another incision is made in the abdomen for abdominal forceps, which are used to lift the tubes or ovaries for viewing, or for sterilization (see page 198). In addition, the doctor can manipulate the uterus with the aid of a uterine cannula inserted through the vagina.

laparoscope

abdominal forceps

light beam

uterine cannula

abdomen filled with gas

bowel

All of these treatments involving the use of high doses of estrogen and/or progesteronelike compounds initially cause swelling and edema of the tissue implants. For this reason, relief of symptoms may not be noticed until the swelling subsides and the implants actually begin to shrink and atrophy, usually by the third month of treatment. Even where there is a favorable response, most doctors advise continuing treatment for six to twelve months. Once medication is stopped, an estimated 60 percent of women may remain comfortable for as long as three to five years.

There are, however, disadvantages to this method of treatment. Some women simply do not tolerate high doses of hormones. Side effects such as nausea, vomiting, and excessive fluid retention may necessitate discontinuing the medication. Among women anxious to conceive, the return of ovulation and regular menstruation may be delayed after the hormones are discontinued. Injections of Depo-provera in particular can delay the return of menstruation for months. The potential risk of blood-clotting problems is another consideration for users of high-estrogen preparations. Equally pertinent, such hormone therapy may fail to relieve the endometriosis, or may even be contraindicated on the basis of other medical conditions.

Recently a new drug approach to endometriosis is proving remarkably effective in many cases. Danazol (Danocrine) is a synthetic hormone (androgen) that creates a menopauselike state by blocking pituitary stimulation of the ovaries. When this drug is taken on a daily basis, the ovaries are put to rest. Ovulation and menstruation cease, and estrogen levels are correspondingly low. In contrast to conventional hormone therapy, areas of endometriosis begin to shrink and atrophy almost immediately once the drug is started. Although therapy usually is continued for six months, Danazol often relieves symptoms within the first month or two of treatment. When medication is stopped, there is a prompt return of ovulation and regular menstrual cycles. This rapid restoration of normal function makes Danazol particularly helpful for women anxious to conceive following treatment for their endometriosis.

Because Danazol does not have any estrogen or progesterone effects, many women can tolerate it better than the conventional hormone preparations. In addition, Danazol does not increase the risk of blood-clotting problems. Any side effects are primarily related to its masculinizing effects from being a weak androgen. In some women, increased oiliness of the skin, acne, and perhaps even deepening of the voice may require discontinuing the drug. Weight gain can occur, but it is usually limited to ten pounds in most women. For others on long-term Danazol therapy, the presence of low estrogen levels may cause hot flashes, sweating, and other menopauselike symptoms. Expense is another consideration. At current pharmacy prices, the cost of one month's supply of Danazol can exceed one hundred dollars, depending upon the dosage used.

Danazol, however, is not a panacea or a cure. Recurrences can and do occur. Surgery, therefore, may still be necessary to treat the endometriosis.

Surgery. As effective as hormone therapy can be, it is not always the solution. Once the medication is stopped, there is always the possibility of recurrence. In other words, once ovulation and menstruation resume, areas of pelvic endometriosis may be restimulated or new areas may even form with the subsequent return of all the old problems. In a woman anxious to become pregnant, for example, hormone therapy would be of little value if scar tissue around the fallopian tubes prevented proper pickup of a released egg. Consequently, where any of these problems may exist, conservative surgery may be the answer.

Conservative surgery is meticulous pelvic surgery performed through a lower-abdominal incision. It seeks to preserve the reproductive organs while ideally eliminating all areas of endometriosis. For example, endometrial implants along the outer walls of the uterus and pelvic ligaments can be excised or cauterized and thereby permanently destroyed. Endometrial implants on the ovaries or even "chocolate cysts" can be removed, leaving as much normal ovary as possible. If the uterus is bound down by scar tissue, it can be freed and resuspended in a more normal position. Similarly, scar tissue around the fallopian tubes can be excised and the normal mobility of the tubes hopefully will be restored. As a further precaution against the recurrence of uterine pain, some gynecologists may strip away the tiny nerve fibers (presacral neurectomy) that carry pain impulses from the uterus.

Where endometriosis is the only known cause of infertility, 40 to 60 percent of women do conceive and carry to term following conservative surgery. When the surgery is performed primarily to relieve pain, results will vary depending upon the extent of the disease. Since it can be difficult to surgically eliminate all areas of endometriosis, temporary hormone therapy after surgery may be necessary to control minor recurrences. Of the women who do undergo conservative surgery, as many as one-third may ultimately need to have their uterus and ovaries removed because of continuing intractable pelvic pain.

The aim of such radical surgery is to bring about a complete cure by eliminating the source of the tissue implants (uterus) as well as the source of their hormonal stimulation (ovaries). If, in addition, the surgeon successfully removes all areas of endometriosis, estrogen therapy for menopausal symptoms can be given without fear of reactivating the disease. Otherwise, a short course of Danazol or other hormonal therapy still may be necessary to permanently eliminate small remaining pockets of endometriosis even after radical surgery. Thereafter, however, estrogen can be given only as needed.

Cancer of the Pelvic Organs

Within the next twelve months, approximately 68,000 women in the United States will develop pelvic cancer. During the same time period, an estimated 22,700 women will die from the following malignancies: 7,600 from cervical cancer; 3,300 from uterine cancer; 10,800 from ovarian cancer; and 1,000 from tubal, vaginal, or vulvar cancer. And yet as awesome as these statistics may seem, more than half of the women who ultimately succumb to pelvic cancer could be saved by currently available methods of early detection and treatment. Cancer is curable. There are thousands of women who can personally attest to that fact.

With the tremendous advances being made in cancer research, more has been learned about the cause,

treatment, and prevention of cancer since 1970 than in the previous five decades. New drugs, new techniques, and super-refined radiation therapy are giving back to many women their rightfully allotted time in which to live full and productive lives. Experts even predict that within our lifetime the mystery of how and why perfectly normal cells become cancerous will be uncovered.

Science and medicine, however, only can go so far. You as an individual woman also must take responsibility for your own health care. Going to your doctor for regular checkups is commendable but it isn't enough. You must become attuned to your own body so that you're aware of what's normal, what's not normal, and when to seek help.

NUMBER OF DEATHS FROM PELVIC CANCER PER YEAR
As shown in the diagram below, approximately 68,000 American women develop pelvic cancer each year, and about 22,700 women die from the disease: 10,800 from ovarian cancer; 7,600 from cervical cancer; 3,300 from uterine cancer; and 1,000 from tubal, vaginal, and vulvar cancers combined.

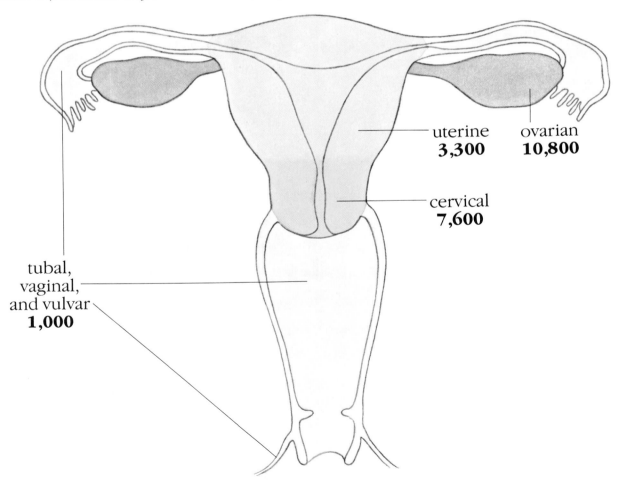

uterine
3,300

ovarian
10,800

cervical
7,600

tubal,
vaginal,
and vulvar
1,000

Cancer Incidence and Death by Site and Sex

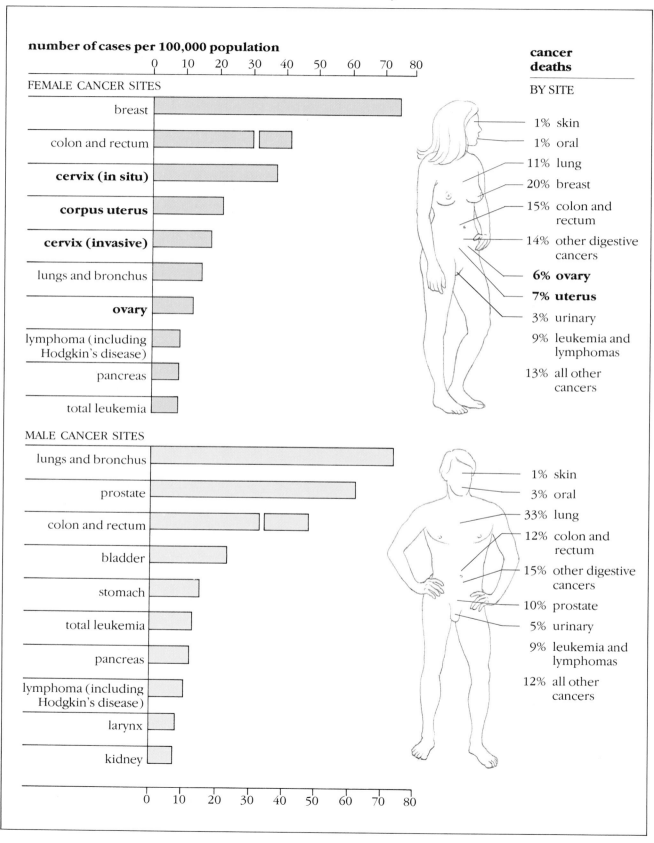

number of cases per 100,000 population

FEMALE CANCER SITES

- breast
- colon and rectum
- **cervix (in situ)**
- **corpus uterus**
- **cervix (invasive)**
- lungs and bronchus
- **ovary**
- lymphoma (including Hodgkin's disease)
- pancreas
- total leukemia

MALE CANCER SITES

- lungs and bronchus
- prostate
- colon and rectum
- bladder
- stomach
- total leukemia
- pancreas
- lymphoma (including Hodgkin's disease)
- larynx
- kidney

cancer deaths

BY SITE

- 1% skin
- 1% oral
- 11% lung
- 20% breast
- 15% colon and rectum
- 14% other digestive cancers
- **6% ovary**
- **7% uterus**
- 3% urinary
- 9% leukemia and lymphomas
- 13% all other cancers

- 1% skin
- 3% oral
- 33% lung
- 12% colon and rectum
- 15% other digestive cancers
- 10% prostate
- 5% urinary
- 9% leukemia and lymphomas
- 12% all other cancers

Cancer of the Cervix

The cervix is the lowermost portion of the uterus (womb). It is also known as the mouth of the womb or the neck of the uterus. Most women can feel their own cervix simply by inserting a finger as deeply as possible into the vagina. The cervix is that firm, rounded, knoblike structure (about an inch or so in width) that projects into the far end of the vagina.

In 1930, cancer of the cervix was the most common cause of cancer death among American women. Today, thanks to the routine use of Pap smears and more regular pelvic examinations, the number of deaths from cervical cancer has decreased dramatically. Despite this encouraging trend, however, the overall incidence of cervical cancer is steadily rising. In 1977, doctors diagnosed 20,000 cases of invasive cervical cancer, and detected an estimated 40,000 preinvasive cancers. Currently, estimates are that 2 to 3 percent of American women ultimately will develop cervical cancer.

Women at risk. Cancer of the cervix may one day be considered a venereal disease. Studies have repeatedly shown that there is a significant relationship between early and continuing sexual activity and the development of cervical cancer. For example, the teen-age girl who has her first intercourse by age 15 and continues to be sexually active runs a considerably greater risk of developing cervical cancer—and developing it before age 40—than the woman who delays intercourse until after age 20 and limits herself to one or two partners. Interestingly, cancer of the cervix is exceedingly rare among nuns, other celibate women, and lesbians.

Some experts believe that cancer of the cervix may be linked with a sexually transmitted virus (Herpes Simplex Virus Type II). The fact that a significant number of women with cervical cancer have had genital herpes lends support to the theory. There also has been speculation about the role of chronic cervical irritations and vaginal infections in predisposing women to cervical cancer.

Birth control pills have not been implicated in the development of cervical cancer. Nonetheless, widespread use of the pill, in addition to allowing greater sexual freedom, has significantly replaced the diaphragm and condom as contraceptive methods. Although difficult to prove, the risk of cervical cancer may be lessened if the cervix is protected from direct penile contact during intercourse by either a condom or a diaphragm.

Development of cervical cancer. The development of cervical cancer is a gradual process that can extend over a period of years. At first it causes subtle changes involving the superficial cells of the cervix. These changes then become more atypical and progress to dysplasia (a premalignant condition of the cervix). If untreated, dysplasia can progress to preinvasive cancer of the cervix and ultimately to invasive cervical cancer.

Symptoms. There are no symptoms in early (preinvasive) cancer of the cervix (Stage 0). This lack of warning signs during the preinvasive phase has been one of the stumbling blocks to early diagnosis. Women without symptoms often postpone routine pelvic examinations on the assumption that all is well. As a result, curable cancers can become advanced malignancies. Equally deceiving, a cervix with beginning malignant changes may look completely normal to the naked eye. Detection of preinvasive cervical cancer therefore relies primarily on a Pap smear (see page 474).

If the cancer remains undetected during this early phase, the malignant cells will gradually invade the deeper layers of the cervix (Stage I). In some women, this may be a fairly slow process, perhaps taking as long as four to ten years or even longer. Among others, and for unknown reasons, an early cancer can become rapidly invasive within a two-year period. Even then, however, symptoms may be absent until the tumor begins to erode tiny blood vessels within the cervix. At this time, a thin, pale, watery, pink or brown vaginal discharge may occur. Other complaints may include spotting after intercourse, spotting after douching, or painless irregular bleeding not related to either activity. This bleeding may be so slight that it doesn't even require a pad. Bleeding episodes also may be separated by several days. Proper treatment of this Stage I cancer (still confined to the cervix) can save four out of five women.

If still undiagnosed, the cancer eventually spreads beyond the confines of the cervix to other pelvic organs. Ultimately the vagina, the upper uterus, bladder, ureters, and even the rectum are invaded by the growing cancer. The cure rate for these relatively late stages drops precipitously, and well over 50 percent of women die from their disease. Unlike the early stages of the disease, which can progress relatively slowly and without pain, advanced cervical cancer usually moves rapidly. If untreated, the time lag between the onset of symptoms and incurable disease is frequently not longer than two or three years.

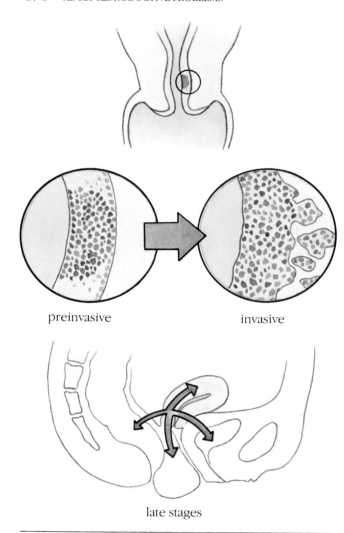

preinvasive   invasive

late stages

DEVELOPMENT OF CERVICAL CANCER

Early or preinvasive cervical cancer is localized and has not begun to spread. There are no symptoms at this beginning stage, but the cancer usually can be detected on a Pap smear (see opposite page). Gradually, usually over years, the cancer becomes invasive, with malignant cells growing into deeper layers of the cervix. The symptoms at this stage are a thin, pink or brown vaginal discharge. Proper treatment at this stage can save four out of five women. If not detected, the cancer eventually spreads to other pelvic organs such as the vagina, bladder, and ureters. The cure rate for late-stage cancers is less than 50 percent.

Diagnosis of preinvasive cervical cancer. When doctors speak of early cervical cancer, they are referring to preinvasive cancer, also known as carcinoma *in situ* of the cervix or Stage O cancer. Preinvasive cancer is still confined and localized to the *surface* cells of the cervix. Without signs and symptoms to alert either the patient or the doctor, detection of preinvasive cancer of the cervix depends primarily on a Pap smear.

The Pap smear is a screening test in which cells that are normally shed from the cervix, upper vagina, and the uterine cavity are collected, stained, and then examined under a microscope. Unlike normal cells shed from these areas, malignant cells have a totally different appearance. Their nucleus or central core is usually larger, and stains a darker color when exposed to certain laboratory dyes. The tissue source of any suspicious cells also can be identified. For example, malignant cells shed from the cervix look different than malignant cells shed from the uterine lining. Therefore the Pap smear also is helpful in pinpointing the location of a possible malignancy.

To take a Pap smear, your doctor must first insert a speculum into the vagina. By gently dilating the vaginal canal, the speculum permits the doctor to examine the inside of the vagina as well as the cervix. Once the cervix is exposed, cells are sampled from three areas: the secretions normally found in the upper vagina, the surface of the cervix, and the area just inside the cervical opening (endocervical canal). To collect cells from the surface of the cervix, most doctors will gently scrape the cervix with a tongue blade or a small wooden spatula. Cell samples from vaginal secretions and the endocervical canal may be collected on a cotton-tipped applicator, a wooden spatula, or a small pipette much like an eyedropper. All three samples are then separately smeared onto a glass slide, which is immediately sprayed with a fixative or immersed in a solution containing a preservative. The Pap smear procedure is not painful. Discomfort, if any, is usually related to the insertion of the speculum. Where a speculum cannot be inserted because of a too-snug vaginal opening, the doctor can obtain a Pap smear (albeit a less accurate one) by inserting a cotton-tipped applicator and swabbing the upper vagina.

When properly taken, Pap smears can be 95 percent accurate in detecting an early preinvasive cancer of the cervix. For the 1 to 5 percent of early cancers that may be inadvertently missed by the Pap smear, studies have shown that a subsequent Pap smear usually will reveal the abnormality. The Pap smear, however, is merely a screening test. While it does not prove or disprove the presence of cancer, it does alert your doctor to the need for further diagnostic studies.

Pap smears usually are reported as belonging to one of five classes. Most Pap smears will be Class I negative, which means that all the cells surveyed were normal in every respect. A Class II Pap smear also is reported as negative, but in this case, some of the cells were abnormal or slightly atypical, probably as a result of a vaginal or cervical infection—rarely because of cancer. Such a smear usually will revert to Class I following appropriate treatment. A Class II Pap smear is no cause for alarm, but it does require a follow-up smear, usually within three to six months. A Class III Pap smear lies in the gray zone and is reported as suspicious. On further testing, women with a Class III Pap smear may prove to have a premalignant condition of the cervix known as dysplasia. A Class IV Pap smear is interpreted as positive—a possible malignancy. A Class V Pap smear also is reported as positive—a probable malignancy.

Biopsy of the cervix. Pap smears reported as suspicious or positive for malignant cells require a tissue biopsy to confirm or disprove the presence of cancer. If there is an obvious ulcer, sore, or other suspicious area on the cervix, a portion of tissue (biopsy) from that area is removed for microscopic examination. In cases where the cervix looks perfectly normal, staining it with an iodine solution can help outline areas of abnormal cells. Normal cells stain a dark mahogany brown, whereas abnormal cells do not pick up the stain and can then be biopsied.

The colposcope also has been helpful in outlining abnormal areas for biopsy purposes in an otherwise normal-looking cervix. The colposcope is essentially a low-power microscope that can stereoscopically magnify the surface of the cervix. With this instrument, abnormal areas previously undetected frequently can be pinpointed and selectively biopsied without damaging surrounding normal tissue. Such tissue biopsies usually can be performed in the doctor's office and without anesthesia. Among young women with premalignant conditions of the cervix (dysplasia) as well as preinvasive cancer of the cervix (carcinoma *in situ*), the use of the colposcope has sometimes eliminated the need for more extensive tissue biopsies.

THE PAP SMEAR PROCEDURE

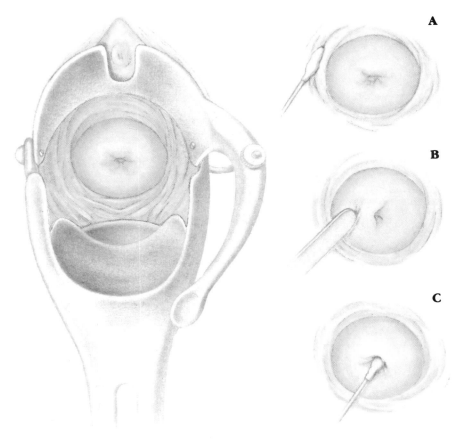

A

B

C

To take a Pap smear, the physician inserts a speculum into the vagina, exposing the mouth of the cervix. Once the cervix is exposed, the doctor takes cells from three areas and examines them under a microscope for signs of preinvasive cancer.

A *A sample of secretions in the upper vaginal area.*

B *A sample from the surface of the cervix.*

C *A sample from just inside the cervical opening.*

Pap smears, when properly taken, can be 95 percent accurate in detecting early preinvasive cancer of the cervix.

At other times, however, hospitalization for a cone biopsy of the cervix is still necessary to establish a definite diagnosis. A cone biopsy of the cervix is the removal of a cone-shaped section of cervix, including tissues from the surface of the cervix and from the inside of the endocervical canal. This is a hospital procedure that requires anesthesia. Because the amount of tissue removed is relatively larger than that removed by small "punch" biopsies, healing time may take up to six weeks. In certain cases, a cone biopsy also may be considered as treatment for early cancer of the cervix (see opposite).

Diagnosis of invasive cancer of the cervix also requires a tissue biopsy. The appearance of the cervix, however, can vary widely depending upon the extent of the cancer. At times, the cervix may appear almost normal, whereas in other instances an obvious tumor or ulcer may be present.

Treatment of cervical cancer depends primarily on the extent of the disease, the age of the woman, and her general physical condition.

If the cancer is diagnosed in its preinvasive stage while it is still confined and localized to the surface of the cervix, the traditional treatment has been hysterectomy—removal of the cervix and uterus. The ovaries need not be removed, as the hormones produced by the ovaries (estrogen and progesterone) apparently have no effect on cervical cancer. When performed for preinvasive cancer (carcinoma *in situ* of the cervix), hysterectomy has a cure rate close to 100 percent.

Not too long ago, preinvasive cervical cancer was usually diagnosed in relatively older women (over age 37). Today the majority of women with preinvasive cancer and dysplasia of the cervix are under 30. These abnormal cervical changes also are being seen with greater frequency among teen-agers. Since these women are young and are deeply concerned about preserving their childbearing function, alternate treatments are becoming more commonplace. Cone biopsy of the cervix (as previously discussed) can be definitive treatment for preinvasive cancer provided, of course, that the edges of the specimen removed are cancer-free. This would imply that the excised segment of tissue was ample enough to remove all of the malignant cells and a margin of normal tissue as well.

More recently, cryosurgery or the destruction of abnormal tissue by the application of extreme cold has emerged as a promising new treatment for preinvasive

cancer. Cryosurgery is an office procedure and does not require anesthesia. The cryosurgical equipment looks somewhat like a "gun" fitted with a probe and a small metal tip, through which a coolant flows. The doctor places the metal tip firmly against the abnormal tissue and allows the coolant (usually carbon dioxide or nitrous oxide) to circulate through the apparatus. Within a matter of seconds, the temperature of the metal tip drops to sub-zero readings and literally freezes the abnormal tissue and that immediately adjacent to it.

Such rapid freezing of the cellular protein destroys the abnormal cells and tissue. The process is then repeated until all of the abnormal areas have been treated. If necessary, an entire cervix can be treated within a few minutes. Cramping sometimes may be noticed, but the procedure is essentially painless, and cold in itself is a good anesthetic agent. For two to three weeks following cryosurgery, there will be a profuse watery vaginal discharge caused by the sloughing of the devitalized cervical tissue. Afterwards, normal cervical tissue rapidly regenerates, and within ten weeks healing is usually complete. Cryosurgery also is being used to treat benign cervical conditions as well as cervical dysplasia (a premalignant condition of the cervix).

Regardless of treatment, however, there is always the possibility of recurrence. This means that all women with an original diagnosis of preinvasive cancer of the cervix must be closely followed. Although the risk of recurrence is almost nonexistent among women treated by hysterectomy, regular pelvic examinations and Pap smears of the upper vagina still are necessary.

Women who've been treated with either a cone biopsy or cryosurgery are at high risk of a possible recurrence. Repeat Pap smears and pelvic examinations should be conducted every three months during the first year, and at least every four to six months thereafter. Such close follow-up enables early recognition of recurrent disease so that appropriate therapy can be started promptly if necessary. Many women who've undergone cone biopsy or cryosurgery will later elect to have a hysterectomy after their family is completed.

Invasive cervical cancer is treated somewhat differently. If the cancer has extended into the deeper layers of the cervix (Stage I), there is the possibility that tumor cells may already have spread to adjacent pelvic lymph nodes. The choice of treatment in this stage is radiation therapy or radical hysterectomy, which implies removal of the uterus plus the surrounding pelvic lymph nodes. Although each treatment has its advantages and disadvantages, therapy must always be individualized. Five-year survival rates for Stage I cancers run 75 to 95 percent.

Advanced cancers that extend beyond the limits of the cervix are treated by radiation therapy or by super-radical pelvic surgery.

Endometrial Cancer

Endometrial cancer is a malignancy that involves the lining of the uterus. It is the most common type of uterine cancer, and is currently the most prevalent pelvic cancer among women. In 1977, approximately 27,000 new cases were diagnosed. Only 5 percent of endometrial cancers occur in women under 40, making the disease predominantly one of menopausal and postmenopausal women.

Women at risk. The women most apt to develop endometrial cancer are over 50, and have a history of previously irregular periods, sporadic ovulation, difficulty in becoming pregnant, and bleeding problems during the menopausal years. Included in this high-risk group would be:
● women with past infertility as a result of the Stein-Levinthal syndrome (polycystic ovarian disease)
● women with a history of endometrial polyps or other benign growths of the uterine lining
● women who tend toward obesity, high blood pressure, and diabetes.
A few reports of endometrial cancer occurring in families lead some experts to speculate that genetic and metabolic factors may be involved in the development of this disease.

Since 1975, various articles in magazines and newspapers have focused on yet another possible risk factor—estrogen replacement therapy in menopausal and postmenopausal women.

Estrogen therapy and endometrial cancer. One of estrogen's normal physiological functions is to stimulate the growth of the uterine lining. In 1947, it was already known that certain types of overactive endometrial tissue could be produced by continuous estrogen stimulation. Recent reports now suggest that in predisposed women, the use of continuous estrogen over a period of time may cause premalignant tissue changes and ultimately even cancer of the uterine lining. According to these studies, the risk of developing endometrial cancer appears to increase with the dosage and duration of estrogen therapy. In one particular survey, women who had been on estrogen for seven years or longer were 13.7 times more apt to develop endometrial cancer than women who did not take estrogen. In contrast, the risk of endometrial cancer was negligible in women who had taken estrogen for less than six months. More long-term comprehensive studies undoubtedly will clarify many issues and hopefully will determine once and for all whether there is a cause-and-effect relationship between estrogen therapy and endometrial cancer.

BIOPSY OF THE CERVIX

If a Pap smear indicates the presence of malignant cells, the doctor will cut a piece of tissue from the cervix to confirm or disprove the presence of cancer. If there is a suspicious sore on the cervix (pink), tissue is removed from that area. The removal of a small amount of tissue by the "punch" method requires less healing time than the more extensive cone biopsy. To perform a cone biopsy, the doctor removes a cone-shaped section of the cervix, including tissue from the endocervical canal. This is done in a hospital under anesthesia, and healing time may take up to six weeks.

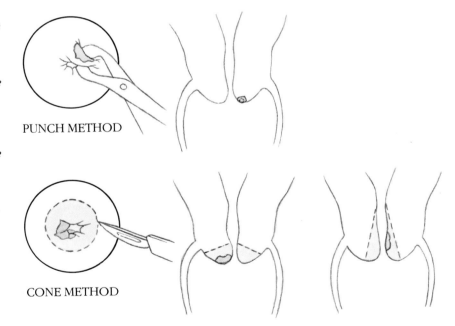

PUNCH METHOD

CONE METHOD

If you are taking estrogen replacement therapy, however, you should be aware of certain precautions that can minimize any risk:

- Estrogen should be prescribed only for very specific symptoms, such as severe hot flashes and vaginal atrophic changes (thinning and shrinking of the vaginal tissues).
- Only the lowest dose necessary to control the symptoms should be prescribed.
- Therapy should be discontinued when no longer needed.
- Estrogen should be taken cyclically (for example, 25 days on, five days off) rather than on a continuous daily basis.
- Women should have frequent checkups to reevaluate their progress and perhaps adjust estrogen dosage. Women at high risk for endometrial cancer probably should be reexamined every three to six months.
- Prior to starting estrogen therapy, each woman should have a thorough physical, pelvic examination, and Pap smear. Ideally this also should include a biopsy of the uterine lining or similar screening test (see opposite). Some experts would even advise repeating the screening test every twelve months thereafter—particularly for women at high risk.

Equally important in minimizing the risk factor, women on estrogen therapy should promptly report any of the following symptoms to their doctor: bleeding that lasts longer than seven days, periods that recur every 21 days or less, bleeding or spotting after intercourse or douching, or the reappearance of any blood or staining after six months or longer of no bleeding whatsoever.

It should be stressed that these precautions do not apply to oral contraceptives—only to estrogen replacement therapy. Women taking combination birth control pills (a combination of estrogen and progestin) are not at an increased risk of developing endometrial cancer.

Symptoms. Cancer of the uterine lining does not develop overnight from a normal endometrium. It almost always is preceded by premalignant tissue changes that in themselves give early symptoms. In the woman who is still menstruating, grossly irregular periods and/or bleeding or spotting between periods may be the first indication that all is not well. Among women over 40 in particular, excessively long, heavy, or frequent bleeding episodes can represent premalignant changes that, if undiagnosed and untreated, can progress to cancer.

Among postmenopausal women (those no longer menstruating), the occurrence of any spotting or bleeding never should be ignored. The bleeding need not be heavy. Frequently it may be nothing more than an occasional pink stain noticed on the toilet paper after voiding. Staining that lasts only a day or so does not mean that the problem is necessarily less serious than if bleeding were heavy and prolonged. Postmenopausal women on estrogen therapy also should promptly report any bleeding or spotting.

Diagnosis. The first sign of endometrial cancer is usually the occurrence of unexpected or abnormal bleeding. Armed with this information, the doctor then can proceed with appropriate tests.

Unfortunately, the Pap smear is not reliable in detecting endometrial cancer. Malignant cells from the uterine cavity may fail to be shed into the upper vagina. Thus it is not unusual for a woman with endometrial cancer to have a perfectly normal Class I negative Pap smear. Furthermore, the fact that the endometrial cancer arises within the uterine cavity makes it impossible to either see or feel on a routine pelvic examination. Detection of endometrial cancer therefore depends on taking a sample of tissue or endometrial cells from the uterine lining.

There are currently a variety of screening tests for endometrial cancer that can be performed in the doctor's office: endometrial biopsy, endometrial aspiration, and even mini-suction curettage. In taking an endometrial biopsy, the doctor inserts a small curette through the cervical canal and removes a strip of endometrial tissue for microscopic examination. Endometrial aspiration involves flushing out the uterine cavity with a sterile solution and then aspirating the fluid and discarded cells into a special container. The material collected is then examined for malignant cells. Mini-suction curettage removes tissue from the uterine lining by gentle suction.

These office procedures, however, are merely screening tests. An early endometrial cancer still can be missed by any one of them. Therefore, if a doctor strongly suspects the presence of an early endometrial cancer, he will proceed with a D and C (dilatation and curettage) even in the face of a negative screening test. Dilatation and curettage is a minor surgical procedure in which the cervical canal is temporarily enlarged (dilated) to easily permit the passage of a curette into the uterine cavity. The entire uterine lining is then thoroughly scraped. All tissue collected is placed in a preservative and sent to a pathologist for meticulous examination. Since a D and C essentially removes all the tissue lining the uterine cavity, it is highly accurate in detecting any malignant changes.

Treatment. Of necessity, treatment is individualized depending on the extent of the disease and the woman's physical and medical condition. If the cancer is early and still localized to the uterine lining, the treatment of choice is surgery—removal of the uterus and cervix (complete hysterectomy) and removal of the tubes and ovaries (bilateral salpingo-oophorectomy). (See page 480.) The ovaries are removed primarily for two reasons: tumor cells sometimes can spread to the ovaries even in fairly early cases of endometrial cancer; and dormant cancer cells, if any, sometimes can be stimulated by estrogen hormones from the ovaries. For this reason, estrogen replacement therapy is not recommended for women previously treated for endometrial cancer. Nevertheless, if the cancer was localized and believed to have been completely removed surgically, estrogen in judicious doses and under strict medical supervision is occasionally prescribed to control severe menopausal symptoms in younger women.

The treatment for more advanced cases of endometrial cancer is also surgical (removal of the uterus, tubes, and ovaries) but with various combinations of radiation therapy either before or after the operation, depending on the individual circumstances.

If endometrial cancer is diagnosed and treated in an early stage, the five-year survival rates can approach 95 percent. However, the overall five-year survival rate is 60 percent. Many women simply ignore symptoms and fail to seek medical help early enough. And of those women who are treated, many are poor medical risks at the time of diagnosis because of age, obesity, and other chronic physical problems.

Rare Forms of Uterine Cancer

Other uterine cancers, such as sarcoma of the wall of the uterus and sarcoma of the uterine lining, are more rare, as are malignancies (leiomyosarcomas) that arise within a fibroid tumor of the uterus. Unlike cancers, which tend to spread via lymphatic channels, sarcomas usually invade blood vessels at an early stage, and rapidly spread to the lungs and other distant organs. Prognosis generally is poor.

Choriocarcinoma is a rare but highly malignant tumor that may occur following a molar pregnancy (hydatidiform mole) or abortion. The tumor usually begins with the muscular wall of the uterus and rapidly metastasizes to other organs. In recent years, 85 percent of women who acquired this disease died within one year in spite of treatment. But today, various combinations of drugs (chemotherapy) can totally eradicate this malignancy in the majority of cases.

ENDOMETRIAL BIOPSY
Detection of endometrial cancer requires taking a sample of tissue from the uterine lining. The doctor inserts a small curette through the cervical canal and removes a strip of endometrial tissue for microscopic examination. The first sign of endometrial cancer is usually abnormal bleeding. But since malignant cells from the uterine lining do not shed into the upper vagina, a Pap smear will not detect endometrial cancer. The lining biopsy described here still may miss early endometrial cancer. If the presence of cancer is suspected by a doctor, he will thoroughly scrape the uterus, preserve all the tissue collected, and send it to a pathologist for meticulous examination.

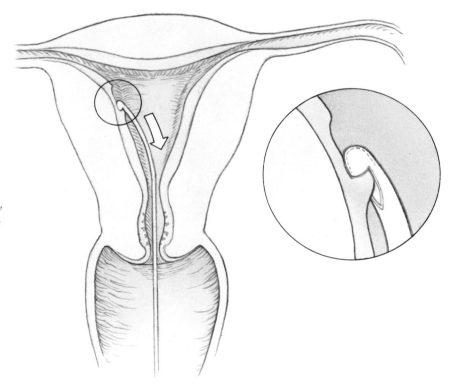

HYSTERECTOMY: SURGICAL REMOVAL OF THE REPRODUCTIVE ORGANS

The most common type of major surgery of the reproductive system is hysterectomy, removal of the uterus. The following definitions are given to aid you in talking with physicians and others. There are three types of hysterectomies.

- **Subtotal hysterectomy** involves surgically removing the uterus only.
- **Total hysterectomy** (also called partial hysterectomy) involves removing the uterus and the cervix.
- **Radical hysterectomy** involves removing the uterus, the cervix, and the pelvic lymph nodes.

In each of the above operations, the ovaries are left intact, so the source of female sex hormones is still present and the menstrual cycle still occurs.

Removal of the ovaries is an operation that may occur independently of hysterectomy or in connection with hysterectomy.

- **Bilateral salpingo-oophorectomy** removes both ovaries and both fallopian tubes (oviducts).
- **Unilateral salpingo-oophorectomy** involves removal of one ovary and one tube.

The major source of female sex hormones is removed when the ovaries are removed, and the result is menopause (premature menopause in a young woman) with its associated symptoms. (For more information, see the chapter on "Menopause," beginning on page 312.)

Careful studies performed in the last decade indicate that between 30 and 40 percent of hysterectomies performed in the United States are either unnecessary or suspected to be unnecessary. Always get at least three opinions, preferably from gynecologists who are not associated, before accepting hysterectomy. Hysterectomy is a major operation, used only for major

THE PELVIC CAVITY PRIOR TO SURGERY

illnesses such as tumors or cancer. Suspect any opinion that prescribes hysterectomy for anything less than one of these diseases.

Hysterectomy, as well as ovary removal, is most commonly done under general anesthesia. A horizontal incision is made at the upper edge of the pubic hair and the organs are removed. The top of the incision is sewn closed, leaving the depth of the vagina the same, so that the operation interferes as little as possible with sexual intercourse.

Hysterectomy has a profound effect on women, both physically and psychologically. If you undergo this operation, or must make a decision as to whether to undergo it, ask detailed questions of your gynecologist. Talk to other women who have had the operation, and consult reading sources (see page 667 and the chapter on "Menopause," beginning on page 312).

NORMAL REPRODUCTIVE ORGANS

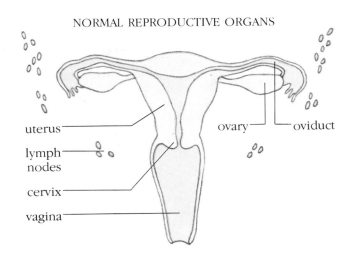

uterus
lymph nodes
cervix
vagina
ovary
oviduct

SUBTOTAL HYSTERECTOMY

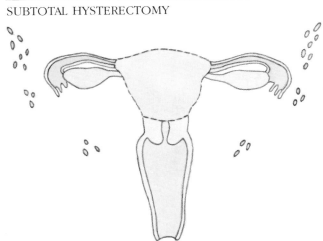

TOTAL HYSTERECTOMY

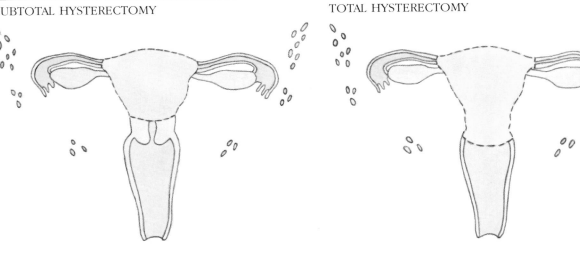

RADICAL HYSTERECTOMY

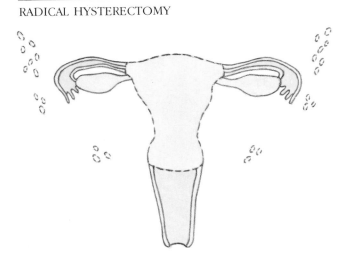

BILATERAL SALPINGO-OOPHORECTOMY

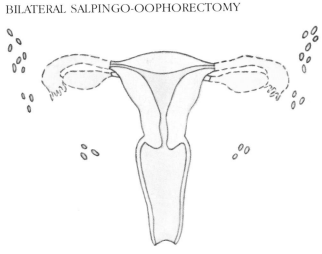

Cancer of the Ovary

Although far less common than either cancer of the cervix or endometrium, ovarian cancer still claims more lives than any other pelvic malignancy. In 1977, approximately 17,000 new cases were diagnosed, and an estimated 10,800 women lost their lives to ovarian cancer. It is currently the fourth most common cause of cancer death among American women—surpassed only by cancer of the breast, large bowel, and lung. Overall five-year survival rates for ovarian cancer are 25 to 30 percent, with over 50 percent of women having advanced disease at the time of diagnosis. Yet when the disease is detected early, five-year survival rates can be as high as 85 percent.

Part of the explanation for these bleak statistics is the nature of the disease. Malignant tumors of the ovary develop rapidly and frequently involve both ovaries simultaneously. Ovarian cancers also tend to seed malignant cells early. This means that tumor cells can be shed and deposited directly onto the surface of nearby organs such as the bowel, bladder, and uterus. Thus, in fairly short order, these newly deposited tumor cells grow and form more tumor masses. Equally important, there are no screening tests for ovarian cancer, and symptoms are minimal and nonspecific in the early stages of the disease.

Women at risk. In addition to being more prevalent in women between 50 and 60, cancer of the ovary also may be linked to other factors. For example, women who've never had children or who have had an infertility problem (or perhaps endometriosis) seem at slightly greater risk of developing ovarian cancer. Otherwise, cancer of the ovary shows no particular predilection for any group of women. Malignant tumors of the ovary have even been reported in children under five and in women over 80.

Symptoms. Lack of definite symptoms (at least initially) makes diagnosis of early ovarian cancer difficult. The first indication may be little more than a vague discomfort in the lower abdomen or a sense of pelvic heaviness. Persistent indigestion or a feeling of fullness after eating small amounts of food are other warning signs. In these instances, women may unsuccessfully resort to self-medication with antacids or other over-the-counter remedies. In premenopausal women, periods frequently remain deceptively normal, and many women thereby neglect their routine pelvic examinations. Bleeding or spotting in postmenopausal women also is uncommon as a sign of ovarian cancer. However, many ovarian cancers produce large amounts of free fluid that cause the abdomen to rapidly enlarge. Thus, a sudden inability to fit into one's clothes may be the symptom that finally prompts a woman to see her doctor. By this time, however, the tumor usually has spread beyond the confines of the ovaries.

Diagnosis. Diagnosing ovarian cancer after it has spread to other pelvic organs is not difficult. The real test lies in detecting the cancer while it is still limited and contained within an ovary. This is not an easy task. To begin with, the ovaries are small prune-sized organs that lie deep within the pelvis. They therefore are much less accessible to thorough examination than the cervix or uterus. Moreover, if the woman is overweight or fails to adequately relax her abdominal muscles during a pelvic examination, it is possible to miss a slightly enlarged ovary. As previously mentioned, there are no screening tests for ovarian cancer. Pap smears are completely worthless in this regard, and even X rays of the pelvis are rarely of value.

Diagnosis of early ovarian cancer therefore depends on the fortuitous finding of a suspiciously enlarged ovary on a routine pelvic examination. Although the ovary can be the site of many different growths, both benign and malignant, any mass that is suspect because of its consistency, shape, or size demands prompt surgical exploration. In postmenopausal women, for example, the finding of an enlarged ovary is never normal. Definite diagnosis of ovarian cancer is done by tissue biopsy at the time of surgery.

Treatment. Treatment is primarily surgical—removal of the uterus, tubes, ovaries, and all obvious tumors wherever possible. If the cancer cannot be completely eliminated by surgery, postoperative chemotherapy and radiation therapy are frequently advised. Some experts are now giving anti-tumor drugs prophylactically even in early cases. The outlook for the individual woman depends upon the type of ovarian cancer, the stage of the disease, and the success of surgery in removing the entire tumor. Age is another factor. Younger women as a group seem to have consistently better five-year survival rates.

Sometimes a slow-growing early cancer of one ovary in an adolescent girl or young woman can be adequately treated by removing only the involved ovary. Certain malignant tumors of the ovary also can be treated by similar conservative surgery, but these cases are indeed rare.

DES and Cancer

There is no longer any doubt that certain rare vaginal and cervical cancers can occur in the offspring of women who took the synthetic estrogen diethylstilbestrol (DES) during pregnancy.

In the 1940s and early 50s, doctors believed that estrogen (DES) could help maintain pregnancies considered at high risk because of previous miscarriage or bleeding problems. As a result, an estimated one to two million women in this country were given DES during pregnancy. In 1954, the effectiveness of estrogen in reducing the risk of miscarriage was discredited, but some doctors continued to prescribe DES in the misguided hope that perhaps it could help. Unfortunately, at that time no one was aware of the possible consequences.

In the late 1960s, the first indication of a possible connection between intrauterine exposure to DES and cancer shocked the medical community. Between 1966 and 1969, eight young women, ages 15 to 22, were diagnosed as having vaginal cancer (clear-cell adenocarcinoma), a particularly rare tumor. But even more startling was the finding that the mothers of seven of the eight young women had taken DES during that particular pregnancy.

To date there have been 333 reported cases of vaginal and cervical adenocarcinoma since 1966, and 68 percent of these cases have been associated with DES taken during pregnancy.

An estimated 70 to 90 percent of women exposed to DES *in utero* also have been found to have abnormal tissue changes, including adenosis of the vagina and cervix. Vaginal adenosis is the replacement of vaginal mucosal tissue by glandular tissue. The extent and distribution of these cell changes varies considerably from woman to woman. Sometimes only a small portion of the vaginal wall is involved. In other instances, adenosis may be present in several areas, including the cervix. Adenosis is not considered a premalignant condition by most experts, but it does represent an area of cellular transformation that does have the potential to become premalignant. For this reason, young women with vaginal adenosis should be closely followed at regular intervals. On the more optimistic side, recent studies indicate that vaginal adenosis may spontaneously regress in the majority of women. Even more comforting is the finding that up to now, not a single woman being followed for proven vaginal adenosis has ultimately developed a vaginal cancer. The actual risk of a DES-exposed woman developing adenocarcinoma of the vagina or cervix has been assessed at about one chance in 1,000. If the disease is diagnosed early, therapy can preserve the ability to have intercourse and bear children.

Currently most doctors are advising that DES daughters be examined at least once or twice yearly, depending on the results of the initial evaluation. Since most cases of DES cancer seem to develop after the menarche (onset of menstruation) with a peak incidence at 19, the first examination should be performed by the age of 14. This would imply a complete physical and careful pelvic examination, with special attention paid to the vagina and cervix. Pap smears as well as special iodine stains to outline suspicious tissue areas for biopsy purposes should be included. Where practical, the use of a colposcope (a magnifying instrument) also could help pinpoint abnormal tissue changes. Among younger DES-exposed girls, the presence of any vaginal discharge or abnormal bleeding should be promptly reported and evaluated.

Male offspring of women who took DES during pregnancy should be examined by a urologist. Although there have been no reported cases of DES-induced cancer among male offspring, there have been scattered reports of testicular abnormalities, epididymal cysts (part of the vas), undersized penises, and low sperm counts.

For the woman who wants more information about DES and cancer, free pamphlets are available. Write to the DESAD Project, National Cancer Institute, Office of Cancer Communication, Bethesa, Maryland 20014.

Other Pelvic Cancers

Vaginal cancers not related to DES are primarily found in women over 50 and represent approximately 1 percent of all pelvic cancers. Symptoms are usually spotting or bleeding after the menopause. Treatment, either by radiation therapy or surgery, depends on the extent of the disease at the time of diagnosis.

Cancer of the fallopian tube is very rare but does occur more frequently in older women. Although it is difficult to diagnose early, abnormal bleeding is present in over half of the cases. Treatment is a combination of surgery and radiation. Five-year survival rates are apt to be poor because of late diagnosis.

Cancer of the Vulva

In the female, the term vulva refers to the entire area between the legs, with the exception of the anus. Thus, the vulva includes the inner and outer lips (labia), the vaginal opening, and the clitoris. Cancer of the vulva can begin in any one of these structures, and accounts for about 3 percent of all pelvic malignancies.

Itching is by far the most frequent early symptom of vulvar cancer. Among women over 50 in particular, any persistent itching, irritation, or inflammation of the vulva should be investigated. Other pertinent signs and symptoms include a mole or freckle that becomes darker, more prominent, or otherwise enlarges or changes. Any lump, bump, ulcer, or other growth of more than two weeks' duration also should be brought to the attention of your doctor.

Treatment is surgical, and five-year survival rates can be excellent, depending on how early the cancer is diagnosed. However, needless procrastination to have symptoms diagnosed allows many vulvar cancers to become relatively advanced before treatment is begun.

Congenital Problems

No discussion of the female reproductive system is complete without a review of genetic and developmental defects of the sex organs. Although some of these conditions may be minor enough never to cause problems, others can have profound effects on a woman's sexual development and reproductive capacity. Parents in particular are invariably disturbed to learn that their daughter may have some abnormality of the sex organs. Particularly stressful is the situation in which the sex of a newborn baby may be uncertain because of the appearance of the external genitalia. In other instances, an adult woman may be unable to carry a pregnancy to term because of an undiagnosed maldevelopment of the uterus. Or, a young teen-ager may fail to develop breasts or have periods like the rest of her girl friends.

But before we can begin to understand some of these complex problems and the factors that control them, we must know something about the process of normal sexual differentiation.

How the Sex Organs Develop

Genetic sex. Each cell in our body normally contains a total of 46 chromosomes, 22 pairs of autosomes (non-sex chromosomes), and one pair of sex chromosomes. In the normal female, these sex chromosomes are XX; in the normal male, XY. In medical shorthand, the symbols for a normal female and a normal male with a full complement of chromosomes are 46XX and 46XY respectively. Genetic or chromosomal sex (XX for female and XY for male) is determined along with the rest of our genetic makeup at the moment of fertilization. If the ovum (which normally carries an X chromosome) is fertilized by an X-bearing sperm, the result is a genetic female, XX. If the ovum is fertilized by the Y-bearing sperm, the result is XY or a genetic male. Since an ovum always carries an X chromosome, the genetic sex of an individual is solely determined by the type of sex chromosome (X or Y) carried by the fertilizing sperm. Thus, the male partner determines the genetic sex of the offspring. But this is only the bare beginning of sexual differentiation.

Ovaries and testes. During the first five or six weeks of pregnancy, the embryo is actually in an indifferent stage of sexual development. In other words, even though the sex of the embryo has already been programmed, there is as yet no ovarian or testicular tissue and no discernible development of internal or external sex organs or ducts. Rather, there are two clusters of cells (the primitive gonads) that have the *potential* of developing into either ovaries or testes. Next to each of these primitive gonads is another mass of undifferentiated tissue that has the potential of developing into either the male internal duct system (epididymis, vas deferens, and seminal vesicles) or the female internal duct system, made up the uterus, tubes, and upper vagina.

At about the sixth week of intrauterine life, the differentiation of each primitive gonad into a testis will begin in genetic males. In females, the development of the ovary occurs somewhat later. Ultimately it is the sex chromosomes (X or Y) that control and direct the differentiation of the primitive gonads into ovaries or testes. The development of a testis depends on the presence of a Y chromosome; the development of an ovary requires two normal X chromosomes. The differentiation of the sex glands (gonads) is usually complete by the twelfth week, but they continue to mature throughout fetal life.

Internal sex ducts. The next stage is the differentiation of the internal sex ducts. As previously mentioned, the mass of undifferentiated tissue lying next to each primitive gonad has the potential to develop into male or female internal ducts. The female component of this tissue (the müllerian duct system) forms the fallopian tubes, uterus, and upper vagina. The male component (the wolffian duct system) develops into the epididymis, vas deferens, and seminal vesicles.

If the fetus is a genetic male (XY), normal male sexual development depends entirely on the secretion of important "masculinizing substances" by the fetal testes. Among these masculinizing substances are an "organizing substance" and various androgen hormones, including testosterone. Beginning at about eight weeks in a genetic male embryo, the organizing substance causes the müllerian or female duct system to disappear, while it also encourages the development of the male or wolffian duct system. The androgen hormones secreted by the fetal testes are necessary for the further development of the male internal sexual ducts (epididymis, vas deferens, and seminal vesicles) and the full development of the male external genitalia (penis and scrotum).

If the fetus is a genetic female (XX), development of the müllerian duct system to form the uterus, tubes, and upper vagina begins near the end of the second month of fetal life. In the normal process of events, the middle and lower portions of the müllerian duct systems (one on each side) fuse to form a single uterus, cervix, and vagina. The upper portions do not join but remain separate and distinct as the fallopian tubes. Any disturbance in the normal development and fusion of these structures can lead to a variety of anomalies.

Also at this time, the wolffian or male duct system in the female fetus begins to regress and disappear. These changes do not depend on or require the presence of a fetal ovary, but occur simply because there are no fetal testes producing masculinizing substances. In other words, without the testicular organizing substance, the development of the duct system is always along female lines. Similarly, female external genitalia will always develop in the absence of androgenic (male) hormone stimulation. To further illustrate this point, individuals who through genetic error have neither ovaries nor testes still will have the internal and external organs and ducts of a female. In effect, a fetus will invariably develop the uterus, fallopian tubes, vagina, and the external genitalia of a female as long as there are no functioning testes to oppose that development. As you will soon see, this basic concept goes a long way toward explaining many problems of sexual identity.

GENETIC DETERMINATION OF SEX

Each cell in our body normally contains a total of 46 chromosomes, 22 pairs of autosomes (non-sex chromosomes) and one pair of sex chromosomes. In the normal female, these sex chromosomes are XX; in the normal male, the chromosomes are XY. Genetic or chromosomal sex (XX for females and XY for males) is determined along with the rest of our genetic makeup at the moment of fertilization. If the ovum (which normally carries an X chromosome) is fertilized by an X-bearing sperm, the result is a genetic female, XX. If the ovum is fertilized by a Y-bearing sperm, the result is XY, or a genetic male.

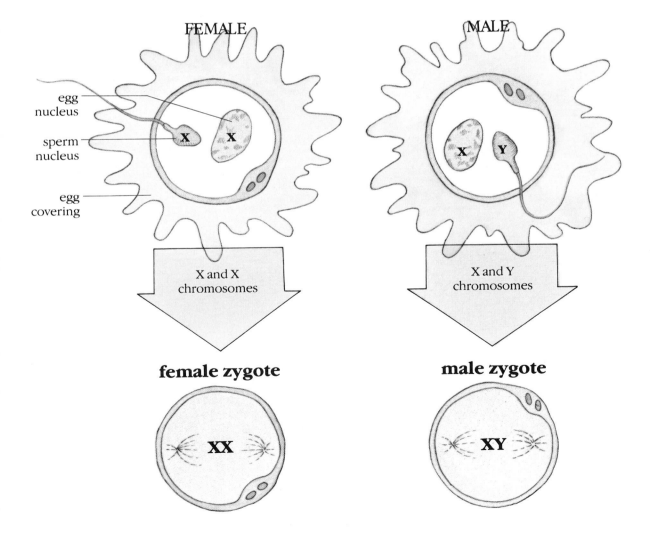

DEVELOPMENT OF THE FEMALE AND MALE REPRODUCTIVE SYSTEMS

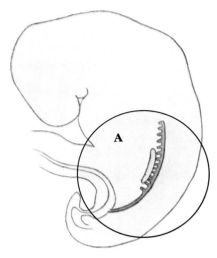

A *At five weeks of age, the future reproductive system of the fetus is in place. At this stage, the paired, primitive gonads appear identical in males and females, although the chromosomal sex is definitely determined (see page 485). The gonads are said to be in the indifferent stage of sexual develop-* ment *because, as yet, there are no ovaries or testes, tubes, ducts, etc. —just the primitive gonads, which are the same in males and females.*
B *An ovary or a testis will develop from the primitive gonadal tissue (yellow) and the other internal sex organs from the primitive duct tissue (adjacent to the gonad).*

7 WEEKS

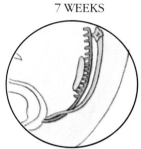

UNDIFFERENTIATED STAGE
(front view at 7 weeks)

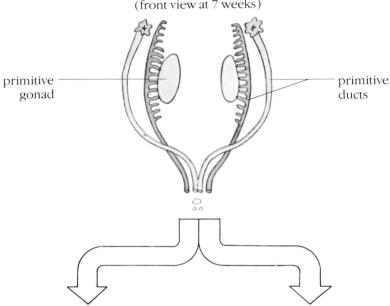

primitive gonad

primitive ducts

male
12 weeks to birth

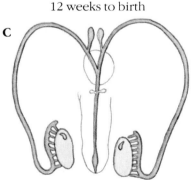

C

female
12 weeks to birth

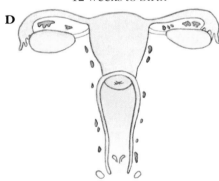

D

The primitive embryonic duct system next to the gonads has the potential of developing into either the male internal duct system (epididymis, vas deferens, and seminal vesicles) (C) or the female internal duct system (uterus, fallopian tubes, and upper vagina) *(D). The differentiation of the ovaries and testes is usually complete by the twelfth week. The other structures of the reproductive system, both internal and external, continue to develop throughout fetal life.*

External genitalia. The external genitalia usually can be identified as male or female by about the twelfth to fourteenth week of intrauterine life. Prior to that time, there is an indifferent stage at which each sex has similar-appearing structures. In the male, the development and growth of the penis (from the genital tubercle), the formation of the scrotum (from the fusion of the genital and labio-scrotal folds), and the placement of the urethra so that it traverses the entire length of the penis all depend on androgenic stimulation from the testes.

In the female, the lack of androgenic hormone stimulation causes the genital tubercle to remain small and become the clitoris. The genital and labio-scrotal folds do not fuse in the midline but instead develop into the labia minora and labia majora. And lastly, separate openings form for the urethra and vagina.

Congenital Maldevelopments

Familiarity with these processes of sex differentiation is important in understanding congenital maldevelopments that affect the female genital tract. For convenience, we will divide the problems into three groups:
• those involving the external genitalia, usually detected in infancy and early childhood
• those affecting menstruation and/or sexual maturation, usually diagnosed during adolescence
• those that can interfere with reproduction, usually diagnosed during the adult years.

Defects of the External Genitalia

One of the most serious of these developmental problems is masculinization of the female newborn. Almost all such cases are the result of prenatal exposure to androgen (masculinizing) hormones, either formed by the fetal adrenal glands themselves or transmitted to the fetus from the mother. The most severe cases of masculinization are usually caused by congenital adrenal hyperplasia.

Congenital adrenal hyperplasia is a complex inherited genetic defect of the fetus in which one or several enzymes necessary for the manufacture or synthesis of cortisol (hydrocortisone) by the adrenal glands is deficient. As a consequence, the fetal pituitary stimulates the adrenals to work harder in an attempt to increase their output of this important hormone, vital to many metabolic processes. In many cases, this pituitary gland overstimulation ultimately does achieve a more normal output of cortisol in the fetus, but at a terrible price: the end result is enlargement and hyperactivity of the adrenal glands, along with a massive overproduction of their androgenic hormones. When the female fetus is exposed to this continuous high output of androgen hormones from her own adrenal glands, the external genitalia begin to develop along male lines.

EXTERNAL GENITAL DEVELOPMENT

A *In the first twelve weeks of life, the future male and female external genitalia appear identical.*
B *At about 12 to 14 weeks of development, male and female characteristics begin to be identifiable. Androgen hormone is secreted in the male fetus, and the penis develops from the genital tubercle (light pink). The scrotum develops from the labio-scrotal folds (yellow), and the urogenital folds (dark pink) fold over to form part of the penis and enclose the urethra so that it traverses the entire length of the penis.*
C *The female genital tubercle remains small and becomes the clitoris (light pink). Instead of fusing in the midline, the urogenital folds develop into the labia minora (dark pink), and the labio-scrotal folds develop into the labia majora (yellow).*

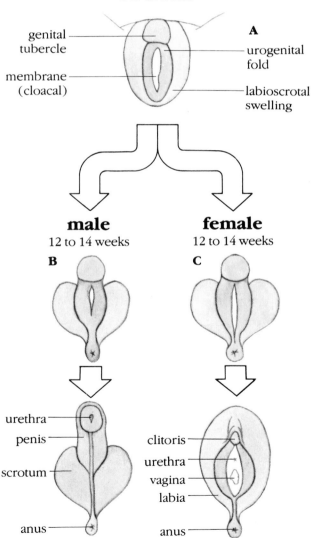

UNDIFFERENTIATED STAGE
0 to 12 weeks

genital tubercle — **A** — urogenital fold

membrane (cloacal) — labioscrotal swelling

male
12 to 14 weeks
B

female
12 to 14 weeks
C

urethra
penis
scrotum
anus

clitoris
urethra
vagina
labia
anus

CONGENITAL ADRENAL HYPERPLASIA

Congenital adrenal hyperplasia is a complex inherited genetic defect occurring in about 15 of every million births. The adrenal gland cannot manufacture sufficient hydrocortisone. As a result, the pituitary signals the adrenal glands to work harder in an attempt to increase their output of hydrocortisone.

The adrenal glands respond by growing larger and indeed do produce more of this important hormone, but also more androgenic (male) hormones. The female, exposed to this output of androgen from her own adrenal glands, begins to develop male sexual characteristics (see page 616).

PITUITARY GLAND

the pituitary gland
overstimulates the
ADRENAL GLAND

the adrenal gland
enlarges and produces
too much androgen

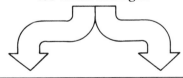

Adrenal hyperplasia

without treatment   with treatment

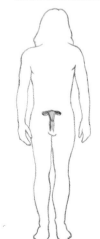 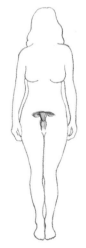

Appearance. Although the appearance of the clitoris and labia can vary considerably from case to case, there are some characteristic changes. The most common deviation from normal is a marked and obvious enlargement and firmness of the clitoris. The labia also may fuse completely in the midline, giving the appearance of a scrotum (albeit an empty one without testes). In extreme cases, the vaginal opening may be obliterated and the urethra actually may traverse the entire length of the clitoris, much as in a normal penis. Is it any wonder that in these instances there may be understandable confusion about the sex of the newborn? Females with congenital adrenal hyperplasia, however, are normal genetic females with two X chromosomes, normal ovaries, and normal internal female structure—uterus, tubes, and upper vagina. As previously discussed, absence of testes and the "organizing substance" still allows normal development of the internal female duct system.

Other complications. Males with congenital adrenal hyperplasia are similarly exposed to high levels of androgen hormones, but in these cases the problem is understandably not obvious at birth. If the condition is not diagnosed and treated, both male and female infants experience progressive and rapid virilization as a result of continuing excessive androgen stimulation. By age two or three, pubic hair frequently appears, followed within months by axillary hair. The clitoris further enlarges and there even may be frequent erections. In male children, the penis can assume adult proportions by the age of five.

In both sexes there is rapid acceleration of long bone growth so that by the age of five or six, these children may have the height of twelve-year-olds. As adults, however, they are shorter than normal because of the premature closure of the growing centers within the long bones. In untreated females, there is no breast development and rarely, if any, menstrual periods. Excessive androgen production blocks the output of the pituitary hormones (gonadotropins) necessary for ovarian function. Ultimately, most untreated females develop marked hirsutism (excessive facial and body hair), deepening of the voice, and a very muscular, stocky build.

In about one-third of all infants with adrenal hyperplasia, the problem also is complicated by a "salt losing" variety of the disorder. These infants are unable to store and conserve sodium (salt), and can rapidly succumb to severe electrolyte imbalance and dehydration. In these specific cases, prompt diagnosis and treatment in the first few days following birth may be lifesaving.

Diagnosis. The first clue in the diagnosis of this condition in female newborns is the appearance of the external genitalia. Interestingly enough, whenever an infant exhibits ambiguous genitalia or genitalia that do not completely conform to those of a normal male or normal female, the most likely diagnosis is congenital adrenal hyperplasia. If this same infant also is shown to be a genetic female (XX) by means of the sex chromatin test—this, too, is confirmatory evidence. But absolute verification of congenital adrenal hyperplasia depends on finding elevated levels of androgenic hormones in the urine.

Treatment. Since this disorder is a lifetime condition, treatment with cortisone or cortisollike compounds to suppress adrenal overactivity must be continued throughout life of the individual. In female infants, surgery also is necessary to correct genital appearance.

The extent of genital plastic surgery depends on the degree of masculinization, but the intent is to restore the appearance and function of normal sex organs. In almost all cases, this requires resection and reshaping of the clitoris to normal female dimensions. At the same time, fused labia can be separated and refashioned into labia minora and labia majora. Where the vaginal opening is covered by a thin bridge of skin, that, too, can be corrected.

These surgical procedures usually are done as soon after birth as possible. Corrective surgery at this early date not only lessens parental anxiety about the appearance of their infant daughter but also helps promote healthy psychosexual development in the child. Since the need for vaginal surgery to redirect or exteriorize the vaginal outlet is less immediate in terms of cosmetic appearance, these procedures, if necessary, can be postponed until just prior to puberty and the advent of menstruation. Thus, with medical treatment and genital plastic surgery, females with congenital adrenal hyperplasia can develop as normal females with the capacity to bear children.

The Sex Chromatin Test

Genetic or chromosomal sex (XX for females, XY for males) can be determined by the study of almost any body tissue, but the simplest screening test—particularly in infants—is the buccal smear test for sex chromatin.

The mucosa along the inside of the cheek is gently scraped with a tongue blade. The material obtained is then spread onto a glass slide and stained with a special dye. The cells are examined under a microscope for the presence or absence of the sex chromatin body, also called the Barr body, after its discoverer. The Barr body is a minute particle of the female X chromosome, and is seen under the microscope as a small dark mass within the nucleus of the cell. Twenty to 90 percent of all somatic or body cells of normal females contain a Barr body or sex chromatin body, and as such are classified as chromatin-positive. Normal males (XY) are classified as chromatin-negative because their cells do not contain any Barr bodies.

The number of Barr bodies found in a human cell always equals the number of X chromosomes minus one. Thus, normal females with the usual two X chromosomes (XX) will have only one Barr body per cell; normal males with the usual XY chromosomes will have no Barr bodies. Individuals with an excess number of X chromosomes as a result of genetic error (for example, XXX, the so-called super female) can have as many as two Barr bodies per cell, but these cases are indeed rare. Where more detailed information concerning genetic makeup is needed, the individual chromosomes can be studied by means of other tests.

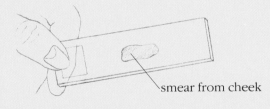

smear from cheek

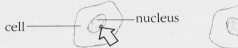

NORMAL FEMALE   NORMAL MALE
one Barr body   no Barr bodies

cell —   — nucleus

GENETIC ABNORMALITIES

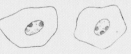

Other causes of masculinization. Synthetic progestogens taken by pregnant women to overcome habitual abortion have been known in some cases to cause masculinization of the female newborn. Although progestogens are not androgens as such, some preparations have androgenic (masculinizing) properties, notably Norlutin and Pranone. And yet, for reasons unknown, surprisingly few female fetuses exposed to these drugs have been affected—fewer than 150 cases have been reported to date.

The extent of the masculinization (when it does occur) is greatly influenced by the dose, duration, and timing of exposure to the androgenic drugs in relation to the development of the external genitalia. Exposure prior to the twelfth week of pregnancy can cause clitoral enlargement and labial fusion. Exposure after the twelfth week usually is limited to clitoral enlargement. Doctors are now careful to avoid prescribing any medication that might cause such masculinizing changes in the female fetus.

In contrast to congenital adrenal hyperplasia, masculinization from androgenic drugs is rarely as extreme. The condition is also self-limiting, which means that once exposure to the androgen ceases, there is no worsening of the problem. Hence, when these children are born, they require no medical treatment, since their own androgen metabolism is perfectly normal. But corrective surgery with restoration of normal-appearing female genitalia is usually required and performed as soon after birth as possible.

On rare occasions, masculinization of the female newborn can result from an androgen-producing tumor of the mother.

Sexual Maldevelopments

Not all congenital maldevelopments are obvious at birth. Many in fact are probably undetected until adolescence or even later, when absence of menstruation or lack of sexual development causes the young woman to seek medical attention.

Imperforate hymen. This is a hymen that completely blocks the vaginal outlet. The condition occurs in about one out of 2,000 women, and usually is not detected until after menarche when blockage and retention of the menstrual flow can cause problems. Initially, most of the menstrual discharge is confined to the vagina, which stretches and distends to accommodate the growing volume of old blood. As each period passes and more and more blood is trapped, the increasing pressure within the vaginal canal causes the blood to back up through the fallopian tubes. The uterus itself can balloon out to the size of a two- to three-month pregnancy. If unrelieved, this causes severe and recurring monthly pain. Cyclic pain plus the lack of menstruation in an otherwise normally developing adolescent are the clues that suggest the diagnosis.

If considerable menstrual blood accumulates within the vagina, the hymen can bulge outward. This condition is corrected by excising the hymen and making sure that all of the retained material drains out. Otherwise, the retention of any old blood or menstrual debris can increase the risk of pelvic infection by providing the perfect medium for bacterial growth. The operation is best done in a hospital rather than a doctor's office, and recovery usually is rapid with no aftereffects.

Other malformations of the hymenal opening also may require surgery. One such example is the cribriform hymen, which has several small perforations instead of a single opening. These small perforations are large enough to allow drainage of the menstrual flow but effectively block penile-vaginal intercourse.

Vaginal transverse septa are simply walls of tissue stretched across the vagina. They too prevent the discharge of menstrual blood (if complete), but unlike an imperforate hymen, they usually are located farther up the vaginal canal. Corrective surgery in such cases can be more complicated, since the tissue can vary considerably in thickness.

Vaginal agenesis is complete or partial absence of the vagina, usually involving the middle and upper vagina. Often the uterus and cervix also are absent or are so poorly developed that menstruation and conception are never possible. Other female organs such as the external genitalia, fallopian tubes, and ovaries usually are uninvolved and are perfectly normal. Hence, breast development occurs as expected, along with other secondary sexual characteristics.

Congenital vaginal defects occur in about one out of every 3,000 women, and are due to incomplete or faulty development of the müllerian duct system. The condition is sometimes diagnosed during infancy, but most cases are unrecognized until the early teen years. Here again, absence of menstruation in a normally developing girl is usually the symptom that prompts an examination, although there have been cases where the problem was not discovered until after marriage. Cyclic monthly pain, however, is uncommon since there is rarely a functioning uterus and thus no retained menstrual flow. On pelvic examination, there may be a very tiny shallow vagina or a dimpling of the skin over the area where the vaginal outlet should be. Since congenital absence of the vagina is frequently associated with anomalies of the urinary tract, an evaluation of the kidneys and ureters should be part of the diagnosis.

Treatment consists of creating a vaginal canal of sufficient depth for sexual intercourse. If there is a functioning uterus, the new vagina would have to connect to the cervix, and the operation would need to be performed prior to menarche to allow external drainage of the menstrual flow. Even though surgery can be successful, these women rarely become pregnant. If the uterus is absent or rudimentary (as is usually the case), the surgery can be postponed until just prior to marriage or anticipated coitus.

Testicular feminization also prevents menstruation, but for an entirely different reason. This unusual congenital problem is believed to be inherited as a sex-linked recessive condition. Individuals with testicular feminization are genetic males (XY) with testes, and yet their appearance is totally female. During infancy and childhood, their external genitalia so closely resemble that of a normal female that the problem is usually unsuspected. At puberty, they become even more feminized, and develop large breasts, rounded hips, and soft, delicate, smooth skin. On pelvic examination, the vagina usually appears quite shallow, and internally there is no uterus, no fallopian tubes, and no ovarian tissue. Sooner or later, lack of menstruation brings these "girls" to the attention of a doctor.

The problem is apparently caused by a lack of androgen sensitivity in target organs and tissues (hair follicles, genital structures, etc.). In other words, tissues and organs that normally respond to androgen stimulation remain unaffected. As a result, there is no masculinization of the genital structures or virilizing effects despite an adequate output of testosterone and other androgen hormones by the testes. Even if these individuals were treated with massive doses of testosterone, they still would not grow a single whisker to mar that soft, velvety skin. Absence of a uterus, tubes, and vagina is caused by the organizing substance secreted by the testes, which in effect prevents the development of the müllerian duct structures (see page 484). Moreover, these testes produce estrogen much like normal testes. Thus it is the estrogen stimulation (unopposed by androgens) that accounts for the breast development and other female physical characteristics.

Since these individuals look completely female and have been raised as females, the sex assignment is always female. The best treatment is therefore to complete the transformation to female (as much as possible). This usually involves fashioning a more functional vagina, at least one of sufficient depth to permit intercourse. The testes (which are usually located in the groin or abdomen) are removed in the late teens, since they can become malignant if left in place. Removal of the testes frequently causes severe hot flashes similar to those experienced by premenopausal women whose ovaries are removed. Following surgery, however, these individuals are maintained on estrogen therapy. This not only eliminates the hot flashes, but also helps prevent premature aging and osteoporosis, and maintains their female appearance.

CONGENITAL DEFECTS OF THE VAGINA

The hymen normally has an opening large enough to allow passage of the flow of menstrual blood when a girl reaches puberty. If the hymen is a solid sheet of tissue (an imperforate hymen), it will block the flow of blood at menarche, causing monthly pain. This condition occurs in about one out of 2,000 women, and is surgically correctable.

A wall of tissue may stretch across the vagina at any point along its length (vaginal transverse septum) causing the same problem and symptoms. Surgery can correct this condition as well.

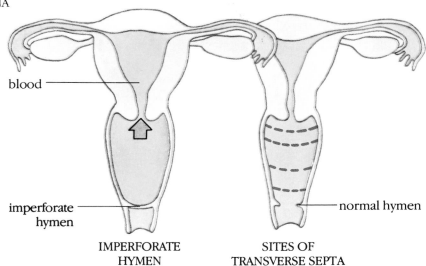

IMPERFORATE HYMEN

SITES OF TRANSVERSE SEPTA

Turner's syndrome is a chromosomal defect in which the ovaries fail to develop. It is also called ovarian agenesis or gonadal dysgenesis. In this condition, the sex chromosome from the sperm fails to be transferred at the moment of fertilization. Thus, these individuals are born with only a single sex chromosome—the X chromosome inherited from their mother. Since it takes two normal X chromosomes to develop ovaries and a Y chromosome to develop testes, they have no sex glands, but they do develop (for reasons previously discussed) a uterus, fallopian tubes, vagina, and the external genitalia of a female.

TURNER'S SYNDROME

Turner's syndrome is a chromosomal defect in which the ovaries fail to develop. The sex chromosome from the sperm is absent, leaving the individual with only a single X chromosome.

Most cases are detected at puberty, for without estrogen stimulation from the ovaries, there is no menstruation and no breast development. Estrogen therapy will cause immediate female secondary sexual development, but since the ovaries are missing, the woman with Turner's syndrome will be unable to have children.

An earlier diagnosis of Turner's syndrome is possible if other symptoms—a slightly thick (webbed) neck and shorter than normal height—are present.

OVARIES FAIL TO DEVELOP

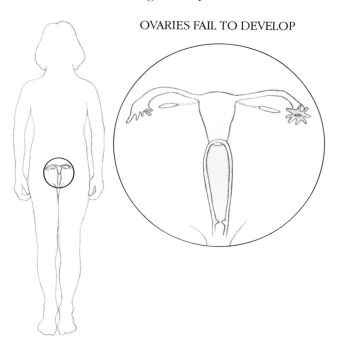

Although most cases are not diagnosed until the teen years, the presence of other associated congenital problems such as cardiac defects, various bony abnormalities, and webbing of the neck may call attention to the condition at an earlier age. Webbing of the neck, when present, can be a conspicuous feature. In extreme cases, the neck is markedly short and wide with a fold of skin extending from the base of the ears almost to the tip of the shoulders. Among others with Turner's syndrome, the only apparent abnormality in the preadolescent years is a retardation in growth resulting in a shorter than average height. An astute mother will probably notice that her daughter is somewhat petite, but if the whole family tends to be short, this may not arouse concern until later.

Without estrogen stimulation from the ovaries, there is no breast development, no feminine contours, and no menstruation. By the time this girl is twelve or even younger, she may well wonder why she isn't developing like her girl friends. Eventually this total lack of sexual development, both in terms of physical appearance and onset of menses, will prompt the girl and her mother to seek medical attention.

The short stature, absence of any sexual development, and lack of periods are the three big clues to the diagnosis. But verification by appropriate hormonal, laboratory, and chromosomal studies still is necessary. Once the diagnosis is confirmed, estrogen therapy is started, usually by age fourteen or fifteen, and is continued for the next thirty to forty years.

Estrogen will have no effect on adult height—most of these individuals will remain essentially four feet seven inches tall—but it will bring about other dramatic changes. Almost overnight the girl will begin to develop breasts and other female secondary sexual characteristics. Estrogen will enlarge and mature the uterus, thus making it possible to establish monthly periods by the cyclic use of estrogen and progesterone. In addition, estrogen will prevent degenerative changes that might otherwise occur earlier than normal. Equally important, in making the girl look more like a female, hormone therapy is of great psychological help. With the exception of being unable to have children, she now can function like any other woman.

Reproductive Conditions

For the most part, these are maldevelopments of the uterus and cervix. As mentioned previously, the development of the müllerian duct structures in the female fetus to form the uterus, tubes, and vagina begins around the end of the second month of fetal life. If conditions are normal, the middle and lower portions of the müllerian ducts (one on either side) fuse to form a single uterus, cervix, and upper vagina. The uppermost portions do not fuse but remain separate and distinct as the fallopian tubes. The entire process takes approximately three months. Any disturbance in the development of these tissues or their failure to fuse properly can cause all sorts of malformations.

At one extreme, there can be complete nonunion, so that each müllerian duct develops independently. The end result is duplication of all structures—a double uterus, double cervix, and double vagina. At the other extreme is the so-called arcuate uterus, with an indentation along its top giving it a heart-shaped appearance. This is perhaps the most common uterine malformation. In between these two extremes, there can be any number of possible variations, as you can appreciate from looking at the few examples illustrated at the bottom of this page.

Uterine maldevelopments probably are present in about one out of every 1,500 women, but their exact incidence is unknown. Many small defects, for example, are never diagnosed for the simple reason that they never cause problems. In fact they are sometimes inadvertently discovered during abdominal or pelvic surgery for nonrelated conditions. Other uterine malformations, however, can cause difficulties.

Pelvic pain, heavy menstrual bleeding, and irregular bleeding are occasional problems that can occur in specific maldevelopments. For example, a woman with two uterine cavities may well have heavier periods. And if she also has cramps with her periods, imagine how many more cramps she will have with two uteri. In rare cases, there may be a uterine horn—that is, an accessory uterine cavity that does not communicate or connect with the vagina. This, of course, would result in trapped menstrual blood, and ultimately would require surgical removal of the uterine horn. For the most part, however, a maldeveloped uterus does not cause infertility. As long as there is a functioning ovary and a uterine lining that responds to hormone stimulation, conception and implantation of the fertilized egg generally proceed normally.

The greatest problems associated with uterine defects actually occur during pregnancy—and the most common complication is spontaneous abortion, usually during the second trimester. The reason is probably insufficient growing room for the baby and/or poor placental growth because of a misshapen or smaller-than-normal uterine cavity. Surprisingly, such abortions are sometimes more likely to happen in a uterus with a comparatively minimal malformation. For example, a woman with a double uterus may breeze through a pregnancy with no complications whatsoever. A woman with a separate uterus or one with a ridge or tissue partially dividing the uterine cavity into two compartments may run into all sorts of problems. In the first example, the uterine cavity is smooth and shaped fairly normally. But in the second example, the cavity is obviously irregular in outline.

If the pregnancy does proceed to term, there are still other increased risks: malposition of the baby (breech or transverse lie); long, difficult labor; poor uterine contractions; and maternal hemorrhage. Developmental defects of the uterus also can cause premature birth, intrauterine fetal death, or may even be a factor in fetal postmaturity with undue prolongation of the pregnancy. Approximately one-third of all pregnant women with a malformed uterus ultimately will lose their babies.

Nonetheless, the presence of a malformed uterus is not necessarily a reason for corrective surgery. Many women have conceived and successfully delivered a healthy baby despite a uterine defect. Corrective surgery, if feasible at all, is therefore reserved for the woman who has had serious difficulties directly attributed to a uterine defect—repeated abortions, late pregnancy complications, or heavy, painful bleeding episodes unrelieved by more conservative measures. If surgery cannot correct the problem and future pregnancies may endanger the woman's life, permanent sterilization is sometimes the best solution.

DEFECTS OF THE VAGINA, CERVIX, AND UTERUS
The development of primitive ducts in the fetus results in the formation of fallopian tubes, uterus, cervix, and vagina (see page 486). Any disturbance of this development in the first two months of fetal life can lead to some of the problems shown below. Defects of the uterus alone occur in about one in every 1,500 women. See the adjacent text for further details of these congenital reproductive problems.

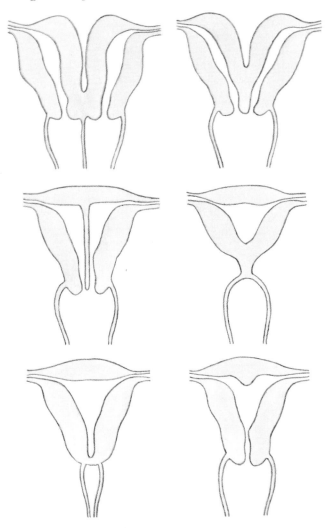

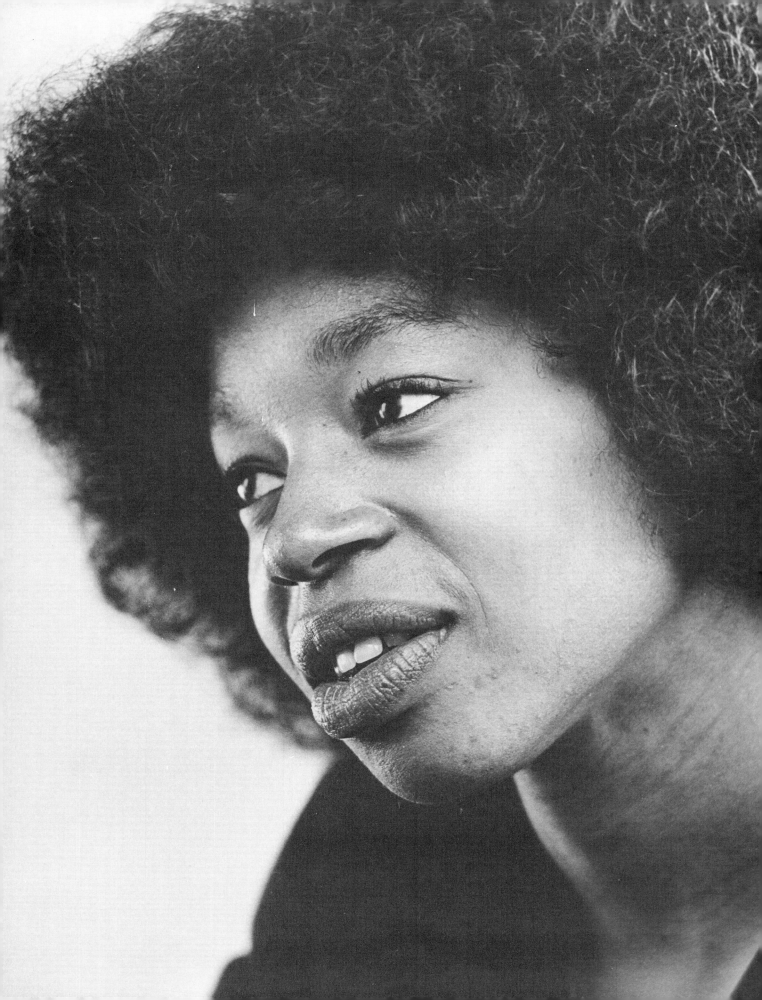

CHAPTER 23

ADOLESCENT REPRODUCTIVE PROBLEMS

S. JEAN EMANS, M.D.

At times, the rewards and challenges of adolescence can seem overwhelming to a young girl even when the transition into womanhood is proceeding normally. But reaching physical and sexual maturity also brings the potential for a variety of infections and problems that can cause a girl and her parents added concern. Many of these actually are minor conditions that eventually will resolve themselves. Other less-common symptoms may require the treatment of a physician.

Adolescent Reproductive Problems

This chapter describes problems that may arise in the transition from childhood to womanhood, the period of adolescence. The normal biology of adolescence and the psychology of adolescence are discussed in some detail in the "Adolescence" chapter. This chapter focuses on the reproductive problems of adolescent development that may require medical intervention. We also will discuss changes of development that may worry you or your child because they seem unusual, but that are in reality only slight variations from normal.

Infancy to Puberty

Female reproductive "problems" are by no means peculiar to adolescents and adults; indeed, even the newborn have them. Before birth, the fetus is exposed to high levels of the hormones estrogen and progesterone, produced by the mother's placenta. As a result, the female newborn baby often exhibits copious whitish vaginal secretions and a small amount of breast development. The infant even may have slight milk production from the breasts, sometimes referred to as "witches' milk." Are these reproductive problems? Certainly not, although many parents have needlessly worried that they were. Actually, the vaginal secretions are normal, and the slight breast development only makes the breast a bit more susceptible to infection. Parents should seek medical intervention only if the breast tissue develops warmth, swelling, and redness (usually on just one side).

Under normal conditions, the small amount of breast tissue gradually disappears within weeks to months. And after the newborn is away from maternal hormones for just two to three weeks, the vaginal secretions begin to disappear. Soon the area around the vaginal opening appears thin and red instead of moist and dull pink. Occasionally, slight vaginal bleeding occurs as the lining of the infant's uterus (womb) is shed in response to the falling estrogen and progesterone levels—the same hormonal shift responsible for the establishment of periods during adolescence (see page 128).

From infancy to puberty, the child increases in weight and height and develops socially, psychologically, and intellectually—but the breasts, vagina, and uterus remain immature. In fact, the appearance of breast development, pubic hair, or periods before eight years of age is sufficient reason to visit the child's physician for prompt evaluation.

Prepubertal Gynecological Problems

Vulvovaginitis. The gynecological problems most frequently seen in prepubertal girl children include bleeding, discharge, and injury. Young girls are particularly susceptible to infections around the opening of the vagina, a condition called vulvovaginitis. At three to six years of age, little girls take bubblebaths and begin to wear brightly colored nylon underpants and hot nylon tights, both of which commonly contribute to vulvovaginitis. Bubblebath soap may be extremely irritating to the vaginal area and cause an itchy rash, and tights and nylon panties may cause a heat rash, particularly in overweight girls.

But most important to the young girl is careful toilet hygiene. When it's toilet time, the four-year-old child usually asserts, "I'll do it myself." And if her mother is at all uncomfortable about looking at or touching her daughter's genitals, the child's independence may be encouraged. The little girl may get her way—at the expense of not being taught the importance of wiping correctly. Although mothers usually know the importance of correct wiping after toilet functions—from front to back, or from the vulva area to the anus—a little girl may wipe the opposite of her mother's teaching, spreading bacteria into her vulva and causing infection. Mothers can help minimize the chance of infection by teaching their daughters how to gently wash the vulval folds when bathing.

Poor toilet hygiene is just one cause of vulvar symptoms. Vaginal discharges may occur in conjunction with other illnesses, including strep infections, chickenpox, and measles. Whitish secretions (smegma) may accumulate in the folds of the vulva and cause irritation. And pinworms—frequently spread in schools—can cause itching at the anal area, where scratching may spread bacteria to the vagina.

In many cases, the discharge and irritation will disappear if the child avoids bubblebaths and harsh soaps, soaks her bottom two or three times a day in warm water, and wears white cotton underpants and loose fitting skirts or pants. If the irritation does not improve in a week or two, *or* if the discharge is excessive, greenish, or bloody, it's time to visit a physician.

Monilial vulvovaginitis. Although most cases of vulvovaginal infection are related to poor hygiene and a bacterial infection from the bowels, other organisms that require specific treatment also may be present. For example, an itchy vaginal discharge can occur after taking a course of antibiotics for an ear or throat infection. The antibiotics alter the bacterial flora of the vagina, resulting in an overgrowth of monilia, a common fungus. Monilial vulvovaginitis is also common in diabetics, and occasionally is the first clue to a diagnosis of the disease.

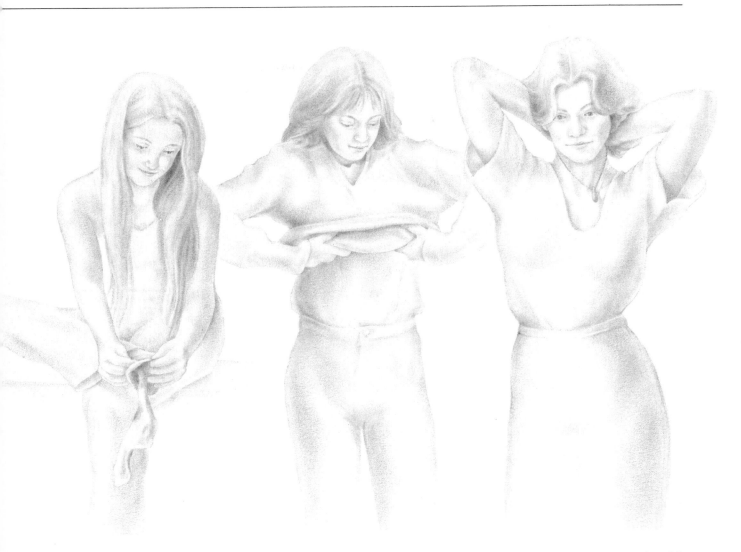

Gonorrhea (see page 457) is a less-frequent cause of vaginal infection in little girls. Because of the possibility of sexual abuse in these cases, cultures of family members can be important in determining the source of the infection. Often a member of the family, a baby-sitter, or an acquaintance is involved, and either the child fails to understand the implications of the sexual encounter or is afraid to tell her mother or physician. A few cases of gonorrhea probably are acquired by close nonsexual contact.

A bloody discharge also requires prompt medical evaluation, although only rarely does it indicate a tumor or an early period (precocious puberty). More often it's the result of injury. A fall on a seesaw, swing, rocking horse, or bicycle may cause profuse bleeding—or perhaps just a few drops of blood on the child's underpants. Sexual abuse is sometimes a cause, and should be considered when there is no clear-cut indication of trauma. If the bloody discharge is also foul smelling, the little girl may have inserted toilet paper or other objects into her vagina.

Mothers and some physicians may feel uncomfortable about discussing or touching the genitals of little girls. This clearly prevents them from dealing in a straightforward manner with the total health care of their child or their patient. As a mother, if you sense that you are uncomfortable in this area, see a counselor or therapist for discussion and aid. A mother should always be the one who undresses her young child completely at the doctor's office, and should explain that the doctor is going to take a look at her bottom and touch her, if that is the case. If a young girl accepts a brief look at her bottom as part of a normal physical checkup, she is less likely to feel embarrassed or upset by the same examination when she reaches adolescence.

Common Problems of Puberty

Sometime between the ages of nine and thirteen, most girls note the early signs of puberty—a spurt in height, breast development, a few wisps of pubic hair, and increased fat on thighs and hips. These signs are modulated by hormonal changes, as described and illustrated in the "Adolescence" chapter. The changes discussed in this section are also normal, but still may be causes of concern to a developing girl.

Asymmetrical Breast Development

The normal stages of breast development are shown on page 152 of "Breasts." Estrogen production at puberty is responsible for breast development, as well as for maturation of the vagina and uterus. Although many girls develop both breasts at the same time, it is not unusual for breast development to begin in a single breast—as a hard, tender lump underneath the nipple. It may be six to twelve months before the other breast begins to change. Full breast development takes four to five years.

GENITAL EXAMINATION OF A YOUNG GIRL

A physician may examine a young girl's genital organs routinely, or only when some problem arises such as itching or injury. If a young girl accepts a brief look at her bottom as part of a normal physical checkup, she is less likely to feel embarrassed by the same examination when she reaches adolescence.

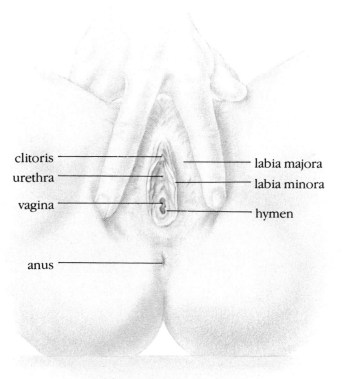

clitoris ———————— labia majora
urethra ———————— labia minora
vagina ———————— hymen

anus ————————

Many girls have breasts that are asymmetrical, meaning that one breast is smaller than the other. Asymmetry may be present only in the early stages of breast development, or it may last throughout adulthood. Although asymmetrical breasts are perfectly normal in function, girls and their mothers may worry about the size differences and focus on asymmetry as a problem. Asymmetry does not indicate a hormone imbalance or deficiency, as many women fear. Check with your physician at your next regular checkup if you are concerned. If the physician finds that your breasts are normal, the simplest solution to a temporary difference in size is a bra pad. Knowing that this is not an uncommon problem should be reassuring to an adolescent girl. Breasts, after all, were meant for nursing children, and almost all breasts are adequate for this function, no matter what their size.

White Vaginal Discharges

A young girl entering puberty may begin to experience a sense of wetness in the vaginal area, or may notice a white vaginal discharge in her underpants. Far from a cause for alarm, this discharge, often called "leukorrhea," is actually a healthy sign that estrogen is stimulating the vagina to produce more cells. In early adolescence, estrogen influences the vaginal area to grow and change from a thin layer of cells into a thicker, more moist layer of cells. As more cells are added to the vaginal wall, some are shed along with mucus secretions, resulting in a characteristic white discharge. This is the same discharge seen in the newborn who has been stimulated by the high hormone levels of her mother's placenta.

Since this shedding is perfectly normal, no treatment is necessary—other than frequent baths or showers and absorbent cotton underpants.

An adolescent girl should, however, be watchful for any itching, odor, or discharge characterized by a green or yellow color. These are possible signs of vaginitis (see pages 445 and 446) that should be evaluated by the adolescent's physician.

Delayed Menarche

The first period, or the beginning of the menstrual cycle in adolescence, is called menarche. Several investigators have suggested that the age of initiating periods is influenced by weight or more exactly, by body fat composition. An average weight of 103 pounds has been measured in girls at the time of menarche. This does not mean that every girl must weigh 103 pounds to start her periods. The short girl may weigh less than 103 at menarche, since the most important factor seems to be body fat composition. However, a girl who is underweight for her height may need to gain 10 to 15 pounds before her periods will begin.

The part that weight plays in menarche is well illustrated by the example of a girl who began her pubertal development at age ten. Development proceeded normally for two years, and at 12, when she weighed 105 pounds, she experienced leukorrhea (white vaginal discharges). Menarche was expected within the next six to 12 months. Then, after her brother commented that she was "fat," she promptly lost 15 pounds by dieting. Further development temporarily ceased. The leukorrhea disappeared because her hypothalamus stopped sending messages to the pituitary gland, which in turn stopped sending pubertal levels of FSH and LH to the ovaries. Estrogen production also declined. After a year, which included medical evaluation and counseling, the girl regained the weight and subsequently her development returned to its normal course. Her periods started at 15. Although in many such cases, a sudden weight loss may be the result of psychological problems or dieting, medical advice still should be sought to rule out organic illness.

Another factor in determining when a given youngster will begin her periods is the family history of age of menarche. For example, a mother who started her periods at 18 may have a daughter who has her menarche at 16.

Delayed menarche has many causes. Chronic illnesses such as bowel and blood diseases, cystic fibrosis, and diabetes, and psychological and family problems can all be responsible. A tumor in the pituitary or hypothalamic area, a genetic problem causing inadequate ovarian function, imperforate hymen (see page 503), and congenital absence of the vagina or uterus are very rare causes of lack of periods (amenorrhea).

When should a girl consult her doctor about delayed menarche? Since periods usually start about 2½ years after the beginning of breast development, a girl of adequate weight who has not had a period within 3½ to 4 years of pubertal development should be evaluated to make sure that her hymen, vagina, and uterus are normal. Similarly, if no breast development or pubic hair is evident by age 13 or 14, medical evaluation also should be sought. Nevertheless, if a teen-ager feels anxious about her periods, she certainly need not wait until some arbitrary age to have a brief examination and discuss her concerns.

Irregular Periods

During her first year or two of menstruation, an adolescent girl usually produces no eggs (ovulation does not occur). This is because the pituitary and the hypothalamus signal the ovaries to produce varying amounts of estrogen (see page 501). As levels rise, the lining of the uterus thickens; as the levels fall, part or all of the lining is sloughed off as a menstrual period. The variability in hormone levels and in the thickening and sloughing-off cycle results in irregular menstrual periods. Menstrual cycles may occur every two weeks, four weeks, three months, or six months. Periods may be light or extremely heavy to the point of true hemorrhage, and may last one or two days, six to seven days, or occasionally for weeks. Such periods are usually not accompanied by menstrual cramps, bloating, irritability, or mood swings. To add to the irregularity of these early periods, stresses, such as an upcoming exam or a new boarding school, may further increase or decrease their frequency.

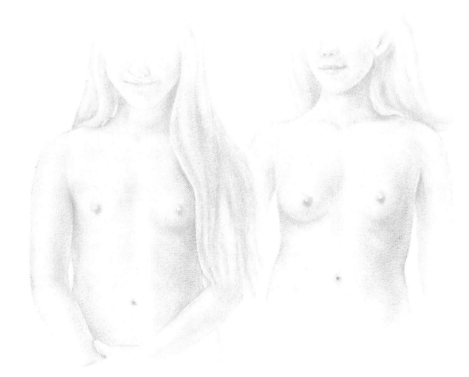

ASYMMETRICAL BREAST DEVELOPMENT
Many girls develop both breasts at the same time. It is not unusual, though, for one breast to develop before the other. This is a perfectly normal event in breast development, and the breasts usually even out by late puberty. Check with your physician if you are concerned about your breasts.

A physician should be consulted if periods begin to occur every two to three weeks (counting from the first day of one period to the first day of the next period); if a period lasts longer than eight or nine days; or if the bleeding seems excessive, especially if large clots are present. In most cases, treatment will restore the teen-ager to normal cycles. A well-kept menstrual record is very helpful to the physician in evaluating the problem. See page 398 for suggestions on keeping such a record.

Although many adolescents have regular cycles with only mild cramps, others either continue to have irregular periods beyond the first year or two of cycles, or suddenly begin to have irregular periods in their middle to late teens. Usually these period problems are the result of stresses—such as taking exams, going to college, or worrying about a boyfriend or the possibility of pregnancy—or gaining or losing weight (even five to ten pounds). The hypothalamus and pituitary are sensitive to these minor alterations in life-style. With lack of ovulation, the uterus again responds to fluctuating estrogen levels. The result may be similar to the first year or two of periods, with flow every two to three weeks or no periods for three to four months. A young woman should consult her physician to make sure that the irregularity is caused by an upset rather than a medical problem.

Treatment may consist of medication, if indicated. Or, the doctor may wait to see if the periods will become more regular before prescribing medication. In cases of heavy frequent periods, birth control pills are often prescribed for one or two months to promote complete sloughing of the endometrium. In cases of less severe bleeding or infrequent periods, pills such as medroxyprogesterone acetate (Provera) taken for five to ten days every one to three months will stimulate normal ovulatory cycle action.

Premenstrual Symptoms

Unlike the painless, often unexpected periods that a girl may have experienced when she was not producing eggs, the hormonal changes associated with ovulation may cause bloating, breast soreness, increased acne, and mood swings the week before a period. These feelings are called premenstrual symptoms and are probably related to the rise in estrogen and progesterone levels before the period begins. Diuretics and tranquilizers, which are sometimes prescribed for those with severe symptoms, may give only slight relief.

Menstrual cramps are probably the most common unpleasant premenstrual symptom. Fortunately, most girls experience only mild cramping the first day of a period. Some teen-agers, however, experience moderate or severe cramps in the abdomen, back, or thighs a few days before a period begins and/or for the first one to three days thereafter. Some girls experience diarrhea, vomiting, malaise, and headaches.

The exact cause of cramps is unknown, but recent evidence suggests that substances known as prostaglandins, released during the period from the uterine lining, cause the uterus muscle to contract and may result in vomiting, diarrhea, headache, and dizziness. Progesterone, produced by the corpus luteum after ovulation, seems to sensitize the lining of the uterus, resulting in vigorous uterine contractions that can be especially uncomfortable for adolescent girls. This is because the opening from the uterus to the vagina, the endocervical canal, may be fairly narrow in girls who have not had a baby. Delivering a baby may substantially relieve the cramps.

Girls and their mothers often experience anxiety about the meaning of these cramps, and this may even contribute to the symptoms. They should be reassured to know that such cramps usually are a normal menstrual symptom. Often simple medications such as aspirin, Empirin, or Midol will relieve uncomfortable cramping, and many girls find that a heating pad is helpful. Although an old-fashioned remedy is a shot of orange brandy, some parents and adolescents oppose the use of alcohol for this purpose. According to one study, girls in overall good physical shape seem to experience fewer cramps than their less-conditioned peers, but exercise on the day of actual cramps is not always helpful.

If the cramps are not relieved by simple over-the-counter medications, if vomiting prevents the use of any medicines, or if absences from school or work are numerous, a girl should consult her physician. Although cramping is normal in 95 percent of adolescents, the physician may prescribe stronger medication (such as the antiprostaglandin drugs Motrin and Naprosyn) to relieve it.

Birth control pills (see page 167) are often suggested for girls who are unable to take other medicines because of vomiting or girls who also need contraception. Birth control pills reduce cramping by preventing ovulation and causing a scantier flow. The pill is often prescribed for three to six months, after which a trial period off medication is attempted. If cramps again become severe, pill use may be resumed. In this way, the young teen-ager is not committed to continuous use of the pill for relief of menstrual cramps. After one to two years of this program, cramps may be less of a problem and are more responsive to antiprostaglandin medications taken only at the time of the period. Adolescents should realize that although cramps are somewhat of a nuisance, in most individuals they are a healthy sign of ovulation.

PHYSICAL CHANGES AT ADOLESCENCE

messages from brain

cause the hypothalamus to release hormones which stimulate the pituitary gland to release **LH and FSH**

estrogen from ovaries

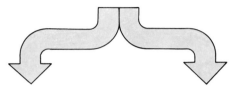

maturation of uterus and vagina   **development of breasts**

Puberty begins around age ten and continues to around age 18. Although the exact event that starts the body changes of puberty is not known, it works by causing the hypothalamus to release hormones that stimulate the pituitary. The pituitary in turn releases luteinizing hormone and follicle-stimulating hormone, which flow in the bloodstream to the ovary and stimulate the secretion of estrogen, the female sex hormone. Estrogen stimulates maturing of the vagina and uterus and development of breasts. The growth of pubic and axillary hair is largely the work of androgens, or male sex hormones, small quantities of which are produced in the adrenal glands.

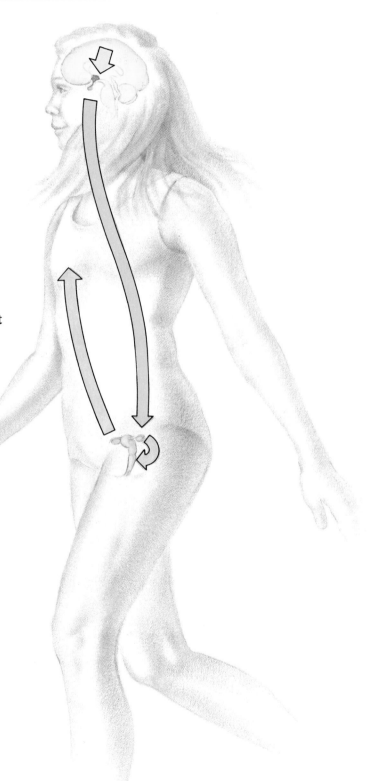

Adolescent Medical Care

Choosing a Personal Physician

An adolescent's primary-care physician may be a pediatrician, internist, or family doctor. Although some pediatricians refer adolescents to another doctor after age 12, many pediatricians continue to see their patients through the late teens and early twenties. Some adolescents, however, request a change of physicians. One girl may wish to see a female physician, another may be unhappy sitting in the waiting room with "all those babies," and still another may feel uncomfortable seeing her mother's doctor. Whatever the choice, it cannot be overemphasized that an adolescent needs a comfortable and confidential patient-doctor relationship. Just like eating well, exercising, and avoiding bad health habits, choosing a personal physician is another way in which a girl can take responsibility for the care of her own body.

The First Gynecological Examination

During adolescence, the annual visit to the doctor usually includes measurements of height and weight, and examinations of the eyes, ears, nose, throat, heart, lungs, breast, abdomen, and genitalia. A rectal or vaginal examination also may be done if the physician feels that it is indicated. Sometimes a physician may suggest an examination by a gynecologist. More often, though, a girl is left to decide for herself when to have her first gynecological examination.

Opinions vary, but probably the best advice for an adolescent is to make an appointment for an examination whenever she has a problem, when she needs contraceptive advice, or at 17 or 18 years of age. Any teen-ager with an abnormal discharge, bleeding, unexplained pelvic pain, or a history of DES (see page 506) certainly should be examined. Sexually active teen-agers should be seen at least once a year for a Pap smear and gonorrhea culture; teen-agers using oral contraceptives generally are examined twice a year. If a young woman has not started her periods by age 15 or 16, or if her hymenal opening appears abnormally small to her family physician, a gynecological examination is in order.

The details of a pelvic examination are included in the chapter on "Choosing a Doctor." Small specula are now available that enable the physician to adequately view the cervix of a virginal teen-ager. As can be seen at right, a narrow speculum about the size of a tampon is used for pelvic examinations of teen-agers. The illustration compares this speculum with the specula commonly used for infants and adults. It is a common misconception that the vagina is totally covered by the hymen and that the examination will alter the hymen in a virginal girl. In actuality, the speculum can be inserted without discomfort and without altering the hymen (see opposite page) in most virginal adolescents, especially if tampons have been used for menstrual periods.

The various hymenal openings common in young women are illustrated on the opposite page. A teen-ager with no opening in the hymen (an imperforate hymen) will not have periods; a normal opening must be made surgically as soon as the problem is discovered. Although a small hymenal ring is common in many virginal adolescents, many other virgins have a normal, wider opening that allows easy insertion of tampons and the larger Pederson speculum. There is no medical way to state unequivocally whether or not a patient with a large hymenal opening is a virgin. For most young women, the trauma of bleeding at first intercourse is a myth; only young women with an unusually tight opening experience this.

Girls who cannot insert tampons should consult their physicians. In most cases, the problem represents the teen-ager's ill ease with touching her opening or, in fact, even finding it. Many girls spend one to two hours with a mirror before successfully inserting the first tampon. In some cases, the hymenal opening is genuinely very small or has a septum and requires a minor surgical procedure to enlarge it. The procedure, a hymenotomy, is elective if menstrual flow is adequate. Since using tampons is a personal choice rather than a medical necessity, a young adolescent may choose to delay the operation. For older adolescents, the inability to have a routine pelvic examination or intercourse (without trauma) may prompt earlier intervention. In deciding on either choice, a young woman always should consult a gynecologist.

Adolescent Medical Problems

Vaginal Discharges and Infections

Vaginal discharge is a common problem for adolescents. In many cases, the discharge is normal—the so-called leukorrhea described earlier in this chapter. With the beginning of menstrual cycles, this normal vaginal discharge assumes a cyclic pattern. During the first half of the cycle, it is whitish and slightly watery; at mid-cycle with the high level of estrogen, the discharge may be profuse and slippery. During the second half of the cycle under the influence of progesterone, it often is scantier and slightly sticky.

THE PELVIC EXAMINATION IN ADOLESCENCE

A young girl usually has her first pelvic examination in a physician's office at around age 14. The physician uses a special adolescent speculum for viewing the cervix. This speculum, about the size of a small tampon, does not cause discomfort in virginal girls, when the hymen does not totally close off the vaginal opening. The inset drawing compares the size of the adolescent speculum to that of infant and adult specula. See page 402 for drawings of a pelvic examination using a speculum.

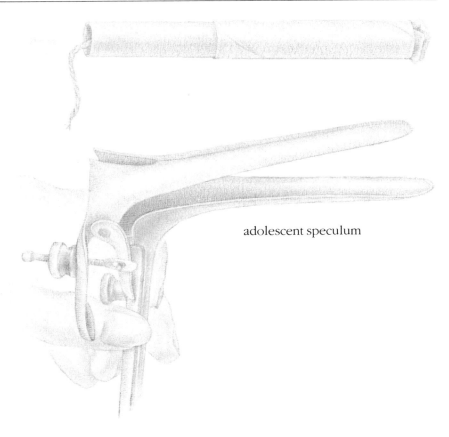

adolescent speculum

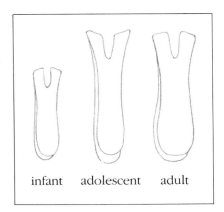

infant   adolescent   adult

TYPES OF HYMENS

The hymen is a membrane of tissue that covers and partly closes the opening of the vagina. Before a girl has sexual intercourse, the hymen usually has a rather small opening (A), although sometimes the opening may be as large as that shown in drawing B. Tampons or a speculum can easily be inserted into a virginal vagina. Most young women do not bleed at first intercourse because the hymen is not that tight. The trauma of pain and bleeding at first intercourse is unusual and most commonly associated with a

tight hymenal opening. If the opening is very small (C and E), minor surgery to enlarge the opening is recommended. If the hymen has no opening (D), it is called an imperforate hymen. With such a hymen, menstrual flow cannot be discharged and the teen-ager will not have periods. A teen-ager who suspects that she has an imperforate hymen should see her gynecologist so that an opening can be made surgically. Girls who cannot insert tampons also should consult a physician.

A　　　**B**　　　**C**　　　**D**　　　**E**

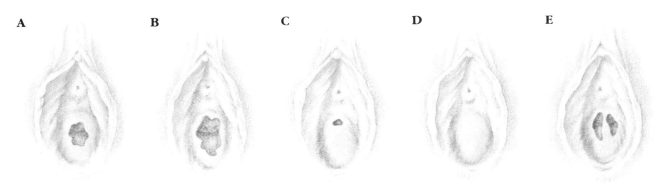

Growth of the Reproductive Organs

CHILDHOOD 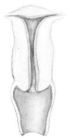 PUBERTY 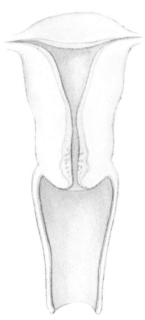 ADULTHOOD

uterus

lining

cervix

vagina

During the period of adolescence, sex hormone secretions cause the vagina to lengthen, the uterus to increase in size, and the lining of the uterus to thicken, as shown above.

● Under the influence of estrogen, the vaginal lining loses the thin, red appearance of childhood and becomes the thicker, pink, moist lining of adolescence and adulthood.

● The lining of the uterus also thickens, and about two to three years after the first signs of breast swelling appear, menstruation begins. The uterine lining detaches from the uterine wall, discharging cells and blood through the cervix and vagina.

Common Problems that May Require Medical Treatment

Even when adolescent development and menstruation are normal, problems such as cramps and irregular periods can arise. These conditions— shown in yellow—are normal, and do not necessarily require medical attention.

● Other conditions—shown in pink—are signs that you should see a physician. Infections (including venereal disease), developmental problems, and pregnancy always require prompt medical evaluation and treatment.

LATE CHILDHOOD

- Mild vulvovaginitis
- Other infections
- Gonorrhea
- Foreign objects in the vagina

EARLY PUBERTY AND LATE PUBERTY

- Irregular periods
- White discharge
- Mild premenstrual symptoms
- Asymmetrical breasts

- Severe cramps
- Pregnancy
- Imperforate hymen
- Pelvic inflammatory disease

- Delayed menarche
- Venereal disease
- Urinary tract infections
- Other infections

A teen-ager should consult a physician if the vaginal discharge is itchy, foul-smelling, yellow, frothy, blood-tinged, or just worrisome. Sometimes a teen-ager will delay telling anyone about the discharge because of embarrassment—especially if she has been raped, if she feels guilty about her first sexual experience, or if she fears venereal disease. Although a check for VD is indicated in such patients, the discharge often is found to represent a yeast infection and is not at all related to sexual activity.

Trichomonas vaginitis. Trichomonas is a small parasite that causes a yellow, frothy, itchy, and often foul-smelling discharge. The infection it causes occurs both in virginal and sexually active teen-agers. The examining physician usually can see this organism on a microscopic slide at the time of the visit. In other cases, however, the cytologist detects Trichomonas in the lab when the Pap smear is read. The physician then may send a prescription for medication several days or weeks after the examination. The parasite also may be present without any symptoms.

The usual treatment in the nonpregnant woman is metronidazole (Flagyl). During the course of treatment, the patient should not drink alcoholic beverages, since the combination of Flagyl and alcohol may cause vomiting. For the sexually active woman, a prescription also is given to her boyfriend because the small organism may be harbored in the man's prostate gland without causing symptoms. Treating the man thus reduces the possibility of reinfection for the woman.

Monilial vaginitis. Monilia (or Candida) is a common fungus that causes an itchy, whitish discharge, sometimes described as "like cottage cheese." It is particularly common in women who have just taken a course of antibiotics (which may alter the bacterial flora of the vagina), in diabetics, during pregnancy, and in patients taking birth control pills. A physician will prescribe a variety of vaginal creams and suppositories for this problem.

Hemophilus vaginalis. H. vaginalis is a small bacteria that causes a gray, foul-smelling (fishy) discharge. After an examination, the teen-ager will receive a prescription for an antibiotic. If the young woman is sexually active, her boyfriend also should be treated to prevent reinfection.

Gonorrhea is a common infection in teen-agers. Since about 75 percent of infected women exhibit no symptoms, it is important for sexually active teen-agers to have a culture of the cervix taken every six to 12 months. A cervical culture may be done by a girl's gynecologist or during a routine physical at her pediatrician's office. Contrary to popular belief, "nice girls" do get gonorrhea, and boys may have the infection without showing any symptoms.

Gonorrhea can cause different kinds of infections with different symptoms. These include cervicitis (infection of the cervix with a profuse yellow discharge), endometritis (infection of the uterus), salpingitis (infection of the fallopian tubes), and arthritis (infection of the joints). Inflammation of all the pelvic organs (uterus, fallopian tubes, and lining of the pelvic cavity) is termed pelvic inflammatory disease or PID.

PID is caused by the gonococcus bacteria in about half of patients, and by a variety of other organisms (Strep, E. coli, Chlamydia, Mycoplasma) in the remaining half. Symptoms include abdominal pain, fever, chills, vaginal discharge, and pain on urination. The major problems that follow this disease are recurrent abdominal pain, tubal pregnancies, and infertility (because of scar tissue in the tubes). Contracting PID can have quite serious consequences—all good reasons for avoiding casual sex. The condom is the only form of birth control that offers some protection against VD.

Two other genital infections, herpes and warts, are discussed in detail on pages 445 and 464. In addition, the teen-ager should remember that a foul-smelling, sometimes-bloody discharge may result from accidentally leaving a tampon in the vagina for days or weeks at the end of a period. If a young woman notices this kind of discharge, she should immediately check to see if a tampon is still in place. Although the string may be high in the vagina, the teen-ager usually can extract the tampon herself. If not, she should see a physician.

Urinary Tract Infections

Urinary tract infections are common among adolescent girls, especially among those who have recently become sexually active. Because the female urethra is short, bacteria may easily enter the urethra and travel upward to the bladder, causing cystitis (see page 530). In some individuals, infection may travel up to the kidneys and cause a kidney infection (pyelonephritis). Teen-agers who have had one urinary tract infection are prone to subsequent infections.

Symptoms of cystitis include frequency of urination accompanied by pain or burning sensations, blood in the urine, and cloudy or foul-smelling urine. Kidney infections also may exhibit these symptoms, as well as fever, chills, and flank pain, and it is often difficult to distinguish between kidney and bladder infections. In addition, an infection may occur without any symptoms and still cause damage to the kidneys.

If symptoms suggestive of a urinary tract infection develop, the teen-ager should consult her physician. She will be asked to void a clean urine sample at the doctor's office or a local laboratory. This urine is then tested to determine the amount and type of bacteria present. Depending on the lab test results, the doctor will prescribe a specific antibiotic. It is crucial that the adolescent not take any leftover antibiotic pills before she has voided this urine sample.

Treatment includes antibiotics and fluids. Emptying the bladder at least every two hours during the day is helpful, since delaying urination allows the number of bacteria in the bladder to increase. Because of the possibility of reinfection—often without symptoms—cultures should be repeated at periodic intervals. After one or two infections, an IVP (kidney X ray) is usually done to rule out any underlying problems.

There are other causes of painful urination and urinary frequency besides urinary tract infections. A vaginal infection such as Trichomonas or gonorrhea can cause urethritis (inflammation of the urethra), and tissues that are inflamed by monilia or herpes infection may burn as urine passes over them. Diabetes mellitus also may cause increased frequency of urination, especially at night. Thus, the only way to be sure that a urinary tract infection is present is to see your physician and have a culture taken so that proper treatment and follow-up can be arranged.

Exposure to DES

An explanation of how a child can become exposed to the drug diethylstilbestrol (DES) during the mother's pregnancy is of great importance to many mothers and their daughters. The facts need to be stated clearly, since articles in many newspapers and magazines have tended to sensationalize the risk of cancer and have caused tremendous fear.

Beginning in the late 1940s and continuing through the 1950s and 1960s, DES and several other related medicines were given to mothers during their pregnancies to prevent miscarriage (see opposite page). Not until the early 1970s was it evident that the daughters born to mothers who took this drug during pregnancy might have certain problems of the vagina, cervix, and uterus. Although the incidence of a rare malignant vaginal cancer (clear-cell adenocarcinoma) is increased by intrauterine exposure to DES, the risk remains extremely low. To date, about 350 cancers have been reported in the estimated one million girls exposed. Clinical studies show that the risk is less than four in 1,000 among exposed daughters, and that the occurrence of this vaginal cancer seems to depend on when the mother was first exposed to DES.

The most common problem observed in girls whose mothers took DES is an abnormal vaginal condition called adenosis, a benign (noncancerous) lesion. Adenosis is the presence of "glandular" cells in certain areas of the vagina and cervix that are normally covered by squamous (flat) cells. Tissues, such as the skin and the lining of the vagina, usually consist of squamous cells; the lining of the intestines and the uterus is made of glandular (columnar) cells. In girls exposed to DES, 40 to 90 percent have been found to have small areas of this glandular epithelium on the cervix and in the vagina. In some cases, the glandular epithelium gradually changes to squamous epithelium; in others, treatment of the glandular cells with cold cautery is the recommended procedure.

Unfortunately, medical authorities do not know whether there are any long-term problems such as cancer or infertility associated with these areas of glandular cells that are exposed to vaginal bacteria and pH. These tissue abnormalities have not been shown to interfere with intercourse, contraception, or pregnancy.

Most medical experts recommend examining a girl exposed to DES as soon as she has started having periods or at age 14, whichever comes first. Use of tampons makes the exam easier, as indicated on page 502. Of course, a girl should be examined at once anytime abnormal bleeding or discharge develops.

Besides the presence of adenosis, studies have shown a difference in the shape of the cervix and uterus in some women exposed to DES. Thus, depending on the results of the pelvic examination, a special X-ray examination of the uterus may be done in selected young women with pregnancy losses. If the shape of the uterus is abnormal, the young woman may then need more careful monitoring during pregnancy. It should be emphasized that this is preliminary information; each patient should discuss this matter with her physician. The National Cancer Institute is funding several major studies to determine the incidence and natural history of genital changes and cancer in DES daughters, and more data on this important subject is forthcoming.

What type of physician should the teen-age girl see? Because of the complex nature of DES health effects and the difficulty of diagnosing changes in the squamous cells lining the vagina and cervix, the best recommendation is a gynecologist who is interested in adolescents exposed to DES. Many medical centers and community hospitals have set up special clinics to examine teen-agers. At these examinations, the procedures should be completely explained to the teen-ager to help her feel comfortable with the situation. During the regular speculum examination, a special stain (Schiller's stain) is often wiped on the cervix to help the physician locate abnormal areas. In addition, many gynecologists look through a special microscope (a colposcope) to examine the cervix and vagina more adequately than is possible with the naked eye. This special examination may take a few additional minutes, but is essentially the same as the routine examination and is not painful.

What is DES?

Diethylstilbestrol (DES) is a synthetic estrogen that was prescribed for women with a history of problem pregnancies during the late 1940s through the 1950s and 1960s. An estimated four to six million Americans (mothers, daughters, and sons) have been exposed to DES.

The drug has been prescribed under a variety of names, as listed below.

Comparatively little DES has been prescribed for pregnant women since 1971, when the Federal Food and Drug Administration required product labeling to state that DES was contraindicated for use in the prevention of miscarriage. The drug is used today for a variety of other purposes though, including estrogen replacement for treatment of hormone deficiency and menopause-related problems, and for cases of advanced breast and prostate cancer. DES also is used as a postcoital contraceptive in some cases, although its use for this purpose has not as yet been approved by the FDA.

DES-type drugs that may have been prescribed to pregnant women

NONSTEROIDAL ESTROGENS

Benzestrol	Estrosyn	Palestrol
Chlorotrianisene	Fonatol	Restrol
Comestrol	Gynben	Stil-Rol
Cyren A.	Gyneben	Stilbal
Cyren B.	Hexestrol	Stilbestrol
Delvinal	Hexoestrol	Stilbestronate
DES	H-Bestrol	Stilbetin
DesPlex	Menocrin	Stilbinol
Diestryl	Meprane	Stilboestroform
Dibestil	Mestilbol	Stilboestrol
Dienestrol	Methallenestril	Stilboestrol DP.
Dienoestrol	Microest	Stilestrate
Diethylstilbestrol	Mikarol	Stilpalmitate
Dipalmitate	Mikarol forti	Stilphostrol
Diethylstilbestrol	Milestrol	Stilronate
Diphosphate	Monomestrol	Stilrone
Diethylstilbestrol	Neo-Oestranol I	Stils
Dipropionate	Neo-Oestranol II	Synestrin
Dethylstilbenediol	Nulabort	Synestrol
Digestil	Oestrogenine	Synthoestrin
Domestrol	Oestromenin	Tace
Estilben	Oestromon	Vallestril
Estrobene	Orestol	Willestrol
Estrobene DP.	Pabestrol D.	

NONSTEROIDAL ESTROGEN-ANDROGEN COMBINATIONS

Amperone	Metystil	Tylandril
Di-Erone	Teserene	Tylosterone
Estan		

NONSTEROIDAL ESTROGEN-PROGESTERONE COMBINATION

Progravidium

VAGINAL CREAM SUPPOSITORIES WITH NONSTEROIDAL ESTROGENS

AVC cream with Dienestrol	Dienestrol cream

What to do if you have been exposed to DES or similar drugs.

If you suspect that you were exposed to DES-type drugs before you were born, try to verify this by medical records from the attending physician or the hospital where you were delivered. It is very important that DES-exposed daughters be screened early and then followed up to detect vaginal abnormalities or cancer. Early diagnosis also will improve the effectiveness of treatment.

The screening procedure should include a thorough pelvic examination, a Pap smear, and tissue inspection (by iodine staining of the cervix and vagina). DES daughters should be examined at least once a year, and more frequently if there are extensive or unusual epithelial changes. In view of the limited information on the long-term effects of estrogens in women exposed, the use of oral contraceptives should be carefully discussed with a doctor.

A relationship between DES and increased risk of breast or gynecologic cancer in mothers who took the drug is not yet established, but it is still important for women to advise their physicians if they have taken the drug. As for all women, a DES mother's routine health care should include an annual pelvic examination and a monthly breast self-examination.

Sons exposed to DES *in utero* should have a physical examination to ascertain genital abnormalities, although medical studies of male infertility and cancer are as yet inconclusive.

For more information on DES, contact your state or local health department or American Cancer Society chapter.

Before the first examination for DES effects, the young adolescent should understand why she is going to see a gynecologist. It is important that her mother reassure her that although she is starting examinations two or three years before some of her friends, some of her other friends may already have seen a gynecologist for the same problem or for vaginal discharges or abnormal bleeding. Appropriate counseling will help the teen-ager understand her mother's concern over these examinations, and will remind her that the DES was only prescribed to keep her mother from losing the pregnancy. Otherwise, some adolescents become very angry at their mother and the physician, focusing on this minor problem as a major defect in body image and becoming overly fearful about the risks of cancer and infertility. Likewise, a mother also may feel angry or guilty, and overlook the need to communicate reassurance to her daughter. Keeping the matter a secret or insisting on an examination under a false pretext is never advised.

Teen-Age Sexual Activity

Opinions vary and feelings are often extremely intense on the subject of teen-age sex. Although one might wish that teen-agers were not sexually active—especially the 11- to 15-year-old-group—the data are to the contrary. Of the about 21 million teen-agers in this country (both male and female), 11 million are estimated to be sexually active (see page 511). In a recent study of a broad cross-section of teen-agers, it was found that of 16- to 19-year-olds, 57 percent had had intercourse, and of 13- to 15-year-olds, 30 percent had had intercourse. Of non-virgins, 11 percent of the 13- to 15-year-old group had been pregnant, compared to 28 percent of the 16- to 19-year-old group. The data may be slightly misleading in that many teen-agers have sex only once or twice and then decide against further intercourse. On the other hand, sexual activity among teen-agers seems to be increasing. Although many teen-agers are having regular sexual relations, it has been shown that most view these relationships as serious and steady. In the study mentioned, 86 percent of the teen-agers viewed their relationships as "close"; only a small percentage were reported having intercourse with multiple partners.

The Issue of Birth Control

Many adolescents now expect to have relationships in which intercourse is defined as the major expression of love. Parents, doctors, nurses, and teachers often feel ill at ease with this change in morality and feel that discussion of contraception in schools, churches, and physicians' offices—and the availability of contraceptive devices—supports this change in behavior. One must recognize the bind: to promote birth control information and availability may imply approval of a particular standard of sexuality; to deny it may result in unwanted pregnancies.

There is no easy solution to the problem. However, one would hope that in deciding to be sexually active, the teen-ager would carefully examine the relationship and the meaning of the sexual expression. In addition, any prescription of birth control hopefully would be preceded by a discussion of the responsibility the teen-ager is undertaking, the problems inherent with some contraceptive methods, and the risks of venereal disease and other infections.

Choosing Not to be Sexually Active

Even though she may believe that all of her friends are sexually active, the virginal teen-ager should know that 40 to 50 percent of young women have not had intercourse by their nineteenth birthday. Since peer pressure to be sexually active is often particularly intense in boarding schools and colleges, counselors and physicians need to offset the pressure with the reassurance that "it's O.K. to wait." One would hope that parents also would talk with their children about their thoughts and feelings about sexuality. Unfortunately, many teen-agers' exposure to sex education focuses only on good contraceptive techniques and the mechanics of how to avoid pregnancy. Most young people are interested in much more than this—how to get along with parents and peers, how others feel, and how they can develop caring relationships in which intercourse may or may not be involved. Sometimes it is actually more difficult for a teen-ager to establish a relationship based on conversation and activities rather than sex. Small discussion groups that focus on factual information as well as feelings and issues of behavior are most helpful to the teen-ager, especially if they are led by a person trained in group dynamics and human sexuality. Unfortunately, few school systems have yet undertaken this type of program.

Contraception for Teen-Agers

What is the best form of contraception for the sexually active teen-ager? Some of the many considerations include the the type of relationship, frequency of intercourse, the teen-ager's medical history, and the ease she has in dealing with her own sexuality. The range of alternatives must be examined carefully for each individual. A mechanical form of contraception may seem ideal for the teen-ager who has intercourse only very rarely, but it must be used to be effective. Because teen-agers frequently feel the need to be spontaneous, they may fail to use any form of contraception, and particularly those that require motivation at the time of intercourse. The diaphragm often remains in the pocketbook, and the condoms and foam are never purchased.

Many adolescents feel uncomfortable inserting something into the vagina. Condoms and foam are accepted by some couples, but often a girl is unable to insist that her boyfriend use them. In spite of their sexual intimacy, the adolescent girl and boy often find it difficult to discuss sex openly because of embarrassment or the girl's fear of losing her boyfriend; unfortunately, such problems may persist into adult relationships as well. Health professionals can help young women to examine their own feelings and needs, and their responsibility to protect themselves from pregnancy and VD.

The chapters on "Birth Control" and "Abortion" contain valuable information and advice about contraception. In these chapters, you also will find information on groups, counselors, and books that offer further assistance and support for teen-agers making decisions about contraception and their own sexuality.

The IUD (see page 173) is used by some teen-agers, but the side effects remain a problem for 20 to 30 percent. The increased incidence of cramping for an adolescent who already has moderate to severe menstrual cramps is a major drawback. Other problems include irregular bleeding, expulsion of the device, uterine perforation, and infection. Although the infection rate is quite low, the risk may be greater in women who have never had a baby than in those who have had a baby. Since a pelvic infection may result in significant medical problems, young women must be aware of this potential side effect.

The birth control pill is the most commonly selected form of contraception for adolescents. The pill substantially relieves menstrual cramps and does not require motivation at the time of intercourse. The pregnancy rate is low if the pill is taken correctly; unfortunately, remembering to take a pill every day is a problem for some adolescents. Certain risks also are present, but fortunately, the serious complications such as blood clots, strokes, heart attacks, and benign liver tumors are rare, and are even less common among the youngest pill users. Minor side effects include menstrual irregularity, weight gain, and headaches. For further side effects of the pill, see the "Birth Control" chapter, beginning on page 164. All side effects must be balanced against the risks of an unwanted pregnancy. Problems should always be reported to the health care professional who prescribed the pill.

It should not be assumed that if a 15-year-old begins taking the pill, she will continue it for her entire fertile life. Undoubtedly she will not. A teen-ager may stay on the pill for around five years, either continuously or starting and stopping when relationships change. Then, after using a diaphragm for several additional years, she may decide to have children in her late twenties. In her thirties, she may select an IUD or a diaphragm or some new method of contraception not yet available. In addition, many men and women now request permanent sterilization. In short, an adolescent's decision to take the pill is probably a temporary one, something to consider when weighing its risks.

Less effective birth control. Unfortunately, a large percentage of teen-agers still use no contraception, or an ineffective method. The withdrawal or rhythm methods are often used by adolescents because they require no paraphernalia, doctor visits, or planning. But even when the male climaxes outside of the vagina, sperm may leak out before ejaculation and cause unwanted pregnancy. In addition, the menstrual cycles of adolescents are particularly susceptible to changes from stress. Not only is it difficult for an adolescent to know when she may ovulate, but it may be difficult for her to regularly enforce the necessary abstinence. The scientific ways of utilizing the rhythm method require an even greater degree of motivation.

Ideally, each teen-ager should have a good relationship with an adult to whom she can turn for help and discussion of when to become sexually active and what kind of birth control to use. A teen-ager's perception of her relationship with her family physician also may influence how freely she is able to discuss her sexual concerns. Some teen-agers elect to use a VD clinic or family planning clinic because they fear the family doctor may disapprove or tell their parents. Sometimes the perception is real, and the physician may strongly disapprove of sexually active teen-agers. In other cases, the teen-ager is projecting her own disapproval of her behavior onto an authority figure. Parents can be helpful to their children (boys and girls) by being open and willing to discuss these matters, as well as encouraging their child to have a confidential patient-doctor relationship during the adolescent years.

Teen-Age Pregnancy

With the establishment of ovulatory cycles, the sexually active adolescent is at risk of becoming pregnant. While the birth rate among the United States population as a whole is decreasing, the teen-age birth rate is increasing. Of the about three million babies born in the United States each year, nearly 600,000 are born to teen-agers. And of the over one million abortions performed in 1977, nearly 300,000 terminated teen-age pregnancies (see page 208).

Why Teen-Agers Become Pregnant

Lack of motivation as well as lack of information contribute to the problem of teen-age pregnancy. Teen-agers may find it difficult to plan ahead and to accept that pregnancy is the consequence of unprotected intercourse. Many say, "I've had sex before and I didn't get pregnant," or "I just didn't think it would happen to me." Many girls fail to use contraception because they really believe that they cannot become pregnant. Or perhaps they feel they need proof that they really are adult women.

Although the majority of pregnant teen-agers are neither promiscuous nor disturbed, many do have worries that may have led indirectly to the pregnancy. For example, pregnancy may follow a divorce or the death of a parent, and the teen-ager may subconsciously view it as a replacement of that loss. Sometimes the teen-ager has a difficult time identifying with her home or family and sees the pregnancy as a way to start a new life. If the pregnancy is a means of testing whether the teen-ager's mother really does love her, it may be a call for help and support. Sometimes a pregnancy represents the daughter's desire to give her mother a "gift" after the mother has had a hysterectomy or gone through the menopause. In other cases, the pregnancy represents contraceptive failure. Of course, some pregnancies are well-planned by a responsible, loving couple; unfortunately, during adolescence this is the exception rather than the rule.

Effective counseling can clarify these issues, and is essential to alleviate guilt and anxiety and reduce the long-term problems of a teen-ager's pregnancy.

A Pregnant Teen-Ager's Decisions

The alternatives available to a pregnant teen-ager must be examined very carefully, and always in light of the teen-ager's plans for the future. It may be the first time that a teen-ager has been faced with a decision that will affect the rest of her life. With the options of abortion and adoption, she must work through feelings of guilt and loss. The teen-ager who elects to keep her baby may be emotionally unprepared to cope with the demands of childcare. She most likely will drop out of school and become dependent on family or welfare for support. Some marry, but most of these marriages end in divorce within a few years.

Not infrequently, teen-agers deny a pregnancy until quite late because of fears about where to turn for help, what parents will say, and how to deal with the crisis. Younger teen-agers often have unrealistic feelings about pregnancy and motherhood, and their decisions may be related to angry feelings toward parents. The older teen-ager is usually able to weigh the consequences of her action and consider the choices available. Since ambivalence about an unwanted teen-age pregnancy is common, good counseling is essential.

The parents' role. Unfortunately, teen-agers are often afraid to discuss the problem with their parents. Sometimes a mother may suspect the pregnancy, and sometimes she may find out during counseling or when the pregnancy begins "to show." If the teen-ager is mature, she may want to take care of the problem herself. But parents often are much more supportive than the teen-ager thought possible. Although a mother's initial reaction may be anger, she can be very helpful during the stress of an abortion or delivery. A counselor usually can establish "who wants what" and help reconcile the differences between mother and daughter. It is also very important for the parent and teen-ager to discuss birth control after the crisis is resolved. The attitude that it won't happen again is dangerous, and repeat pregnancies are common—especially if underlying emotional concerns have not received adequate attention.

Discovering the pregnancy. The symptoms and diagnosis of pregnancy and the details of abortion and delivery are discussed in the "Pregnancy" and "Abortion" chapters. The major difference with adolescent pregnancy arises because teen-agers often deny the possibility of pregnancy. Although some teen-agers do recognize that a missed period, morning nausea and/or vomiting, dizziness, and fatigue may represent pregnancy, others either do not experience these symptoms or relate them to the flu, mononucleosis, or just an irregular period. Even teen-agers who have thought of the possibility may go to the doctor with a sore throat or an earache, hoping to have the pregnancy discovered.

Parents, too, may deny the pregnancy even though the daughter is getting "fatter and fatter." On the other hand, parents should not accuse their daughter of pregnancy every time her period is late. In addition, it should be noted that a teen-ager who has ambivalent feelings about whether or not she wants to be pregnant may develop all the symptoms of pregnancy when in fact she is not pregnant at all. If the communications between parents and teen-agers are honest and open, both parties are likely to be able to deal with the problem more realistically. If the pregnancy is discovered early, there is more time for constructive counseling and decision making.

Keeping the baby. Of the many teen-agers who do elect to continue their pregnancy to term, the overwhelming majority keep their babies. Medical problems among pregnant teen-agers include an increased incidence of toxemia (see page 590) and low birth-weight babies; the latter is probably a result of poor nutrition. Thus it is important for the adolescent to receive good prenatal care with an emphasis on education about nutrition, delivery, newborn care, and contraception. Over 200 special programs are currently helping the pregnant adolescent deal with the problem of becoming a mother while she is still sorting out the important issues of adolescent development.

Teen-Age Sexual Activity and Pregnancies

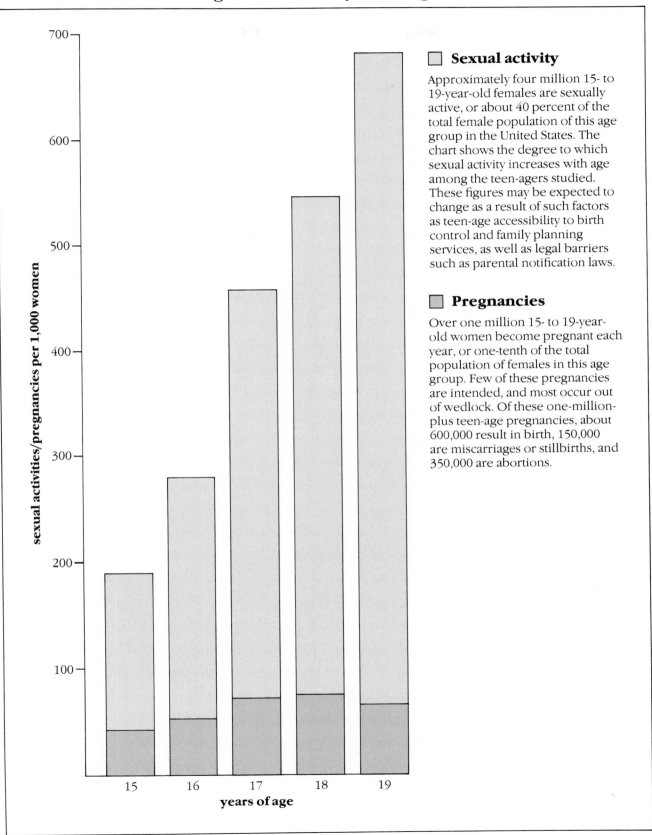

sexual activities/pregnancies per 1,000 women

years of age

Sexual activity

Approximately four million 15- to 19-year-old females are sexually active, or about 40 percent of the total female population of this age group in the United States. The chart shows the degree to which sexual activity increases with age among the teen-agers studied. These figures may be expected to change as a result of such factors as teen-age accessibility to birth control and family planning services, as well as legal barriers such as parental notification laws.

Pregnancies

Over one million 15- to 19-year-old women become pregnant each year, or one-tenth of the total population of females in this age group. Few of these pregnancies are intended, and most occur out of wedlock. Of these one-million-plus teen-age pregnancies, about 600,000 result in birth, 150,000 are miscarriages or stillbirths, and 350,000 are abortions.

CHAPTER 24

INFERTILITY

ALBERT DECKER, M.D., F.A.C.S., F.A.C.O.G.

Most women assume that they will be able to become pregnant and bear a child at any time in their reproductive lives. If you have unsuccessfully tried to become pregnant or have failed to carry a pregnancy to a live birth, you probably are bewildered and perhaps are dismayed. Beyond the physical inability to reproduce, infertility can pose a complex life crisis for the couple who is unable to fulfill their desire for children.

Because of our increased understanding of infertility, many couples no longer keep their barren condition a secret. And because infertility often is a treatable disorder, many of these childless couples are being helped to achieve their goal of having a family.

Infertility

Sir William Osler, the renowned Canadian physician, once proclaimed, "The natural man has two primal passions, to get and to beget." Nevertheless, there are at all times in the United States six million couples who are able to experience only one of those desires. These involuntarily childless men and women are infertile. And their condition—beyond the physical inability to reproduce—can pose a complex life crisis that also threatens psychic and emotional stability.

These couples often are relentless in their efforts to achieve parenthood, and increasingly are seeking help from physicians trained in the management of infertility. Treating infertile couples has become a growing specialty of gynecologists and urologists—for a number of reasons.

Foremost among them is the increased difficulty of adopting a child. In the past two decades, fewer babies have been available for adoption simply because fewer were born. Later marriages, birth control, increased availability of abortion, and effective publicly funded programs to control fertility—all have had the effect of reducing the birth rate in this country. In fact, population control has received such serious private and public attention that the United States now experiences a near-negative population growth.

Happily, many couples no longer keep their infertility a secret. No longer do they consider their childless state to be a reflection on their sexuality or human qualities. Instead, we see them appearing on television programs or giving press interviews to inform others about the nature and treatment of their problem. They've realized that there is simply no reason to think of infertility as a sign of being sexless, unfeminine, unmasculine, or—with today's treatments—untreatable.

Fertile, Infertile, Sterile

Fertility is the ability of a male or female to participate in the production of a live child. Infertility often is incorrectly defined as a state of being sterile or barren. Actually, physicians who treat childless couples use the term "infertile" for a conception failure that can be reversed so that fertility is restored. They reserve the term "sterile" for a barren state that is permanent and irreversible. From a medical standpoint, a couple is considered to be infertile if they are unable to conceive a pregnancy after a year of trial without contraception (see opposite page).

It is estimated that 10 to 15 percent of all married couples in the United States are unsuccessful in their attempts to have a child. About 35 percent of these failures are traceable to abnormalities in the man. And in cases involving the woman, the problem may be an inability to carry a pregnancy to a live birth. This is an important factor in infertility; an estimated 10 percent of all pregnancies are spontaneously aborted. A significant number of these "silent abortions" occur very early in pregnancy and are sometimes mistaken for delayed menstrual periods.

A woman reaches her maximum fertility or greatest reproductive potential between the ages of 25 and 26. Before that time, twelve months of unsuccessful efforts to conceive can be considered proof that some problem exists in either husband or wife, or perhaps in both. Between the ages of 26 and 32, female fertility and the chances for successful pregnancy decrease moderately. If a couple is trying to conceive and pregnancy does not occur within six months, the couple may well suspect some reproductive inadequacy. After age 33 to the end of her fertile years, a woman should seek medical advice if she is unable to conceive.

The Major Causes of Infertility

Hormonal defects in men and women 15%
- Usually pituitary inadequacy

Defects of the male partner 30-35%
- Low sperm count or no sperm
- Undescended testicles
- Kleinfelder Syndrome
- Antibody factor

Defects of the fallopian tubes 30-35%
- Occlusion
- Adhesions
- Endometriosis
- Scarring from previous infection

Defects of the uterine cervix 20%
- Failure to produce mucus antibody

This chart shows the occurrence rates of the major causes of infertility. Often, there are multiple defects, and defects in both partners.

The Routine Fertility Survey

The first step for couples who seek professional help for infertility problems is a careful and thorough "fertility study" to determine why pregnancy does not occur. It should begin with an orientation interview with both husband and wife. All records and results of previous examinations and tests should be made available to your physician at this first session.

The First Appointment

The interview begins by recording the age of each partner, past marital history, number of years married, use of contraception, previous pregnancies by the present or former spouse, and duration of infertility. The couple then will be given the opportunity to discuss any sexual, marital, social, or economic problems they may have.

Previous surgical or medical treatment of both partners will be noted, and, whenever possible, medical records of these events will be secured for review.

Careful inquiry should be made at this time concerning the possibility of thyroid and ovarian disease, and about any instances of tuberculosis or diabetes in the immediate family. The physician will certainly ask about the use of alcohol and drugs, and the interview should include a description of each partner's diet and exercise program. The man's history will include questions about any past complications of mumps, venereal disease, or whether there are any abnormalities of the genital organs.

A complete physical examination of the woman will be made at this time, including examination of the pelvic organs, thyroid, breasts, and abdomen, as well as blood tests, a urinalysis, and a Pap smear. The woman will be shown how to record her basal body temperature on a chart to determine her fertile days (see page 518), and how to time coitus with ovulation.

After this examination and interview, the physician will be in a better position to express his opinion concerning the probable cause for a couple's infertility. He should then outline all the tests he plans to do, describing each one carefully and explaining why it is necessary to confirm or deny his tentative diagnosis.

Average Times Required for Conception

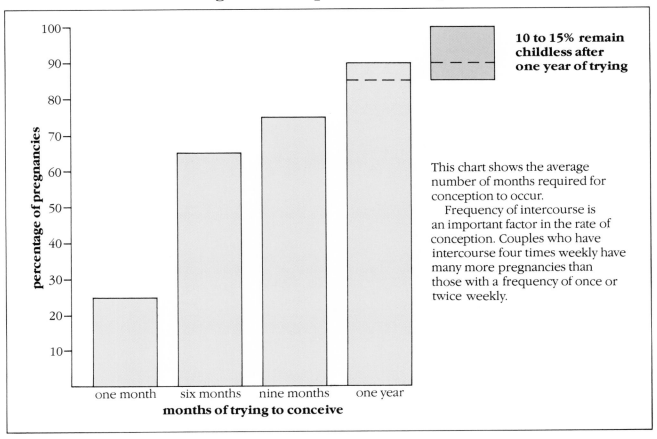

10 to 15% remain childless after one year of trying

This chart shows the average number of months required for conception to occur.

Frequency of intercourse is an important factor in the rate of conception. Couples who have intercourse four times weekly have many more pregnancies than those with a frequency of once or twice weekly.

Examination of the Man

Each element in the reproduction process is called a "factor" in the fertility examination. In the man, for example, the sperm is a factor—the seminal factor. Each factor is identified by a name and is examined by a specific test.

Infertility in men results from the inability of the sperm to reach and penetrate the egg (see opposite page). This may be because a man is unable to deposit sperm in the vagina due to impotence, premature ejaculation, or some other problem. (Behavioral problems or problems of sexual dysfunction are discussed on page 521 and in the "Sexuality" chapter.) Or, the man's sperm may be abnormal, or of a low concentration in the semen. Medical tests of the male, then, are primarily examinations of the semen and sperm to determine whether adequate numbers of sperm are being produced, whether they are of normal form and activity, and whether they stay alive long enough to reach and fertilize the egg.

As mentioned, men are responsible for the reproductive problems in about 35 percent of all cases of infertility or sterility. Even though a man may be strong and healthy with no apparent sexual problems, he may produce sperm of poor quality. And although he may not be completely sterile, if his deficiency is matched by a minor defect in his spouse, the combination of problems may be significant.

A semen analysis is the first step in the examination of the male (see below left). The semen specimen should be obtained in a clean, dry, glass container. If the analysis shows that the man produces active sperm in adequate numbers, he is probably not contributing to the couple's inability to conceive. A further check of the potency of his sperm and their ability to survive in the woman's reproductive tract is determined by the postcoital test.

The postcoital test is done in a doctor's office four to six hours after intercourse to determine, among other things, whether active, normal sperm are present in sufficient numbers at the cervix, and whether they have survived for at least several hours.

The Semen Analysis

A semen analysis is usually the first step in determining why a couple cannot conceive. For a semen analysis, the man produces a sample of semen, usually by masturbation. The ejaculate should be collected after two days of abstinence from intercourse, and all of the sample should go directly into a clean glass tube provided by the physician or clinic. The specimen must be delivered to the lab within two to four hours, and must be kept "cool" (about 64 degrees F.). Even normal body heat is hostile to sperm and may kill them.

The following sperm factors are studied at the lab:
- **Volume in cc; number of sperm in each cc**
- **Total sperm number in the ejaculate**
- **Motility or rate and direction of sperm movement**
- **Morphology of the sperm**
- **Percentage of sperm that appear abnormal, with large heads, small heads, or long tails.**

The normal sperm count is as follows:
- 2 to 6 cc total volume of semen
- 20 to 200 million sperm
- 60 to 80 percent of the sperm still active two hours after ejaculation
- 60 to 80 percent of sperm with a normal shape or morphology.

Examination of the Woman

The routine fertility examinations take longer for the woman because the female factors influencing fertility are so numerous (see opposite page). Time, patience, and perseverance are often required before the problem can be identified.

Ovulation tests and postcoital tests are made to determine whether ovulation is occurring and whether the sperm is normal and active after being deposited in the vagina at the time of ovulation.

Four tests are used to determine if and when ovulation is occurring. They are:
a) the basal body temperature chart
b) Fern and Spinnbarkeit tests of the cervical mucus
c) Endometrial biopsy
d) Blood test for progesterone.

The ovulation test to determine if ovulation is occurring is normally made on Day 12 to 14 of a regular 28-day cycle. Women with irregular menstrual cycles are examined on days determined by the basal body temperature chart.

The cervix is the entrance portal to the womb through which sperm pass on their way to meet an egg. The cervix must produce mucus at the time of ovulation, and the mucus must be of sufficient quantity and consistency to permit sperm to survive and travel through the cervix into the uterus and finally into the fallopian tube.

CAUSES OF INFERTILITY IN MEN

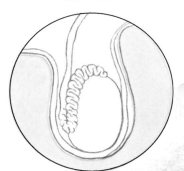

Abnormalities of the testes

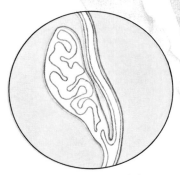

Obstruction of the seminal tract

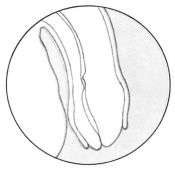

Urethral abnormalities

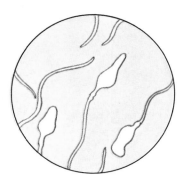

Abnormalities of the sperm

CAUSES OF INFERTILITY IN WOMEN

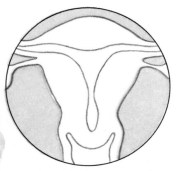

Congenital abnormalities of the uterus or vagina

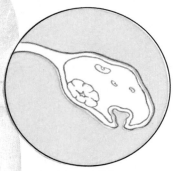

Disorders of the ovary and ovulation

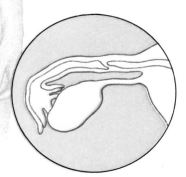

Tubal obstructions

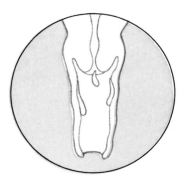

Changes in cervical mucus

INFERTILITY IN MEN
In the male, fertility involves production of a sufficient number of normal sperm in the testes, their unobstructed passage through the seminal tracts, and their deposition high within the vagina at the mouth of the cervix during intercourse. Each of the problems illustrated at left can prevent this process.

INFERTILITY IN WOMEN
The union of a healthy egg with a healthy sperm is the basis of fertility. Anything that interferes with this process, and the implantation of the fertilized egg in the wall of the uterus, can cause infertility. Some of the causes of infertility in women are illustrated at right.

The Fern test and Spinnbarkeit test can determine whether the cervical mucus is normal (see below). The tests are simple and do not cause any discomfort. Later tests will determine if the cervical canal is open and free of infection.

If the mucus is normal at the time of ovulation, it is assumed that the woman is ovulating normally. This can be confirmed by a basal body temperature chart, and a woman should bring the charts she has been keeping at the time the mucus tests are done (see below).

The appointment for the mucus tests (Fern and Spinnbarkeit tests) should be made a few days after the tubal test and on a day calculated to be at or near the time of ovulation. The couple will be instructed to have intercourse four to six hours before the appointment.

For the test, a sample of cervical mucus is removed with a swab. Normally, the mucus at this time is thin and almost liquid. Ovulation is suspected when the Fern and Spinnbarkeit tests are favorable. Another drop of mucus is examined under the microscope to determine whether it contains sperm. This is the postcoital test. If the mucus contains many normal, active sperm, it

probably is normal and is not inhibiting the sperm, and the man is presumed to be normal. If the sperm are dead, the mucus may be hostile—a condition that can be due to a hormone imbalance or an infection in the glands of the cervix. Rarely is it caused by an antibody reaction in which certain specific substances produced in the cervical mucus destroy the sperm.

If the woman's menstrual cycles are irregular, the day of ovulation may be missed. So even if the test is negative and the mucus does not indicate ovulation, the woman should be retested during another cycle or on another date. Positive tests occurring after Day 18 indicate delay or failure of ovulation to occur.

The tubal test or Rubin test is done to determine if the fallopian tubes are open and free for the passage of sperm and fertilized eggs. It's also called the tubal insufflation test (see page 520). The modern equipment shown in the illustration permits this test to be completed with very little discomfort. The appointment for the tubal test should be made after the cessation of menstrual bleeding and before ovulation, as indicated by your basal body temperature chart.

TESTS FOR NORMAL FUNCTION OF THE MENSTRUAL CYCLE

A basal body temperature chart is shown below, along with the cyclic changes that occur in the cervix and its mucus. These three factors change in response to the levels of estrogen and progesterone in a woman's body, and reveal whether or not she is ovulating normally. Changes in temperature on a basal body temperature chart help establish when and if ovulation is occurring.

During ovulation, the cervix moves forward and opens slightly. The mucus becomes slippery and stretchy, and when seen under a microscope, it creates a fern pattern. Mucus tests (Fern and Spinnbarkeit tests of cervical mucus) that show this normal pattern indicate that ovulation is occurring and the approximate time it is occurring.

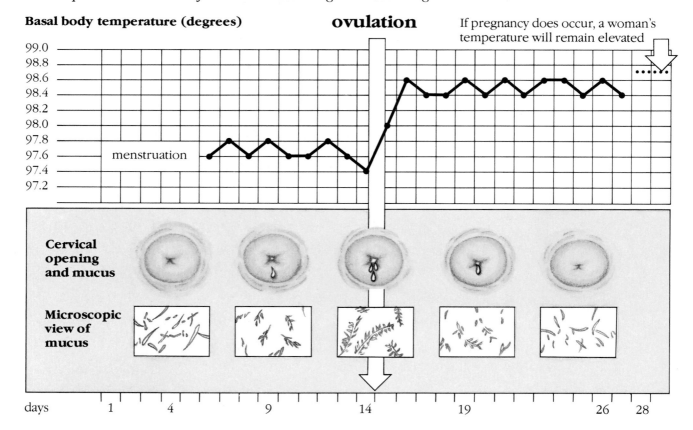

Basal body temperature (degrees)   **ovulation**   If pregnancy does occur, a woman's temperature will remain elevated

menstruation

Cervical opening and mucus

Microscopic view of mucus

days   1   4   9   14   19   26   28

The X-ray examination is scheduled during the seventh to tenth day of the menstrual cycle. If there is any doubt that the cavity of the uterus is open and normal, or that the fallopian tubes have a clear and normal central, hollow channel, X rays of the uterus and tubes will confirm it. This test is called a hysterosalpingogram or X-ray exam (see page 520).

Because it is the cavities of these organs that must be examined, they are filled with a radiopaque fluid that makes them visible as pale gray areas on the X-ray film (see page 520). As the opaque fluid is introduced into the uterus and tubes through the opening in the cervix, it completely fills the cavities and pinpoints any defects with considerable accuracy. Even so, some minor but important abnormalities are not discoverable by X rays alone, and require other tests.

The endometrial biopsy is one of the most important, although uncomfortable, of such tests. Its purpose is to examine the lining of the uterus to determine if it is ready to receive and implant a fertilized egg. Indirectly, this test also reveals whether the ovary is producing hormones for this phase of the reproductive cycle. The endometrial biopsy may be made during the second or third menstrual cycle after fertility testing begins, usually between the twenty-first and twenty-fifth days of a regular 28- to 30-day cycle. Although the endometrial biopsy is unlikely to affect very early pregnancy, most physicians ask couples to avoid intercourse during the fertile period of the cycle being tested.

In order to test the endometrium, the doctor removes a small sample of tissue from the lining of the uterus. The procedure for an endometrial biopsy is described on page 477. The tissue is then treated with various stains and is examined under a microscope. This test accurately reveals the degree of hormonal response of the endometrium, as well as its ability to receive and nourish a fertilized egg. This in turn reflects the degree of hormonal activity of the ovaries during the development of the egg.

Endocrine system tests can determine whether the hormones necessary for a normal reproductive cycle are being produced in the proper quantity at the right times. Some tests are relatively simple; others require a specially equipped laboratory. And in the detective work necessary to establish the cause of defective ovulation or infertility, these tests may be very useful.

Upon completion of the endocrine tests and the tests preceding, the physician can explain in some detail the condition of the couple's reproductive systems, and may make a fairly accurate prognosis as to why the couple is unable to conceive. At this point, the physician and the couple will discuss possible treatments, and may decide on a course of action. If the prognosis is for continued infertility, adoption procedures may be considered at this time.

Laparoscopy and culdoscopy. Sometimes it is not possible to determine the exact cause for a failure to obtain pregnancy, even after extensive testing of both partners. Perhaps the results of the tests are indefinite, or maybe they indicate normalcy even though pregnancy does not occur.

Conception can be prevented or delayed by minor disease processes or defects in the pelvis that cause no other symptoms and that may not be revealed by routine tests. The defect may be the result of some previous infection, a previous operation for appendicitis, or some viral infection. Infertility also may result from that frequently occurring pelvic condition, endometriosis (see page 521).

To look for defects inside the pelvis that may not have shown up to this point, a procedure called laparoscopy is performed (see page 199). The doctor introduces a lighted telescope through the abdomen at the navel in order to examine the pelvic organs. The procedure is quick and simple, and has proven to be extremely useful in discovering certain "occult" causes of infertility problems. It is performed in the hospital, sometimes under general anesthesia.

Basal Body Temperature and Infertility

The information recorded on a basal body temperature chart is extremely important for infertility treatment. If you take your temperature first thing every morning before getting out of bed and record it accurately on a chart, you will know exactly when ovulation has occurred.

Because of estrogen production, your body temperature will remain lower for about two weeks after the first day of your menstrual period. The temperature reaches its lowest point right before ovulation, after which there is a sharp rise in temperature on the day of ovulation.

When basal body temperature is used as a method of birth control, you must avoid intercourse around this time. Likewise, if you are trying to become pregnant, you should have intercourse as close as possible to the day of ovulation. The same chart that assists birth control also is helpful when you are trying to have a baby. See page 188 in the "Birth Control" chapter for information on how to keep a basal body temperature chart.

The menstrual cycle and changes in the cervical mucus can be recorded along with basal body temperature changes for a complete fertility chart. This record is important for your doctor to examine when you have fertility problems, and only you can provide it.

THE RUBIN TEST OF THE FALLOPIAN TUBES

The tubal test or Rubin test determines whether the fallopian tubes are open and free for the passage of sperm and fertilized eggs. The illustration shows carbon dioxide gas being passed through the cervical area into the uterus and tubes. On the left, there is no pressure buildup, and the gas escapes into the peritoneal cavity. The gas can be heard escaping with a stethoscope. On the right, blocked tubes prevent the gas from escaping, and the pressure buildup is registered on a gauge. Unfortunately, this test does not show if only one tube is blocked, or if there is only partial blockage. There is little discomfort with this test. The appointment for the tubal test should be made after the cessation of menstrual bleeding and before ovulation, as indicated by your basal body temperature chart.

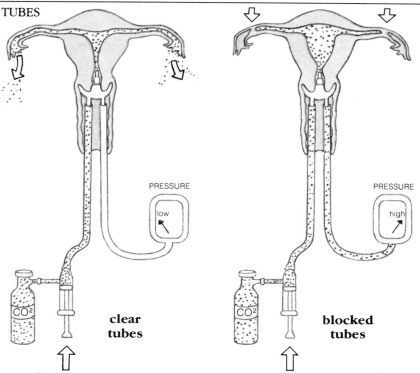

clear tubes

blocked tubes

X-RAY EXAMINATION OF THE FALLOPIAN TUBES

The X-ray examination is scheduled during the seventh to tenth day of the menstrual cycle. If there is any doubt that the cavity of the uterus is normal, or that the fallopian tubes have a clear and normal central, hollow channel, X rays of the uterus and tubes, called a hysterosalpingogram test, will be needed.

Because the cavities of these organs must be examined, the cavities are filled with a radiopaque fluid that makes them visible as pale gray areas on the X-ray film. As the opaque fluid is introduced into the uterus and tubes through the opening in the cervix, it completely fills the cavities and pinpoints any defects with considerable accuracy. Even so, some minor but important abnormalities are not discoverable by X rays alone and require other tests.

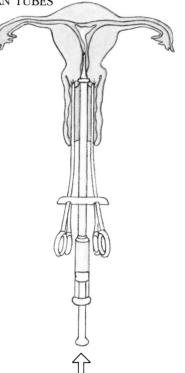

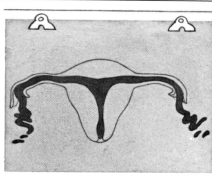

clear tubes

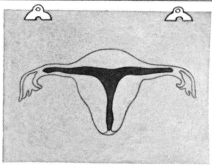

blocked tubes

The pelvis also can be inspected directly by inserting a Culdoscope (a lighted telescope) through the thin vaginal wall. This examination, called culdoscopy, is pictured on page 201. Although slightly uncomfortable, culdoscopy is actually painless since it is done under a local anesthesia. Culdoscopy permits direct visual inspection of the uterus, tubes, ovaries, and even the appendix, and can pinpoint even minute defects. While the doctor inspects the tubes, he will pass a blue solution through them and observe its travel. The pressure of the fluid alone may be enough to overcome minor obstructions. If not, the tube will swell at any narrowing or area of blockage.

The mouth of the fallopian tube, with its delicate tubal fimbriae, also may be stuck together in some way that effectively narrows it.

Of infertile women who are examined by the Culdoscope, 80 percent exhibit some minor defects, and half of that number are shown to have endometriosis. When discovered early, endometriosis can be effectively treated by medication (see page 522).

Summary of the Tests

After completing all the necessary tests and analyzing the basal body temperature charts, the physician will give the couple a detailed explanation of the results and of which organs or functions of the reproductive process are defective. He or she will be able to arrive at a fairly accurate prognosis so that the couple can decide about necessary treatment or consider the possibility of having no children, adopting children, or resorting to artificial insemination or even *in vitro* fertilization.

Sexual Dysfunction

Just as physiological factors can exert a broad range of effects on human fertility, so can emotional and psychological factors. We know that the hypothalamus of the brain regulates the secretion of certain hormones vital to the cyclic function of all reproductive organs (see page 128). In women, this cycle is particularly complex and subtle, and certain emotional states can effectively upset the balanced hormonal cycle.

Human fertility, as well as human sexuality, involves an interplay of the physiological lives of men and women, both individually and as partners. Certainly, psychological conditioning can affect our physical responses to sexuality, and impeded fertility may be one result. Just as important as an examination of the physiological factors that impede reproduction is the exploration of possible psychological factors.

Here the notion of multiple causation has special significance due to the ultimately delicate, complex ways in which people—and certainly sexual partners—relate with and react to one another. The actual physical manifestation of a psychologically induced sexual problem may exist in only one partner, but its solution lies in the active, shared sensitivity of both partners with their physician.

Common forms of sexual dysfunction that result in infertility are well known and treatable. In the male, they are:
- Premature ejaculation—a condition in which ejaculation occurs so early in intercourse that effective deposit of sperm in the woman is impossible. This is the most common of all forms of male sexual dysfunction.
- Impotence—the inability to achieve erection or the loss of erection after insertion into the vagina, preventing orgasm.
- Retarded ejaculation, or the inability to complete an ejaculation during orgasm.

In the female, the common forms of sexual dysfunction include:
- Dyspareunia or painful intercourse.
- Vaginismus, or muscular contraction of the vagina that prevents entrance of the penis.
- Aversion to intercourse and complete avoidance of any form of sexual contact.

All of these dysfunctions obviously impede the completion of satisfactory intercourse, both in terms of pleasure and fertility.

In the realm of strictly physiological infertility factors, emotional phenomena such as frustration, guilt, resentment, and hostility crop up as effects of being "infertile," and may be real barriers to treatment. But in the case of sexual dysfunction, these phenomena—together with possible past trauma and conditioning in the couple's psychological history—contribute as both causes and effects. This is a "chain reaction" process that can only be broken through sensitive, open communication between the partners themselves and together with their physician. With proper counseling, all of these forms of sexual dysfunction can be successfully treated. See the "Sexuality" chapter for a further discussion of the treatment of sexual problems.

Treatment of the Wife

Endometriosis

This curious disease occurs with greater frequency among women of childbearing age than appendicitis, yet few women have heard of it. It is a curious disease simply because it can cause infertility and sterility. In fact, infertility even promotes its development. But should pregnancy occur in the presence of the disease, it acts as potent therapy for the condition, and may even cure it. Endometriosis is discussed in the chapter on "Adult Reproductive Problems," but because it ranks high as a cause of conception failure, we will also describe its effect on the problem of infertility.

What Is Endometriosis?

The endometrium, the cells that line the uterus, are cast off each month with the menstrual blood. But on some occasions and for various reasons, some menstrual blood and many endometrial cells are forced back through the fallopian tube into the pelvis. Once in the pelvis, they act almost like a skin graft, attaching themselves to various pelvic structures: the ovaries, the bowel, the outside of the uterus, the rectum, the bladder, and the delicate lining of the pelvis. Their final resting place seems to be purely a matter of chance.

Although the implants are tiny at first, they often manage to survive in their new environment. And when the command to multiply and prepare for a fertilized ovum comes to these cells from the ovaries (transmitted via the hormones estrogen and progesterone) the displaced endometrial cells respond just as if they were in the uterus. However, unlike their uterine counterparts, they are unable to separate and be cast off during the following menstrual period, but instead may bleed a little. Once the menstrual cycle is over, the endometrial implants heal somewhat, only to be stimulated again during the next menstrual cycle.

The growing, bleeding, and healing cycles result in scarring and adhesions about the tubes and ovaries, and especially around the delicate tubal fimbriae. Adhesions also can fix the ovary and tubes in a manner that interferes with the transfer of ova from the ovary to the fallopian tube.

The growing endometrial cells eventually may invade the tough covering of the ovary where, once they dig in and multiply, they often collect large amounts of blood. This results in an ovarian blood cyst that can attain the size of a hen's egg or even an orange. With time, the blood becomes dark brown, which is why these cysts are sometimes called "chocolate cysts."

Severe menstrual pains, sometimes beginning in the teens, often are suggestive of endometriosis. Unfortunately, the condition can be overlooked because many people, including doctors, believe that discomfort during menstruation is natural. Painful periods may or may not be a sign of endometriosis, but as the condition worsens, periods become progressively more uncomfortable. Endometriosis also can cause pain during intercourse.

Diagnosis is easy if the endometrial growths are extensive; the masses have a characteristic lumpy consistency and are extremely tender to the touch. However, when the cysts are small and the discomfort negligible, diagnosis is not that simple since identical symptoms are associated with a great variety of gynecological disorders. One way to confirm these minor degrees of endometriosis that may be responsible for infertility is with a Culdoscope or a laparoscope. Even the smallest bit of endometrial tissue can be seen when examined with instruments that carry their own light source.

Treatment of Endometriosis

Treatment of endometriosis depends on several factors—notably, the degree of discomfort, the size of the endometrial growths, and the age of the patient.

Because the condition is clearly related to the cyclical hormonal stimulation associated with menstruation and is suppressed during pregnancy (which often cures the condition permanently), treatment consists of inducing a state of pseudopregnancy. This is easily done today with birth control pills that contain both estrogen and progesterone. The procedure usually takes six to nine months and will relieve many of the symptoms, but normally does not prevent the adhesions and scarring left by the disease.

If endometrial growths are extensive and if they interfere with conception or pleasurable intercourse, it is usually advisable to surgically remove as much of the endometrial tissue as possible. The surgeon must carefully cut out all endometrial growths, scar tissue, and adhesions on the ovaries, on the outside wall of the uterus, on the fallopian tubes, or wherever else the endometrial cells have spread. Smaller growths often are destroyed by heat (cauterization). The surgery must be performed with great care in order to enhance the patient's chances for future pregnancy; if necessary, the surgeon also will replace the reproductive organs in their normal position.

Surgery for endometriosis can be extensive, but need not be. Sometimes small endometrial implants can even be removed during exploratory culdoscopy. To facilitate surgery, it is sometimes preceded by hormone therapy to shrink the endometrial tissue and soften the adhesions that surround the growths. Menstruation is suppressed with birth control pills both before and for a number of months after the operation.

Endometriosis also can be treated with male hormones that suppress the growths of endometrial tissue. Unfortunately, these have a masculinizing effect, and doctors generally agree that infertility problems in which endometriosis is the primary cause are more successfully treated with surgery than with hormonal therapy. Danazol, a new synthetic male hormone, apparently has a minimum of masculinizing side effects, and has now been approved for general use. As in the treatment with progestins and estrogen (birth control pills), Danazol treatment is unable to dissolve the adhesions that have formed because of the endometriosis, or for that matter, to reposition the pelvic organs in a manner more conducive to conception.

After menopause when the endometrial implants are no longer cyclically stimulated by sex hormones, endometriosis is rarely troublesome.

Treatment of the Fallopian Tubes

Complete closure of the fallopian tubes, the result of inflammation, requires surgical treatment (see below). Fortunately, most defective conditions of the tubes that prevent or delay pregnancy can be corrected by simple procedures. Partial or incomplete blockage often can be corrected by pressure, as in the tubal insufflation tests. Cases in which blocked or partially blocked tubes are the result of muscular spasm can be remedied by proper medication.

Sometimes tubal sterility is caused by adhesions outside the tube or between the delicate fimbriae at the funnel end of the tube. This condition can be corrected by a simple surgical procedure (see below). Minor adhesive bands that delay pregnancy can be satisfactorily removed during a culdoscopic examination.

Every physician is aware that a woman can possibly become pregnant soon after she has abandoned as hopeless her serious striving for motherhood. The assumption is that changes in her life resulting in an improved emotional condition and a relaxed attitude have somehow improved fertility. However, many women with stable emotional qualities who have not made serious attempts to improve fertility have required from three to ten years to achieve pregnancy. Clearly, these results cannot be attributed to an improved mental state.

SURGERY FOR BLOCKED TUBES

Doctors use several techniques to reconstruct damaged fallopian tubes—a procedure called tuboplasty.

Tubal implantation is done when the tube is blocked at its connection to the uterus. The blocked portion is cut away, and a new canal to the uterus is formed. A

tubal anastomosis is useful when the blocked area can be cut away, allowing the remainder of the tube to be joined end-to-end. Salpingostomy frees the tube from adhesions. The tubes and ovaries must be able to move freely for conception to occur.

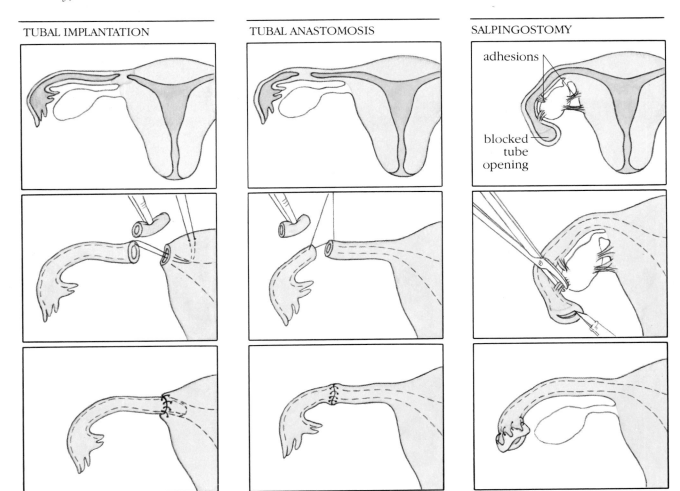

TUBAL IMPLANTATION

TUBAL ANASTOMOSIS

SALPINGOSTOMY

adhesions

blocked tube opening

Many of these women have minor defects of the delicate fimbriae at the ends of the fallopian tubes, reducing the fimbriae's ability to sweep an egg from ovary to tube. By rare chance, an egg *may* be transferred into the fallopian tube, so technically, these women are not completely sterile. They may become pregnant within six months, or fail to become pregnant for ten years. And having achieved pregnancy once, they may never succeed in becoming pregnant again. If the defects of the tubal fimbriae are minor, they can be corrected by comparatively simple surgical methods (see page 523).

Treating Defective Ovarian Function

Many women fail to conceive because they do not ovulate, or because they ovulate at irregular intervals. Failure to ovulate regularly is always associated with irregularity of menstruation, or even failure of menstruation to occur at all.

Low follicle-stimulating hormone. Ovulation is prevented when the pituitary gland produces an insufficient amount of follicle-stimulating hormone (FSH) to start or continue the reproductive ovarian cycle. The ovaries do not function normally under reduced amounts of pituitary hormones. This type of ovarian deficiency can now be treated with remarkable success by the drug Clomid (clomiphene), which is taken in tablet form for a period of five days.

If the pituitary gland does not produce the necessary amounts of FSH to sustain ovarian activity, treatment with a natural hormone, Pergonal, is very successful. This remarkable substance is produced by older women whose health is normal. The pituitary gland of women in their early menopausal years produces excessive amounts of FSH in an unsuccessful effort to sustain ovarian activity. This excess FSH, eliminated from the body in the urine, is recovered, purified, and furnished to physicians under the trade name Pergonal. When it is injected into women with defective ovarian function, it causes their ovaries to produce one egg, or even two or more eggs. Because Pergonal treatment has resulted in multiple births, it has received considerable publicity, and patients must be selected with great care. Only women who produce inadequate amounts of FSH should receive Pergonal therapy.

Polycystic ovaries. Abnormal ovarian function may cause many incompletely developed follicles to accumulate in the ovaries. This condition is termed polycystic ovaries, or Stein-Leventhal ovaries, and accounts for about 4 percent of all infertility cases. Polycystic ovaries are two to five times larger than normal size. A woman with this condition will stop

menstruating or will menstruate erratically, will gain weight, and may develop excessive facial or body hair. Once such a woman discovers that she has polycystic ovaries, she should seek treatment, whether or not she plans to have children.

Treatment with Clomiphene—a drug that induces the pituitary to produce more FSH—is often successful. This extra follicle-stimulating hormone seems able to assist the ovaries in maturing and releasing the "stuck" ova. Rarely, stubborn cases that do not respond to this drug are treated by removing some of the cysts through "wedge resection" of the ovaries. In this surgical operation, the doctor makes a wedge-shaped cut in the ovaries, allowing them to release eggs from the ovarian capsule, which has grown tough.

Other hormone disorders. Shortage of thyroid hormone, or estrogen and progesterone, also may reduce fertility. In some cases, replacement of these hormones has allowed a woman to achieve and maintain pregnancy. Abnormalities of ovulation, the result of abnormal functioning of the adrenal glands, can be improved by cortisone medication.

Treatment of the Uterus and Cervix

Tumors. Abnormal menstrual bleeding may be due to tumors of the uterus or abnormal activity of the endocrine glands. Large fibroid tumors may exist without ever interfering with conception or pregnancy. However, when they cause pain or abnormal bleeding, they are easily detected and can be surgically removed without removing the uterus. Even small fibroid tumors may interfere with conception and pregnancy if they impinge on the cavity of the uterus.

Developmental abnormalities. Malformation of the uterus may result from a congenital deformity (see page 493). During embryonic development, the female pelvic organs grow in pairs: one tube and ovary and one-half of the uterus and cervix develop on each side of the pelvis. During fetal growth, the two sides normally join together to form a perfect uterus. Occasionally, however, they fail to unite, resulting in two separate uteri. A less serious abnormality is partial division, known as a bicornuate uterus.

Each of these abnormal conditions can interfere with conception and pregnancy. In each case, a trial pregnancy should be attempted before surgical repair is considered. Many women with malformed uteri have borne children. In fact, women with double uteri have even borne a child in each uterus at the same time.

Endometrial problems. A common uterine defect exists when the lining of the uterus (endometrium) does not develop sufficiently to support an implanted, fertilized egg. Even if implantation is successful, the poorly developed endometrium may cause an early spontaneous abortion. Often, this condition is due to progesterone deficiency or simply to poor general health. Treatment with special hormones and measures to improve general health are frequently successful.

ARTIFICIAL INSEMINATION

A fertile woman who is married to a sterile man may choose to become pregnant by artificial insemination with donor semen. Artificial insemination, sometimes referred to as "therapeutic" insemination and also as A.I.D., has been used with increasing frequency in this country during the last half-century.

In artificial insemination, sperm are introduced into the vagina with a syringe or some mechanical device rather than through the penis. The illustrations below show two methods of artificial insemination. In this country, it is estimated that as many as 10,000 babies are born each year by this means.

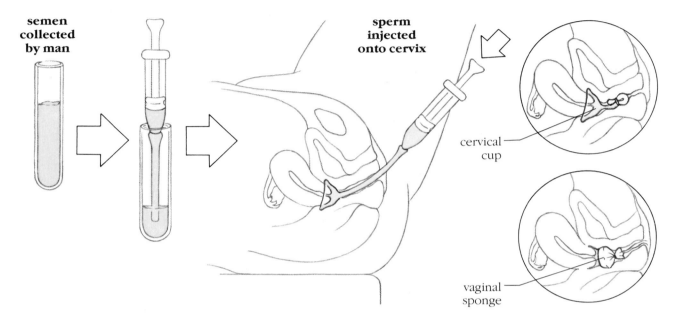

semen collected by man

sperm injected onto cervix

cervical cup

vaginal sponge

Treatment of the Cervix

Sometimes conditions in the cervix or uterus prevent sperm from moving through the cervical canal to meet the egg. Inflammation of the cervical canal may block sperm by producing a thick plug of mucus. Doctors can remove such a plug by suction and then treat the cervix with antibiotics or cauterization. Other defects in the cervical mucus result from ovarian deficiencies (see page 449).

In some cases, the cervical mucus may contain antibodies that destroy the sperm. When the human body is exposed to bacteria or other foreign substances, it produces antibodies in the blood serum to destroy the invaders. It is suspected that some women inadvertently produce such antibodies against their husband's sperm. These antibodies in the cervical mucus may destroy sperm before an ovum can be fertilized. However, if the wife is not exposed to her husband's semen for several months, the immunity ceases. Treatment therefore requires either sexual abstinence or the use of condoms for six months, after which a couple should resume sexual relations without contraceptives only at the time of ovulation. This therapy has met with some success.

Treatment of the Husband

Infertility in the male usually results from an inadequate number of sperm, or sperm that are inactive or sluggish. Testes that have lost their ability to produce sperm because of disease or congenital defects cannot be improved by any method of treatment known at present. But when the quality of the sperm is only relatively decreased, several methods are used to increase the chances of conception.

Of these, medications and "hormone shots" have been the least successful. Medications that have improved ovulation in women just haven't been successful in treating men.

A different problem exists when sperm are produced in adequate quantities but are unable to escape because of blocked ducts. This may be the case even when a normal amount of seminal fluid is ejaculated. In many instances, surgery can correct this condition.

Another problem arises if the semen contains an insufficient number of sperm that are sluggish in activity. This may result from reduced blood circulation in the testes caused by varicose veins in the scrotum—a condition termed varicocele. When the defective veins are surgically removed, blood circulation and the quality and activity of the sperm often improve.

Some institutions are helping men with low sperm concentration by collecting samples of semen from them at different intervals. Each specimen is frozen and stored until a satisfactory concentration is attained for artificial insemination.

Artificial insemination. A fertile woman who is married to a sterile man has the choice of adopting a child or becoming pregnant by artificial insemination with donor semen. Artificial insemination, sometimes referred to as "therapeutic" insemination and also as A.I.D., has been used with increasing frequency in this country during the last half-century.

In artificial insemination, sperm are introduced into the vagina with a syringe or some other mechanical device rather than through the penis. The illustrations on page 525 show two methods of artificial insemination. In this country, it is estimated that as many as 10,000 babies are born each year by this means.

In some instances, the husband's sperm can be successfully used for artificial insemination if it is collected by the "split ejaculate" method. Because the first ejaculation of semen always contains a greater concentration of sperm, it is collected separately and used for insemination.

The Test-Tube Pregnancy

It has long been considered impossible for a pregnancy to occur without at least one normal fallopian tube. Diseases of the fallopian tubes account for 35 to 40 percent of all infertility problems. This dynamic organ makes possible all the essential processes required to make an ovum available for fertilization by a sperm, leading to successful pregnancy.

The end of each fallopian tube is equipped with tiny fingerlike structures (fimbriae) that pick up an ovum at the moment of ovulation and deliver it into the tubal lumen. There, the delicate lining of the tube secretes special fluids to nourish the sperm and prepare them for penetration and fertilization of the ovum.

After the ovum is fertilized in the outer end of the tube, it grows rapidly by cell division, first into two cells, then four, eight, sixteen, and so on. During this growth period, gentle tubal activity transports the ovum through the length of the tube and deposits it in the uterus for implantation and growth into a fetus.

How In Vitro Fertilization Takes Place

In vitro fertilization is a complex and often unsuccessful procedure, although the idea is a simple one. To date, only two babies have been born using this method. To fertilize and grow an egg outside the body, the following ingredients are needed: a ripe (mature) egg, some sperm, and a "soup" in which to mix them that will allow fertilization and will support the embryo.

In the first step of this procedure, a woman is given the hormone human chorionic gonadotropin (HCG) at exactly the right moment to cause her ovaries to prepare a ripe egg or eggs for release.

Thirty-three to thirty-four hours later, the woman is put under general anesthesia for laparoscopy to remove the ripe egg from the ovary surface. This timing is precise, for even a few hours later, the egg will spontaneously burst from the ovary and be swept into the fallopian tube. The doctor makes a small incision in the abdomen (see page 198), inserts the laparoscope, and views the ovaries directly. He looks for a bulge on the surface of the ovary, indicating the ripe egg about to pop out, and uses a suction tube to suck the egg out of the ovary. If there is more than one bulge, he may collect more than one egg. The eggs are immediately pipetted into the nutrient medium (highly specialized to duplicate the fluid in the fallopian tubes) in a small glass dish called a petri dish.

Meanwhile, sperm is collected from the woman's husband and put into a solution that dilutes it and causes it to undergo the chemical changes necessary to penetrate the coat around the egg (see page 485). The eggs are then carefully lowered into the sperm suspension using a special technique to keep eggs and sperm together in a small amount of fluid.

Union of the egg and sperm (fertilization) occurs within a few hours. The embryo is then placed in a special fluid in a chamber with precise mixtures of oxygen and carbon dioxide. The embryo divides into eight cells by day two, and into approximately 100 cells by day four after fertilization. At this point, the embryo is inserted into the mother's uterus. To complete this final maneuver, the embryo is once again drawn up into a pipette (a cannula), the tip is inserted into the uterus through the cervix, and the embryo is gently blown out into the uterine cavity. Several days before, the mother was treated with hormones to help the uterine endometrium prepare for implantation. Now the embryo must settle and implant itself on the wall of the uterus.

Even minor defects of the tubal fimbriae may delay or prevent conception. Diseases that narrow the tubal lumen can destroy the delicate lining or cause closure of the tube, resulting in sterility. Although many defects of the tubes and fimbriae can be repaired surgically, some cannot be improved by presently known methods.

The procedure by which an ovum can be removed from an ovary by an endoscope (Culdoscope) and transferred directly into the uterus was perfected many years ago. Now it is possible to fertilize an ovum removed from the ovary. To accomplish this, it is necessary to reproduce in a culture medium conditions that are similar to those in the fallopian tube. On two occasions, Drs. Steptoe and Edwards of England have been able to mimic the conditions that occur naturally in the fallopian tube and achieve normal pregnancies. The adjacent box explains their methods.

Qualifying for *In Vitro* Fertilization

To qualify for an *in vitro* procedure, a woman must be under 36 years of age and in good health, and must ovulate regularly or have ovaries that respond to ovulation stimulants. Her tubes must be absent or hopelessly occluded. In addition, her husband must produce semen adequate to achieve fertilization, or both husband and wife must consent to use donor semen for fertilization of the recovered ovum.

Physicians in the United States who perform this procedure will abide by the required principle of informed consent. Patients will be carefully screened to assure emotional stability in facing the possibility of many failures, with only a low probability of success at the first trial. At present, there have not been enough successes to suggest that the procedure is infallible or even practical.

Following removal of the ovum, its fertilization in the test tube or glass dish, and its deposition back into the uterus, the ovary may fail to complete its proper function and the fertilized ovum may not implant on the uterine wall. In this case, spontaneous abortion will occur. This also is the fate of 10 percent of normally conceived pregnancies.

Some fertility services are making plans to establish a service for *in vitro* fertilization to accommodate patients who meet the requirements. Special equipment and facilities are required that must meet rigid standards, and such services will require funding to keep the cost at the $3,000 fee suggested for each procedure. Physicians and the research community are moving cautiously on *in vitro* fertilization. After only two live births of apparently healthy babies, there can be no assurance that the *in vitro* procedure does not contain hazards for other children conceived in this manner.

Where to Go for Infertility Problems

For information on clinics and doctors in your community who specialize in treating problems of infertility, contact—RESOLVE, Inc., a national, nonprofit organization with chapters in many states. It provides counseling, referral services, and support groups for men and women with infertility problems.

RESOLVE, Incorporated
P.O. Box 474
Belmont, Massachusetts 02178

An increasing number of physicians, clinics, and university medical centers specialize in treating infertility problems. The following is a partial list of some of these resources.

Boston Hospital for Women
Fertility and Endocrine Unit
221 Longwood Avenue
Boston, Massachusetts 02115

Fertility Clinic
610 North 19th Street
Milwaukee, Wisconsin 53233

Louisville General Hospital
Infertility Clinic
323 East Chestnut Street
Louisville, Kentucky 40202

New York Fertility Research Foundation
1430 Second Avenue
New York, New York 10021

Stanford Medical Center
Stanford, California 94305

Tyler Clinic Research Foundation
921 Westwood Boulevard
East Los Angeles, California 90024

University of North Carolina Medical School
Department of Obstetrics—Gynecology
Chapel Hill, North Carolina 27514

University of Texas Medical School
P.O. Box 20708
Houston, Texas 77025

Yale-New Haven Hospital
Fertility Clinic
789 Howard Avenue
New Haven, Connecticut 06504

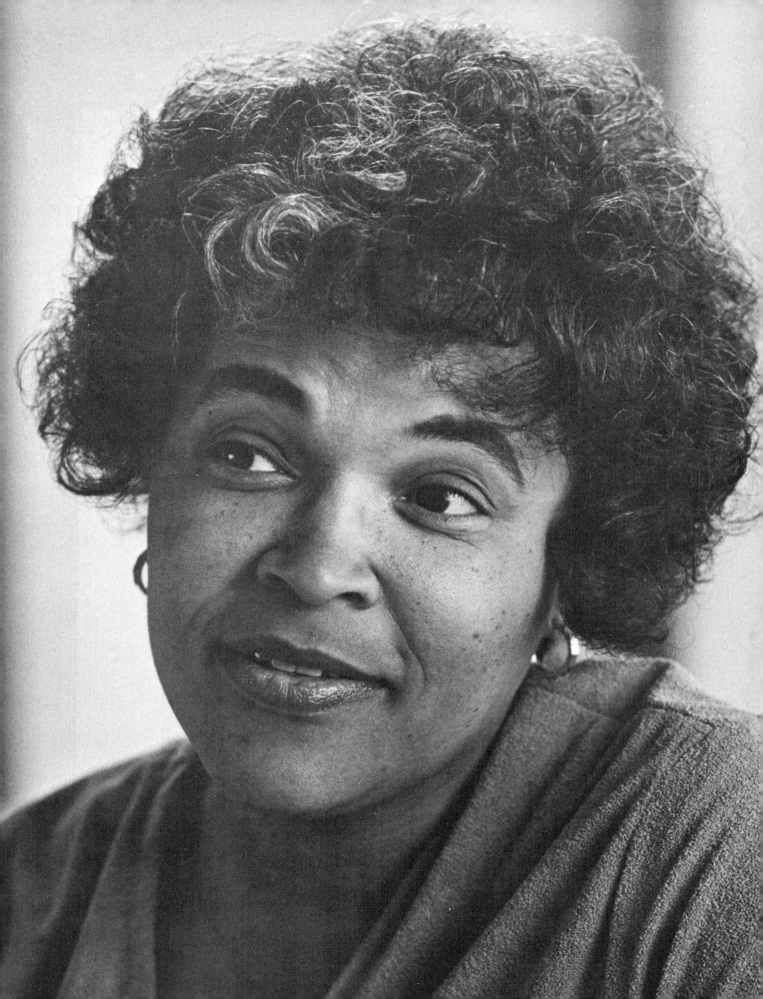

CHAPTER 25

URINARY SYSTEM DISORDERS

LUCIENNE T. LANSON, M.D., F.A.C.O.G.

Urinary tract infections are common problems with women, and some experts estimate that all women experience urinary pain at some time in their lives. Sometimes urinary problems are related to sexual intercourse, or occur during pregnancy or labor and delivery. Others don't arise until later in life, when disorders of the pelvic support system result in incontinence. Fortunately, there are preventive measures women can take to minimize the incidence and severity of many of these common problems.

Urinary Disorders

If you have urinary frequency or recurrent bladder infections, or feel that your vagina is overly large for your sexual partner, you might find consolation in knowing that many of these problems can be corrected and sometimes even prevented.

Sexual intercourse, pregnancy, childbirth, and aging all stretch and strain vaginal tissues and pelvic organ supports. Gradual estrogen depletion in the post-menopausal years can further weaken these pelvic supports, and in some cases, ultimately lead to organ prolapse such as a dropped uterus or sagging bladder. Moreover, the unique anatomy of the female genitourinary system predisposes women to a variety of bladder disturbances. For some women, this can mean intermittent urinary incontinence or the embarrassing loss of a few drops of urine when laughing or sneezing. For others, bladder irritations and infections recur with annoying regularity.

Urinary Tract Infections

Bladder infection (cystitis) is without a doubt one of the most common medical problems of women. It can occur as a single acute infection or as chronic, recurrent infections that linger into the postmenopausal years. Women are considerably more vulnerable than men to such infections, partly because of the relatively short female urethra. The male urethra measures approximately eight inches from the tip of the penis to the bladder. It evacuates urine from the bladder and acts as a channel for the passage of sperm and seminal fluid. In contrast, the female urethra is a scant 1.6 inches long, and serves only to evacuate urine. The close proximity of the female urethra to both the vagina and the anus also facilitates the introduction of vulvar and fecal bacteria into the urethra and bladder. Many women probably acquire their first urinary tract infection through such urethral contamination. For other women, sexual intercourse can precipitate acute and recurrent bladder infections.

In a woman just beginning an active sex life, so-called honeymoon cystitis may well be the first encounter with a urinary problem. Although any woman is vulnerable (whether or not she's on her honeymoon), a woman with a relatively snug vaginal opening is most susceptible. For her, intercourse in the conventional male-dominant position will automatically direct the penis along the roof of the vagina and against the floor of the overlying urethra and bladder. The thrusting motion of the penis in this position can irritate these urinary structures as well as push bacteria from the vulva into the woman's urethra and bladder. Repeated acts of intercourse over a short time span are particularly prone to elicit honeymoon cystitis. Since bacteria introduced into the bladder normally take a day or so to establish themselves, symptoms of acute cystitis usually don't begin until about 36 hours following the initial precipitating intercourse. Honeymoon cystitis is a serious bladder infection that requires treatment and supportive care.

Pregnant women also are more vulnerable to urinary infections because of hormonal, chemical, and physiological changes associated with pregnancy. Bladder tone, for example, is normally reduced during pregnancy, allowing the bladder to fill and retain more urine before a woman feels the need to void. As a consequence, less-frequent voiding can lead to urinary stasis and an increased chance of infection. This situation is in sharp contrast to the urinary frequency many women experience during early pregnancy as a result of pressure from an enlarging uterus.

As many as 10 percent of pregnant women have an asymptomatic and unsuspected bladder infection. Since these "silent" bladder infections during pregnancy can lead to pyelonephritis and kidney damage, they must be detected and treated as soon as possible. This is one of the reasons for routine urinalysis during pregnancy.

Other factors that predispose a woman to urinary tract infections include diabetes, obstructions to the flow of urine (stones, strictures, tumors, etc.), bladder disturbances because of nerve damage (for example, spinal cord injuries), and even catheterizations or instrumentations of the urethra and bladder. But regardless of the cause, the symptoms of a urinary tract infection depend on the specific location of the infection within the urinary tract.

Symptoms. In contrast to pyelitis or another acute kidney infection, most bladder infections exhibit rather mild symptoms. Women with cystitis complain primarily of frequent voiding, urgency, and a burning, stinging pain along the urethra during and immediately after voiding. They experience occasional cramping pain over the pubic area, but fever, if any, rarely exceeds 100 degrees. If the cystitis is especially severe, the urine may be blood-tinged or grossly bloody because of marked irritation of the bladder lining.

ANATOMY OF THE PELVIC ORGANS

This side view of the pelvic organs shows their openings to the exterior of the body. The lower bowel or rectum opens through the anus. Next, moving toward the front of the body, the vagina opens through the *vaginal opening. The bladder empties urine through the urethra. These openings may be seen from another view on page 444. The pubic symphysis is the firm band of cartilage joining the pubic bones.*

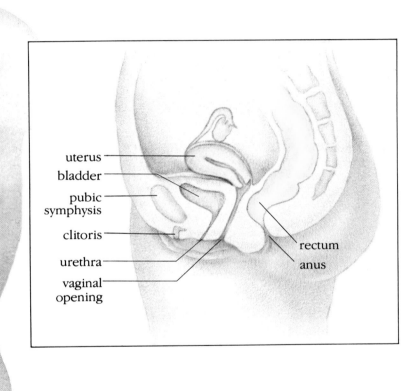

uterus
bladder
pubic symphysis
clitoris
urethra
vaginal opening
rectum
anus

uterus
bladder

These symptoms, however, can be misleading. Not all painful urination should be blamed on an acute bladder infection. Vaginal infections, vulvar irritations, and gonorrheal involvement of the urethra also can mimic acute cystitis.

Urethritis or inflammation with or without infection of the urethra also causes burning, stinging pain that can be both severe and persistent. In urethritis, the urethral mucosa is frequently red and swollen, and may produce a discharge. Painful urination—especially if it occurs shortly after intercourse—may be caused by trauma to the urethra during coitus. In a woman with inadequate vaginal lubrication or a snug vaginal opening, friction of the penis against the floor of the urethra and bladder can be responsible. In a postmenopausal woman, the relative thinness of the vaginal walls makes the overlying urinary structures even more vulnerable to injury during coitus. But a sexually inactive older woman also can experience pain on urination from urethral atrophy and irritation that result from lack of estrogen. In addition, such urethral tissue changes can cause stress incontinence in postmenopausal women (see page 533).

Symptoms of a kidney infection can be dramatic and develop rapidly over a 24- to 48-hour period. Characteristically, they include a high fever (usually over 102 degrees), often with shaking chills and aching pain in one or both flanks. Patients also may experience nausea and vomiting, as well as the symptoms of cystitis. Although it is sometimes impossible to determine how the kidney infection started, bacteria that spread to the kidney from the bladder are probably the most common cause. Bacteria also can travel through the bloodstream to the kidney from other sites of infection—for example, the tonsils in tonsillitis.

Diagnosis of urinary infections. Although the patient's history and symptoms are of great value in diagnosing urinary tract infections, doctors rely primarily on microscopic examination of the urine for the presence of bacteria and white blood cells (pus cells). Since the vast majority of bladder infections are caused by E. coli, a colon bacteria that responds to most bladder medications, your doctor probably will order a routine urinalysis simply to confirm the presence of bacteria and pus cells. If this is your very first bladder infection, your doctor may order no other urine studies before starting treatment.

But if your urine contains a significant number of bacteria and pus cells even after therapy, or if you have had recurrent flare-ups of cystitis, your doctor may ask for a urine culture and sensitivity test. A urine culture is a laboratory procedure that specifically identifies the bacteria responsible for the infection. It also can gauge the severity of the infection by specifying the number of bacteria present per cc. (cubic centimeter) of urine. More than 100,000 organisms or bacteria per cc. is considered significant. The urine sensitivity test goes one step further by testing the bacteria's resistance or sensitivity to the most common antibiotics and bladder medications. In other words, a urine culture and sensitivity test will tell your doctor what bacteria are causing your infection, how severe the infection is, and what medicine will work best against it.

It goes without saying that if the diagnosis and treatment of your infection depend on a urine examination, you should know the proper way to collect a specimen. Although urine is sterile and contains no bacteria under normal and healthy conditions, it is susceptible to contamination with bacteria from the vulva or vaginal areas. Short of using a catheter, the only reliable method of collecting a clean, uncontaminated urine specimen is the "midstream, clean-catch method." Gently wash the outside of the urethral and vaginal areas. If you are menstruating, block the vaginal opening with a tampon or tissue to avoid contaminating the urine with blood. While holding the urine receptacle in one hand, spread the labial lips with the other hand and begin voiding. As soon as you are certain that your urine stream is not deflecting off the vulva, simply catch the urine in the container. Make certain that the container does not come into contact with the vulva. Collecting urine in this manner is best done while standing. If you are having just a routine urinalysis, a clean, dry jar with a screw top makes an adequate container. Specimens for urine cultures require sterile containers that usually are provided by the laboratory.

Doctors use a new urine test—the FA or fluorescent antibody test—to help distinguish an infection confined to the bladder from one that involves the kidney and upper urinary tract.

Treatment of any urinary tract infection must be individualized. This includes checking for possible contributing factors such as obstructions due to stones, diabetes, and even inadvertent contamination of the urethra by faulty hygiene habits. In a young healthy woman with an uncomplicated bladder infection, there are many effective antibiotics and antibacterial drugs. The sulfonimides (Gantrisan, Gantanol) are an old and reliable group. Among the antibiotics, Furadantin, Macrondantin, Ampillin, and Tetracycline are commonly used. Equally important, you should increase your water intake by at least four to six glasses a day. This dilutes the urine and flushes out bacteria by encouraging more frequent urination.

After treatment is completed, your urine should be rechecked. If symptoms recur, another course of therapy will be needed. This may mean changing to a different antibacterial drug, depending on the results of a new urine culture. An examination of the urethra and the interior of the bladder (cystoscopy), and possibly an IVP (intravenous pyelogram) also may be indicated. These studies can give important information about possible obstructions or abnormalities that could contribute to continuing urinary problems.

But regardless of the medication your doctor orders, it is important to follow instructions closely. Your symptoms may disappear within one to three days, but you should continue taking your medicine as prescribed. This will prevent flare-ups and avoid the risk of the infection ascending into the kidney. Most bladder infections require at least ten to fourteen days and sometimes as long as three to five weeks to eradicate; some may even take months.

For women who have recurrent bladder infections, these suggestions may prevent another bout with cystitis. First always empty your bladder before intercourse. An empty bladder is not readily infected, and even though bacteria may be milked into the bladder during coitus, infection is unlikely unless sufficient urine is present to stimulate bacterial growth. Second, drink plenty of water and fluids—especially during the hot summer months. This dilutes the urine, and lowers its potential bacterial count. Even if urine is present in the bladder during intercourse, the more dilute it is, the better your chances of avoiding infection. The color of your urine is a good guide to your fluid intake. If you are drinking enough water, your urine should be pale yellow to almost colorless. Third, empty your bladder after intercourse and drink at least two glasses of water. This ensures adequate bladder volume to effect proper voiding, and dilutes the urine. You will undoubtedly have to get up during the night to urinate, but that's what it's all about—flushing out the bacteria before they can cause trouble. Some urologists suggest substituting showers for tub baths as another way to reduce the incidence of bladder infections. Where recurrences of cystitis are frequent despite conscientious efforts, a small dose of an antibiotic taken on a regular basis prior to intercourse has helped some women remain symptom-free.

Problems of Urinary Control

As adults, most of us take urinary control for granted. And yet, it is one of the body's most complicated functions. Urinary continence, or the ability to control one's urine, requires a normal nervous system, an intact urinary system, and well-toned pelvic muscles and tissues that support the bladder and urethra in their proper anatomical positions. Disturbances in any one of these areas can result in temporary or permanent loss of urinary control. Here again, because of our anatomy and childbearing capacity, women are particularly susceptible to such disturbances. Although urinary incontinence can take many forms, two of the most common types are stress incontinence and urge incontinence.

Stress incontinence. If you've ever lost a few drops of urine while laughing or sneezing, then you have experienced stress incontinence—the sudden and involuntary expulsion of urine when pressure rises within the bladder. Stress incontinence is sometimes normal if you happen to have a full bladder. But for some women, it is a constant and embarrassing problem. In severe cases, any strain, bearing-down effort, sneeze, cough, or laugh can cause a sudden small loss of urine.

Stress incontinence usually results from a weakening and thinning of the muscles and connective tissues that support the bladder and urethra. Furthermore, the angle at which the urethra joins the bladder is of critical importance in maintaining urinary control. Therefore, any weakness in these support tissues that allows the urethra to sag, thus changing its normal position in relation to the bladder, can bring on stress incontinence. The fact that women with this problem are rarely incontinent while lying down (even if they sneeze) is further evidence that stress incontinence is mainly a problem of inadequate pelvic support.

Since most cases of stress incontinence are specifically caused by inadequate urethral support or a sagging urethra (urethrocele), the urethra must be resuspended in its normal position to bring relief. Depending on the severity of the problem, this can be accomplished by surgical correction or by retraining and strengthening the pelvic muscles.

Surgical correction. Even in long-standing and severe cases of stress incontinence, vaginal plastic surgery can successfully reposition the urethra and return normal urinary control in a high percentage of women. The operation, which is performed entirely within the vaginal canal, repairs any defects in the muscles and connective tissue supports. If necessary, the procedure also can include a snugging-up of an overly stretched vagina. Another fairly common approach to resuspending the urethra is the Marshall-Marchetti operation. Unlike the vaginal operation, this procedure is performed through a lower abdominal incision. Of course, the selection of either operation is individualized and is based on a thorough evaluation of the urinary problem or disturbance.

Exercise programs for stress incontinence.

Women with mild to moderate stress incontinence can improve or even overcome their problem with special pelvic exercises that strengthen the pubococcygeus muscle. The pubococcygeus muscle is one of the most important muscles you possess as a woman. It forms the floor of the pelvic cavity and helps support the pelvic organs. In essence, it is a broad band of muscle tissue that stretches like a taut hammock from the pubic bone in front to the coccyx or tailbone behind. You might think of it as an internal sling that stretches between the legs from front to back. In a normal and healthy state, this muscle encircles the urethra close to where it joins the bladder, surrounds and supports the middle third of the vagina, and encompasses the rectum just above the anal opening. Contracting the pubococcygeus muscle will therefore cause a tightening sensation from the urethra to the rectum. Some women describe the feeling as a "drawing up" or a "pulling together" of the external genitalia.

You can exercise this muscle in any position—while sitting, lying down, or even walking—and you needn't contract any other muscle group at the same time. All too often, women will squeeze their buttocks together, hold their breath, make terrible facial grimaces, or worse yet, push down as though they were having a bowel movement. Contracting the pubococcygeus muscle does just the opposite of pushing down. It draws the anus closer to the urethra, tightens the rectal sphincter, and prevents the inadvertent escape of flatus (gas). To be sure you're contracting the correct muscle, check yourself by alternately stopping and starting your urine stream the next time you go to the bathroom. To stop voiding on command requires a strong contraction of the pubococcygeus muscle; relaxing the muscle allows you to resume voiding. Contracting this muscle will also tighten the vaginal canal. For confirmation, insert one finger into your vagina. As you contract the pubococcygeus muscle, your vagina should tighten and squeeze your finger.

EXERCISES FOR THE PUBOCOCCYGEUS MUSCLE

The pubococcygeus muscle is one of the most important muscles you possess as a woman. It forms the floor of the pelvic cavity and supports the pelvic organs. By strengthening it, you learn to control the opening and closing of the urethral opening, increase the muscle tone of the vaginal canal, and avoid incontinence, sagging pelvic organs, and a loose rectal sphincter.

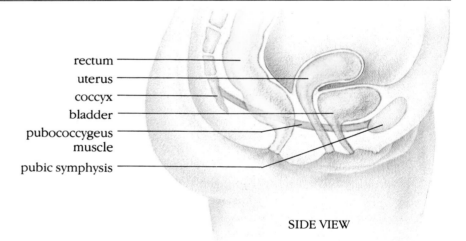

rectum
uterus
coccyx
bladder
pubococcygeus muscle
pubic symphysis

SIDE VIEW

TOP VIEW

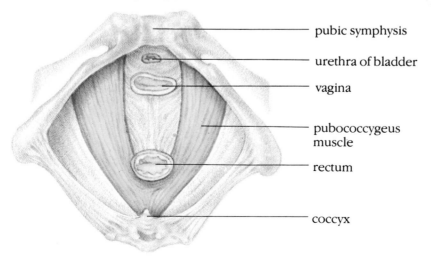

pubic symphysis

urethra of bladder

vagina

pubococcygeus muscle

rectum

coccyx

Exercising the pubococcygeus muscle is simple. Just contract the muscle, drawing the anus closer to the urethra. Repeat this contraction, holding it for three seconds, 100 times a day. See above for complete instructions.

As with any exercise program, you'll have to be conscientious to get results. Muscles don't increase in bulk and strength overnight. If you have never consciously used or contracted this muscle, these exercises may initially be difficult. But stay with them. Women with only mild stress incontinence should notice some improvement within two months.

An effective exercise program should include at least 100 contractions per day. Hold each contraction for a full three seconds and make it as forceful as possible. Relax between contractions for another three seconds. If this seems like a lot of effort on a daily basis, remember that you can exercise this muscle anywhere, in any position, and without anybody being the wiser. Many women do their "daily 100" while driving or riding public transportation.

A regular exercise program such as this also promotes healthier and firmer vaginal tissues by increasing the blood flow through the pelvis. As you will recall, the pubococcygeus muscle encircles and supports the middle third of the vagina. Loss of tone or slackness in this middle area—whether from childbirth, aging, or lack of exercise—will gradually make the vagina shorter and wider. Such a vagina is no longer able to ensheathe the penis snugly during intercourse or properly contract or expand. A woman with this problem often complains of a lack of vaginal sensation during coitus; her partner may complain that his penis seems virtually lost inside the vagina. Proper exercise can help restore shape and tone to this middle third of the vaginal canal, with noticeable improvement after two to three months

Urge incontinence refers to involuntarily losing a small amount of urine whenever the urge to urinate suddenly strikes. Unless a bathroom is near, a woman with this problem may inadvertently wet her underwear. This condition is considerably less serious than stress incontinence, and can result from inflammation and irritation of the urethra or bladder. Sometimes the problem can be linked to an obvious urinary infection. In postmenopausal women, an estrogen deficiency can aggravate and even cause urge incontinence.

Correcting the condition depends on finding and treating the cause. But since urge incontinence frequently occurs with a full bladder, a woman can minimize the problem if she takes the time to void at regular intervals throughout the day.

Complete urinary incontinence. Constant and uncontrollable leakage of urine is usually due to fistula formation. A fistula is an abnormal opening, passageway, tract, or connection between two organs or structures. In women, such fistulas can form between the urethra and vagina, between the ureter and vagina, and between the bladder and vagina. The most common is the so-called vesico-vaginal fistula, an abnormal passageway between the bladder and vagina. If the fistula or passageway is very small, urine loss from the bladder through the vagina may be slight and intermittent. Where the fistula is large, however, urine drainage is usually constant.

A large vesico-vaginal fistula is one of the most intolerable and miserable of all female urinary problems. Women who suffer this condition exhibit redness and inflammation of the vulva and upper thighs, which frequently are covered with pustules or caked with deposits of urinary salts. Although such fistulas are relatively rare in this country, they are not uncommon in other parts of the world. Most vesico-vaginal fistulas are caused by prolonged obstructed labors and injuries during childbirth, but they also can result from operative accidents during difficult pelvic surgery. Less commonly, they may appear following extensive radiation therapy for cancer of the cervix or uterus.

Treatment is, of course, surgery to close the fistula. Results are predictably better when the woman's vaginal tissues already are in good condition and the area is free of scar tissue.

Other causes of urinary incontinence may be spinal cord injuries, anatomical defects such as spinabifida (a congenital defect of the vertebral column) and neurological diseases that affect bladder control, such as multiple sclerosis, brain or spinal cord tumors, and diabetes. Incontinence also can occur in women with severely disturbed mental and emotional states.

Urinary retention is just the opposite of urinary incontinence—the inability to urinate and empty one's bladder. Although this problem is more common in men because of an enlarged prostate, women also are susceptible under certain circumstances. Acute inflammation and swelling of the urethra from a genital herpes infection is certainly one of the most common causes of acute urinary retention. Voiding also may be impossible for a woman whose bladder has become overly stretched and distended with urine. This type of urinary retention is sometimes seen in the postpartum period—particularly among women who have had regional anesthesia (epidural or spinal anesthesia) and intravenous fluids during childbirth. Under these circumstances, the anesthesia causes a temporary lack of bladder sensation for the need to void. This, coupled with increased fluid intake, leads to a full bladder and urinary retention. These problems are fortunately short-lived and promptly respond to catheterization, usually for one to two days. Where urinary retention is caused by a tumor or cyst that blocks the urethra, surgery may be necessary to correct the problem.

PELVIC SUPPORT PROBLEMS

NORMAL VIEW

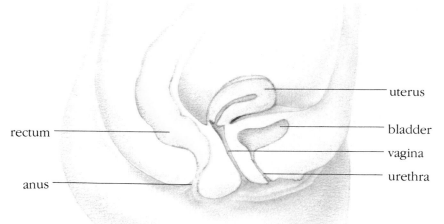

rectum

anus

uterus

bladder

vagina

urethra

URETHROCELE

A urethrocele is a ballooning or prolapse of the urethra, the tube from the bladder to the outside.

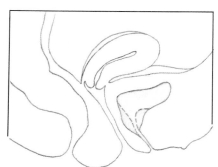

Pelvic Support Problems

Women are uniquely vulnerable to pelvic support problems. Conditions such as a sagging urethra, a sagging bladder, or a dropped uterus all can be explained by inadequate pelvic support. Although some women seem naturally predisposed to weak pelvic muscles and ligaments, most prolapse problems result from unavoidable trauma and injury to these tissues during childbirth. Obesity places additional strain on these supports, as does excessive coughing from a lung condition. Chronic constipation with bearing-down efforts during defecation can further weaken these supports. But a common cause that none of us can avoid is aging. As previously discussed, aging and estrogen depletion can severely aggravate the situation. A woman with a slightly dropped uterus at age 45 may have a serious prolapse problem by age 65.

Specific symptoms depend on the organ involved and the severity of the problem. What originally may have started as a slight weakness in the pubococcygeus muscle and connective tissues (see page 225) can develop into an actual defect. In other words, the weakened tissues may become so stretched and thin that the fibers begin to separate and tear. Eventually, as more muscle and connective tissue fibers separate, a hole or defect is created—much the way a hole wears through the heel of a sock.

Urethroceles. Without proper support, the pelvic organs begin to prolapse or herniate through the defect, and in time, bulge down and into the vaginal canal. The urethra, instead of being tucked against the pubic bone, visibly sags downward. This condition is called a urethrocele and can lead to stress incontinence, as previously discussed. Similarly, the bladder, rectum, and uterus also can prolapse and protrude into the vaginal canal.

A cystocele is a protrusion or prolapse of the urinary bladder into the vaginal canal. Small cystoceles don't usually cause symptoms, but larger ones can be troublesome. Most women with a large cystocele will complain of a heavy dragging sensation, as though their pelvic organs were falling out. They also may notice a lump or bulge just inside the vaginal opening. This lump, which is actually the cystocele, is particularly noticeable in the standing position, when the weight of any urine forces the bladder to protrude even further. If a woman examines herself with a mirror while standing, she may well mistake that rounded pink lump for a dropped uterus or even a tumor.

With progressive enlargement of the cystocele over a period of time, urinary difficulties usually develop. The most common of these is the inability to completely empty the bladder. Marked prolapse of the bladder causes a large portion of the organ to sag below the level of the urethral outlet. Consequently, trying to empty the bladder completely is somewhat like trying to urinate uphill; some urine is retained even after voiding. For this reason, a woman with a large cystocele will feel the need to void even after she has just been to the bathroom. This type of distress is particularly common at bedtime. A woman who has just been to the bathroom may be overcome with the urge to void as soon as she lies down.

CYSTOCELE

A cystocele is a protrusion or prolapse of the urinary bladder into the vaginal canal.

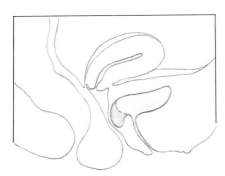

RECTOCELE

A rectocele is a protrusion or prolapse of the rectal wall into the vaginal canal.

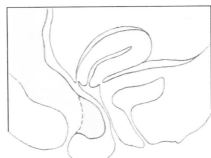

UTERINE PROLAPSE

A uterine prolapse is the descent of the uterus from the pelvic cavity into the vaginal canal.

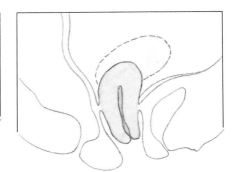

Some women have discovered that they can empty their bladder by inserting a finger into the vagina and pushing up on the "bulge." As helpful as this maneuver can be, it still does not solve the problem.

In addition, the residual urine that is retained in the bladder at all times makes a perfect breeding ground for lurking bacteria. Women with cystoceles are therefore more apt to develop chronic and recurrent bladder infections. Persistent bladder floor irritation also can cause urge incontinence (see page 535).

Diagnosis of a cystocele is usually made during a pelvic examination by identifying the telltale bulge along the roof (anterior wall) of the vagina. But treatment is seldom undertaken unless there are symptoms. Exercises for the pelvic muscles are unfortunately of little or no value in correcting a cystocele. The bladder bulge and weakness in the vaginal wall must be corrected by surgery. Since this area cannot be reached through an abdominal incision, the operation is done vaginally.

A rectocele is a protrusion or prolapse of the rectal wall into the vaginal canal. Unlike other sagging organs, a rectocele causes few if any problems—except, possibly, in a woman with chronic constipation. In this instance, a stool may collect and harden in the pouched-out rectal wall just above the anus. As more stool accumulates in this area, it may become increasingly difficult to have a bowel movement. Some women facilitate evacuation by placing a finger in the vagina and pushing against the bulging rectal wall. Keeping stools soft and improving bowel habits may help, but the only permanent solution is surgery to resupport the sagging rectal wall in its proper position.

Prolapse of the uterus. Although special ligaments help maintain the normal position of the uterus, its support also depends on the pubococcygeus muscle and pelvic connective tissue. Any weakening of these supports can lead to a prolapse or descent of the uterus into the vaginal canal—the so-called dropped uterus. A few cases may be due to inherent weakness of the supporting tissues, but most probably stem from tissue trauma as the result of childbirth.

Symptoms usually depend on how far the uterus has actually descended into the vaginal canal. With minimal descent, there may be no discomfort whatsoever. With a more perceptible uterine prolapse, a woman's sexual partner may be the first to notice the problem. As the uterus gradually descends into the vaginal canal, it can block deep penile penetration during intercourse. Women who are accustomed to douching may complain that something is blocking the vagina. As long as the cervix does not protrude beyond the vaginal opening, the prolapse is classified as a first-degree prolapse. In a second-degree prolapse, the cervix can actually appear outside the vaginal opening; in a third-degree uterine prolapse, the entire uterus protrudes outside the vaginal opening. Long before this happens, however, most women will sense that their uterus is dropping.

PROLAPSE OF THE UTERUS

The normal support of the uterus depends on the pubococcygeus muscle (see page 534) and pelvic connective tissue, as well as special ligaments that help maintain the normal position of the uterus.

NORMAL UTERINE SUPPORT

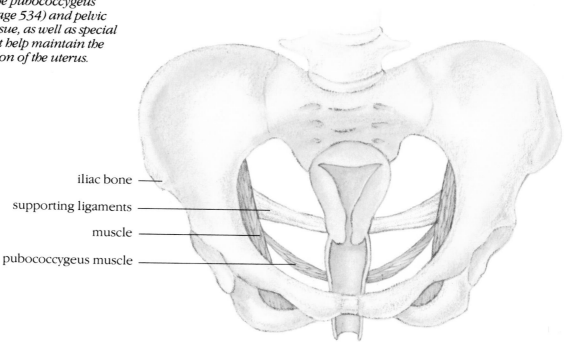

iliac bone

supporting ligaments

muscle

pubococcygeus muscle

Uterine prolapse can occur due to a breakdown of the supporting ligaments and poor muscle tone.

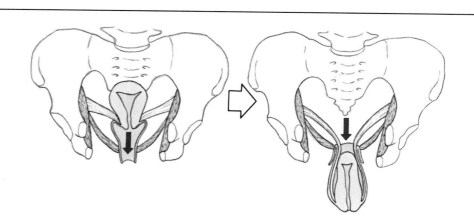

Uterine prolapse also occurs when both the ligaments and the pelvic floor support fail (collapse of the pubococcygeus muscle).

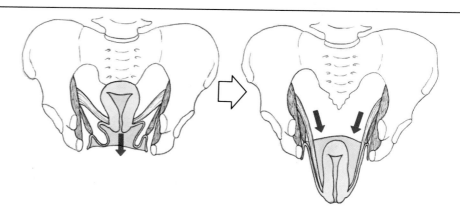

Prolapse of the uterus also interferes with blood circulation through the pelvis. Congestion and engorgement of the uterine vessels can cause a heavy, dragging sensation and low backache. Since a dropped uterus can pull and exert traction on the bladder and urethra, urinary difficulties such as straining to void and repeated infections because of retained urine are fairly common.

If a dropped uterus is causing sufficient distress, most doctors will suggest a vaginal hysterectomy—the removal of the uterus through the vagina. At the same time, any sagging of the vaginal walls, urethra, bladder, or rectum also can be corrected. If prolapse of the uterus develops in a younger woman who desires another pregnancy, surgery usually will be delayed until she has completed her family.

Sometimes, however, surgery is not always the best solution for a prolapsed uterus or sagging vaginal walls. For example, elderly women with severe cardiac conditions or respiratory insufficiency generally make poor candidates for surgery. For symptomatic relief, these women may be fitted with a vaginal pessary to keep sagging organs tucked up.

Vaginal pessaries are appliances made of hard rubber or plastic. In contrast to contraceptive diaphragms worn solely for birth control purposes, vaginal pessaries are designed to help support the uterus and vaginal walls in their normal position. Since they come in a variety of shapes and sizes, each woman must be individually fitted, depending upon the extent of her uterine prolapse and vaginal wall relaxation.

Vaginal pessaries do have their drawbacks, however. Any device left in the vagina tends to create an irritating and malodorous discharge. Regular douching and the use of vaginal creams are necessary to decrease discharge and odor formation. The pessary also should be removed, cleaned, and replaced periodically. Since this is usually done professionally, it requires a visit to the doctor at least every two to four months. In elderly women, even a properly fitted vaginal pessary can rub and irritate the thin vaginal mucosa. In sexually active women, a pessary also can interfere with normal intercourse by limiting the depth of penile penetration. Fortunately, however, with improved anesthesia and

monitoring methods during surgical procedures, more and more women who were previously resigned to wearing a pessary are now safely undergoing corrective vaginal surgery.

In addition to these advances in surgical techniques, the past several years have made both doctors and women more acutely aware of preventive measures. Factors such as proper nutrition, good general health habits, competent obstetrical care, and exercise of the pubococcygeus muscle can substantially minimize prolapse problems and urinary disturbances. So although the human female will still be vulnerable to these conditions because of her anatomy, much can be done and much is being done.

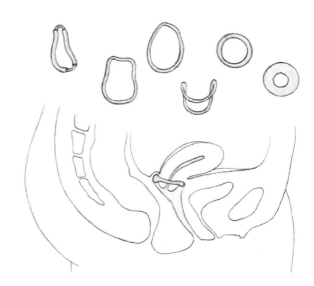

VAGINAL PESSARIES FOR UTERINE PROLAPSE

Vaginal pessaries may be fitted to help support sagging pelvic organs. Pessaries are made of hard rubber and come in a variety of shapes and sizes so that each fitting is individual. Corrective surgery is usually the best remedy for uterine prolapse, but pessaries may be useful to women who, for some reason, cannot undergo surgery.

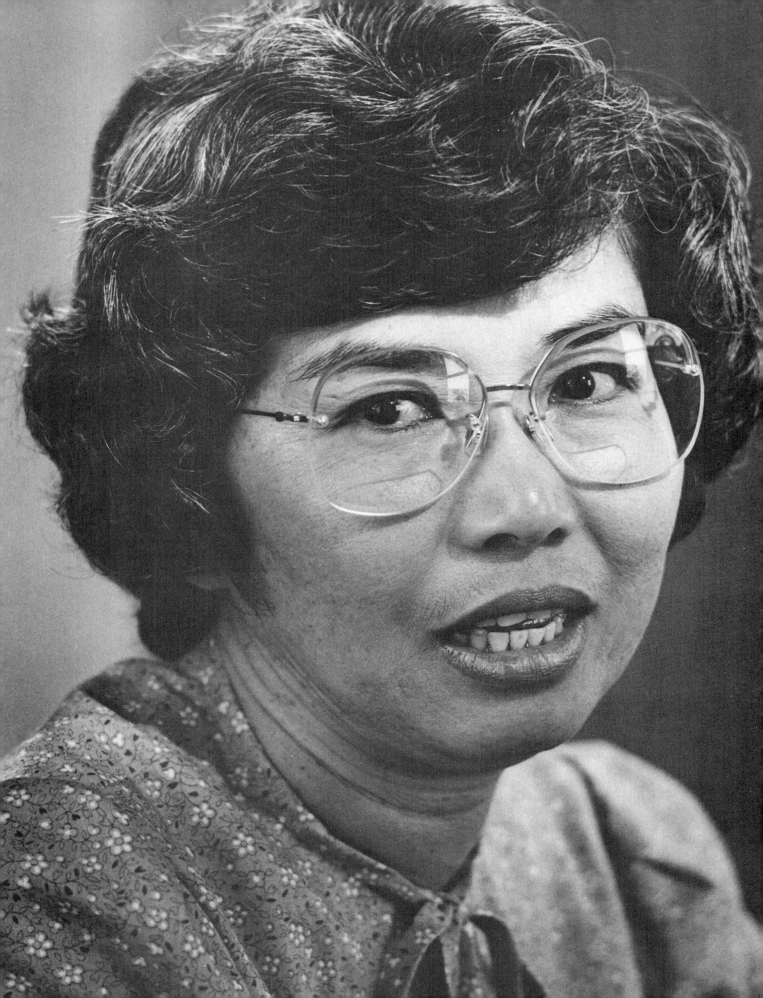

CHAPTER 26

BREAST DISEASE

JUSTIN J. STEIN, M.D., F.A.C.R., F.A.C.S.

The term "breast disease" has immediate connotations of breast cancer for many women. Yet, benign, non-cancerous conditions are, by far, the most common breast problems diagnosed by physicians. Learning about the normal structure of the breast and the differences between benign breast conditions and breast cancer can be reassuring.

Still, it is a distressing fact that the death rate for breast cancer patients has remained the same for many years, regardless of all of the treatment procedures used. Each case of breast cancer requires very individual diagnosis and treatment. A woman who faces decisions regarding breast disease needs all of the information and counseling she can get in order to make a rational, confident choice about her treatment.

Breast Disease

For most women, breast disease is a fearful topic. In fact, the greatest physical fear that some women have is that they might develop breast cancer. Many women equate any lump in the breast with cancer, while, in fact, most lumps are not cancerous. Yet at some time in your life, you may well develop breast symptoms of some kind that will cause you concern. Knowledge of the structure and function of the breast in general, and of your own breasts in particular, will go a long way toward protecting you from diseases of the breast and from the fear of breast cancer.

The Structure of the Breast

In order to understand the types of diseases that affect breasts, it's important to understand the specialized structure of the breast that enables it to function as a milk-producing gland.

The breast is composed of 15 to 25 lobes of glandular tissue, each of which opens into the nipple. The lobes are surrounded by fat, which gives mass and a smooth contour to the breast. Fibrous connective tissue binds the lobes together and provides support and protection for the delicate glandular tissue. Each of the lobes contains a duct system of branching channels capable of conducting milk to the surface of the nipple. Only during pregnancy does the glandular tissue develop fully enough to produce milk. The individual lobes vary in size, and during pregnancy, usually fewer than half enlarge to begin milk production.

We can compare the duct system to the streams and tributaries that flow into a river—a river that then flows into a lake or reservoir. This comparison should be evident by looking at the drawings on the opposite page, which illustrate the structure of the breast responsible for producing milk.

In the lobes themselves, the milk is produced in tiny structures called *alveoli,* and flows from each alveolus into the smallest channels of the duct system. Comparable to the smallest streams in our river system analogy, these smallest channels flow into larger channels which, in turn, flow into the main duct. The main duct in each lobe enlarges to form a reservoir (called a *lactiferous sinus*) where milk is pooled. This reservoir is located directly behind the areola (the dark area surrounding the nipple). Finally, the main duct again narrows, forming a channel that takes the milk to the surface through the nipple.

The actual glandular tissue in the lobes of the breast extends further than the exterior contour of the breast suggests. This tissue usually extends into the armpit and may extend as far toward the center of the chest as the breastbone, as high as the collarbone, and as low as the region beneath the breastbone where the rib cage curves.

Changes in the Breast

Even when milk is not being produced, the breasts undergo constant changes that are regulated by the body's endocrine system. For example, many women are aware of breast swelling and tenderness preceding the menstrual period. These changes are caused by the buildup of fluid and fibrous tissue in the breast as one aspect of the monthly cycle of body changes that prepares women for pregnancy. When pregnancy does not occur and the menstrual period begins, the excess fluid and tissue are broken down by special cells in the lymph system, and are then drained from the breast and reabsorbed by the body.

The lymphatic system is a series of ducts and channels that extends throughout the body; the fluid that fills these channels is called lymph. It is this system of ducts that is responsible for draining excess fluid and dissolved tissue from the breast during the menstrual cycle.

Throughout the lymphatic system are lymph nodes (or glands) into which the fluid drains (see the opposite page). Most of the lymphatic drainage from the breast is received by the lymph nodes located in the axilla (armpit). Lymph nodes located beneath the breastbone, in the breast tissue itself, and near the collarbone also receive lymphatic drainage from the breast. As we shall see, the lymphatic system plays a vital role in breast health and disease.

Some of the changes that breasts undergo are associated with disease. Breast diseases can be classified into two types: benign (non-cancerous) conditions and malignant (cancerous) conditions.

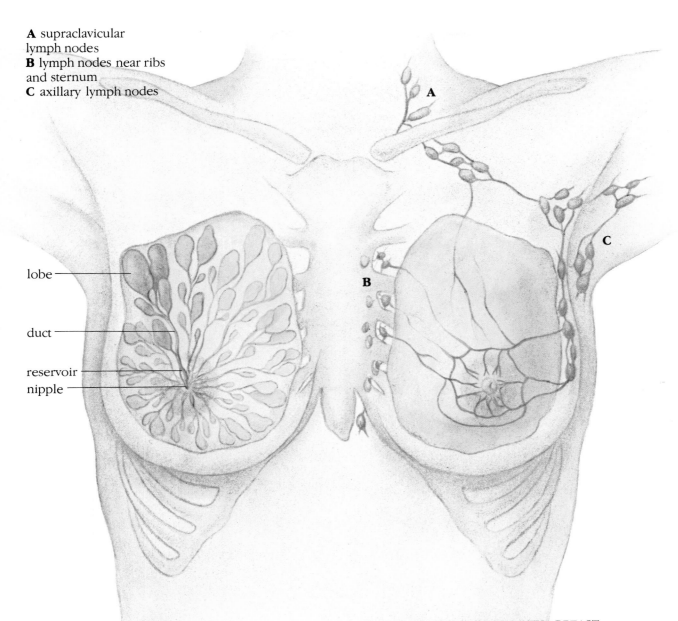

A supraclavicular
lymph nodes
B lymph nodes near ribs
and sternum
C axillary lymph nodes

lobe

duct

reservoir
nipple

THE STRUCTURE OF THE BREAST

*The breast is composed of 15 to 25 lobes of glandular
tissue, each containing a duct system of branching
channels capable of conducting milk to the surface of
the nipple. The main duct in each lobe forms a reservoir
near the nipple where milk is pooled. The reservoir
opens through a small duct into the nipple.*

THE LYMPHATIC SYSTEM OF THE BREAST

*The lymphatic system plays a vital role in breast health
and disease. The lymph ducts and nodes collect extra
fluid and cell debris, and defend the body against
disease. Monthly, extra fluid and cells from
premenstrual swelling are carried away through the
lymph ducts. Under special conditions, such as breast
cancer, cells in the lymph nodes destroy cancer cells that
escape from the breast cancer site.*

BENIGN CONDITIONS OF THE BREAST

FIBROADENOMA

Fibroadenoma, a benign tumor, is a firm lump that is easily felt. It may be removed surgically.

FIBROCYSTIC DISEASE

In fibrocystic disease, there are a small number of cysts—small sacs of fluid surrounded by fibrous, thickened breast tissue.

INTRADUCTAL PAPILLOMA

An intraductal papilloma is a small, harmless growth inside a duct. The benign disease causes a watery or pink discharge from the nipple.

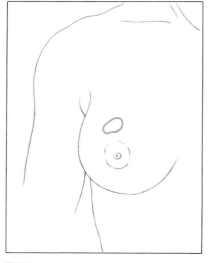

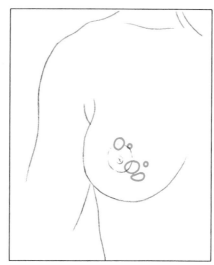

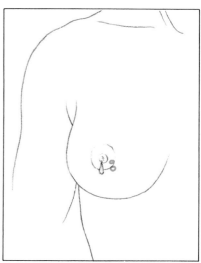

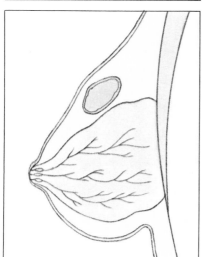

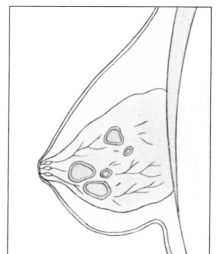

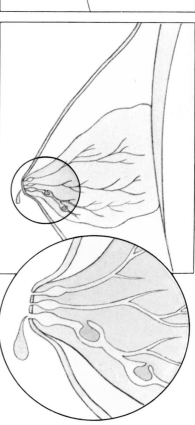

In intraductal papillomas, small, benign growths appear in the ducts, usually just beneath the nipple.

Benign Breast Conditions

Benign conditions are, by far, the most commonly noted states of the breast. The majority of lumps brought to the attention of physicians are found to be benign. This information should calm the fears of women who believe that most lumps are malignant. Because of the possibility that a lump may be malignant, however, it's important that a diagnosis be made by a physician.

More and more, women are the first to find a lump in the breast. A woman who examines her own breasts every month and is thoroughly familiar with their normal cyclic changes is far more likely to detect an abnormal lump or thickening than is her physician. See page 158 for a step-by-step guide to breast self-examination.

If you discover a lump in your breast, you immediately should have the presence of the lump confirmed by a physician. Tissue from the lump may then be examined under a microscope to determine whether it is malignant. If the lump is diagnosed as malignant, the prognosis will be far better if it's detected in the early part of its growth phase, when small in size and confined to one place in the breast (see page 548).

Even when diagnosis has determined that a lump is benign, many women still feel alarmed or anxious. It should be emphasized that benign conditions are harmless. They represent not a disease state, but one of a wide range of normal variations that occurs in breast tissue. The names and descriptions of common breast conditions that are classified as benign are listed for you below. Don't hesitate to ask your physician for the medical term ascribed to any lump that is detected, and to pursue whatever questions you have.

Fibroadenomas are the most common benign tumors in female breasts. They rarely ever become malignant, and are most prevalent among women in their reproductive years. In most cases, a single lump is found; however, there may be several lumps. In a small percentage of cases, both breasts may be involved.

The lumps themselves are firm, non-tender, and of varying sizes. They are characterized by firm borders that can be distinguished from the surrounding breast tissue. In addition, fibroadenomas do not attach to the overlying or outer breast skin, so they move relatively freely under the fingers. These distinguishing characteristics make diagnosis fairly simple for a physician. In most cases, the physician can diagnose a fibroadenoma simply by feeling (palpating) the breast.

Most physicians advise removing such lumps through a simple surgical procedure that requires from one to three days' hospitalization. The operation usually requires only local anesthesia at the site of the cut. Understandably, while your physician may consider this a simple procedure, you may be frightened by any breast surgery that requires hospitalization. However, the procedure is recommended for two main reasons. First, *unless a tumor is removed and subsequently examined in the laboratory under a microscope, it is impossible to be absolutely certain that it is not malignant.* Second, although fibroadenomas do not invade or destroy breast tissue, it's possible for the tumor itself to grow quite large, deforming the contour of the breast in some cases.

Fibrocystic disease is another common benign condition of the breast. Like fibroadenoma, this condition occurs most often during the reproductive years. Fibrocystic disease affects 30 percent of all women, and appears to be related to the cyclic estrogen stimulation of breast tissue. Typically, both breasts will develop a number of small cysts — small sacs of fluid surrounded by fibrous, thickening breast tissue. A woman with this condition may notice breast tenderness, especially preceding the menstrual period.

Fibrocystic disease should be diagnosed and treated by your doctor. Needle aspiration, a procedure that can be performed in the physician's office, is the treatment most often used. The doctor inserts a needle into the cyst and withdraws some fluid. If the fluid is yellowish or brownish and not bloody, and if the lump disappears after aspiration, it's clear that it was, indeed, a cyst. Further examination of the cells under a microscope is not necessary in these cases.

An intraductal papilloma is a small, harmless growth inside a duct. Frequently the growth cannot be felt, but a watery or pink discharge may be found on the bra, or may appear when the duct and nipple areas are palpated. Even though less than 4 percent of breast cancers are associated with a bloody or watery discharge, the physician will order a microscopic study of the secretion, and may also request a mammographic examination (see page 548) to rule out the possibility of cancer.

Most physicians recommend that these growths be surgically removed by a procedure, again, considered simple. Since papillomas are typically found just beneath the nipple, a small incision can be made around the nipple so that the operation does not deform the breast in any way. The procedure does require hospitalization, however.

Hematoma (sometimes called fat necrosis) is caused by an injury to the breast. A bruised area will appear on the skin of the breast with an associated lump beneath the skin, as is common with many bruises or injuries.

Important Facts About Breast Cancer

- Ninety percent of breast cancers occur in women over 39 years of age.
- Breast cancer is very rare in women under 20 years of age, and relatively rare up to age 25.
- With increasing age, the chances of developing breast cancer steadily increase.
- The cause of breast cancer is not known.
- Cancer is most likely not caused by a virus.
- Cancer is most likely caused by a number of factors, rather than any single factor.
- It is very unlikely that repeated injuries or a single blow to the breast can cause cancer.
- There is no evidence to indicate that women who nurse their infants are protected against breast cancer.
- Women who have never had children have a greater chance of having breast cancer than women who have had a child.
- Less than 4 percent of breast cancers involve a bloody discharge from the nipple.
- Few breast cancers are signaled by breast pain.
- The first full-term pregnancy, especially for women 18 or younger, seems to afford considerable protection against breast cancer.
- Women who have had both ovaries removed prior to age 35 have a greatly reduced risk of developing breast cancer. (However, it certainly would not be desirable to remove both ovaries prior to 35 just to reduce the chances of developing breast cancer.)

Who Risks Developing Breast Cancer?

WOMEN WHO HAVE...
- A past history of breast cancer themselves
- A family history of breast cancer in close female relatives: mother, sisters, or daughters
- Nipple discharges (while neither pregnant nor lactating)
- Begun menstruation prior to age 12
- Not delivered a live infant prior to age 30
- Reached age 40 without having had a full-term pregnancy.

These factors indicate only a small risk when taken alone, but when combined, they indicate that a woman should be examined more frequently and more thoroughly than other women.

The lump beneath the skin is the blood clot that has collected at the place where the breast was injured. The area around the clot may swell and become painful or tender to the touch, and remain that way for a few days to several weeks. Special treatment is not necessary for the bruise if the lump is getting smaller and the blood clot is obviously being absorbed. But if the hematoma does not reabsorb and turns into a lump, or if the blood of the hematoma becomes surrounded by a capsule and forms a fluid-filled lump, surgical incision is recommended to drain the fluid or remove the lump.

Malignant Breast Conditions

Breast conditions that are malignant are commonly called breast cancer. One cancer specialist has described breast cancer as "the most feared ..., the most frequently self-discovered, and the most controversially treated of all cancers." It ranks first among cancers in number of surgical procedures, in radiation therapy treatments, and in number of hormone and chemotherapy administrations. And in cancer diagnosis, it is the first in number of biopsies.

Little wonder that a Gallup poll requested by the American Cancer Society revealed that fear of cancer, and especially of breast cancer, was the greatest health concern of women over 18. However, the poll also revealed that most women do not regularly practice monthly breast self-examination, nor do most physicians regularly examine the breasts as part of a general checkup.

Discovering Breast Cancer

Approximately 95 percent of the time, breast cancer is accidentally detected by a woman who feels a lump or thickening in her breast in the process of bathing or dressing.

Only a very small number of breast cancers are detected by routine office or hospital examination when the patient is admitted for problems not specifically related to her breasts.

Guarding Against Breast Cancer

The cause of breast cancer is unknown, and it's impossible to predict very accurately who will be affected. Still, there are two things women can do to allay their fears and protect themselves from breast cancer as much as possible.

● Learn the facts. Misinformation and myths about breast cancer abound. Learn the facts about breast cancer by reading and by asking questions of your physician (see page 393). Remember that breast cancer can be cured if it is detected and treated early.
● Take action. Become familiar with your own breasts through learning the technique of breast self-examination (see page 158). Practice self-examination regularly once a month. Visit your physician annually, or more often, for a complete examination. And if necessary, remind your doctor of his or her professional obligation to thoroughly examine your breasts as part of your overall examination. Describe any changes in your breasts to your doctor, and ask questions about anything you don't understand.

What Is Breast Cancer?

Although we don't know at this time what causes breast cancer, we do have information about how it looks and how it behaves.

Cancer cells can be reliably differentiated from normal cells by an expert. This reliable recognition is the reason biopsies are performed. In a biopsy, a section of tissue is removed from the lump in question and is examined under a microscope by a specialist called a pathologist (see page 394). Only through direct examination of tissue and cells under a microscope can the pathologist conclusively determine whether or not cancer cells are present.

Cancer cells, also called malignant cells, invade and destroy normal tissue. This destruction proceeds at different rates depending on the type of cancer present.

Primary cancer. Cancer confined to a single organ is primary cancer, or localized cancer as it is also called. As long as breast cancer is primary, it is found only in one place in the breast and only the tissue of the breast itself is damaged. The rest of the body is not endangered.

Secondary cancer. Cancer that spreads to other organs is secondary cancer. The secondary cancer, also called a metastasis, always spreads out from the site of the primary cancer. This spreading process, called metastasis, is what makes cancer so difficult to control and cure. Once the cancerous cells begin to spread through the body via the blood system or lymph system, they may be present and growing at a site in the body for some time before they are detected.

If the cancer is detected early, and if treatment is carried out to remove or kill the cancerous cells confined to the breast, then a woman can expect to be cured and to live out her normal life-span. That is, if primary cancer is removed before it metastasizes, a woman will *not* develop secondary cancer. And such a woman is no more likely than anyone else to develop another *primary* cancer in another organ. However, she is at greater risk of developing cancer in her other breast.

How Breast Cancer Spreads

Because of the role the lymphatic system plays in transporting cancer cells from the primary site to secondary sites, it's important to know how the lymphatic system works in order to understand how breast cancer spreads.

INCIDENCE OF CANCER IN SITES OF THE BREAST

The most common breast site for a tumor to develop is in the upper outer quadrant. About half of breast cancer originates here, 17 percent in the nipple area, 15 percent in the upper inner quadrant, and 11 percent and 6 percent in the outer and inner lower quadrants.

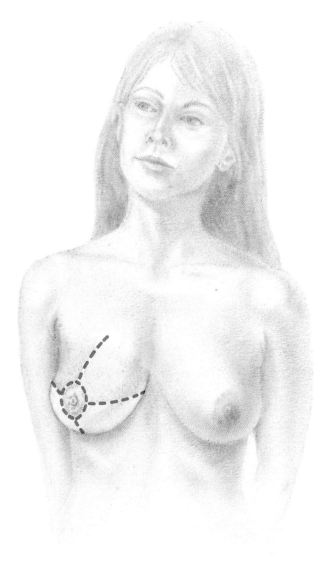

Lymph ducts are channels filled with a fluid called lymph. Throughout the lymphatic system are lymph nodes (or glands) into which the fluid drains (see page 543). Together, lymph ducts and nodes collect extra fluid and cell debris, and defend the body against disease. Cancer spreads when cancer cells enter the lymph ducts and are carried to other parts of the body in the lymph fluid. In the lymph nodes, special cells called lymphocytes destroy cancer cells that "escape" from the breast's primary cancer site.

After a time, though, the lymphocytes cannot maintain their protective function. The length of time that the defenses hold is different for every woman, but when the defense system breaks down, cancer cells then grow in the new site. The breakdown of this defense system is simply not understood at the present time.

About 75 percent of the lymphatic drainage from the breast is received by the lymph nodes located in the armpit (axilla). As a result, the axilla nodes are the ones most likely to be involved when breast cancer is present (see page 543).

The most common site in the breast for a tumor to develop is in the upper outer quadrant (see page 547), from which the cells usually spread to the axillary lymph nodes. However, cells from a tumor also tend to spread to the lymph nodes closest to the tumor. So tumors in the inner half of the breast —those located near the nipple — typically spread to the nodes beneath the breastbone (see page 543). Remember, though, that the lymphatic system is a network of connecting ducts throughout the body, so its cells can spread to almost any lymph node in the body regardless of where the tumor is located.

Early Detection of Breast Cancer

When a tumor is found to be malignant, the treatment that follows will depend on:
- The size of the tumor
- The cell type of the tumor
- The extent of metastasis of the tumor.

The size of the malignant tumor or breast cancer is important in that, generally, the larger the cancer, the more likely it is that the lymph nodes in the armpit (axilla) will be involved.

The cell type of the malignant tumor is important because breast cancers are medically classified by the type of cells that make up the tumor. Some common types of breast cancers are tubular carcinomas (tumors), lobular carcinomas *in situ,* and non-invasive ductal carcinomas. The pathologist should exercise meticulous care in preparing and identifying these cells, as some tumors, such as lobular carcinomas *in situ,* contain cancerous cells that look very much like benign cells (see page 547).

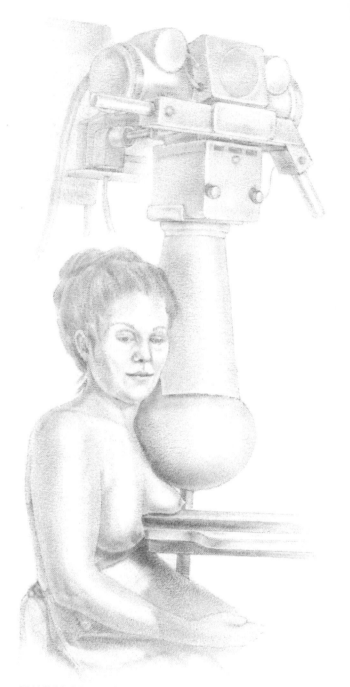

MAMMOGRAPHY

Mammography is an X-ray procedure in which radiation produced in a mammogram machine passes through your breast. The image produced on film, called a mammogram, shows internal breast structures and any abnormal growths. Cancers so small that they cannot be felt can be located precisely, but it is important that you be screened by a skilled technician, using the lowest possible X-ray dosage.
The end of the shaft that conducts the X rays is fitted with a soft, air-filled balloon that presses firmly on the breast from the top. The X-ray film is placed on a table beneath the breast. Then the breast is flattened slightly between the balloon and the film for one exposure.

The extent of metastasis of the tumor is important in predicting a patient's chances of recovery. A woman has about an 85 percent chance of being alive and well five years later if the cancer is found to be strictly limited to the breast — that is, if the malignant tumor has not metastasized or spread to other sites of the body.

There is a good deal of scientific evidence to indicate that the majority of breast cancers or malignant tumors began as groups of cells in one place — the primary site. These cells may remain there for a long period of time before they begin to migrate and spread to other parts of the body. In a small percentage of cases, however, metastasis may occur early in the development of the tumor.

Though it's very important to discover breast tumors as early as possible, cancer cannot be detected until the cancerous cells form very small groups of cells referred to as *minimal cancers*. These cancers are less than one centimeter in diameter and are too small to be felt by you during your breast self-examination, or by the physician who examines your breasts. These very small tumors can be detected, however, by the X-ray technique called mammography. This technique can detect some very small tumors or carcinomas up to two years before they can be felt by you or your physician.

It should be stressed that women using self-examination and skilled physicians performing palpating breast exams often detect lumps that are small. Because of breast self-examination, the number of women who discover breast cancers in the early stages is increasing every year. And, women are beginning to use new screening techniques for detecting cancers too small to be felt on a manual examination.

Screening and Diagnosis

The screening processes for breast cancer include:
- Self-examination by palpation (touch)
- A physician's examination by palpation
- Thermography
- Mammography
- Xeromammography.

The only accurate diagnostic procedure for breast cancer is biopsy.

Breast self-examination is detailed on page 158.

Breast examination by your physician is discussed on page 400.

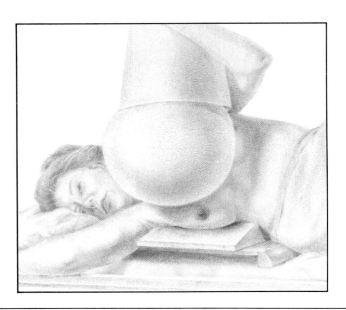

To ensure that all internal breast structure is surveyed, at least two mammograms are taken of each breast from two different angles. You will be asked to lie on your side for a second exposure. In this position, the breast is gently pressed between the X-ray shaft and the film plate. A foam rubber wedge may be used to lift the breast for a better exposure of internal structures.

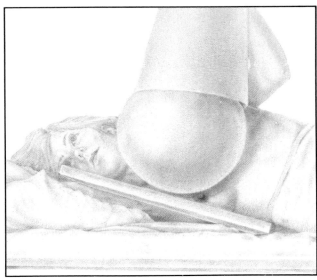

Women with small, flat breasts may require an additional mammogram. Supporting the film plate with one raised arm while the breast is pressed gently from above by the balloon allows the best picture.

Thermography is a screening process for breast cancer that measures the patterns that come from your natural body heat. When a heat sensor is placed near your breast, it picks up heat waves and translates the waves into a heat photograph. There is no radiation from the machine involved in this procedure.

A cancer located in the breast may raise the temperature in that area one degree centigrade higher than the temperature of the surrounding tissue. The malignant tumor will then form a distinctive pattern in the heat photograph.

The advantages of this procedure are that it is painless, simple, and involves no radiation. The disadvantages are that it cannot pick up small, very early cancers. For that reason, it is not used alone, but in conjunction with mammography and xeromammography.

Mammography is the screening technique most likely to be suggested by your physician. It is currently the most well known and widely acclaimed method of breast cancer detection because it can detect tumors of very small size and locate them accurately.

Mammography is an X-ray procedure that uses very small amounts of radiation to produce a film image of the breast. This image, called a mammogram, shows details of internal breast structure.

Xeromammography is a form of mammography that transfers the film image of the internal breast structure to a special paper. Otherwise the procedure is the same as that for a mammogram. The procedure you must go through for these breast X rays is quick and painless, as shown in the illustrations on page 548.

Some of the advantages of mammography and xeromammography are:
• Cancers so small (3 or 4 millimeters in diameter) that they cannot be felt, even when their location is precisely known, can be detected and pinpointed.

FOUR TYPES OF BREAST-TUMOR BIOPSIES

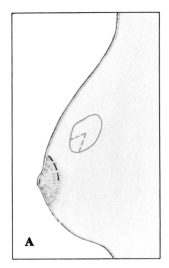
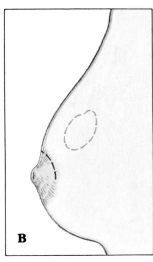

Once a suspicious lump is detected in the breast, a biopsy is recommended. A biopsy is a surgical procedure involving removal of a piece of breast lump tissue for study under a microscope. Cancer cells look different from normal cells, and the microscope makes positive identification possible. This test is the only way to determine conclusively if cancer cells are present in the breast tissue. In this instance, the woman whose breast is to be biopsied has a lump in the upper half of her breast. The placement of the biopsy incision is indicated by a dotted line.

A *Excision of a portion of the lump for examination is the usual method of biopsy. After local anesthesia is administered, a small cut is made at the edge of the areola where less visible scarring of the breast will occur. The tissue removed is sliced very thin, the cells of the tissue are stained to make them visible, and the cells are examined in the microscope to determine whether they are normal or cancerous.*

B *Excision of a complete, small lump for biopsy is a less frequent procedure than excision of a portion of the lump or tumor.*

• The entire breast can be evaluated. (Breast cancer is often multicentric, with one or more areas of involvement.)
• If very small lesions are detected, the pathologist can locate the precise area from which to take tissue for "specimen radiography" (use of X rays to detect cancer in a biopsy specimen).
• The procedure prevents unnecessary biopsies —especially important for women who have multiple lumps in both breasts.

The disadvantage of mammography and xeromammography is that exposure to radiation can and has caused cancer, even though the amount used in these techniques is very small. Concern about the cancer-causing risk of mammography has resulted in the establishment of regulations that limit the dose of X rays to one rad (a unit of absorbed radiation) to the midpoint of the breast in a two-film examination. Yet there are experts who consider any dose to be unsafe.

Many specialists believe that all women over the age of 50 should have mammogram screening for breast cancer every year. Certainly, women who are between the ages of 40 and 50 and who have a greater than usual chance of developing cancer must carefully consider the risks of radiation against the risks of an undetected breast tumor.

The decision as to whether you should undergo regular cancer screening using the mammography procedure should be made by both you and your physician. Continual improvement in equipment, the use of low-dose films, and the better training of radiologists have considerably reduced the risk factor in mammographic examination. However, you should ask the radiologist what type of equipment will be used, when it was last calibrated, and the amount of absorbed radiation exposure you will receive to the breasts. If the absorbed dose is above one rad to the midpoint of the breasts, you should seek the examination elsewhere.

Mammography and xeromammography offer the best methods we now have for diagnosing small breast cancers early in their development. However, you must weigh the benefits with the risks, and keep in mind that professional opinion on this subject is still divided.

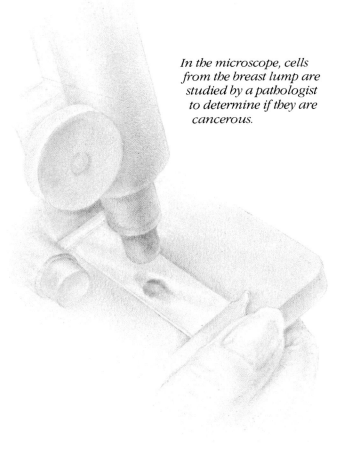

In the microscope, cells from the breast lump are studied by a pathologist to determine if they are cancerous.

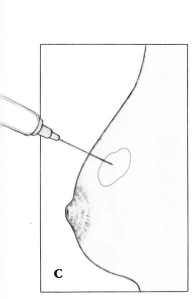
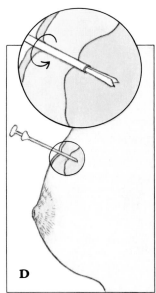

C *Needle aspiration of a breast cyst that is fluid-filled is also performed under local anesthesia. The fluid contains cells that are examined under the microscope.*
D *A needle biopsy of the breast under local anesthesia uses a special needle with a hollow core. The needle is passed into the tumor mass, and a tiny cutting blade is advanced down the hollow core of the needle and into the lump. When the blade is rotated, it cuts a core from the lump or tumor. The tissue is then retracted with the blades and thin-sliced for study in the microscope.*

A biopsy involves the removal of a thin section of the breast tumor for microscopic study. The cells of the breast tumor are studied by a specialist (a pathologist) who is skilled in determining whether the cells under study are malignant or normal. This is the only method for accurate diagnosis of cancer.

Once an abnormal lump or mass is discovered during an examination, whether by the woman herself or by one of the procedures just discussed, a biopsy usually is ordered immediately by a physician. The biopsy often is performed under local anesthesia in a minor surgery room of the hospital where the patient can wait for the final report. The patient and the surgeon often know within minutes whether the tissue is malignant.

If the tissue is malignant, a woman should take all the time she needs to evaluate the risks and benefits involved in the various types of treatment available for breast cancer. She may wish to begin such an evaluation immediately by discussing with her physician what treatment he or she recommends. But under no conditions should she rush into operative procedures without carefully considering all the information and alternatives available to her.

For years, it was standard to perform biopsies using general anesthesia so that radical surgery, should it be indicated, could be accomplished at the same time. This procedure has come under severe criticism in the last few years for a variety of reasons. Patients are demanding more control over decisions regarding breast cancer treatment, and many specialists feel that treatments such as radiation therapy and chemotherapy, with perhaps less extensive surgery, may be effective in the treatment of some breast cancers.

Treatment of Breast Cancer

Statistics. Before we begin a discussion of treatment, we must face some startling facts. The breast is the leading site of cancer incidence and death among women. Breast cancer is the leading cause of all deaths among women 40 to 44 years of age. *And there has been no change in the mortality rate due to breast cancer in the past fifty years.* To put it another way, none of the treatments or screening procedures have had any effect on the death rate due to breast cancer.

Some slightly more heartening statistics from the American Cancer Society are as follows:
• The five-year survival rate for breast cancer patients has increased from 53 percent for cases diagnosed in the 1940s to 65 percent for diagnoses in the 1970s.
• The percentage of breast cancers diagnosed in the localized (non-metastasized) stage has gradually increased from 38 percent to 47 percent during the period from 1940 to 1970.
• The five-year survival rate for localized breast cancers was 85 percent for cases diagnosed in the 1970s, compared to 78 percent for cases diagnosed in the 1940s.

It's distressing that the death rate for cancer patients has remained the same for many years, regardless of all the treatment procedures used. Fewer than 50 percent of all patients treated survive for ten years. We know that once the cancer has spread beyond the local lymph nodes (see page 547), it is very difficult to cure the disease. So the aim of treatment at this time is to control the disease and prolong life as much as possible. Again, the greatest hope for cure lies in early detection and treatment, while the cancer is still localized in the breast.

Preliminary treatment. Should a woman be diagnosed as having breast cancer, it's vitally important that she play an active role in determining her therapy. In the past, a woman who detected a lump in her breast would see her physician, receive a cursory examination, and be sent to a hospital. There, she would be prepared for surgery, only to wake up the next morning with her breast removed. Fortunately, this traumatic experience need no longer occur.

No one method of treatment is suitable for all breast cancers or for all women. From the physician's point of view, it would be far simpler to know the type of treatment to recommend and how aggressive it should be were it possible to precisely determine the extent of the disease at any given time. Knowing that the cancer is localized in the breast and has not metastasized, for example, would make it clear whether we should undertake aggressive "curative" surgery, radiation therapy, or some combination of the two.

One of the first things that must be discovered, then, is whether the disease is still localized in the original or primary site, or whether the disease has spread to lymph nodes near the breast. If any lymph nodes are enlarged, a lymph node biopsy may be performed to determine if the lymph nodes also have cancerous cells. Because the axillary lymph nodes are the first line of defense against most breast cancers, those are the ones examined in the lymph node biopsy. If no cancerous cells are present, then the tumor is said to be localized at the primary site in the breast (if the cancer is located in the outer half of the breast).

If the nodes are involved, then there is reason to suspect that the malignant cells may have spread to other parts of the body as well. A chest X ray will be required to see whether or not the lungs are free of disease and are functioning normally.

If the woman has bone pain, bone scans and/or bone X rays are done to determine whether the cancer has spread to the bones. In some cases, a liver scan also may be requested to find out whether metastasizing cells have reached that organ. And a brain scan will be performed if headaches indicate that the brain may be involved.

Determining the extent of metastasis is important before surgery, because once a woman knows the extent of the cancer spread, she is better able to make a decision about her chances of recovery and to participate fully in choosing lines of treatment.

Decisions about further treatment. If you've gone this far in the treatment of a breast lump, if the biopsy indicates that the lump is indeed cancer, and if you've determined the extent of metastasis, then you're faced with life-and-death decisions that will require great strength and resourcefulness.

You don't have to make a decision immediately. Usually you have from one to several weeks to consider all the treatment alternatives and to make your choice. Use that time to ask tough questions, both of your physician and of yourself.

The woman facing a decision regarding surgical procedures has a very real problem. The fact that medical opinion on surgery is divided doesn't make her decision any easier, nor is it comforting that there are no accurate means of precisely assessing the extent of the disease in a particular woman. Each woman who faces such a decision will have to make it on the basis of the existing evidence and the counsel of her physician. She must draw on all her strength and intelligence to participate fully in following the results of each test and in evaluating the treatment recommended by her physician.

If you face making a decision about breast cancer treatment, feel free to seek second and third opinions of the diagnosis and treatment of your disease. It's important that each physician explain the proposed treatment, the alternatives available, and his or her opinions regarding the relative advantages of each approach. You should ask whatever questions will enable you to arrive at a final decision, and you must give your written consent before any procedure can be performed.

Currently, surgery and radiation therapy (see page 556) are used alone or in combination for the treatment of breast cancers. Hormone therapy and chemotherapy provide relief of symptoms, but they do not cure cancer.

Surgical Treatment

The various surgical procedures used in cancer treatment are listed and explained below.

Lumpectomy means the excision of the tumor. This procedure is used to remove the tumor itself, along with some of the surrounding breast tissue.

Subcutaneous mastectomy involves removal of all underlying breast tissue, leaving intact the overlying skin and the nipple. A silicone implant then can be inserted to minimize the deformity and to restore roundness and fullness to the contours of the breast (see page 655).

Partial mastectomy involves removal of the entire tumor along with whatever amount of surrounding breast tissue is necessary to ensure complete removal of the tumor. As much as one-third to one-half of the breast tissue may have to be removed. Reconstructive surgery also can be performed at the time of the partial mastectomy surgery to restore the contours of the breast.

Simple mastectomy involves removal of the entire breast and perhaps some of the axillary lymph nodes, but not the chest muscles. If the overlying skin is preserved, reconstructive surgery can partially restore breast contours (see page 655).

Modified radical mastectomy involves removal of the entire breast as well as removal of the axillary lymph nodes. Usually the lowest and middle lymph nodes are removed from the axilla on the same side as the breast. By leaving the chest muscles intact, the full range of movement in the arm is preserved and the deformity of breast size and shape is less than with a radical mastectomy (see page 555).

Radical mastectomy has been a standard operation since it was first introduced by the surgeon William Halsted in the 1880s. This operation, used almost as a ritual for many years, is no longer recognized as the only operation to be used for all operable breast cancer patients. The radical mastectomy procedure involves removal of the entire breast, muscles of the chest wall, and all of the lymph nodes from the axilla.

Studies that have been conducted on the survival rates associated with the surgical procedures just described reveal the following:

• There is no difference in survival rates after five and ten years regardless of whether the operation is a simple, modified radical, or radical mastectomy.

• 85 percent of women will survive five years regardless of whether the operation performed is a radical, modified radical, simple, or partial mastectomy, so long as the cancer has not spread to an axillary lymph node.

Clearly, this information points to using the most simple operative procedure possible. But at this time, the controversy continues as to whether to operate at all, and if so, how extensive the operation should be.

SURGERY FOR BREAST CANCER

LUMPECTOMY

A small incision is made near the areola, and the tumor is removed with a minimum of breast tissue.

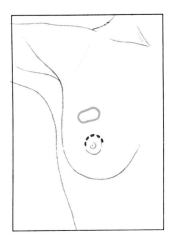 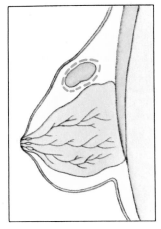 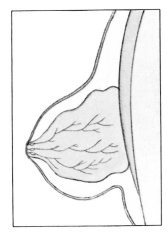

PARTIAL MASTECTOMY

A small incision is made near the areola, and the tumor is removed with as much as one-half of the breast tissue.

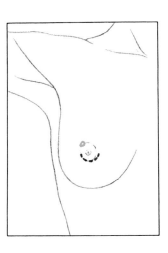 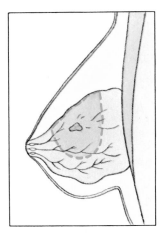 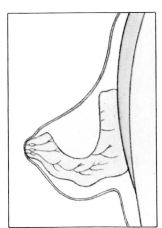

SUBCUTANEOUS MASTECTOMY

A large incision is made under the breast, and all of the breast tissue is removed, leaving the overlying skin and the nipple intact.

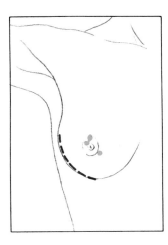 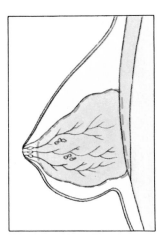 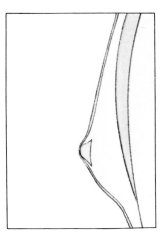

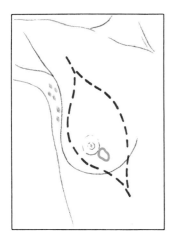
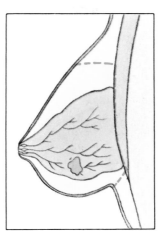
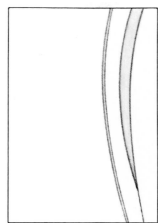

SIMPLE MASTECTOMY

The entire breast is removed, along with some of the axillary lymph nodes, but not the chest muscles. Some overlying skin may be preserved.

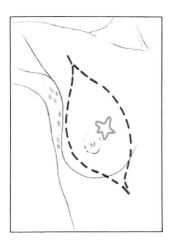
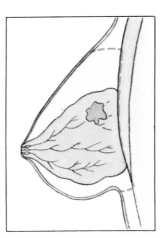
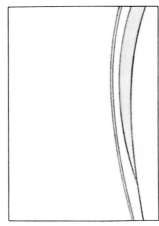

MODIFIED RADICAL MASTECTOMY

The entire breast is removed, with more axillary lymph nodes than in the simple mastectomy. Chest muscles may be left intact, or the minor pectoral muscle may be removed.

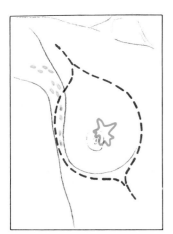
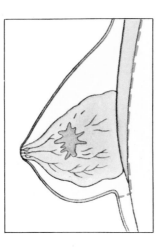
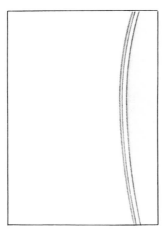

RADICAL MASTECTOMY

Radical mastectomy involves removal of the entire breast, the muscles of the chest wall, and all of the lymph nodes from the axilla. This operation is performed less frequently.

Radiation Therapy

For many years, women were offered only surgical treatment for breast cancer. But during the past ten years, there has been increasing interest in the treatment of breast cancer by radiation therapy combined with surgery, or by radiation therapy alone.

What is radiation therapy? Radiation therapy uses a large machine to generate a high-energy electrical beam that is focused on the tissue to be irradiated. Some machines use cobalt as an energy source. Radiation therapy also may be administered by surgically implanting in the breast a small device that emits radioactivity. The beam of energy damages all the cells that it touches, both healthy and malignant. It is known from careful research studies that normal cells grow back more quickly than malignant cells. The expectation from radiation therapy treatment is that normal cells will grow back, but that malignant cell growth will slow or cease.

At the present time, radiation therapy is used almost exclusively to treat breasts that already have been operated on to remove tumors. The patient who chooses radiation therapy after her operation probably will be treated five times a week for a period of five to six weeks.

The tissue irradiated will vary with each woman's particular case, but usually the breast that has been operated on will be irradiated in the area that contained the cancerous growth. If the cancer has spread to the lymph nodes of the axilla, they, too, will be irradiated, as well as lymph nodes in the clavicle area and the internal mammary lymph nodes (see page 543).

When is radiation therapy recommended? Radiation therapy has been most successful in controlling the metastasis or spread of cancer. If breast cancer has spread to the axillary lymph nodes, there is a good chance that the cancer also may spread to the nodes above the clavicle and beneath the breastbone (see page 543). In a high percentage of such cases, scientific evidence indicates that the spread of the disease can be controlled if the patient is given radiation therapy postoperatively.

Radiation therapy also may be used for the control of cancer that for some reason cannot be operated upon, or for those patients who simply choose radiation therapy instead of surgery. It is usually recommended in conjunction with chemotherapy for the treatment of acute inflammatory breast cancer—a serious, rapidly progressing form of cancer that is diffused throughout the breast.

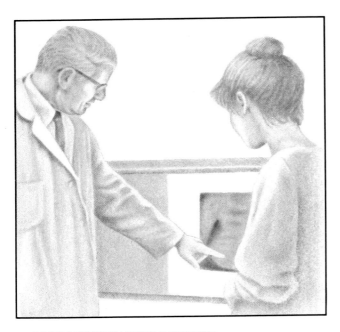

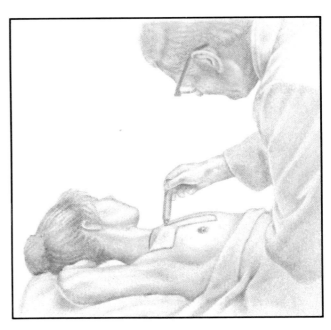

RADIATION THERAPY PROCEDURE

A woman with breast cancer consults with her doctor about radiation therapy procedures. The specialist is pointing out the area of her chest to be treated with radiation. The X-ray film of her breast was just made, and the area to be treated is marked off by the doctor.

The doctor draws the exact area to be irradiated on the patient's chest with a felt pen. A machine that uses light rays, instead of irradiation, is now placed over the patient. This is called a simulator machine, because the light rays are focused exactly on the area to be irradiated, simulating the radiation machine. Then readings for setting the radiation machine are taken from the simulator so that only the area of diseased tissue and lymph nodes will be carefully irradiated.

Concerns about radiation therapy. Since we know that radiation can induce cancer, much concern has been expressed that irradiating the entire breast and the lymph nodes may be causing the very disease it is supposed to cure.

There are patients still living 15 to 20 years after receiving full courses of radiation therapy for breast cancer. And there is no definite evidence that the radiation therapy has resulted in new cancer in the cells or organs located in the field that was irradiated.

There is some skin cell death from the radiation treatment. The skin of the breast may become reddened, similar to a sunburn reaction, but this will usually disappear in three to six weeks.

An additional concern for the woman who retains part or all of her breast tissue or one who plans reconstructive surgery (see page 654) is to keep the breasts soft and pliable. This will require careful calibration of the radiation dose — too high a dose will cause the breast to become shrunken in appearance due to the fibrous masses that form on the interior of the breast. In cases where a high dose of radiation is recommended for a primary tumor area, a radioactive implant may be used. This implant is left in the breast for several days until the proper radiation dose has been delivered. This method of radiation eliminates the skin reactions that lead to the formation of scar tissue and contraction of areas of the breast.

Prospects for the future. Many radiation therapists believe that with the use of modern radiation therapy, breast cancer can be controlled after a minimal operation.

There is an expectation that as techniques improve, it may be possible to treat some breast cancers entirely by radiation therapy. However, much more data must be collected before the exact effectiveness of this treatment can be assessed.

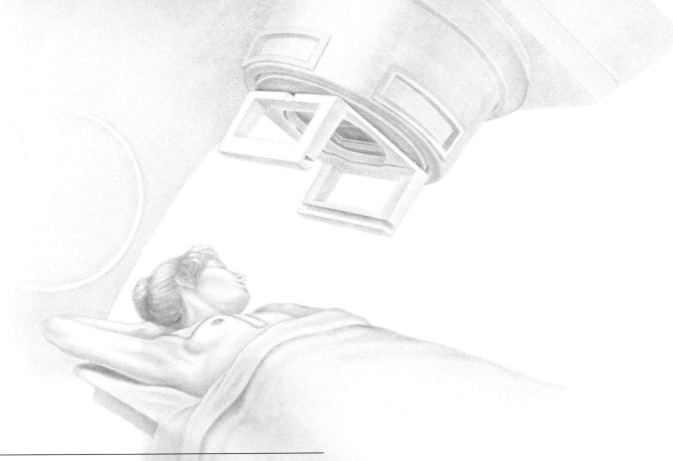

Once the settings are determined for the machine that delivers the radiation, the woman is rolled under the machine. Once again, a beam of light is used to simulate the radiation. The light falling on the chest is adjusted to the exact area marked with the pen. Only after the doctor and the technician are satisfied that the beam will fall exactly on the area to be treated is the actual radiation delivered to the chest.

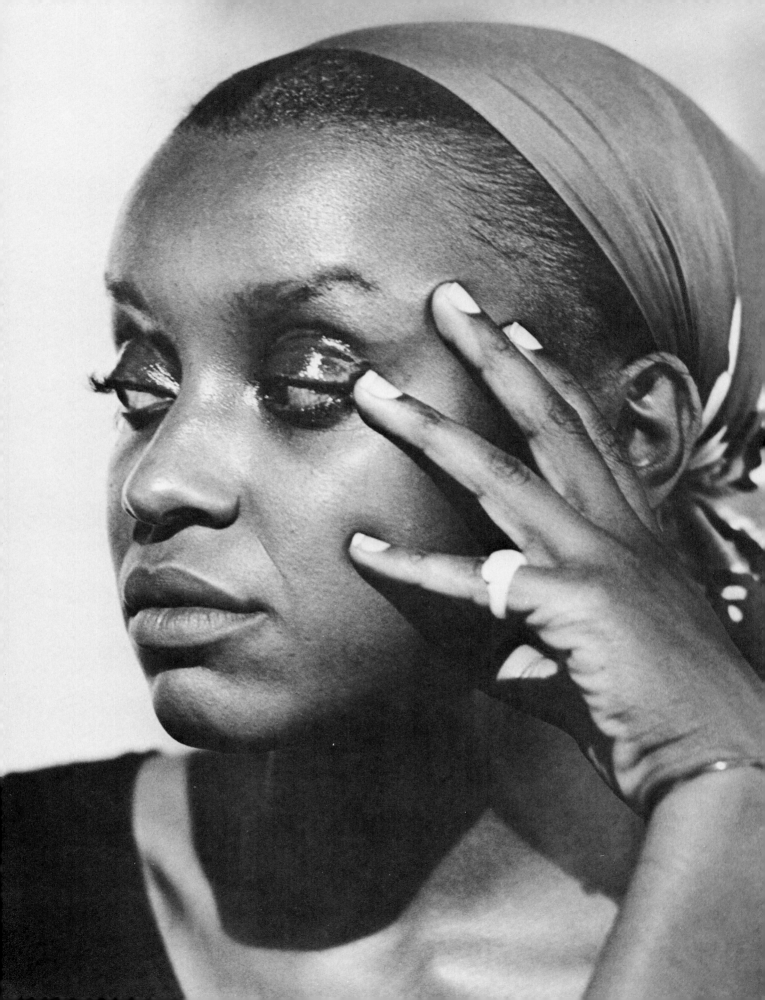

CHAPTER 27

SKIN PROBLEMS

CARY E. FEIBLEMAN, M.D.

Perhaps no organ of our bodies plays a more important social and aesthetic role than our skin. Our health, our femininity, and our personality are at once mirrored in the appearance of our skin. But aside from its social and cosmetic functions, the skin performs many essential services for us. As the largest organ of the body, it protects us from the external environment, excretes waste materials, acts as a sensory organ, and tells us much about the outside world through sensations of pressure, pain, heat, and cold.

Because of the skin's visibility and importance, even minor skin problems—often ones that quickly disappear—may cause us great concern. Likewise, it is important to recognize more serious disorders that may require treatment by a physician.

Skin Problems

Your skin is the one organ of your body that is in constant contact with the external environment. And many of the diseases and problems that affect the skin are caused by direct exposure to the outside world. Sunburn, frostbite, and poison ivy are common examples of what happens when the environment and living tissue come together with less than favorable results. It follows that many skin problems could be prevented by avoiding conditions in the environment that harm the skin.

This chapter, then, will stress those environmental factors that might make skin conditions better or worse. It treats normal skin first, and then common problems that occur in skin, as well as a few rare diseases that particularly affect women.

Normal Skin

Few people realize that the skin is one of the largest organs in the body, with a complex structure and many functions. At its thickest point, it is one-quarter of an inch thick, while at its thinnest point where it covers the eyelid, it is one-sixteenth of an inch thick.

The outer layer of the skin, the *epidermis,* grows constantly and renews itself every thirty days. The epidermis varies from six to fifteen cells thick, depending on the region of the body it covers. The outermost layer of the epidermis is dead and constantly sheds. This outer layer acts as a two-way barrier to prevent body fluids from leaking out and external fluids from seeping in. If not for this layer, we would swell like balloons every time we bathed.

The *dermis,* the layer beneath the epidermis, consists of a strong supportive structure of fibrous tissue, blood vessels, nerves, and glands. The fibers that make up the dermis interweave to give strength to the skin. Elastic fibers, a specialized form of resilient fibrous tissue, act like an elastic band in clothing to prevent gaping and puckering of sites such as the elbow that constantly stretch and bend.

The dermis also contains blood vessels that supply the skin with nutrients and oxygen, and remove wastes. When the skin reddens, it is because these blood vessels are dilating; when the skin pales, the vessels have contracted. Nerve fibers in the dermis allow us to perceive pressure, temperature, and pain, and just below the dermis, the fatty layer (subcutaneous tissue) insulates the inner structures of the body from excessive heat or cold. The fatty layer also serves as a source of stored energy. Hairs are rooted in this deep dermis and fat, with a small wisp of muscle attached to each one. It is the action of this muscle that makes hair stand erect when a person experiences "goose flesh."

Eccrine glands (sweat glands) are present throughout the dermis. Apocrine glands, which

THE STRUCTURE OF THE SKIN

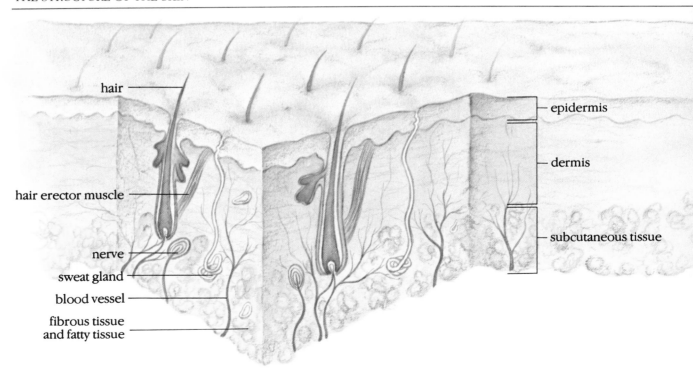

produce a thicker secretion, are found in the axillae, nipples, pubic area, external ear canal, and eyelids. Sebaceous glands emit an oily secretion and occur on the face, scalp, upper chest, back, and areolae.

Pores

Pores are the openings in the skin surface that allow moisturizing oils produced in the dermis to reach the surface. Dilated (enlarged) pores are part of the normal spectrum of genetically determined skin features. While scarcely noticeable to most of us, to the woman who stares at them in the mirror each morning, they may seem as prominent as craters. There is no way to permanently decrease their size, although astringents and makeup will make them somewhat less noticeable.

Sweating

Sweating is an annoyance to many people — so much so that an entire industry has been spawned to repress it. Actually, sweating is a beneficial, protective measure that keeps the body from overheating. The body's internal metabolism generates heat, much like a combustion engine. When the body sweats and the sweat on the skin evaporates, this heat is released. Nearly everyone has observed this reaction during the drenching sweats that accompany a fever. When a

person is no longer able to sweat, the body temperature soars, as happens in heat stroke.

Eccrine (sweat) glands are distributed all over the body and are in highest concentration on the palms and soles. Eccrine secretions are salty and odorless, although occasionally the scent of garlic or onions pervades the sweat after these foods are eaten.

It is the apocrine glands, however, that have captured the attention of the deodorant industry. These glands are predominantly in the armpits (axillae) and ano-genital region. Odors from these body regions occur when bacteria on the skin interact with the secretions of the apocrine glands. The warm, moist environment of these regions, coupled with eccrine secretions, encourages bacterial growth and probably contributes to the odor. Thus, deodorants containing antibacterial ingredients are successful in eliminating these odors.

The most common cause of increased sweating is an exaggerated response to emotional stimulation, a reaction beyond conscious control. Rarely, a person will have excessive underarm (axillary) sweating to the point that it drenches the clothing almost daily. A more common problem, often beginning in childhood, is excessive sweating of the palms and soles. Increased sweating in these areas may be treated with repeated application of glutaraldehyde. This treatment may cause light brown discoloration of the skin on some people, however.

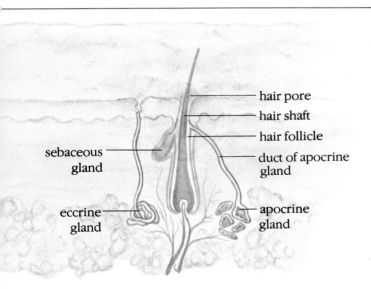

sebaceous gland

eccrine gland

hair pore
hair shaft
hair follicle
duct of apocrine gland
apocrine gland

The skin has a complex structure. The outer layer of the skin, the epidermis, grows constantly and renews itself every thirty days. This outer layer acts as a two-way barrier to prevent body fluids from leaking out and external fluids from leaking in. The dermis is the layer beneath the epidermis, and consists of a strong supportive structure of fibrous tissue, blood vessels, nerves, and glands. Just below the dermis, the fatty layer or subcutaneous tissue acts to insulate the inner structures of the body. Hairs are rooted in the deep dermis and fat.

There are two types of sweat glands present in the skin. Eccrine glands, whose sweat secretions are salty and odorless, are distributed throughout the body and are in highest concentration on the palms and soles. Apocrine glands open into hair follicles, and are found predominantly in the underarm, genital, and anal regions. Apocrine gland secretions interact with bacteria on the skin to produce body odors.

SKIN PIGMENTATION

Skin color is directly related to the number of pigment-producing cells, called melanocytes. About every tenth cell at the base of the epidermis is a melanocyte.
FRECKLED SKIN contains a collection of overactive melanocytes that produces more pigment than normal skin when they are exposed to sunlight (arrows).
SUNTANNED SKIN develops when ultraviolet light from the sun stimulates melanocytes in the skin to increase

their production of brown pigment for distribution to other cells in the skin. This pigmentation accumulates in the skin, producing a darker or tan color.
SUNBURNED SKIN occurs after a person receives an excessive amount of ultraviolet light. The melanocyte does not make pigment fast enough to protect the skin, and the dermis and blood vessels swell. Sunburn is usually a first-degree burn.

melanocyte

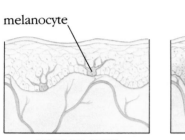

NORMAL SKIN

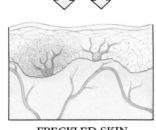

FRECKLED SKIN

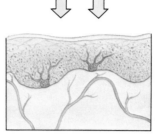

SUNTANNED SKIN

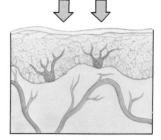

SUNBURNED SKIN

Total inability to sweat is a serious and, fortunately, rare problem. But temporary blockage of the sweat glands can occur anytime clothing or bedding blocks sweat secretions. The heat and moisture caused by this blockage make the sweat-duct openings swell shut, preventing further sweating and resulting in a heat rash. The swollen glands cause fine bumps, and mild inflammation causes the red color change. To resolve the problem, uncover the area and air it.

Deodorants prevent offensive odors either by masking them with stronger inoffensive ones or by controlling the growth of bacteria that contribute to odor production.

Antiperspirants actually suppress sweat production. It is uncertain whether they cause the sweat gland openings to temporarily close or whether they cause the entire gland mechanism to stop functioning. Research data suggest the latter. Compounds containing aluminum, benzalkonium, and zirconium are used most frequently. The length of the effect is related to the concentration of the compound in the antiperspirant.

Most deodorants and antiperspirants are mixtures of many fragrances, stabilizers, and preservatives, any one of which can cause irritation to the skin. Early signs of such irritation are itching, slight tenderness, and a pink color change in the skin. In severe reactions, there is inflammation with swelling, oozing, and red discoloration. Whenever such irritation occurs, stop using the product in question. When the skin heals, try applying other brands on small test areas of the skin.

Pigmentation

Skin color is directly related to the number and activity of the pigment-producing cells (melanocytes) in the body. Approximately every tenth cell at the base of the epidermis is a pigment cell. These cells account for racial color, hair color, and individual reactions to the sun.

Racial color variations are due to the way the pigment is made and how it is dispersed, rather than differences in the number of pigment cells. Melanocytes produce "packages" of pigment which, in dark-skinned people, are simply larger than in the white population. These pigment packages are broken down into small pigment particles and are spread throughout the upper cells of the epidermis. In Caucasian skin, the pigment stays in large clumps, with little spread to other cells.

Freckles

Freckles are small, light brown spots that occur on sun-exposed skin, particularly on blue-eyed, fair-skinned persons with light-colored hair. The face, neckline, and arms have the greatest number of freckles, and freckles are more prominent in the summer than in winter. That's because each freckle contains a collection of overactive pigment cells that produces more pigment than normal skin when exposed to sunlight. Thus, avoidance of sunlight is the only way to prevent freckles from forming, although the application of sunscreens prior to sun exposure may help. Makeup can be used to make facial freckles less noticeable.

Hair

With few exceptions (the palms, soles, lips, and labia minora), all areas of the body are covered by at least some hair. The largest hairs are terminal hairs that form on the scalp, eyebrows, and eyelashes. The rest of the body is covered with fine, soft, vellus hairs that, in many people, can be seen only with a magnifying glass. The hairs in the underarm and pelvic regions are vellus hairs until puberty, when hormonal changes bring about their replacement with terminal hairs. The differences in hair distribution between men and women also are based mainly on hormonal differences between the sexes (see page 123).

Each hair shaft has a finite life-span and a unique growth rate. The living part of the hair bulb is located about one millimeter below the surface of the skin (see page 560). From it, the hair shaft passes through pores on the skin's surface at the rate of one inch every six to eight weeks, depending on its location on the body. Hairs on the crown grow faster than those on the side of the head, and hair may grow for three to eight years before entering a resting stage of no growth. (At any given time, one out of eight scalp hairs is in its resting stage of hair growth.) After several months, the hair shaft sheds and a new hair starts to grow from the hair-bulb base; from 50 to 150 hairs can be shed each day. Because all hairs have a set or predetermined life-span, hair growth has a maximum limit, with potential hair length related to its location on the body.

As a person ages, hair growth slows, as do many metabolic processes. Women often notice mild to moderate thinning of their scalp hair and a slight recession of the hairline, although neither of these changes is as pronounced in women as in men. Eating a balanced diet and washing your hair when it feels oily are the best ways to ensure healthy hair growth; treatments, lotions, salves, or vitamins can do nothing to increase hair growth. Brushing hair helps to distribute the oils secreted by the scalp and adds sheen to the hair; however, excessive brushing may cause unnecessary hair loss. One hundred brush strokes at night might be too much for the scalp of one woman, while another may tolerate five hundred strokes. Notice how much hair you lose in your brush and adjust your strokes accordingly.

Shampooing removes excess oil and dislodges older layers of skin that would normally shed but have been trapped by the hairs. Normal and medicated shampoos work best if allowed to remain in the scalp for at least five minutes prior to rinsing. Sun, wind, heat, hair cosmetics, and chlorinated water all cause varying degrees of damage to hair, and blow-drying with excessive heat can permanently frizz the hair. To repair this damage, try using moisturizers and rinses that add oil to the hair and help damaged hair feel softer and more flexible. Protein shampoos add a residue of protein that gives the appearance of added body until it is washed away with the next shampoo. Permanent dyeing, waving, and straightening do little damage provided the chemical solutions are not left on too long. Occasionally, however, a woman may develop an allergic reaction to one of the solutions used in these processes.

Moderate hair loss also can occur after delivering a child, following a serious illness, or with malnourishment. Tight hairdos that place the hair in traction, such as braids, buns, and corn rows, also can cause loss of hair at the sides, front, and back of the scalp. Fortunately hair loss due to illness, childbirth, or traction is not permanent and the hair usually will grow again.

Nails and Nail Problems

Nails protect the exposed ends of the fingers and toes. They form from a highly specialized and compressed form of protein called keratin. The outer layer of the epidermis is composed of a more loosely organized form of this same protein. The area of active growth of the nail — the "living" part of the nail — is found below and behind the cuticle. As with hair, what is visible is "dead." It takes approximately six months for a fingernail to totally regrow. Toenails grow much more slowly, and may take as long as 18 months for full regrowth.

Brittle nails, as defined by a physician, are nails that fragment at the end with the slightest amount of trauma. The major causes of brittle nails are unknown, but they may occur as a result of iron deficiency, anemia, and poor circulation. Severe iron deficiency can cause the nails to become concave and resemble the bowl of a spoon. Constant immersion of the nails in water with a high alkaline content also can contribute to brittleness.

Nail discoloration has many causes. The entire nail may discolor when in contact with hair dyes. Some nail products themselves produce permanent nail discoloration, and everyone has seen the discolored nails of heavy tobacco smokers. Bacterial and yeast infections can produce yellow-green discoloration and painful swellings filled with pus at the sides of the nails. Many of the above conditions also can cause the nail to separate from the finger.

Although the nails seem very hard and impervious to damage, nail growth is easily affected by trauma. Tight-fitting shoes that constrict or severely rub the toes can cause abnormal toenail growth. A hematoma (blood blister) may form under the nail following such a pressure-induced injury. The blister forms because small blood vessels are ruptured, as in a bruise. Often the nail sheds because the blood blister breaks the attachments of the nail bed to the nail. If the blood is released soon after injury, the nail often can be saved. A very hot paper-clip tip will melt a hole through the nail and release the pressure.

Serious illnesses often cause a line of transverse thinning across the nail. One can estimate the time lapse since the sickness by the location of the line on the nail. A penetrating injury to just one portion of the deep skin behind the cuticle can cause a permanent longitudinal line that grows out to the end of the nail. Small white spots in the nails are normal, but if the nail in the white spot becomes crumbly, a fungus infection may be present.

Constantly immersing the hands in dishwater and detergent cleaning solutions can cause irritation that may lead to a chronic infection at the sides of the nails. Irritation usually precedes the infection, which is called a "paronychia." Treatment consists of draining the pus and treating the nail with antibiotics.

Injury, incorrect nail cutting, and poorly fitting shoes can cause small fragments of the toenails to separate at the edges and grow into the skin. Treatment of such an ingrown toenail consists of freeing the nail so that it can grow out over the skin rather than into it. Toenails should be trimmed short and cut straight across, not curved.

Common Skin Conditions

All of us notice changes in the appearance of our skin from time to time. Some of these changes represent skin conditions that are common to people of all ages. Others are temporary and relate to specific states, such as pregnancy. Still others are primarily associated with normal aging, or result from an injury to the skin.

Most people experience a number of such conditions during their lifetimes, but many of us are not aware of the causes or the remedies of some of these common skin conditions.

Skin Conditions Common to All Ages

Acne is the most common disease seen by dermatologists. While most cases start and resolve in the teen-age years, some persist into adulthood, while still other cases flare up again in the 20s or later. Acne is associated with the increased production of hormones that occur at puberty. As more sebum (an oily secretion) is produced by the sebaceous glands, the lining cells of the pores adhere to one another as they shed, causing small plugs to form and block the pores. When the plugs occur near the skin surface, they are called "blackheads." The color is not dirt; rather it represents trapping of skin pigment that normally would be shed. When the plug occurs deeper in the pore, a "whitehead" forms. Some of the deeply plugged pores trap normal skin bacteria and subsequently become inflamed, forming nodules and pus-containing cysts.

HOW ACNE DEVELOPS

Acne starts in the hair follicle where a tiny sebaceous gland manufactures sebum, a natural moisturizing oil that, under normal conditions, keeps the skin supple. Sebum moves up past the hair shaft and out the hair pore to the skin surface.

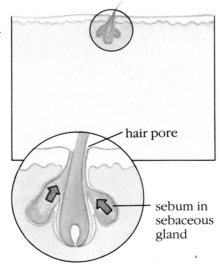

hair pore

sebum in sebaceous gland

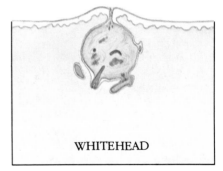

WHITEHEAD

WHITEHEAD *The oily sebum may be produced in such quantity that the skin becomes too oily — usually during periods of life such as adolescence when hormone production increases, or during phases of the menstrual cycle when hormone balances shift. The excess oil then moves up the hair follicle*

Many factors aggravate acne — emotion, high temperatures, humidity, certain garments, greasy cosmetics, etc. — but the specific mechanism through which each acts is unknown. There is no data to support the long-held notion that certain foods aggravate acne; nevertheless, some people may notice a flare-up of acne a few days after eating nuts, greasy foods, milk, or chocolate. It is wise for these people to avoid the offending foods and whatever else seems to make their acne worse. Oil-based cosmetics are another major culprit because they plug the pores. Although makeup can disguise the acne, it also encourages its development. Water-based cosmetics will not cause acne. A woman in doubt about a product's composition should rub it between her fingers; a water-based substance will not feel greasy.

For unknown reasons, many women experience a flare-up of acne during their 20s, sometimes occurring only on the chin. This may be due to use of cosmetics. Acne often is worse a few days before the menstrual flow, most likely because of the surge of progesterone levels at that time. In the same way, birth control pills that contain high levels of progesterone can aggravate acne, whereas estrogen-containing pills may allow some improvement.

Sunlight often is beneficial to acne, which explains why a person's skin may clear totally in the summer, only to flare up again in the fall. Treatment of acne has improved significantly in the last ten years with the development of medications containing benzoyl peroxide or retinoic acid. Once-a-day application of creams or gels containing these ingredients helps dissolve existing plugs and prevents new ones from forming. The antibiotics tetracycline and erythromycin fight infection and redness that sometimes complicate simple acne. In the future, medications may incorporate these antibiotics into solutions that can be applied directly to the skin.

Red marks left by resolving acne eventually fade to a normal skin color. In cases where acne scars are severe and disfiguring, dermabrasion can be helpful (see page 659). In this treatment, the superficial layers of skin are removed, thus decreasing the apparent depth of the acne pits. Some physicians now inject the deepest pits with a nonabsorbable polymer that fills the cavities to match the surface contour.

Dry skin, or xerosis, is a simple problem with a complex cause. When it occurs on the arms and legs, the limbs may look as if they were lightly dusted with chalk. The dry, fine scaling of xerosis is easily differentiated from the oily, thicker scales of seborrheic dermatitis. Extreme dryness of the skin causes severe itching.

Many factors contribute to dry skin, and they can be external or internal in origin. External environmental factors are the drying actions of low humidity, wind, temperature extremes, and excessive sun exposure. Frequent washing and bathing with strong soaps that remove nature's moisturizers also exacerbate the condition. Finally, some women are born with skin that always seems to need added moisture; subtle abnormalities in the outer layer of the epidermis may allow too much moisture to evaporate. Internally, female homones contribute to the control of skin moisture. At menopause, any existing dry skin problem becomes worse, presumably because of decreased hormone production. A diet deficient in vital nutrients also can cause dry skin.

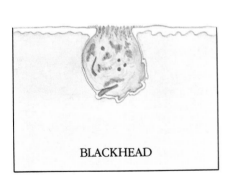

BLACKHEAD

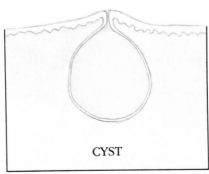

CYST

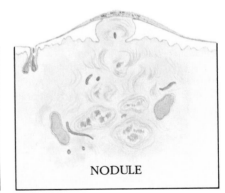

NODULE

and out the skin pore. If, on the way, it begins to mix with skin debris and dead cells, a stiff, waxy plug forms and blocks the pore. The resulting whitehead is visible at the surface of the skin. The hair follicle begins to degenerate, and pus forms, causing a bump on the skin surface.
BLACKHEAD *As the tip of a plug*

forces its way through the skin pore, the plug traps skin pigment and becomes black in color.
The blackhead also has a pus-filled cavity beneath it containing the remains of the hair follicle.
CYST *When the cavity beneath the whitehead or blackhead becomes enlarged and entirely pus-filled, it is*

referred to as a cyst.
NODULE *In its later stages, acne becomes red and swollen, and the sebaceous gland may rupture. This causes bacterial infection and pus to spread under the skin surface, spreading the acne and resulting in skin discoloration. This is the nodule stage of acne.*

Treatment consists of minimizing and correcting any obvious external factors, and frequently applying a moisturizing cream or salve. Simple petroleum jelly is more effective than many of the expensive lotions and products on the market. Less frequent bathing and use of warm rather than hot water helps prevent loss of natural oils. And, cool-air humidifiers may be helpful in seasons of low humidity.

Itching, or pruritus, is a symptom of many different skin diseases and conditions. Itching is a sensation directly perceived through the skin, and dry skin is probably its most common cause. Itching often results in frequent rubbing, which thickens the skin and, for reasons unknown, causes it to itch more. The itching that accompanies contact dermatitis (see page 576) is presumed to be due to the release of granules contained in the white blood cells that migrate from the blood system to the affected area. Antihistamines are effective for this type of itching.

Genital and anal itching are also common problems, particularly because these areas are moist and thus are favorable environments for bacterial growth. In addition, folded and occluding skin surfaces in these areas prevent normal friction that usually assists in rubbing away superficial layers of dead skin that contribute to itching. Daily cleansing of these regions minimizes the potential for discomfort.

Treatment of any itching problem must be based on curing the underlying condition and then treating the residual itching.

Folliculitis is a condition that affects most people at one time or another. It usually occurs on the buttocks, thighs, or upper arms as small, pinpoint, tender red bumps around a fine hair shaft. Because sitting for long periods of time restricts circulation and prevents evaporation of water from the skin's surface, secretaries and desk workers frequently have this problem. Intense athletic activity and humid climates also play a role. Tight-fitting clothes not made of "breathing" fabrics such as cotton can add to the problem, and women with acne may be even more susceptible. Loose clothing, frequent changes of position, frequent bathing, and porous cushions all help to prevent or minimize the problem.

Excess body hair (hypertrichosis) is a common cosmetic problem, and one that is inherited; ethnic background and race greatly influence the degree of body hair. As mentioned earlier, the number of hairs on every person is constant; their differences in appearance are determined by the number of terminal hairs versus vellus hairs. Body hair is least noticeable in Asians, and is quite apparent in some Mediterranean cultures.

In a few rare cases, women may have an elevation of male hormones in the body that contributes to excess hair. Laboratory tests for hormone levels allow a physician to evaluate whether an excess of male hormones is present.

Should you wish to remove body hair, there are several treatments available. Shaving the hair is an obvious and common solution, but not a permanent one. Bleaching dark hair is often used cosmetically to make it less noticeable; depilatory creams also may be useful. Electrolysis is a tedious procedure for individually killing each hair root; however, it is the only permanent way to remove undesirable hairs.

Moles (nevi) are small, flat, pigmented spots or gentle bumps that can appear anywhere on the skin. Moles usually are benign and need not be removed *unless* they seem to grow, change color, or bleed spontaneously (see page 580). Many moles begin life as flat spots that, as a woman ages, constrict like a ring at the base, causing the mole to look like a balloon on a string; eventually such moles may fall off. Moles often are mistaken for skin tags (see page 569).

Moles that measure one to two inches in diameter at birth should be watched carefully for any change. Most authorities recommend having the larger ones removed because of the risk of their becoming malignant.

Warts are small, rough-surfaced bumps on the skin. They are caused by a virus that stimulates local growth of skin and *not,* as myth has it, by toads. Warts do not become malignant or cancerous. The wart virus easily spreads and produces smaller warts nearby — on adjoining fingers or toes, for example. Rubbing and scratching the wart on a toe can spread it to a finger.

The average life-span of a wart is from one to three years. Almost all warts will resolve spontaneously if given enough time, but for many people they are an ugly nuisance. Furthermore, warts can infect other people as well as other parts of one's own body. When warts occur on the sole of the foot, they are very painful. Occasionally, bothersome warts occur in the vagina and rectum; if you notice warts in these areas, have them treated by a doctor in their early stages of development.

Treatment of warts, except those on mucosal surfaces (the vagina, rectum, and mouth), consists of daily application of a solution containing salicylic and lactic acids. You may apply this treatment yourself, a drop to the wart each day, and then scrape off the dead skin that develops. The wart becomes so soft that it can be scraped with a butter knife. Because this process takes about one month of daily applications, the patient really must do it herself.

Plantar warts (those on the sole of the foot) can be treated similarly with adhesive felt pads that contain 40 percent salicylic acid. The pads are applied to the wart and are taped in place every day. Again, a butter knife is used to slowly remove the disintegrating wart. In order to satisfactorily treat such warts, the pad should be slightly larger than the wart, even though the medicated pad also will affect normal tissue in the surrounding area.

Alternative treatments for warts are a 20-second application of liquid nitrogen, or electrocautery that coagulates the virus. These treatments are potentially painful and may have to be repeated two or three times in order to effect total removal of the wart.

Stretch marks are annoyances for many women who have been pregnant or who have gained and lost considerable weight at one time or another. When the elastic fibers of the skin are stretched, the skin becomes thin, and the small blood vessels in the dermis are prominent through this very thin epidermis. There is no danger of an actual tear in the skin, however. If multiple stretch marks start to appear on a person who is not pregnant, she should see her doctor. Misuse of strong steroid creams on the armpits, groin, and ano-genital regions also can cause stretch marks, and on the face, they can stimulate acne. Plastic surgery is the only way to remove stretch marks.

THE STRUCTURE OF MOLES AND WARTS

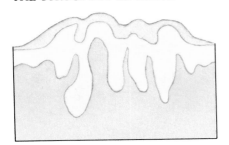
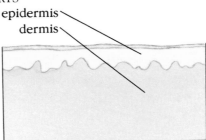
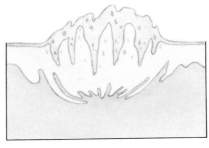

epidermis
dermis

THE STRUCTURE OF A MOLE
Moles are pigmented, roughly circular patches of skin in which normal skin cells and normal pigment cells have overgrown to produce a dark, slightly raised bump. Moles may be large or small, flat or raised up off the skin surface, and smooth or hairy. They vary in color from yellow-brown to black. The color of a mole is produced by cells containing pigment that are scattered throughout the epidermis and dermis. Moles rarely become malignant, but those that grow, bleed, or change color should be examined by a physician.

NORMAL SKIN

THE STRUCTURE OF A WART
Warts are roughly round overgrowths of skin that never become cancerous. Warts are caused by a virus (red dots) that stimulates skin growth, and that may spread through the skin to produce other warts. Warts seem to come and go spontaneously, with or without treatment.

mole

wart

Telangiectases are small, fine, dilated blood vessels that occur on the face, neck, and shoulders, and sometimes look like small red spiders. Excessive sun exposure may increase their number and make them more prominent, and they may be more noticeable in pregnancy and before menstrual periods. Telangiectases occur when small vessels from the dermis penetrate to the epidermis and become visible. Pressure on the center of the telangiectasia makes the vessel disappear temporarily. For cosmetic purposes, a doctor can decrease the size of telangiectases by administering a slight electric current to the center of the vessel.

Hemangiomas are red, purple, or blue bumps on the skin that look as if they are filled with blood. In fact, they are. Because of their appearance, they are called "portwine stains." They consist of small interweaving collections of dilated blood vessels, and occur most commonly on the chest and back. In rare instances, a large flat hemangioma can occur on the face and cause considerable disfigurement. Hemangiomas occur at birth; some increase in size with age, while others disappear.

Hemangiomas are usually harmless, and treatment is done for cosmetic purposes only. In the past, this treatment has not been universally successful. Some physicians have had success with liquid nitrogen, while others use injections. Some resort to plastic surgery, while still others prefer laser treatment.

Skin Conditions and Pregnancy

Pregnancy produces a variety of skin changes, some of which have been noted previously. Many such skin conditions have been attributed to the elevated levels of female hormones at this time. The majority of pregnant women experience "flushing," which occurs most prominently as red palms and increases as pregnancy passes into the third trimester. Most pregnant women also develop scattered telangiectases, usually no wider than the diameter of a hair shaft, which increase toward term and decrease almost to the point of disappearing completely in the months following delivery.

Marked itching occurs in 20 percent of women during the last trimester. All women experience some degree of hair loss three months after delivering a child. In most women it is minimal, but in many cases the loss is quite significant. The hair regrows within a few months, however. Pregnancy also causes nipples, genitals, and moles to darken.

Stretch marks occur where the tissues are particularly stretched during pregnancy — the breasts and abdomen. And if there is a general weight gain, such marks may appear in other places as well. Stretch marks do become somewhat smaller after delivery, but usually persist throughout life. Although there is no known way to prevent their development, they become pale with age.

VARICOSE VEINS

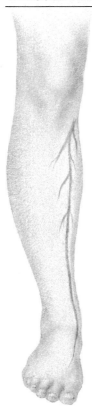

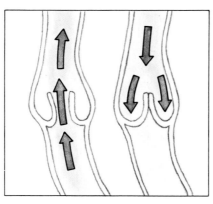

NORMAL VEINS
Normal veins have small one-way valves every few inches. A surge of blood from below (arrows) forces blood through the valve toward the heart. As the blood tends to flow backward due to the force of gravity, the valve closes. The valves of the veins, then, only allow blood to move toward the heart.

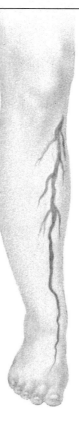

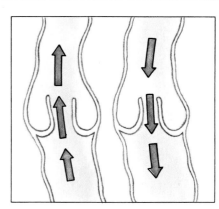

VARICOSE VEINS
In varicose veins, the valves do not close completely, and the force of gravity causes blood to pool in the legs, enlarging the veins.

Pregnancy causes two types of skin infections to worsen—venereal warts on the labia and vagina, and yeast infections. On the other hand, some skin conditions improve—psoriasis, atopic dermatitis, and in some cases, acne.

Pregnant women frequently develop blotches of light brown pigment on eyelids, cheeks, and chin. This condition is called chloasma or "the mask of pregnancy." Intense sunlight may deepen the coloration of these spots, but they usually fade after delivery. Occasionally birth control pills bring on the condition as well.

Skin Conditions Associated with Aging

Wrinkles are a normal feature of aging and appear as the elastic fibers in the skin gradually break down with time. Much of this deterioration is unavoidable; nevertheless, overexposure to sunlight markedly hastens such changes, as does wind damage. Plastic or cosmetic surgery is the only treatment for wrinkles and, because it serves to remove the slack in the skin only temporarily, it may have to be repeated every five years (see page 658). Fortunately, most people consider wrinkles to be a natural, distinguished sign of aging that marks the face with character.

Lentigines (liver spots), though often mistaken for freckles, are actually darker and larger; lentigines do not fade in the winter and they increase in number as a person ages. Many people are born with a few scattered lentigines, which differ from most moles (nevi) in that they are totally flat. Lentigines consist of a localized collection of active pigment cells that increase in number during a lifetime of sunshine and outdoor exposure. They have no relation to the liver and are best treated, for cosmetic purposes, by liquid nitrogen freezing. They do not become skin cancers.

Skin tags are small, thin, harmless threads of normal skin that occur in most people in the armpits, the sides of the neck, and the upper trunk. They increase in number with age, but may become irritated or nicked while shaving; therefore, patients often ask doctors to remove them.

Varicose veins are abnormally dilated veins beneath the skin of the legs. Many women and men inherit the tendency to develop varicosities, and some women notice this condition after pregnancy. Leg veins also become more prominent in persons holding jobs that involve considerable standing. And sometimes a severe injury to the leg can alter the blood flow to the extent that varicose veins occur.

Normal veins have small valves every few inches that help blood flow to the heart against the pull of gravity. When the varicose vein dilates, the valves no longer close together and the force of gravity causes the blood to pool in the legs. The same problem may occur when a disease process permanently damages these valves.

Tight support stockings are helpful because they exert pressure that compresses the veins, thus helping to close the valves and force blood to the heart. Some people undergo vein-stripping operations in which the dilated veins are removed and all of their branches are tied off. In about half of such cases, however, the remaining leg veins are abnormal, and new varicose veins arise within two years of surgery.

Skin Conditions Associated with Injury

Sunburn. Ultraviolet light in sunlight stimulates the skin to make more pigment, which accumulates in the skin to produce a darker or "tan" color. Long-wave ultraviolet light produces primarily tanning, whereas shortwave ultraviolet light can produce sunburn and tanning.

A suntan develops because ultraviolet light from the sun stimulates the pigment cells in the skin to increase production of brown pigment to distribute to other cells in the skin. As this occurs, a tan appears. The freshly made pigment absorbs ultraviolet light, and therefore helps prevent burns. Sunburn occurs after a person receives an excessive amount of UV light. The amount that will produce a burn varies from person to person; however, freckled and fair-complected people tend to burn rather than tan.

A sunburn is an actual burn on the skin that can blister, just as a finger touched to a burner on the stove. Sunburns occur within hours, rather than within the days needed for the evolution of a tan. The waves that cause sunburn are most intense between 10 a.m. and 2 p.m., and they are strongest at high elevations. Care also should be taken to avoid burning when you are on sand or snow, since both surfaces reflect light from the sun.

In our society, a dark suntan has been considered a sign of good health, affluence, and beauty. But we know today that the sun has more harmful than helpful effects. Overexposure to the sun's rays can cause wrinkles, dry skin, seborrheic keratoses, actinic keratoses, and even skin cancer. In addition, the harmful effects of the sun are additive and irreversible; the skin remembers every ray of sunlight to which it has been exposed. Unfortunately, the harmful skin changes that warn us of too much sun only begin to show late in life. At this point, protection is long overdue.

Using caution is the best way to prevent sunburn and sun-related skin damage. The season's first exposure to the sun should be no longer than 15 minutes for the most sensitive, and one hour for dark-complected people. The best times of the day for this first sun exposure are morning and late afternoon. Time spent in the sun can be increased by 15- to 30-minute increments each day thereafter.

Sunburn prevention has come a long way from the days of tanning butters and baby oil. Great advances have been made fairly recently with the finding that para amino benzoate and benzophenones *will* prevent sunburn and still permit tanning. These compounds absorb harmful ultraviolet rays at the skin's surface before they penetrate further. Preparations containing these ingredients are called sunscreens.

If a sunburn develops, apply cool compresses to the skin and take two aspirins every four hours to soothe the discomfort and reduce inflammation. Severe burns require medical evaluation, however. Sun lamps also can cause severe burns; for home use, a sun lamp must have an automatic timer that will turn off the lamp if you should fall asleep.

Burns. Injury by heat is dependent on the intensity of the heat and the duration of contact with the skin. A burn caused by the steam spray of an iron produces more injury than a short splash of hot water, because steam is usually hotter than boiling water. The depth of injury determines whether a burn is first-, second-, or third-degree. Sunburns and common household burns are almost always first-degree. They may cause painful redness, but heal without blisters or scars. Second-degree burns produce blisters as well as some damage to the dermis lying below the dead epidermis. Minimal scarring may occur, depending on the depth of the burn, but mild to moderate hair loss and skin color change may result. Third-degree burns are the most serious. They kill the epidermis, the dermis, much of the fat, and sometimes extend to the muscle and bone. Because third-degree burns destroy the nerves, no subsequent pain is felt from this level of burn, even though surrounding tissue, perhaps second-degree burned, can be painful.

In the past, treatment of burns has varied from the application of butter to use of the mucin of the aloe plant. The best home treatment for first- and second-degree burns is immediate immersion into a bath of ice water, which both numbs the pain and slows the inflammation. Any blister that forms should be left intact as long as possible, for it acts as nature's bandage while the skin is healing. If the blister is on a pressure surface (a sole or buttock), a sterile needle can be used to drain the fluid.

It is important to avoid infection, which complicates many second-degree burns and all third-degree burns. In fact, most deaths of patients with third-degree burns are due to infection and the loss of body fluids through the oozing burned surfaces. Burns of this severity should be treated by a doctor. Extensive third-degree burns require special treatment available only in burn-treatment centers.

Bruises occur when a blow causes sufficient damage to the capillaries that they leak blood. The capillaries quickly heal, but it takes a long time for the body to remove the blood pigments that have leaked into the tissues. Initially the bruise is red-purple, but as it heals, it changes to yellow-brown and then disappears.

People who have had thrombophlebitis are frequently put on anticoagulants — "blood-thinning" medicines that prevent the formation of dangerous blood clots. If too much of such medication is taken, bruising may become so excessive that the slightest blow can cause a bright red bruise. This condition is called an *ecchymosis.* When the same process occurs but the spot is less than one-half inch in diameter, it is called *purpura.* The smallest bruises, such as those occurring in stasis dermatitis (see page 577), are called *petechiae.*

Petechiae occur when the platelets in the blood —the initiators of clotting — are low. Widespread petechiae can occur on the lower legs of healthy women for no apparent reason. Normal bruising occurs on surfaces repeatedly exposed to bumping:

TYPES OF BURNS

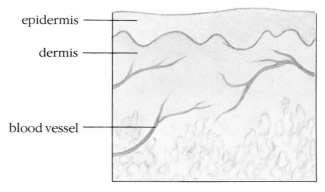

NORMAL SKIN

the shins, forearms, shoulders, elbows, knees, and breasts. However, one should be suspicious if bruises occur suddenly in other areas without apparent cause.

Scars occur whenever the skin heals after being cut through to the dermis. Scarring occurs only when the dermis and the bottom layer of the epidermis are damaged. The actual scar forms because the space between the skin surfaces is replaced by cells that produce fibers to draw the skin together and hold it in place. When cuts in the skin do not penetrate that deeply, there is no need for strengthening fibers to be produced; consequently, the epidermal cells merely reproduce themselves to fill the open space left by the injury.

Disfiguring scars can be treated in any of several ways. Nodular scars can be injected with steroid medications that slowly cause them to flatten. Depressed scars can be injected with a nonabsorbable substance that raises the depressed area to match the surrounding surface. Some scars cannot be "beautified" without surgical excision and careful resuturing, however.

Frostbite is an injury to the skin and underlying structures caused by severe cold, or moderate cold combined with wind. Unprotected fingers, the nose, and the ears are most susceptible. At first, the exposed skin turns white and becomes numb. The skin becomes white because blood that normally supplies the outer skin is preferentially transferred to the inner parts of the body to warm the important internal organs. Because blood flowing through the

skin is its sole source of warmth, the skin becomes even more susceptible to cold after this stage. The next step is actual freezing of the skin. Here, the degree of damage depends on the amount of underlying tissue that becomes frozen, and the duration of exposure.

If a frostbitten area is discovered while you are outside, cover it immediately with a protective scarf, glove, or sleeve, and, if possible, seek shelter. The next step is to place the injured part of the body in a basin of warm water. Washcloths and towels soaked in warm water can be used for the face. Although the intention is to rapidly rewarm the frozen tissue, do *not* use hot water. Look for a return of pink color to the skin — usually occurring within 30 minutes; further warming is of little value. Do not rub the frozen surfaces, since rubbing injures the skin. Once rewarmed, the frostbitten surfaces will throb painfully, and a blister may form. Treat the frostbitten area as you would a burn.

Ear piercing has long been fashionable. One method of piercing ears is to make a small hole in the lobe and place a metal post (preferably of 22-karat gold) in this hole. Once this is done, the post is rotated every day and the earlobe is dabbed with alcohol. After one month, the skin should be well healed around the post if the treatment of rotation and alcohol application is carried out faithfully. During this one-month period, the gold posts should be worn constantly. After healing, the posts can be removed and other earrings inserted.

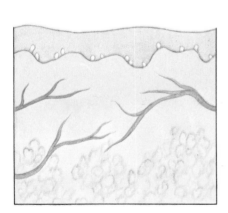

FIRST-DEGREE BURN
Sunburn and common household burns are almost always first-degree burns. They cause painful redness, but heal without blisters or scars. In a first-degree burn, small holes form at the base of the epidermis. There is swelling in the upper dermis, and vessels dilate.

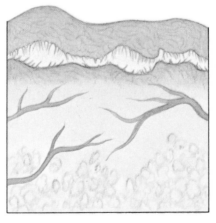

SECOND-DEGREE BURN
In second-degree burns, the epidermis is badly damaged; the little holes become big holes filled with fluid (blisters). The upper dermis is damaged, the dermis swells considerably, and the blood vessels dilate. The epidermis peels off and some scarring may occur.

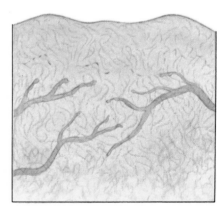

THIRD-DEGREE BURN
In third-degree burns, the epidermis and dermis cells are killed. Much of the fat and sometimes muscle is destroyed, as are nerves and blood vessels. The burn becomes inflamed, and fluid can rapidly leave the skin through the unprotected surface.

Three problems may arise in women who have had their ears pierced: contact dermatitis, infection, and keloids. Contact dermatitis occurs frequently because as many as one in forty women are allergic to nickel, which is used in almost all jewelry for its added strength. Those with a nickel allergy will develop itching, crusting, and "weeping" around the post and earrings. Those who have a past history of being unable to wear a wristwatch or who develop skin irritation under rings should be on guard for similar reactions to earrings. Changing to jewelry made with 22-karat gold will solve this allergy problem for many women.

Infection can arise from the initial post placement or may occur subsequently, particularly when the earlobes are not dressed with alcohol. If significant infection occurs, the posts must be taken out and the ears treated with an antibiotic.

Keloids are a rare problem, but are somewhat more common in blacks than Caucasians or Asians. Keloids are hard, thick scars that occur after the earlobe hole has healed. Most women know from childhood accidents or subsequent surgeries whether they have the tendency to form large nodular scars after their skin has been cut. These women should not attempt to have their ears pierced.

Bugs

There are a number of irritating skin conditions caused by a variety of tiny bugs. With all of these conditions, the "cure" lies in the eradication of the little creatures.

Scabies are mites that have caused a minor epidemic in recent years. They live only on humans and cause intense itching of the fingers, web spaces, wrists, breasts, waist area, and portions of the genitalia. The feature shared by all of these areas is their relative hairlessness. The rash often starts as small water blisters that are scratched so quickly that they may never be seen. The itching is often more noticeable at night when the distractions of daytime activities are no longer present to divert attention from the itching. Although dog scabies can temporarily infect humans, it is a rare occurrence. One problem that makes infestation difficult to eradicate is that the itching does not start until a person has had the infection for one month; as a result, the mite has had ample opportunity to spread to numerous other people before the infected person experiences the first symptoms. The itching is so intense that the small water blisters and red bumps may be scratched until they bleed and form scabs.

Because infants and children have less body hair, the mite spreads diffusely over their entire body. Infection of the shoulders, neck, and feet is common in young children.

Fortunately, there are several lotions available that will cure the infection within 24 hours. The lotions may contain crotamition, gamma benzene hexachloride, or sulfur. Adults should rub the lotion on every square inch of skin between the neck and the ankles. Children's feet also should be treated. The lotion should be left on for 24 hours and then washed off. Although this single treatment should kill all the organisms, many authorities recommend repeating the treatment a week later. Every member of the family and anyone with whom an infected person has had close contact should be treated. Otherwise, a single non-itching infected person can reinfect others.

Bedbugs bite humans, frequently leaving their bite marks in a row on parts of the body not covered by bedding, such as the face, neck, and forearms. They may live in bedding, under floor boards, or actually travel from outside the house at night to feed. Insecticides for bedbugs must be sprayed on the sites where they live.

Body lice cause small pinpoint red marks that start to itch after one week. They frequently live in the seams of clothing and should be sought there.

Pubic lice are the largest of all the mites that infest humans. The crab louse measures one millimeter in diameter and, with the aid of a magnifying glass, can be seen to have an obvious crablike shape. The mite spreads by direct contact and is killed by selective louse-killing lotions.

Lice produce egg sacs on the hair that look like dandruff, but do not flake loose since they are cemented to the hair shafts. The louse bites the scalp, neck, and shoulders, producing crusted red bumps that may look like scabies. The egg sacs frequently occur on the hairs above the ears. Both scalp lice and pubic lice also may be found on the eyelashes. Treatment for the hair is to shampoo with lotions used to treat scabies. The eyelashes should be treated with physostigmine drops or salve.

Mites have plagued civilization for thousands of years. Some attribute the "seven-year itch" phrase to a sufferer of mite infection. Mites are selective about whom they infect. Animal mites seldom attack humans beyond their first bite, which tells them that human flesh is not to their liking. They also claim "territorial" rights in the body: mites in the scalp will not infect the groin, and mites that infect the hairless parts of the body never infect the more hirsute areas.

Infections of the Skin

Infection of the skin may be caused by a fungus, a virus, or by various kinds of bacteria. Whatever the cause, these infections can result in conditions that are irritating and sometimes painful.

Fungus Infections

Fungus infections are, for unknown reasons, more common in men than in women. Fungal infections (ringworm) of the scalp occur almost exclusively in children. The fungus produces a red, round, scaling patch that itches. As the hairs become infected, they fall out causing a "moth-eaten" appearance of multiple bald spots. The fungus lives in the dead, outer layers of the skin and the hair shafts. Often the hairs are destroyed flush with the scalp surface, leaving only the hair bulbs. In dark-haired people, this pattern of disease is called "black-dot ringworm." This disease can be shared from child to child, or from an infected cat or dog to a child. An antibiotic called griseofulvin will cure a fungal infection in six to eight weeks. Trimming the hair helps to keep the scalp and hair clean, but there is no longer any need to shave the scalp bald and to wear a stocking cap as was once done.

Fungal infections on the feet occur frequently in the web spaces between the toes, with the web space next to the smallest toe the most common site. Itching and scaling of the skin are the major signs of fungal infection, and the rash is often worse in the summer. In susceptible people, fungi cause a dry, scaling rash all over the sole of the foot. Twice-a-day application of tolnaftate, haloprogin, or miconazole will cure most of these infections in a month; however, recurrences of the infection are frequent.

Fungal infections of the nails are difficult to treat. As the nail becomes infected, it develops a yellow-brown discoloration and becomes thick and crumbly at the edges. Since toenails take up to 18 months to grow out, curing toenail fungi requires 18 months of continuous treatment. Griseofulvin cures the fungal disease, but there are side effects and 50 percent of those cured will relapse.

RINGWORM INFECTION

Ringworm is a fungal infection of the scalp that occurs almost exclusively in children. The fungus (brown in the inset drawing) lives in the epidermis of the skin and in hair shafts. The typical ringworm patch is red, round, itchy, and scaling. If the hair shafts are infected, hair falls out of the patch areas.

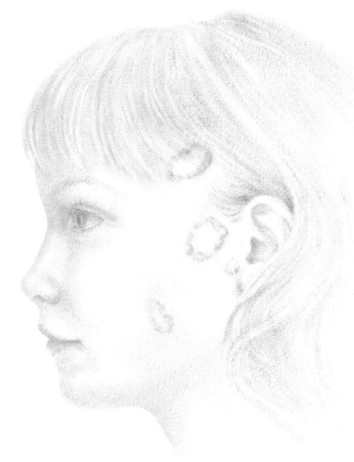
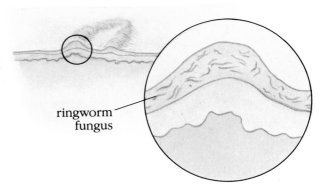

ringworm fungus

Yeast infections (Candida) have a characteristic appearance, depending on the region of the body that is infected. Vaginal infections produce a cheesy discharge; infections in the mouth and on the tongue show small patches of creamy white material that has a red base when removed. Nail-bed infections cause considerable redness and swelling at the base of the nail. Pus may exude from behind the nail, and nail growth may be markedly abnormal. Infections in the groin, under the breasts, and in the axillae (armpits) cause a beefy red rash with a sharp border. Just beyond the border are small, pinhead-size eruptions that have a small central white pus collection on a red base. The finger and toe web spaces may be infected.

Candida is a normal inhabitant of the skin and the gastrointestinal tract, and it only causes an infection when the yeast organisms markedly increase in number. Many infections start in the ano-genital region and are then spread to other parts of the body. People who are overweight seem to be more susceptible to Candida occurring in the occluded skin folds where moist warmth seems to encourage Candida growth. Other people who are susceptible to Candida infections are people on broad-spectrum antibiotics and those with diabetes. Housewives, waitresses, and laundry workers whose hands are often in water develop Candida infections in the web spaces between the fingers. The painful infections at the base of the nails are called Candida paronychia.

Candida can be treated with an anti-yeast cream applied three times a day for two to three weeks. Ano-genital infections additionally require pills to lower the population of yeast in the intestines. Vaginal yeast infections are decidedly uncomfortable, but respond to anti-yeast medication in the suppository form (see page 447).

HERPES SIMPLEX

DISTRIBUTION OF
TYPES I AND II

TYPE I
Above the waist

TYPE II
Below the waist

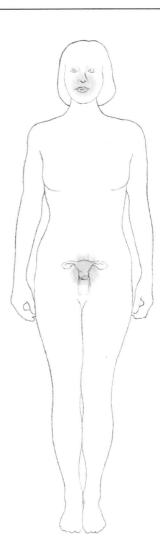

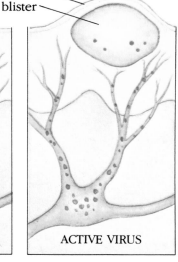

skin surface
blister

DORMANT VIRUS   ACTIVE VIRUS

Herpes simplex is a virus that causes painful, clear, fluid-filled water blisters. The blisters usually appear around the mouth as cold sores in Type-I infections, and around the genitals in Type-II infections.

HOW BLISTERS FORM IN HERPES SIMPLEX
You become infected with herpes simplex by actual contact with the virus of an infected sore. Thereafter, the virus remains stored in your skin's nerve cells, for this disease can be treated but not cured. Once the proper stimulus is presented, the dormant virus (red dots) travels through the nerves causing blisters to form. Virus particles move into the blister area and are found in the open sores and broken blisters of the skin.

Tinea versicolor is caused by a mild fungus present on everyone's skin. It produces asymptomatic, finely scaling flat spots on the trunk and upper arms that are either lighter or darker than the surrounding uninvolved skin. Although the fungus is present on everyone's skin, only susceptible people develop this widespread rash. It is a mild condition, but often difficult to eradicate. Daily application of 20 percent sodium thiosulfate or lotions containing selenium sulfide for four weeks, then every other day for four more weeks, will cure most conditions. When the scale is gone, the condition is cured, but it takes many months for the pigment alterations to return to their normal state.

Viral Infections

Herpes simplex is the name of the virus that causes fever blisters and cold sores. There are two types of herpes simplex virus. Type I causes the painful, clustered, clear-fluid-filled water blisters that occur at the corner of the mouth and on the lips. Attacks of these blisters occur in times of stress, at menses, accompanying fevers, and after long sunlight exposure. A flare-up preceding a wedding has been the bane of generations of brides. A day of tingling and burning usually occurs before the outbreak of blisters, and the condition usually runs its course in two weeks. Water blisters occasionally occur in small groups randomly distributed on the body.

Herpes simplex Type II virus causes a similar-appearing infection, but is limited to the genital region. The lesions may be obvious on the labia majora or on the thighs, but frequently they are hidden in the vagina, the urethral orifice, the cervix, or on the labia minora. Intense burning pain may be the only symptom. On rare occasions, inflammation near the urethra (urinary tract opening) can be so severe that the orifice swells shut, requiring a catheter to allow urination.

Many people are immune to developing herpes, while others are highly susceptible. The mate of a herpes sufferer can go through life without ever contracting it. Others, particularly those with atopic dermatitis and those who are on medication for cancer treatment, may develop severe, widespread infections in which their entire body is covered with herpes simplex blisters.

Once a person is infected, the virus travels up the nerves that supply the infected part of the skin. It then remains dormant in the nerve until a stimulus causes the virus to travel down the nerve and cause blister eruption. While we know the course of the infection, little is known about why it acts in this manner.

As may be expected, herpes Type II infections can be spread by intercourse. A woman with active genital herpes infection should avoid sexual intercourse until the blisters heal. Newborns have no resistance to herpes, and it can be lethal to a child delivered through a vagina in which there is an active herpes sore. An obstetrician should evaluate a genital herpes infection, particularly if it occurs at delivery.

Treatment of herpes remains inadequate. Because it is caused by a virus rather than a bacterium, antibiotics have no effect, and so far, no vaccines or drugs have been developed that prevent or cure the disease. The best treatment at present is to rupture the blisters and dab the sores with alcohol or ether. Although a painful procedure, it encourages drying and thus hastens crust and scab formation so that healing can begin.

Herpes zoster (shingles) is a painful viral infection that looks like a collection of herpes simplex water blisters (vesicles) occurring most commonly in a straight line starting at mid-back and encircling the chest under the breast to the sternum (breastbone). The reason for the configuration is that herpes zoster infections also follow the distribution of nerve fibers on the skin. These nerves originate in the spinal column, extend laterally on each side of the back, wrap around, and end in the middle of the chest, on the face, and in the midline on the front of the chest. Nerves also extend down the limbs to the fingers and toes. Stabbing or burning pain may precede the skin changes by a few days.

Herpes zoster is a disease whose virus also causes chicken pox (varicella). Scientists believe that a few virus particles lie dormant in the nerve roots after recovery from a childhood case of chicken pox and, at some later time in adult life, the zoster virus descends down the nerve fiber, infecting the skin along its path. Since the virus particle is the same, children who have never had chicken pox can sometimes develop active cases of chicken pox from a person with herpes zoster. Since each nerve tract only supplies half of the body, zoster infections occur on only one half of the body. Usually only a single nerve is involved. The herpes zoster virus is related to the herpes simplex virus, but is not identical.

Most herpes zoster attacks resolve in two to four weeks. Wet soaks and pain-killing medications are the usual treatment. Severe infections causing intense discomfort, or those occurring in the elderly, may benefit from a course of strong cortisone-type medication. Occasionally, pain will linger after the infection has resolved, but recurrences are very rare. Infections on the face that involve the eye should be seen by an ophthalmologist to prevent permanent damage to vision.

Impetigo is a superficial skin infection that may occur anywhere on the body. It consists of a honey-colored patch, crusted and itching. The infection is caused by staphylococcus and streptococcus bacteria, and may occur in a simple cut or following an episode of folliculitis (inflammation of the hair follicles). Transmission from one person to another often occurs, particularly when people share shaving instruments, washcloths, and towels. It is common in children, and usually the first outbreak is on the leg. Antibiotic tablets rapidly cure the disease, and symptomatic relief can be had by applying warm compresses soaked in Burow's solution, available in tablet or powder form at any drugstore.

Intertrigo produces a dull, pink, sharply defined inflammation in skin folds that also may itch. Intertrigo is most notably found under the breasts and in the groin. The two surfaces that are in constant touch with one another are involved equally. Women who are overweight or who have pendulous breasts seem to be most bothered by this problem. The exact mechanism of intertrigo is unknown. The moist environment produced by the two opposing surfaces prevents aeration, and normal friction can lead to trapped secretions and dead cells, all of which add to the potentially irritating milieu. Aerating the skin surfaces and appying hydrocortisone cream help heal the condition.

Bacterial Infections

Boils and abscesses occur when bacteria on the skin invade the deeper portions of the skin and cause a localized infection. As with many infections, early signs are redness, localized warmth, and tenderness. At this stage, the body's defense mechanisms mount an attack against the rapidly dividing bacteria, and pus accumulates as the bacteria and surrounding infected tissue are destroyed by the white blood cells. Boils are the early inflammatory state and can turn into abscesses — collections of pus — if untreated.

The staphylococcus bacterium is the most common cause of abscesses. Time-honored home remedies are effective for early treatment of these skin infections. Warm soaks in plain tap water, or in water mixed with Burow's solution, repeated at least four times a day for periods of 30 minutes help soothe the inflammation, cause more blood to flow to the area to fight the infection, and encourage a "head" of pus to form. Spontaneous drainage usually follows, although doctors often prescribe antibiotics like erythromycin, dicloxacillin, or tetracycline to speed resolution.

Diseases of the Skin

Some skin conditions result from specific diseases of the skin itself. Some of these diseases — such as dermatitis — are relatively common and may cause only minor discomfort. Other diseases — such as melanoma — are rare and life-threatening.

Dermatitis

Dermatitis is an inflammation of the skin. Four types of dermatitis are discussed in this section —contact dermatitis, irritant dermatitis, seborrheic dermatitis, and stasis dermatitis.

Contact dermatitis is a condition affecting more than 10 million people in the United States. The manifestations of the disease are itching, crusted, red raised patches frequently occurring at body sites that come into contact with a particular substance or object. The five most common agents causing contact dermatitis are: poison ivy (as well as oak and sumac), paraphenylenediamine (used in hair dyes, fur dyes, leather processing, and rubber manufacturing), nickel (in jewelry, wristwatches, zippers, and bra clasps), rubber compounds, and ethylenediamine.

Many other agents and substances also cause contact dermatitis. The only way to prove a contact allergy is to apply a very small amount of the substance to the skin and see if a reaction develops. If the reaction occurs in the armpits, the cause may be deodorants and antiperspirants. If it is on the neck and behind the ears, it may be perfumes. If it is limited to the earlobes, suspect nickel-containing earrings. If it is in the mid upper back, think of the metal in bra clasps. If the rash has sharp borders and follows the area covered by a particular piece of clothing, consider the chemicals and dyes used in manufacturing clothing. Rings and watches produce obvious, well-localized rashes. The same condition on the tops of the feet suggests leather-tanning products. Rashes on the sides and bottom of the feet may be due to the rubber and glues used in shoe manufacturing. A person who suspects any of these conditions should see a dermatologist or allergist for testing, since contact dermatitis and fungus infections can be easily confused.

Irritant dermatitis can occur in normal women whose skin dries out easily or who subject their hands to solvents, strong detergents, and constant hand washing. The resultant condition may look and feel like the scaling, fissuring, red eczematous conditions described opposite. Minimizing or eliminating exposure to the irritating elements speeds recovery. The skin beneath wedding rings is a common site for irritant dermatitis since water and detergents can become trapped under the ring and cause irritation.

Seborrheic dermatitis is characterized by yellow-pink patches that are scaly and slightly greasy in appearance. They appear on the areas of distribution of the sebaceous glands — the scalp, face, ears, and chest — and the condition usually is milder in women than in men. When it occurs on the scalp, it frequently causes dandruff. It is easy to treat, however, because the excessive dandruff associated with seborrheic dermatitis usually responds to a medicated shampoo or to hydrocortisone cream. Although the condition is likely to recur, it usually responds to the same medications.

Stasis dermatitis is a condition that predominantly affects the ankle. It occurs in people who stand much of the day, and in those who are overweight or who have had heart failure or a leg injury causing abnormalities in circulation.

In its mildest form, stasis dermatitis causes mild itching, superficial flaking, dry skin, and sometimes slight redness. Altered pressure relationships between the arteries, veins, and lymphatics (vessels that convey lymph) presumably play a major role. As the abnormalities progress, leakage of blood occurs from the weakest vessels, the capillaries, producing pinpoint, painless bruises on the skin called *petechiae*. As the petechiae heal, the red-purple color changes to light brown. Severe stasis dermatitis causes ulcers near the ankles. The ulcers are usually painless unless they become infected.

The dryness, chapping, and mild inflammation of stasis dermatitis can be treated with hydrocortisone cream and lubricating salves. In addition, patients should wear support stockings. Indeed, any woman who works at a job that requires considerable standing should wear support stockings, regardless of her age. The only type of support stockings of any value are those available from a surgical supply house or a special retail outlet. Those advertised on television and available in supermarkets do not supply enough support. Women with stasis dermatitis, as well as those working in jobs that demand standing for long periods of time, also should take regular breaks during which they elevate the legs.

Eczema

Eczema is a condition that is frequently used synonymously with dermatitis. They both refer to a variety of conditions that may be subdivided into many categories. In some cases, a known irritation precedes development of the rash, while in others, it is a seasonal occurrence that heralds the beginning of winter or a drop in the humidity. In still other people, it is a constant problem that always involves the same area of the skin throughout life. Generally, the rash consists of dry patches, redness, cracking, crusting, and thickened skin, or it may be signaled by occasional small water blisters.

Atopic eczema is a unique form of exzema. It characteristically starts in infancy with an itching rash on the cheeks, arms, and legs. In childhood, the rash may localize at the back of the legs behind the knees and in a similar location on the arms at the inner side of the elbow. Severe cases involve the eyelids, waist, neck, and trunk. Atopic eczema is usually worse in the winter, and those with the disease frequently have hay fever and asthma as well. The condition is often inherited from a parent, and all the siblings may develop it. Atopic eczema usually resolves by puberty.

Although most patients with the condition are very healthy in every other respect, a rare atopic will suffer repeated skin infections and be in need of frequent antibiotic therapy. Cataracts sometimes can occur.

Of gravest concern, however, is protection from viral infections. Herpes simplex infections and smallpox vaccinations can cause serious, extensive, viral infections in the skin that may spread to the internal organs. For this reason, people with atopic eczema should not be given smallpox vaccinations, nor should they come in contact with anyone who recently has been vaccinated. Spouses or close relatives of atopics also should *not* receive smallpox vaccinations. There are rare occasions, however, when the benefits of vaccination outweigh the risks.

Essential to eczema treatment is the replenishment of moisture in the skin and judicious use of steroids, salves, and creams while the condition is active. Antihistamines help suppress the itching associated with eczema. People afflicted with atopic eczema should use mild soap that does not remove natural skin moisturizers; for the same reason, they should bathe less frequently to prevent skin dryness. It is also helpful to avoid wool fibers, harsh chemicals, and strong detergents, and to use moisturing creams.

Dyshidrotic eczema produces itching symptoms similar to atopic eczema, but the condition is limited to the hands and feet. This form of eczema is characterized by small water blisters deep on the sides of the fingers, sometimes involving the palms and soles. The blisters occur deep in the skin, and because the skin is so thick in these areas, cause just a pinhead-size collection of fluid. Itching is usually intense and sufferers are unable to avoid scratching.

The condition is often worse in the summer, with "attacks" lasting for over a month, but then resolving for no apparent reason. There are no connections with other types of eczema, but treatment consists of applying strong steroid creams with overnight use of cotton gloves to increase absorption of the medicine.

Nummular eczema is the name given to small round, itchy patches of eczema that have the same surface characteristics as atopic eczema. Treatment is exactly the same as for atopic eczema. Nummular eczema can occur in any person, but many atopic individuals who seem to have "outgrown" their atopic disease continue to get patches of nummular eczema.

Psoriasis

Psoriasis is a noncontagious common disease characterized by itchy, thick, silvery scales on top of reddened skin, which are called plaques. Psoriasis frequently occurs on the elbows and knees, although the same thick scaling plaque can occur on the scalp, where it may be mistaken for dandruff or seborrheic dermatitis. The exact cause of the disease is unknown, but inheritance seems to play a major role.

The course of the disease is variable and unpredictable. The first attack of psoriasis may follow a streptococcal throat infection, and appear as a shower of ¼-inch-diameter small red spots, all of which have a fine white scale. In active cases,

psoriasis may occur following a scratch or nick in normal skin. This is called the "Koebner phenomenon," a condition that may clear with treatment and not return for years. More commonly, however, the disease will recur after a variable length of time. The small spots may be replaced by sparse, larger plaques in the characteristic areas mentioned above, or occur at almost any other site of the body. Severe cases, with over half the body covered with psoriasis, may require hospitalization.

In psoriasis, the skin grows five times faster than normal. This phenomenon produces considerable scale that is dead and unable to shed naturally. Consequently, the more successful treatments appear to be those that actually slow down skin reproduction.

SKIN CANCER

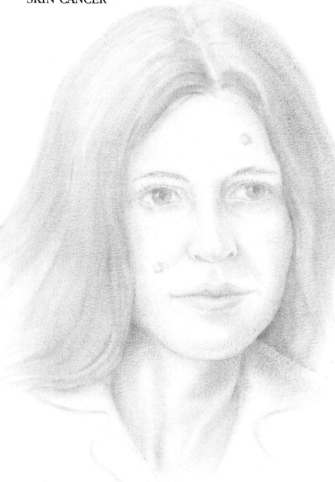

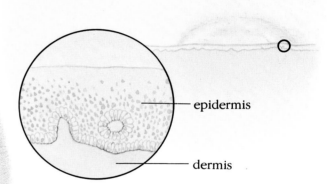

BASAL-CELL CARCINOMA *is the most common type of skin cancer, and may start as a ⅛-inch to ¼-inch skin-colored bump. Over a period of a few years, the bump grows to form a pearl-colored ring with a central depression and a scab in the center.*

SQUAMOUS-CELL CARCINOMA *is usually noticed when it is quite small—⅛ to ¼ inch in diameter. This skin cancer is round with an irregular, raised, dark pink border and a central ulcer or scab.*

The enlargements indicate that the two types of cancer look quite different under the microscope. Both are generally treated by surgical removal.

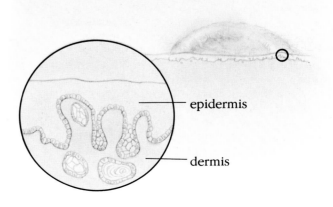

Methotrexate, used for severe cases, is a potent drug that slows down division of cells. Unfortunately, it is not selective for skin cells and thus affects all tissues of the body. For this reason, the benefits of the drug must be weighed against its liabilities.

For less-severe cases, psoriasis is treated with steroid creams and ointments supplemented with coal-tar preparations and ultraviolet light. The use of crude coal tar is unappealing, yet it has a significant healing property that is noticeable within one week. Special ultraviolet light boxes, generally only available to physicians, also speed resolution of the disease. The ultraviolet lamps and light bulbs generally available for home use do not generate enough ultraviolet light to be of much benefit. A new experimental treatment, abbreviated PUVA, consists of taking a drug that increases the beneficial effects of ultraviolet light. Many people who have never responded to any treatment have totally cleared with PUVA. Generally speaking, persons with psoriasis find that their skin heals in the summer and worsens in the winter, and those who live in or vacation in the sunbelt do better than those living in the cloudier regions of the country.

Keratosis

Actinic keratoses are small pink-tan rough spots that occur on the face, the backs of the hands, the upper chest, and back, and are caused by many years of excess sunlight. Starting as small areas of dilated blood vessels, they become homogeneously light pink and scaly, although thinner than the scale of seborrheic keratoses (see below). Women with fair complexions and red or blond hair may develop actinic keratoses as early as their twenties, but they usually occur in the 50-to-60 age group. If untreated, a small percentage of these keratoses will turn into slow-growing skin cancers.

Like seborrheic keratoses, actinic keratoses can be treated with liquid nitrogen and with daily application of "5-FU" (5-fluorouracil) for three weeks. After several days of treatment, this medication causes the sun-damaged skin to become inflamed and to form crusts. As the skin heals, the actinic keratoses are replaced by normal skin. Many women who have led lives full of outdoor activities have this treatment when they reach their early sixties. But prevention with a good sunscreen is the best treatment.

Seborrheic keratoses are gray-tan to dark brown spots that commonly occur on the face, neck, upper back, chest, and arms of women in their fifties. The spots vary in size from one-half to one inch in diameter. Although initially flat, the spots gradually thicken to an elevated surface that is often shiny, scaly, and greasy, with the appearance of being pasted onto the skin. Sunlight-induced damage contributes to the growth of these lesions; however, they are benign growths that scrape off easily after being frozen with liquid nitrogen. Despite treatment, some growths will recur months or years after treatment.

Alopecia Areata

Alopecia areata is a disease in which, for reasons as yet unknown, the body attacks its own hair follicles. Hair falls out in round patches, leaving one or many totally bald areas on the scalp. The process may evolve over many months, and usually resolves with renewed hair growth. When it occurs in adults, there is a good chance of total recovery without the need of medications. But when it occurs in children, regrowth is paradoxically less likely, and many affected children develop extensive bald areas.

Skin Cancer

Basal-cell carcinoma is the most common type of skin cancer. It occurs in the same distribution as do actinic keratoses (see opposite), but most commonly on the face. People who sunburn easily are most susceptible to this condition, and women with fair skin who spend a great deal of time in the sun increase their risk of developing basal-cell tumors.

These skin cancers first start as a ⅛-inch to ¼-inch normal skin-colored bump that may have telangiectases (see page 568). Over a period of a few years, the bump slowly grows to form a pearl-colored ring that has a central depression with a scab in the center. Basal-cell cancers are easily removed. If treated early, they do not spread through the body as do most internal malignancies. It is important, however, to remove the tumors when small, because they will continue to grow and to cause damage to surrounding tissues. People susceptible to cancers, and certainly those treated, should always use sunscreens prior to sun exposure.

Squamous-cell carcinoma is the second most common skin cancer. Like basal-cell carcinoma, it occurs on sun-exposed skin in fair-complected people. Individuals who have received X-ray treatments to the head and neck for acne are also at risk of developing these tumors.

Squamous-cell carcinomas usually go unnoticed until they measure ⅛ inch to ¼ inch in diameter, when they will have an irregular, raised, dark pink border with a central ulcer. The cancer may bleed spontaneously and have a central scab with surrounding inflamed and thickened skin. These tumors are often treated by local excision. They grow faster than basal-cell carcinomas, but only rarely spread to nearby structures. Women who have had these cancers should use the same sun precautions as those who have had basal-cell carcinomas.

Melanomas are highly malignant skin cancers that can be mistaken for common moles; it is sometimes impossible for a layman to differentiate a melanoma from a nevus (mole). The features that suggest that a pigmented bump or spot is a melanoma are: change in color to black, dark red, or dark blue; spontaneous bleeding; and increase in size. They occur most frequently on sun-exposed skin in pale-complected, blue-eyed Anglo Saxons. Dark-skinned people have a considerably lower incidence of melanoma, while the fair-skinned English of Celtic origin have the highest incidence in the world. Also, those living in the southern latitudes of the United States have a higher incidence than those in the north.

In women, the lower legs are the most frequent site for the cancer to develop. Next in frequency are the arms and head. A dermatologist should see any mole that fits one or more of the above criteria or that concerns the patient. Fortunately, the vast majority of nevi brought to the attention of dermatologists are benign. Melanomas removed in the early stages can result in a total cure, but if the melanoma invades ⅛ inch into the skin, it may be lethal. The mortality rate for such an invasion is 50 percent.

Pityriasis Rosea

Pityriasis rosea is a disease consisting of multiple, minimally itchy, pink-fawn flat patches that occur on the trunk. They are usually oval, with the more pointed ends pointing to the sides or center of the body, rather than up or down. There is no known cause for the eruption, but many suspect it is due to a virus; more cases are seen in the spring than in the fall. The rash lasts from four to six weeks. Two to three minutes of ultraviolet exposure may induce a speedier recovery, and hydrocortisone creams can be applied to soothe any mild itching.

Rosacea

Rosacea is a disease occurring in 30- to 50-year-old women and causes redness, bumps, and tiny dilated blood vessels in the middle of the face. Occasionally, the dome-shaped bumps have pus in the center. The course of rosacea is unpredictable, and its cause is unknown, however stress and fatigue may worsen it. Tetracycline and drying creams are often helpful in treating this condition.

THE DANGER SIGNALS OF MELANOMA

It is sometimes difficult to see the difference between a mole and a melanoma. A change in color to black, dark red, or dark blue; spontaneous bleeding; or increase in size are all signals to have a mole examined by your doctor. Melanomas removed in their early stages of development can result in a total cure.

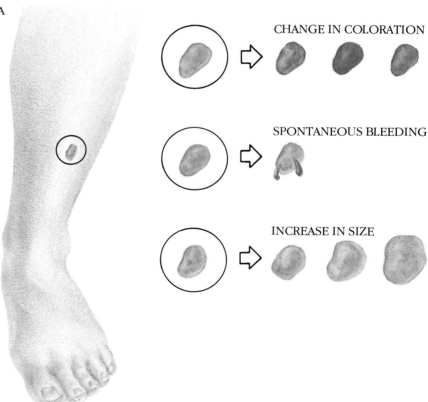

CHANGE IN COLORATION

SPONTANEOUS BLEEDING

INCREASE IN SIZE

Skin Conditions and Disease

Skin conditions also may be manifestations of disease elsewhere in the body. Several such diseases and their skin manifestations are discussed below.

Hives (urticaria) are slightly elevated white-pink, smooth-surfaced, itchy bumps on the skin. They may be as small as ¼ inch or as large as several inches. At least one out of every five women has an episode of urticaria at some time in her life, lasting from minutes to hours. Allergies to medicines, particularly to aspirin and penicillin, are among the most common causes of urticaria. Foods such as nuts, eggs, shellfish, chocolate, and certain fruits frequently can cause urticaria in susceptible individuals. Some infections, hepatitis, and other internal medical conditions also cause hives, and in rare cases, pressure, cold, heat, and anxiety can cause attacks.

A woman who has had several episodes of urticaria should conduct a thorough examination of her environment, assessing what she has eaten, what types of fabrics she wears, what medications she takes, and new pets and cosmetics. Unfortunately, documentation of the specific urticaria-inducing substance is made in only a quarter of cases. Antihistamines and soothing lotions are used to help treat the condition.

Gonorrhea is a bacterial infection usually spread by direct sexual contact. Although the infection can cause considerable damage, the gonorrhea organism is fragile, dying quickly when exposed to air or deprived of body warmth. For these reasons, the mucous membranes of the vagina, rectum, and throat are ideal sites for infection. No distinctive lesions appear on infected surfaces as with the person who has hives or acne. Instead, gonorrhea may cause a foul-smelling yellow discharge that occurs within one to two weeks of infection. If not diagnosed and treated at this stage, many infections spread to the fallopian tubes and ovaries, causing painful abdominal disease that results in sterility. A small percentage of infections spread through the blood to cause arthritis and a distinctive rash. The rash consists of ¼-inch-wide pink spots having a purple central dot. There are usually less than ten of these spots and they occur over joints infected with gonorrhea organisms, particularly the wrists, fingers, ankles, and feet.

Syphilis is the third most common venereal disease. The characteristic skin lesion of primary syphilis is a small, relatively painless ulcer that has firm borders and a sharply defined "punched-out" appearing center. The syphilitic ulcer forms ten days to four weeks after initial exposure, and almost always heals without antibiotics. There is no discharge as in gonorrhea. The bacterialike organisms thrive in the ulcer and will infect the skin that comes in contact with it. The fact that the ulcer can occur on any part of the genitalia can make discovery difficult. However, the syphilis organism has already entered the bloodstream and is growing in the body by the time an ulcer is discovered.

Two months to a year pass before the majority of untreated patients develop the signs of secondary syphilis. In this stage, there are widespread red-brown, round patches occurring on both flanks, palms, soles, and on the mucosal surfaces. Syphilis has been called "the great imitator" because its symptoms mimic those of other diseases. In addition to the flat red patches just described, there may be widespread small red bumps no more than ¼ inch in diameter. Women and men can develop a pink, warty growth on the genitals called condylomata. Small red bumps and flat patches on the palms and soles may form a scale, and there may be loss of scalp hair in diffuse patches.

Many doctors routinely test for syphilis and gonorrhea as part of the regular medical examination of any person in their sexually active years. Since treatment is very effective and infections are often inapparent, cautious doctors perform these tests as preventive measures. Most of the antibiotics used to treat gonorrhea are also effective against syphilis, but dosages and the length of treatment are different.

Necrobiosis is a skin lesion that occurs in diabetics. In this condition, small red bumps form oval, scarred patches with depressed yellow centers and purple borders. The diabetic should see a dermatologist for treatment of necrobiosis.

Systemic lupus erythematosus (lupus) (see page 642) is a much rarer disease than skin cancer, predominantly affecting women in their twenties and thirties. It is eight times more common in women than in men. The most characteristic feature of the disease is a red rash with telangiectasia (see page 568) occurring under both lower eyelids onto the upper cheeks. A sudden long exposure to sunlight may bring out the rash which, because of its distribution, is nicknamed a "butterfly rash." Quite often the cutaneous signs of SLE are very subtle, and are frequently accompanied by diffuse joint pains, fever, and lethargy. Nevertheless, the signs and symptoms are quite diverse so that lupus is often mistaken for seborrheic dermatitis, arthritis, or the flu. Simple blood tests can confirm the diagnosis of lupus. Strong steroid medications are used to control the disease in order to prevent permanent damage to the skin and internal organs.

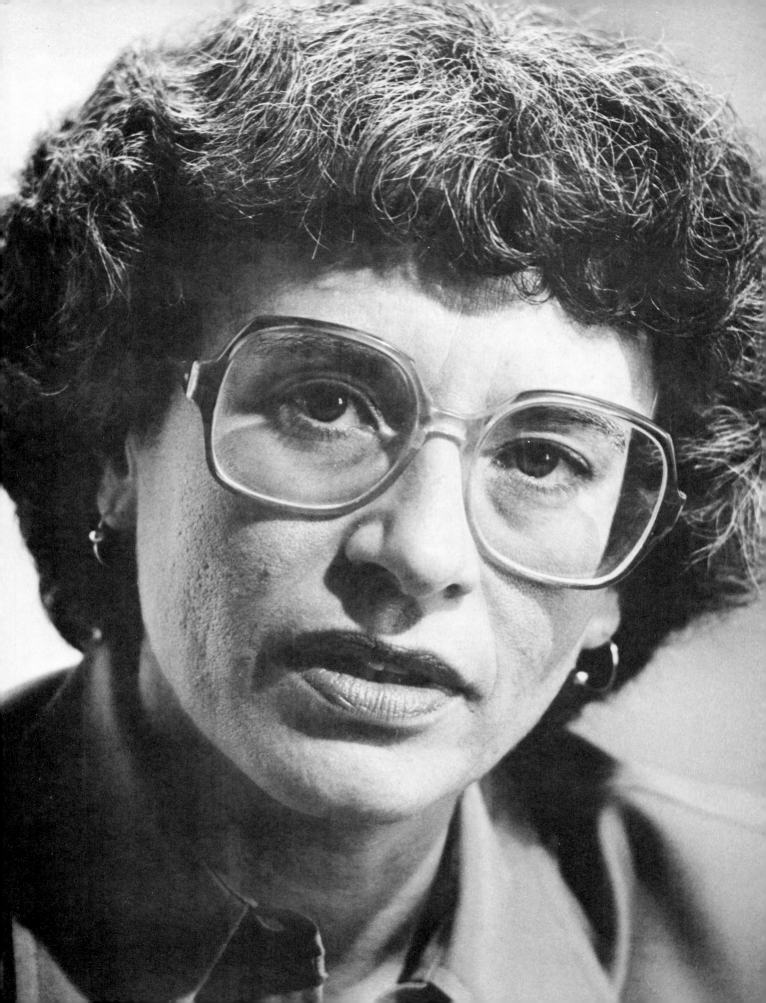

CHAPTER 28

CIRCULATORY DISORDERS

DORIS GOODMAN, M.D.

Blood and the system that circulates it throughout our bodies are essential to life. Though we may be barely conscious of the sound of our heartbeat, it is a vital sign that indicates life or death.

The circulatory system is a series of closed pipelines that carries blood in a circular path around the body. It is the heart that furnishes the pressure to keep the blood moving. And this small organ, about the size of your fist and weighing less than a pound, must be kept healthy if you value your health and your life.

Circulatory Disorders

More than cancer, more than accidents—your chances of dying from heart disease are greater than the risk you run from any other cause of death. Ailments of the heart and blood vessels do not discriminate between men and women when they strike. With a few notable exceptions, they affect both sexes, have the same causes, and require similar treatments. But they don't affect both sexes equally. Deaths and death rates for diseases of the heart are higher for men at all ages. And in women, certain types of cardiovascular disease have a more benign course, occur later in life, and do less damage to other vital organs.

In discussing various diseases of the cardiovascular system, this chapter will point out those aspects that are unique to women, and will emphasize the different approaches to managing cardiovascular problems.

The Heart and Circulation

The heart is a "sexless" organ. It is a pumping muscle with the relatively simple function of distributing blood and nutrients to the entire body through a network of blood vessels. These blood-transporting channels can be likened to a tree trunk that branches off into progressively smaller limbs. The trunks or distributing blood vessels are called arteries, and the final twigs of the arterial system are the capillaries that supply blood to the periphery of the body—for example, the skin surface of the fingers and toes.

Blood returns from the periphery to the heart through the veins, which follow the branching pattern in reverse, returning "used" blood to the heart through progressively larger trunks. This "used" blood is replenished with oxygen as it circulates through the lungs (see page 589), after which it is then ready to be recycled through the arteries. The arteries and veins are aptly called the vascular tree, and together with the heart, comprise the circulatory system.

The heart itself gets oxygen from its own supply system, the coronary arteries (see page 589). It pumps ceaselessly, about seventy times each minute, delivering blood as needed—whether it be to the body of a top-form marathon runner or to that of a pregnant woman whose uterus must support the circulation of one or more unborn infants. For example, to accommodate the increased needs of pregnancy, the mother's blood volume increases significantly and her heart muscle fibers become thicker and longer during the period of most rapid fetal growth.

The heart and the vascular tree function as a unit in health and disease, although both parts of the circulatory system may not be equally affected when dysfunction occurs. In addition to defining common cardiovascular problems, this chapter also describes other conditions that mimic heart disease, as well as certain harmless heart signs and symptoms that may cause needless worry or unnecessary restriction in individual behavior and life-style.

Types of Heart Disease

Cardiomyopathy

Cardiomyopathy simply means "diseased heart muscle" and is a rather vague category covering a multitude of ills. Its causes may be known or unknown. The list of known causes of cardiomyopathy includes drugs, endocrine diseases (such as diabetes and thyroid disorders), hereditary illnesses (sickle-cell anemia and muscular dystrophies), and hypertension. In our society, alcoholism is another significant cause of cardiomyopathy. Alcohol is toxic to the heart muscle, poisoning various enzyme systems (the energy-manufacturing elements of heart muscle cells) and weakening the pumping ability of the heart. An alcoholic heart patient will show symptoms that usually include a stretched, flabby heart, irregularities of heartbeat, the tendency to retain fluid, and clot formation.

Other drugs and chemicals known to damage heart muscle cells include certain anti-cancer drugs, tranquilizers, and mood elevators; nicotine and caffeine irritate the heart muscle and cause "skipped beats." While amphetamines (such as "diet pills") do not act on heart muscle cells directly, they may have the effect of a shot of adrenaline, speeding heart rate and increasing pumping so that the heart is constantly driven to work harder and faster—a condition analogous to running a race standing still. In addition to stressing the heart, these stimulants cause nervousness, tremors, and insomnia, and reduce the ability to concentrate. In short, they exact a severe price for their weak effect of suppressing the appetite and giving the illusion of energy.

In cardiology as in other fields, we now know that all drugs have side effects, and that the perfectly "safe" drug is a myth.

Congenital Heart Disease

This category includes heart or vascular defects that are present at birth. These defects include deformed heart valves (valves that are too tight or that leak), holes between heart chambers, underdeveloped heart muscle tissue, misplaced or deformed blood channels leading to or from the heart, or combinations of these defects. Some hearts may be so seriously deformed that the infant survives only a short while after birth. Other congenital malformations are not life-threatening if treated, although they may severely limit the child's activity. Congenital heart disease affects both sexes equally, and "blue babies," those suffering from lack of oxygen in the blood due to congenital heart problems, can be either male or female.

Don't confuse congenital heart disease with inherited heart abnormalities. An example of congenital heart disease might be an infant born with a malformed heart because its mother had rubella (German measles). On the other hand, an infant may have heart disease because it was born with genes that cause sickle-cell anemia. These genes were, of course, inherited from the infant's parents, making this hereditary cardiomyopathy.

Acquired Heart Disease

The majority of heart ailments are neither congenital nor hereditary, but are acquired, and their list of causes is almost endless. Drugs, poisons, infections, hypertension, anemia, diabetes, an over- or underactive thyroid, and aging blood vessels all take their toll on the cardiovascular system. There are still other external factors whose effects on the heart remain controversial. Most cardiac specialists agree that severe prolonged emotional stress probably is detrimental to heart function. Less agreement exists about the effects of hard physical labor on a healthy heart. Does hard work hurt you? Evidence suggests that strenuous physical activity on a *regular* basis may actually protect a normal heart from degenerative changes.

Two types of acquired heart disease affect women only and are related to pregnancy and delivery.

Postpartum cardiomyopathy is a serious heart muscle weakness that develops rather suddenly from one day to several weeks following an apparently normal delivery. The first signs may be a sudden, dramatic heart enlargement resulting from a stretched, flabby muscle that has lost its pumping efficiency. The patient may complain of shortness of breath, severe fatigue, swelling of the abdomen and legs, and palpitations. X-ray studies will confirm the heart's enlargement and the fluid accumulations in the lungs, abdomen, and legs. The muscle contracts poorly and the heart rhythm may be irregular.

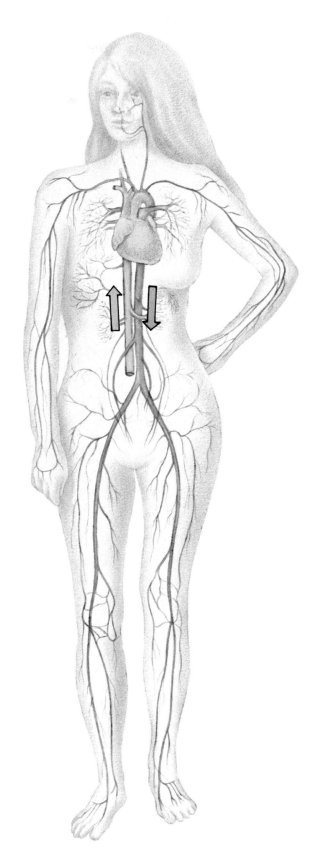

The Ten Leading Causes of Death for Men and Women

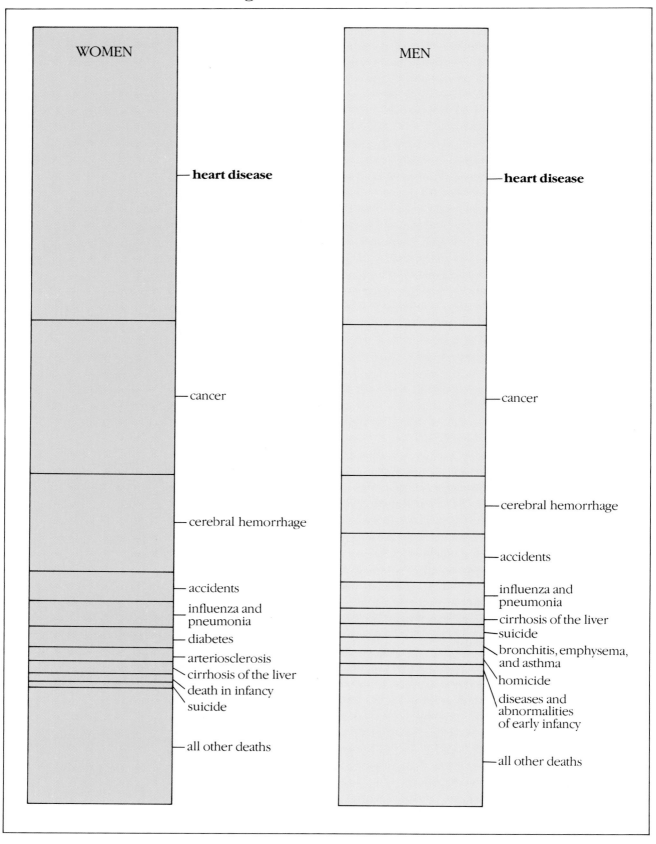

WOMEN

— **heart disease**

—cancer

—cerebral hemorrhage

—accidents

—influenza and pneumonia

—diabetes

—arteriosclerosis

—cirrhosis of the liver

—death in infancy

—suicide

—all other deaths

MEN

— **heart disease**

—cancer

—cerebral hemorrhage

—accidents

—influenza and pneumonia

—cirrhosis of the liver

—suicide

—bronchitis, emphysema, and asthma

—homicide

—diseases and abnormalities of early infancy

—all other deaths

Deaths and Death Rates for Diseases of the Heart

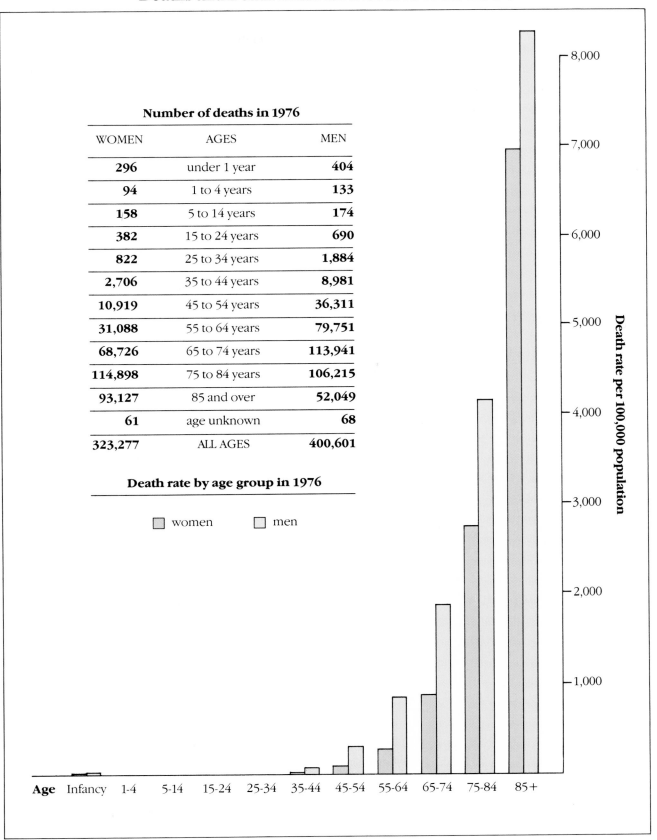

Number of deaths in 1976

WOMEN	AGES	MEN
296	under 1 year	404
94	1 to 4 years	133
158	5 to 14 years	174
382	15 to 24 years	690
822	25 to 34 years	1,884
2,706	35 to 44 years	8,981
10,919	45 to 54 years	36,311
31,088	55 to 64 years	79,751
68,726	65 to 74 years	113,941
114,898	75 to 84 years	106,215
93,127	85 and over	52,049
61	age unknown	68
323,277	ALL AGES	400,601

Death rate by age group in 1976

☐ women   ☐ men

Death rate per 100,000 population

Age   Infancy   1-4   5-14   15-24   25-34   35-44   45-54   55-64   65-74   75-84   85+

THE HEART

The heart is located between the breasts in the center of the chest, and has its own cavity, called the pericardial cavity. Here it is protected by the sternum and the rib cage. Blood flows from the body into the heart's right atrium (RA), passes through valves into the right ventricle (RV), and then is pumped out through the pulmonary artery (PA) to the lungs. Freshly oxygenated blood returns to the heart from the lungs, enters the left atrium (LA), and flows through valves into the left ventricle (LV), where it is pumped through the aorta (A) to the rest of the body.

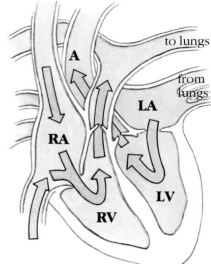

☐ oxygenated blood

☐ deoxygenated blood

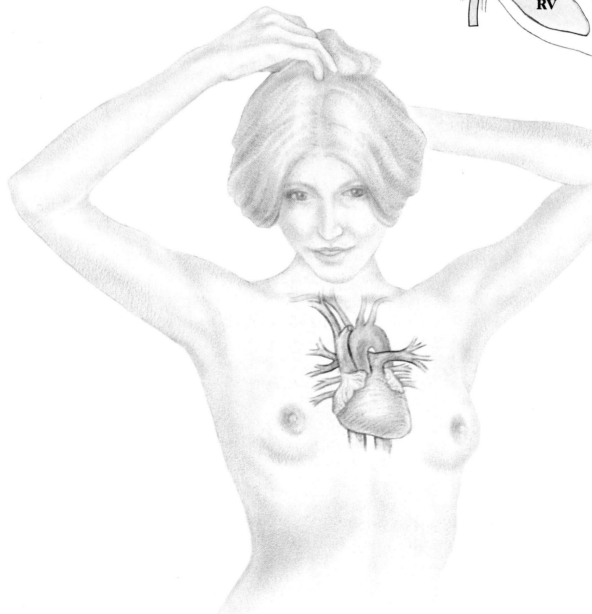

BLOOD CIRCULATION FROM THE HEART TO THE LUNGS

Blood from the body returns to the heart depleted of oxygen and carrying waste carbon dioxide. This "used" blood is pumped immediately to the lungs (follow arrows below), where the carbon dioxide passes from *the blood to the lungs and is exhaled, and oxygen enters the blood. The oxygenated blood then returns to the left atrium of the heart and is pumped out the aorta to the various organs of the body.*

RIGHT LUNG

LEFT LUNG

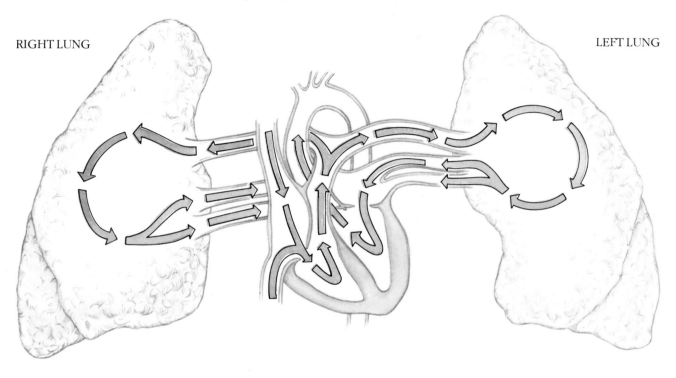

CORONARY BLOOD SUPPLY

The first organ to receive freshly oxygenated blood is the heart itself, for the coronary arteries exit right at the base of the aorta. The heart gets its greatest flow of blood when the ventricles relax from a beat (diastole). When the heart contracts (systole), flow through the coronary arteries is greatly reduced. This situation is unique to the *heart; other organs behave exactly the opposite, getting their greatest blood flow during heart contractions.*

Coronary arteries branch into arterioles and capillaries. After the blood leaves the capillary beds in the heart musculature, it flows into veins and returns to the right and left atria.

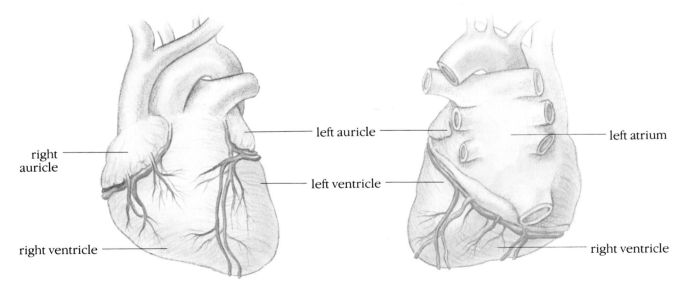

right auricle

left auricle

left atrium

left ventricle

right ventricle

right ventricle

With proper treatment, the condition may improve partially or completely. Some women, however, develop chronic heart failure that is unresponsive to any known treatment, and die.

As in many cardiomyopathies, the cause of postpartum cardiomyopathy is unknown. One theory states that an unknown substance present in the body during delivery may act as a toxin to the individual's own heart tissue: an "allergy to self" phenomenon. If a woman survives postpartum cardiomyopathy, she should undertake further pregnancies with great caution or not at all. The chances of the disease recurring at another pregnancy are great.

Toxemia of pregnancy is another acquired cardiovascular disease whose most dramatic effects are on the arteries. A previously healthy woman with no blood pressure problems may suddenly develop sky-high blood pressure during active labor. The danger here is doubled. In the mother, the dangerously high blood pressure levels may cause hemorrhage in the vessels of the eyes, brain, and kidneys, and possibly even convulsions or coma because of oxygen-deprived brain tissues. The deranged circulation also may deprive the infant of blood and oxygen through the placenta, resulting in damage to the child, or even the infant's death.

Toxemia of pregnancy is a medical emergency requiring the constant attendance of an experienced doctor and nursing staff. Heroic efforts must be made to bring the mother's blood pressure down to safe levels in order to save two lives. Once the baby is born either by natural or obstetrical means, the toxemia condition is considered to be "cured."

The cause of toxemia, also known as preeclampsia and eclampsia in its more severe stages, is still unknown. It occurs in 6 to 7 percent of all pregnancies, and is more common in cases of twins or triplets, and when the mother is diabetic. About 75 percent of toxemia cases occur in first pregnancies.

The earliest noticeable signs of toxemia are increased blood pressure, excessive weight gain, excessive swelling, and the presence of albumin in the urine. Severe persistent headache, drowsiness, amnesia, vertigo, and visual disturbances also are signs that the disease is becoming dangerously severe.

Mild toxemia can be controlled by diet, rest, and sedation. However, if the eclampsia threatens to become severe, early induction of labor or a cesarean section may be necessary.

In the United States, toxemia causes about one-third of all maternal deaths from pregnancy, and about 30,000 stillbirths or neonatal deaths per year.

Valvular Heart Disease

Valvular heart disease may be congenital or acquired. The acquired type is usually caused by a childhood case of rheumatic fever, a disease that is said to "lick the joints and bite the heart." Rheumatic fever is a disease of the connective tissue that follows strep infections. It is most damaging when it scars the heart muscle or valves, producing rheumatic heart disease. The inflammation in the heart heals after weeks or months, and the child is thought to be cured. However, healing proceeds to scarring, and over many years there is a gradual thickening, stiffening, and deformity of the heart valves. The process is slow and insidious, and symptoms of valve dysfunction may not appear until middle-age.

In the United States, rheumatic fever in children is definitely on the decline. However, cardiologists still see enough adults with heart valve problems to indicate that these individuals sustained the initial inflammation 20, 30, or more years previously.

Commonly, the two left-sided heart valves are affected. These are the mitral valve (the inlet valve to the left side of the heart) and the aortic valve (the outlet valve from the left side of the heart to the body). Either or both valves may disrupt blood flow if they are too tight (stenosis) or if they leak (insufficiency).

Despite the fact that boys and girls get rheumatic fever in about equal proportions, adult women get rheumatic heart disease more often than adult men. The usual patient with mitral valve stenosis is a middle-aged woman who comes to the doctor with complaints of fatigue, weakness, shortness of breath, palpitations, cold hands and feet, and nervousness. Many such women are written off by their doctors as being "just nervous" or depressed, and the diagnosis is easily missed without a careful examination. Valvular disease also may first show up during pregnancy, when added strain aggravates any congenital weakness.

Aortic valve disease is the type more commonly seen in middle-aged or older men. Although childhood rheumatic fever may be the culprit, the most common cause here is a congenital deformity of the aortic valve that progressed to scarring as years passed. Both types of valve disease may occur in both sexes, and good treatment is available.

Mitral valve disease, especially stenosis, lessens the amount of blood available for distribution to other organs—including the nourishing organ for the fetus, the placenta. Pregnant women with mitral valve disease have a great tendency to form blood clots within the heart that may detach and travel via the circulation to other body sites. The medical treatment for this clotting tendency includes drugs (anticoagulants) that render the blood less coagulable and protect against clot formation. As with most medications, these drugs have undesirable side effects. Patients taking anticoagulants are at greater risk of abnormal bleeding—a highly dangerous state during pregnancy and delivery for both mother and unborn child. The impaired cardiac function of the mother also may worsen with the added stress of supporting two circulations.

NORMAL HEART VALVES

SEMILUNAR VALVES *The semilunar valves are located at the entrance to the aorta and at the entrance to the pulmonary artery. Viewed from the top, each valve has three one-way flaps tightly closed when the heart is relaxed so that no blood can flow backward into the heart. When the ventricles contract, these flaps fly open in response to the pressure of the blood flow.*

Many children are born with deformities of these valves. Diseases such as rheumatic fever also can affect valve function (see the opposite page).

ATRIOVENTRICULAR VALVES *The atrioventricular valves lie at the opening between the atria and the ventricles in the heart. These valves have flaps of membrane (cusps) that are held in place by fibers called chordae tendinae. These fibers connect the flaps to the papillary muscles, which are anchored in the heart wall. When the heart contracts, these valves close, preventing the blood from flowing from the ventricles to the atria. When the heart is relaxed, they open, allowing the blood to flow from the atria into the ventricles.*

TOP VIEW OF SEMILUNAR VALVE

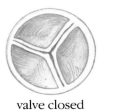
valve closed

valve open

TOP VIEW OF ATRIOVENTRICULAR VALVE

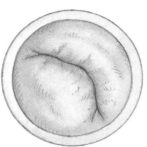
valve closed

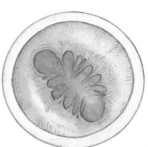
valve open

aorta

pulmonary artery

semilunar valves

atrioventricular valves

A pregnant woman with mitral valve disease must be followed closely, often by a cardiac consultant working along with her obstetrician, and especially near term and at delivery. Some women have required emergency valve surgery during pregnancy to lessen the risk for both mother and child.

Aortic valve disease, particularly stenosis, is especially dangerous during pregnancy; fortunately it is rare in women of childbearing age. The tight aortic valve limits the ability of the heart to deliver adequate amounts of blood to vital organs during the great circulatory stress of delivery. Because this may lead to sudden death of the mother, experienced cardiologists recommend terminating the pregnancy in a woman who is known to have aortic valve disease.

Coronary Heart Disease

The greatest thrust of current heart research is directed toward improved understanding and treatment of coronary heart disease—the most common cardiovascular affliction in humans. Basically the problem is one of aging blood vessels, or atherosclerosis of the heart's own arteries. The atherosclerotic or hardening process begins in infancy and progresses throughout life; all arteries undergo it.

The progress begins when fatty and fibrous deposits form on the inner walls of the coronary arteries. At first these crucial blood vessels show only some roughening and decreased elasticity. But with time, buildup of the deposits occurs and the channels may become narrowed and even completely blocked (see the opposite page). The effect is to deprive the heart muscle of its needed pathway for delivery of oxygen. The narrowed arteries still may be able to deliver enough blood through networks narrowed to only one-quarter of their original size, but further narrowing becomes critical when demand outstrips supply.

The oxygen-starved heart muscle signals its distress in the form of chest pain, called angina pectoris. Prompt resting or certain drugs may relieve the temporary state of oxygen lack and allow the muscle to continue pumping. But with severe or prolonged oxygen lack, the affected portion of heart muscle may not recuperate. The symptoms of such death of muscle tissue are severe chest pain lasting an hour or more, sweating, and fear of impending doom. This is the so-called "coronary attack" or myocardial infarction, a most significant cause of death in the United States today. Indeed, coronary heart disease causes one-third of all deaths in this country.

Survivors of a coronary attack may do well if the remaining heart muscle is able to carry the work of the dead tissue. But if tissue destruction has been extensive, even mild activity may bring on pain and other complicating symptoms.

There is a dramatic difference in the incidence of coronary disease between the sexes. In the 30- to 50-year age range, the victims are men by almost ten to one. After the fifth decade, however, both sexes are affected nearly equally.

Many reasons have been suggested to explain the favored status of women who enjoy protection from coronary disease in their early years. The premenopausal woman has significant levels of female hormones that are thought to be protective. After menopause, estrogen levels decline and nearly approach those of men, possibly increasing women's vulnerability to disease.

Prior to the current trend of more women working outside the home, there was a much larger difference in rates of coronary heart disease between the sexes. It would seem that the stresses of homemaking and child-rearing did not hasten the atherosclerotic process in the vascular tree as much as outside employment did. The proponents of this theory now point to the apparent earlier onset of coronary heart disease in business and career women.

And numerous other factors abound. Cigarette smoking is now known to cause earlier coronary disease, just as proper diet, weight control, and exercise are known to forestall it. Future medical research will lead to a better understanding of these and other factors that affect coronary disease.

Our present state of medical knowledge is firm on one point, however. There are two disorders that definitely nullify the protection from coronary events enjoyed by premenopausal women: hypertension and diabetes. Both hasten the aging of blood vessels. Women who suffer from one or both of these diseases lose their age-related advantage and can expect to be at earlier risk of coronary attack. Indeed, their risk is equal to that of men in the same age groups. Adequate medical and surgical treatment is available for high blood pressure, but whether this treatment may restore some of the odds in women's favor is unknown.

Hypertension and Circulation

Along with coronary heart disease, hypertension (high blood pressure) is a significant threat to the life and health of many Americans. The disease involves the medium-sized and small arteries throughout the body, which become abnormally constricted and deprive vital organs of their necessary blood supply. Checking blood pressure is a simple but important part of every physical examination, and patients should request such a check whenever they visit their doctors. Even a routine gynecologic examination is incomplete without a blood pressure check.

HOW ATHEROSCLEROSIS CHANGES CORONARY ARTERIES

A *A normal vessel.*
B *Deposits begin to form on the inner walls of the artery.*
C *Plaque finally forms, narrowing or completely blocking the channel.*
D *Angina pectoris (a "coronary") may result, leading to death of muscle tissue in the heart, or if severe enough, to death of the individual.*

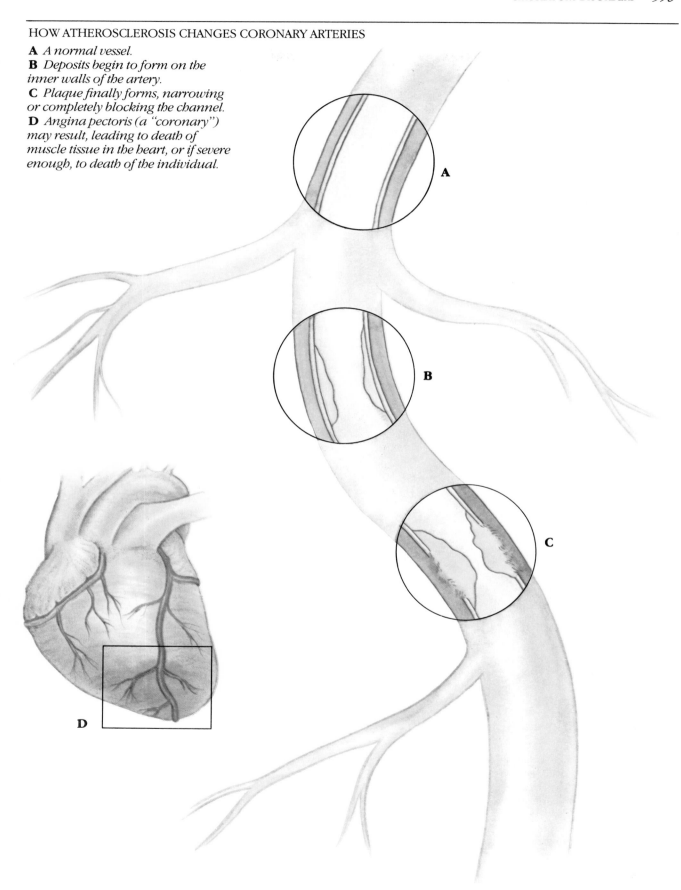

Women and Hypertension

Hypertension (high blood pressure) is a major cause of disease and death in the United States. One out of every five adult white women, and one out of every three adult black women, have some elevation of blood pressure.

While hypertension can be detected by a simple test (opposite page) and controlled effectively, many cases of high blood pressure go untreated, and result in stroke, heart failure, kidney failure, or coronary artery disease.

Hypertension is a silent killer. Its presence usually is not obvious because symptoms are often absent. Thus, many women are unaware that they have high blood pressure—especially if they are young and in good health. *All* women should have their blood pressure checked regularly, especially if they are in the following high-risk groups:

Black women. Hypertension is much more prevalent in black women than in either white women or white men, and also is more serious.

Hypertension Prevalence by Sex and Race: 1976

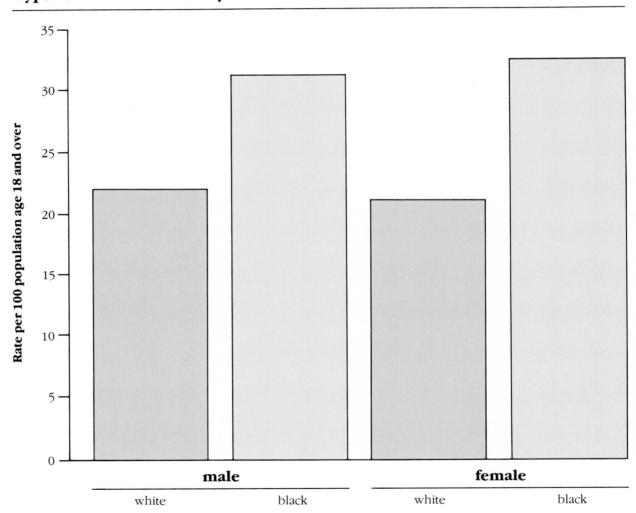

Pill users. High blood pressure has been associated with oral contraceptives, especially when taken by women with other risk factors (such as overweight or a family or personal history of hypertension). Women should have their blood pressure checked before starting the birth control pill and at least twice yearly thereafter.

Pregnant women. Pregnancy often is a time when high blood pressure develops rapidly—both in women who have never had high blood pressure and in those who have. Untreated hypertension can be dangerous to both maternal and fetal health and well-being.

Menopausal women. Menopause increases a woman's chances of getting high blood pressure; in fact, hypertension is more prevalent among elderly women than elderly men.

Women with a history of hypertension. Individuals whose parents or close relatives have had high blood pressure are more likely to be hypertensive. If this is the case, their children also are at greater risk of having high blood pressure and should be checked regularly as well.

While the causes of hypertension are not well known, there are preventive measures an individual woman can follow to minimize her risk of high blood pressure and resulting health problems. These guidelines are especially important for women in the high-risk groups described above.

● Have your blood pressure checked regularly and follow prescribed treatment.

● Watch your weight and diet. Reduce your intake of saturated fats. Ask your physician to measure the amount of cholesterol in your blood (serum cholesterol) by a simple blood test.

● Exercise regularly.

● If you smoke cigarettes, quit. If you don't, avoid the habit.

● Reduce stress as much as possible in your daily life—meditate, practice yoga, or jog to relax.

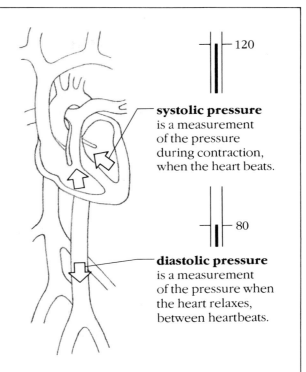

systolic pressure is a measurement of the pressure during contraction, when the heart beats.

diastolic pressure is a measurement of the pressure when the heart relaxes, between heartbeats.

The Measurement and Meaning of Blood Pressure

Blood pressure is measured by a simple test. An inflatable rubber cuff (sphygmomanometer) is placed on your arm to take two measurements. The first reading, the systolic pressure, is taken when your heart beats, and is a measurement of how hard your heart works to pump blood. The second reading, the diastolic pressure, is taken between heartbeats, and measures the pressure the arteries exert on the blood as it flows through them. A reading of about 120/80 is normal for most people, although this varies with different factors such as age.

Your doctor will determine what is normal for you and may prescribe a non-drug treatment (such as reduced salt intake or weight loss) or medications to control hypertension.

Blood pressure readings consist of two numbers—an upper (systolic) reading and a lower (diastolic) reading. The latter is most important in determining how severe any hypertension problem may be, and should not exceed 90. Nervousness at the start of an examination may cause blood pressure to rise transiently, and so it may be wise to repeat the reading after the patient becomes more relaxed.

The heart plays only a secondary role in the early stages of this disease. But later, after months or years of pumping against the resistance of the constricted blood vessels, the heart muscle weakens because of its increased work load and may stretch and fail. The arteries of the brain may be affected by the constant pounding of the increased pressure and "blowouts" or hemorrhages can result. In long-standing hypertension, the kidneys will invariably suffer oxygen deprivation. The inevitable result of untreated hypertension is death from kidney failure. In addition, persons with high blood pressure are about three to five times more likely to suffer heart trouble or stroke than are persons without this condition.

Again, women are somewhat favored when it comes to the ill-effects of hypertension. In addition to this sex difference, there is also a racial difference; blacks have much higher rates of hypertension than other racial groups. Thus, blacks and males are most susceptible to the severe complications of hypertension, while whites and women seem to suffer them less often. Hypertension in black men may even become malignant, with rapid progression to convulsions, coma, brain damage, strokes, heart attacks, kidney failure, and death. At the other end of the spectrum, white women may have the disease for years and experience few side effects.

Again, there are many conjectures but few solid facts to explain these differences. Dietary factors, hereditary susceptibility, and differing stresses have been mentioned, but all remain unproved.

At least 90 percent of the time, the cause of elevated blood pressure in any given person cannot be determined. In a few cases, medical testing will reveal endocrine disease, rare tumors, congenital narrowing of a large artery, or kidney abnormalities. However, most persons found to have high blood pressure do not show these abnormalities and their hypertension is assumed to be "essential" or of unknown cause.

Contrary to popular opinion, hypertension rarely signals its presence by symptoms. Headaches, dizziness, and nosebleeds are rare, and victims never suffer pain while the pressure is silently doing its damage. In some patients, there may be fleeting attacks of blindness, speechlessness, or paralysis—all warning signals that a stroke may be pending. In others, the first symptoms of hypertension may be those of a full-blown stroke or severe chest pain, signaling a coronary attack.

Fortunately, excellent drugs are now available to treat essential hypertension, but unfortunately, they are often unused or misused. A keystone of treatment is a drastic reduction of salt in the diet. Large amounts of salt can worsen high blood pressure and cancel out any good effects of medications. Women who cook for a family member with hypertension can help in an important way by cooking *without* salt. This will benefit the person with high blood pressure without greatly inconveniencing other family members, who can season their food to taste at the table.

Recently an intensive radio and television campaign has begun to inform the public of the dangers of uncontrolled hypertension. It stresses the importance of taking prescribed medication regularly, and of getting blood pressure checks. Blood pressure checks are readily available to practically everyone (see below), and patients who have the disease can easily learn to check their pressures at home if they wish. Although hypertension is not curable, regular treatment can make the difference between prolonged health and severe disability or untimely death.

High Blood Pressure Screening

High blood pressure (hypertension) is a major public health problem affecting more than 20 million people in the United States. Screening and early treatment is important in reducing the incidence and severity of kidney, heart, and brain damage associated with progressive hypertensive disease.

A number of community health resources—both public and private—provide high blood pressure screening and treatment services. For information and referral on such programs, contact your community chapter of the American Heart Association or the American Red Cross, or your local public health department. You also may purchase your own sphygmomanometer—the device used to measure blood pressure—and regularly check your blood pressure at home.

Benign Signs and Symptoms

Chest Pain

Since ancient times, society has placed an almost magical importance on the fist-sized organ located beneath the breastbone in the front cavity of the chest. The magic seems to persist today, and the heart is the foremost concern of people who experience discomfort anywhere from the waist to the neck. In reality, there are numerous causes of chest pain that are not always easy to pinpoint.

The pain of oxygen lack or angina pectoris has been described previously. Heart pain is classically distinct. It is centered beneath the breastbone, is pressing or squeezing in nature, and also may travel to the left arm, hand, shoulder, or jaw. It characteristically comes on with exertion and is relieved with resting. The problem arises when the pain doesn't match the textbook description. Pains "around the heart," in or under the left breast, under the collarbone, or on the left side may not be related to the heart at all.

Chest pain may arise from any structure that makes up the chest cage, such as ribs, muscles, and nerves. These structures can give rise to muscle soreness, arthritis, and neuritis in the chest just as they do elsewhere in the body. Pneumonia and pleurisy also commonly cause chest pain, as do cystic breasts. Arthritis of the neck vertebrae may compress nerves that supply chest and arm muscles and result in pain. Neck X rays can be taken to confirm this condition.

One of the most important causes of chest pain in women is called costochondritis. This is an inflammatory condition of the cartilages where the ribs and breastbone join that can be quite painful and disabling. If pressure is applied to these rib-breastbone connections by an examiner's finger, the pain is reproduced and the patient winces. One can be quite certain that this pain, which is similar to arthritis, is unrelated to the heart; heart pain is never located on the surface of the chest and cannot be brought on by pressing, pounding, or squeezing the chest structures.

Although also seen in men, costochondritis seems to be more common in women, especially those of stocky build. Often the physician can elicit a history of repetitive arm and chest motions that may have brought it on. Carrying heavy loads (books or a baby) with the left arm, as right-handed women are prone to do, is a common cause. Heavy-breasted women with inadequate brassiere support also may suffer from this type of chest pain. Prolonged or repetitive pressure or weight on the front chest wall exerted by a heavy sexual partner is another common cause. Treatment of costochondritis is similar to that of other arthritic or muscle strain conditions. Agents such as aspirin and a heating pad usually work wonders.

Our discussion would be incomplete without mentioning that anxiety also can cause many symptoms, including chest pain and tightness. Often, a keen physician can detect anxiety or fear in a patient, especially if the patient has a family member or friend with a heart condition. Explanation and reassurance are the best medicine for such symptoms, and heart medications are to be avoided.

Heart Murmurs

One of the most common misconceptions about heart disease is that the presence of a heart murmur automatically indicates heart disease. Nothing is further from the truth. A large percentage of young people of both sexes have murmurs and no evidence of cardiac problems. Unfortunately, many of these youngsters have been needlessly restrained from "doing their thing" because of them. Boys and girls have been prevented from pursuing athletics, and women have been warned that pregnancy would be disastrous.

It is estimated that almost half of all infants are born with heart murmurs that disappear as they mature. These murmurs usually arise because of vigorous youthful circulation, oddly-shaped chest cages (such as a depressed or sunken breastbone), or causes totally unrelated to the heart. They are called "functional" or "innocent" murmurs, and their chief significance is that they may be confused with murmurs of organic heart defects. A careful examination by an experienced cardiologist, including a chest X ray and possibly an electrocardiogram, is usually sufficient to make the distinction. In puzzling cases, further studies such as cardiac catheterization may be necessary. In this procedure, dye is injected into the circulatory system and various measurements and films are taken to determine pressures within the heart chambers, the pathways of blood circulation, the shape and function of the heart valves, and the pumping action of the heart muscle.

Such a procedure is certainly not indicated in all cases and should be considered only when the patient's health and life-style may be compromised without such a definite diagnosis. Catheterization should not be attempted during pregnancy because the procedure requires significant exposure to X rays; other special tests can be substituted.

Although innocent murmurs are usually soft, they may become louder in anemic states, during fever, and during pregnancy. It is greatly reassuring to an informed patient to know that his or her murmur will become softer when these conditions abate.

Healthy persons with heart murmurs should find consolation in knowing that if a murmur is significant, it will usually "show itself" in the form of symptoms; until then no meddling should be done. Exceptions to this practice should be undertaken only on the advice of a qualified cardiologist.

Therefore, affected children should be allowed to do any activities they can perform without difficulty, unless, of course, an innocent murmur is proved to be organic in nature.

The Effects of Estrogen

It is now almost twenty years since estrogen-containing birth control pills were first marketed, and this important form of contraception has played a major role in the changing status of women all over the world. It also has brought attention to the benefits and risks involved with female hormones. The benefits are obvious; the risks, formidable. Although the major ill effects of "the pill" and estrogens have been on the cardiovascular system, we now know that other organs also are affected.

Birth Control Pills

The earliest reported side effects of birth control pills were reported in 1968 and concerned thrombosis and embolism (blood clots). Since then, these complications have remained foremost in frequency and importance. It was clear to investigators that the female hormones contained in the pill increased blood coagulability, leading to clot formation in veins and arteries, and that the probability of clotting was directly related to the dose used. Extensive research has verified the exact action of the hormones on certain blood-clotting factors and specialized cells called thrombocytes or platelets. These small corpuscles normally circulate freely, but under certain stimuli they become sticky and form clumps in the vascular tree, causing obstructing clots. The clots may attach to the inner vessel walls and enlarge, much as a snowball enlarges when more snow particles aggregate on its surface. Then they may break away from their attachments and travel (embolize) to other locations in the body.

The most common site for clot formation is the leg veins, where clots can cause phlebitis, a disease characterized by pain, swelling, warmth, and redness of the legs. Clots may break off and travel to the lungs, causing destruction of oxygen-bearing lung tissue. Lung clots, or pulmonary emboli, may be so serious as to cause severe pain, massive spitting-up of blood, and even death. Clots traveling to the brain may cause transient or permanent strokes, and those tiny enough to lodge in the eye vessels can cause hemorrhage and blindness. If clots travel to the coronary artery system, they may occlude (close off) small arteries and permanently damage the heart muscle.

Long-term use of oral contraceptives has now been shown to cause decreased arterial circulation to the legs, as well as severe obstruction of the blood supply to the intestinal tract. This last condition can "kill" segments of the small intestine, requiring their surgical removal.

These coronary manifestations have been particularly well studied and reported in medical literature. Clearly, there have been numerous cases of coronary attacks in young women who were taking oral contraceptives. As mentioned earlier, women enjoy a sex advantage as far as coronary heart disease is concerned, developing it later and in a less severe form than men. But this female advantage is obliterated by risk factors such as diabetes, hypertension, smoking, increased blood cholesterol, menopause, aging—and as we know now—birth control pills.

In young (age 30 to 39) users of birth control pills, the estimated risk of coronary attacks is *at least* twice that of nonusers. In the 40- to 44-year age group, the risk in users escalated five times. In the majority of oral contraceptive users who have suffered a coronary attack, at least one other risk factor was implicated in their backgrounds. Interestingly, cigarette smoking was the most important one.

Many of these coronary survivors have undergone catheterizations and other special studies after recovery. Surprisingly, their coronary arteries have not shown the expected atherosclerotic deposits, but have shown areas of oxygen-deprived heart muscle, even though the vessels appeared open and smooth. This is clearly a different form of coronary heart disease from the most common form—that due to aging blood vessels.

Hormone Therapy

A particularly revealing study involved both men and women aged 40 to 70 who were on estrogen treatment for various reasons. Some of these people also had diabetes and hypertension. This group of 51 subjects underwent exercise electrocardiograms before and during their estrogen treatment, and again after estrogens were discontinued. Electrocardiographic changes denoting oxygen-deprived heart muscle were particularly noted. When the electrocardiograms were abnormal *before* the patients started estrogens, they became worse *during* treatment. Some patients even developed angina pectoris while on the hormones. Six weeks after discontinuing treatment, however, the patients' electrocardiograms improved to their original level. If a patient's starting electrocardiogram was normal, no subsequent changes occurred during estrogen treatment.

HOW THE HEART BEATS

The sinoatrial node is the pacemaker of the heart. This tiny island of tissue generates a rhythmical electrical impulse that spreads as an electrical wave through the muscle of the atrium. This impulse is then picked up by another node, the atrioventricular node, which passes it along to the atrioventricular bundle and into both ventricles of the heart.

It is in the sinoatrial node that an automatic rhythm is maintained. The primary center for control of this rate is the cardiovascular regulatory center in the medulla oblongata, at the base of the brain. This center is stimulated by other parts of the brain during states of anger, fear, excitement, and other emotional disturbances to effect changes in the heart rate.

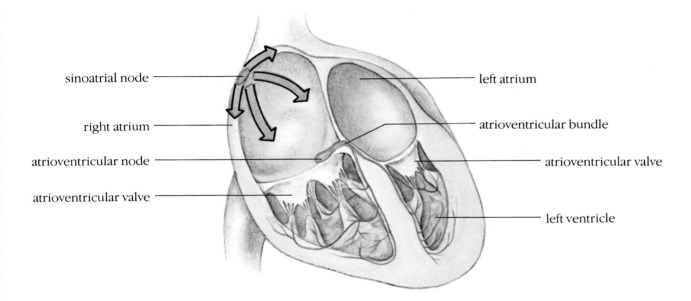

sinoatrial node — left atrium

right atrium — atrioventricular bundle

atrioventricular node — atrioventricular valve

atrioventricular valve — left ventricle

The electrocardiographic changes indicated that estrogens seemed to further decrease oxygen supply in hearts where the supply was already diminished. The cause was felt to be spasm or further narrowing of coronary arteries already compromised by atherosclerosis, and the hormone was the apparent culprit.

The effects of female hormones on blood clotting are fairly well understood at present. Other effects are more speculative. The blood pressure-raising effects of estrogens and contraceptive drugs are well known, and may be due to their "tightening" effect on medium- and small-sized arteries. Even women without previous history of hypertension have developed the disease while on the drugs, although in many cases, the hypertension was cured when the drug was stopped.

Another poorly understood effect of hormones is their tendency to increase blood cholesterol and other fats. Along with diabetes, hypertension, and smoking, these chemicals are widely held to be risk factors in cardiovascular disease.

In addition to adverse cardiovascular effects, hormonal therapy has been linked with the development of diabetes, cystic breasts, migraine, skin eruptions, and vitamin deficiencies. The major controversy concerning a causal relationship between uterine cancer and estrogens is still unsettled, but the evidence of a positive link is exceedingly strong.

On the positive side, estrogens have proved extremely helpful in treating severe menopausal symptoms. Hot flashes and sweating (both manifestations of skin vascular instability) are completely controlled by small replacement doses of estrogens, as are the itching and dryness of skin and mucous membranes in the genital areas. They are extremely effective in slowing down the thinning and brittleness of bones associated with aging in postmenopausal women. (For a discussion of estrogen and postmenopausal women, see page 317.)

The message is clear. The indications and contraindications in the use of oral contraceptives must be clearly defined, and the relative risks of the medication weighed against the potential disease it may cure. Improved pills using smaller estrogen dosages or modified chemical structures also must be sought. And women on long-term administration should be checked at regular intervals for early signs of the complications known to threaten health and life.

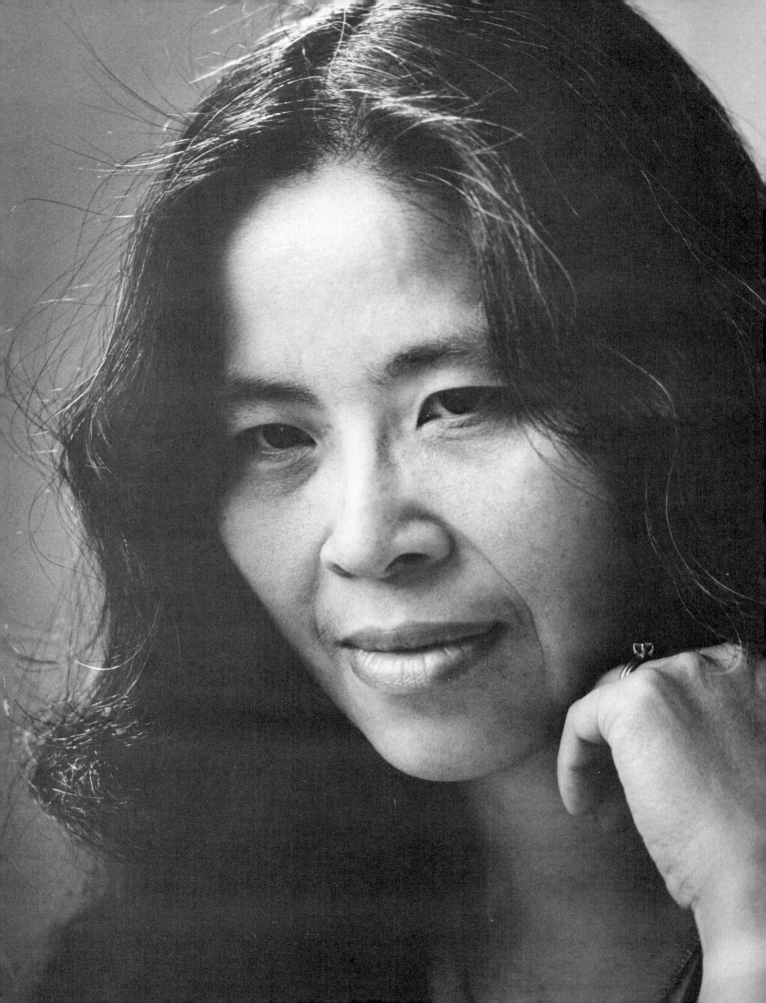

CHAPTER 29

ENDOCRINE GLAND AILMENTS

F. ALLAN HUBBELL, M.D.

The endocrine glands produce hormones—the messengers and directors of the body. Our reproductive systems, especially, are governed by hormones. They regulate the beginning, end, and duration of menstruation. They manage pregnancy and the growth of the embryo, and toward the end of the pregnancy, they stimulate milk production in the breasts and set off the muscle contractions that initiate the beginning of labor.

But beyond producing hormones, the endocrine system also determines important aspects of our personality and behavior—and our behavior, in turn, affects our secretion of hormones. Finally, the endocrine system is responsible for the size of our bodies, their growth rate, and many of the metabolic functions that keep us alive.

Endocrine Gland Ailments

Endocrinology is the science dealing with the endocrine glands and their secretions, which are called hormones. Hormones are chemicals that are secreted into the bloodstream by one cell or a group of cells, and that exert a physiological effect on other cells of the body. These hormones are responsible for the characteristics that differentiate men and women, and just as important, they affect the activity of every cell in the body and influence every activity of daily life.

Diseases of the endocrine glands usually result from either an excess or a deficiency of hormones, as will become evident in this chapter.

Female Endocrine Function

Most women are aware of endocrine functions in their body through their monthly menstrual cycles and through staying in touch with body and mood changes accompanying menstruation. Both men and women also are aware that somehow their sexuality is dependent on hormones. But few of us have considered that men and women share the same hormones, except for some placental hormones that only women possess. It is the *amount* of these hormones that differs in men and women. Except for the all-important reproductive structures, the ovaries in women and the testes in men, men and women have the same endocrine glands. However, the hormones secreted by the reproductive organs are the same in both sexes. It is the great differences in the amounts of hormones that distinguish the sexes.

The hypothalamus is both a part of the brain and of the endocrine system. It is important to realize that the brain controls hormone release, and that some of that release may be under conscious control. For whatever the brain registers—whether emotion or thought—may affect the hypothalamus, which in turn secretes hormones that activate all other glands of the body. Of the nine hypothalamic hormones, oxytocin most strongly affects female functions. Produced in the hypothalamus and stored in the posterior pituitary, oxytocin increases uterine contractions in childbirth. As the fetus moves against the uterine wall, oxytocin is released into the bloodstream. When the baby is born and begins to suck at the breast, oxytocin controls the "letdown" of milk (see page 155). The hypothalamus also signals the onset of puberty (see page 501 and page 118).

The pituitary, controlling activities such as growth, metabolism, and milk secretion, takes orders directly from the brain's hypothalamus. Hormones of the pituitary integrate menstrual cycle activities (see page 128), control egg production (see page 127), stimulate the secretion of milk (see page 155), and influence sexual development at puberty (see page 118).

The thyroid, under directions from the pituitary, controls the rate of metabolism, or the basal metabolic rate as we have come to call our measure of this function. As far as we know, there is no difference between men and women in the function of this gland.

The parathyroids regulate the mineral metabolism of the body, particularly the amount of calcium released into the bloodstream.

The adrenal glands, located on top of the kidneys, secrete the steroid hormones, which control body metabolism; the male sex hormones; androgens; and adrenaline, which assists the body in coping with emergencies.

The pancreas secretes enzymes, which are important in regulating the metabolism of blood sugar or glucose. The hormones are insulin and glucagon.

The ovaries produce the female sex hormones, estrogen and progesterone, which are responsible for the sexual characteristics of women: breasts, more delicate body structure, broader hips, special fat deposits, and the development of ovaries, fallopian tubes, the uterus, and the vagina. The original instructions for femaleness were contained in the X chromosomes that determined female sex at the moment of conception.

Estrogen is responsible for the development of the female secondary sexual characteristics (see page 120); progesterone causes the changes in the uterine wall that allow the fertilized egg to implant and grow. Birth control pills contain various combinations of estrogen and progesterone (see page 167).

The placenta, once it is established in early pregnancy, produces hormones called gonadotropins, similar to FSH and LH produced by the pituitary. One of these hormones, called human chorionic gonadotropin or HCG, is secreted into the urine. The pregnancy test checks for the presence of this hormone. Finding it indicates pregnancy, since HCG can come only from the placenta. Later in pregnancy, the placenta begins to secrete estrogen and progesterone.

Menstrual fluid and seminal fluid contain the most recently discovered hormones called prostaglandins. They appear to be produced all over the body by cell membranes, and their known effect in women is to cause contractions of the uterine wall. As a result of this discovery, prostaglandins are being studied as a possible birth control method. If taken early in pregnancy, they could conceivably induce menstruation or a very early abortion.

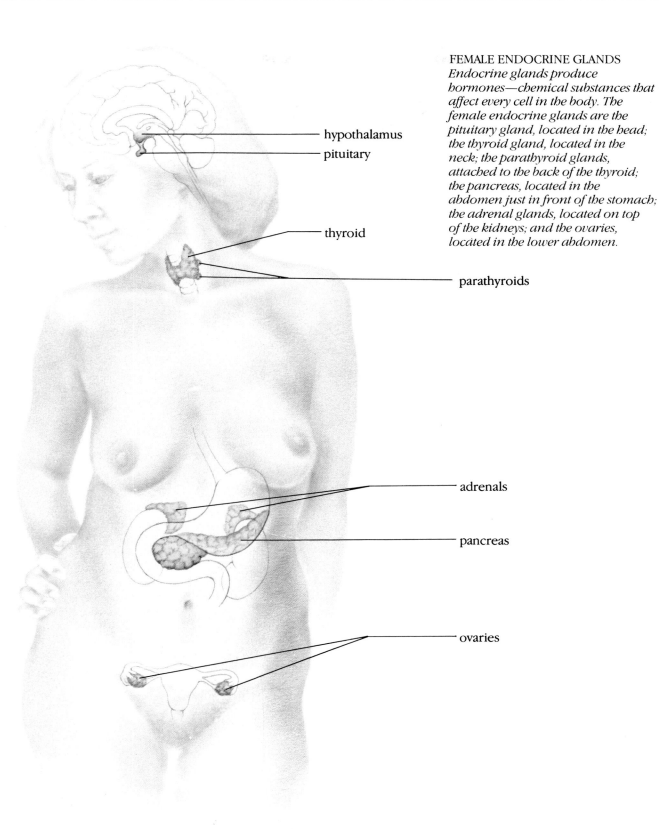

hypothalamus

pituitary

thyroid

parathyroids

adrenals

pancreas

ovaries

FEMALE ENDOCRINE GLANDS
Endocrine glands produce hormones—chemical substances that affect every cell in the body. The female endocrine glands are the pituitary gland, located in the head; the thyroid gland, located in the neck; the parathyroid glands, attached to the back of the thyroid; the pancreas, located in the abdomen just in front of the stomach; the adrenal glands, located on top of the kidneys; and the ovaries, located in the lower abdomen.

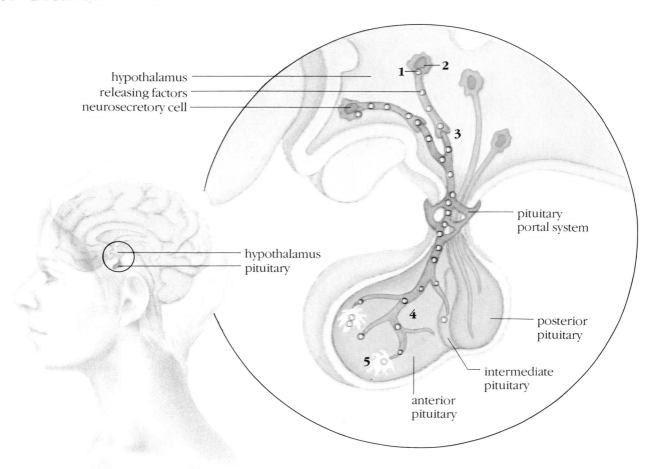

hypothalamus
releasing factors
neurosecretory cell

hypothalamus
pituitary

pituitary
portal system

posterior
pituitary

intermediate
pituitary

anterior
pituitary

THE HYPOTHALAMUS

The hypothalamus plays a crucial role in the function of the endocrine system and is the main mediator between the external world and our hormonal levels. Information from our environment is processed in the brain, where the hypothalamus senses the emotional states aroused by this information—states such as fear, anger, and sexual arousal. The hypothalamus, in turn, has a direct effect on the master endocrine gland, the pituitary. Through this connection, information or stimuli from the external world directly affect the reproductive system, the cardiovascular system, the respiratory system, and the digestive system.

THE PITUITARY

The pituitary gland lies at the base of the brain. It is divided into an anterior portion and a posterior portion, which are connected by an intermediate lobe. The hypothalamus coordinates the mind and the hormonal system by regulating the pituitary through chemicals made in nerve cells (neurosecretory cells) and released into the circulatory system (pituitary portal system). Chemicals called releasing factors (1), which are secreted by nerve cells (2) in the hypothalamus, enter the bloodstream (3), and flow directly to the pituitary (4), activating the secretion of specific pituitary hormones (5).

The Hypothalamus

The hypothalamus is an extremely important part of the brain, even though it is very small, comprising only about 0.3 percent of brain volume. It looks something like the meat of a walnut. Among its many functions is the regulation of the pituitary gland to which it is connected. Scientists believe that the hypothalamus produces a hormone that controls the secretion of each of the hormones produced by the anterior pituitary gland, although only three of these hormones have been identified. These three hormones are thyrotropin-releasing hormone (TRH), which stimulates thyroid-stimulating hormone (TSH) release from the anterior pituitary; luteinizing-hormone-releasing hormone (LHRH), which causes luteinizing hormone and follicle-stimulating hormone release from the pituitary; and somatostatin, which inhibits the release of growth hormone. The other postulated hypothalamic hormones are corticotropin-releasing factor (CRF), which stimulates ACTH production; growth-hormone-releasing factor, which stimulates growth hormone; prolactin-inhibiting factor and prolactin-releasing factor, which regulate prolactin secretion; and melanocyte-stimulating factor and melanocyte-inhibiting factor.

Diseases of the Hypothalamus

There are several rare diseases that are caused by abnormalities in the hypothalamus.

Inadequate production of TRH can cause hypothyroidism, which is discussed on page 611. Since TRH stimulates release of TSH from the pituitary gland, and because TSH stimulates release of thyroid hormone from the thyroid, a lack of TRH ultimately leads to decreased production of the thyroid hormones and results in hypothyroidism.

Physicians have discovered a deficiency of growth hormone, causing growth failure, in patients with diseases affecting the hypothalamus, such as tumor and meningitis. They now think that the cause of decreased growth hormone in these individuals may be lack of growth-hormone-releasing factor. Likewise, they have observed a lack of luteinizing-hormone-releasing hormone (LHRH) in some women who have delayed sexual development.

Decreased production of prolactin-inhibiting factor causes increased production of prolactin by the pituitary and is responsible for some cases of galactorrhea (milk secretion) at times other than immediately after the birth of a child. Galactorrhea is discussed further on page 608.

The Pituitary Gland

The pituitary gland is sometimes called the master gland of the body, since it controls the functions of many of the other endocrine glands. It lies at the base of the brain in a cavity called the sella tursica, and is divided into an anterior and a posterior portion, which are connected by an intermediate lobe. The anterior pituitary produces seven hormones: growth hormone (GH), thyroid-stimulating hormone (TSH), follicle-stimulating hormone (FSH), luteinizing hormone (LH), prolactin, melanocyte-stimulating hormone (MSH), and adrenocorticotrophic hormone (ACTH). The posterior pituitary stores antidiuretic hormone (ADH) and oxytocin (see page 155).

The pituitary gland is very important in the development of secondary sexual characteristics during adolescence. The normal maturation of the ovaries and the regulation of menstrual cycles depend on FSH and LH. FSH causes the ovaries to produce estrogen, which stimulates the development of breasts and the maturation of the vagina, uterus, and fallopian tubes. The onset of sexual development in women is between the ages of 8½ and 13. As a person grows older, the pituitary gland decreases in size; in the elderly, it is about 80 percent of its former size.

Diseases of the Anterior Pituitary

Growth hormone, one of the seven hormones released by the anterior pituitary, has a generalized effect on all tissues and organs of the body. It is necessary for growth in children and is important in maintenance of the body stores of calcium, phosphorus, sodium, potassium, and nitrogen in adults. Its effects are opposite those of insulin in that it elevates blood sugar. Normal blood levels of growth hormone in women are always higher than in men.

Acromegaly. Growth hormone imbalances can cause rather spectacular symptoms. For instance, the tallest person for whom accurate measurements exist had a growth hormone disorder called acromegaly. He was nearly nine feet tall. This disease is caused by an increase in the production of growth hormone—usually as the result of a pituitary tumor. When acromegaly occurs after puberty, the extreme height is usually not present, but the disease causes enlargement of the hands, feet, and head—usually noticed because of an increase in glove, shoe, or hat size. Other features include arthritis, emotional instability, and diabetes.

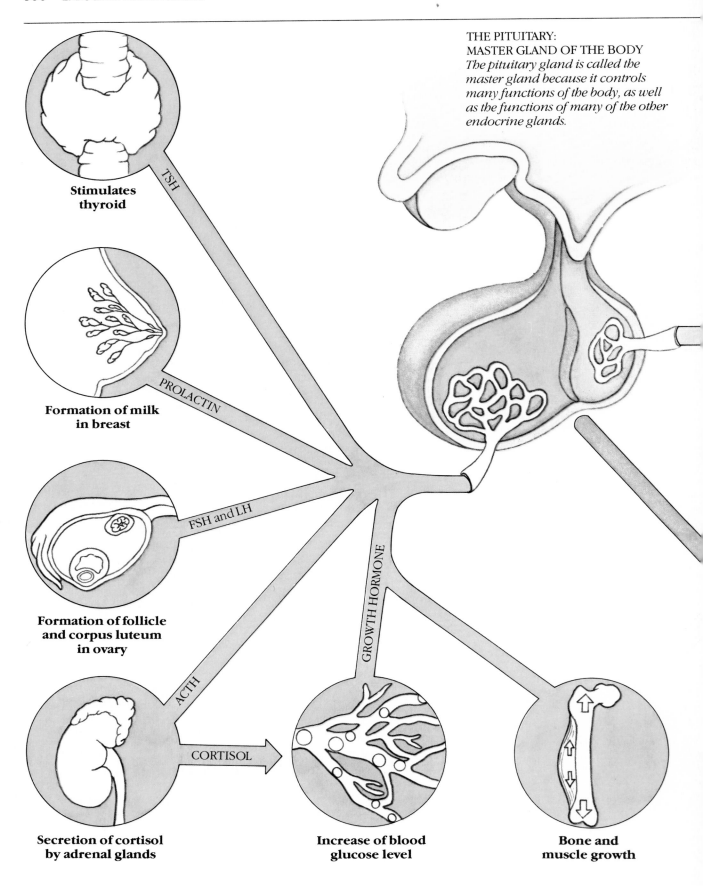

Stimulates thyroid

TSH

Formation of milk in breast

PROLACTIN

Formation of follicle and corpus luteum in ovary

FSH and LH

ACTH

CORTISOL

Secretion of cortisol by adrenal glands

GROWTH HORMONE

Increase of blood glucose level

Bone and muscle growth

THE PITUITARY:
MASTER GLAND OF THE BODY
The pituitary gland is called the master gland because it controls many functions of the body, as well as the functions of many of the other endocrine glands.

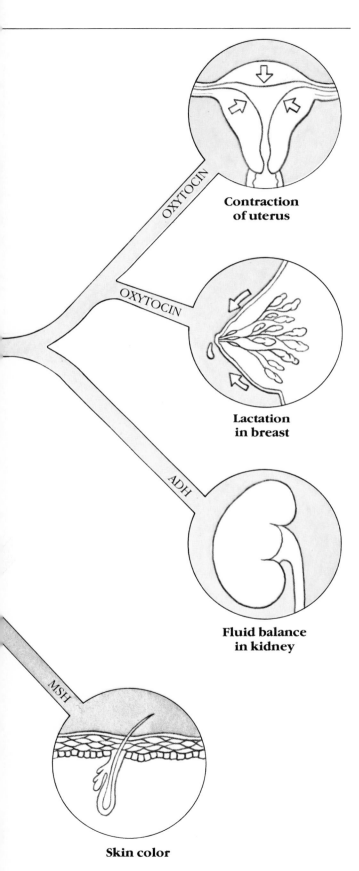

**Contraction
of uterus**

**Lactation
in breast**

**Fluid balance
in kidney**

Skin color

Lab studies reveal an increased level of growth hormone in the blood, and X rays show an enlarged sella tursica (the cavity in which the pituitary gland lies).

Treatment consists of destroying the pituitary tumor either by radiation therapy or by surgical removal. Hypopituitarism (lack of pituitary hormones) is often a complication of treatment, and is corrected by hormonal replacement.

Pituitary dwarfism. At the opposite end of the scale is a disease recognized in childhood that is due to a lack of growth hormone secretion. Pituitary dwarfism may be hereditary or be caused by a pituitary tumor, but most often its cause is not known. Boys are affected more commonly than girls. The condition is easily recognized: a child has short stature but normal body proportions and normal mental development. Growth hormone levels in the blood of such children are very low—even under conditions that normally cause elevation, such as hypoglycemia.

Treatment of pituitary dwarfism involves replacement of the deficient growth hormone, as well as any other pituitary hormones that may be lacking.

Thyroid-stimulating hormone (TSH) causes increased production and secretion of the thyroid hormones. The amount of TSH secreted by the pituitary is regulated by the hypothalamus through production of thyrotropin-releasing hormone (TRH), which stimulates its release, and by the amount of circulating thyroid hormones already in the bloodstream. With increased levels of thyroid hormone, less TSH is produced; with decreased levels of thyroid hormone, more TSH is produced in an attempt to keep the blood level of thyroid hormone normal. Rarely, pituitary tumors produce TSH and may cause hyperthyroidism with the symptoms described on page 613.

FSH, LH, and prolactin. Follicle-stimulating hormone (FSH) and luteinizing hormone (LH) regulate the development and reproductive functions of the ovaries and testicles, and prolactin stimulates milk production from the breast. These three hormones are known as gonadotropins, meaning that they stimulate the reproductive glands. FSH and LH are regulated in the female in part by the amount of circulating estrogen—the primary female sex hormone produced mainly by the ovaries. When estrogen levels increase, FSH and, to a lesser extent, LH levels are suppressed. Conversely, when estrogen levels decrease, FSH and LH levels are increased. This accounts for the high levels of FSH and LH in postmenopausal women and in those who've had surgical removal of the ovaries, since estrogen levels are markedly decreased in both of these instances. The other controlling factor of LH and FSH production is luteinizing-hormone-releasing hormone. There are no known pituitary disorders associated with increased levels of FSH or LH.

Galactorrhea is the syndrome of milk secretion from the breast at times other than postpartum. One cause of galactorrhea is an increased prolactin level, usually caused by a pituitary tumor. However, all women with increased prolactin levels do not develop galactorrhea. Other causes include histiocytosis, sarcoidosis, and certain drugs—including birth control pills, usually occurring after the pills have been stopped. The treatment of galactorrhea depends on the cause.

Adrenocorticotrophic hormone (ACTH). The principal effect of ACTH is to cause secretion of hydrocortisone from the adrenal gland. Increased levels of hydrocortisone in the blood cause a decrease in ACTH production. The other controlling substance is corticotropin-releasing factor (CRF), which is produced by the hypothalamus.

Cushing's disease may be caused by increased levels of ACTH, and is discussed on page 617.

Melanocyte-stimulating hormone (MSH) is produced by the same cells that produce ACTH, and causes increased pigmentation of the skin. Very rarely, pituitary tumors also secrete MSH.

Panhypopituitarism. When there is a lack of all of the anterior pituitary hormones, the resulting disease is panhypopituitarism. It is sometimes caused by a cyst or tumor of the pituitary gland, and less commonly by head injuries, meningitis, sarcoidosis, or Hans Schuller Christian's disease.

A disease called Sheehan's syndrome occurs in women after the birth of a child, and is caused by blood clots in the area of the pituitary. The symptoms occur because of a lack of pituitary hormones, and include failure to secrete milk and failure to menstruate within the usual time after delivery—from six weeks in a non-nursing mother to 18 months in a nursing mother. Later, intolerance to cold, loss of sex drive, and loss of pubic and axillary hair develop. Decreased heart rate, low blood pressure, and shrinking of the breasts and genitalia also may occur.

Blood tests reveal diminished levels of TSH, ACTH, GH, estrogen, thyroid hormone, and cortisol.

The logical treatment of panhypopituitarism would be the replacement of the missing pituitary hormones. However, many of these hormones are not available in a suitable form for long-term use. Therefore, the hormones that the pituitary hormones stimulate are given instead. These include thyroid hormone, cortisol, and estrogen.

Diseases of the Posterior Pituitary

The posterior pituitary produces two hormones—oxytocin and antidiuretic hormone (ADH). Oxytocin causes an increased force of contraction of the muscles of the uterus, and is particularly important during the final stages of labor. It also causes milk secretion from the breast.

ADH helps conserve body water. As with most other pituitary hormones, the body requires a delicate balance of ADH. Too much or too little causes disease.

Inappropriate ADH. The syndrome of inappropriate ADH is so named because the posterior pituitary secretes ADH at times when it is not appropriate, such as when there is already too much fluid in the body. Cancers of many types produce ADH—lung cancer (oat-cell cancer) being the most common. Other lung diseases such as tuberculosis and pneumonia also can cause increased production of ADH, as can insults to the brain such as skull fractures, strokes, and meningitis. Some medications also cause ADH secretion. Among these is Diabenase, a common drug used to treat diabetes. Still other causes include systemic lupus erythematosus, porphyria, and even physical or emotional stress.

Symptoms of inappropriate ADH include weight gain, lethargy, mental confusion, and in severe cases, convulsion and coma. Lab studies reveal a low sodium level and a high ADH level in the blood.

Initial treatment of the disease is directed toward correcting the blood sodium level, since a low sodium level can cause convulsion and death. In mild cases, restriction of fluid intake may be all that is necessary. In more severe cases, high concentrations of sodium solution must be given intravenously. The final treatment of the disease depends upon the specfic underlying cause.

Diabetes insipidus is caused when the posterior pituitary produces insufficient ADH. People with this disease produce enormous quantities of urine. If this fluid is not replaced by drinking, serious dehydration can occur.

Causes include cancer in the area of the pituitary, severe head injuries, and surgical procedures in the region of the pituitary. Sometimes diabetes insipidus is idiopathic, meaning that its cause is not known.

Increased frequency of urination (sometimes every 30 minutes to one hour), excessive thirst, and excessive water intake are the usual symptoms. When the person with diabetes insipidus has access to plenty of fluids, dehydration does not occur. But if for some reason fluids are not available, severe and dangerous dehydration may develop.

Treatment involves replacement of body fluids and ADH. Until recently, ADH had to be given by injection; however, it is now available in a nasal spray form that is quite effective.

HOW ENVIRONMENT AFFECTS THE ENDOCRINE SYSTEM

Physicians have long known that environmental factors such as emotional stress, smells, and sights affect the body, particularly the secretion of hormones. But only recently have we understood through experimental work that the brain has a direct connection to the hormonal system through chemicals released from the hypothalamus into the pituitary gland.

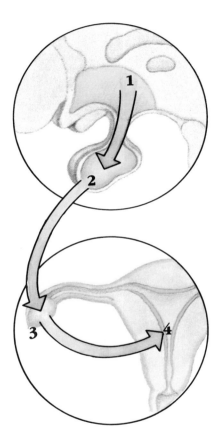

Environmental Stress

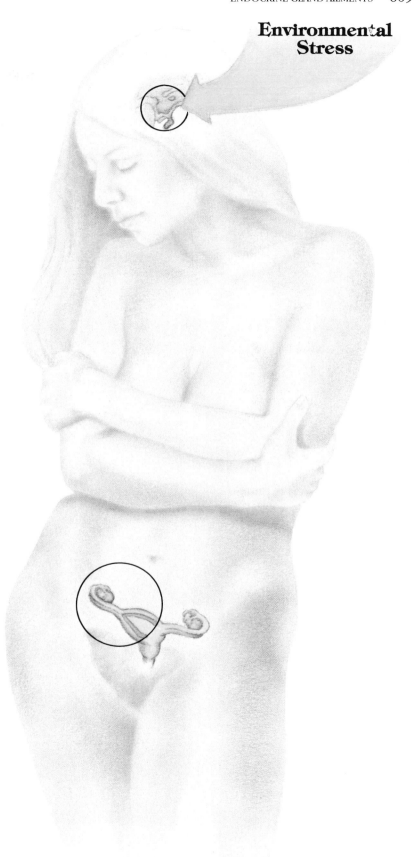

HOW ENVIRONMENT AFFECTS THE REPRODUCTIVE SYSTEM

An environmental factor such as the loss of a loved one, or a crowded, unhappy work condition can affect the brain, arousing complex emotions that activate the hypothalamus. This stimulates the pituitary, which in turn stimulates the ovaries, which stimulate the uterus. The result, in this particular case, may be that menstrual flow ceases.

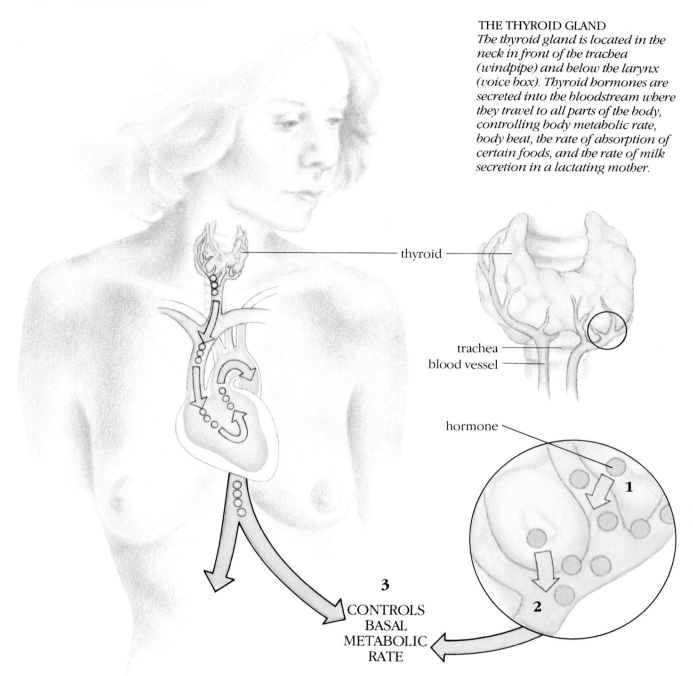

THE THYROID GLAND
The thyroid gland is located in the neck in front of the trachea (windpipe) and below the larynx (voice box). Thyroid hormones are secreted into the bloodstream where they travel to all parts of the body, controlling body metabolic rate, body heat, the rate of absorption of certain foods, and the rate of milk secretion in a lactating mother.

thyroid

trachea
blood vessel

hormone

1

2

3
CONTROLS
BASAL
METABOLIC
RATE

The Thyroid Gland

The thyroid gland is located in the neck in front of the trachea (windpipe) and below the larynx (voice box), and cannot easily be felt except by experienced persons, unless it is enlarged. The gland is composed principally of a substance called colloid, in which the thyroid hormones are produced. Iodine is necessary for the production of these thyroid hormones. Because lack of iodine was at one time a common cause of goiter (see below), iodine is often added to foods—particularly bread and salt.

The thyroid hormones, thyroxine (T4) and triiodothyronine (T3), perform diverse functions. They influence the metabolic rate of the body, body heat, the rate of absorption of certain foods, and the rate of milk secretion in a lactating mother. They also are necessary for maintenance of a normal menstrual cycle and fertility.

The thyroid gland begins to make thyroid hormones at about ten weeks' gestation, and normally functions adequately even in very elderly persons. There are, however, certain changes that occur with age. The gland becomes increasingly fibrous and nodular. And although there is a gradual decrease in production of T4, there is also a decrease in the rate of destruction of the hormone, so the blood level remains normal.

Thyroid disorders in general occur much more frequently in women than in men, and this may be due to a relationship between thyroid function and ovarian function. In pregnancy, the thyroid gland becomes enlarged but usually returns to its normal size within six weeks after delivery. The thyroid hormones are increased, as is the basal metabolic rate, but these too return to normal after delivery.

Thyroid function is regulated by the pituitary gland and, in a way that's not well understood, by the thyroid itself. The pituitary gland produces a substance called thyroid-stimulating hormone (TSH), which causes the thyroid to secrete more hormone. The pituitary in turn is regulated by the hypothalamus through thyrotropin-releasing hormone (TRH). In a normal person, when there is too much thyroid hormone circulating in the blood, the pituitary gland produces less TSH and the thyroid produces less thyroid hormone until the blood levels once again become normal.

Diseases of the Thyroid Gland

Once again, the symptoms of thyroid disease are usually caused either by too much or too little circulating thyroid hormone.

Nontoxic goiter. An enlargement of the thyroid gland is known as a goiter. When a goiter does not result from a tumor or inflammation, and when it is not associated with hyperthyroidism or hypothyroidism, it is known as a nontoxic goiter.

Such a goiter results from the inability of the thyroid to produce enough hormone to meet the needs of all the tissues of the body. In an attempt to meet these needs, the thyroid enlarges. If the demands of the body for thyroid hormone cannot be met, hypothyroidism results and the goiter is no longer "nontoxic." For unknown reasons, goiters seem to occur more often in adolescence, during pregnancy, and during menstrual periods.

The thyroid's inability to produce sufficient hormones may stem from inherited abnormalities in production; transmission of antithyroid drugs or iodine from the mother to her fetus during pregnancy; iodine deficiency; certain drugs, including para-amino-salicylate, iodine, and phenylbutazone; and Hashimoto's disease, a condition in which white blood cells infiltrate the thyroid gland.

The symptoms of a nontoxic goiter include swelling of the neck because of the increased size of the thyroid gland, and sometimes difficulty breathing or swallowing because of displacement of the trachea (windpipe) or esophagus by the enlarged gland. In nontoxic goiter, the blood level of the thyroid hormones T3 and T4 is normal.

Treatment seeks to decrease the size of the gland by providing enough thyroid hormone in tablet form to suppress the thyroid. If iodine deficiency is the cause, oral doses of iodine are given. Early goiter, in which the whole gland is involved, responds very well to oral thyroid hormone treatment, and the goiter usually disappears within six months. When the goiter is nodular, meaning that small lumpy masses may be felt within the gland, the response to treatment is not as good. Thyroid hormone replacement is required for prolonged periods of time. Surgery is not indicated for treatment of nontoxic goiter unless there is compression of the trachea or esophagus that does not respond to thyroid hormone replacement.

Hypothyroidism ("hypo" meaning "less than normal") is the result of too little circulating thyroid hormone. There are many causes of hypothyroidism, the most common being the surgical removal of the thyroid gland or its destruction by radioactive iodine in the treatment of hyperthyroidism. Hashimoto's disease, an autoimmune disease of the thyroid gland, is another common cause. Other less-frequent causes include iodine deficiency; certain drugs, such as lithium carbonate (used in the treatment of some depressive states) and paramino-salicylic acid; inherited abnormalities in the production of thyroid hormones; and rarely, pituitary or hypothalamic disorders that cause decreased production of TSH.

Hypothyroidism from birth is known as cretinism. A baby with hypothyroidism usually exhibits a hoarse cry, constipation, and feeding problems. In adulthood, the condition may be recognized by short stature, a protruding tongue, a flat nose, wide-set eyes, and mental retardation.

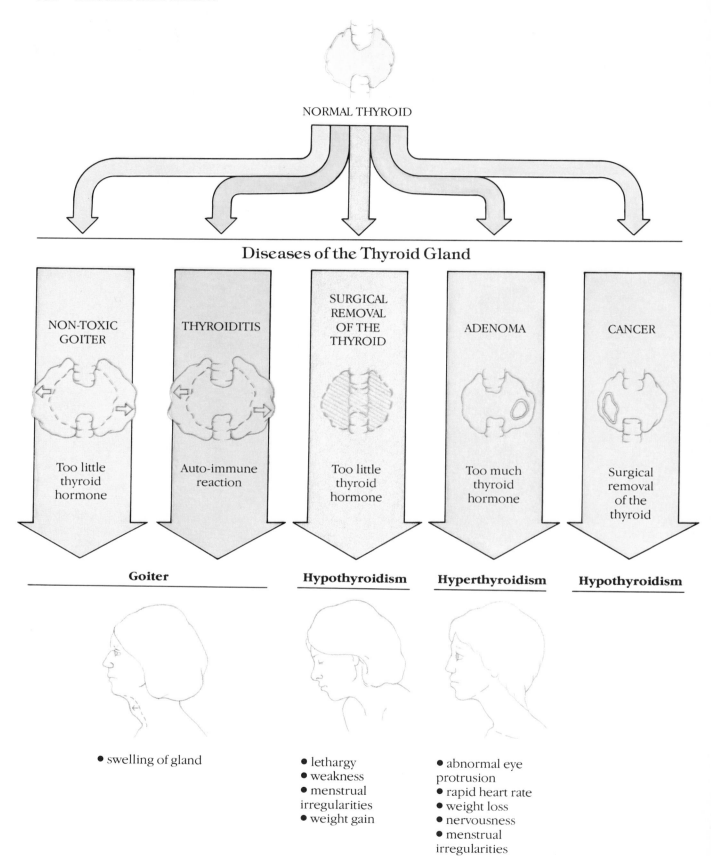

NORMAL THYROID

Diseases of the Thyroid Gland

NON-TOXIC GOITER	THYROIDITIS	SURGICAL REMOVAL OF THE THYROID	ADENOMA	CANCER
Too little thyroid hormone	Auto-immune reaction	Too little thyroid hormone	Too much thyroid hormone	Surgical removal of the thyroid

Goiter   **Hypothyroidism**   **Hyperthyroidism**   **Hypothyroidism**

- swelling of gland

- lethargy
- weakness
- menstrual irregularities
- weight gain

- abnormal eye protrusion
- rapid heart rate
- weight loss
- nervousness
- menstrual irregularities

The adult woman with hypothyroidism may have few if any symptoms early in the disease. Later, common complaints include lethargy, constipation, cold intolerance, lack of appetite, and menstrual irregularities—including increased or decreased amount of blood flow or lack of periods altogether.

Women with hypothyroidism also have a diminished libido, impaired fertility, and increased rate of miscarriage when they become pregnant. When the disease is very severe, it is known as myxedema, which can lead to coma and death. Blood tests show that the thyroid hormone levels are lower than normal.

Doctors treat hypothyroidism by replacing the missing thyroid hormones. This is accomplished by taking daily doses of one of many different kinds of thyroid extracts available in tablet form.

Hyperthyroidism ("hyper" meaning "excessive") is caused by the opposite condition—too much circulating thyroid hormone. Grave's disease is a type of hyperthyroidism that produces a goiter, a particular type of skin problem (dermopathy), and eye problems (ophthalmopathy), although a person with Grave's disease does not necessarily have all three. The disorder is much more common in women than in men, and its cause is unknown.

Symptoms of hyperthyroidism include goiter, excessive sweating, rapid heart rate, palpitations, weight loss associated with increased appetite, and increased anxiety and nervousness. There also may be abnormalities in the menstrual cycle, including decreased frequency and duration of menstrual periods or complete lack of periods. Fertility is decreased, and, as with hypothyroidism, the rate of miscarriage is increased in women with hyperthyroidism.

The eye problems associated with Grave's disease include protrusion of the eyes, and often less-obvious abnormalities, such as infrequent blinking and failure to wrinkle the forehead when looking upward. The skin is usually thickened and itchy, particularly on the shins.

Blood tests reveal elevated thyroid hormone levels, and, when sensitive methods are used, almost 100 percent of patients with Grave's disease will have an antibody called thyroid-stimulating immunoglobulin. Doctors believe this protein is partially responsible for the symptoms of the disease.

There are three major ways to treat hyperthyroidism. The first is with antithyroid drugs, such as propylthiouracil, that block the production of thyroid hormone. This blockage lasts only as long as the drug is administered.

The second mode of treatment uses radioactive iodine to permanently destroy thyroid tissue. The disadvantage here is that the opposite condition, hypothyroidism, often develops, which is why some physicians recommend thyroid hormone replacement for all patients who receive radioactive iodine. There is no current evidence of increased risk of cancer in patients treated with radioactive iodine, but because this possibility has not been completely excluded, many doctors reserve radioactive iodine treatment for patients over 40 years of age.

The third treatment of hyperthyroidism is partial removal of the thyroid (subtotal thyroidectomy). This formerly was the treatment of choice; however, it is now used mainly in younger patients and in those in whom antithyroid treatment has been unsuccessful.

When hyperthyroidism is present during pregnancy, doctors disagree about how to treat it. However, most doctors do agree that the use of antithyroid drugs such as propylthiouracil is preferable to surgery, at least during the first and third trimesters of pregnancy.

Toxic multi-nodular goiter. A complication of a simple goiter can be a toxic multi-nodular goiter. This disease differs from simple goiter in that the goiter has masses of tissue known as nodules that produce too much thyroid hormone and can cause hyperthyroidism. This disease normally occurs in elderly individuals, and its cause is unknown. The symptoms are those described opposite, although symptoms usually are less severe than those seen in Grave's disease. The thyroid is enlarged and nodular. Eye problems are uncommon.

Blood tests usually reveal increased thyroid hormone levels. The disease is treated with antithyroid drugs and radioactive iodine.

Thyroiditis is an inflammation of the thyroid gland. There are four types of thyroiditis, the first two of which are extremely rare.

Pyogenic thyroiditis is caused by an infection of the thyroid gland. It is usually the result of infection in other parts of the body, and is treated with antibiotics.

Riedel's thyroiditis is a type of inflammation that causes scar formation of the thyroid gland and the tissues that surround it.

Subacute thyroiditis is caused by a virus. It usually produces pain in the area of the thyroid gland and sometimes the symptoms of hyperthyroidism. Aspirin, or in more severe cases, corticosteroids are given to relieve symptoms until the disease subsides on its own.

Hashimoto's thyroiditis is a chronic inflammation of the thyroid that leads to hypothyroidism. It occurs most often in middle-aged women, and its cause is unknown. Doctors believe that it is one of the so-called auto-immune diseases. Autoimmunity occurs when antibodies, which are normally produced by the body to fight various infections, attack normal body cells—in this case, the thyroid gland—instead of cells foreign to the body. Two of these antibodies frequently found in Hashimoto's thyroiditis are the antithyroglobulin and antimicrosomal antibody.

Symptoms include a goiter and, later in the course of the disease, signs of hypothyroidism. The treatment is thyroid hormone replacement.

Tumors of the Thyroid

Thyroid adenomas are benign (benign, when used in reference to a tumor, means that the tumor does not spread to other parts of the body) growths of thyroid tissue that do not respond to the usual control mechanism of the thyroid. The adenoma continues to produce thyroid hormone even when there is an abnormally large amount of thyroid hormone already in the blood. This, of course, can lead to hyperthyroidism.

Depending on whether or not too much thyroid hormone is made, the disease may cause no symptoms, or the symptoms of hyperthyroidism. Thyroid adenomas are treated with radioactive iodine or surgical removal.

Thyroid cancers are classified according to the cell type most prevalent in the tumor. The most common tumor is called papillary carcinoma, which is very slow growing. Anaplastic carcinoma, which has no distinct cell type, is the most deadly, and is usually found in elderly patients. The other types of thyroid cancer are follicular carcinoma and mixed papillary and follicular carcinoma.

These cancers are more frequent in people who have had X-ray treatment of the head or neck in childhood, and are usually discovered when a non-tender mass is noted in the area of the thyroid. Thyroid scans (special X rays of the thyroid gland) also often reveal the tumor.

When a diagnosis of thyroid cancer is made, doctors recommend surgical removal of the thyroid gland. Radioactive iodine is then given to destroy any remaining thyroid tissue that might contain cancer cells. After surgery, patients must take thyroid tablets, since no thyroid gland remains to produce thyroid hormone.

The Parathyroid Glands

The parathyroid glands are located just behind the thyroid gland. There are usually four glands, although there may be more or fewer in some people. The parathyroid glands produce parathyroid hormone (PTH), which causes increased levels of calcium in the blood. The amount of PTH they produce is governed by the level of calcium already in the blood. When the calcium level goes down, PTH is released to help bring the level back up to normal; when the calcium level is elevated, less PTH is secreted by the parathyroid glands. PTH works in three ways: first, it dissolves calcium in bone, which then gets into the bloodstream; second, it decreases the amount of calcium that enters the urine through the kidneys; and third, it causes more calcium to be absorbed in the intestines.

As a person grows older, PTH levels in the blood and the density of the bones decrease slightly. In women, the decrease in bone thickness may be due in part to the lower levels of estrogen after menopause. PTH seems to have less effect on bones in premenopausal women, possibly because of a protective effect of estrogen. After menopause, when this protective mechanism is presumably lost, there is an increase in hyperparathyroidism.

Diseases of the Parathyroid

Hyperparathyroidism is divided into two categories—primary and secondary. Primary hyperparathyroidism is caused by a primary disease of the parathyroid glands that causes them to produce too much PTH. Secondary hyperparathyroidism occurs when PTH levels increase in response to other diseases, such as chronic kidney disease, osteomalacia, and pseudohypoparathyroidism.

Primary hyperparathyroidism occurs most often in adults from age 20 to 50. Approximately 85 percent of all cases are caused by a tumor of the parathyroid gland (only about 5 percent of these tumors are malignant); the other 15 percent of hyperparathyroidism cases are caused by enlargement of the glands, a condition known as hyperplasia. An increased PTH level leads to an increased calcium level in the blood, and the symptoms of hyperparathyroidism are secondary to this high calcium level. These symptoms include calcium deposits in the kidneys, kidney stones, bone resorption, personality disorders, nausea, abdominal pain, and muscle weakness. There also is an increased incidence of ulcers and pancreatitis in patients with hyperparathyroidism.

Tumors of organs other than the parathyroid, especially lung cancer and kidney cancer, can produce a substance that is very similar to PTH and that causes the same symptoms described earlier. Blood tests reveal an increased level of PTH and an increased level of calcium. Angiograms (X-ray studies of the arteries that supply the parathyroid with blood) may be necessary to pinpoint the parathyroid tumor.

Treatment depends on the specific cause of the high parathyroid hormone levels. If a tumor is found, it should be surgically removed. If there is hyperplasia of the glands, three glands and part of the fourth gland can be removed. When a parathyroid tumor is malignant, removal usually cures the disease. Still, it is important for hyperparathyroid patients to have a blood calcium check once a year. This is because even if the tumor was benign, it may recur.

Hypoparathyroidism is caused by diminished levels of PTH in the blood or by body resistance to the effects of PTH. The most common cause is removal of or damage to the parathyroid glands during surgical treatment for hyperparathyroidism, thyroid disorders, or cancer of the neck. Radiation to the neck is a rare cause of this condition. In addition, infants born to hyperparathyroid mothers may suffer a transient lack of parathyroid hormone.

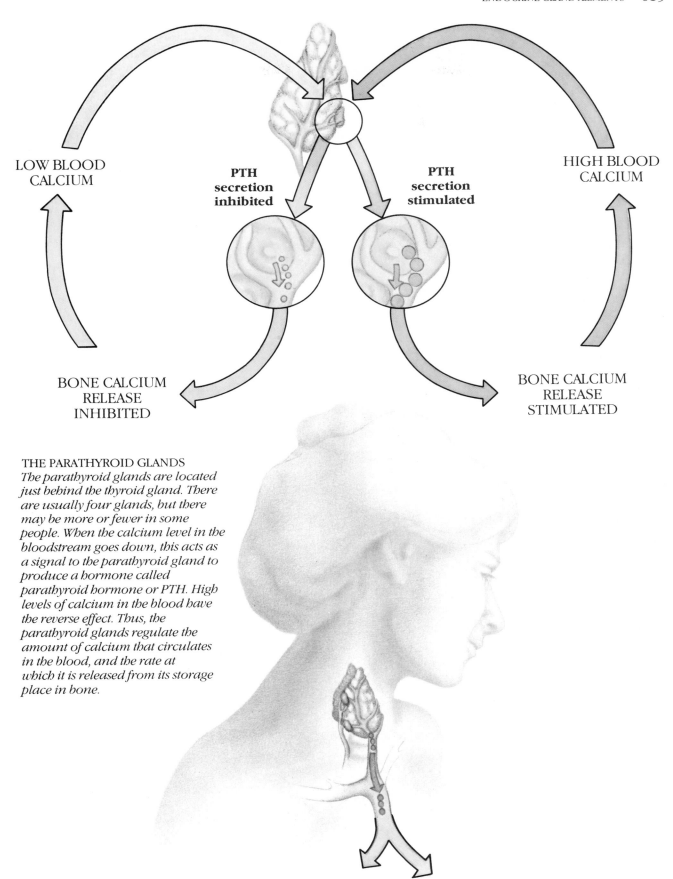

LOW BLOOD
CALCIUM

**PTH
secretion
inhibited**

**PTH
secretion
stimulated**

HIGH BLOOD
CALCIUM

BONE CALCIUM
RELEASE
INHIBITED

BONE CALCIUM
RELEASE
STIMULATED

THE PARATHYROID GLANDS
*The parathyroid glands are located
just behind the thyroid gland. There
are usually four glands, but there
may be more or fewer in some
people. When the calcium level in the
bloodstream goes down, this acts as
a signal to the parathyroid gland to
produce a hormone called
parathyroid hormone or PTH. High
levels of calcium in the blood have
the reverse effect. Thus, the
parathyroid glands regulate the
amount of calcium that circulates
in the blood, and the rate at
which it is released from its storage
place in bone.*

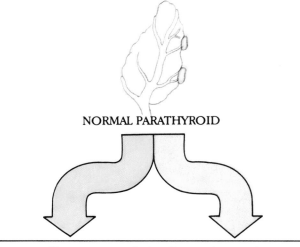

NORMAL PARATHYROID

Diseases of the Parathyroid

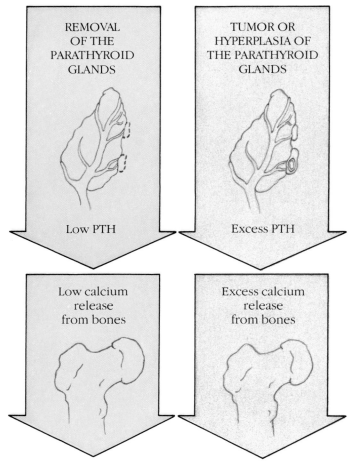

REMOVAL
OF THE
PARATHYROID
GLANDS

TUMOR OR
HYPERPLASIA OF
THE PARATHYROID
GLANDS

Low PTH

Excess PTH

Low calcium
release
from bones

Excess calcium
release
from bones

Hypoparathyroidism

- muscle spasms or tetany
- begins as numbness of hands & feet
- convulsions

Hyperparathyroidism

- kidney stones
- bone resorbtion and brittleness
- personality disorders
- muscle weakness

Hypoparathyroidism causes decreased blood calcium levels—the end result of inadequate PTH. The symptoms of hypoparathyroidism are due to these low levels of calcium, and include tetany, which begins as numbness and later spasms of the hands and feet, and sometimes convulsions. Calcification of the skin and muscles also may occur.

Blood tests reveal increased phosphorus, decreased calcium, and decreased parathyroid hormone associated with decreased calcium.

Treatment attempts to restore the blood calcium level to normal. To accomplish this, patients take calcium tablets and vitamin D tablets (vitamin D causes increased absorption of calcium from the intestines). Hypercalcemia (excess calcium in the blood) is a complication of hypoparathyroidism treatment, and must be guarded against. After the best dosages of vitamin D and calcium have been established, patients should have their blood levels of calcium checked three or four times per year.

The Adrenal Glands

The two adrenal glands are located in the abdomen just above the kidneys. These glands are divided into the outer layer, or cortex, and the inner layer, or medulla. The cortex in turn is divided into three layers, each responsible for the production of different hormones. The zona glomerulosa is the outermost layer of the cortex, and produces aldosterone, which has two major activities: the regulation of fluid volume in the body and the regulation of potassium metabolism. The remaining two layers, the zona fasciculata and the zona reticularis, produce cortisol, corticosterone, and the adrenal androgens. Cortisol and corticosterone have many activities, including regulation of the metabolism of fats, carbohydrate, and protein; inhibition of inflammatory reactions; regulation of loss of body water; and elevation of blood sugar. The adrenal androgens are responsible for the development of male secondary sexual characteristics. Adrenal production of androgens is trivial compared to that of the ovaries and testes; however, women with certain adrenal problems may exhibit an increase in body hair, lack of menstrual periods, decreased breast size, deepening of the voice, acne, and increased muscle strength and size.

The cortex of the adrenal glands uses cholesterol to produce these hormones. The hypothalamus releases corticotropin-releasing factor, which causes the pituitary gland to produce ACTH, which in turn causes the adrenal glands to produce the hormones.

The inner portion of the adrenal gland, the medulla, secretes epinephrine (adrenaline) and norepinephrine. These chemicals increase heart rate, blood pressure, alertness, and metabolic rate in stressful situations.

The appearance of the adrenal glands doesn't change markedly as a person grows older, although their hormone secretions decrease.

Diseases of the Adrenal Glands

Addison's disease results when the adrenal glands can't produce enough of the adrenal hormones to allow the body to function normally. About 90 percent of the gland must be destroyed before symptoms of adrenal insufficiency appear. In the past, tuberculosis was the most common cause of Addison's disease, but doctors now believe the condition is an autoimmune disease. Occasionally, Addison's disease results from a fungal infection, adrenal tumor, amyloidosis, or sarcoidosis.

Common symptoms include weight loss, weakness, loss of appetite, and increased pigmentation of the skin and mucous membranes. Very low blood pressure and low blood sugar also are frequently present. Blood tests reveal low sodium, low bicarbonate, and high potassium levels, and decreased cortisol production.

To treat Addison's disease, doctors replace the missing hormones—the most important of which are cortisone and aldosterone. Anyone with Addison's disease should carry a medical identification card, since without treatment the disease is fatal. But the prognosis is good when patients are well-informed about the condition and receive treatment.

There are various diseases associated with an excess of each of the adrenal hormones. An increased level of cortisol results in Cushing's disease; increased aldosterone results in aldosteronism; and increased androgen results in adrenal virilism. A rare tumor of the adrenal glands causing increased production of catecholamines is called a pheochromocytoma (see page 619).

Cushing's disease results from excessive glucocorticoids in the blood. The majority of cases are caused by hyperplasia (enlargement) of the glands due to too much ACTH produced by the pituitary. Other causes are benign adrenal tumors called adenomas, malignant adrenal tumors (adrenal carcinoma), adrenal tissue located outside the adrenal glands, pituitary tumors, non-adrenal tumors (such as a certain type of lung cancer known as oat-cell carcinoma), pancreatic carcinoma, cancer of the thymus gland, and glucocorticoids (steroids) given by doctors to treat other diseases.

Symptoms include a peculiar type of body build that people with Cushing's disease acquire. The face becomes red and round (moon face), a lump develops in the back of the neck (buffalo hump), and excessive fat accumulates in the trunk of the body. Other common symptoms are weight gain, weakness, high blood pressure, and in women, increased body hair, acne, loss of menstrual periods, and enlargement of the clitoris. Personality changes are prominent, and diabetes develops in about 20 percent of patients.

Many complicated laboratory studies can confirm the diagnosis of Cushing's disease, but increased cortisol production in the absence of stress is the most frequent indicator of the condition.

THE ADRENAL GLANDS

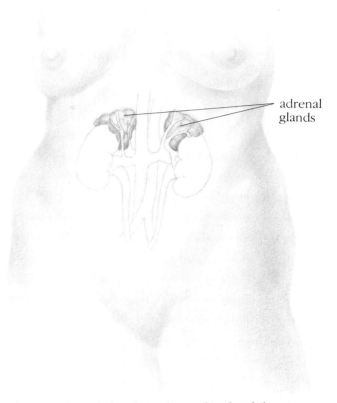

adrenal glands

The two adrenal glands are located in the abdomen just above the kidneys. Cortisol and corticosterone hormones produced by the adrenals regulate food metabolism and loss of body water, to name only two of their functions. A small amount of androgen, or male sex hormone, also is produced by the adrenals. Aldosterone, a major adrenal hormone, regulates fluid volume in the body and potassium metabolism. Adrenaline (epinephrine) and norepinephrine are secreted by the inner portion of the adrenal gland during stressful situations, when they increase alertness, heart rate and blood pressure, and metabolic rate.

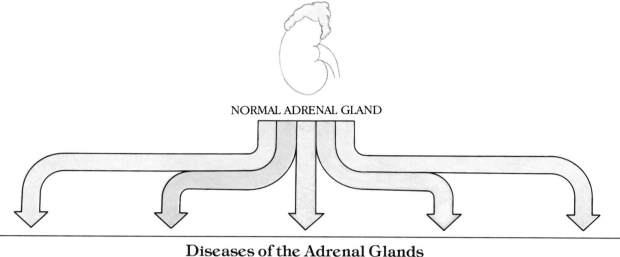

NORMAL ADRENAL GLAND

Diseases of the Adrenal Glands

GLAND DESTROYED	ENLARGEMENT OF GLAND	ADENOMA	ADENOMA	TUMOR OF THE MEDULLA
Too little adrenal hormone	Too much cortisol	Too much aldosterone	Excessive adrenal androgens	Too much nor-adrenaline

Addison's Disease	**Cushing's Disease**	**Aldosteronism**	**Adrenal Virilism**	**Pheochromocytoma**
• weight loss • appetite loss • weakness • increased pigmentation of skin • low blood pressure	• red, round, moon face • hump at back of neck •fat gain in trunk • high blood pressure • personality change	• high blood pressure • muscle weakness • fatigue	In women: • increased body hair • deepening voice • baldness • acne • increase in muscle size • decrease in breast size	• very high blood pressure • palpitation of the heart • excess perspiration • tremors • nervousness • flushing

The treatment of Cushing's disease depends on the cause. When an adrenal tumor is found, it is surgically removed. If the tumor is malignant, chemotherapy also may be necessary. When adrenal hyperplasia is the cause, there are two ways of treating the disease. One is total surgical removal of both adrenal glands, with oral replacement of the missing hormones. The other method is destruction of the pituitary gland with irradiation to stop the abnormal production of the ACTH. If a pituitary tumor is present, the tumor is removed by surgery or irradiation. When a non-pituitary tumor is producing the ACTH, that tumor is removed.

Aldosteronism is associated with increased production of aldosterone, which, as you recall, is important in the maintenance of body fluids and potassium levels. Primary aldosteronism is usually caused by an adrenal adenoma (benign tumor) that produces aldosterone. Occasionally a malignant adrenal tumor is the cause. For unknown reasons, the disease is twice as common in women as in men.

The most common symptom of aldosteronism is high blood pressure. Although a rare cause of high blood pressure, it is important to discover since it is curable. Aldosterone causes the body to retain sodium and lose potassium. This low potassium level is responsible for many of the other symptoms, including muscle weakness, fatigue, and even transient paralysis. Lab studies reveal a low blood potassium level and high aldosterone levels that are not lowered by the usual factors that cause aldosterone secretion to be decreased, such as increased blood volume.

The adrenal tumor may be located by adrenal angiography and venography. In these techniques, dye is injected into the arteries and veins that supply blood to the adrenal glands. Treatment then consists of surgical removal of the adrenal tumor.

Adrenal virilism is due to increased production of adrenal androgens, which are converted to testosterone—a potent male hormone. Hyperplasia (enlargement) of the adrenal glands, adrenal adenoma, or adrenal carcinoma is the usual cause of adrenal virilism.

Since the symptoms of this disease are due to excessive male hormones, adrenal virilism is much more easily recognized in women than in men. In the adult woman, the symptoms include increased body hair (hirsutism), acne, baldness, deepening of the voice, increase in muscle size and strength, decrease in breast size, and increased sex drive.

Diseases of the ovaries also can cause virilism in women, and must be differentiated from adrenal virilism. The simplest lab study for diagnosis is measurement of 17-ketosteroids in the urine. Ketosteroids are formed when the testosterone is metabolized.

Treatment is the surgical removal of the tumor. Since the tumor is often malignant, chemotherapy is frequently necessary. Unfortunately, long-term survival rates are disappointing.

Pheochromocytoma is the rather cumbersome name for a tumor of the adrenal glands, and sometimes other regions of the body, which produce the catecholamines epinephrine and norepinephrine, discussed on page 616. As you might expect, the symptoms of this tumor are caused by excess catecholamines. The most common of these is high blood pressure—sometimes to extremely high levels. Other symptoms of this tumor are palpitations of the heart, excessive perspiration, nausea, tremors, nervousness, and occasionally, chest pain, shortness of breath, flushing, numbness, and visual blurring.

This tumor can occur from childhood through old age. Lab tests that help make the diagnosis of pheochromocytoma include urine studies for catecholamines and their breakdown products. Adrenal angiography and venography are again helpful in locating the tumor, which is then surgically removed.

Diabetes Mellitus

Diabetes mellitus is a very common disease—there are over four million diabetics in the United States, and probably another two million with undiagnosed cases. The disease results from a relative or absolute lack of insulin production by the pancreas, the cause of which is unknown. Since the body's cells require insulin to extract glucose (one of the blood sugars) from the blood, lack of insulin causes an elevation in blood glucose (hyperglycemia). This increase in blood glucose can lead to a severe condition called diabetic ketoacidosis, discussed later. Many of the other complications of diabetes are caused by its effect on blood vessels throughout the body, such as premature atherosclerosis, hardening of the arteries.

The symptoms of diabetes depend on when the disease develops. In juvenile-onset diabetes, the child suddenly has increased thirst, drinks and eats more, and urinates more frequently. Weight loss, loss of strength, and marked irritability follow. If untreated, children with diabetes are likely to develop ketoacidosis.

In adult-onset diabetes, symptoms may be the same as those seen in children, or early in the disease, there may be no symptoms at all. Symptoms due to the effects of diabetes on blood vessels may lead to the eventual diagnosis. These include blurred or decreased vision (or even blindness) due to eye involvement, numbness, lack of sensation, ulcer or (later) gangrene of the legs and feet due to decreased circulation, and extreme fatigue and anemia due to kidney involvement. Since there are blood vessels in all parts of the body, diabetes is far-reaching in its effects.

Diabetes may first become apparent during pregnancy. After pregnancy, the blood glucose level may return to normal, but frequently rises later and becomes permanent diabetes.

Ketoacidosis is a condition that develops in some people with severe diabetes, particularly in those who have not been taking their prescribed insulin, and is caused by increased acids in the blood. As mentioned previously, insulin is necessary for the body to use glucose for energy. When glucose cannot be used because of lack of insulin, fats are used for energy instead, and acids are produced as a by-product. When too many of these acids accumulate in the blood, ketoacidosis develops. Symptoms include vomiting, abdominal pain, heavy breathing, confusion, and later coma. When these symptoms occur in a diabetic, she should immediately be taken to a hospital for emergency treatment.

Laboratory studies on diabetics reveal an increased fasting blood glucose level or abnormal glucose tolerance test in which blood glucose levels are determined *before* and ½ hour, 1 hour, 2 hours, and 3 hours *after* the patient drinks 100 grams of glucose. Glucose is also found in the urine, and all diabetics should be taught how to test for glucose in the urine.

Diet is the most important part of treatment for mild diabetics, and is extremely important for all diabetics. Blood glucose levels in obese diabetics may return to normal when ideal body weight is reached. A woman can get a rough idea of her ideal body weight by determining her height, allowing 100 pounds for the first five feet and 4 to 5 pounds for each inch above five feet. Thus, a five-foot five-inch woman should weigh 120 to 125 pounds. The purpose of dietary treatment for diabetics is to reach and maintain ideal body weight, and to reach and maintain normal blood glucose levels. In most diabetics, these goals require that the patient eat a diet with restricted caloric intake. However, in diabetics who are underweight, a high-calorie diet is necessary. A well-balanced diet consists of about 40 to 50 percent carbohydrates, 15 to 20 percent protein, and 35 to 40 percent fat. A diabetic diet should be similar in content. The American Diabetes Association and the American Dietetic Association publish an extensive booklet on diabetic diets that is quite helpful in planning meals. Many people with adult-onset diabetes mellitus may be treated with diet alone.

When diet alone does not control the diabetes, two other means of treatment are available: oral agents and insulin. Oral agents (medications that can be taken by mouth) such as Orinase work mainly by stimulating pancreatic secretion of insulin. Since 1970, when a large study by the University Group Diabetes Program evaluated the various modes of treating diabetes, much controversy has surrounded the use of oral agents. In this study, no clear-cut benefit from the oral agents Orinase (tolbutamide) or phenformin could be found. In fact, death rates from cardiovascular disease were increased in patients, mostly women, who took the medication. Some physicians now feel that no one should be given oral agents.

Others feel that there were flaws in the study and that the oral agents such as Orinase and Diabinase are needed in certain diabetics. Currently, these medications are recommended only for adult-onset diabetics who are non-ketotic (meaning that they are not prone to develop ketoacidosis) and for whom diet has failed, insulin treatment is unacceptable, or only short-term medication is needed. Most physicians now feel that DBI (phenformin) should not be used in any diabetic.

Insulin treatment is necessary in juvenile-onset diabetics and in adults in whom diet alone does not control blood sugar levels. The major drawback to the use of insulin is that it must be injected. There are several types of insulin that differ mainly in the length of time in which they are active in the blood. Crystalline or regular insulin is fast acting, with a duration of about six hours, and is used in emergency situations. The two most common long-term types are NPH and Lente insulin. Both last about 24 hours, with their peak effect at about 8 to 12 hours after injection. Therefore, one injection per day will serve most diabetics.

There are certain complications that may arise from insulin use. Hypoglycemia results from excessive insulin, and is recognized by visual disturbances, headaches, uncontrollable yawning, mental confusion, and—if it persists—coma. Sometimes increased heart rate, palpitations, irritability, and hunger also are present. A diabetic should learn to recognize the symptoms of hypoglycemia and immediately eat candy, sugar, orange juice, or some other food high in carbohydrates. Because the symptoms of hypoglycemia may simulate those of alcohol intoxication, diabetics should carry a medical identification card at all times.

Other complications of insulin include redness and swelling around the site of injection, which usually disappear after a few days or weeks; lipodystrophy, which is either formation of a mass or loss of fat at the area of insulin injection; and insulin resistance. Insulin resistance is present when large doses of insulin—over 200 units daily—are required to control blood sugar.

All diabetics should be well-informed about their disease. They should know how to check their urine for sugar and how to adjust insulin dosages accordingly. And, they should carry a medical identification card at all times. Insulin-requiring diabetics also should have lumps of sugar or a candy bar readily available for episodes of hypoglycemia. Proper diet with maintenance of ideal body weight is the cornerstone of treatment in all diabetics.

Hypoglycemia

Hypoglycemia (low blood sugar) is a relatively rare disorder. Because the symptoms may be vague and because so much has been written about hypoglycemia, many women may mistakenly think that they have this problem. Hypoglycemia is of two types—reactive hypoglycemia, which occurs within one to five hours after eating a meal, and fasting hypoglycemia, which occurs during the fasting state. The causes of reactive hypoglycemia include functional (unknown) cause, mild diabetes, prior surgical removal of the stomach, and several hereditary enzyme deficiencies. The causes of fasting hypoglycemia are usually more obvious. They include islet-cell tumors of the pancreas (which secretes insulin), non-endocrine tumors, hypopituitarism, malabsorption, starvation, alcoholism, adrenal insufficiency, cirrhosis of the liver, necrosis of the liver, renal tubular acidosis, and certain drugs, including insulin and oral hypoglycemic agents.

The symptoms of hypoglycemia usually do not occur until the blood glucose level is less than 45 mg, which is about one-half of the normal fasting value. These symptoms include sweating, shakiness, palpitations, rapid heart rate, nervousness, weakness, fatigue, nausea, vomiting, and hunger. Other symptoms that may be present include headache, lightheadedness, blurred vision, yawning, and speech difficulty. In severe cases, stupor, coma, and death may occur.

Lab studies should include a glucose tolerance test, which requires the patient to drink a measured amount of glucose with blood sugar determination made before and each ½ hour for 4 to 5 hours after the glucose ingestion. If the blood glucose drops below 45 mg and symptoms occur, then the diagnosis is confirmed. Blood glucose and insulin levels can be determined after a 72-hour fast to test for fasting hypoglycemia. In a normal individual, blood glucose levels will not drop below 45 mg even after a prolonged fast. If fasting hypoglycemia is present, then other tests are done to determine the cause.

If the hypoglycemia is functional or due to prior surgery on the stomach, a diet low in carbohydrates and high in protein often will relieve symptoms. If mild diabetes is the cause, a diabetic diet is the treatment. Some patients later develop more severe diabetes.

Endocrine Causes of Obesity

Obesity is defined as excess fat in the body. In men, a fat content of more than 25 percent of body weight is considered excessive; in women, more than 30 percent is excessive. Obesity is the most common metabolic disorder in countries where food is abundant. It is estimated that up to 45 percent of the United States population over 30 years of age is at least 20 percent overweight. In women, the excess fat is distributed mainly in the hips, arms, and legs. In men, the fat accumulates in the abdomen and upper trunk.

The hypothalamus governs food intake, and contains both a satiety center and a feeding center.

Although rare, there are several endocrine disorders that contribute to obesity.
- Sheehan's syndrome (see page 608) is associated with weight gain.
- Hypothyroidism is one of the more common endocrine causes of obesity.
- Cushing's disease causes the moon face, buffalo hump, and obesity discussed on page 617.
- Diabetes mellitus is often accompanied by obesity, and obesity is a predisposing factor in the development of diabetes.
- Diseases that cause an increase in insulin production also lead to obesity by causing hypoglycemia and increased food intake to combat the low blood sugar. Among these disorders is the islet-cell tumor of the pancreas.
- Deficiency of the sex hormones testosterone and estrogen also is associated with obesity. Menopause is often accompanied by weight gain, possibly due to decreased level of estrogen.

To treat obesity in individuals who do not have the endocrine abnormalities outlined above, caloric intake must be reduced. Because prolonged fasting can be dangerous and is most often ineffective in the long run, a modest reduction in calories is best. To maintain ideal body weight, some permanent restriction of diet is necessary. Exercise is an excellent means of burning up calories, and in motivated individuals can be quite effective in weight reduction, particularly when combined with decreased caloric intake.

Amphetamines and similar drugs are commonly used to treat obesity, but they may be habit forming and have dangerous side effects, including increased blood pressure and heart rate.

When an endocrine cause for obesity is found, specific hormone treatment is indicated. Hypothyroidism is treated by replacing thyroid hormones. Thyroid hormones are sometimes used by doctors to treat obesity when there is no thyroid disorder. They increase the basal metabolic rate, which burns more calories. Unfortunately, low doses of thyroid hormone do not increase the basal metabolic rate, and larger doses often lead to hyperthyroidism.

Obesity related to Cushing's disease, Sheehan's syndrome, and islet-cell tumors should respond to the previously discussed treatments of these diseases.

Obese diabetics should be treated with diabetic diets—the most important part of treatment for adult-onset diabetes.

If obesity is caused by sex hormone deficiencies, the treatment is replacement of the sex hormones.

One last method of managing obesity is the surgical removal of large portions of the intestine. However, this procedure is not recommended except in extreme circumstances when obesity endangers a patient's life.

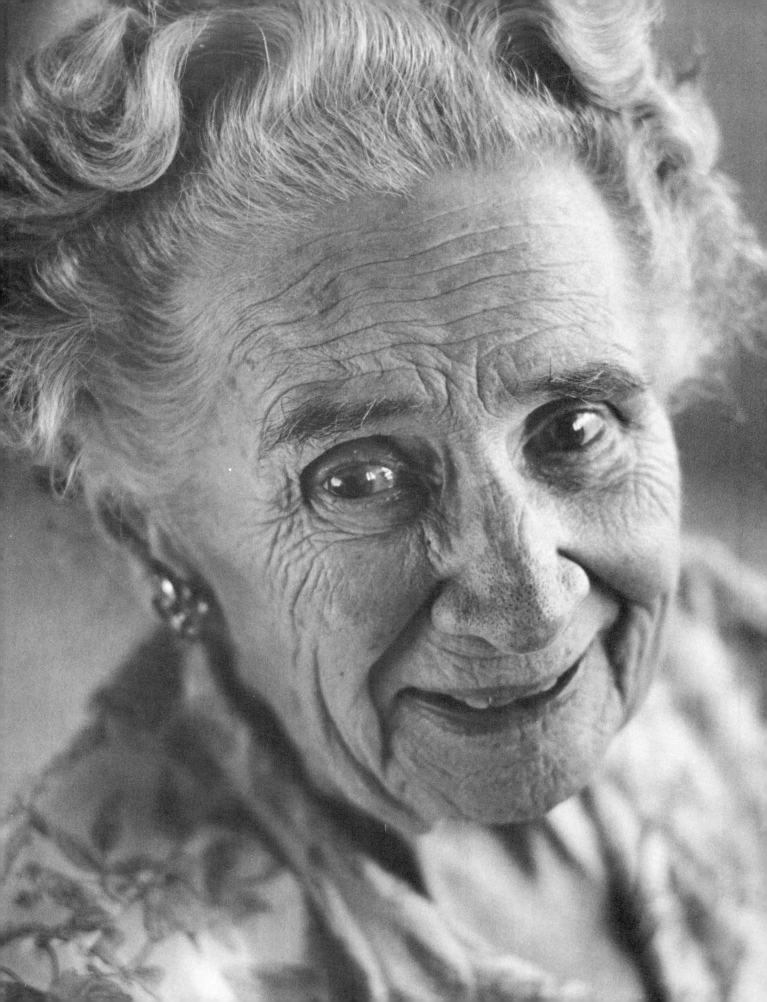

CHAPTER 30

ARTHRITIS AND RHEUMATISM

ROBERT D. FRIEFELD, M.D.

Aches and pains in our joints affect every one of us at some time in our lives. Perhaps this is why arthritis has been called "everyone's disease." Essentially, arthritis is any inflammation of a joint that shows itself as pain, heat, swelling, and redness. Rheumatoid arthritis is probably the most severe form of the disease, but there also are many other kinds of arthritis.

Arthritis and Rheumatism

Joints are involved in every move we make. If part of a joint begins to malfunction, we feel it right away as an ache, a crunch, or a sharp pain. Wear and tear on the joints produce the aches and pains that many of us refer to as "rheumatism." And when a joint becomes swollen or inflamed, we feel the pain and restricted movement of "arthritis." Actually, what we commonly call arthritis and rheumatism are known to the medical profession as varieties of a larger disease classification — rheumatological diseases.

Rheumatological disorders not only affect the joints or the tissue around the joints, they also may affect connective tissue anywhere in the body. The specific disorder called degenerative joint disease, commonly referred to as "arthritis," occurs only in joints. But rheumatoid arthritis, or "rheumatism" as it's popularly called, may affect not only the joints, but also the connective tissues around the joints and elsewhere in the body — including, for example, the lining of the heart and blood vessels.

In a survey done in the 1960s, more than 16 million Americans, two-thirds of them women, stated that they suffered "arthritis." Actually, they may be suffering from either degenerative joint disease or rheumatoid arthritis.

This chapter will present the various kinds of rheumatological diseases, their symptoms, and treatments. You may appreciate that classifying rheumatological diseases is difficult because a person may suffer from several of them at once. The malfunction of a joint due to injury may weaken the adjoining connective tissue, or an aching joint (degenerative joint disease) may overlap with inflammation of adjacent connective tissue (rheumatoid arthritis). So before proceeding to the diseases, it will be most useful for our overall understanding to learn something of the anatomy of joints and connective tissue, as well as to understand some details of the immune system.

Anatomy

Each bone in the body is joined to the bone next to it by a joint. Joints work in conjunction with other connective tissue structures—such as bones, tendons, and ligaments—to support the body, protect internal organs, and provide mobility.

Joints

Three types of joints connect the bones of the skeleton, each in a manner appropriate to the necessary function of the particular bones and joints. For example, the bones, joints, and connective tissue in the skull provide protection for an internal organ — the brain. The joints in the skull, called *fibrous joints,* are immovable because bone movement would endanger the brain.

Sometimes restricted motion is desirable to provide flexibility as well as structural support, as with the disks between the 26 jointed bones of the spine. Such restricted motion is provided by *cartilaginous joints.*

The free movement necessary for the function of the knee and the hip is provided by *synovial joints.* The majority of the joints in the body are freely movable—some in only one or two directions, and others in many. These movable joints have two opposing surfaces that are covered by cartilage and are enclosed in a fibrous capsule that fits like a tight sleeve. A specialized lining of the capsule (the synovium) produces a lubricating fluid (synovial fluid). In considering how the joint is held together, the interrelationship of bone, muscle, ligaments, and the joint mechanism itself becomes clear. The sleevelike capsule holds the joint together while allowing movement. Ligaments bind and strengthen the capsule with the additional support of muscles working across the joint. Tendons that pass through the joint, with their own synovial lining, serve to transfer muscle power.

The joint surfaces come in contact only over a small area; otherwise, they would bind and lock. In the knee, for example, the synovial fluid lubricates the joint and nourishes the outer layers of cartilage so the surfaces can spin, slide, and roll across each other.

Joint cartilage has its collagen fibers arranged in arches, forming a smooth, slightly compressible surface that acts as a cushion to absorb shock. Cartilage has no blood vessels of its own, but depends on the force of alternate compression and relaxation to pump in nutrients provided by blood vessels in the bone. The underlying (subchondral) bone also is slightly compressible and helps absorb shocks.

Connective Tissue

Connective tissues are the structural substances of the body, consisting of a matrix of varying proportions of cells, fibers, and an amorphous glue called *ground substance.* Loose connective tissue —such as that of the breast, for example — has relatively more cells and fewer, thinner fibers than dense connective tissue, such as that of the joints.

TYPES OF JOINTS IN THE BODY

Joints work in conjunction with other connective tissues—bones, tendons, and ligaments—and skeletal muscles to protect internal organs, to support the body, and to provide mobility.

In the drawing, the major joints of the body are indicated by colored circles. There are three types:

FIBROUS JOINTS
These joints connect parts of the skull and are immovable, as they are part of the structure that protects the brain.

CARTILAGINOUS JOINTS
Found in the spine between vertebrae, these joints are flexible, yet are so restricted in motion that they provide structural support for the body.

SYNOVIAL JOINTS
These joints are found at such places as the knees, shoulders, elbows, hips, fingers, and toes. The majority of joints in the body are synovial and are freely movable.

Three kinds of fibers are present in connective tissue: collagen, reticulin, and elastin. Collagen, the most plentiful protein in the body, forms strong interlacing bundles, particularly in tendons and ligaments. Reticulin is somewhat finer and forms supportive networks around vessels, nerves, muscle cells, and other tissues. Elastin, as its name suggests, is elastic and is a major component of large arteries and stretchable ligaments. All connective tissue is metabolically active—rather than inert like the structure of a building—because there are living cells within it.

The Immune System

The immune system is the body's main defense against invading microbes (bacteria, viruses, fungi), but it also may react to pollens, foods, drugs, or transplanted tissues. Ordinarily, the body must recognize a substance as "foreign" in order to evoke an immune response. The type and magnitude of this response varies with each individual.

Substances evoking an immune response are called *antigens,* and are recognized by the immune system by their "foreign" molecular structure. Sometimes the body itself is mistakenly recognized as "foreign," perhaps because of a breakdown in the normal recognition system, accidental cross-reaction (as is thought to occur in rheumatic fever), or alteration of the body by foreign substances (perhaps virus particles or food products). An immune response against one's own body is called *autoimmunity.*

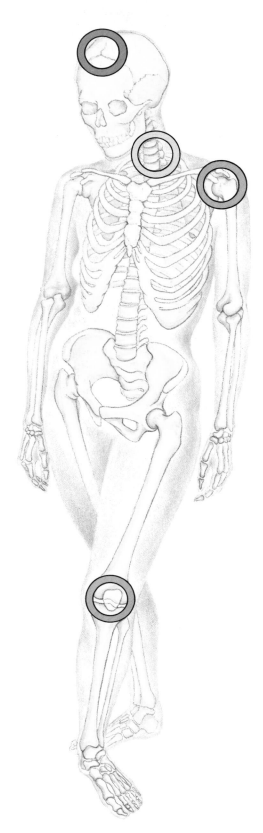

THE STRUCTURE OF A SYNOVIAL JOINT

Synovial joints are found between two bones (5). The two opposing bone surfaces are covered by cartilage (4). The joint capsule (1) encloses the joint. A specialized lining of the capsule called the synovium (2) produces synovial fluid (3) to lubricate the joint and to provide nourishment to the outer layers of cartilage.

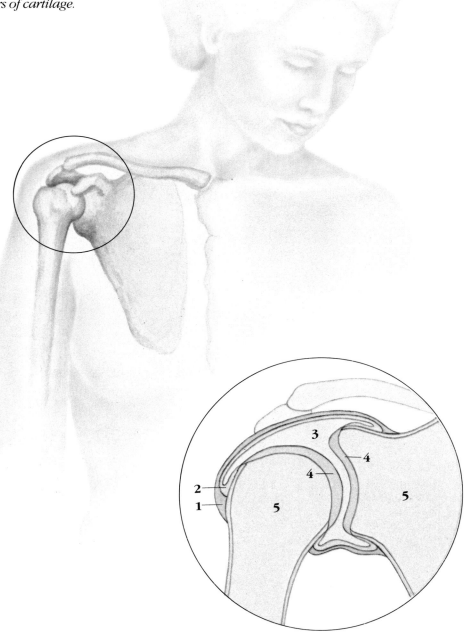

HOW MUSCLES SUPPORT SYNOVIAL JOINTS

Bone (5), joints (6), muscles (7), ligaments (8), and tendons (9) work together to provide skeletal stability and mobility. The joint capsule holds the joint together while allowing movement. Ligaments bind and strengthen the capsule, with the additional support of muscles working across the joint. Tendons passing through the joint, with their own synovial lining, serve to transfer muscle power.

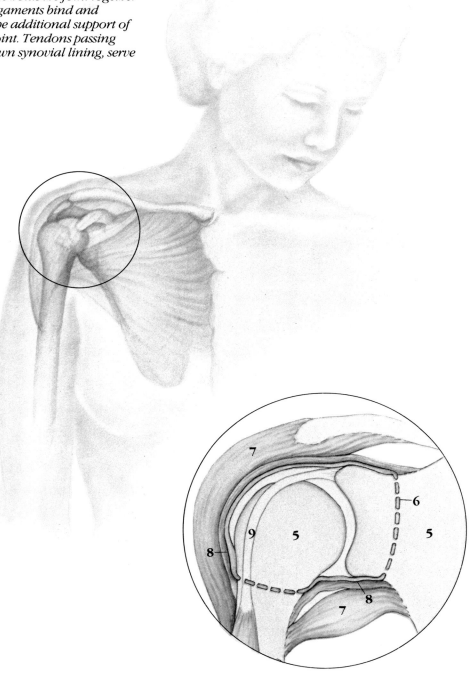

THE NOURISHMENT OF CARTILAGE

Joint surfaces come into contact only over a small area; otherwise they would bind and lock. The joint cartilage is bathed and cushioned by synovial fluid at the contact area. This cartilage, which contains no blood vessels, depends on joint movement to receive proper nourishment and remove wastes, as shown in the following enlargements.

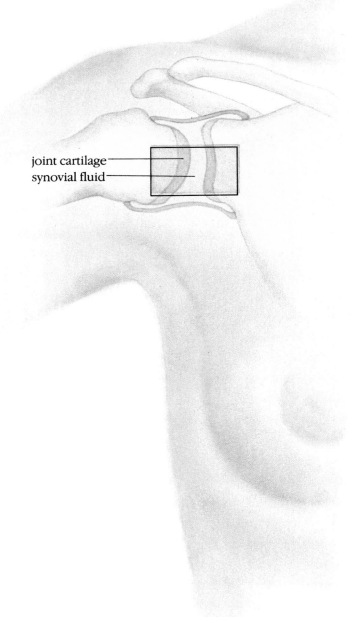

joint cartilage
synovial fluid

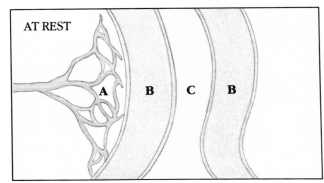

In this enlargement of a joint, cartilage (B) forms a smooth, slightly compressible surface that acts as a cushion to absorb shock to the bones and joints. Synovial fluid (C) cushions the outer layers of cartilage. Blood vessels (A) in the bone extend only as far as the inner edge of cartilage.

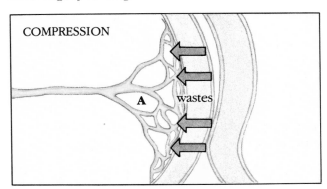

Since the cartilage contains no blood vessels, it is dependent on the blood vessels in the bone (A). When the joint is compressed, some wastes are forced into these blood vessels from the cartilage.

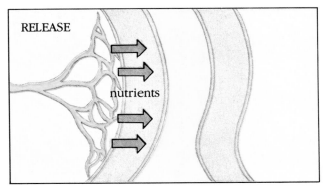

When the compression of the cartilage is released, nutrients move from the blood vessels into the cartilage. This alternate compression and release of the shock-absorbing cartilage pumps nutrients from the bone's blood vessels into the cartilage, and in turn forces wastes from the joint capsule into the blood vessels.

The inflammatory response begins when an antigen is taken up by a cell called a macrophage (big eater), which processes it and presents it to small white cells called lymphocytes (cells from the lymph system). Some lymphocytes then become factories producing *antibodies*. These antibodies (gamma globulins) are specially tailored to match the structure of the antigen, much the way a key fits a lock, and form antibody-antigen combinations called immune complexes. Certain white blood cells, called neutrophils, engulf the immune complexes and whatever they're attached to (for example, the wall of a bacterium), destroy them, and release sacs of digestive enzymes. They are aided by complement, an enzyme system in the blood that attracts more neutrophils and antibodies to the area, sticks everything together, and punches holes in the walls of cells under attack. This process is highly destructive of invading cells, whether working normally to destroy "foreign" cells or malfunctioning to destroy "self" cells. We're aware of it only as a local inflammation that produces warmth, tenderness, swelling, redness, and pus.

Under some circumstances, immune complexes in the circulatory system are deposited in the kidneys, along vessel walls, or in the joints. If the immune reaction occurs in these places, the damage is done to innocent tissues that were not involved in the initial immune reaction.

Autoimmunity seems to play an important role in connective tissue diseases. Often the presence of increased levels of gamma globulin in the blood and *autoantibodies*—one autoantibody is the rheumatoid factor (see page 631), another is the anti-DNA antibody—are found in conjunction with connective tissue diseases. In addition, the presence of immune complexes at sites of injury and evidence of complement depletion further suggest that autoimmunity is related to connective tissue disease. As additional evidence, we know that connective tissue diseases respond favorably to drugs that inhibit immune reactions.

Preventing Joint Dysfunction

As we take up a discussion of each disease in this chapter, preventive measures will be mentioned for each one. But first, here are some general guidelines you can follow to maintain normal joint function.

Joints must be used if they're to maintain their function. The mobility of your body depends on the formation of loose connective tissue in all areas where motion occurs. The more movement, the looser the meshwork of connective tissue becomes. With restricted movement, however, the meshwork becomes tighter until it's tough and dense.

What happens to this meshwork of loose connective tissue if you become immobilized for some time? Bed rest or confinement in a cast has a debilitating effect on the connective tissue, which reorganizes itself into a scarlike formation called a *contracture*. A contracture, like a tight scar, will hold a joint in its flexed position. While the formation of a contracture may be caused by immobilization, the condition can be worsened by poor circulation, inflammation, injury, or edema fluid, which acts like a glue in the connective tissue. Normal activity will prevent the formation of a contracture, but if one begins to form after prolonged immobilization, bone and cartilage will be affected. The bone will then become demineralized, the cartilage will be invaded by blood vessels and nerve endings, and the joint will become very painful.

Stretching exercises. When prolonged bed rest is necessary, contractures can be prevented by performing regular stretching exercises. Continued mild tension, as in exercise, tends to break up and loosen the matrix of the contracture, making tightened tissue more elastic.

With your pillow removed, lie flat and place your hands behind your neck for 30 minutes to straighten your back. Now lie prone with pillows under your chest for 15 to 30 minutes, stretch your arms up, and pull your feet against the end of the mattress. This moves all joints through their full range of motion without forcing them. Repeat these movements at regular intervals for maximum benefit.

Isometric exercises. Loss of muscular strength can be minimized with isometric exercises. It is especially important to maintain quadriceps muscle strength to stabilize the knee.

The quadriceps muscle in the thigh is the muscle that straightens the knee. To set this muscle, straighten your leg and tense your thigh or push your knee against the bed. Hold this position, relax the leg, and repeat the exercise five times.

During pregnancy, low backache is a common problem. The exact cause is unknown, but normal loosening of cartilaginous joints to accommodate the growing fetus, and the change in weight distribution may be contributing factors. Back-strengthening exercises begun early in pregnancy may prevent backache and are a regular part of most prenatal training classes (see page 296).

AVOIDING JOINT DYSFUNCTION WHEN BEDRIDDEN

STRETCHING EXERCISES

When prolonged bed rest is necessary, contractures can be prevented by performing regular stretching exercises that move joints through their full range of motion without force. Repeat the following exercises once daily.
A *Without a pillow, lie flat with your hands behind your neck for about 30 minutes to expand the chest and straighten the back.*
B *Lie prone with pillows under the chest and abdomen for 15 to 30 minutes, stretching the arms up and pulling the feet against the end of the mattress.*

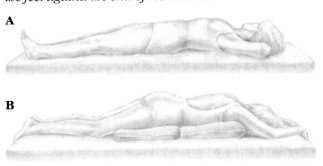

ISOMETRIC EXERCISES

Loss of muscular strength when bedridden can be minimized with isometric exercises. It is especially important to maintain quadriceps muscle strength to stabilize the knee.

To set the quadriceps muscle, straighten your leg, tense your thigh, and push your knee down against the bed. Hold for several seconds and then relax. Repeat this straightening-tensing-relaxing cycle five times.

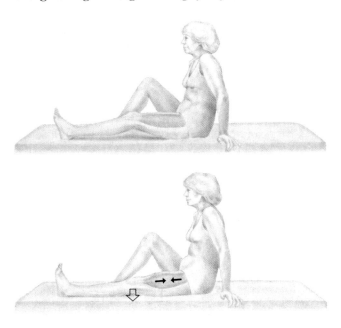

Chronic lower back pain is one of the most common complaints of women, and is almost always the result of poor posture and lack of proper exercise. The problem can be alleviated only by regular back-strengthening exercises that eventually correct posture (see page 296). Acute back strain occurs when a person with a poorly aligned back undergoes some unaccustomed activity. Strain of the back muscles then initiates a vicious cycle of spasm, pain, and more spasm. The best treatment then is flat-on-the-back bed rest and pain-relieving drugs.

Rheumatoid Arthritis

Rheumatoid arthritis (RA) is a chronic systemic disorder of unknown cause. The course of the disease varies greatly from person to person, but ends in severe joint deformity in only a minority of cases. Tissue damage is produced primarily by inflammation. A characteristic of RA is its tendency to flare up and then become quiescent in an irregular pattern. While no cure is known, treatment can effectively reduce the pain and suffering.

Susceptibility

Rheumatoid arthritis is the most common of the severe rheumatic diseases; in the United States, it is estimated that 3 percent of the population suffers from some form of RA. Rheumatoid arthritis can start at any age, but most commonly it begins between the ages of 30 and 60, with women affected three times as often as men. RA does not seem to run in families or even in identical twins, and it has no strong relationship to climate, location, race, or culture.

Signs and Symptoms

In the majority of cases, the onset of RA is insidious and is characterized by fatigue, general weakness, and a vague aching and stiffness in the muscles and joints. After a few weeks, joint pain becomes a prominent symptom, along with warmth, swelling, tenderness, and stiffness after inactivity of the joint. In rare cases, the onset may be abrupt and widespread.

Although only one or two joints may be involved initially, RA progresses into a multiple-joint disease with a tendency to affect the same structure on both sides of the body (for example, both hands rather than just one hand). The structures affected are the hands, wrists, elbows, shoulders, knees, ankles, and sometimes the hips, jaw, and neck. Muscle weakness and wasting is due to the direct muscle involvement in the disease, but tendons also become inflamed and may rupture.

The active phase of rheumatoid arthritis with its characteristic symptoms and "hot" joints may last weeks to months and then subside with little functional impairment. In recurrent or unremitting cases, there is more permanent disturbance in joint function. Chronically involved joints become enlarged, lose stability, and may become contracted or even dislocated. Chronic involvement of the hand produces a characteristic deviation of the fingers to the side opposite the thumb (ulnar drift) and incomplete dislocation of the joints. Once RA has caused joint damage, secondary degenerative arthritis can develop. A major source of disability is flexion contractures (see page 629) of the knees and hips that occur if joint involvement causes disuse or immobilization. When the upper neck is involved, a serious complication of spinal-cord pressure may result.

Extra-articular manifestations. As a systemic connective tissue disease, RA is sometimes evident at sites other than joints. These extra-articular manifestations of the disease sometimes require special treatment.

Rheumatoid nodules are hard, painless lumps that occur most often at pressure points along the underside of the forearm. They are virtually unique to RA and are present in about 25 percent of all cases. The nodules come and go, and seem to parallel the activity of the disease. If rheumatoid nodules form in the eye, they can cause an inflammatory reaction.

Mild anemia is also an extra-articular manifestation and is very common, except in inactive cases. The anemia is due to failure of the bone marrow to produce enough new red cells to make up for the ones destroyed. Iron supplements do not correct the problem. Less commonly, the white cell count may be reduced and the spleen may enlarge.

The lungs also may develop rheumatoid nodules and fibrosis, and an associated shortness of breath accompanies severe cases. Inflammation of the lining of the lung (pleurisy) sometimes produces sharp pains that are worsened by deep breathing. The sac surrounding the heart (pericardium) may become inflamed, and if the heart muscle itself is weakened, congestive heart failure may result. There is often a circulatory insufficiency manifested by red palms and cold, tingly hands. Nerve entrapment may result in the carpal tunnel syndrome (see page 641) caused by tendon sheath swelling. Kidneys, liver, intestines, and other organs are usually spared, however.

Vasculitis is inflammation of the connective tissue in arteries, leading to wall weakening or obliteration. If small arteries are affected, there may be small brown spots at the nail folds or finger pulp. Skin ulcers, particularly in the lower legs, are common. Other manifestations include skin rashes, Raynaud's phenomenon (see page 642), numbness due to interruption of the blood supply to nerves, and bleeding intestinal ulcers. When large arteries are affected, there can be massive hemorrhage. Vasculitis is the most serious complication of RA, and may be life-threatening. Fortunately, it is not common.

Cause and Effect

The cause of RA has not been discovered. While viruses, bacteria, and other infectious organisms can cause arthritis, so far no one has isolated one of these from patients with RA. It may be that a susceptible individual is sensitized by a viral particle to which her immune system is especially vulnerable. Other theories abound, including the notion that RA is a psychosomatic illness, or the result of food allergies.

Immune mechanisms, as outlined previously, are important elements in producing tissue damage. In the early stages, the synovial fluid distends the joint capsule; this is called an *effusion*. The fluid is cloudy, watery, and loaded with neutrophils that are producing destructive enzymes. In this way, the synovial fluid loses its normal nutritional and protective function. In advanced stages of the disease, the synovial membrane increases greatly in size because of infiltration of inflammatory cells, and forms folds that eventually encroach upon and adhere to the cartilage. This "pannus" is responsible for much of the destruction of cartilage and the erosion of underlying bone. As inflammation subsides, the pannus thickens and limits joint movement.

There are no specific laboratory tests that can diagnose RA. Rheumatoid factors (RF) are autoantibodies present in 85 percent of people with RA, as compared to about 4 percent of the rest of the population. RFs also may be present in other connective tissue diseases and in chronic infections in which there is no arthritis. Very high concentrations (titres) of RFs in the blood tend to accompany more severe cases. In addition, the sedimentation rate or ESR (erythrocyte sedimentation rate) — a nonspecific indicator of inflammation based on the rate at which red blood cells settle out of a prepared blood specimen — is elevated in active RA, but drops as disease activity wanes. X rays show bone erosion and loss of cartilage as these conditions develop.

Course and Prognosis

Statistics regarding the eventual outcome of RA are biased in the negative direction because many people with mild cases do not seek medical care. Therefore, statistics reflect the more severe cases. Even so, there is considerable room for optimism. After 10 to 15 years, about 20 percent of patients will have had remission, and 50 to 70 percent remain capable of full-time employment. After 15 to 20 years, only about 10 percent of patients are invalids.

Some factors associated with a poorer prognosis are the presence of rheumatoid nodules or high titres of rheumatoid factors, onset of the disease before age 30, persistent active disease without a letup for more than a year, and extra-articular manifestations other than anemia. Some individuals have recurrent attacks but fail to develop joint damage (palindromic rheumatism). However, the average person will undergo episodes of active disease and remission leading, over a period of years, to some disability.

Treatment

RA is a treatable disease, and the fact that there is no specific cure need not lead to despondency. A combination of physical measures and medications is used to relieve symptoms, preserve function, and prevent deformity. These treatments result in a far better prognosis than if a patient remains untreated, but a continued commitment to self-help is vital. Such a commitment comes in part from understanding the disease, as well as understanding the purpose of every aspect of the treatment.

All persons afflicted with a chronic condition must yearn for a "miracle cure," one with minimum emphasis on waiting and invested time and effort. An entire industry exists to feed these inevitable hopes with quack remedies. Unfortunately, none of these "miracle cures" have stood the test of time.

Since RA is an inflammatory disorder, the aim of treatment is to reduce inflammation. Pain is a result of the inflammation and will be relieved as treatment achieves its goal. To settle for pain relief as an end in itself is to stop short of the full benefits of available treatment. The basic program is comprised of (a) rest, (b) physical therapy, (c) analgesic drugs, (d) suppressive drugs, and (e) readjustment. More dramatic therapies may be added when their benefits outweigh their risks. The following discussion covers the aims, rationale, methods, and risks of treatments that have been developed with experience.

In following the activity of disease and the response to treatment, your doctor will ask routinely about the duration of morning stiffness, the time of onset of afternoon fatigue, and the medication needed to reduce pain. He may make serial measurements of joint swelling, body temperature, grip strength, or the time needed to walk a standard distance. He also will measure sedimentation rate (ESR), rheumatoid factors, and other factors dictated by your individual case. And, he should work with you in planning your particular treatment program.

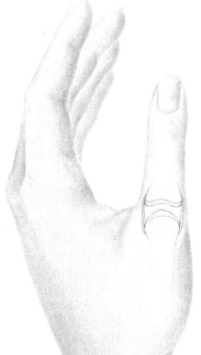

Rheumatoid arthritis commonly occurs in the synovial joints of the hand. The following enlargements of the thumb joint show the changes that occur in the joint as rheumatoid arthritis progresses.

JOINT CHANGES IN RHEUMATOID ARTHRITIS

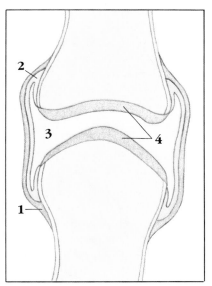

In a normal synovial joint, the joint capsule (1) fits like a sleeve. A fluid-filled space (3) enclosed by the synovial membrane (2) exists between the opposing bones, which are covered with smooth cartilage (4).

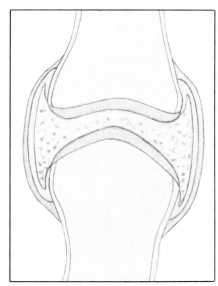

In the early stages of rheumatoid arthritis, excess synovial fluid swells the joint capsule. The fluid becomes cloudy, fills with neutrophils, and loses its normal protective and nutritional function. Symptoms at this stage are joint pain, warmth, swelling, and stiffness after inactivity.

Physical Measures

The aim of physical therapy is to help relieve symptoms, shorten disability, prevent or correct deformities, and improve function. The exact methods used depend on individual evaluation and prescription. Then a physical therapist initiates treatment and most importantly, teaches the patient what she can do on her own.

Rest vs. activity. At one extreme, the patient who takes permanently to bed and feels that "it's no use" will have little pain but may become severely crippled. At the other extreme, the patient who feels she must "keep going no matter what" will suffer unnecessary pain and joint damage. Obviously, a balance must be reached.

During episodes of active RA when joints are inflamed and prominent systemic symptoms persist, rest quiets the disease. Continued activity during this phase makes the disease worse and may decrease the chance of a remission. In milder cases, partial bed rest of 12 hours at night and two half-hour rests during the day (sleep unnecessary) combined with reduction of everyday activities will be adequate. With multiple joint involvement, especially that of weight-bearing joints, complete bed rest is needed. Rest must be continued until significant improvement has been sustained for one to two weeks. Initially, it may be a good idea to enter a hospital to obtain freedom from extraneous responsibilities and distractions. When symptoms subside sufficiently, rest may be continued at home.

When in bed, you should be in a comfortable position, but not all curled up. It will be best to use a firm mattress with a plywood board underneath. Lie on your back most of the time, use only a small pillow, and avoid support under the knee. The feeling of increased stiffness following rest periods, called gelling, is not a sign that joint injury is occurring, and this symptom decreases as the rest program continues. Individual joints can be rested with specially designed splints.

Exercise is movement to preserve or increase the range of motion, prevent muscle atrophy, maintain patterns of joint motion, and achieve maximum function. Exercise should begin immediately — even during bed rest. It is extremely important to *prevent* the development of contractures. Contractures occur when joints are not moved through their full range because of pain or because the body, and therefore the joints, are maintained in a flexed position, as with prolonged sitting in a chair (see page 629).

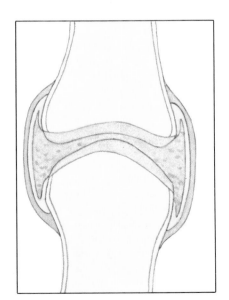

Joint spaces become narrow, resulting in limitation of movement.

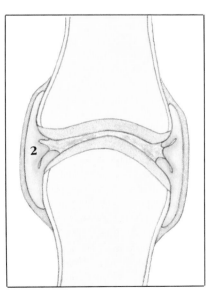

In advanced stages of the disease, the synovial membrane (2) increases greatly in size due to inflammation. It forms folds that encroach upon and adhere to the cartilage.

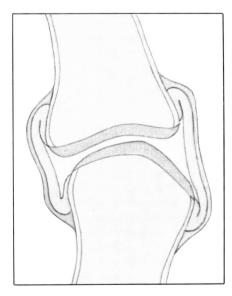

The swelling of the joint may subside, but the joint has lost stability and becomes contracted or even dislocated. The thickened synovial membrane remains.

Joint function depends on motion of the joint. And joint stability depends on muscular strength. Therefore, muscle exercise is most important in RA treatment. Exercises are classified as follows:

Passive exercise. The patient does nothing but relax, perhaps with the help of heat applications, while a helper or therapist moves her limbs. Passive range-of-motion exercise helps prevent adhesions and muscle shortening, and is preliminary to active movement.

Isometric exercise. Muscles are tensed (see page 630) but there is no motion of the joint. This helps maintain strength when the part of the body or the limb cannot be moved.

Active exercise. The patient moves the part herself, with or without assistance.

Resistive exercise. The patient moves against weights or against a helper. This is good exercise for strengthening specific muscle groups.

Increased pain can be expected during exercise and is not a reason to stop exercising. However, if the pain persists more than an hour after exercise, decrease the amount of exercise you perform in any given time. If you are bedridden, perform the exercises outlined on page 630 of this chapter. As disease activity abates, more and more active exercise is possible. The exercise regime adopted by a patient and her physician or physical therapist must be done regularly to be beneficial in relieving RA symptoms.

Heat and cold. Heat application is probably the oldest and most commonly used form of therapy for RA. Heat has several effects:
• Heat reduces stiffness through reducing the viscosity of synovial fluid (like heating maple syrup).
• Heat increases blood flow as well as local metabolic activity.
• Heat increases the stretchability of collagen fibers.
• Heat reduces muscle spasm by decreasing nerve sensitivity to stretching.
• Heat gives mild sedation and a sense of well-being.

Too much heat may make a severely inflamed joint worse, however. Heat should not be used on areas of the body where the blood supply is poor or on areas that are numb.

Superficial heat may be applied with a hot water bottle or hydrocollator pack heated to about 175 degrees F. and placed over layers of terry cloth. The maximum effect occurs in about ten minutes, after which the increased blood flow generated by the heat carries the heat away from the affected area. Shortwave diathermy and ultrasound are good for deep heating. Paraffin baths work well for heating small joints of the hands or feet. They can be prepared at home with simple equipment using a mixture of canning-grade paraffin and mineral oil. Heated water tanks in which you can immerse your whole body at about 105 degrees F. have the advantage of permitting active exercise with the buoyant support of water. Radiant heat from lamps also is useful at home. Half an hour in a warm tub at home is perhaps the easiest way to relieve morning stiffness.

Cold has well-known anesthetic effects. Cold packs may provide the most relief during acute inflammation. Usually, a five-minute application is enough to provide relief.

Massage. Gentle stroking massage warms the skin, stimulates nerve endings, and brings about a muscle-relaxation reflex. Massage also is soothing, giving a general sense of well-being. When combined with exercise, it decreases adhesion formation.

Splinting. When joints are swollen and painful to move, they need protection. In mild cases, an elastic bandage may be adequate support. In more severe cases, traction applied to the hips and knees puts the joints at rest and relieves muscle spasm. However, neck traction should not be used for rheumatoid neck disease. Finally, the limb can be casted with plaster or fiber-glass splints. The cast is cut into halves so that it can be removed, and is wrapped with elastic bandages when in place. During periods of immobility, splints are particularly useful in maintaining joints in a position required for optimum function. While the limb is splinted, isometric exercises can be used to maintain strength.

Surgical Measures

A number of different surgical procedures have been developed to improve the functional abilities of people with RA.

Joint surgery is not done during the acute stage of arthritis. Patients who have been bedridden for years are poor operative candidates because their tissues heal poorly and because they have little chance of becoming active enough to benefit from the surgery. The objective of reconstructive surgery is to obtain a functionally useful joint and not to achieve normality. For example, a stiff straight knee is more functional than one that is unstable or contractured in a flexed position. In all cases, the surrounding muscles must be strengthened by exercise for several weeks before surgery, and postoperative rehabilitation must start as soon as the wound is sufficiently healed. Usually surgery is withheld until a trial of more conservative therapy has failed.

Synovial membrane removal (synovectomy) has been performed for a number of years with the idea that dysfunctional synovial tissue is responsible for much of the joint damage that occurs. Synovectomy does effectively relieve pain, but it is not certain how successful the operation is at reducing eventual joint damage or at what point in the progression of the disease it should be done. The best results have been obtained on patients whose knees were operated on before they were severely damaged.

With more severe joint disease, a variety of reconstructive procedures, including total joint replacement, may be helpful. The total hip prosthesis has been the most successful of these. Finger joint replacement often has been successful as well, but knee, ankle, elbow, and shoulder prostheses are not yet perfected. More conservative treatments include osteotomy (trimming bones to improve angulation) and arthrodesis (fusing joints in a functional position).

Manipulation of joints is considered a useful treatment when the deformity is chiefly due to adhesions or contractures. Under a general anesthetic (for total muscle relaxation), the joint is stretched and then casted in the improved position. The procedure can be repeated at weekly intervals and produces good results. Contractures may be released by lengthening and resewing the joint capsule and the tendons.

Occupational Therapy

Functional occupational therapy attempts to retrain the patient to perform such vital daily tasks as eating, bathing, and handling tools through specific activities. It is most valuable in developing or maintaining movement of the upper extremities. Exercise in the form of projects is especially helpful in showing patients what they can accomplish. Morale building is one of the major goals of occupational therapy, and includes vocational retraining and guidance.

Activity should not be tiring or painful. The therapist will work with the patient in designing special aids to increase functional capacity. After corrective surgery, occupational therapy is particularly valuable in retraining fine movements.

Medical Therapy

A large variety of useful drugs is available for the treatment of RA. They fall into three categories:
● Analgesic (pain-relieving) drugs such as acetaminophen (Tylenol) are always helpful for temporary relief of RA pain symptoms. Codeine and other narcotics should be avoided because they can lead to a tolerance and addiction with prolonged use.
● Anti-inflammatory agents (a list follows) do not appear to influence the eventual outcome of RA. Their purpose is to relieve symptoms by reducing joint swelling, pain, and morning stiffness. These agents also have a separate analgesic effect.
● The third category includes drugs with specific activity in RA. They are more effective than anti-inflammatory drugs, and seem to fundamentally alter the disease process. These drugs retard the progression of joint damage, improve extra-articular manifestations, and reduce the sedimentation rate and serum rheumatoid factor. They cannot reverse joint damage that has occurred, however. Since these drugs are slow-acting and tend to have the most damaging side effects, they are usually reserved for more severe cases of RA.

Corticosteroids are in a class by themselves. They are anti-inflammatory (not analgesic), nonspecific, highly toxic, and have a controversial role in the management of RA, despite their great value in treating certain other conditions.

Salicylates (aspirin). Aspirin (acetylsalicylic acid) is often regarded as the mainstay in the medical treatment of RA. Analgesic effects are noticeable at the low doses prescribed for common aches and pains, but the more important anti-inflammatory effects do not become apparent until much larger doses are taken. Your doctor will prescribe the dosage appropriate for your particular case.

The usefulness of aspirin is limited by the inability of many people to tolerate it. At effective anti-inflammatory doses, it can be very hard on the stomach. The most common gastric symptom is indigestion. It usually helps to take each dose with meals and snacks or with a liquid antacid. Specially buffered or coated preparations may be better tolerated but are less effective. Salicylates have a definite tendency to produce serious stomach ulceration that may lead to hemorrhage. (Watch for black, tarlike stools as a sign of heavy intestinal blood loss.)

As the blood level of aspirin approaches the toxic range, central nervous system side effects occur. Most patients first notice a ringing in the ears (tinnitus) that may disappear if the daily dose is lowered by as little as one tablet per day. At dangerous levels, symptoms of headache, dizziness, difficulty in hearing, nausea, vomiting, hyperventilation, sweating, thirst, lassitude, confusion, and coma may occur. Under these circumstances, the medication must be stopped and a doctor contacted. Some individuals have an allergy to aspirin manifested by skin rashes, nasal congestion, or wheezing.

Aspirin should not be used by people with an active peptic ulcer or an aspirin allergy.

Anti-inflammatory agents—non-steroidal. Partly because of the problems with aspirin, a number of other anti-inflammatory agents have been developed. Their therapeutic actions are very similar to those of aspirin, but they differ as to degree of toxicity.

Ibuprofen (Motrin) compares with aspirin as a pain reliever but is a weaker anti-inflammatory agent. Nausea and upset stomach are usually less severe, and intestinal bleeding is uncommon. The usual effective dose is 400 mg three times daily.

Fenprofen (Nalfon) is approximately as effective as aspirin, and is less likely to cause gastric disturbances. It is more toxic than ibuprofen. The usual starting dose is 600 mg three or four times daily, which may be reduced once a response is achieved.

Naproxen (Naprosyn) is also as effective as aspirin, but with more gastrointestinal side effects than ibuprofen. An advantage of naproxen is that it is taken only twice daily for full effect.

Tolmetin (Tolectin) is nearly as effective as aspirin. Gastric intolerance is fairly common, and it may cause rashes, headaches, dizziness, and edema. The usual dose is 1.2 g daily in three divided doses.

Indomethacin (Indocin) is a potent anti-inflammatory drug effective in RA but with greater toxicity than the agents above. With daily administration, indigestion and nausea are common. Headaches, lightheadedness, and confusion also are frequent, but may disappear with a reduced dosage. Peptic ulceration and bleeding may occur as well. The usual dose is up to 150 mg per day in three divided doses. Sulindac (Clinoril) is a newer derivative of indomethacin with fewer side effects. In RA treatment, a dose of 100 mg to 200 mg twice daily is usually required.

Phenylbutazone (Butazolidin, Azolid) and *oxyphenbutazone* (Tandearil) are effective agents in the treatment of RA. Again, gastric side effects are common. Of the drugs so far listed, these have the most serious potential side effects. Bone marrow reactions may cause a drop in the white blood cell count in younger patients. This side effect tends to occur within the first three months of therapy and is reversible by discontinuing the drug. In elderly patients, the marrow may be nearly wiped out with a usually fatal result. Elderly patients also may develop heart failure from fluid retention. These complications are quite rare but *do* occur. The drugs should not be taken for minor conditions or when other agents will do, and in no case for longer than three weeks.

Chloroquine (Aralen) and *hydroxychloroquine* (Plaquenil) are anti-malarial drugs that are minimally effective in RA. They were used as alternative drugs for a long time, but now have been largely abandoned because they can cause partial or complete blindness. Persons taking these drugs should have an exam by an ophthalmologist every six months.

The drugs so far listed have roughly similar effectiveness in large groups of patients. The key to their use is individual variation in response to treatment and individual occurrence of side effects. What works for one person may be useless for the next person. Since the objective is relief of symptoms, side effects and risks must be kept to a minimum. It makes sense to start with the safest and best-tolerated drugs and then to move to more potent ones if needed.

An anti-inflammatory drug should be used at full dose for about two weeks before concluding that it is ineffective or safe to tolerate. While analgesic effects start immediately, anti-inflammatory action takes several days to reach a peak, and side effects also should be apparent by then. If effective, a drug should be continued on a long-term basis, perhaps at reduced dosage. Improvement is not a sign that a drug is no longer needed but that it is working. As the activity of the disease enters remission, only intermittent therapy may be needed. However, if the drug is not effective, there is no point in continuing it, and others should be tried in succession. There is no advantage in combining several of these drugs except, in some cases, when night supplements of indomethacin may prove effective.

The long-term side effects of the newer drugs are, of course, not known. None of them should be taken during pregnancy.

Corticosteroids are the most potent anti-inflammatory agents known. The ones in use today are synthetic analogues of cortisol, a steroid hormone produced by the outer layer (cortex) of the adrenal glands. This hormone plays an essential role in regulating the body's metabolism and response to stress. Their oral use in RA is limited to the treatment of serious extra-articular manifestations or occasional treatment in cases of severe RA that have not responded to other therapy. Although they can produce rapid and dramatic relief of symptoms, prolonged use inevitably produces debilitating side effects. Meanwhile, the underlying disease process is unaltered. The problem is that they may do more harm than good in most cases.

When needed, steroids are employed in the lowest dose that will ameliorate symptoms. Experience has shown that beneficial effects tend to be temporary unless the dose is made larger and larger. On the other hand, once started, the drugs are difficult to discontinue because the RA may then flare up, perhaps even worse than before.

Therapeutic steroid doses suppress the body's normal ability to release internal steroids in situations of stress. Without an adrenal response, stresses such as illness, accident, or surgery may produce a shock state. So it is essential not to miss doses (by forgetting or running out) and to taper the dose slowly when discontinuing a steroid drug. The adrenal suppression effect lasts up to a year or two after a course of steroids. It is a good idea for patients in that situation to wear a bracelet alerting emergency care personnel so that supplemental doses of corticosteroids may be administered if needed.

The major side effects, all dose-related, are weight gain (cheeks, abdomen, "buffalo hump"), fluid retention, diabetes, high blood pressure, fragility of the skin, accelerated osteoporosis (decrease in bone mass) with concomitant bone fractures, and increased susceptibility to all types of infection. Corticosteroids probably do not cause peptic ulceration. In high doses, they may cause a psychosis or aggravate an underlying psychiatric condition. The powerful anti-inflammatory effect may result in poor wound-healing or may mask the signs of a serious illness such as a perforated appendix.

Gold compounds have been an important adjunct in the therapy of RA for over 50 years. Recently, it has been realized that gold may be one of the very few drugs to have a specific beneficial effect in RA beyond relieving symptoms. Gold is used principally when early, progressive RA has not been controlled by more conservative therapy. In patients with long-standing disease, it may be beneficial if inflammation is still active.

Gold must be administered by intramuscular injection (an oral form is in an experimental stage) once a week until a response occurs, or until a maximum dose has been reached. This takes several months, but once the response occurs, it tends to be long-lasting. Then injections can be continued at longer intervals and at lower doses indefinitely. Unfortunately, only about half of RA patients benefit from or can tolerate gold therapy. Its mechanism of action is unknown, and it works in only a few other arthritic conditions.

The problem with gold, aside from the inconvenience, is the high incidence of side effects and serious toxicity. It commonly produces skin rash, sore tongue, ulcers in the mouth, and a metallic taste, but these effects are often transient. Gold may damage the kidneys, and frequently there is a small amount of protein in the urine that goes away when treatment is temporarily discontinued. However, sometimes severe nephritis occurs. Gold also may decrease blood platelets resulting in an increased chance of bleeding. In rare cases, bone marrow activity may be suppressed. This effect may be temporary in some cases, but is fatal in others.

When a blood count and urinalysis are performed every two or three weeks, signs of serious toxicity can be picked up early, and the hope is that morbidity will be minimized. When side effects clear, therapy can usually be resumed, except in the case of bone marrow depression, nephritis, or severe skin rash. Overall, about one-third of patients treated with gold will have some side effects, but three-fourths of those side effects will be inconsequential. Gold therapy can be uniquely effective but requires close monitoring by a rheumatologist.

Penicillamine (Cuprimine). Penicillamine has been used for some time in the treatment of other disorders and recently has been found to be approximately as effective as gold for RA. It, too, seems to have a specific anti-RA effect. It is chemically related to penicillin, but it has no antibiotic effect, and can be used by individuals who are allergic to penicillin. Penicillamine is administered orally on a daily basis. If improvement occurs, it takes four to six months to reach a peak improvement level.

Symptoms of toxicity include skin rash, loss of taste for sweet and salt, nausea, kidney damage, and bone marrow suppression. Skin rashes may be treated with antihistamines, but more serious reactions will require discontinuation of treatment. As with gold treatments, your rheumatologist will take regular blood counts and urinalysis tests during therapy.

Intra-articular steroid injections. There are several corticosteroid preparations that can be injected directly into a joint with minimal absorption and, hence, no side effects of the type seen with systemic use. When disability is due to disease in only a few joints, injections are practical and temporarily effective in suppressing inflammation. But since the steroids may eventually damage cartilage, the number of injections that should be taken in one joint is limited. It is important to make sure that no bacterial infection is present in the joint because the suppressive effect of the steroid is strong enough to knock out the body's normal defensive inflammatory mechanism.

Psychological Factors

It is a common but not universal experience among people with rheumatoid arthritis to feel the first signs and symptoms of illness during a period of stress or emotional shock. For many people, such stresses are present each time the disease recurs, and often ups and downs in life crises seem to parallel the ups and downs of the illness. However, at the present time, there is no clear-cut evidence that psychological stress causes rheumatoid arthritis.

Once an individual has been diagnosed as having rheumatoid arthritis, the patient's willingness to follow a prescribed course of treatment — that is, the actual *positive motivation* to become well — is the most important factor in improvement. The patient's self-motivation to overcome the disability of rheumatoid arthritis will be the determining factor in reducing the degree of disability suffered.

Climate and Spas

Climate does not seem to affect the incidence of rheumatic disease, yet nine out of ten people with arthritis have a varying degree of sensitivity to changes in the weather. It is a common experience for them to forecast changes in the weather by noting variations in their symptoms. This relationship between weather and arthritis symptoms was verified experimentally in 1961 with a device called a climatron. Volunteers were enclosed in a room for up to a month while temperature, humidity, barometric pressure, ionization, and airflow were varied singly and in combination. No definite effects on the symptoms of arthritis were noted except when a rapid fall in pressure was combined with a rise in humidity, as might occur before a storm. All but one of the volunteers with RA experienced a worsening of symptoms under these conditions. An explanation may be that scarred tissues are less able to extrude fluids under these circumstances and so become distended and painful. Normal tissues respond to such a change in the vapor and pressure in the environment by losing water.

Mild, dry climates with stable temperatures and humidity may provide some benefits to RA sufferers. Arizona and New Mexico have been recommended despite their large day-to-night temperature change, and the West Indies also are in good repute.

From ancient times, people suffering various maladies have visited healing waters in an attempt to relieve their symptoms. Spas are health resorts where you may devote prolonged periods to rest, diet programs, regular walks and exercise, adequate sleep, and various water treatments. Spa therapy often includes physical therapy in combination with drug therapy, prescribed by attending physicians.

Water does provide a soothing treatment for RA patients; the exact reasons for this are unknown, but sulfur-containing waters are said to be the most beneficial for rheumatoid arthritis. The temperature of the water is most important, and is individually prescribed at the spa. The usual spa program involves a short thermal bath (at 98 to 107 degrees F.) to test

JOINT CHANGES IN DEGENERATIVE JOINT DISEASE

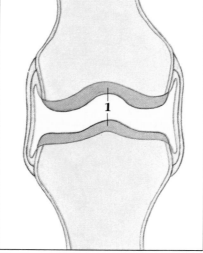

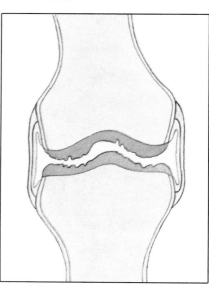

The knee joint is most frequently affected by degenerative joint disease (DJD), the cause of which is not known. The following enlargements of the knee joint show changes in the joint as the disease progresses.

Repeated minor injury may cause micro-fractures and hardening of underlying bone, subjecting the cartilage (1) in the normal knee joint to increased stress.

In the first stage of DJD, the cartilage becomes rough and pitted, and the joint space narrows. You may hear or feel a crackling sensation when you move your knee, and experience pain and aching as well.

the patient's tolerance, progressing to daily baths of increasing temperature and duration. Once begun, the treatments must be applied for one to two months to be of benefit. Peloids (mud baths) also may be applied at spas. Mud baths provide a steadier and more uniform heat than water baths.

The spa treatment is best for early illness, and is much less beneficial for those people disabled and confined to wheelchairs. Spas are not recommended during the acute phase of rheumatoid arthritis.

A trip to a spa may have considerable benefits for a patient's emotional and psychological state of mind as well. The natural, organic ritual of healing and bathing soothes, relieves, and relaxes, making spa treatment highly valuable as a simple comfort during the course of rheumatoid arthritis.

Pregnancy and RA

Often women find that pregnancy has suppressed the symptoms of rheumatoid arthritis. Improvement usually begins in the first trimester and gradually reaches a maximum in the third trimester. The reason remission sometimes occurs is unknown, but it is presumably related to changes in cellular immunity known to occur during gestation. After delivery, a relapse is common within two to six months.

The aims of treatment during pregnancy are the same as at other times, but special caution must be taken with drugs because they pose the possibility of damage to the fetus.

Degenerative Joint Disease

Degenerative joint disease (DJD), also called osteoarthritis, is a wear-and-tear disorder affecting the joints that bear the most body weight or do the most work. Although 90 percent of people over age 40 have some joint degeneration, only about 10 percent exhibit any symptoms. Degenerative joint disease is a chronic condition affecting only a few joints in the body, and does not have the implication of crippling disability of some other rheumatological diseases.

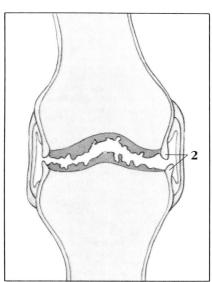

Under this changing pattern of stress, the bone reshapes and develops irregular protuberances called spurs (2) at the joint margin.

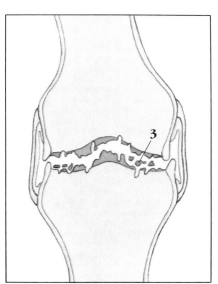

As DJD progresses, cartilage begins to break up (3). Under severe stress, fragments of cartilage may actually break loose, irritating the synovial lining. Such irritation may cause joint warmth, tenderness, and pain, and result in fluid accumulation.

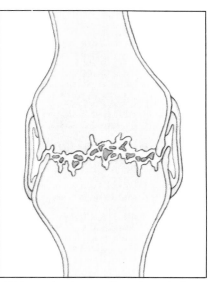

Ultimately, the cartilage is entirely worn away, leaving only bone against bone.

Signs and symptoms. The typical patient is middle-aged or elderly and in otherwise good health. Symptoms usually start when a degenerated joint is mildly stressed, resulting in an acute reaction with pain, swelling, and warmth. When the acute phase subsides, there may be a continued aching pain that becomes worse with motion or with weight bearing on the joint. Affected joints may ache at night and tend to feel stiff after rest.

The knee is the joint most frequently affected by DJD. Often the joint will have a crackling feeling on motion. If pain leads to disuse, the thigh muscles weaken and the knee becomes unstable and more easily injured. Degenerative disease of the hip may produce pain in the groin or down the inner thigh to the knee, but not usually at the side. The back and neck also are commonly involved. In severe cases, there may be pain that radiates down a limb.

A variant of DJD occurring in women of middle age involves the joints at the ends of the fingers. Characteristic nodules (Heberden's nodes) that appear at these joints may be soft and tender initially, but eventually become hard and painless. This form of osteoarthritis tends to run in families.

Cause and effect. The actual cause of DJD is not known. Possibly, repeated minor injury causes micro-fractures and hardening of the underlying bone. With loss of bony cushioning, the cartilage is subject to increased stress. The cartilage may become roughened, then pitted, and finally worn away, leaving bone against bone. Under the changing pattern of stress, the bone remodels and develops spurs and irregular protuberances at the joint margins. On X ray, these spurs are easily seen, along with joint-space narrowing resulting from loss of cartilage. Fragments of cartilage irritate the synovial lining and may cause an acute synovitis manifested by warmth, tenderness, and fluid accumulation. However, the degenerative process is not inflammatory.

Degeneration may be accelerated by abnormal stress. This includes obesity, congenital malformations (particularly of the hip), previous injury, or repetitive excessive usage.

DJD is usually slowly progressive within an affected joint, but does not move from joint to joint. An optimistic outlook is therefore appropriate. The most serious disability occurs when hip disease is severe enough to cause immobilization.

Treatment includes physical therapy, medication, and sometimes surgery. No cure is achieved, but the prognosis for retarding the disease and relieving pain is good.

When symptoms of pain and swelling are acute, the joint should not be actively exercised; overuse will aggravate the reaction and cause further deterioration. At this stage, immobility is less likely to cause stiffness of the joint than persistent activity. Isometric muscle contractions at the joint will help prevent muscle wasting, and local heat will relieve pain and lessen muscle spasm. Heat application is best limited to 20 to 30 minutes at a time. In the acute stage, while pain and swelling are most severe, some people find ice packs more helpful.

Joint conservation measures are aimed at reducing the wear and tear on involved joints. Excessive walking, standing, and stair climbing should be avoided and difficult as it is to achieve, weight reduction may be very helpful. Good posture also helps to keep joint surfaces in optimal alignment. And since most people have slightly unequal leg length —a condition that may increase joint stress, as can a flat arch — special shoes may be needed to relieve the stress. Finally, a cane can take weight off of a bad knee or hip.

Under the direction of a physical therapist, neck pain resultant from DJD is often relieved by heat and gentle traction. The best treatments are exercises that strengthen muscles and those that move the neck through a range of motion. Such exercises serve to maintain joint function and stability.

Analgesic (pain-relieving) drugs are most effective when taken regularly. Aspirin or acetaminophen is often adequate, but indomethacin may be of more benefit for some people. Many of the newer anti-inflammatory drugs, particularly ibuprofen, also have analgesic effects and often are better tolerated by the stomach. Steroids taken orally should be avoided for treatment of DJD. Although they relieve symptoms, the side effects are much worse than the disease, and they may even aggravate the degenerative process. However, steroids injected directly into the affected joint are effective for temporary pain relief.

Orthopedic surgery can be extremely helpful in some cases of severe DJD. As a prerequisite, the patient must be physically and emotionally prepared to cooperate with postoperative rehabilitation. Surgery does not repair a damaged joint but enables the patient to regain some use of it. For instance, removal of a wedge of bone (osteotomy) can realign joint surfaces to take pressure off worn cartilage. Surgery may be necessary to relieve nerve-root pressure from DJD of the spine after more conservative physical measures have failed.

Total hip-joint replacement was perfected by Dr. John Charnley in England about 20 years ago, and now about 75,000 operations are performed yearly worldwide. The surgery requires removal of the diseased joint and its replacement with a shallow plastic dish cemented to the pelvis. This, in turn, fits a metal ball-and-stem cemented into the thigh bone. The prosthetic joint permits good motion and is free of pain in about 85 percent of cases. Middle-aged and elderly people can perform normal activities with no limp or extra support. About 80 percent of Charnley's first patients still had a good result after ten years.

The most frequent complication has been loosening of the metal stem, perhaps more common in heavy patients. Infection is a serious complication because it is usually necessary to remove the implant, leaving a shortened leg. Antibiotic-impregnated implants designed to lessen infection are in the experimental stage. Other complications that occasionally have arisen include fractured or weakened bone, dislocation of the prosthetic joint, and reactive new bone formation that results in a decreased range of motion of the hip joint.

The knee is a much more complex joint. Artificial knees used in the early 1970s have had a high rate of failure, and orthopedists presently recommend delaying total knee replacement as long as possible to allow time for development of better designs. Artificial elbows have met with a similar high failure

rate, and new designs are being developed. Ankle and shoulder prostheses also are short of perfection at the present time.

Carpal Tunnel Syndrome

The carpal tunnel syndrome is a common cause of tingling and loss of strength in the hands during pregnancy or after menopause. The first sign of this disorder is a tingling or burning pain that may occur during the night. These sensations often can be relieved by shaking the wrist. There also may be numbness of the thumb and first two fingers. As the disease progresses, wasting and weakness of the muscles at the base of the thumb can develop.

The symptoms are caused by compression of the median nerve, one of the three nerves serving the hand. The nerve is vulnerable where it passes through a tunnel between the bones of the wrist, along with tendons that curl the fingers. Any increase of pressure within this tunnel affects the softer nerve before it affects the tendons. Some of the things that can lead to such an increase in pressure include swelling due to water retention in pregnancy, or a local injury to the wrist. In addition, inflammation of the tendon sheaths may occur from overuse or from infection, or from rheumatoid arthritis. Frequently there is no obvious cause at all.

CARPAL TUNNEL SYNDROME

A *The carpal tunnel syndrome is a common cause of tingling and loss of strength in the hands during pregnancy or after menopause. The first sign of this disorder is a tingling or burning pain, but there also may be numbness of the thumb and the first two fingers.*
B *The symptoms are caused by compression of the median nerve (1), one of the three nerves that serve the hand. The nerve is vulnerable where it passes through a tunnel between the bones of the wrist (3) along with tendons (4) that curl the fingers.*
C *Any increase of pressure within this tunnel (2) affects this softer nerve before it affects the tendons, resulting in tingling, burning, and numbness of areas to which the nerve passes. Your physician will test for carpal tunnel syndrome by tapping the wrist where the median nerve passes through the bony tunnel.*

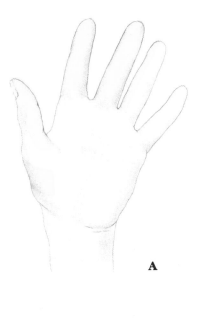

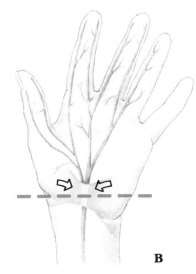

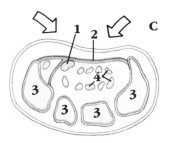

Your physician will test for a classic physical sign by tapping the wrist where the median nerve passes through the carpal tunnel. This tapping point is located between the radial pulse (the underside of the wrist toward the thumb) and the midline of the wrist. If carpal tunnel syndrome is present, the tap will greatly increase the symptoms of tingling or burning pain. Your doctor can confirm the diagnosis of carpal tunnel syndrome by measuring nerve conduction with an electromyograph (EMG).

The disorder is usually temporary, resolving a few weeks after pregnancy. In mild cases when neither edema nor tendon inflammation is present, the only treatment needed is a splint to keep the wrist straight at night. If edema is present, a diuretic may be helpful, and if the tendons are inflamed, local steroid injections may be used. Finally, surgical decompression can be performed, usually with excellent results.

Raynaud's Phenomenon

Raynaud's phenomenon is a disorder characterized by spasms of the superficial vessels in the hands. In a typical attack, cold exposure or strong emotion causes the hands to blanch and then to turn a dusky blue. On recovery, the fingers become bright red and often tingle, swell, and throb painfully. Some people also have these symptoms in their toes, ear lobes, chin, or nose. Raynaud's phenomenon may be primary (not associated with any other disease) or secondary (occurring in association with another disease). The primary form is the most common, and most often affects young women.

Cause and effect. The initial pallor in the hands is a result of decreased blood flow due to spasm of the small arteries of the hand. The blue phase occurs as small veins dilate to allow more blood to remain in the tissues (venous, deoxygenated blood looks bluish). On removal of the stimulus, the arteries open way up, allowing fresh blood to flow in. The cause of this arterial overreaction to cold or emotion is unknown.

In rare cases of Raynaud's phenomenon, circulation may be permanently impaired. In such cases, the fingers become slim and tapering, with smooth, shiny skin and slowly growing nails. If an artery is blocked completely, there may be a small, painful area of gangrene at the fingertip that heals slowly. Finger amputation is very rarely necessary, however.

Raynaud's phenomenon may be secondary to other conditions such as connective tissue disease, particularly scleroderma or rheumatoid arthritis. It also may follow repeated trauma, especially vibration such as typing or piano playing. An overdose of ergot compounds or methysergide, drugs used in the treatment of migraine, may be a cause of secondary Raynaud's phenomenon.

Treatment. In most cases, the most effective treatment of Raynaud's phenomenon is to protect the hands from cold by wearing loose-fitting gloves outdoors or even when removing items from the refrigerator. Since emotional upsets also can cause attacks, sedatives or tranquilizers may be needed. Use of tobacco, which causes constriction of arteries, compounds the symptoms of Raynaud's phenomenon.

For those with more severe cases, many drugs have been tried in an attempt to dilate the arteries, but none have been really effective. Reserpine in small doses may decrease the frequency and severity of attacks, and pit-viper venom has been employed to lower blood viscosity. A treatment suggested may be medication to block the affected nerves in the hand. This procedure can relieve symptoms dramatically, but they often return in two to five years. Surgical interruption of the sympathetic nerves may be warranted in extreme instances.

Systemic Lupus

Systemic lupus erythematosus (SLE) is a chronic systemic inflammatory disease of unknown cause. The usual manifestations are skin rashes, joint pains, fever, muscle aches, and pleurisy. Serious cases involve the kidneys, heart, or nervous system. Immune system abnormalities, some occurring only in this disorder, are important causes of tissue injury, but the majority of patients have a good prognosis.

Susceptibility

SLE is predominantly a disease of young women in their 20s and 30s but may occur at any age in either sex. The prevalence is about one case per 20,000 people, and it is about three times more common in black women than in white women. Immune system abnormalities are common in blood relatives and household members of persons with SLE, but the disease is not contagious.

Signs and Symptoms

The "classic" presentation of SLE is in a young woman with fever, loss of weight, fleeting aching pains in the joints, and a "butterfly" facial rash. Although easily recognizable, this picture is not the usual one. Often, the cumulative combination of seemingly unrelated abnormalities finally suggests the diagnosis. The most common features of the disorder are listed below.

Almost all patients have joint aches (arthralgias) involving the hands, feet, and large joints at some time. The onset may resemble rheumatoid arthritis, with fever, fatigue, malaise, and multiple-joint arthritis. However, the joint destruction so common in RA is rare in lupus.

Skin eruptions of various types occur in about 70 percent of cases. Most commonly there is a reddish rash on the face, neck, elbows, palms, or fingertips, particularly on sun-exposed areas. The "butterfly" rash over the nose and cheeks is less common. Hair loss is characteristic and usually temporary. Discoid lupus is a skin disorder with scaly lesions of the head and arms that heal as depressed scars. Some people with discoid lupus later develop SLE. Raynaud's phenomenon and a variety of other skin and mucous-membrane disorders also occur.

About half of lupus patients have kidney involvement, which can be the most serious aspect of the disease. If the kidneys are involved, a urinalysis may detect protein and perhaps red and white cells in the urine. Severe lupus kidney damage (nephritis) results in edema, high blood pressure, and uremia.

In addition, about half of patients have pleurisy or sharp pain when they breathe. This is a sign of inflammation of the lining of the lung (pleuritis) and may be associated with a fluid accumulation (pleural effusion). Sometimes the lung itself is involved, causing coughing and shortness of breath — a picture resembling pneumonia. Involvement of the sac enclosing the heart (pericarditis) may be another cause of chest pains. Most patients have abnormalities on the electrocardiogram (ECG) from pericarditis or inflammation of the heart muscle itself. Only in rare cases will heart involvement become serious.

About one quarter of patients have nervous system involvement. It may result in seizures, bizarre behavior, psychosis, stroke, palsy, or paralysis. These abnormalities may be mild and transient, but also occur in patients with severe disease needing maximum treatment.

When tested in the laboratory, most patients exhibit mild anemia and often have a low white blood cell count as well. Substances in the blood that interfere with clotting may cause a bleeding tendency, and many persons have painless enlargement of the lymph nodes, spleen, or liver.

Prognosis

SLE may be a mild disorder with limited symptoms; most individuals have remissions and relapses of variable length over a period of years. Severe cases are usually obvious within the first year, when most of the disease fatalities occur. With our present knowledge and treatment, more than 90 percent of lupus patients survive ten years or longer. But the outlook for survival is grave in patients with severe renal, nervous system, or heart involvement.

Treatment

No cure is available for SLE, but appropriate treatment helps to suppress flare-ups and prolong life. The type of treatment depends on the severity of the illness in each individual case. Those individuals with mild symptoms may require no treatment. Arthritis, arthralgias, muscle aches, and fever may respond to rest and anti-inflammatory compounds. Patients with skin rashes should protect themselves from the sun. Women with SLE probably should not use birth control pills. Rest and medication also are applicable to SLE patients.

In more severely ill patients, corticosteroids are the mainstay of treatment and often produce dramatic responses. Patients with renal, nervous system, or heart involvement in SLE are often given these drugs. Initially, patients are given high doses, typically 60 mg per day of prednisone; improvement may occur in 48 hours. If there is no response, the dose may be increased. Once improvement has occurred, the dosage is tapered over a period of weeks or months to the lowest level that will control the disease. If a flare-up occurs, a small increase in the dose is prescribed.

SLE and Pregnancy

There is a definite tendency for SLE to first appear or to flare up during the last trimester of pregnancy or shortly after the birth of a child. These exacerbations are usually treated in the same way as for nonpregnant women. Women with SLE should consult a physician immediately upon becoming pregnant. Therapeutic abortion is a possible choice if the disease is active, as pregnancy may be extremely hazardous for those women with more severe heart or kidney involvement.

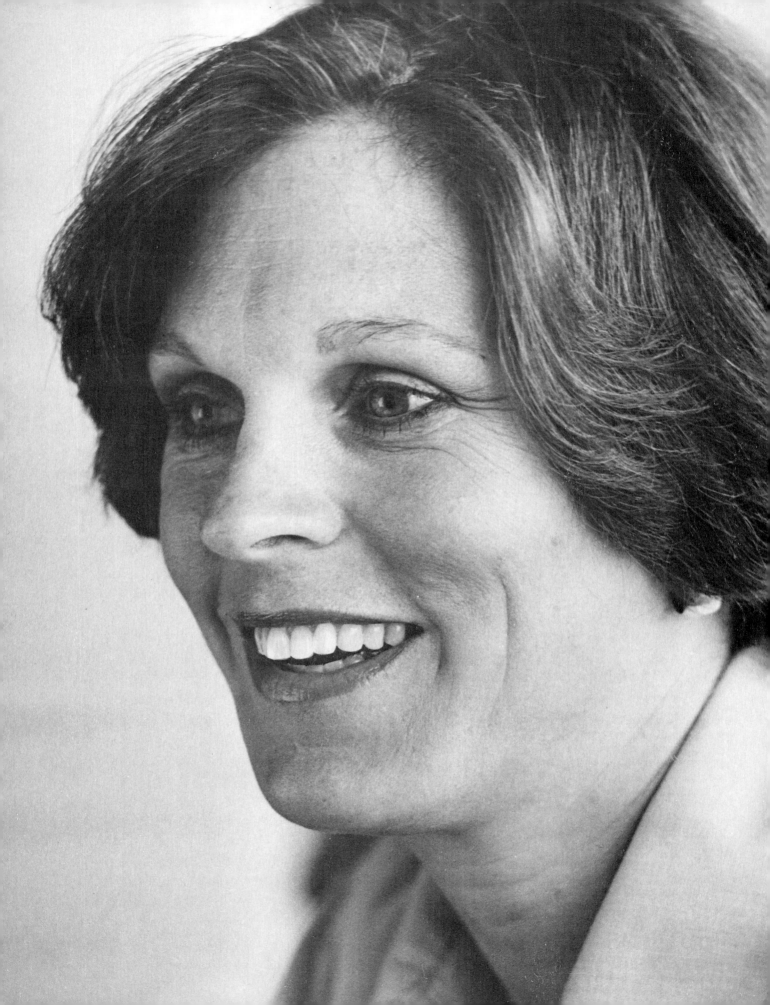

CHAPTER 31

PLASTIC SURGERY

PATRICK H. BECKHAM, M.D., F.A.C.P.S.

When we speak of plastic surgery, we usually think of cosmetic surgery, which helps a person who already looks fine to look even better. Another type, reconstructive surgery, helps to correct deformities resulting from birth defects, burns, disease, and injuries.

In recent years, the field of cosmetic surgery has grown so rapidly that 40 percent of all plastic surgery now performed is done for aesthetic reasons. If you are considering some type of cosmetic surgery, thoroughly discussing your motives and expectations with your plastic surgeon will help you achieve the most satisfactory results.

Plastic Surgery

The term "plastic surgery" was coined long before man synthesized the substance called plastic, but was derived, rather, from the root meaning of the word, which is "moldable" or "shapable." Molding and shaping were precisely what the early plastic surgeons learned to do with living tissue, transferring it from one place to another to reconstruct defects caused by war injuries or cancer. The synthetic substance plastic also is moldable or shapable when hot, hence its name. It is only coincidence that this manufactured substance, in the form of silicone implants, also has been used in the specialty of plastic surgery.

Plastic surgery developed as a specialty around the time of World War I when surgical techniques were maturing and when there was a great need for facial reconstruction because of the devastating injuries resulting from a trench war. More extensive dental reconstruction also was being done at that time, using surgical techniques to mold available skin. The entire range of present-day reconstructive and elective procedures has developed from these early efforts.

The specialty of plastic and reconstructive surgery is only partly understood by most people. It is not a specialty that is confined to a particular region of the body, nor is it confined to a particular organ system. Rather, it is a specialty of techniques that can be applied to tissues all over the body. Although it deals primarily with surface problems and skin surgery, it often involves surgery on bones, cartilage, nerves, muscles, and occasionally, internal organs as well.

Choosing a Plastic Surgeon

In choosing a plastic surgeon, it is first helpful to pinpoint the specific nature of the problem, if possible, and then to consult the physician most knowledgeable and best trained for that problem.

Pinpointing the Problem

Determining the nature of the problem in terms of the appropriate medical specialty may not always be an easy task. Nevertheless, one of your first decisions may involve the question of whether a plastic surgeon or another type of surgical specialist is appropriate for your particular problem.

Because a well-trained plastic surgeon covers so many areas of the body, there is considerable overlap between the work of plastic surgeons and that of other surgical specialists. For example:
• A person with a fractured nose and resultant breathing problems might justifiably seek an ear, nose, and throat surgeon to improve the airway. But in addition, a plastic surgeon might be needed to improve the outer shape and appearance of the nose (rhinoplasty).
• Similarly, dermatologists treat a myriad of skin problems and operate very successfully on some of them. But other problems involving more extensive skin removal and more complex reconstruction are often referred to a plastic surgeon.
• Some oral surgeons also have been trained to correct jaw deformities as well as to perform dental surgery, and, in the same way, cross paths with the plastic surgeon who reconstructs jaw and facial deformities.
• In hand injuries, both orthopedic and reconstructive surgeons have common interests in rebuilding bone as well as correcting tendon, nerve, blood vessel, and skin injuries.
• Plastic surgeons and urologists share a common field of interest in dealing with birth defects of the genitourinary tract.
• Finally, plastic surgeons and neurosurgeons are jointly concerned with several aspects of peripheral and facial nerve injuries.

Plastic surgeons perform a large number of surgical operations to improve facial and body appearance. If your goal is to improve your appearance, you may decide to contact a plastic surgeon directly for your problem.

In selecting a plastic surgeon, you should seek the recommendation of your family physician and check with others who have been patients of that surgeon.

Find out whether or not the surgeon under consideration is board-certified. The American Board of Plastic Surgery certifies those with sufficient training — preliminary general surgery training and a plastic surgery residency. To be board-certified, the surgeon must have passed a two-part examination.

Your county medical society generally lists the board certifications of all physicians practicing in the county. There is also such a listing in the *Directory of Medical Specialists* in most local libraries. And, if no other source of information is available, the American Board of Plastic Surgery may be contacted directly.

It is also possible to check a physician's membership in county, state, and national medical societies as other indications of his or her reputation, or to scan local hospital staff appointments to see if the surgeon is active in the local medical community.

Plastic Surgery Techniques

The techniques of plastic surgery include the use of grafts, flaps, and implantable materials; microsurgery and free tissue transfer; and organ transplantation.

Grafts and flaps are the two most common terms for the transfer of skin from one part of the body to another. A graft is formed from tissue that is completely detached and transferred to a new location. Skin may be transferred in varying thicknesses — a shave-thickness (split-thickness) graft or a somewhat thicker (full-thickness) skin graft. The term flap indicates that some part of the transferred tissue retains its connection to the original blood supply, at least until it can create new attachments for survival in the new location. For some reconstructive problems requiring thick padding, the underlying muscle is moved with the skin.

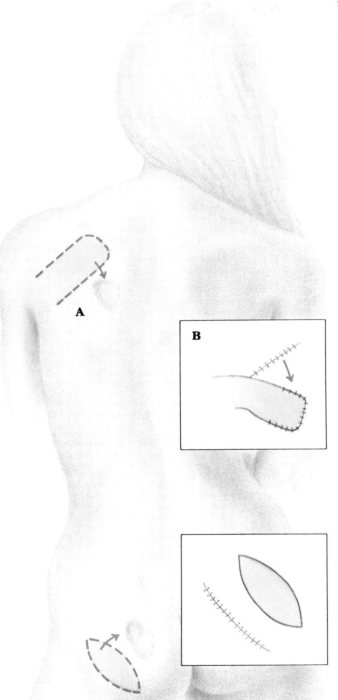

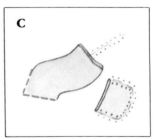

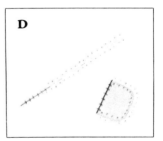

TECHNIQUES FOR SKIN TRANSFER

SKIN FLAP

A *The incision is made to form a flap.*
B *The free end of the flap is stitched over the defect. The site of flap removal is closed with stitches.*
C *After the new attachment is complete, the flap is detached.*
D *The incisions of the donor and defect sites are closed.*

SKIN GRAFT

Tissue from the donor site is completely detached and transferred to a new location.

The implantation of synthetic material, such as silicone, has been a relatively recent addition to plastic surgery techniques. These implants may be used to reshape or to enlarge parts of the body.

Microsurgical techniques — surgery under magnification — is another recent development, one that makes it possible to connect small blood vessels, thus permitting the transfer of tissue to entirely new locations with an instant blood supply. While the technical problems in this type of surgery are formidable, the procedure is increasingly successful. Similar techniques also have been used in transplanting whole organs, such as the kidney.

Restoring Use and Appearance

The techniques of plastic surgery are designed to restore both function and appearance. The plastic surgeon uses these techniques in a variety of ways to correct problems as diverse as severed tendons and facial wrinkles. The types of surgery performed can be divided into two categories — reconstructive and elective plastic surgery.

Reconstructive plastic surgery refers to procedures that are performed to restore the function and appearance of a missing or damaged part of the body. A part of the body may be missing or malformed due to a birth defect, an injury, or disease.

Elective plastic surgery (also called cosmetic or aesthetic plastic surgery) concentrates on improving appearance when no functional problem exists.

Reconstructive Surgery

Reconstruction can apply to almost any area or organ of the body. The most common conditions calling for reconstructive surgery are congenital deformities of the face, hands, and genitalia; burns and other scars of the face and hands; skin cancers; vascular ulcers or other skin losses due to skin disease; and arthritis of the hand.

Birth defects involving the face. *Cleft lip and palate* problems have plagued mankind as long as medical records have been kept. The incidence of such deformities ranges between one in 800 and one in 1,000 births.

Sometimes the lip and nose are affected, and the upper jaw and palate remain intact. The reverse also can be true, with the hard and soft palate divided and the lip, nose, and jaw properly developed. The most difficult conditions to correct are those involving the lip as well as the palate. Sometimes both sides of the face are affected. Lip repair is usually done somewhat earlier than palate repair because of their differential growth characteristics. Specifically, it is important that the lip sides are together to properly align the upper jaw as it grows. If the lip is not repaired and remains divided, the jaw parts will often grow wider apart.

Generally, the first surgery is performed on the lip at the age of two or three months, after the baby shows good signs of growing and thriving. Very often, at the time of surgery, small polyethylene tubes are placed in each eardrum to prevent middle-ear infections.

Ear infections are common in cleft-palate children in the first two years of life because the muscle connection across the palate does not allow the eustachian tube (the air vent to the middle ear) to open properly in the throat. Because of this problem, it is important to feed a cleft-palate baby with the head and shoulders propped up about 45 degrees from the flat position so that liquid food doesn't enter the ear passages during swallowing.

Cleft-lip repair involves repositioning the lip and attaching the two sides, as well as attempting to reposition the base of the nose. The nose repositioning can be the hardest part of the operation, and both the lip and the nose may require additional correction as normal growth changes occur.

The palate surgery is usually delayed until an infant is eighteen months old because earlier surgery tends to cause more scarring deformity in the development of the upper jaw. Because the child already has begun to develop speech habits in the first eighteen months, many speech-control patterns may have to be broken and relearned.

With modern methods of palate closure, about three-fourths of the children operated upon for cleft palate do not require further surgery, although a good many of them do need speech therapy. If necessary, further surgery in the throat may improve the sound of the voice. With additional speech therapy, most of these patients will develop acceptable speech.

Both the lip and palate operations require general anesthesia and about five days of hospitalization after surgery. Their discomfort is probably similar to that associated with a tonsillectomy.

More complex facial deformities can involve the jaws, the ears, or sometimes the whole facial structure. A team of surgical specialists, including a neurosurgeon, has recently developed techniques for rearranging the facial bones, as well as the eye sockets and the front part of the skull.

FEEDING A CLEFT-PALATE BABY

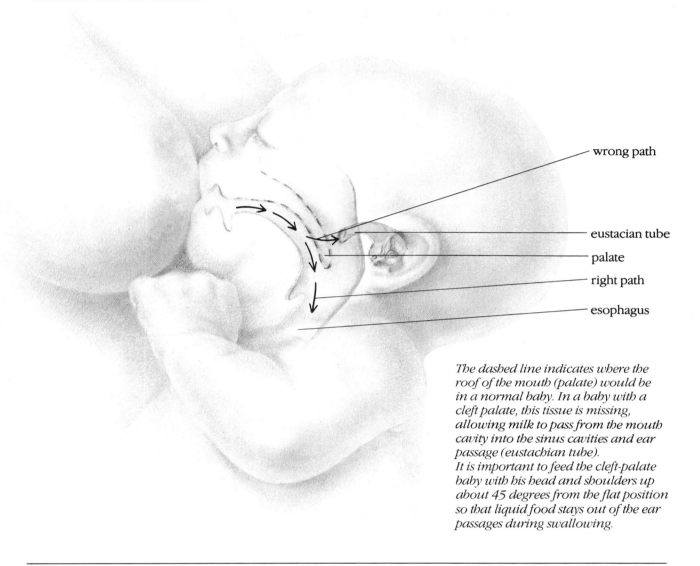

wrong path

eustacian tube

palate

right path

esophagus

The dashed line indicates where the roof of the mouth (palate) would be in a normal baby. In a baby with a cleft palate, this tissue is missing, allowing milk to pass from the mouth cavity into the sinus cavities and ear passage (eustachian tube).
It is important to feed the cleft-palate baby with his head and shoulders up about 45 degrees from the flat position so that liquid food stays out of the ear passages during swallowing.

REPAIR OF A CLEFT LIP

Cleft-lip repair involves repositioning the lip, attaching the two sides, and repositioning the base of the nose.
A *A cleft lip before surgery.*
B *An incision is made, and the lip is repositioned.*
C *The incision is closed with sutures.*

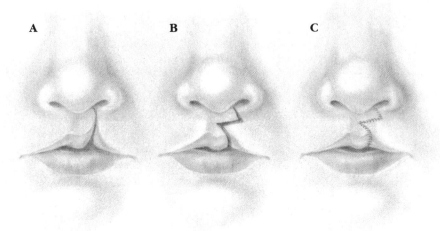

A   B   C

Less complicated deformities include severe variations of the outer ear or the complete absence of the outer ear. Surgical correction usually involves several stages of shifting cartilage and skin into the appropriate area to make a replacement for the ear. A silicone frame may be successfully substituted for cartilage, but it is quite difficult to make a completely natural-looking ear. In some cases, an external prosthesis — a false ear made of silicone rubber and attached by surgical cement that must be reapplied every few days — remains the best solution for cosmetic purposes.

Vascular tumors (hemangiomas and lymphangiomas) about the face cause discoloration and can invade surrounding tissue (see page 568). While many will fade spontaneously, others must be removed surgically with appropriate graft or skin-flap replacement. Vascular tumors in later stages often require removal of small remnants of the tumor subsequent to surgery. Sometimes other forms of treatment beyond surgery are required; presently underway is experimental work with laser beams.

Large moles on the face and sometimes those on the body require extensive removal and skin grafting. Because a certain percentage of heavily pigmented moles becomes cancerous, these dark moles must be watched very closely. Often it is recommended that they be removed and replaced with skin grafts.

Hand deformities. Birth defects resulting in deformities of the hand occur about as frequently as those resulting in facial deformities. *Webbed fingers,* the most common hand deformity, can be successfully reconstructed by the plastic surgeon, even though the webbing may extend all the way to the fingernails.

Webbed fingers are separated in order to allow the fingers to work individually. The techniques used to accomplish this goal include the application of skin flaps and skin grafts. Skin flaps from the back of the hand are combined with full-thickness skin grafts from the groin area to produce a hand that is more functional and more nearly normal in appearance. However, there will be considerable scarring. If the webbing extends to the fingernails, there may remain some deformity of the nail area as well.

The hospital stay for such a procedure may be as short as two or three days. But it is still necessary to wear a cast on the hand for about two weeks thereafter in order to prevent hand movement until the grafts are satisfactorily healed.

Extra fingers are the result of abnormal fetal development and can be removed or shortened at an appropriate time — usually before the child starts the first grade. Sometimes it is necessary to proceed much earlier if the deformity is such that it obstructs the normal growth of the hand.

Abnormal genital development can involve the bladder as well as the vagina. Bladder problems are surgically corrected early, but a congenital absence of the vagina need not be corrected until adolescence.

The absence of the vagina may be treated in one of several ways. The most common procedure creates a vault lined with thin (split-thickness) skin grafts. Since these skin grafts have some tendency to shrink, changing the size of the vault, it may be necessary to wear a packing device for a few months until the tendency for shrinkage has vanished. Once the vault has matured, the functional capacity is usually satisfactory.

Other disturbances in genital development involve sexual abnormalities. In some cases, an infant's external genitalia are not clearly male or female. Such cases usually require abdominal surgery to determine the true sex of the patient. If surgery reveals the

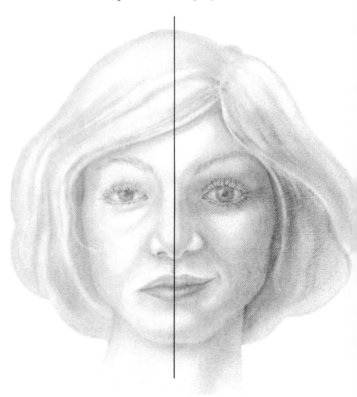

REPAIR OF THE FACIAL NERVES

Facial paralysis, as shown on the right side of the woman's face, can result from a laceration causing damage to the facial nerve. If damaged nerves can be found and repaired under magnification, the chances of recovering muscle function are good.

presence of ovaries, for example, the patient's "true sex" is female.

In cases of mixed sexual development, it is more common to reconstruct existing female structures. Occasionally, endocrine therapy is helpful in the later stages of development, as is social and behavioral support to reinforce appropriate psychosexual development as a female. In cases of sexual anomalies of this magnitude, it is most important that the sexual determination be made as soon as possible, before male or female behavior patterns are established in the formative years.

Injuries. Reconstructive surgery following injury is a major concern of plastic surgery. Most injuries requiring reconstruction occur on the face, and include the trauma of lacerations and fractures.

Lacerations of facial skin, lips, and eyelids are especially demanding for the plastic surgeon. To obtain the best result, reconstruction of missing tissue often must be performed in stages.

One of the primary complications of a face laceration is damage to the facial nerve, which controls the muscles used in facial expressions. Division of the facial nerve near the lower part of the ear results in

facial paralysis. Smaller branches toward the front of the face also can be damaged.

When muscles are paralyzed after a laceration, it is important to locate and reconstruct the small nerve branches. If the nerve branches can be found and repaired under magnification, the chances of recovering muscle function are usually good.

Another important structure in the cheek area is a rather large salivary gland with a duct leading from the corner of the jaw into the side of the mouth. If this passageway is injured by a deep laceration and continues to leak, healing is very difficult and may not occur because of the continued drainage of saliva. Repair of the duct should prevent this problem.

Damage to the eyelid—with its cartilage, inner lining, and lashes—often cannot be completely restored. Bony fractures about the rim of the eye socket usually require repositioning and sometimes supportive wiring of the eyelid. If the floor of the eye socket is fractured at a position inside the rim but the rim remains intact, it is still possible for the eye contents to be wedged into this area due to the pressure of the injury. In such cases, surgery is usually necessary to restore unhampered eyeball movement.

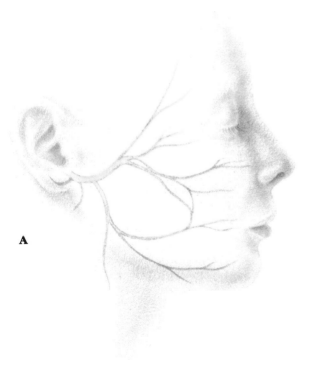

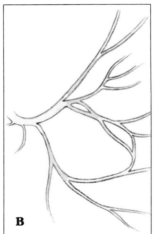

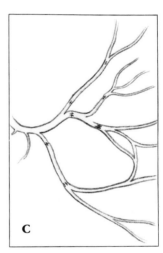

The side view of the face above (A) shows the position of the facial nerves. In the boxes are close-ups of the normal facial nerves (B) and damaged facial nerves that have been repaired (C).

Fracture of the nose, a common facial injury, should be repaired within a week or ten days, or the bones will heal in their dislocated positions. For four or five days following surgery, packing must be used inside the nose to support the proper inner position, and a stiff cover—such as a malleable metal disk or a plaster mold—is worn for about two weeks to maintain the proper outer position. At that point, the nose is likely to stay in position, but for about another month, it could be dislodged by a blow.

Hand injuries are challenging to reconstruct because they often involve tendons, nerves, blood vessels, and missing skin as well as nail-bed injuries.

Tendons usually can be repaired at the time of injury. Different tendon-repair techniques are used depending, in part, on the location of the injury. But the operation is only the first step. Most of the work of recovery is done by the patient who must undergo appropriate physical therapy in order to recover full use of the hand.

REPAIR OF TENDONS

The reconstructive surgeon uses a number of different surgical techniques for tendon repair, depending upon the zone of injury. The anatomy or structure of the tendons makes repair more complicated in some zones than in others.

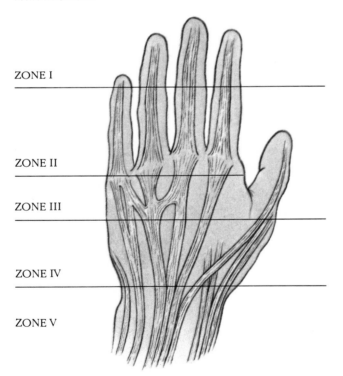

ZONE I

ZONE II

ZONE III

ZONE IV

ZONE V

Nerve injuries in the hand can be repaired by microsurgery techniques. Microsurgery also permits reattachment of small arteries and veins, even to the extent of replacing a completely severed finger. Even when circulation is restored, however, tendons, nerves, and bones still create significant obstacles to satisfactory function of the hand, and recovery takes several months. Nevertheless, reconstruction is often very effective.

Skin loss over the hand usually occurs from burns, but also can result from a severe scraping injury such as that sustained in a motorcycle accident. It is important that skin coverage be restored early so that the patient can exercise the hand and joints, which tend to stiffen very quickly in a swollen hand.

Scars following the treatment of second- and third-degree burns are often thick and sometimes show strong tendencies to shrink and contract. Because a contracted scar can respond to constant stretching and flattening pressure, it is possible to wear elastic garments on the extremities that provide constant, gentle, uniform pressure to the thickened scars.

If the contracture interferes with joint motion, it may be necessary to use elastic splinting to restore as much motion as possible. Exercising is beneficial, but the constant pressure of an elastic splint seems to be of primary importance in bringing about improvement.

Badly thickened scars sometimes must be removed or rearranged quite late in the course of burn care when freer function and better joint motion are needed. In fact, the care of severe burns usually extends into a period of several years.

Reconstruction following disease. Disease also causes conditions that require reconstructive surgery. Perhaps the most common of these is skin cancer.

Basal-cell carcinomas are the most common skin cancers, and they do not tend to spread to any distant site. If left unattended, however, they can spread locally and burrow into underlying tissue. A complete removal of the cancer will usually control it, and if the cancer is large, a skin graft or local flap is sometimes used. Sun exposure is a major causative factor of basal-cell carcinomas.

Squamous-cell carcinoma commonly develops on the lower lip. Such carcinomas are not only aggravated by sun exposure, but also by smoking. In these cases, it is usually necessary to remove a wedge or a triangle of the lower lip. Lip tissue is sufficiently elastic that a rather large wedge can be removed and the rest of the lip will stretch to make up the difference. It is possible for squamous-cell carcinomas to spread by way of lymphatic vessels and sometimes by way of blood vessels to lymph nodes or other organs in the body. Such cases may require surgery to remove the nearby lymph nodes, and possibly radiation therapy as well.

Malignant melanoma is another type of skin cancer that may occur on the face, but it more commonly occurs on the extremities or on the back. These cancers usually arise in a mole, and are usually signaled by a darkening in color or a change in size (see page 580).

Melanomas have a great tendency to migrate by lymphatic or blood channels, and therefore may require removal of wider sections of tissue than squamous-cell carcinomas. Covering these open areas properly usually requires skin grafting.

Arthritis can severely deform joints, resulting in loss of function (see page 632). The reconstructive surgeon may perform hand surgery to realign joints that have tilted out of position from the destruction of the joint lining. The tendons in the hand may also need to be repositioned, reinforced, or reattached.

The operation to remove inflamed linings and to straighten the direction of the joint is called arthroplasty. When the joint is so severely deformed that it cannot be repaired, it is possible to cut out the joint section and to place a flexible silicone rubber shaft into the space. Such devices are designed to keep the finger better aligned and to allow some degree of motion. This operation could be called "replacement arthroplasty" but it is more commonly referred to as a "joint implant operation."

Ordinary arthroplasty can achieve better alignment of the fingers, and hopefully, more useful motion with less pain. But secondary problems in the smaller joints of the fingers sometimes cannot be helped to a great extent.

Replacement arthroplasty usually does not restore the full range of motion of the joint, but in some cases, the operation does allow a much improved range of motion and less pain.

Varicose veins usually are treated by either a general surgeon or a vascular surgeon (see page 569). Sometimes, however, varicose veins result in a degeneration of circulation around the ankle to such an extent that ulcers appear in the skin. In this instance, the reconstructive surgeon may be called upon to assist in restoring skin coverage.

The ulcers (called venous stasis ulcers) cannot be corrected until the varicose veins are corrected. Otherwise, the vein pressure at the ankle would be so great that circulation essentially would stop and the skin would not heal.

The basic mechanism involved in causing the problem is the overstretching of the leg veins so that the internal check valves cannot operate (see page 568). These valves, in stepladder fashion, segment the standing column of blood and prevent the total pressure from bearing down on the veins in the ankle.

JOINT REALIGNMENT IN ARTHRITIS

The reconstructive surgeon may perform hand surgery to realign joints that have tilted out of position from the destruction of the joint lining. The tendons in the hand may also need to be repositioned, reinforced, or reattached.

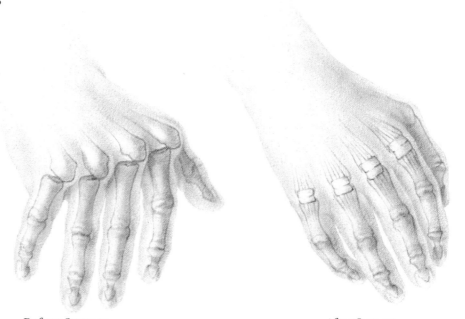

Before Surgery   After Surgery

Once the circulation problem has been corrected, the reconstructive surgeon uses skin grafts to cover the ulcerated area. It is easy to achieve healing if the patient is kept flat in bed with the legs elevated. After grafts have healed, elastic stockings can be worn to correct the back pressure and perhaps prevent a recurrence.

Pressure ulcers (bed sores) are not caused by any specific disease; rather, they result from the condition of being ill and are brought on by the effects of physical pressure on circulation.

Patients who are paralyzed, who have lost sensation because of nerve injury, or who have diseases such as diabetes, feel no pain from constant pressure. When the pressure is constant in areas of bony prominence, skin death is likely to occur. Bedridden patients, for example, commonly develop pressure ulcers over the hip bone as a result of lying on one side for extended periods of time.

Pressure ulcers can be prevented by arranging for frequent changes in position, as well as by cushioning and distributing the pressure away from those points most likely to ulcerate. If ulcers do occur, the reconstructive surgeon can use the techniques of grafts and flaps to repair the affected area.

Reconstruction often demands that rather large flaps of skin and subcutaneous fatty tissue be shifted into the area of ulceration after the ulcer itself has been completely removed. A thinner graft is used to repair the distant area uncovered by the shift of the flap. Although immobilization is very important until solid healing has occurred, a gradual weight-bearing program must be begun in order to prevent the same problem from recurring.

Cancer of the breast is discussed extensively beginning on page 546. Breast cancer represents another area in which the general surgeon and the plastic surgeon frequently consult. In fact, when a woman desires reconstruction, it is of primary importance that these surgeons work together in order to obtain the best result.

Planning for reconstruction must begin *before* any breast tissue is removed. If you are faced with the possibility of the removal of all or part of your breast, and if you would like information about breast reconstruction, it is crucial that you seek it prior to the initial surgery.

The goal of reconstruction is to restore a breast that is as nearly normal in appearance as possible. Factors influencing the outcome of the reconstruction include the amount of tissue removed and whether or not the nipple is removed.

In the simple mastectomy (see opposite page) where the nipple, the breast, and some skin are removed, it is fairly easy to regain some fullness of contour by placing a breast implant under the remaining skin, and sometimes under the pectoralis (chest) muscle.

In a radical mastectomy, the chest wall muscles are removed, and insertion of an implant is difficult because so little tissue remains. It may be necessary to move thicker skin, usually taken from the side of the ribs, to the breast area. Once this skin has been transferred, an implant can be placed under it to restore better contour.

As in any breast operation involving the insertion of an implant, there is the potential problem that the skin will not adequately cover the implant, and/or that scar tissue will form around the implant, shrinking and tightening the skin in such a way that it creates unwanted firmness. The problem can be so severe that the tissue eventually separates and exposes the implant. Reconstruction procedures can be used to place the implant more deeply into the cavity, thereby securing the skin covering and maintaining the improved contour.

If the nipple is removed, it is difficult, but possible, to rebuild a new one. The nipple may be simulated by grafting skin that tends to darken after transfer. Or, if enough skin is spared, the surgeon can place a circle of sutures underneath it to simulate the protrusion of the nipple. The areola can be simulated by tattooing the area around the nipple.

Severe fibrocycstic disease (see page 545) that has not developed into a cancerous stage may still require a mastectomy because removal of the glandular tissue will often relieve the severe unrelenting pain associated with this disease. In this operation, all of the glandular tissue is removed, and the overlying skin is left in place. The placement of a breast implant under this thin skin is not as successful as the ordinary augmentation. There is also more than the usual amount of scarring associated with this type of breast gland removal.

To rebuild some satisfactory shape, an implant may be placed under the pectoralis muscle either at the time of the breast gland removal or at a delayed operation. Whether or not the nipple itself needs to be removed and rebuilt depends on the likelihood of cancer being present in the nipple. This operation is sometimes performed after cancer has been found in the opposite breast. It is not a guarantee that cancer will not reappear since it is impossible to remove all the breast tissue cells while leaving sufficient skin for a satisfactory reconstruction.

BREAST RECONSTRUCTION FOLLOWING MASTECTOMY

LUMPECTOMY

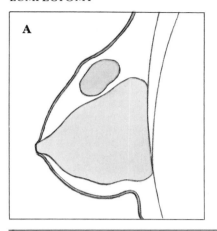
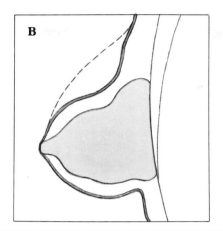
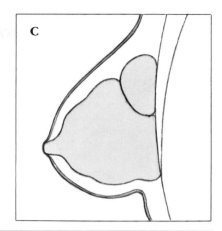

PARTIAL MASTECTOMY

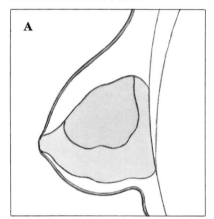
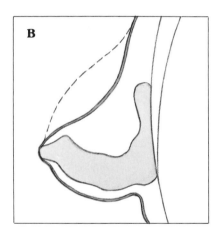
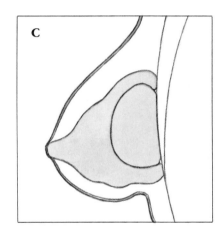

SIMPLE MASTECTOMY

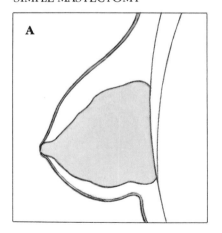
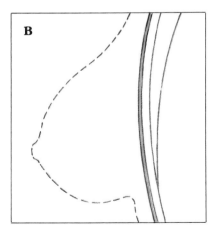
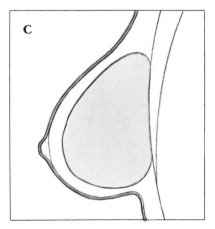

A *The shaded area shows the breast tissue to be surgically removed in each of the three operations shown.*

B *The dashed line shows the shape of the breast before mastectomy. The solid pink line shows the skin remaining after the breast tissue has been removed.*

C *A soft, pliable silicone implant (in yellow) is used to restore normal contour to the breast. The implant is placed between the remaining breast tissue and the chest-wall muscles.*

Elective Plastic Surgery

In addition to the reconstructive techniques mentioned, the plastic surgeon offers a large number of surgical procedures designed to improve appearance where there is no functional problem present. These operations have sometimes been labeled "cosmetic surgery," but plastic surgeons generally refer to them as "aesthetic surgery."

Some of the conditions that the plastic surgeon treats are those that have been present since birth, those that result from aging, and those cosmetic problems that result from disease or injury.

Congenital problems commonly treated include minor abnormalities of the face, such as a hump nose or a receding chin. Women who feel that their breast size or shape is abnormal also seek help from the plastic surgeon. One woman may consult the plastic surgeon about breasts that have been small since puberty, while another woman may want to change the shape of breasts that have begun to sag as she has grown older. Other conditions that may be related to aging include "bagginess" in the arms, thighs, and abdominal skin. Scars caused by injury and by disease also may be improved by aesthetic surgery.

Elective surgery for congenital variations. *Rhinoplasty* (plastic surgery of the nose) is one of the more complex aesthetic surgery operations, and the results may be unpredictable.

The basic plan is to lift the skin off the framework of the nose through hidden internal incisions, to reshape the bone and cartilage framework, and then to drape the skin over the new shape until healing has occurred. Dramatic improvements can be made, but since the bone and cartilage are living material, they tend to react to the injury of surgery in ways that may not be predictable prior to healing. Sometimes this reaction is reflected in a warpage of the cartilage or in the growth of a new hump where the bone heals. The effect is similar to the bump that results from a cracked tree branch as it heals.

Another complicating variable is the thickness of individual nose skin. Thicker skin is more difficult to reshape. In addition to this problem, it may be necessary to make external incisions at the base of the nostril on either side to prevent the nostril walls from looping outward if they are too long for the new shape of the nose. In spite of these potential difficulties, the surgery usually results in a very worthwhile improvement.

Rhinoplasty is almost always done under local anesthesia and fairly heavy sedation. The inner lining of the nose is deadened by a cotton or gauze packing moistened with a contact anesthetic and inserted into the nasal passages. (This procedure also tends to control bleeding.) A local anesthetic solution is then injected all around the nose to numb the entire area.

It is usually necessary to work on bone as well as cartilage, although sometimes only the tip cartilage requires reshaping. The bone can be repositioned and reduced by sawing, rasping, or chiseling it to the desired size and shape. It may seem unnerving to remain conscious during this type of work, but if the patient is sufficiently sedated and highly motivated to

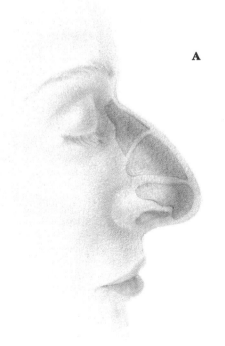

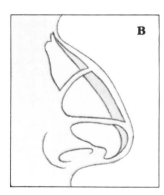 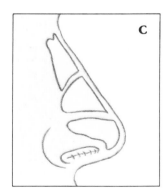

CORRECTIVE NOSE SURGERY

A *Hidden incisions allow the skin to be lifted off the framework of the nose.*
B *The bone and cartilage are reshaped.*
C *The skin is draped over the new shape and stitched.*

have the surgery done, the procedure usually is tolerated quite well.

After surgery, the inner passages of the nose are packed to stabilize the position of the replaced parts. The inner packing is usually left in place for a few days. The outer surface is shielded with a rigid splint of metal or plaster that is worn for about two weeks.

If the bones were repositioned, there will be considerable bruising and swelling about the nose and eyes. These reactions should diminish within two weeks. If discoloration persists longer, it usually can be covered with makeup until it fades completely.

One month after surgery, the bones should be strong enough for most normal activities, although they do not regain full solidity for about six weeks. And since the cartilage and bone undergo a healing process, the final result of rhinoplasty may not become apparent for six months or so. Often, some minor corrective procedure will then be necessary.

A receding chin is commonly associated with a large nose. Quite often, when surgery is used in such cases, the best balance can be achieved by reducing the nose as well as adding to the profile of the chin.

Chin reconstruction is usually done under local anesthesia on an outpatient basis. An incision is made underneath the chin in a horizontal crease, or across the inside of the lower lip. A molded silicone rubber implant can then be inserted. Some surgeons prefer a type of silicone rubber foam that can be sculptured to the individual chin shape of each patient.

When nose reduction is done concurrent with chin reconstruction, some surgeons use the bone and cartilage removed from the nose area to mold the chin, provided there is enough available.

Elective procedures about the face. These procedures usually concern themselves with the removal of sagging skin and wrinkles that result from aging. The larger wrinkles can be stretched out fairly well by shifting the skin upward and backward toward the ears. Smaller wrinkles, particularly around the lips, cannot be removed by stretching, however. For these areas, other procedures, such as chemical peeling or dermabrasion, might be used.

The face-lift operation (rhytidectomy or meloplasty) can be done under local or general anesthesia. The basic incision begins in the temple on either side and extends down in front of the ear, then curls under the earlobe to the back of the ear before passing into the hair of the mastoid area behind the ear. The skin of the neck, jaw, and cheek can be loosened and elevated upward and backward, permitting the excess to be trimmed away and the remaining skin to be reattached.

Sometimes the fatty tissue directly under the chin cannot be removed by tightening the skin, and requires a separate incision in the chin crease. Similarly, forehead wrinkles or wrinkles between the eyebrows can be flattened somewhat, but most efforts at dealing with these particular wrinkles are not as permanent as one would like.

The swelling, discoloration, and bruising associated with face-lift surgery generally last up to two weeks. Occasionally, these aftereffects last longer, but they can be covered with makeup.

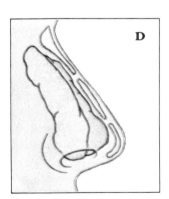
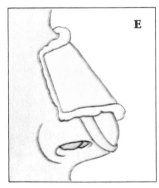
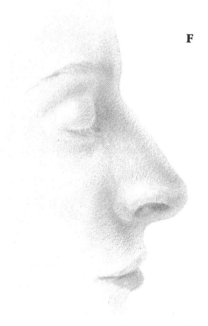

D *The inner passages of the nose are packed to maintain the new shape.*
E *A splint is placed on the nose.*
F *The packing and the splint are removed.*

Some residual swelling may last considerably longer if bleeding resumes under the elevated skin flaps after surgery. Bleeding and clotting are particularly dangerous in patients with hypertension. In all cases when bleeding is significant, the clot should be surgically removed and the skin sutured again. A compressive wrap is usually applied about the face to minimize the occurrence of this complication. Smaller clots can be left to dissolve gradually. A clot may leave a firm area that can be felt for a few months, but eventually this, too, should disappear completely.

Besides bleeding, another potential complication of facial surgery is injury to the facial nerve or its branches. This nerve activates the muscles in the face, and its loss would leave an area of the face weak or droopy. Since the nerve is located just under the skin, the surgeon must be very careful in lifting the skin tissue. It is fairly common to notice temporary weakness after surgery due to stretching or bleeding around a nerve branch, and these transient symptoms may take a few days to a few weeks to resolve. Symptoms persisting after that time are still very likely to correct themselves within a few months. If necessary, the surgeon can begin reconstructive procedures, or perhaps attempt to repair the nerve at a later stage.

The face-lift reportedly lasts from five to seven years or even longer, but this determination is relative since individuals vary in their view of what is acceptable. Although it is possible to repeat a face-lift, there is some tendency for the skin to lose its elastic properties, and after more than one procedure, it may develop some unnatural texture. Yet some patients have undergone face-lifts several times with good success.

Reduction of loose skin and puffy tissue around the eyes is often done along with the face-lift operation. The two procedures are separate in that the eyelids do not benefit from the face-lift, and the skin of the face cannot be helped by treating the eyelids.

When done alone, eyelid surgery can be performed easily under local anesthesia, although many patients prefer general anesthesia. The incision is made along the crease formed by the opening and closing of the eyes. A rather large amount of skin usually can be taken from the upper eyelid. The muscle tissue is split, and some fatty tissue often is removed at the same time. The incision is closed so it lies within the normal crease formed when the eyelid opens.

The lower eyelid must be treated somewhat differently. It is difficult to remove very much lower-lid skin without causing the edge of the lower lid to roll outward, away from the eyeball. To avoid this tendency, the surgeon usually shifts the skin laterally to remove wrinkles here.

Puffy tissue in the area of the lower eyelid is caused by fat that is meant to cushion the eyeball within the eye socket. This fat is normally kept in place by a curtain of fibrous tissue within the layers of the lower eyelid. In certain families, and with age, this curtain tends to weaken to the extent that fatty tissue behind the lid bulges forward. The bags are particularly prominent when a person is most relaxed.

To correct this problem, an incision is made about three-sixteenths of an inch below the lower eyelashes and is extended in a slight downward curve over the outward bony rim of the eye socket. The skin is lifted so that the underlying muscle is exposed. Penetrating openings are then made through the muscle, and the curtain of fibrous tissue is pierced so that excessive fatty tissue can be removed. Bleeding is controlled, and the skin is shifted so no excess skin remains.

After the usual ten days to two weeks, resultant bruising has usually cleared up, and the eyelids are considerably improved in appearance. Some surgeons prefer to keep the eyelids closed under some pressure for several hours in order to minimize the

THE FACE-LIFT OPERATION

The incision, shown in red in the drawings below, follows the pattern indicated.

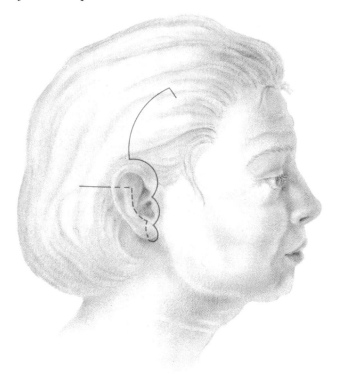

swelling. This can be rather alarming, and can cause the eyelids to swell shut for a day or two.

Chemical peeling, like any other plastic surgery technique, has the potential for substantial benefits as well as for complications. This procedure is often used in conjunction with the face-lift and may be done at the same time, but usually not in areas that are undermined by the face-lift. Chemical treatment of those areas should be postponed for at least several days until the initial incisions are well healed.

As might be expected, the chemicals used are caustic to the skin and create a more or less "controlled" chemical burn. After chemical application, the face is taped with waterproof adhesive that is removed after about two days. The exposed "weeping" surface is caked with powder that turns into a type of thin cast. Patients inclined to claustrophobia are sometimes bothered by this powder cast.

When the cast dries and flakes off after several days, the fresh pink skin must be protected from excessive sunlight. (Because pigmentation of the skin is aggravated by early sun exposure, winter is a better time to plan for chemical peeling or dermabrasion.) The skin returns to its normal color within several weeks and usually has a tighter, smoother texture.

Possible complications associated with chemical peeling are excessive scarring in areas where the chemical might have burned deeper than desired, new pigment in the skin treated by the chemicals, and rarely, symptoms of internal toxicity (poisoning) resulting from absorption of the chemical. The amounts used by most surgeons do not cause internal problems, however.

Dermabrasion is the mechanical counterpart of chemical peeling and achieves most of the same results. The relatively simple office procedure is often used for small areas that need treatment. A local anesthetic is injected into the area to be treated, and it is then abraded by a motor-driven wire brush or diamond head to remove the upper layers of skin.

Mechanical abrasion is a little safer to use but may not achieve quite the uniform result of chemical peeling. While it is possible to dermabrade to such a depth that scarring will occur, this should not happen with reasonable care.

Skin that has been treated by dermabrasion requires somewhat less aftercare than chemically peeled skin—usually remaining in a dry environment is sufficient to promote healing. A scab forms from this process but peels off after about seven days. As with chemical peeling, new skin should be protected from the sun.

It is a bit risky to apply makeup to freshly healed skin. The components of makeup may soak in and cause body allergies, skin rashes, or swelling.

The skin of the neck, jaw, and cheek is loosened and elevated upward and backward.

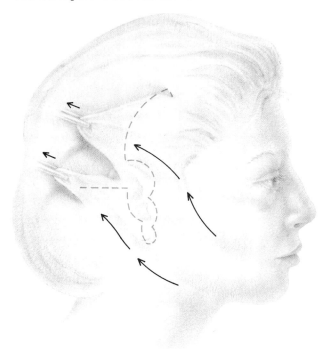

The excess skin is trimmed away, and the remaining skin is reattached.

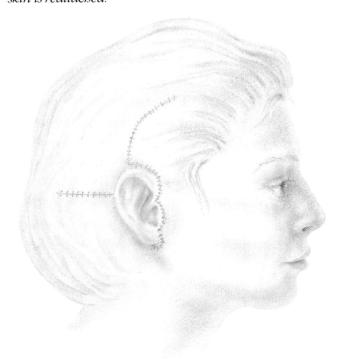

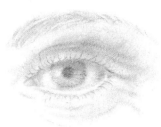

COSMETIC SURGERY FOR THE EYES

Loose skin and puffy tissue may be present on both the upper and lower eyelids.

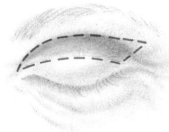

For the upper eyelid, the incision is made along the creases formed by the opening and closing of the eyes, as indicated by the dashed lines.

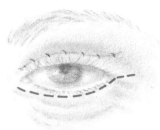

Loose skin and some fatty tissue are removed from the upper eyelid. Sutures along the crease of the upper eyelid close the incision.

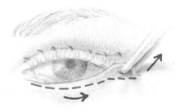

An incision is then made beneath the lower eyelid. The skin is shifted to the side to remove wrinkles.

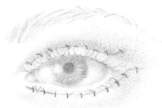

The incision is closed.

Elective procedures to improve scars. The plastic surgeon frequently is consulted about scars, particularly those on the face. Scarring may result from injury to the skin, or from a disease of the skin such as acne.

Ordinary scars take about six months to mature and lose their redness. If they have not enlarged by that time, they probably won't enlarge further. Consequently, improvement of a scar is usually delayed until it is clear that the scar is completely healed.

Contracted scars can sometimes be camouflaged by revision surgery using an accordion-type design. This sawtooth pattern, called a "Z-plasty," can be elaborated into a series of interlocking notches.

Scars that are surrounded by roughened areas may benefit from a combination of excision, rearrangement, and surface abrasion. Dermabrasion may improve the texture of the scar and help to mask the surgical excision.

Facial scarring caused by acne has brought a number of young people to the plastic surgeon. Success in these cases is quite limited, however. Before surgery is considered, the active acne should be controlled, and a reasonable period of time should be allowed for the tissue to lose its inflammation. Acne scarring can be divided into two general types: scars that are rather shallow and broad, and those that are pitted and quite deep.

Dermabrasion (see page 659) is the surgical method most commonly used, but this procedure cannot be carried to deeper skin layers to remove pitted scars. Sometimes small areas with several pits simply can be removed by excision and closure; dermabrasion may then be effective on the surrounding areas.

More shallow scars seem to respond better to surgical treatment, although in either type, dermabrasion may have to be repeated three or four times at intervals of a few months. To attempt the entire treatment in one session invites the risk of creating new scars.

Although the degree of enhancement after dermabrasion is sometimes remarkable, it is hard to depend on more than 60 to 70 percent improvement. In some patients, no more than 20 to 30 percent improvement is possible.

Other methods of improving the severe forms of acne scarring include dermaplaning, chemical peeling, and face-lifting techniques.

Dermaplaning uses a cutting blade that is carefully gauged to remove a thin, shaved layer of skin. If carefully used on the face, dermaplaning can speed up the ultimate result, and in some cases, achieve a better appearance than dermabrasion. Dermaplaning does involve additional risks, however.

Chemical peeling (see page 659) is sometimes used with acne scarring, although by nature, chemicals do not differentiate between the higher and lower surfaces of the irregular skin.

In somewhat older patients, the presence of loose or wrinkled skin makes acne scarring appear more severe. In such cases, perhaps only a face-lift procedure can effectively stretch and flatten the skin to achieve the desired improvement.

Unfortunately, the ideal remedy for acne scarring has not yet been found. Experimental efforts to add bulk by inserting bits of clotted blood with chemical additives, or substances derived from dissolved scar tissue may prove fruitful.

Elective breast surgery. Plastic surgery may be performed both to increase the size of the breast (augmentation mammoplasty) and to decrease the size of the breast (reduction mammoplasty).

Augmentation mammoplasty is often requested by a woman who has perceived herself to be small-breasted since puberty. A woman also may want to increase the size of her breasts if she has a dramatic shrinkage in breast size after pregnancy.

In most cases, the procedure used for increasing the size of the breasts has proved successful, from both the patient's and the physician's viewpoints. The anesthesia used for breast augmentation may be local or general. Many surgeons do all of their breast augmentations under local anesthetic, whereas others accommodate the needs and wishes of the individual patient. In the past, it was customary to keep the patient in the hospital for a few days; it is now common practice to do breast augmentation as an outpatient procedure.

Incisions for breast augmentation are most commonly made in the area under the breast near the natural fold at the chest wall. Many surgeons also make the incision in a curved fashion around the edge of the nipple area. This procedure necessitates dissection through some additional breast tissue, but if the scar heals well, the incision is very inconspicuous. On the other hand, should the incision heal improperly, the scar would be difficult to improve. Another attempt to minimize the difficulties of scarring entails making the incision in the underarm. While considerably more difficult, this approach also has its proponents.

Augmentation is accomplished with the aid of an implant. The most common type of implant used is a soft, round, gel mass covered by a thin elastic envelope of silicone rubber. The consistency of the silicone gel creates a low mound that feels like youthful breast tissue. Many surgeons prefer to use a silicone envelope filled with saline solution. Either implant can give excellent results, but either may fall short of the desired result as well.

Some slender women with very little "natural padding" may be happier with an implant placed *under* the pectoralis major muscle (the muscle arising from the ribs and extending to the shoulder) rather than on top of the muscle. In any case, the implant is placed behind or underneath the breast glandular tissue so that the function of the breast is not hindered, and a woman can lactate and breast-feed despite the presence of implants.

Complications can arise with any implant procedure. The most common of these is the formation of a scar tissue membrane around the implant. The formation of scar tissue is a normal reaction of the body, but it may become too thick and tend to shrink. It can then trap the contents of the implant, creating a certain amount of external pressure. When this happens, the implant begins to feel like a firmer mass than it really is. In extreme cases, this firmness can feel "unnatural" and can be somewhat uncomfortable to lie on.

Certain precautions can be taken to avoid this firmness, however. Shortly after surgery, the patient should be instructed to shift the implant to all sides of its pocket by applying pressure in each direction and holding it for a little while. The goal is to keep the internal pocket expanded so the scar tissue membrane remains thin, pliable, and roomy. This procedure is performed several times a day and is usually continued for several months after surgery.

Should contraction of the tissue capsule begin, the surgeon can forcibly expand it using manual squeezing—sometimes vigorously enough to require sedation of the patient.

Should these efforts fail, it may be necessary to surgically remove the thickened scar capsule, at least over a large portion of the implant pocket. The original size of the pocket can then be restored or the implant can be exchanged for a different type or a different size, depending on considerations the surgeon will discuss with the patient. Some surgeons believe that adding a small amount of cortisone inhibits membrane contracture. Others believe that oral doses of Vitamin E may help.

A thickened scar capsule also may form when significant bleeding occurs in the implant pocket after surgery. Although bleeding is meticulously controlled at the time of the operation, significant bleeding may resume after the surgery. The surgeon will then advise a return to the operating room in a few days to remove any existing clot and check continued bleeding before the incision is closed.

In any of the above procedures, the patient may experience some decrease in feeling around the nipple area of the breast. This is not a common reaction, although there is sometimes an unavoidable division of sensory nerves leading to the nipple area. Even when this happens initially, the feeling usually returns to a satisfactory degree.

BREAST AUGMENTATION

A *The incision is made near the crease beneath the breast (dashed line).*
B *Before augmentation, breast tissue (in pink) is located in front of the chest-wall muscle and rib cage.*

C *A soft, pliable silicone implant (in yellow) is placed over the chest-wall muscle.*
D *In very slender women, the implant may be placed under the chest-wall muscle for a more natural look.*

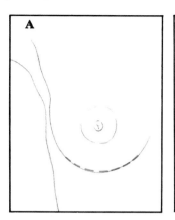
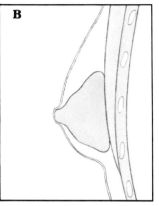
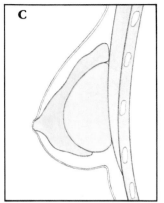
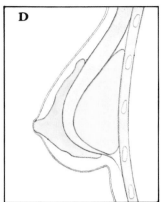

Following surgery, the breast area is usually fitted with some type of compressive dressing for a few days. Then the woman is fitted with a brassiere. An implant patient should always avoid brassieres with wires, bones, or stays, all of which cause a constant outside pressure point that can thin the skin cover and cause unnecessary problems.

Physical activity after surgery is usually limited moderately for about two weeks, and slightly for four to six weeks. Since the object subsequent to surgery is to keep the implant fairly mobile, it is not necessary to severely restrict one's activity.

Reduction mammoplasty may be requested to correct oversized breasts resulting from hormonal imbalance, pregnancy, or overweight.

As with the undersized breast, the oversized breast also may become a problem around puberty or, more commonly, may be associated with pregnancy and aggravated by overweight.

Virginal hypertrophy is a condition that begins at or around puberty in which the breasts develop rapidly and may continue to grow to rather massive proportions. Hormone therapy as well as surgical reduction may be recommended. In extreme cases, it may be necessary to remove all breast tissue and replace it with a breast implant for contour. Generally, however, breast tissue can be reduced surgically, and further growth can be controlled with hormones.

A woman with very large breasts may experience secondary symptoms such as backache, partial numbness in the hands associated with a tingling sensation, and even an unsteady posture noticeable in such activities as going up and down stairs.

Surgery for reducing the size of the breasts must deal with the mass of tissue as well as skin coverage. Usually in a reduction operation, the nipple also will have to be relocated. In other words, the surgeon must do more than simply amputate a section of the breast and sew it back up again. Several intricate patterns of internal and external incisions have been developed for such operations, but generally, the incision encircles the nipple area and extends straight downward to the crease below the breast gland. The closure at the crease extends to the left and right for a variable distance, depending upon the amount of skin and breast gland removed. In extremely large breasts, it may be necessary to simply remove the nipple tissue, reduce the entire breast to an appropriate size, and then replace the nipple as a free skin graft. Although there is always some chance that the graft will not "take," this method seems to work dependably in most cases.

Reduction surgery is usually done under general anesthesia in the hospital. Because of the mass of tissue removed and the bleeding encountered when large areas of raw surface are exposed, blood transfusion may be necessary. Recovery is quite rapid, however, and the patient usually is in good condition within two or three days after surgery.

Sagging breasts represent another problem dealt with by the plastic surgeon. In such cases, the amount of breast tissue present may be appropriate, but there simply may be too much skin, or the breasts may lack a firm contour. To correct this condition, the glandular tissue is preserved and relocated at a higher level. This operation can be done on an outpatient basis under either local or general anesthesia.

BREAST REDUCTION

A *The incision encircles the nipple area and extends straight down to the crease beneath the breast.*
B *The shaded area shows the breast tissue to be removed. The nipple will be transferred as a skin graft.*

C *The closure at the center and the crease extends to the left and right for a variable distance, depending on the amount of breast tissue removed.*
D *The nipple is replaced to complete the reduction.*

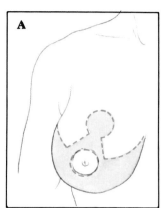
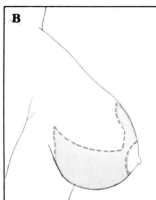
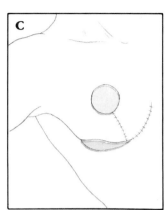
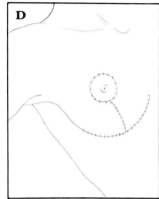

PLASTIC SURGERY FOR SAGGING BREASTS

A *The incision is made in the pattern indicated by the dashed line. It continues in a wedge shape beneath the nipple, and then follows the crease beneath the breast.*

B *The nipple is moved to the higher area indicated.*
C *The incision beneath the nipple is closed next.*
D *The incision in the crease below the breast is closed.*

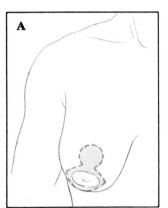
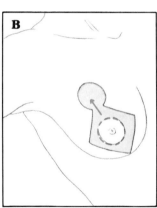
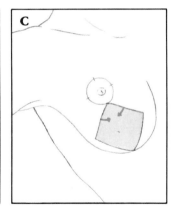
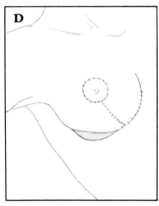

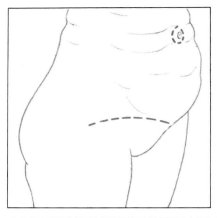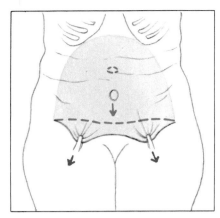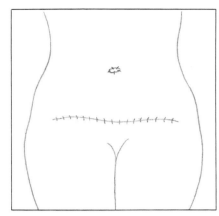

COSMETIC SURGERY FOR THE ABDOMEN

A wide lateral incision is made along the lower abdomen just above the pubic area.

Excess tissue is pulled across the incision, and is removed.

The incision is closed and a small "window" is made for the navel, which is stitched in place.

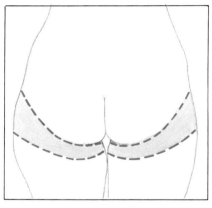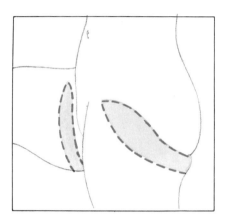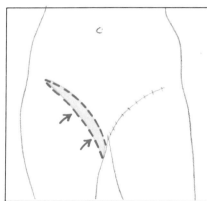

COSMETIC SURGERY FOR THE THIGHS

This initial view shows the dashed incision lines below the buttocks.

An incision is made from the groin to the buttock, passing high in the crotch area.

Excess skin is lifted toward the inner thigh, and the incision is closed.

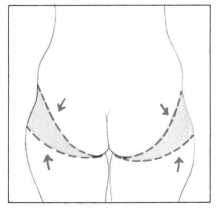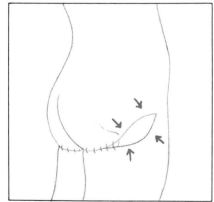

COSMETIC SURGERY FOR THE BUTTOCKS

An incision is made in the crease of the buttock.

Flabby tissue is removed, and the incision is closed.

Elective procedures on the lower body. Most surgery in this area of the body is performed to remove excess skin and fat that may result from pregnancy, extreme loss of weight, or aging.

The removal of excess skin and fat from the abdominal wall is becoming increasingly popular. As our society becomes more conscious of physical fitness, many patients have begun to jog, play tennis, bowl, and exercise at home. In spite of these efforts, skin and fatty tissue that have been stretched out of shape by pregnancy often do not recover their former tightness and elasticity. In other words, it is possible to bring the muscles of the abdominal wall into excellent shape without affecting the sagging, loose skin that covers them.

Best results are achieved when the undermining of the abdominal wall tissue is extensive. The incision is usually made in the lower abdomen as a wide lateral cut just above the pubic area and extending into the groin on each side. The placement of the incision is such that wearing a brief swimsuit will conceal the resulting scar.

The plastic surgeon loosens the skin from the point of the incision all the way up to the ribs. A rather tight pull brings the excess tissue across the incision so that it can be removed. A small "window" in the skin is then made for the navel, which is sutured in its new position.

This operation requires hospitalization. The patient must remain in bed in a flexed position for a few days until the healing tissue has made new attachments. Because of the massive undermining involved, blood transfusion is sometimes necessary.

Removal of folds of skin draping from the upper arm is accomplished in a procedure similar to the abdominal operation. In the upper arm, it is possible to remove a rather large spindle-shaped portion of skin and fatty tissue that runs from the underarm area to the inner point of the elbow.

The resulting scar will not be seen with the arms in their usual resting position, but it will be visible when short-sleeved blouses are worn in postures of activity. If the scar remains thin, this should be no great problem. Occasionally, however, scars "build up" in spite of all precautions.

The reduction of extra tissue in the thigh area sometimes can be accomplished by making an incision from the groin to the buttock, passing high in the crotch area, and then lifting the loose skin toward the inner thigh. If the loose skin is so positioned that tissue must be taken in a circumferential direction, then an additional scar must be carried downward on the inner side of the thigh. This scar will show when wearing a bathing suit, of course, but the scar in the crotch usually can be hidden. Thigh surgery requires a rather long recovery, and patients usually are hospitalized. Transfusion also may be necessary.

For some patients, the main problem is flabby tissue in the buttocks. A less-drastic procedure performed in the crease of the buttock often can correct this condition.

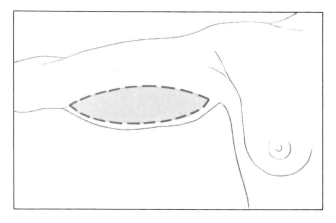

COSMETIC SURGERY FOR THE UPPER ARM

The shaded area indicates the portion of skin and fatty tissue that can be removed. The scar may be visible when short-sleeved blouses are worn and the arm is raised.

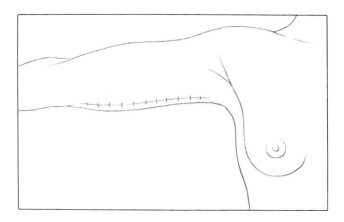

Heavy padding in the lateral part of the hip area usually cannot be removed without making direct incisions to remove the thickened tissue. This procedure results in scars on the hips that are quite visible. In addition, an incision in the upper thigh area presents a potential problem: it may interrupt the lymphatic channels and some of the larger veins to the leg. This interruption may cause temporary swelling of the leg that can necessitate wearing elastic stockings until the swelling subsides.

REFERENCES

NUTRITION

Page 47—Ideal Weights for Women
Source: The Metropolitan Life Insurance Company
Page 57—Dietary Needs of Pregnant and Lactating Women
Source: California State Department of Health, *Nutrition During Pregnancy and Lactation,* 1975.

FITNESS

Page 71—Ten Sports: How They Promote Fitness
Source: The President's Council on Physical Fitness and Sports, 1978.
Pages 78-79—Exercise During and After Pregnancy
Adapted from R. C. Benson, *Handbook of Obstetrics and Gynecology,* 5th ed. (Los Altos, California: Lange Medical Publications, 1974).

SELF-AWARENESS

Page 110—Physical Relaxation Exercises
Adapted from Edmund Jacobson, *You Must Relax* (New York: McGraw-Hill Book Co., 1962).

PREGNANCY

Page 237—Down's Syndrome and Maternal Age
Source: Robert L. Brent and Maureen I. Harris, eds. *Prevention of Embryonic, Fetal, and Perinatal Disease,* Fogarty International Series on Preventive Medicine, Volume 3 (National Institutes of Health, U.S. Department of Health, Education, and Welfare, 1976), p. 223.
Page 244—Risks of Taking Drugs During Pregnancy
Adapted from K. L. Moore, *The Developing Human,* 2nd ed. (Philadelphia: W. B. Saunders Company, 1977).

AGING

Page 326—The Aging of America
Source: The Commission on Population Growth and the American Future, Demographic and Social Aspects of Population Growth (Washington, D. C.: U.S. Government Printing Office, 1972), pp. 52-53.

HEALTH RESOURCES

Page 370—Community Health Resources
Source: National Center for Health Statistics, *Health Resources Statistics: Health Manpower and Health Facilities,* 1972-73 (Washington, D. C.: U. S. Government Printing Office, 1973).
Page 383—Personal Consumption Expenditures by Type of Product in the United States, 1975.
Source: U. S. Department of Commerce.

DEATH AND DYING

Page 362—Quotation
Source: Kahlil Gibran, "On Death," in *The Prophet* (New York: Alfred A. Knopf, 1923), p. 190.

CHOOSING A DOCTOR

Page 393—Reasons to Go to a Doctor
Adapted from Mike Samuels, M.D. and Hal Bennett, *The Well Body Book* (New York: Random House, Bookworks, 1973).
Page 395—A Patient's Bill of Rights
Source: Marvin S. Belsky, M.D. and Leonard Gross, *How to Choose and Use Your Doctor* (New York: Arbor House Publishing Company, 1975).
Page 405—Quotation
Source: Donald M. Hayes, M. D., *Between Doctor and Patient* (Valley Forge, Pennsylvania: Judson Press, 1977).

DEPRESSION

Page 415—Quotation
Source: Reverend Richard Baxter, *The Practical Works of the Reverend Richard Baxter,* ed. W. Orme (London: James Duncan Publishing Co., 1830), pp. 235-285.

BREAST DISEASE

Page 547—Incidence of Cancer in Sites of the Breast
Adapted from Gunther Kern, *Gynecology* (Chicago: Year Book Medical Publishers, Inc., 1976).

CIRCULATORY DISORDERS

Page 586—The Ten Leading Causes of Death
Source: U. S. Department of Health, Education, and Welfare, Public Health Service, National Center for Health Statistics. *Facts of Life and Death,* November, 1978.
Page 587—Deaths and Death Rates for Diseases of the Heart
Source: U. S. Department of Health, Education, and Welfare, Public Health Service, National Center for Health Statistics. *Facts of Life and Death,* November, 1978.
Page 594—Women and Hypertension
Based on The American Heart Association, *Heart Facts, 1979.*

ARTHRITIS AND RHEUMATISM

Page 629—Stretching exercises and isometric exercises
Source: Joseph Hollander, ed. *Arthritis and Allied Conditions* (Philadelphia: Lea & Febiger, 1972).

FURTHER READING

WOMAN'S BODY

Benson, Ralph C. *Current Obstetric and Gynecologic Diagnosis and Treatment.* Los Altos, California: Lange Medical Publications, 1978.

The Boston Women's Health Book Collective. *Our Bodies, Ourselves.* New York: Simon & Schuster, Inc., 1971.

Diagram Group. *Woman's Body.* New York: Paddington Press, Ltd., 1977.

Langman, Jan. *Medical Embryology: Human Development—Normal and Abnormal.* Baltimore, Maryland: Williams & Wilkins Co., 1975.

Notman, Malkah T. and Nadelson, Carol C., eds. *The Woman Patient: Medical and Psychological Interfaces.* New York: Plenum Press, 1978.

Ruzek, Sheryl Burt. *The Women's Health Movement.* New York: Praeger Publishers, 1978.

Schlossberg, Leon, ed. *The Johns Hopkins Atlas of Human Functional Anatomy.* Baltimore, Maryland: The Johns Hopkins University Press, 1977.

WOMAN'S PSYCHOLOGY

de Beauvoir, Simone. *The Coming of Age.* New York: Warner Paperback Library, 1973.

Friday, Nancy. *My Mother /Myself.* New York: Delacorte Press, 1977.

Fuchs, Estelle. *The Second Season.* Garden City, New York: Anchor Press, 1978.

Hamalian, Linda and Hamalian, Leo, eds. *Solo: Women on Woman Alone.* New York: Dell Publishing Company, Inc., 1977.

Konopka, Gisela. *Young Girls: A Portrait of Adolescence.* Englewood Cliffs, New Jersey: Prentice-Hall, Inc., 1976.

Lerner, Gerda, ed. *Black Women in White America.* New York: Vintage Books, 1973.

Lopata, Helene. *Widowhood in an American City.* Cambridge, Massachusetts: Schenkman Publishing Co., Inc., 1973.

Rich, Adrienne. *Of Woman Born: Motherhood as Experience and Institution.* New York: W. W. Norton & Co., Inc., 1977.

Rush, Anne Kent. *Getting Clear: Body Work for Women.* New York: Random House, Inc., 1973.

Williams, Juanita H. *Psychology of Women: Behavior in a Biosocial Context.* New York: W. W. Norton & Co., Inc., 1977.

NUTRITION

Barrett, S. and Knight, G. *The Health Robbers.* Philadelphia: George F. Stickley Co., 1976.

Berland, Theodore and the editors of *Consumer Guide. Rating the Diets.* Skokie, Illinois: Publications International Limited, 1976.

Burton, Benjamin T. *Human Nutrition.* 3rd ed. New York: McGraw-Hill Book Co., 1976.

Stare, F. and McWilliams, M. *Living Nutrition.* 2nd ed. New York: John Wiley & Sons, Inc., 1977.

Stare, F. and McWilliams, M. *Nutrition for Good Health.* Fullerton, California: Plycon Press, 1974.

Stare, F. and Whelan, E. *Eat OK—Feel OK.* Christopher, Massachusetts: Christopher Publishing House, 1978.

Stare, F. and Whelan, E. *Panic in the Pantry: Food Facts, Fads, and Fallacies.* New York: Atheneum Publishers, 1975.

FITNESS

Anderson, James L. and Cohen, Martin. *The West Point Fitness and Diet Book.* New York: Rawsons Associates, Publishers, 1977.

Cooper, Mildred and Cooper, Kenneth. *Aerobics for Women.* New York: Bantam Books, Inc., 1977.

Folan, Lilias. *Lilias, Yoga, and You.* New York: Bantam Books, Inc., 1976.

Hittleman, Richard. *Yoga: 28-Day Exercise Plan.* New York: Workman Publishing Co., Inc., 1969.

Kahn, Manya. *Body Rhythms.* New York: E. P. Dutton, 1977.

(continued on next page)

FITNESS (continued)

Kuntzleman, Charles T. and the editors of *Consumer Guide. Rating the Exercises.* New York: William Morrow & Co., Inc., 1978.

Lumiere, Cornel and the editors of *World Tennis* magazine. *Book of Tennis: How to Play the Game.* New York: Grosset & Dunlap, Inc., 1970.

Matthews, Donald K. and Fox, Edward L. *The Physiological Basis of Physical Education and Athletics.* Philadelphia: W. B. Saunders Co., 1976.

Noble, Elizabeth. *Essential Exercises for the Childbearing Years.* Boston: Houghton Mifflin Co., 1976.

Editors of *Runner's World* magazine. *The Complete Woman Runner.* Mountain View, California: World Publications, 1978.

Rush, Anne Kent. *The Basic Back Book.* New York: Simon & Schuster, Inc., 1979.

Editors of *Sports Illustrated* magazine. *Sports Illustrated Swimming and Diving.* Philadelphia: J. B. Lippincott, Co., 1973.

Ullyot, Joan. *Woman's Running.* Mountain View, California: World Publications, 1976.

Zane, Frank and Zane, Christine. *The Zane Way to a Beautiful Body Through Weight Training for Men and Women.* New York: Simon & Schuster, Inc., 1979.

MENTAL HEALTH

The Boston Women's Health Book Collective. *Our Bodies, Ourselves.* New York: Simon & Schuster, Inc., 1973.

Corea, Gena. *The Hidden Malpractice: How American Medicine Treats Women as Patients and Professionals.* New York: William Morrow & Co., Inc., 1977.

Janeway, Elizabeth. *Man's World, Woman's Place.* New York: Dell Publishing Co., Inc., 1972.

Miller, Jean Baker. *Toward a New Psychology of Women.* Boston: Beacon Press, Inc., 1976.

SELF-AWARENESS

Benson, Herbert. *The Relaxation Response.* New York: Avon Books, 1975.

Friedman, Meyer and Rosenman, Ray H. *Type A Behavior and Your Heart.* Greenwich, Connecticut: Fawcett Book Group, 1974.

Jacobson, Edmund. *You Must Relax.* New York: McGraw-Hill Book Co., 1962.

LeShan, Lawrence. *How to Meditate: A Guide to Self-Discovery.* Boston: Little, Brown & Co., 1974.

Luce, Gay Gaer. *Your Second Life.* New York: Delacorte Press, 1979.

McQuade, Walter and Aikman, Ann. *Stress.* New York: Bantam Books, Inc., 1974.

Miller, Eddie. *Stress.* Chicago: Blue Cross Association, 1974.

Pelletier, Kenneth. *Mind as Healer, Mind as Slayer.* New York: Dell Publishing Co., Inc., 1977.

Selye, Hans. *The Stress of Life.* New York: McGraw-Hill Book Co., 1976.

Tulku, Tarthang, *Gesture of Balance.* Berkeley, California: Dharma Press, 1978.

Tulku, Tarthang. *Kum Nye.* Berkeley, California: Dharma Press, 1978.

ADOLESCENCE

Anyan, Walter R. *Adolescent Medicine in Primary Care.* New York: John Wiley & Sons, Inc., 1978.

Conger, John J. *Contemporary Issues in Adolescent Development.* New York: Harper and Row Publishers, Inc., 1975.

Daniel, William A. *Adolescents in Health and Disease.* St. Louis: C. V. Mosby Co., 1977.

Emans, Jean. *Pediatric and Adolescent Gynecology.* Boston: Little, Brown & Co., 1979.

Gordon, S. *Facts About Sex.* New York: John Day Co., Inc., 1973.

Grinder, Robert F. *Adolescence.* 2nd ed. New York: John Wiley & Sons, Inc., 1978.

Jersild, Arthur T. *Psychology of Adolescence.* 3rd ed. Riverside, New Jersey: Macmillan Publishing Co., Inc., 1978.

Kaplan, Helen Singer. *Making Sense of Sex.* New York: Simon & Schuster, Inc., 1979.

Katchadourian, Herant. *The Biology of Adolescence.* San Francisco: W. H. Freeman & Co., 1977.

Kreutner, A. Karen and Reycroft-Hollingsworth, Dorothy. *Adolescent Obstetrics and Gynecology.* Chicago: Year Book Medical Publications, Inc., 1978.

Lieberman, E. James and Peck, Ellen. *Sex and Birth Control: A Guide for the Young.* New York: Schocken Books, Inc., 1975.

Rush, Anne Kent. *Moon, Moon.* New York: Random House, Inc., 1976.

Schowalter, John W. and Anyan, Walter R. *The Family Handbook of Adolescence.* New York: Alfred A. Knopf, Inc., 1979.

Shenker, I. R., ed. *Adolescent Medicine: Selected Topics.* Vol. I. New York: Stratton Intercontinental Medical Book Corp., 1978.

Sorensen, R. C. *Adolescent Sexuality in Contemporary America.* New York: World Publishing, 1973.

Zackler, J., ed. *The Teenage Pregnant Girl.* Springfield, Illinois: Charles C. Thomas Publishers, 1973.

SEXUALITY

Barbach, Lonnie Garfield. *For Yourself: The Fulfillment of Female Sexuality.* Garden City, New York: Doubleday & Co., Inc., 1975.

Comfort, Alex. *The Joy of Sex.* New York: Simon & Schuster, Inc., 1974.

Haeberle, Erwin J. *The Sex Atlas: A New Illustrated Guide.* New York: Seabury Press, Inc., 1978.

Kaplan, Helen Singer. *Disorders of Sexual Desire.* New York: Brunner/Mazel, Inc., 1979.

Kaplan, Helen Singer. *New Sex Therapy: Active Treatment of Sexual Dysfunctions.* New York: Brunner/Mazel, Inc., 1974.

Kaplan, Helen Singer. *The Illustrated Manual of Sex Therapy.* New York: Times Books, 1975.

BREASTS

Pryor, Karen. *Nursing Your Baby.* New York: Pocket Books, Inc., 1976.

Rothenberg, Robert E. *The Complete Book of Breast Care.* New York: Ballantine Books, Inc., 1975.

BIRTH CONTROL

Billings, John. *Natural Family Planning: The Ovulation Method.* Collegeville, Minnesota: Liturgical Press, 1978.

Hatcher, R. A.; Stewart, G. K.; Guest, F.; Stratton, P.; and Wright, A. *Contraceptive Technology, 1978-79.* New York: Irvington Publishers, 1978.

Lanson, Lucienne. *From Woman to Woman: A Gynecologist Answers Questions About You and Your Body.* New York: Alfred A. Knopf, Inc., 1977.

Lauersen, Niels and Whitney, S. *It's Your Body: A Woman's Guide to Gynecology.* New York: Grosset & Dunlap, Inc., 1977.

Shapiro, Howard I. *The Birth Control Book.* New York: St. Martin's Press, Inc., 1977.

Stewart, Felicia; Guest, Felicia; Stewart, Gary; Hatcher, Robert. *My Body, My Health: The Concerned Woman's Guide to Gynecology.* New York: John Wiley & Sons, Inc., 1979.

STERILIZATION

Nason, Ellen M. and Poloma, Margaret. *Voluntary Childless Couples: The Emergence of a Variant Lifestyle.* Beverly Hills, California: Sage Publications, Inc., 1977.

Planned Parenthood:
Sterilization for Women
Voluntary Sterilization for Men and Women
Vasectomy
These three pamphlets are available from:
Planned Parenthood
Publications Department
810 7th Avenue
New York, New York 10019

(continued on next page)

STERILIZATION (continued)

Sciarra, John J., ed. *Advances in Female Sterilization Techniques.* New York: Harper & Row Publishers, Inc., 1976.

Wylie, Evan M. *All About Voluntary Sterilization.* Berkeley: Berkeley Publishers, 1977.

ABORTION

Denes, Magda. *In Necessity and Sorrow: Life and Death in an Abortion Hospital.* New York: Penguin Books, Inc., 1977.

Gardner, R. F. R. *Abortion: The Personal Dilemma.* New York: Pyramid Books, 1974.

Luker, Kristen. *Taking Chances: Abortion and the Decision Not to Contracept.* Berkeley, California: University of California Press, 1978.

Skowronski, Marjory. *Abortion and Alternatives.* Milbrae, California: Les Femmes Publishing, 1977.

PREGNANCY

American College of Obstetricians & Gynecologists. *Causes and Treatment for Genetic Disorders.* (Information Booklet). Chicago: A.C.O.G., 1977.

Colman, Arthur and Colman, Libby. *Pregnancy: The Psychological Experience.* New York: Bantam Books, Inc., 1977.

Danforth, David N., ed. *Gynecology and Obstetrics.* 3rd ed. New York: Harper & Row Publishers, Inc., 1977.

Gots, Ronald E. and Gots, Barbara A. *Caring For Your Unborn Child.* New York: Stein & Day, 1977.

Lamaze, F. *Painless Childbirth: The Lamaze Method.* New York: Pocket Books, 1972.

Odell, William D. and Moyer, Dean L. *Physiology of Reproduction.* St. Louis: C. V. Mosby Co., 1971.

Whelan, Elizabeth. *The Pregnancy Experience: A Psychological Guide for Expectant Parents.* New York: W. W. Norton & Co., Inc., 1978.

LABOR AND DELIVERY

Arms, Suzanne. *Immaculate Deception: A New Look at Childbirth in America.* New York: Bantam Books, Inc., 1977.

Bean, Constance. *Labor and Delivery: An Observer's Diary.* Garden City, New York: Doubleday & Co., Inc., 1977.

Benson, Ralph C. *Handbook of Obstetrics and Gynecology.* 6th ed. Los Altos, California: Lange Medical Publications, 1977.

Brennan, Barbara and Heilman, Joan. *The Complete Book of Midwifery.* New York: E. P. Dutton, 1977.

Chard, Tim and Richards, Martin. *Benefits and Hazards of the New Obstetrics.* Clinics in Developmental Medicine, No. 64. Philadelphia: J. B. Lippincott Co., 1977.

Donovan, Bonnie. *The Cesarean Birth Experience.* Boston: Beacon Press, Inc., 1977.

Feldman, Silvia. *Choices in Childbirth.* New York: Grosset & Dunlap, Inc., 1978.

Goodlin, Robert C. *Care of the Fetus.* New York: Masson Publishing U. S. A., Inc., 1978.

Hassani, N. *Ultrasound in Gynecology and Obstetrics.* New York: Springer-Verlag New York, Inc., 1977.

Kitzinger, Sheila and Davis, John. *The Place of Birth.* New York: Oxford University Press, Inc., 1978.

McCauley, Carole S. *Pregnancy After 35.* New York: E. P. Dutton, 1976.

Parfitt, Rebecca. *The Birth Primer.* Philadelphia: Running Press, 1977.

Simkin, Penny. *Directory of Alternative Birth Services and Consumer Guide.* NAPSAC, 1978. (Available from: National Association of Parents and Professionals for Safe Alternatives in Childbirth, Box 267, Marble Hill, Missouri, 63764)

MENOPAUSE

Clay, Vidal. *Women, Menopause and Middle Age.* Pittsburgh, Pennsylvania: KNOW, Inc., 1977.

Fuchs, Estelle. *The Second Season: Life, Love, and Sex in the Middle Years.* New York: Anchor Press, 1977.

Reitz, Rosetta. *Menopause: A Positive Approach*. Radnor, Pennsylvania: Chilton Book Co., 1977.

Rose, Louisa, ed. *The Menopause Book*. New York: Hawthorn Books, Inc., 1977.

Seaman, Barbara and Seaman, Gideon. *Women and the Crisis in Sex Hormones*. New York: Rawsons Associates, Publishers, Inc., 1977.

Silverberg, Steven G. *Estrogens and Cancer*. New York: John Wiley & Sons, Inc., 1978.

Weideger, Paula. *Menstruation and Menopause: The Physiology and Psychology, the Myth and the Reality*. New York: Alfred A. Knopf, Inc., 1976.

AGING

Block, Marilyn R.; Davidson, Janice L.; Grambs, Jean D; and Serock, Kathryn E. *Uncharted Territory: Issues and Concerns of Women Over 40*. Silver Spring, Maryland: Center on Aging, University of Maryland, 1978.

Comfort, Alex. *A Good Age*. New York: Simon & Schuster, Inc., 1978.

Hornbaker, Alice. *Preventive Care: Easy Exercise Against Aging*. New York: Drake Publishers, Inc., 1974.

Luce, Gay Gaer. *Your Second Life*. New York: Delacorte Press, 1979.

Papalia, Diane and Wendkosold, Sally. *Human Development*. New York: McGraw-Hill Book Co., 1978.

Puner, Morton. *To the Good Long Life*. New York: Universe Books, Inc., 1974.

Rosenberg, Magda. *Sixty-Plus and Fit Again: Exercises for Older Men and Women*. New York: M. Evans & Co., Inc., 1977.

Zarit, Stephen H., ed. *Aging and Death: Contemporary Perspectives*. New York: Harper & Row Publishers, Inc., 1977.

DEATH AND DYING

Feifel, Herman, ed. *New Meanings of Death*. New York: McGraw-Hill Book Co., 1977.

Green, Betty R. and Irish, Donald P. *Death Education: Preparation for Living*. Cambridge, Massachusetts: Schenkman Publishing Co., Inc., 1971.

Lifton, Robert Jay and Olson, Eric. *Living and Dying*. New York: Praeger Publishers, 1974.

Morgan, Ernest, ed. *A Manual of Death Education and Simple Burial*. Burnsville, North Carolina: Celo Press, 1973.

Kübler-Ross, Elisabeth. *Death: The Final Stage of Growth*. Englewood Cliffs, New Jersey: Prentice-Hall, Inc., 1975.

Kübler-Ross, Elisabeth. *On Death and Dying: What the Dying Have to Teach Doctors, Nurses, Clergy and Their Own Families*. New York: MacMillan Publishing Co., Inc., 1969.

Stoddard, Sandol. *The Hospice Movement*. New York: Stein & Day, 1978.

HEALTH RESOURCES/HOSPITALS AND HOSPITAL CARE

Annas, George J. *The Rights of Hospital Patients: The Basic ACLU Guide to a Hospital Patient's Rights*. New York: Avon Books, 1975.

Chisari, Francis V.; Nakamura, Robert M.; and Thorup, Lorena. *The Consumer's Guide to Health Care*. Boston: Little, Brown & Co., 1976.

Isenberg, Seymour and Elting, L. M. *The Consumer's Guide to Successful Surgery*. New York: St. Martin's Press, Inc., 1976.

Knowles, John, ed. *Doing Better and Feeling Worse: Health in the United States*. New York: W. W. Norton & Co., Inc., 1977.

Kotelchuck, David, ed. *Prognosis Negative: Crisis in the Health Care System*. New York: Vintage Books, Inc., 1976.

Nierenberg, Judith and Janovic, Florence. *The Hospital Experience*. New York: Bobbs-Merrill Co., Inc., 1979.

CHOOSING A DOCTOR

Belsky, Marvin S. and Gross, Leonard. *How to Choose and Use Your Doctor.* New York: Arbor House Publishing Co., 1975.

Corea, Gena. *The Hidden Malpractice: How American Medicine Treats Women as Patients and Professionals.* New York: William Morrow & Co., Inc., 1977.

Hayes, Donald M. *Between Doctor and Patient.* Valley Forge, Pennsylvania: Judson Press, Inc., 1977.

Notman, Malkah T. and Nadelson, Carol C. *The Woman Patient: Medical and Psychological Interfaces.* Vol. I. Sexual and Reproductive Aspects of Women's Health Care. New York: Plenum Press, 1978.

Rosenfeld, Isadore. *The Complete Medical Exam.* New York: Simon & Schuster, Inc., 1978.

Rothenberg, Robert E. *What Every Patient Wants to Know.* New York: Medbook Publications, 1976.

Vickery, Donald M. and Fries, James F. *Take Care of Yourself.* Reading, Massachusetts: Addison-Wesley Publishing Co., Inc., 1976.

DEPRESSION

Arieti, Silvano and Bemporad, Jules. *Severe and Mild Depression.* New York: Basic Books, Inc., 1978.

Knauth, Percy. *A Season in Hell.* New York: Harper & Row Publishers, Inc., 1975.

Nicholic, Armand M., ed. *Harvard Guide to Modern Psychiatry.* Cambridge, Massachusetts: Harvard University Press, 1978.

Plath, Sylvia. *The Bell Jar.* New York: Harper & Row Publishers, Inc., 1971.

Schuyler, Dean. *The Depressive Spectrum.* New York: Jason Aronson, Inc., 1974.

Weissman, M. M. and Paykel, E. S. *The Depressed Woman: A Study of Social Relationships.* Chicago: University of Chicago Press, 1974.

MENTAL ILLNESS

Chesler, Phyllis. *Women and Madness.* New York: Avon Books, 1972.

Franks, Violet, ed. *Women in Therapy: New Psycho-Therapies for a Changing Society.* New York: Brunner/Mazel, Inc., 1974.

ADULT REPRODUCTIVE PROBLEMS

Danforth, David N., ed. *Gynecology and Obstetrics.* 3rd edition. New York: Harper & Row Publishers, Inc., 1977.

Lanson, Lucienne. *From Woman to Woman: A Gynecologist Answers Your Questions About You and Your Body.* New York: Alfred A. Knopf, Inc., 1977.

Silverberg, Steven G. *Surgical Pathology of the Uterus.* Surgical Pathology Series. New York: John Wiley & Sons, Inc., 1977.

ADOLESCENT REPRODUCTIVE PROBLEMS

See the ADOLESCENCE listing.

INFERTILITY

Decker, Albert and Loebl, Suzanne. *Why Can't We Have A Baby?* New York: Dial Press, 1978.

Menning, Barbara Eck. *Infertility: A Guide for the Childless Couple.* Englewood Cliffs, New Jersey: Prentice-Hall, Inc., 1977.

URINARY SYSTEM DISORDERS

Cantor, Edward B. *Female Urinary Stress Incontinence.* Springfield, Illinois: Charles C. Thomas Publishers, 1978.

BREAST DISEASE

American Cancer Society. *Cancer Facts and Figures, 1979.* New York: American Cancer Society, 1979. (Available from the American Cancer Society, 777 Third Avenue, New York, New York, 10017)

Gallagher, H. S. *Early Breast Cancer: Detection and Treatment.* New York: John Wiley & Sons, Inc., 1975.

Gallagher, H. S. ed. *The Breast.* St. Louis: C. V. Mosby Co., 1978.

Kushner, Rose. *Breast Cancer: A Personal History and Investigative Report.* New York: Harcourt Brace Jovanovich, Inc., 1975.

SKIN PROBLEMS

Domonkos, Anthony N. *Andrews' Diseases of the Skin.* 6th ed. Philadelphia: W. B. Saunders, Co., 1977.

Goldstein, Norman and Stone, Robert B. *The Skin You Live In: How to Recognize and Prevent Problems and Keep Your Skin Youthful and Attractive.* New York: Hart Associates, 1978.

Montague, Ashley. *Touching: The Human Significance of the Skin.* rev. ed. New York: Harper & Row Publishers, Inc., 1978.

Schoen, Linda Allen, ed. *Skin Health: The AMA Book of Skin and Health Care.* Philadelphia: J. B. Lippincott, Co., 1978.

Whitlock, F. A. *Psychophysiological Aspects of Skin Disease.* Vol. 8. Philadelphia: W. B. Saunders Co., 1978.

CIRCULATORY DISORDERS

American Heart Association. *Heart Facts 1979.* Dallas, Texas, 1979. (Contact your local American Heart Association chapter or write the national center: American Heart Association, 7320 Greenville Avenue, Dallas, Texas 75231).

Berne, Robert M. and Levy, Matthew N. *Cardiovascular Physiology.* 3rd ed. St. Louis: C. V. Mosby, Co., 1977.

Oliver, Michael F. *Coronary Heart Disease in Young Women.* New York: Churchill, Livingstone, Inc., 1978.

Kazdi, Paul. *You and Your Heart: How to Take Care of Your Heart for a Long and Healthy Life.* New York: Atheneum Publishers, 1978.

ENDOCRINE GLAND AILMENTS

Givens, James R. *Gynecologic Endocrinology.* Chicago: Year Book Medical Publishers, 1977.

Speroff, Leon. *Clinical Gynecologic Endocrinology and Infertility.* Baltimore: Williams & Wilkins Co., 1978.

Vokaer, Roger and DeMaubeuge, M. *Sexual Endocrinology.* New York: Masson Publishing U. S. A., Inc., 1978.

Williams, Robert H. *Textbook of Endocrinology.* 5th ed. Philadelphia: W. B. Saunders Co., 1974.

ARTHRITIS AND RHEUMATISM

The Arthritis Foundation. *Primer on the Rheumatic Diseases.* New York: The Arthritis Foundation, 1977.

Fries, James F. *Arthritis: A Comprehensive Guide.* Reading, Massachusetts: Addison-Wesley Publishing Co., Inc., 1979.

Licht, Sidney, ed. *Arthritis and Physical Medicine.* Baltimore: Waverly Press, Inc., 1969.

McMarty, Daniel J. Jr., ed. *Arthritis and Allied Conditions: A Textbook of Rheumatology.* 9th ed. Philadelphia: Lea & Febiger, 1979.

PLASTIC SURGERY

Brown, William. *Cosmetic Surgery.* New York: Stein & Day, 1978.

Dicker, Ralph L. and Syracuse, Victor R. *Consultation with a Plastic Surgeon.* New York: Warner Books, Inc., 1977.

Educational Foundation of the American Society of Plastic and Reconstructive Surgeons. *Source Book of Plastic Surgery.* Edited by Frank McDowell. Baltimore: Williams & Wilkins Co., 1977.

Georgiade, Nicholas. *Reconstructive Breast Surgery.* St. Louis: C. V. Mosby Co., 1976.

Rosenthal, Sylvia. *Cosmetic Surgery: A Consumer's Guide.* Philadelphia: J. B. Lippincott Co., 1977.

Wagner, Kurt and Gould, Helen. *A Plastic Surgeon Answers Your Questions: A Personal Consultation in Book Form.* Englewood Cliffs, New Jersey: Prentice-Hall, Inc., 1977.

INDEX

O

P